THE CANNABIS GROW BIBLE

4th Edition

The Definitive Guide to Growing Marijuana for Recreational and Medical Use

BY GREG GREEN

GREEN CANDY PRESS

The Cannabis Grow Bible
The Definitive Guide to Growing Marijuana for Recreational and Medical Use, 4th Edition
By Greg Green

PUBLISHED BY GREEN CANDY PRESS
greencandypress.com

ISBN: 978-1-937866-78-5
ebook ISBN: 978-1-937866-79-2

Also by Greg Green, *The Cannabis Breeder's Bible*

Editorial: Virginia Haze and Breda Lezha
Technical Editor for Chapter 18: Craig Flaman
Senior Production Manager: Thomas Whitcomb
Design and illustration: Ian Phillips

Cover photos: Rob Bramhill (top row and bottom left), Dankshire Photography (bottom right)
Back cover photos: Tee Roberts (left), Hip2thecrop (middle), Dankshire Photography (right)
For a complete list of photography credits, see page 885.

This book contains information about illegal substances, specifically the plant Cannabis and its derivative products. Green Candy Press would like to emphasize that cannabis is a controlled substance in North America and throughout much of the world. As such, the use and cultivation of cannabis can carry heavy penalties that may threaten an individual's liberty and livelihood.

The aim of the Publisher is to educate and entertain. Whatever the Publisher's view on the validity of current legislation, we do not in any way condone the use of prohibited substances.

PRINTED IN CHINA BY 1010 PRINTING.
MASSIVELY DISTRIBUTED BY P.G.W.

Acknowledgments

My thanks go to my family and friends. I love you all. I would also like to thank my publisher and editor for their always-welcome words of wisdom and their dedicated efforts in bringing you the best presentation of cannabis cultivation methods possible. They have been instrumental in developing *The Cannabis Grow Bible*. Without them, this book wouldn't be what it is.

I wish to thank cannabis cultivators worldwide for their research and help in developing this book. Without them, I couldn't do it. Also, thank my tutors and professors for helping me with my never-ending biology research.

Freedom is not something we fall out of bed into. We must always strive for it, often against forces that think oppression is a solution. It can never be. Only education and love can occupy that place. This book is dedicated to anyone who accepts that truth and practices it.

Publisher's Acknowledgments

First and foremost, a huge thank you to Greg Green for his unwavering dedication to expanding and sharing his knowledge of the cannabis plant in this fourth edition of *The Cannabis Grow Bible*. A big shoutout to the contributors—The Northern Scrogger, The Rev, Preston, Dinafem Seeds, Father Nature, and Trichome Technologies—for generously sharing their expertise. Your insights have truly enriched this edition. We couldn't have done this without the incredible work of over 100 photographers. Special thanks to Rob, Eric, Trichome Art, Russell-Howland Photography, Bubbleman, David, Tanya, Ryan, Nate, Joe, and all the talented photographers who provided stunning visuals for this edition. Behind the scenes, the amazing team at Green Candy Press—Ian, Virginia, Tom, and Breda—put in tremendous effort and thought to bring this edition to life. This book has been a true collaboration, and it's been an absolute honor to work with such a talented group to bring you the fourth edition of *The Cannabis Grow Bible*.

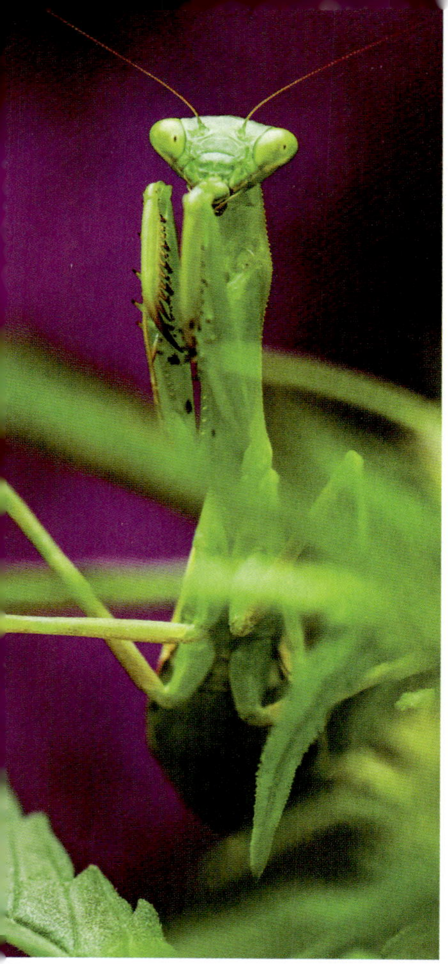
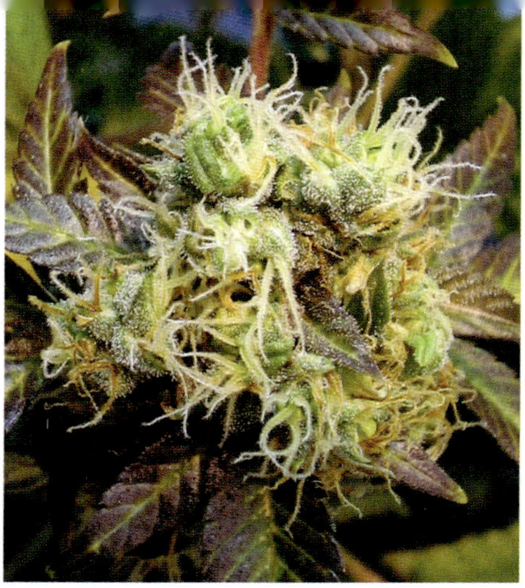
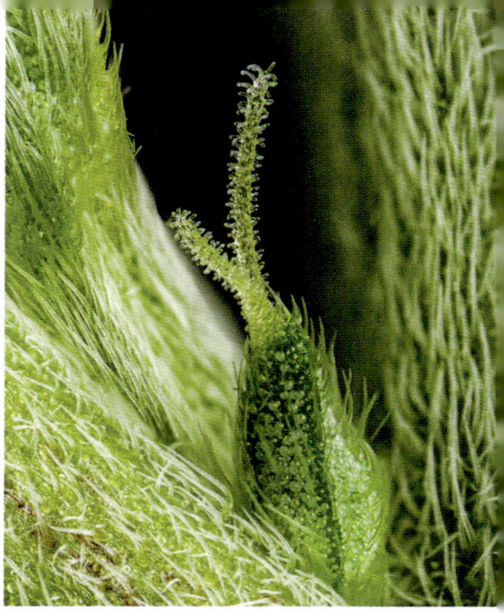
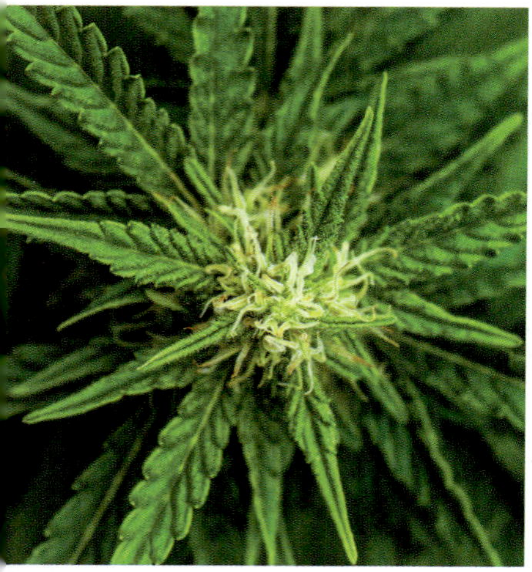
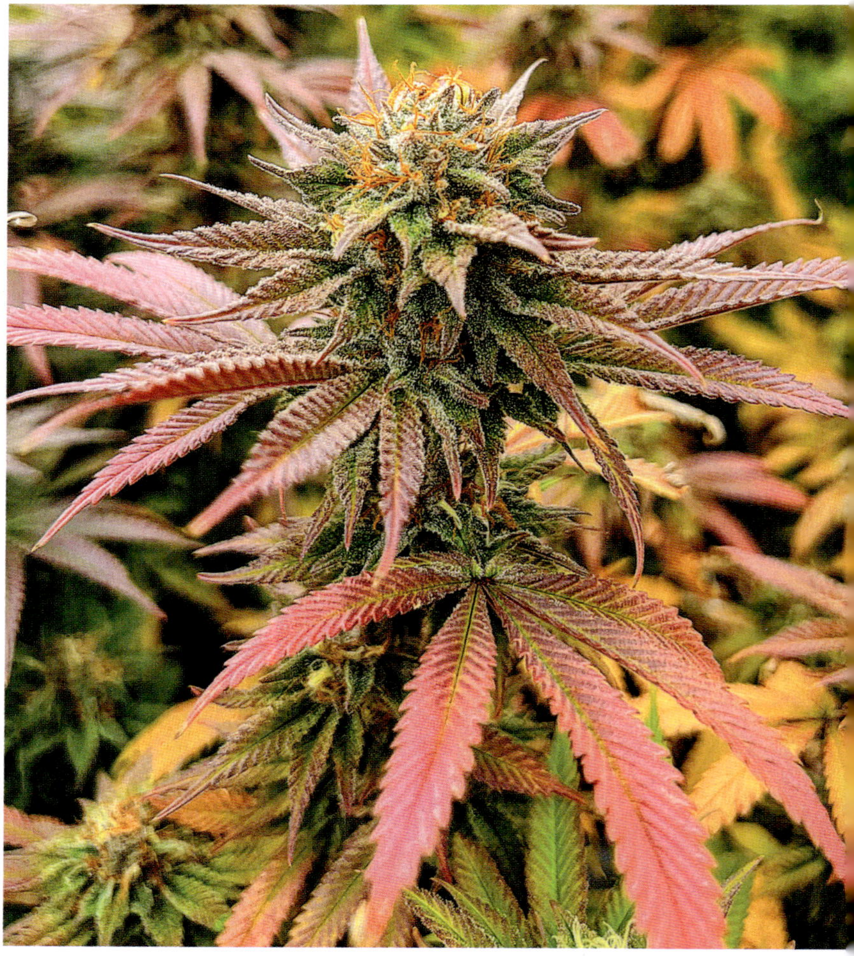
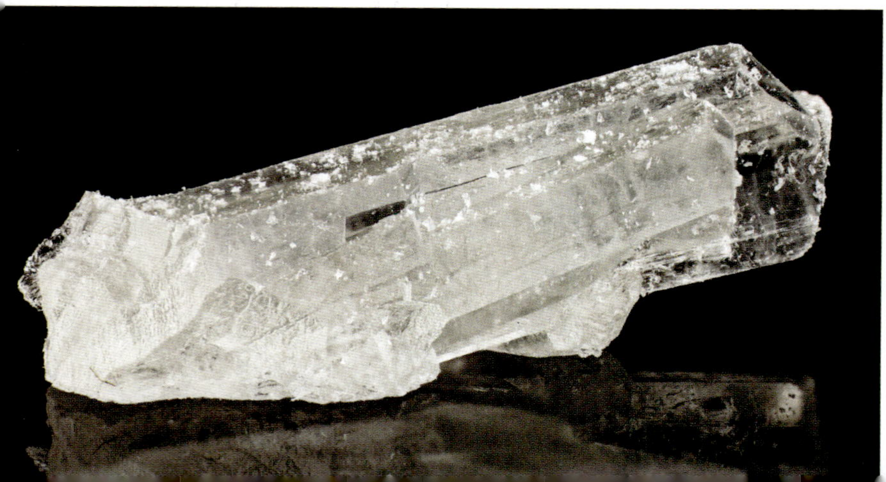
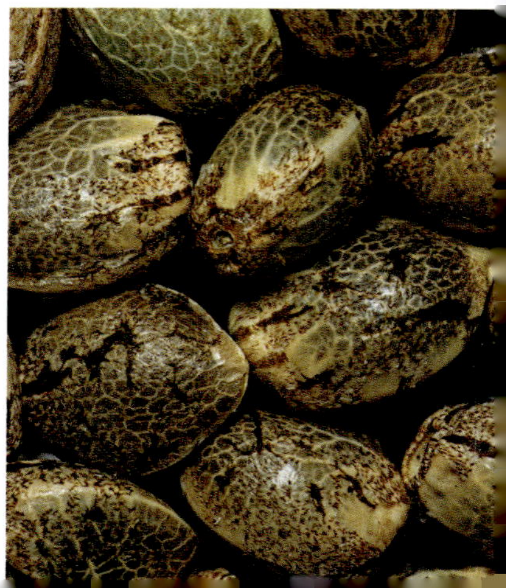

Contents

PHOTOS CLOCKWISE FROM TOP LEFT: ERIC PALMER, ORIGINAL SEEDS, ROB BRAMHILL, TEE ROBERTS, ROB BRAMHILL, TRICHOME ART, ERIC PALMER

Contents

PHOTO: HIP2THECROP

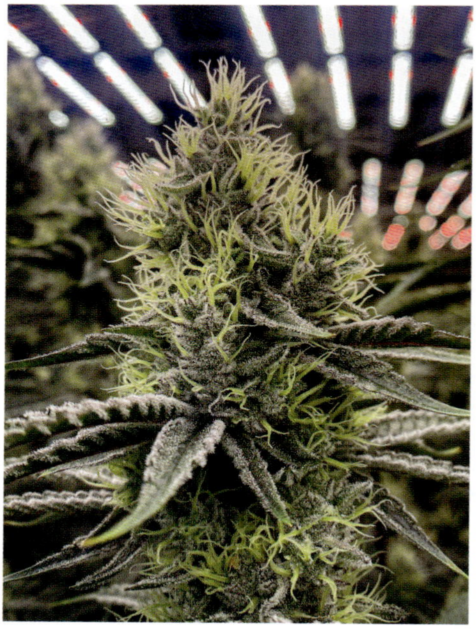

CHAPTER 9

CHAPTER 10

CHAPTER 11

CHAPTER 12

Contents

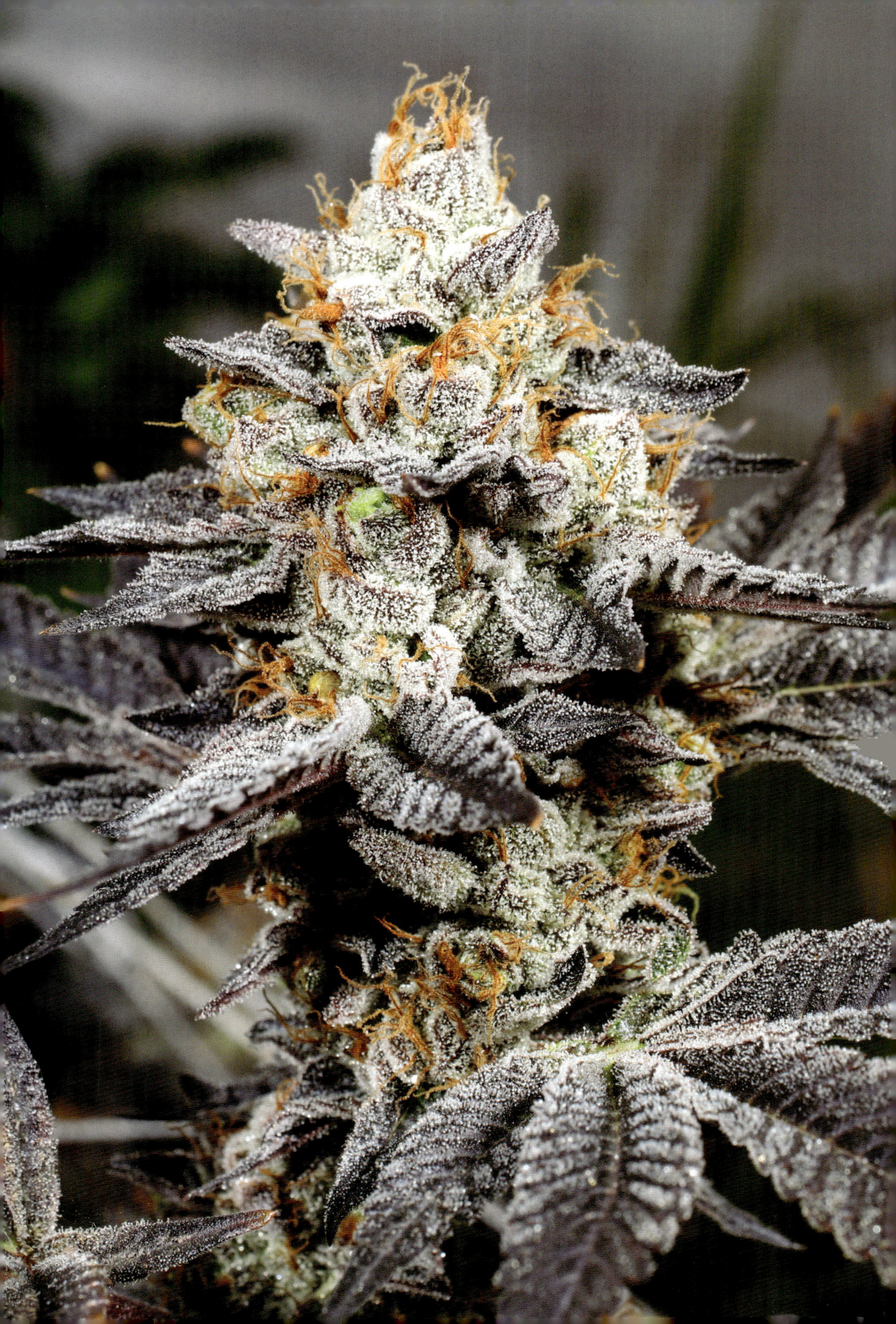

Preface

It's now twenty years since the first publication of *The Cannabis Grow Bible*—and what better way to celebrate than with a fantastic fourth edition? When publishing cannabis grow books, there is a constant need to revise and update previous systems, due to new advancements and progress in the cultivation world. Although this edition does this, it also celebrates the cannabis community itself. Apart from the fact that twenty years have gone by far too quickly, I am thrilled that this publication has managed to enter its fourth edition. In this book's acknowledgments, I thank growers and say this book wouldn't be possible without them. That has never been truer than now.

What you will read in this book is more than just my research. *The CGB* is the work of growers worldwide, pooled together in one understandable volume that will help you grow big, effective buds. We listen to and talk with growers every single day. Imagine I am just the writer, assembling information from large numbers of growers in all different environments with many various strains of cannabis. It can never be about one person or even a few. It is about us all.

Why grow? My answer is mainly found in the reward of self-sufficiency. What's your answer? Why do you want to grow? I love being one with nature and helping a plant develop. What about you? If you don't feel that growing can be very rewarding in many ways, I would like to persuade you otherwise. I don't want to encourage you to grow cannabis if you don't want to, but I would like you to consider, hypothetically at the least, what it might be like. I am not trying to sell you anything. I am not trying to push a magic product or magic system. I am trying to convey that it just might be possible to supply yourself with homegrown cannabis for as long as you want it. Not only is it possible, but it's also better—much better than you could imagine.

In 2003, I introduced what I call a *genetic theory of cannabis cultivation*. That pointed to one fact: You can't get good results if you start with bad genetics, no matter what you do. Growing with bad genetics is like trying to raise a racehorse out of a population of mules. By the second edition's publication in 2009, the global genetic seed base had stabilized sufficiently to compare most genetics to any suitable industrial-grade germplasm. It became possible to improve yields by using new advances in

PHOTO: ANDRE GROSSMAN

our understanding of indoor and outdoor cannabis cultivation practices combined with these stable and high-quality genes.

The second edition was designed to deal with the urgent need to generate productive and efficient grows that instantly met expectations and produced exceptional results the first time. To do this, it took the genetic theory of cannabis cultivation and expanded upon it with improved cultivation techniques. The book was also all-color with professional, high-quality photographs. I still enjoy looking at them today because the photographer was perfectly tuned into the ideas presented in the book. If photographers can learn the specifics of great cannabis growing, so can you.

For the third edition in 2017, we addressed the emergence of medical cannabis growing on an industrial scale, where most of the new data is in post-processing harvested bud into oils, for example. The explanation for the sudden emergence is simple: Cannabis was becoming legal in more civilized places. Science and industry were stepping up to the task, and the stock market was taking note. Cannabis will likely play a part in our economic renewal for its medical value and as an environmental biocomposite product for cars, homes, clothes, and other applications. There is, along with the medical cannabis revolution, a growing hemp revolution that even non-cannabis users should be paying attention to.

What's New in the Fourth Edition?

This fourth edition will contain many new developments, such as how LED lighting has changed nearly everything. In addition, there is a complete overhaul of our understanding of the evolutionary origins of cannabis. Cannabinoid synthesis is better understood, as are the biological pathways governing cannabis sexual expression. The science behind cannabis cultivation has been refined, answering previously unanswered questions. That is quite a development from an already packed third edition, so this entire book underwent deep revision—every page, paragraph, sentence, and word. However, it is still *The Cannabis Grow Bible*, with the same structure and approach to cannabis cultivation through science, experimentation, and application—but even better. Like previous editions, we will address new technologies and include the latest and most effective growing information to achieve consistent results with high-yielding crops at medical and connoisseur quality.

You will not produce good cannabis from bag seed. The same goes for people who spend a lot of money on grow equipment but none on quality genetics. Genetics is where you should focus your time and investment first, then attend to the growing environment after. If you use inferior genetics, your growing environment will always perform subpar, regardless of how much money you throw into it. However, once you know what good genetics are, you can invest effectively in your growing environment. You may think that your lack of a "green thumb" will stop you from succeeding in

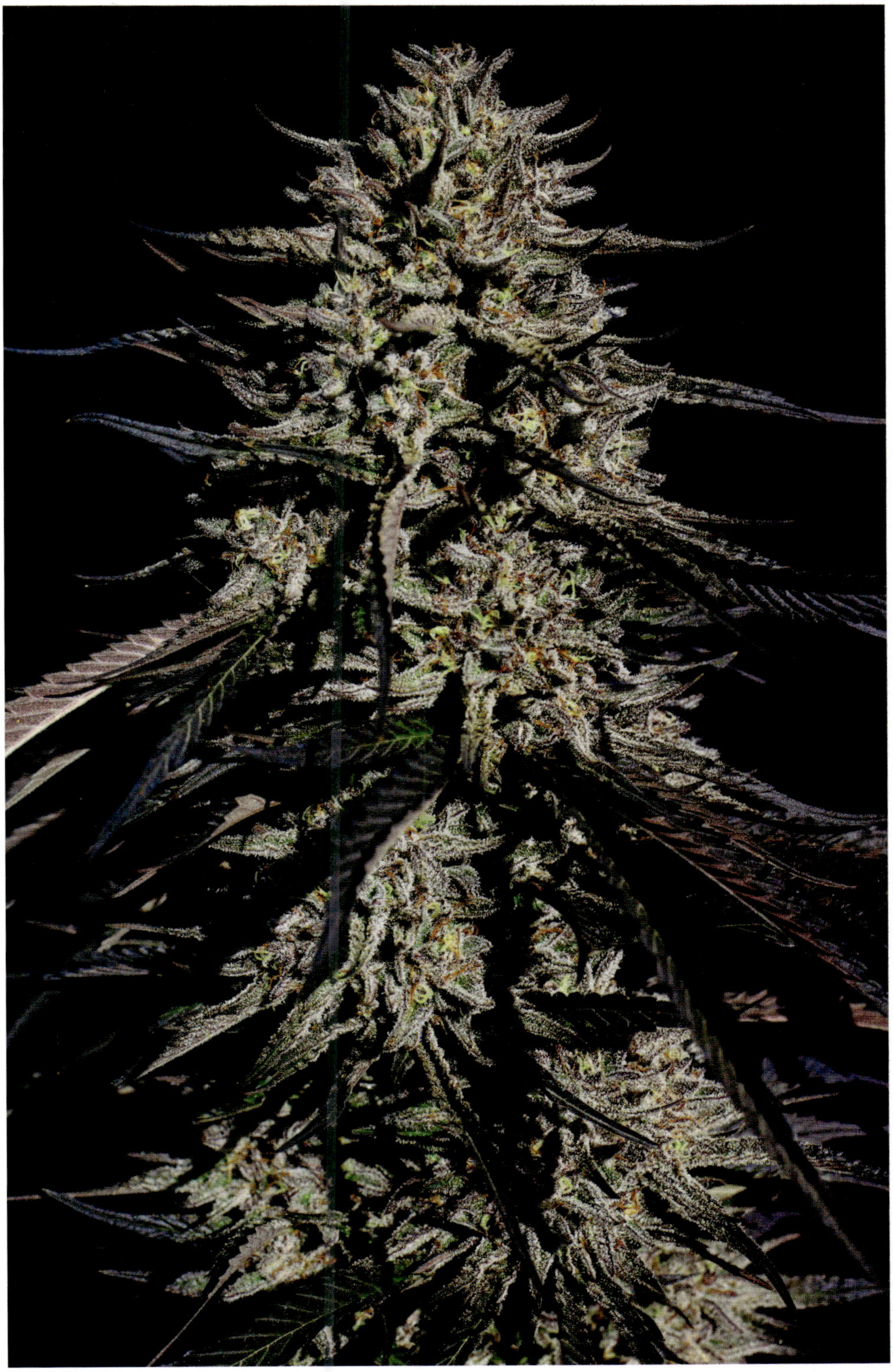

PHOTO: ANDRE GROSSMAN

Plants like this are a result of good genetics and optimal growing conditions.

cannabis cultivation. The problem is not you. In the past, experienced growers failed to communicate their experiences properly. For newer growers to succeed, experienced cultivators must share their methods succinctly and understandably. You have a green thumb within you; everyone does. All you need is the correct information. The strength of this book is its explanatory power. By the end of this book, I hope you have learned insights, tips, and tricks that will save you time, money, and effort. The type of self-sufficiency we talk about here is real, not fiction.

The one thing I can't do is make you read this book. It is up to you to get out your bookmark and cover a few pages daily. Read everything through properly and get to the end. Before you start, however, we should address security and safety again, as we can never talk about this too much. Put your family before your pot, not the other way around. Discussing growing online is not always safe, so use a VPN and browsers that aren't tracking you. Finally, forget websites offering where to buy seeds and ratings; those days are long gone. Due to legalization, much information is now found on social media. Growers, friends, and seed banks connect and give each other reports on how things are going, live, 24 hours a day. Security concerns should be paramount when it comes to social media networking, but it is there because it is the biggest venue for communication. You don't need anything dictated to you by one source or site. Open communities in social media are where you can find out what people are growing today.

This book has cost you less than a pack of 10 reasonably good quality seeds. It will, however, save you a lot more money. If you read this book and apply the methods herein, your cultivation process and results will improve, and you won't waste money. I can promise you that. A little know-how will immediately put you in a position to avoid common mistakes, and you may achieve higher success rates than more experienced cultivators. This book will cover all the groundwork for you.

The information in this book is clear, correct, and coherent. I am not sponsored by brands. I am not selling you some strain or seed line. I do not claim to know everything, but I know what works because I have interacted with many people it has also worked for. Despite what you may have read or heard, there is no particular way to grow. In this book, I use science. I use it because it works. Without science, the world would be much different. No dental hygiene. No vaccines. No central heating. No electricity. Every piece of grow bulb technology has been through several scientists somewhere in its history before it reaches your grow room. Every nutrient product has been developed and tested. Breeders wouldn't know how to create new strains without understanding the basic principles of Mendelian genetics. In science, pure research explains natural facts. Biology is the main branch of science that studies cannabis as a plant. Physics is the branch of science that deals with the principles of light energy. Chemistry and biochemistry deal with plant nutrition. Engineering is the ability to take scientific knowledge and design ways to use it. Cannabis cultivation is an applied science.

Once we can apply the science, get the desired results, and generate enough experience, we can get into the *art* of cannabis cultivation. Then, we can add special touches or whatever we bring to our love and hobby. Aside from science, each grower has their point of view because cannabis use is partially a subjective experience. Our senses and perceptions of smell and taste are used to assign personal values to cannabis, such as "enjoyable" or "unpleasant." These are not scientific values; they are entirely subjective interpretations of a personal experience. However, they exist, and we should respect others' opinions. To continue with this train of thought, being critical of another grower's point of view is not how you become a better grower. The better grower is critical of themselves, not others.

This book is not about me. It is all about you. Learn better growing information, see better growth as a result, and keep a record of what you did. That is a positive feedback loop, and you are part of that loop.

I try to present this data as a case for growing cannabis in the most optimal ways. Our methods are documented and repeatable, providing for the needs of all cultivators, from the small home grower and the outdoor breeder to the modern medical cannabis farm operator. I recognize there is a greater need to be concerned with the home grower, and to this end, I offer plans to get the results you need. Commercial farms, indoor and outdoor, are often a case of just scaling up designs, but we address them also.

Frequently, I include my brief recommendations, but I do so knowing that the work you put in will eventually generate what you need. Take this advice. A good grower is someone who gets into the rhythm of growing well. The fact is that there is no right way—but some ways are better than others for some people.

Find your way. It is your grow. It is your fun. It is your love. Never forget this when people dangle their steroid-pumped-up buds before you. Cannabis cultivation is about enjoying your time. Remember: Growing cannabis without love is never to experience the joys of cannabis cultivation. Some growers with the biggest buds have never truly grown at all! Your homegrown bud will eventually not only match the best quality bud you've ever had, but will surpass it. Your produce will be the best for you.

Greg Green

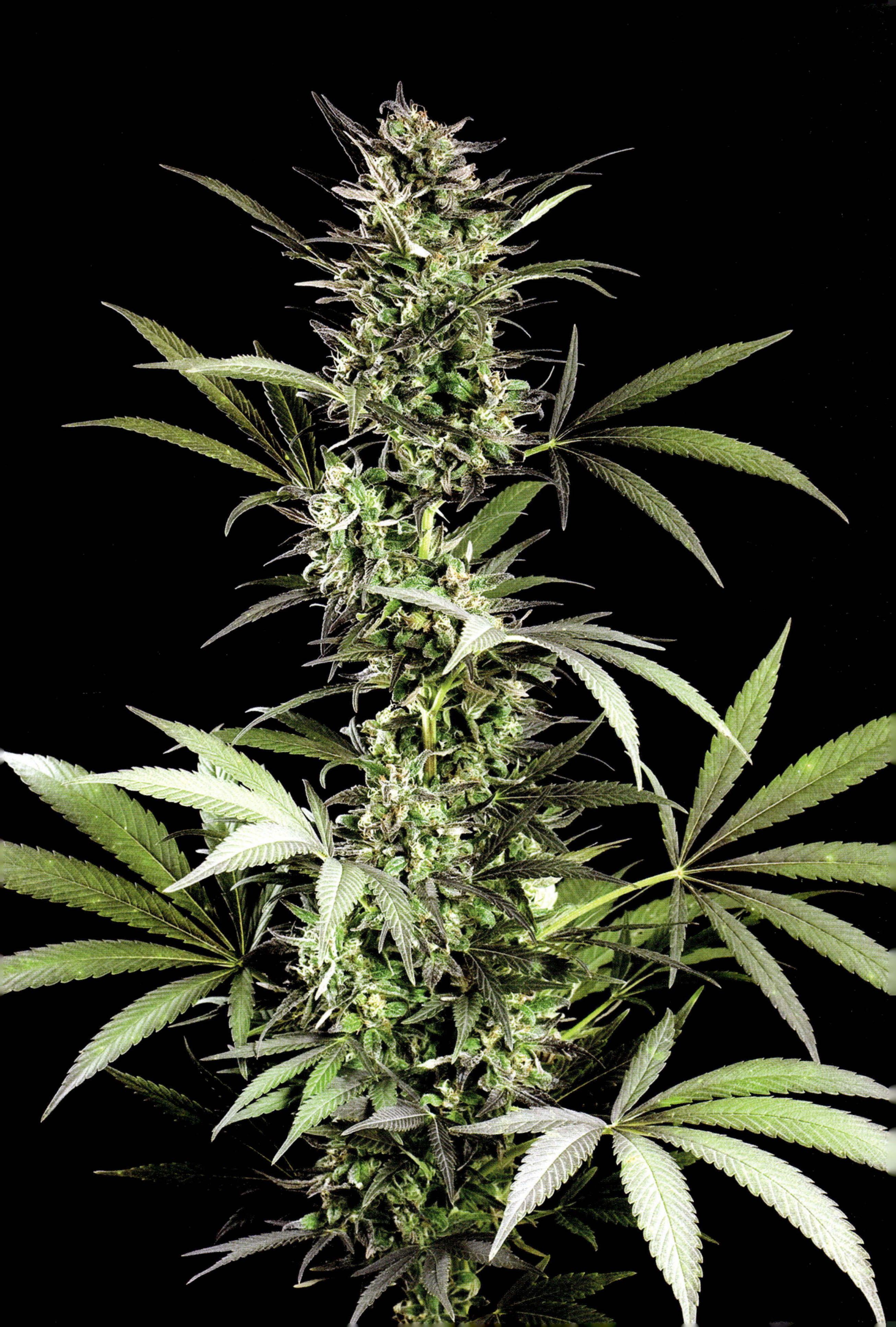

Foreword to the Fourth Edition

Twenty years is quite a story arc, and this fourth edition had a lot of new information to cover. It needed more than defragging and formatting pages, upgrading chapters, patching sentences, and clearing cached words. While the table of contents may seem similar to the third edition, you will see changes. When you turn to those chapters, you will find that almost everything has been redone. If you treat it all as new content, you will find revisions, modifications, and new material. Most of the data is from growers and scientific, peer-reviewed articles. There was an underground ethos due to legality in the past. However, this has changed because cannabis is now more widely recognized as legal, mainly because governments and citizens have realized its commercial potential and that prohibition hasn't worked, is costly, and is politically impossible to defend when pressed with science. The answer is legalization and education. The former puts cannabis back into the hands of law-abiding citizens, reducing organized crime, while the latter will likely have a more significant impact on minimizing risks and use. That statement is level-headed thinking. That is where my politics start and end. Everything else is science. The third edition was close to a textbook, so I kept turning it into one. I hope you enjoy reading and using this fourth edition as much as I enjoyed writing it.

Greg Green

PHOTO: DINAFEM SEEDS

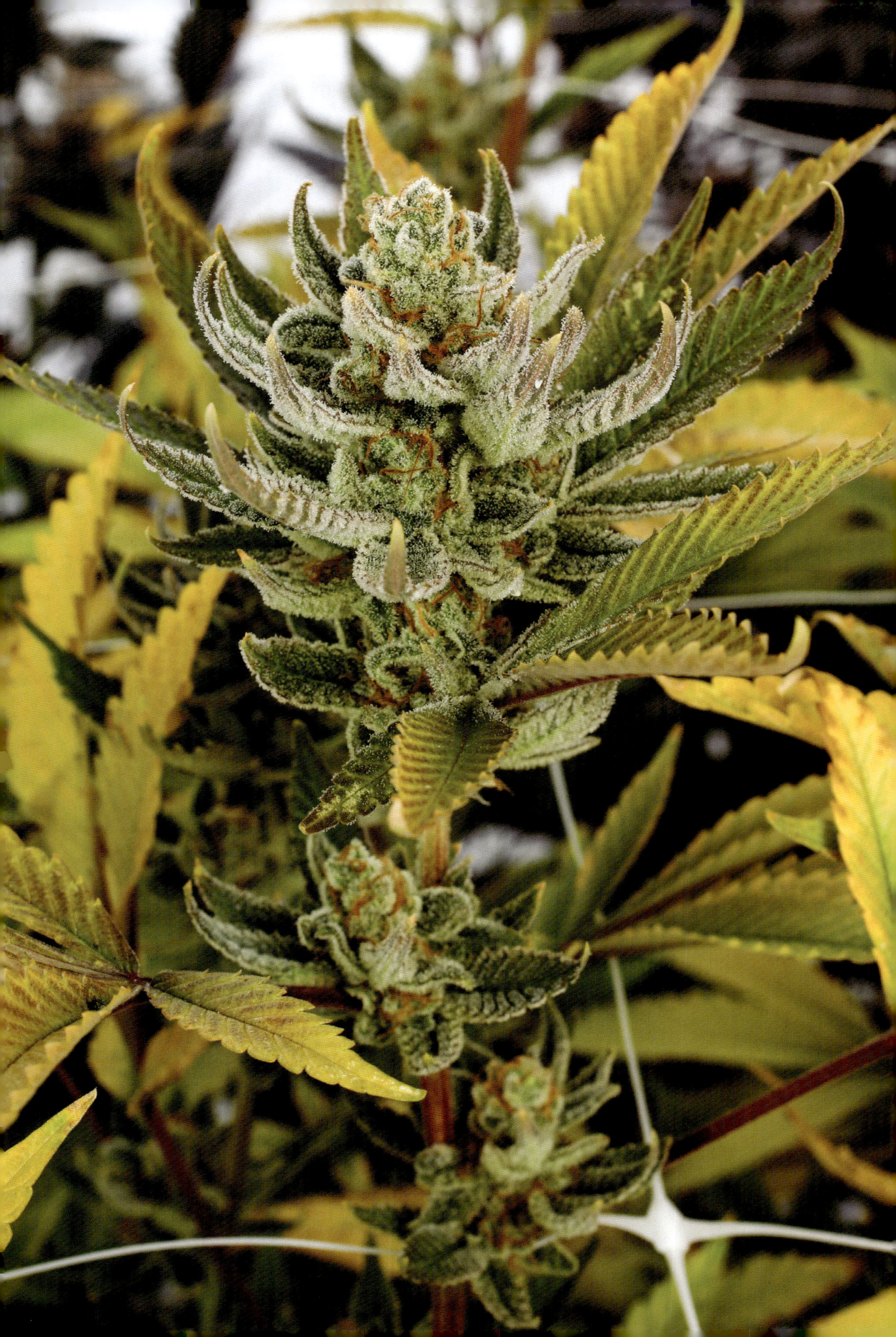

Introduction

The Language of Statistical Cannabis

We are, or at least should be, well acquainted with the boom of the cannabis produce market. As controversies about cannabis were overcome with facts, Wall Street found cannabis registered a solid ten on their Richter scale. Moreover, it was bonafide recession-proof (at least as much as any sector can be), seemingly immune from market turmoil. Why? Because cannabis is a highly robust plant, literally weathering storms, and has enormous potential across a range of markets, from medicine to biocomposites in car panels, much of which has been realized commercially. The stock market is vulnerable to environmental changes that impact crop supply and demand, including overproduction (oversupply). However, the cannabis market stabilizes itself by having such a broad reach across so many sectors that only a massive economic downturn across all those sectors can have a significant impact. When one sector goes down, the others compensate because the foundation for everything cannabis is this highly robust plant. Market analysts, though, don't use the Richter scale; they use graphs that plot the values of commodities over time. The idea that we can quantify something by getting good data and turning it into a presentation like a graph is essential for understanding the cannabis plant. Cannabis can be measured and represented as information for our calculations. There is a solid science behind it.

In Victorian times, the naturalist Richard Owen (1804–1892) contributed the idea of the archetype to the scientific community. By comparing similarities between living things (and also comparing differences) in a move to develop a better classification of these living things in their respective groupings, Owen realized that some biological structures could be seen as *analogous* and others as *homologous*. For example, if we take a seal flipper, a human arm, a horse's leg, an amphibian leg, a bird's wing, and a fish fin, then strip everything from them down to the bones, we see a striking resemblance in the majority of these vertebrate appendages. These commonalities are homologues. However, the fish fin seems substantially different because of the bone arrangement, so we can't call it homologous.

Nonetheless, it is analogous, as is an appendage, to the bird's wing or seal flipper. While this most excellent contribution by Owen certainly raises our consciousness, it also proves to be a mental block. By recognizing homologous and analogous structures,

PHOTO: ANDRE GROSSMAN

we subconsciously infer, through our emotions and thoughts, that these groupings are less perfect examples of their imaginary perfect blueprints. The same goes for cannabis. When we see a species of cannabis, we try to fit it into our perfect version of "indicaness" or "sativaness" or even its "cannabisness." We critique by comparing it to our mental archetype. The problem is that this is a corrupt picture of what is going on with cannabis, and this type of thinking is one of the reasons Owen failed to make the required leap in biological thought that we now embrace in the 21st century. The jump that he needed was the revolution of *Darwinian biological evolution by natural selection.*

Even glancing at the scientific tree of life can give us the impression that modern living things are derived from their ancestral "originals." However, the tree branches only reach so far before cannabis meets a common ancestor from which, for example, a line of modern rose species evolved.[1] Groups that share a common ancestor are called a "monophyletic group."

Table 1: The Scientific Classification for Cannabis

Kingdom	Plantae
Division	Magnoliophyta
Class	Magnoliopsida
Order	Rosales
Family	Cannabaceae
Genus	*Cannabis L.*
Species	*Cannabis sativa L.*

A close cousin of cannabis can be found in the Cannabaceae family (Table 1). Here we will also find (not shown in the table) the Genus *Humulus* (hops) and the Genus *Celtis* (hackberries). Like Owen's example of homologous structures, cannabis shares many traits with hops and hackberries, but their closeness is further substantiated by comparative genetic sequencing. In short, cannabis shares characteristics with hops and hackberries that are both shared derived characters and shared ancestral characters with their respective second and first common ancestors (that are now extinct). If we look at the scientific classification for roses (Table 2) we can probably identify where cannabis begins to differ. Just compare it with Table 1.

Table 2: The Scientific Classification for the Rose[2]

Kingdom	Plantae
Division	Magnoliophyta
Class	Magnoliopsida
Order	Rosales
Family	Rosaceae
Genus	*Rosa*
Species	*(depends)*

As we can see, the change appears at the Family level while Kingdom, Division, Class, and Order remain the same. Cannabis is Cannabaceae, while roses are Rosaceae. In the tree of life, both cannabis and roses, while separate, now would join together in the Order of Rosales. Rosales is an Order that sits alongside similar Orders, all descendants from various common ancestors (Table 3). There we would find a common ancestor from which both are derived.

Table 3: Phylogenic Example from the Tree of Life

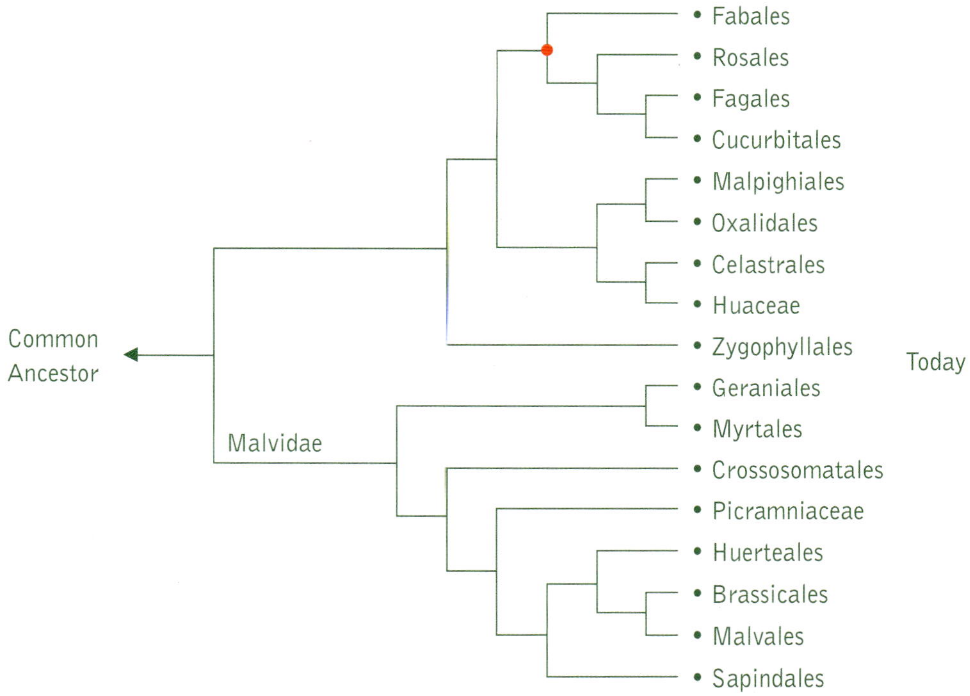

Phylogenic example of where Rosales is in a small section of the tree of life. Trace Rosales back and trace Fabales (above Rosales). Notice where they meet? It is not labeled and is just a branching meeting point. It is marked with a red spot. That would be their common ancestor that no longer exists.[3] You can trace any two back to a common ancestor that no longer exists.

The tree of life shows us something startling. Cannabis enthusiasts will have to suck in the following rational conclusion: Cannabis is no more permanent than *Tyrannosaurus rex*, and there is no template for "cannabisness." Cannabis is no more likely to endure than the cannabis-rose common ancestor was. That ancestor is long gone. Unless humans keep cannabis alive and alter it very little (if humans live that long and natural selection no longer acts on wild cannabis!), cannabis will be a fleeting speck, a millisecond on the cosmic calendar. That, however, does not impede our progress in understanding cannabis. On the contrary, it will enhance it dramatically.

While Owen was stuck on templates of originals derived from "types," which he believed appeared spontaneously and fully complex by the hand of a supernatural designer, Darwin realized a serious flaw in this reasoning.[4] Darwin would tackle this argument by objecting to the *watchmaker argument* that Paley developed. Rev William Paley (1743–1805) suggested that if you were walking along, came across a pocket watch, and examined it, the complexity and apparent suitability for purpose would lead you to assume that a watchmaker was responsible for creating it. Therefore, Paley inferred that if we find complex living things in nature, we should similarly assume that a designer made them. Darwin noted that there are bad "designs" (the term design would eventually be dropped from modern biology) as well as good "designs" in nature. For example, many of us require wisdom tooth extraction, we can choke through the same passage we eat and breathe through, and we have blood vessels passing in front of our retinas, often blocking light.[5] We also see birds with wings that can't possibly fly, like the kiwi (*Apteryx*), and animals with eyes that are blind, like moles (*Talpa occidentalis*).[6] Darwin explained that what we see here are former adaptations now falling into disuse. These show the limitations and constraints of natural selection. Darwin's famous book *The Origin of Species* (1859) showed that evolution by natural selection was a far better explanation of biology.

If species truly were fixed and not transmutable, then there should have existed a *static fossil record* to prove this hypothesis. However, during Darwin's time, the fossil record was starting to emerge as geologists (then revising the age of the Earth because of the slow, gradual formations of mountains and basins they were observing) discovered that the layers of the ground beneath their feet revealed gradual changes in species and also mass extinctions. Later, this would become known as the *transitional fossil record*, replacing the failed static fossil record hypothesis. Most importantly, Darwin had discovered that Paley's watchmaker was unnecessary if biological complexity could arise through natural processes involving the struggle for survival, variation, and reproduction. Today these are scientifically called *reproduction*, *inheritance*, and *variation*. These are the components of natural selection, the mechanism that drives evolution. That is not about abiogenesis or how life first arose; it is about how life evolves complexity after it arises, although we suspect some aspects of natural selection will be involved. If you are interested in abiogenesis, read about it, including panspermia.

The struggle for survival becomes evident when we realize that cannabis plants do not overpopulate the planet.[7] Cannabis plants produce an abundance of seeds, say fifty to a few hundred per plant in their natural habitat. Yet not all germinate, and not all survive. If they did, we would find the Earth covered in cannabis plants in a few decades, thanks to exponential increases.[8] Human males produce approximately one hundred million sperm that compete to reach the female egg, and only one can win. Birds have evolved optimal clutch sizes, increasing the chances of surviving individuals. That paints the picture of a biological war, even at the genetic level. Organisms exhibit fascinating reproductive methods to compete in the struggle for survival. Variation is also apparent when we look at "types" of living things. We notice that not all of them are the same and that there are huge differences or subtle ones. Darwin put two and two together. Organisms compete to reproduce, and variations confer advantages in that struggle. That is Darwin's big idea in a nutshell. It is that simple.

Variations that confer advantages occur again in the next round, and so on. For example, elephants that migrate north after their food or are chased that way by predators will eventually evolve thicker, hairier coats to deal with the cold, because variations in the population for hair length and density will give those elephants a survival advantage. How about the reverse? Mammoths (*Mammuthus*) went south because they were chased that way by predators or were following a food source, and so didn't need their hairy coats anymore because they got too hot.[9] In such a struggle for survival, those with less hair go on to the next round. You get the picture. You can see it elsewhere with other species. Organisms compete to survive, and those with the necessary variations can get their variation into the next round by having offspring. Now, we should be able to see that an elephant is not "better" than a mammoth. They have different adaptations that are suitable for different environments. Mammoths existed in colder climates and elephants in warmer ones, and that's all there is to it. The same goes for species of elephants. An African bush elephant (*Loxodonta Africana*) is no better than an African forest elephant (*Loxodonta cyclotis*) or an Asian elephant (*Elephas maximus*). They have adapted to their environment. The popular term "survival of the fittest" refers not to how fast or strong or stealthy a creature is but how adequately it "fits" its environment.

Now, let's apply all this to cannabis. Indica is no better than sativa; both are adapted to the environment. A strain of cannabis that has been bred for taste is no better than a strain of cannabis that has been bred for high potency. But what if someone introduces a third breed that is both high in potency and tastes great? Wouldn't that trump the other two? If we were breeding to ensure taste and potency, then yes, in a sense, it would. However, we need to be aware of what we are saying. Our preferences give these strains a value that we arbitrarily assign to them. The strains themselves do not inherently have these values. There is nothing intrinsically of value in them. We can't scientifically point to anything about the strain that makes it better than any other, except for reproductive fitness.[10] In our subjective taste for the ultimate cannabis that we find suitable for our needs, we are, however, getting dangerously close to a very un-Darwinian picture again. That is because as we search for the perfect plant, we form the image of the archetype that doesn't exist. The archetype is static. Evolution is not. The archetype doesn't exist. Evolution does. Breeders can try to lock down traits in the strain, but there will always be some variation in population members because the environment also influences the expression of genes. It has a name—the expressed phenotype.

We take a group of 100 bats and inspect them. We will see variations. Let's narrow it down again to bats between four and six years old. Still, we will find variations in other attributes in that group, such as wingspan or weight. Let's add ear length within a range. Choose whatever attribute you want, and we will still find variations within the group with other traits. Therefore when we refer to the group, we are grouping them on some traits they appear to all share. If we start being more precise in our definition, we will find that some individuals won't qualify in large group samples. Something is wrong with that picture. The archetype of the perfect bat haunts us again. So what defines a group in biology? We can ask precisely the same question about cannabis.

When we take our large sample of cannabis and try to describe the cannabis plant grouping, we might find ourselves excluding some cannabis plants as per above. So that can't be right. Instead, we can draw up a table for the distribution of attributes, count how many plants have certain characters, and then show our results in a bar chart.[11] We can also draw up graphs and pie charts for each characteristic. The overall picture is something close to what biologists call "population thinking." Cannabis is a population of shifting values. Likewise, groups of any biological population are shifting values. Values of what? Now we are closing in on something important. To talk about cannabis as a population of shifting values is to say something finally accurate and quantifiable instead of clinging to subjective attributes we give the plant in what we hope to expect from it. Now we are dealing in terms of traits that shift in the population. What exactly is shifting? The answer is genes. Our population thinking has entered the tangible phase of this biological thought called "population genetics."

The Language of Cannabis Genes

Genes are shuffled around in different combinations through a biological process called "meiosis," a type of cell division undergone by sexually reproducing individuals. It allows male and female genes to combine like two sides of a zipper to produce an individual that combines genes from both parents.[12] Genes are DNA sequences transcribed by cell machinery and eventually translated into proteins that build a living thing into what it is.[13] The process is generally ongoing throughout the organism's development. Genes are usually expressed in the form of the *morphology* of the plant, in that they control plant characteristics, but the environment impacts how much they control what they do. That expression of the gene is known as the *phenotype*. We observe, taste, and smell these in our plant populations, but what ultimately controls them is genes and how they react to the environment. These are the hidden values that fluctuate, our shifting values in populations.

When we refer to fluctuating genes, we are talking about the number of genes for that trait in a population. For example, in our sample of bats, a certain percentage will have genes for long ears because longer ears have been conferring an advantage in echolocation. More of these males do better finding insects for food. That means they do better than the ones that have shorter ears. Having food maintains health and fitness for reproduction. So the frequency of longer ear genes in the population increases in the next generation.[14] Now apply that concept to everything about cannabis in terms of anything and everything that goes into making up a cannabis plant. It is all about frequencies of genes shifting to higher and lower values in the population.

The overall cannabis population refers to all the world's currently living cannabis plants. However, cannabis populations can be divided by artificial boundaries (grow room separation) or natural environmental boundaries (mountain ranges). Grow rooms are types of artificial geographical boundaries causing *geographical isolation.*[15] There may also be *reproductive isolation* (pollen sheds too early in one strain before flowers bloom in another, so no hybridization is naturally possible). They form individual *gene pools.*[16] Populations are samples from this larger population; within them, a portion of those genes shift from higher to lower values. The separation can eventually form different strains of cannabis, especially under domestication. In a longer evolutionary timescale, this produces *speciation.* Cannabis has probably not undergone speciation, but there are examples of separation producing highly variable characteristics. Our struggle for survival still applies. Genes can become extinct, never to be seen again. If a gene for blue flowers is unpopular with insects for one year and the insects select yellow flowers instead, blue flower genes can become extinct; only the yellow genes remain. Breeders can intervene and do precisely the same thing. They control the frequencies of genes, deliberately altering them to create a unique population. When sufficient quantities of unwanted genes are replaced with more desired genes, the strain becomes more uniform, with less diversity and variation.

The question "what is cannabis?" *can* be answered: Cannabis is a plant population that consists of shifting values, and these values are cannabis genes that are expressed as phenotypes.

The above is an orientation in biology that has worked for over a century, since the modern evolutionary synthesis. In addition, the technological innovation of gene sequencing has further allowed us to have DNA markers to help us determine what species an organism belongs to. It can also tell us directly about paternity. Whole databases of genetic trees can be stored in computers mapping out living things in terms of population genetics.

Now that we have you up to speed on how biology views any organism, we can proceed with a gene-centered view of cannabis cultivation combined with the best practices of multiple methods for optimal results. In short, we are using proven techniques and great genetics in growing environments that are shown to give the results you see in the photographs advertised in breeder's advertisements and this book!

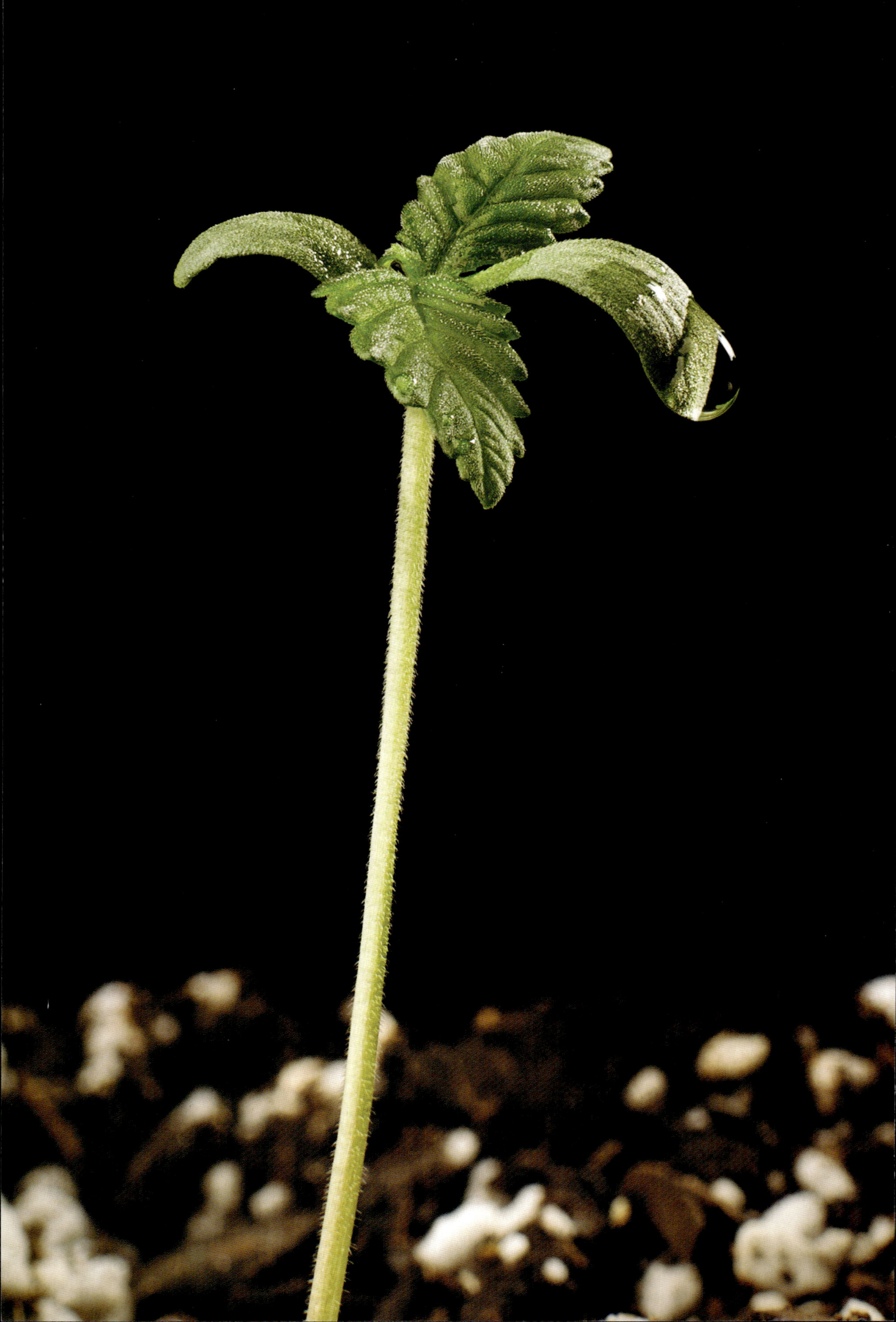

1

A Quick Start Guide

This chapter provides a brief introduction to cannabis cultivation. It will give you an overview of the process and, more importantly, help you get your seedlings sprouting and ready to go.

Before acquiring seeds or clones, consider whether to grow indoors or outdoors. Professional growers typically categorize strains as either indoor or outdoor varieties. You'll also need to decide whether you want to grow an indica for its body-stone effect or sativa for its head-high. Indoor strains tend to be indicas, while outdoor strains are usually sativas. Hybrid strains combine both types to offer a mix of medicinal effects; however, first-time growers should probably avoid new hybrids due to their higher variability. For indica plants, consider strains like Kush, Shiva, Afghani, and Northern Lights. Northern Lights, despite being a hybrid, has been selectively bred for indica traits to the point of having uniform pure indica characteristics. If you prefer sativa plants, look into strains like Haze and Pearl, or African, Mexican, Jamaican, and equatorial strains.

Once you've determined your preferences, the next step is to acquire seeds or find a source for clones. The method for starting is the same regardless of the strain you choose. You don't need to overspend on your first seed purchase as pure strains tend to be more affordable than hybrids. Ensure that you obtain quality genetics and avoid using bag seeds. You'll need around 10 seeds to begin.

While you may be able to visit a local head shop to purchase genetics, many places around the world now offer seed-shipping services to places where cannabis cultivation has been legalized. If you prioritize security, you can maintain anonymity conducting research and transactions online by using a Virtual Private Network (VPN). Keep in mind that while VPNs offer security, your Internet Service Provider (ISP) still has some level of visibility into your online activities. Search terms like "how to make anonymous purchases online" and "buy cannabis seeds with cryptocurrency online" will help enhance your online privacy. Cryptocurrencies are the preferred currencies

PHOTO: RUSSELL-HOWLAND PHOTOGRAPHY

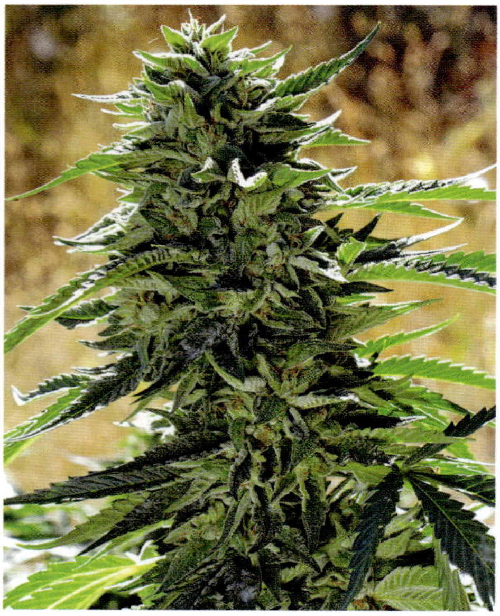

Blatant self-sufficiency is the goal of most growers.

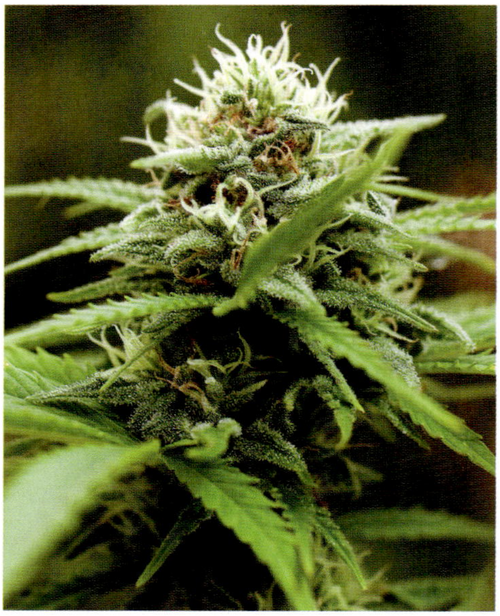

A green thumb is not required. Anyone can grow.

PHOTOS: EMERALD TRIANGLE SEEDS (LEFT), ROYALQUEENSEEDS.COM (RIGHT)

for online transactions, so that you can directly purchase seeds and have them shipped anonymously, although it's crucial not to assume this process is entirely foolproof. Many growers opt to have seeds shipped to an address unrelated to the actual growing location, providing an extra layer of security. Always ensure the seller is trustworthy to reduce the risk of financial loss.

You will likely buy your seeds from a seed bank, so you will want to find a reputable one with a solid trading history. Online searches will help you identify the oldest seed banks, but the most well-established ones may not ship worldwide. Your next best resources for finding a reputable seed bank are social media platforms and online forums with large user bases, where a brief search will reveal which seed banks have a track record of success and which ones do not. The market is vast, but the time and effort invested in research are well worth it.

Once you have chosen a seed bank, place your order, wait for the shipping confirmation via email, and then proceed to purchase the germination materials you'll need for a quick and cost-effective start. For successful germination, you will need:

- seeds
- germination tray (Tupperware, or similar, without the lid can be used)
- small Rockwool cubes
- water
- 15-watt LED grow bulb (the economical type)
- gooseneck lamp for the grow bulb (make sure it matches the bulb socket size)

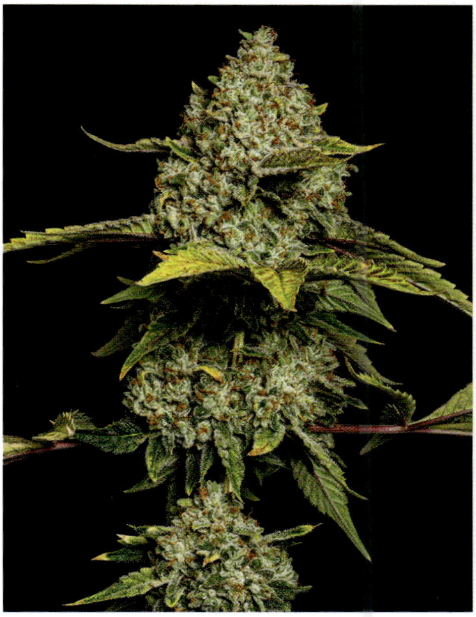

You get top quality by growing it yourself.

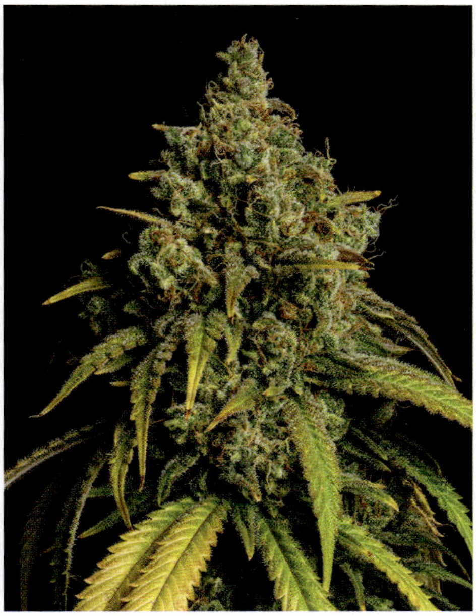

You will never go back to inferior quality.

The ideal LED grow bulb typically has a lamp-like shape, with a flat surface covered in numerous smaller lights in the front. This type of bulb can fit into most lamps, though lamps with a bendable gooseneck are preferred. Some gooseneck lamps don't have a stand, instead featuring a clip, and can be powered via USB. The cost-effective system described in this chapter is primarily designed for starting seeds or maintaining a small number of clones, so there's no need to invest in a full LED array kit just yet. The idea is to learn and gain experience while building a foundation. You can conveniently order all these items online if your local gardening shop doesn't have them in stock.

When purchasing Rockwool, you'll find slabs with either 24 or 150 cubes in two different sizes with premade holes for placing seeds. Rockwool dimensions are stated in length, width, and height (L × W × H for product descriptions), such as 1.5″ × 1.5″× 1.5″ or 3.5 cm × 3.5 cm × 3.5 cm.

Insert your seeds into the holes of the Rockwool cubes and place the cubes in a tray. Water the cubes, but ensure they're neither too wet nor too dry. Within a couple of weeks, your seedlings will begin to germinate. Once the seedlings show their petioles, position a table lamp with the LED grow bulb over them. Maintaining the right distance between the bulb and the seedlings is crucial, especially as they grow taller and closer to the light. You can use your hand to gauge the necessary distance; if the temperature feels too hot, then the bulb is too close to the seedlings. If this distance is managed well, the seedlings will remain compact for easier transplantation into your primary growing area. This is all you need for a quick start to get your seeds on the path to successful growth.

PHOTOS: ROB BRAMHILL

Strawberry Mango Crumble: Seed to Harvest

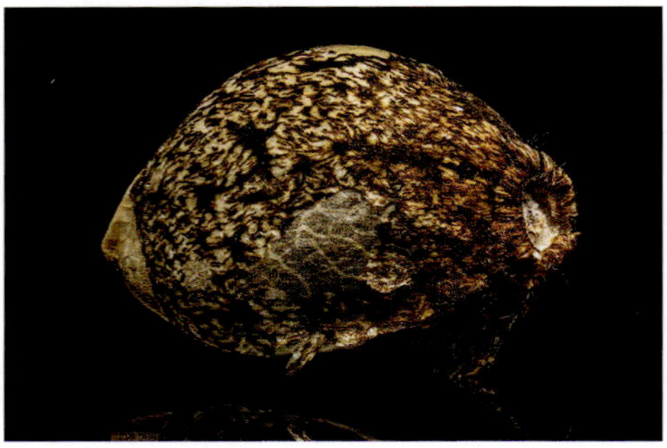

A seed coat testa protects the genetics of the new plant. The code to unlock is 'H_2O'.

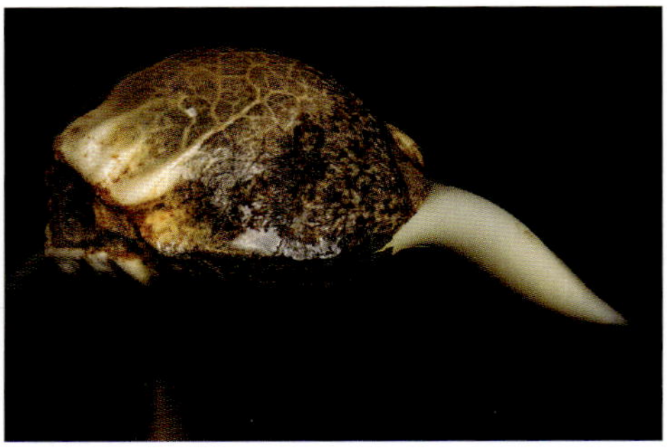

The typical tadpole look of the embryo emerging radicle first for rooting.

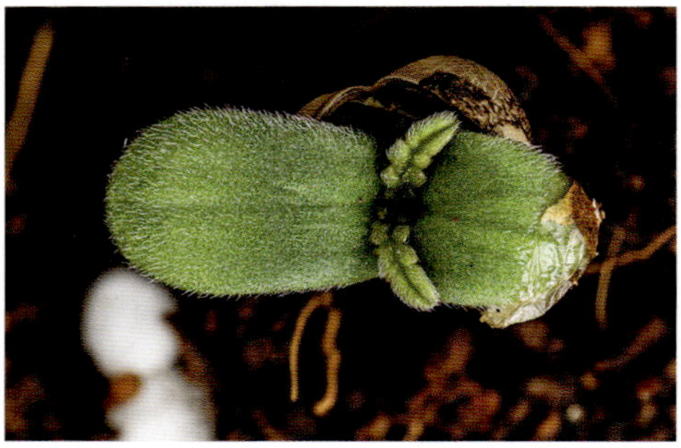

Overhead view of the rooted seedling using its cotyledons to push away the testa.

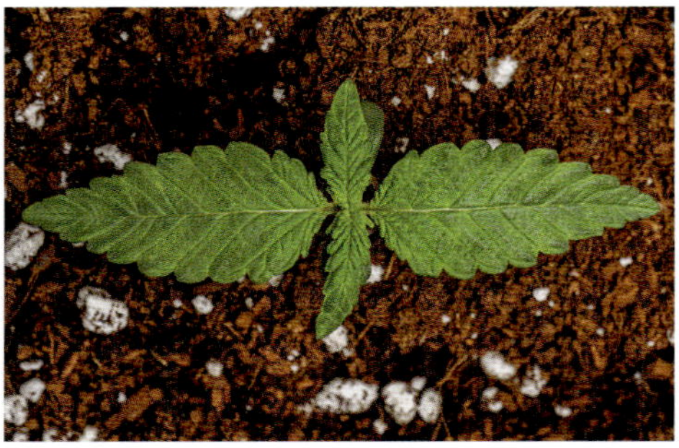

True leaf growth will be serrated but still not the typical cannabis leaf shape.

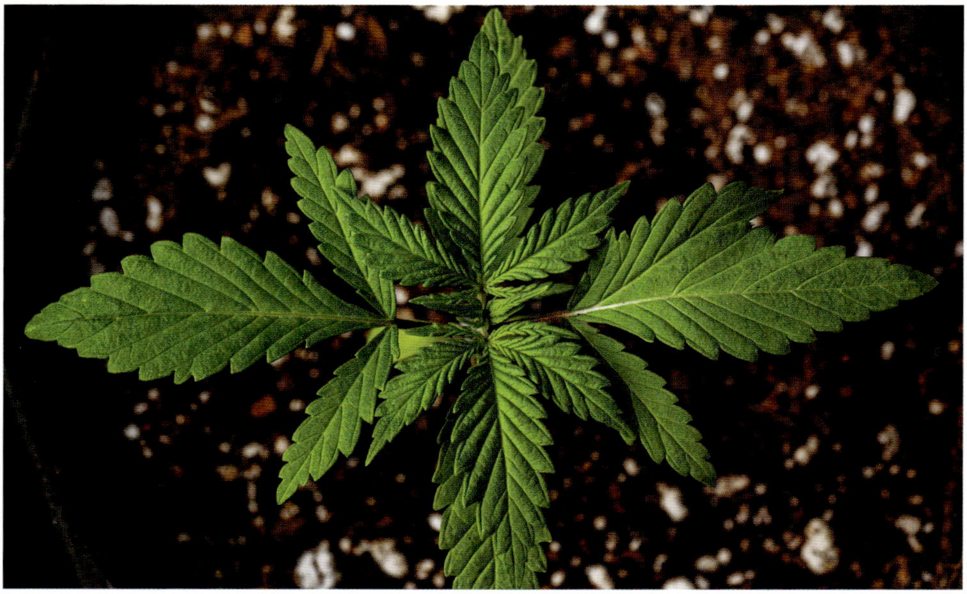

Cannabis leaf morphology is a progression of complexity. Multiple leaflets create the typical cannabis leaf shape. Day 15.

PHOTOS: ROB BRAMHILL

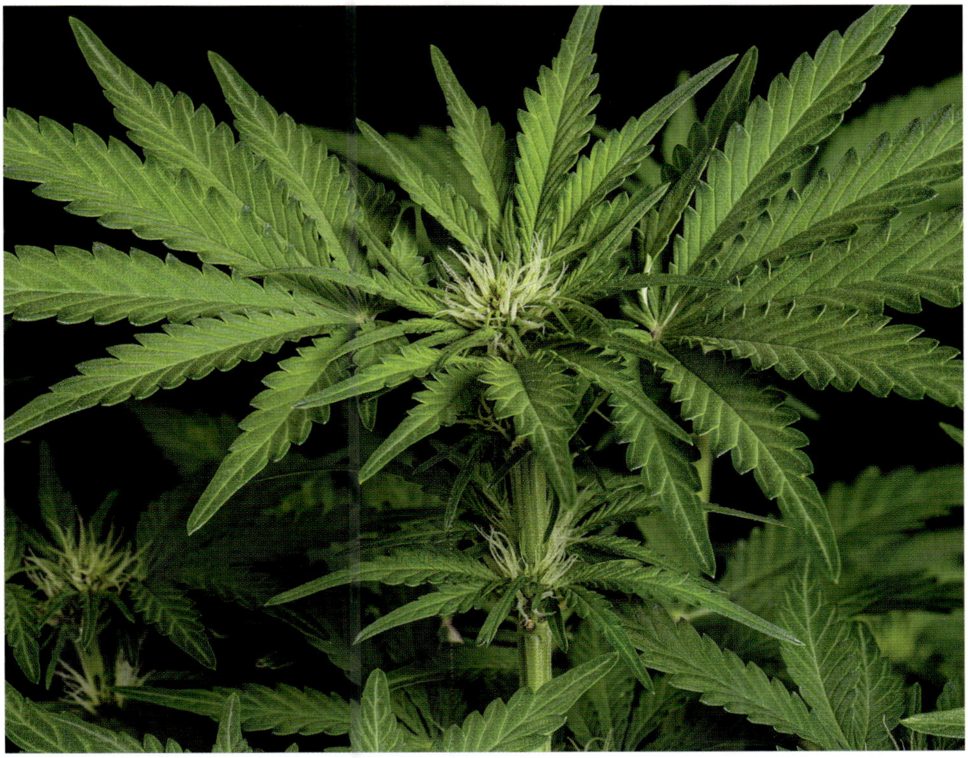

Plant complexity arises due to the duplication of similar properties at different sizes and stages of growth.

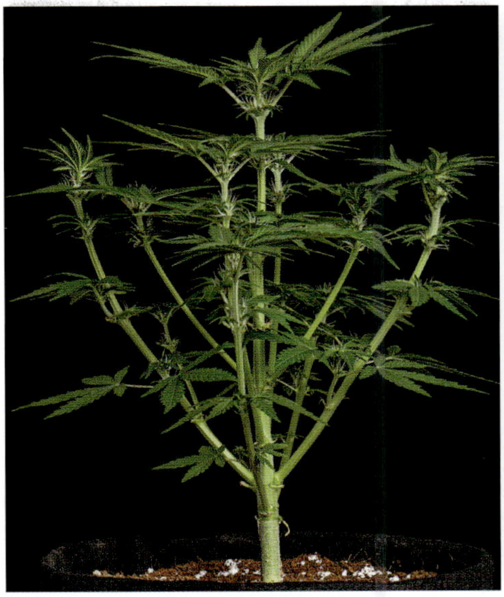

The finished vegetative plant shape is not unlike a candelabra for holding multiple candle sticks.

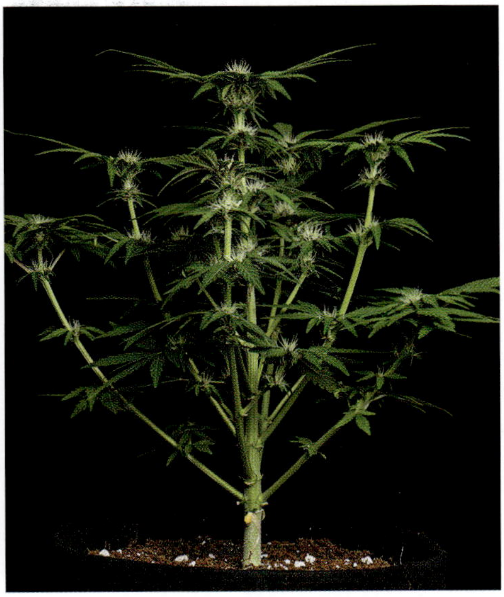

As the flowers bulk, branches will bend outwards with the weight, changing the shape of the plant.

continues...

Strawberry Mango Crumble: Seed to Harvest *continued*

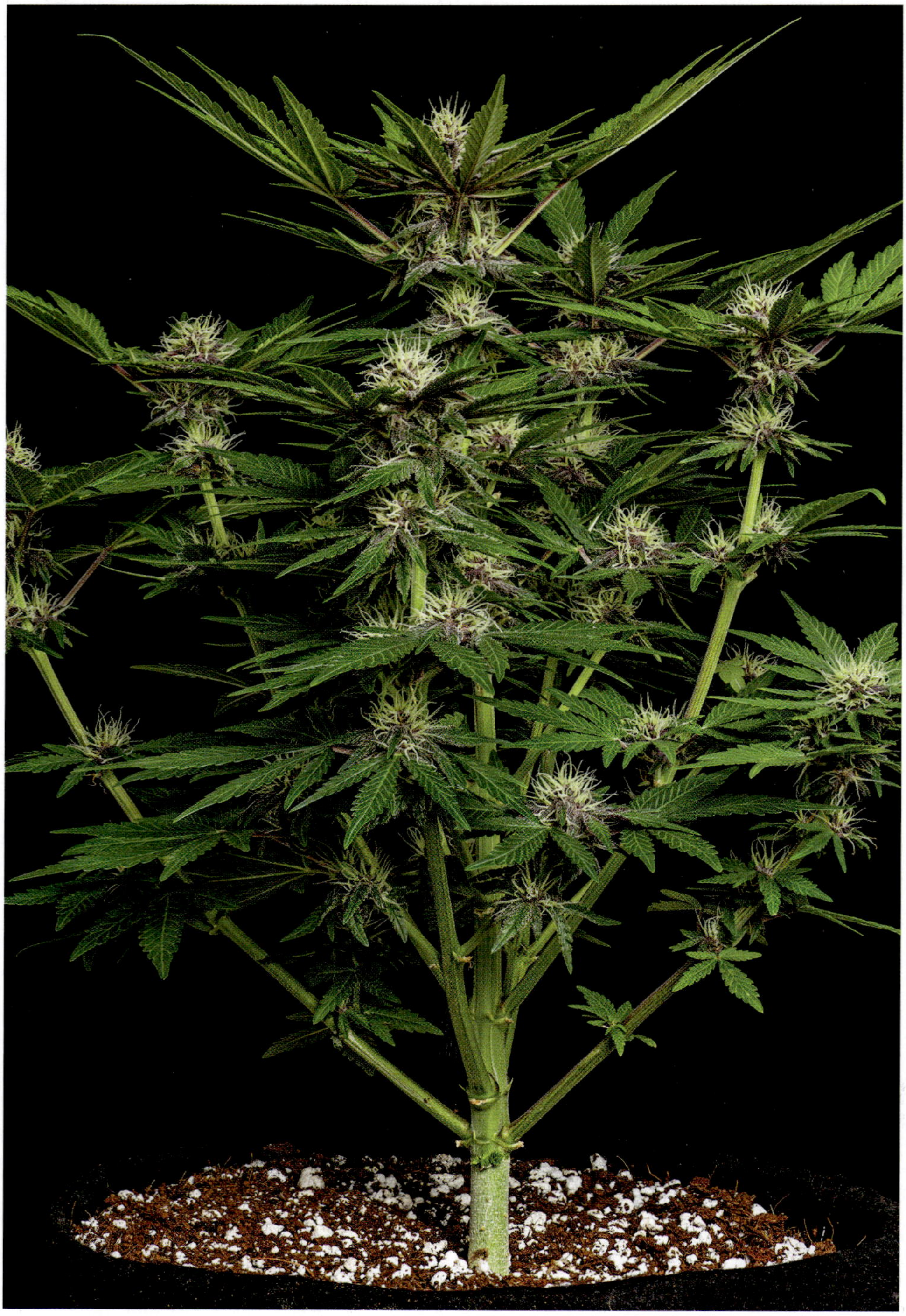

PHOTOS: ROB BRAMHILL

The cannabis plant shape is primarily for keeping flowers upright towards the light. Internodes between flowers are still visible.

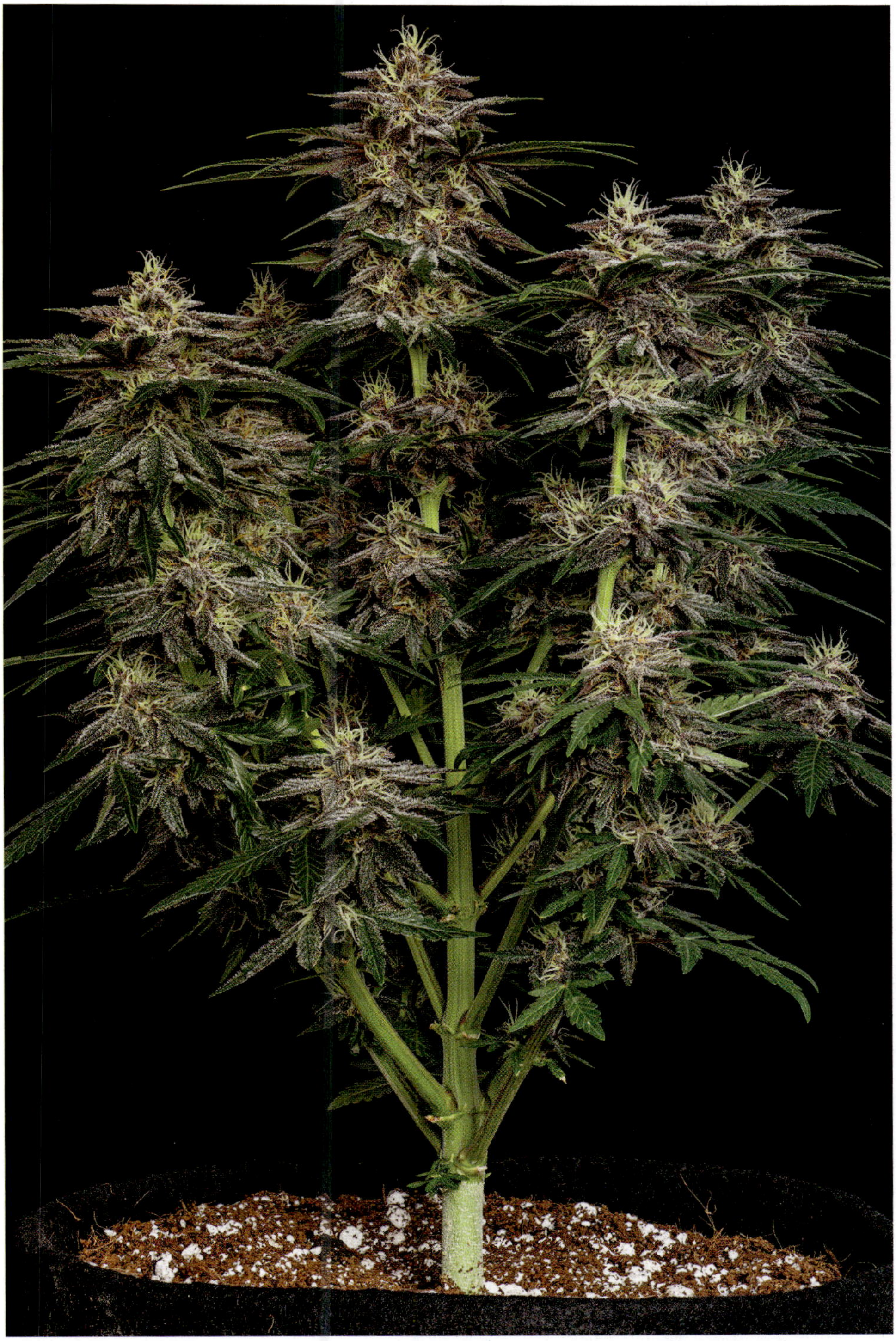

During flowering the plant size will increase and the plant looks bushier, but most notably internodes are filling out with flowers.

continues...

Strawberry Mango Crumble: Seed to Harvest *continued*

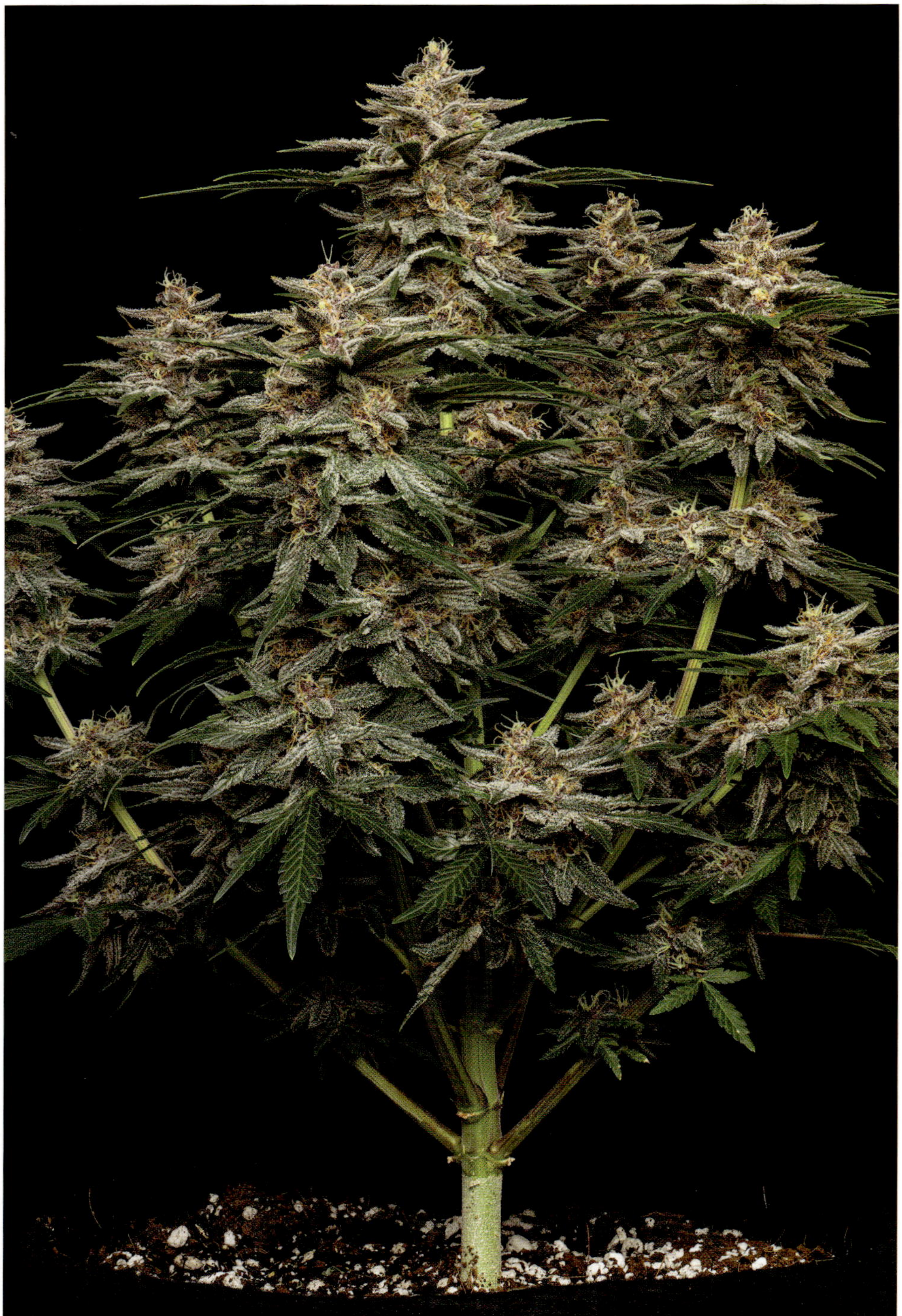

PHOTOS: ROB BRAMHILL

Towards the end of flowering, flowers appear caked with icing sugar. Trichomes produce this effect.

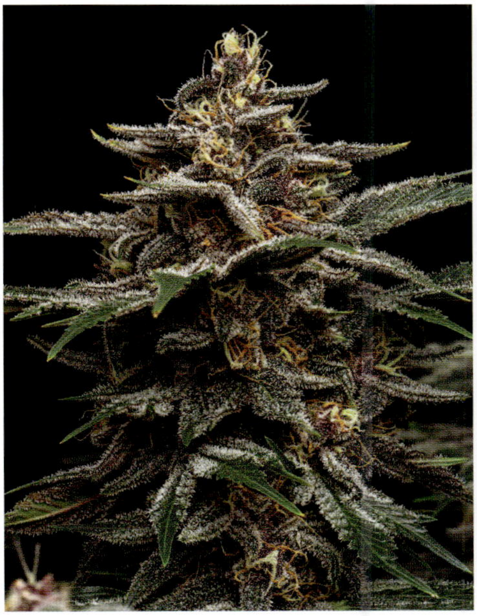

Remember single leaf morphology during the seedling phase? These reappear in flowering within the flowers.

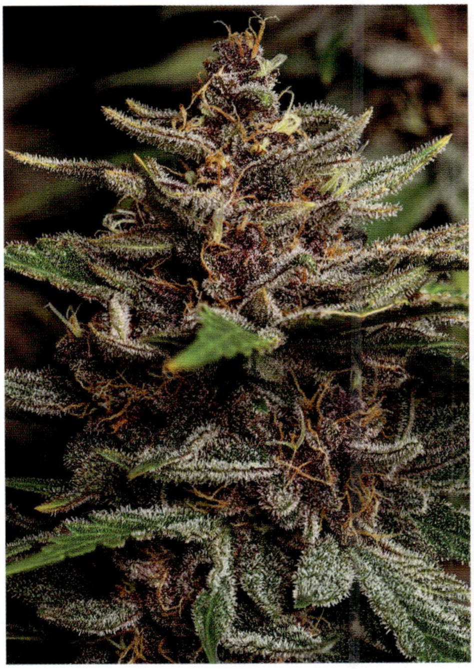

Saturated with resin, flowers are extremely sticky but the bulk of plant matter will be somewhat dense.

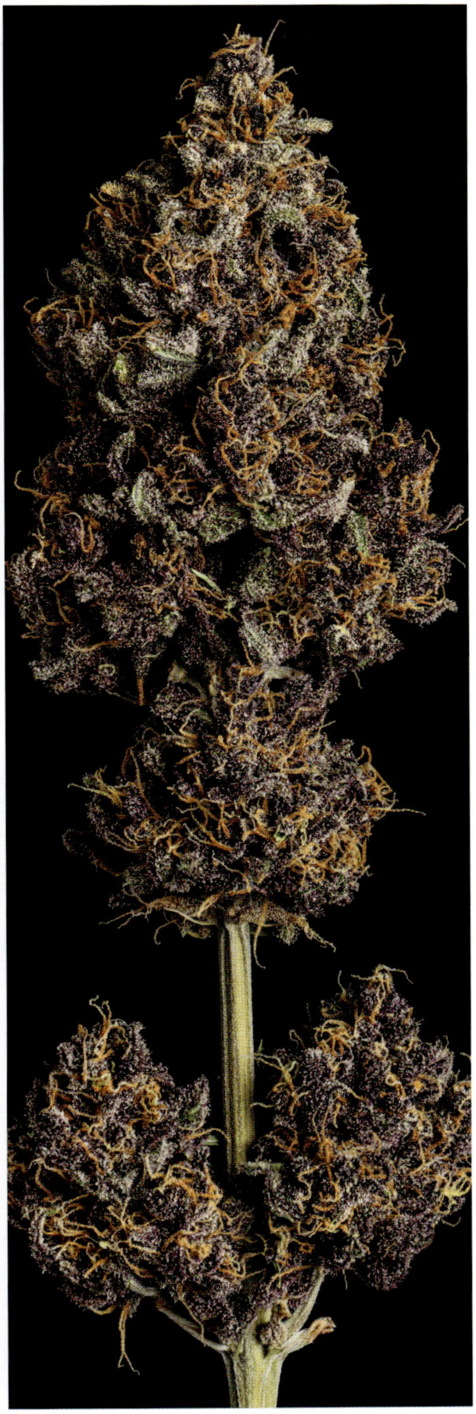

Trimming away the leaves reveals the many colors of flowering clusters, especially after drying.

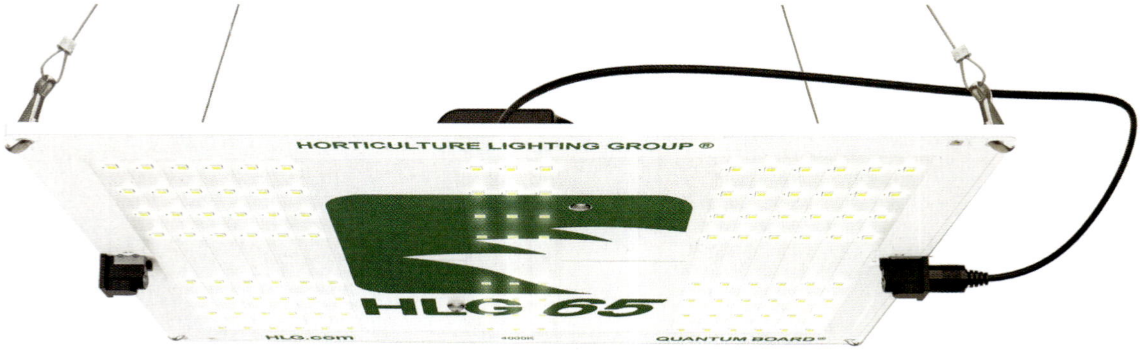

This LED is a great choice for growers who are starting out with seedlings or clones and will easily go through vegetative or a full grow with a single plant. It's a low-cost unit and great value for new growers.

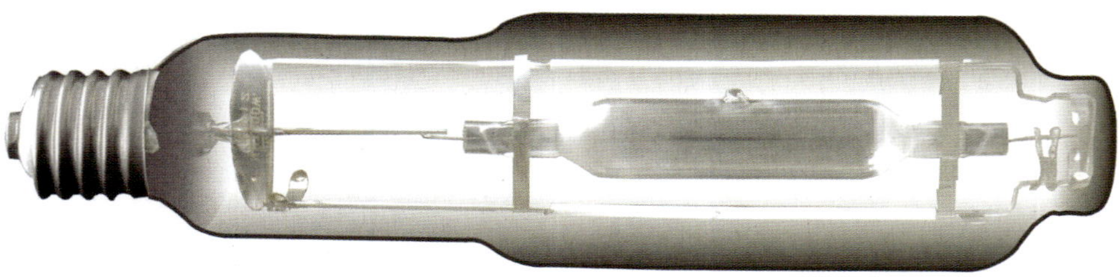

1000-watt MH light is better for vegetative growth.

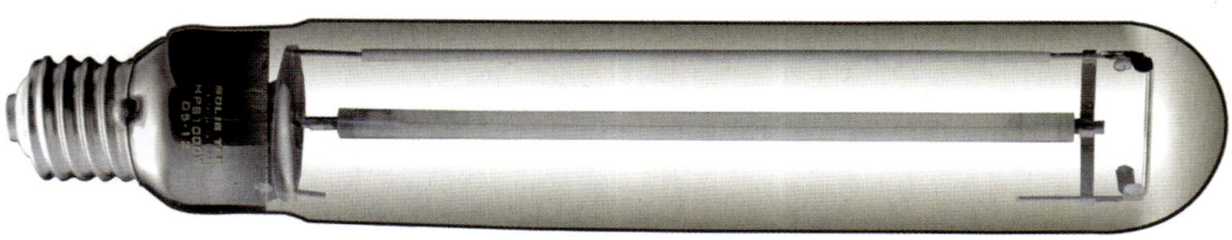

1000-watt HPS light is better for flowering.

PHOTOS: HORTICULTURE LIGHTING GROUP, HLG.COM (TOP), SOLIS TEK (BULBS)

The following section provides a concise overview of the cannabis cultivation methodology and offers valuable insights to quickly familiarize yourself with the fundamentals. Outdoor growers should read both the indoor and outdoor sections, as certain indoor information can also prove useful for outdoor cultivation.

Indoor Quick Start

Lights

LED lighting has revolutionized indoor cultivation, and high-intensity discharge (HID) and fluorescent lights can, mostly, no longer compete. Fluorescents were generally used exclusively with clones and seedlings due to their low wattage and poor color spectrum, which resulted in less-than-ideal yield returns. However, there are now specialized growing fluorescents that can outperform standard domestic fluorescents. HID lights were typically used at low wattages (up to 250 watts) in

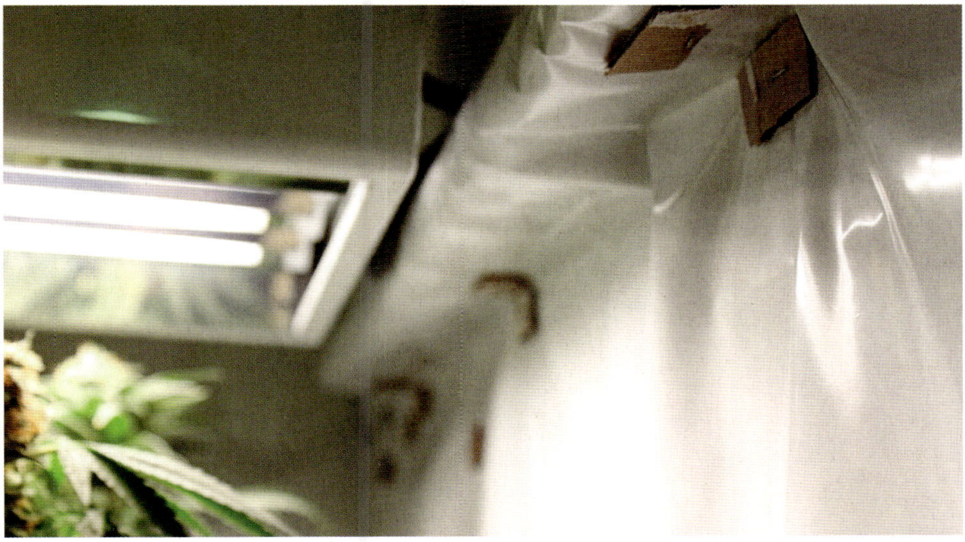

White reflective grow room sheeting can be installed quickly and removed again. Sheets are black on the other side.

well-ventilated grow cabinets, and in larger grow spaces at higher wattages, typically between 400 and 1000-watt, or multiple lights of different wattages. With the emergence of LED lights, HIDs are no longer the first choice. LEDs are more energy-efficient and generate significantly less heat while also achieving the same color spectrum as HIDs, including the intensity needed for rewarding results. This book will cover the different types of LED grow lights, and what you need to know about them.

White Walls or Mylar

Your grow room must maximize light reflection onto your plants. You can improve light reflection by painting the grow room walls white or using reflective grow sheeting like Mylar. Taking this simple step could potentially double your yield.

Soil, Substrates, and Hydroponics

You have the option to grow in soil, another substrate, or a hydroponic system. Soil is recommended for beginners and continues to be used by many advanced growers. Hydroponic and aeroponic systems are better suited for experienced or advanced growers. However, soil-based grows can be just as successful as hydroponic or aeroponic systems. To begin, you'll need some soil, or loam, or another substrate, and approximately 3-gallon (11-liter) pots. Substrates, such as vermiculite or perlite, can replace soil and are often mixed with it. Ensure the loam you buy has the right nutrient content for vegetative growth, as indicated on the packaging. You may also need a medium which physically supports the plant stem and holds roots upright. Some strains of cannabis will need more support than others.

PHOTO: GCP

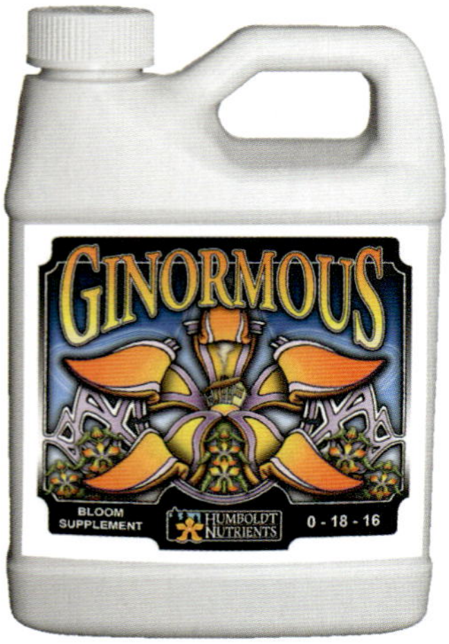

An example of a liquid plant fertilizer specifically designed to promote primary flowering growth.

Nutrients

You will require the following nutrients. Whenever possible, opt for organic nutrients:

- Primary vegetative growth feed in liquid form, with a balanced Nitrogen (N) Phosphorus (P) Potassium (K) ratio such as 5-5-5 or 10-10-10. Ratios with higher nitrogen are acceptable. Only use full-strength nutrients explicitly designed for cannabis grows. Your loam soil should have a similar NPK ratio to a primary vegetative growth feed.
- Primary flowering growth feed in liquid form, with more P than N and K, such as 5-10-5 or 10-20-10. Do not use full strength unless the nutrients are advertised as cannabis nutrients.
- Secondary nutrients bottle containing magnesium, sulfur, and calcium. Use this sparingly.
- Micronutrient bottle. Use this sparingly.

Vegetative Growth

Bring your seedlings into a grow room or tent when they have developed substantial growth. Maintain a light regime of 24 hours of light per day, or 24/0, for the breeder's recommended vegetative growth time. Then feed primary vegetative nutrients

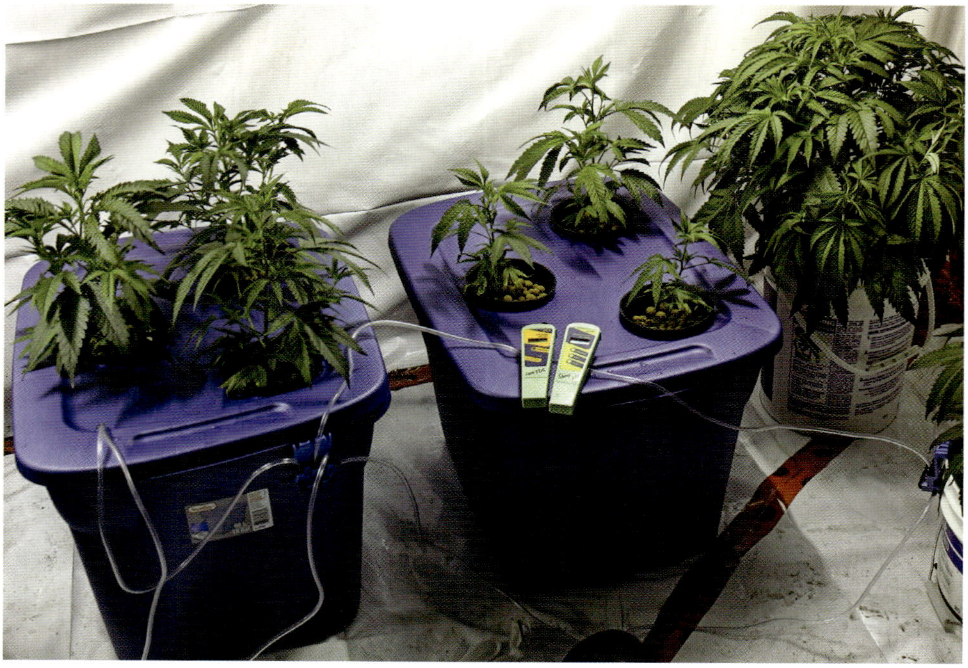

Hydroponic systems with plants in vegetative growth.

PHOTOS: HUMBOLDTNUTRIENTS.COM (TOP), DAVID STRANGE (BOTTOM)

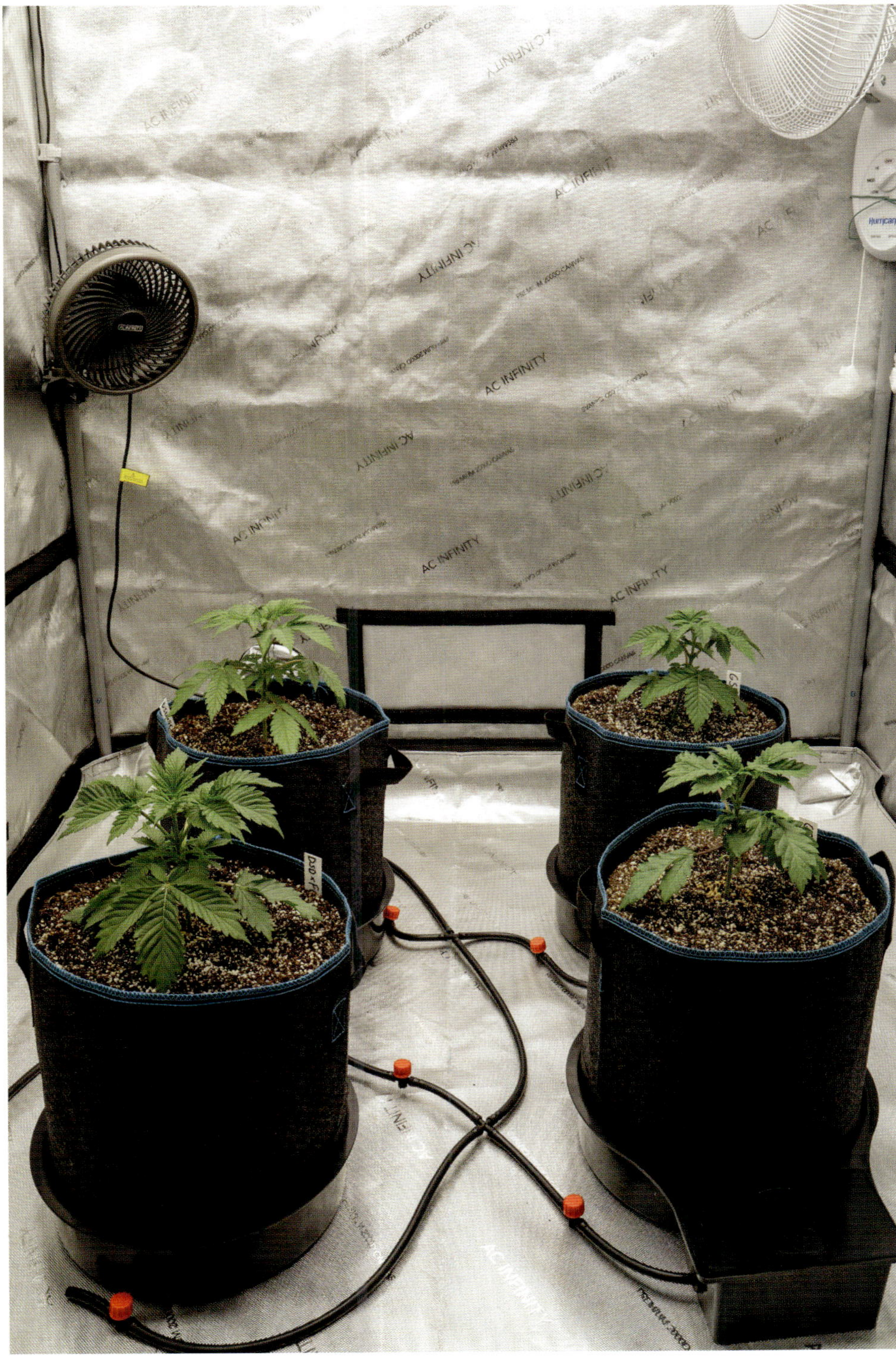

PHOTO: JOE'S CANNA GROWS

A tent goes up, and it can go down again if you want. Tents are a very effective way to turn any indoor area into grow space.

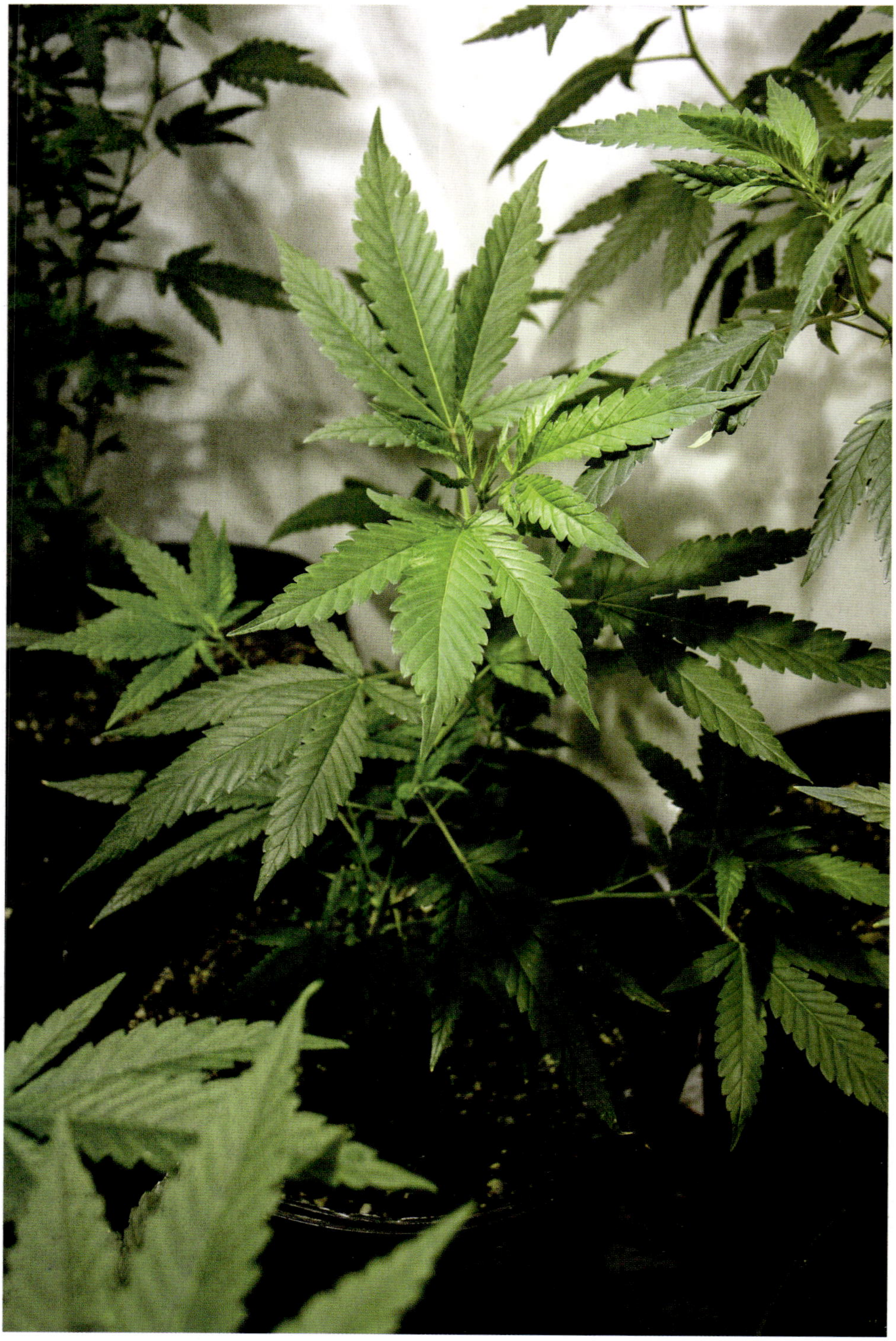

PHOTO: DAVID STRANGE

This hobby can be very enjoyable, and seeing your ability to bring plants to life like this is a reward in itself.

once a week, along with secondary and micronutrients as needed. You'll learn what's required as issues arise; this book covers necessary adjustments for various problems. If you grow the same strain more than once, for instance through clones, you'll become familiar with the nutrient strength and timing needed for that particular strain.

Pre-Flowering

Pre-flowering is not influenced by light, but rather relates to plant maturity. Your goal is to identify calyx development for flowering. This book provides information on flowering and calyx development, complete with images of microstructures to help you identify male and female plants at this stage. Clones are occasionally mature enough to start flowering, so it's essential to monitor them for any signs of this. If they seem to be transitioning into that stage, your priority should be to ensure your 24/0 light cycle is properly set up. This will help maintain them in the vegetative growth stage.

Flowering

Cannabis flowering in mature plants is triggered by changes in the photoperiod, the number of hours of light the plant gets in a day. The exception to this are autoflowering hybrids (ruderalis crosses) that will flower according to age, not the photoperiod change. With regular cannabis, your objective is to initiate flowering when the plants are mature enough and have sufficient vegetative growth. Once you observe pre-flowering calyx development, you can force flowering. For several weeks, maintain a light regime of 12 hours of light per day and 12 hours of total darkness, or 12/12, while feeding your plants primary flowering nutrients once a week, with secondary and micronutrients as needed. Ensure complete darkness is maintained, without any light leaks into the flowering room or tent.

Harvest

The ideal time to harvest can be determined by observing color changes in the flowers. When most of the trichomes have turned amber, the plant can be harvested. Harvest time can also be identified by using a sampling system if you plan to grow the same strain multiple times. Over a two-week period, remove a small bud sample each day, label it with the date or otherwise indicate the number of days in the flowering stage, and note its color. Allow the bud to dry and cure, then compare your samples. Based on the sample you prefer, you can use the number of days it spent in the flowering stage to find your future harvest date for that specific strain.

Curing

Finally, cure your harvest. Curing involves darkness and aeration. Hang your harvested buds to dry in a well-ventilated and completely dark room. Once the plants are sufficiently dry, trim your buds and store them in jars away from light. Regularly inspect your jars for mold and allow them to air out briefly while you inspect your buds.

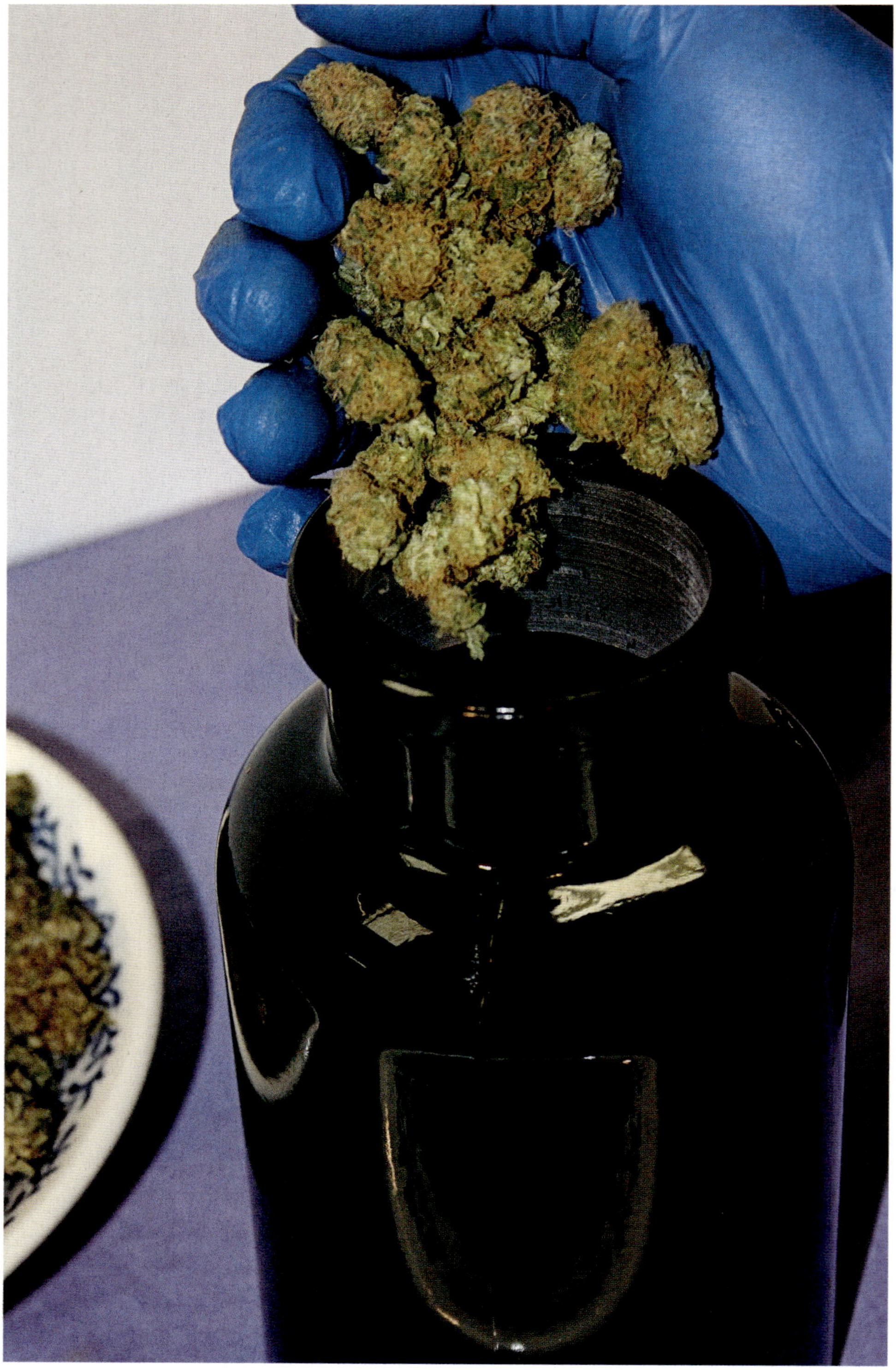

PHOTO: MM JARS

Manicured dried bud is stored in jars away from light. Open now and again to air and check for mold.

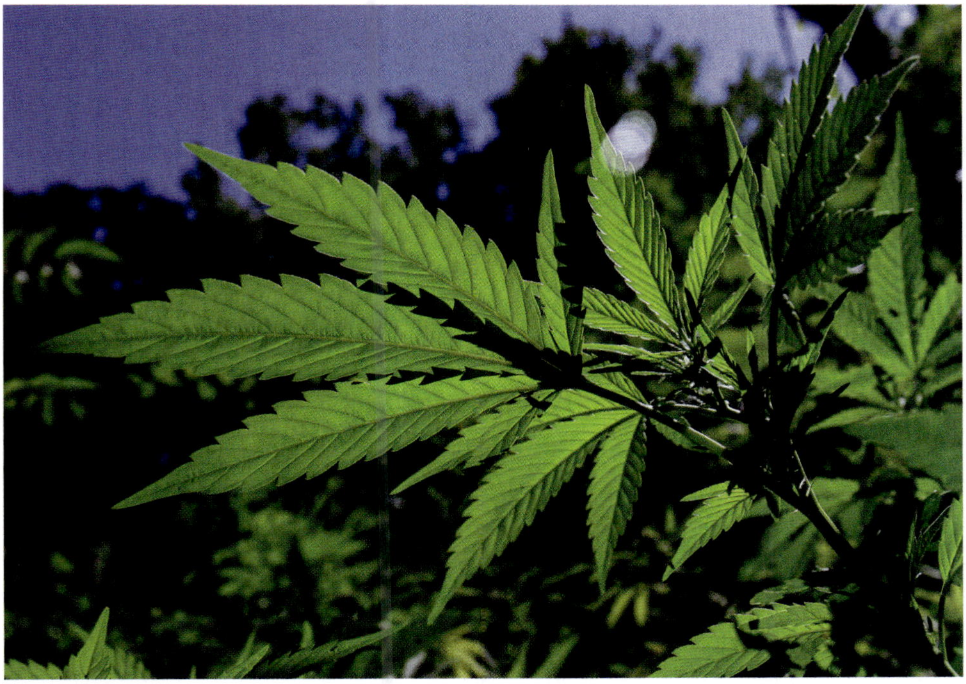

Cannabis is tough and naturally adapted to outdoor environments.

Outdoor Quick Start

Most of the information for indoor growers applies to outdoor growers as well, as outdoor strains are typically started inside before being transplanted outdoors.

Sunlight

Understanding your outdoor environment is crucial because your crop's success depends on fertile soil, stable weather conditions, and adequate sunlight. If you're growing cannabis outside, your light source is the sun. If you don't receive enough sunshine for the longer flowering times required by sativa strains, you can opt for indica or hybrid strains including autoflowering hybrids for earlier flowering.

Medium

Prepare an outdoor plot with store-bought soil, and replace the topsoil with this fresh soil. Refer to the outdoor chapter, which discusses various outdoor soil mixes, or to the organics chapter for information on preparing slow-release organic soil mixes.

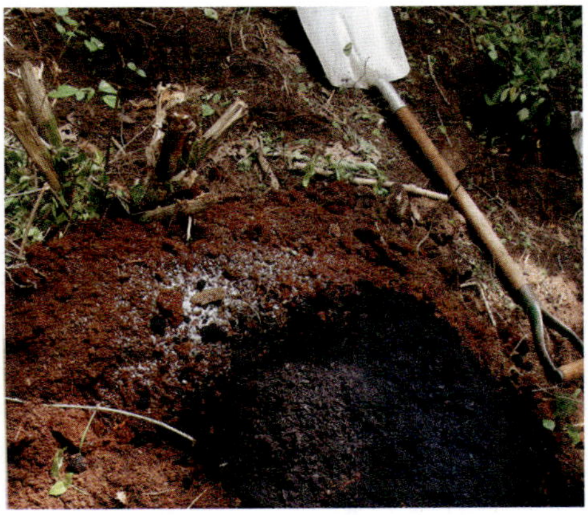

Combining soils gives growers more control over the medium in which their plants will grow.

PHOTOS: DAVID STRANGE

Organic Pesticides

To protect your outdoor plants from wildlife, insects, and mold, consider using organic pesticides only during the vegetative growth stage, as applying pesticides during the flowering stage is not advisable. Inspect the bugs at your outdoor grow site to identify potential threats. Only organic pesticides, which target only pests but leave beneficial insects unharmed, should be used.

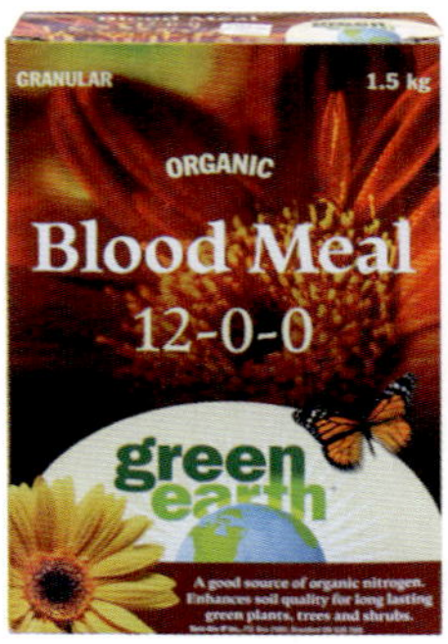

Blood meal for vegetative growth.

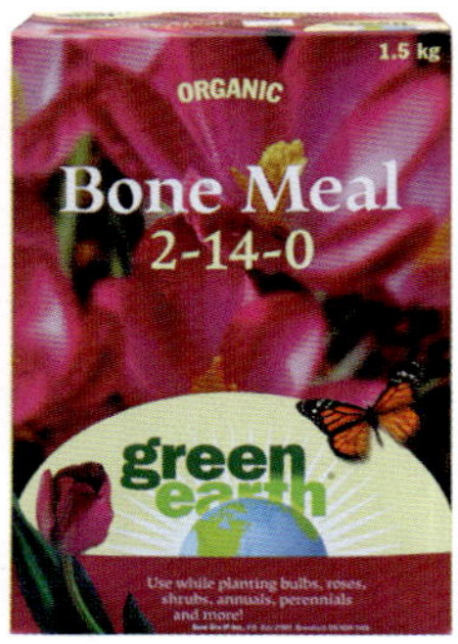

Bone meal for flowering.

Nutrients

You can use the same liquid nutrients outlined in the indoor section of the guide. However, if you incorporate slow-release nutrients into your plot mix, you'll need to reduce the strength and frequency of your weekly liquid feedings to accommodate for nutrients provided through the slow-release method.

Growth

Sunlight provides the light regime for outdoor plants, so you cannot initiate flowering manually. The exception to this rule is with ruderalis hybrids. Your plants will grow, mature, and flower as the seasons change. Feed your plants with primary vegetative nutrients once a week, and secondary and micronutrients as needed during the vegetative growth stage. When flowering begins, switch to flowering nutrients.

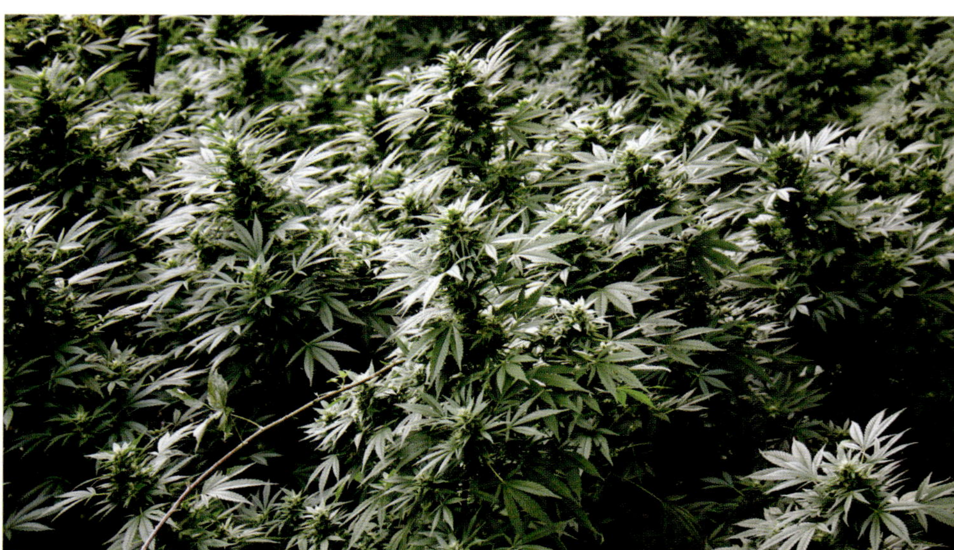

This cluster of Lowryder by the Joint Doctor was grown in a ravine. The light was so-so, but the genetics meant that the plants had a huge yield.

PHOTOS: GCP (TOP) DAVID STRANGE (BOTTOM)

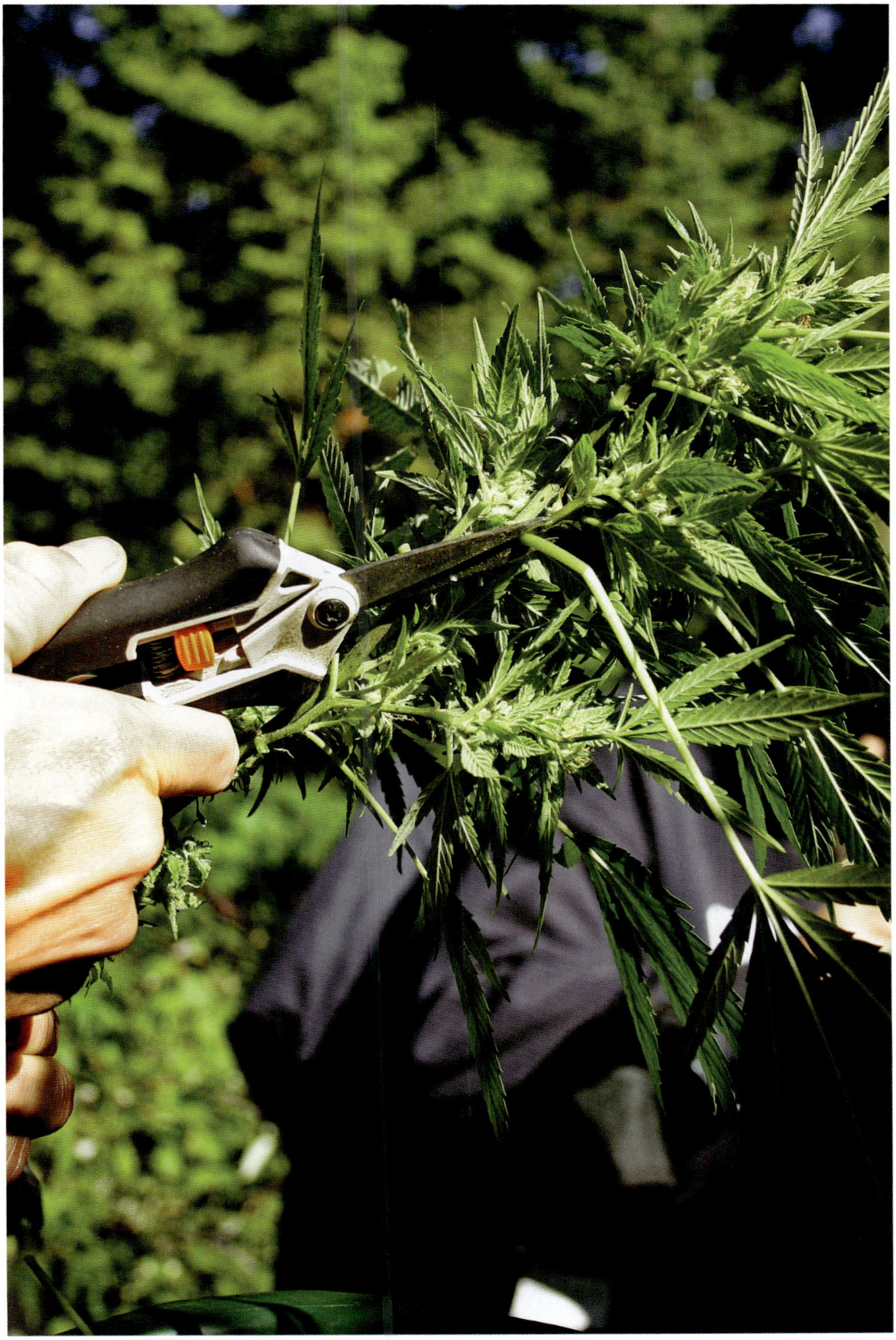

PHOTO: DAVID STRANGE

At harvest, before hanging for drying, trim larger branched leaf stalks (petioles) away to make the harvest lighter and more compact.

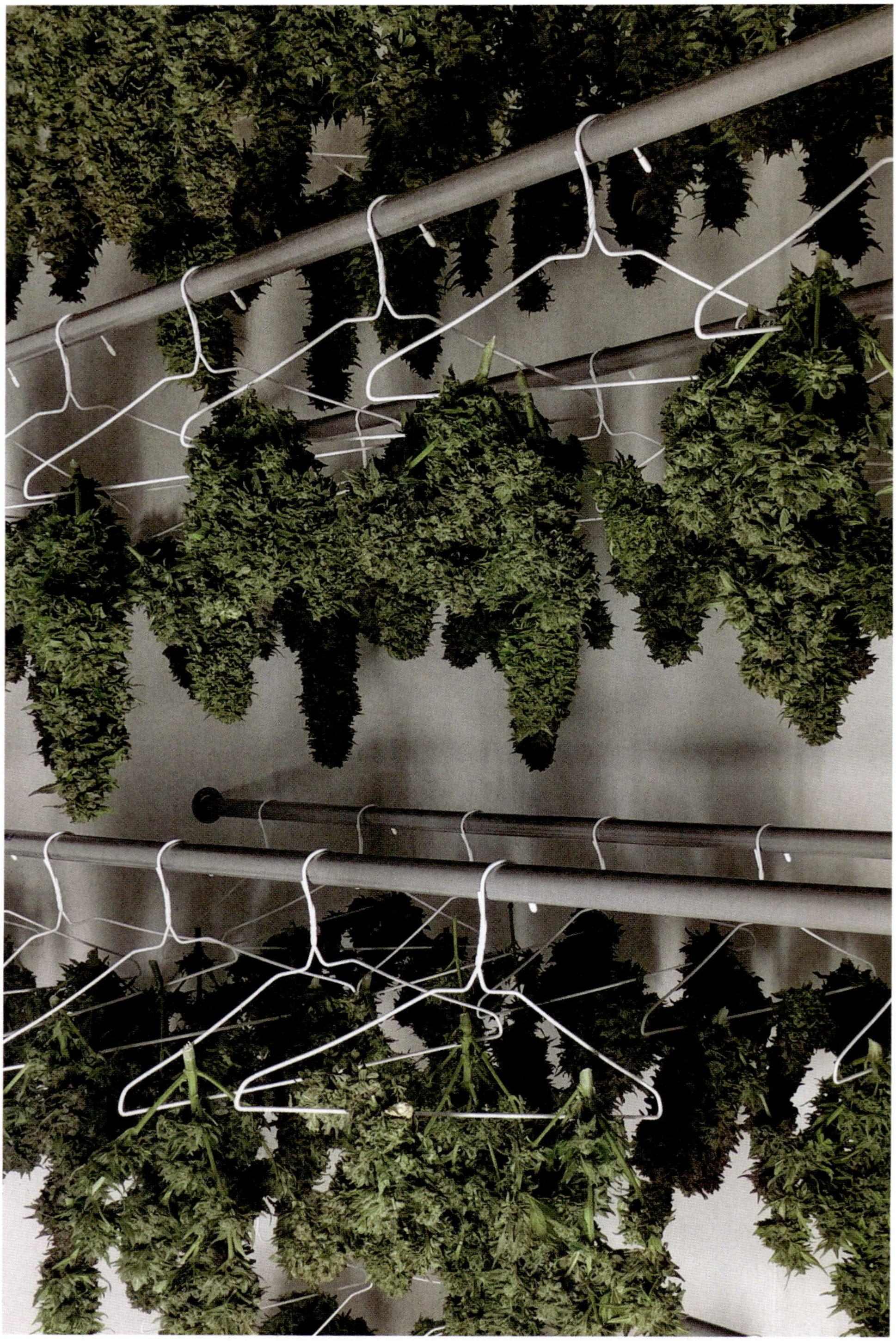

PHOTO: BRENDAN BROWN

White reflective grow room sheeting can be installed quickly and removed again. Sheets are black on the other side.

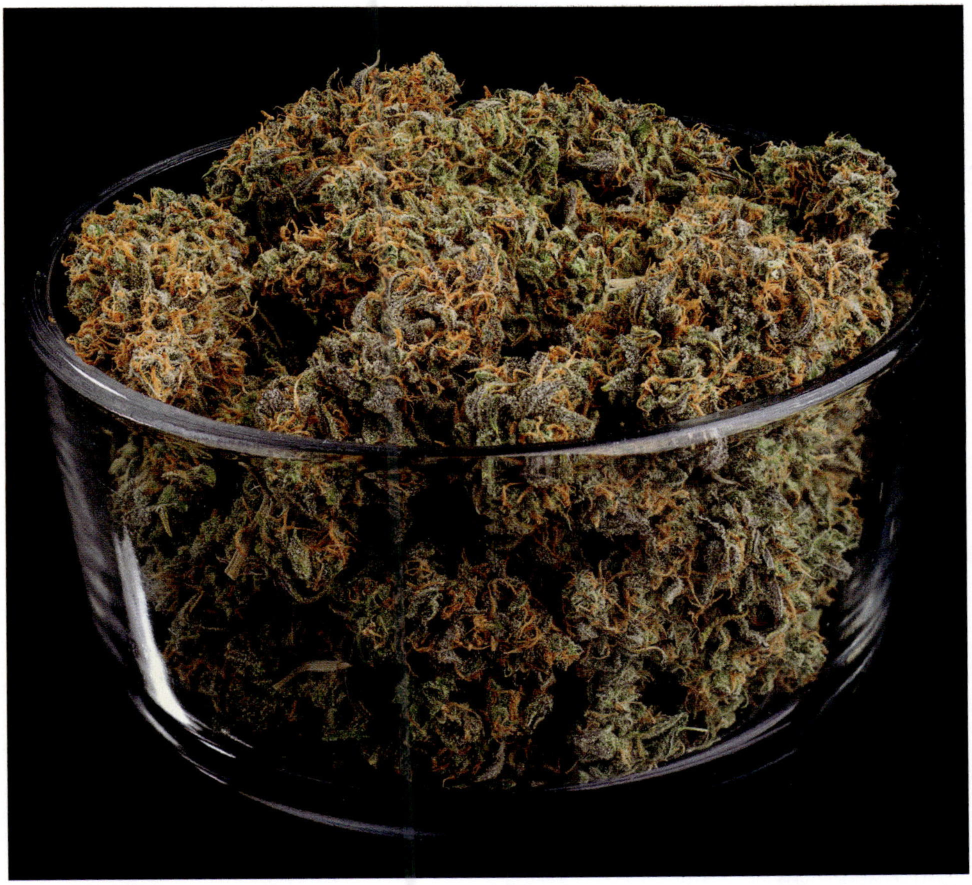

Finished manicured dried buds. In addition to appealing looks, the herb has aromas, flavors and so much more.

Harvest

Before cutting down your outdoor plants, remove any insects that may be present. You'll need canvas spreads for transporting your harvested plants. After cutting, roll the buds up inside the spreads. Avoid using plastic bags, as they tend to trap resin. Hemp canvas is best.

Curing

Lastly, cure your outdoor harvest just like you would an indoor harvest. Inspect it regularly for insects, fungi, and mold. Do not store an indoor harvest alongside an outdoor one, as fungi, mold, and insects can spread from one to the other.

There are various ways to use your results, including processing them into hashish and oils, which will be covered later in this book. The upcoming chapters will provide you with all the information you need to cultivate high-quality buds.

PHOTO: RUSSELL-HOWLAND PHOTOGRAPHY

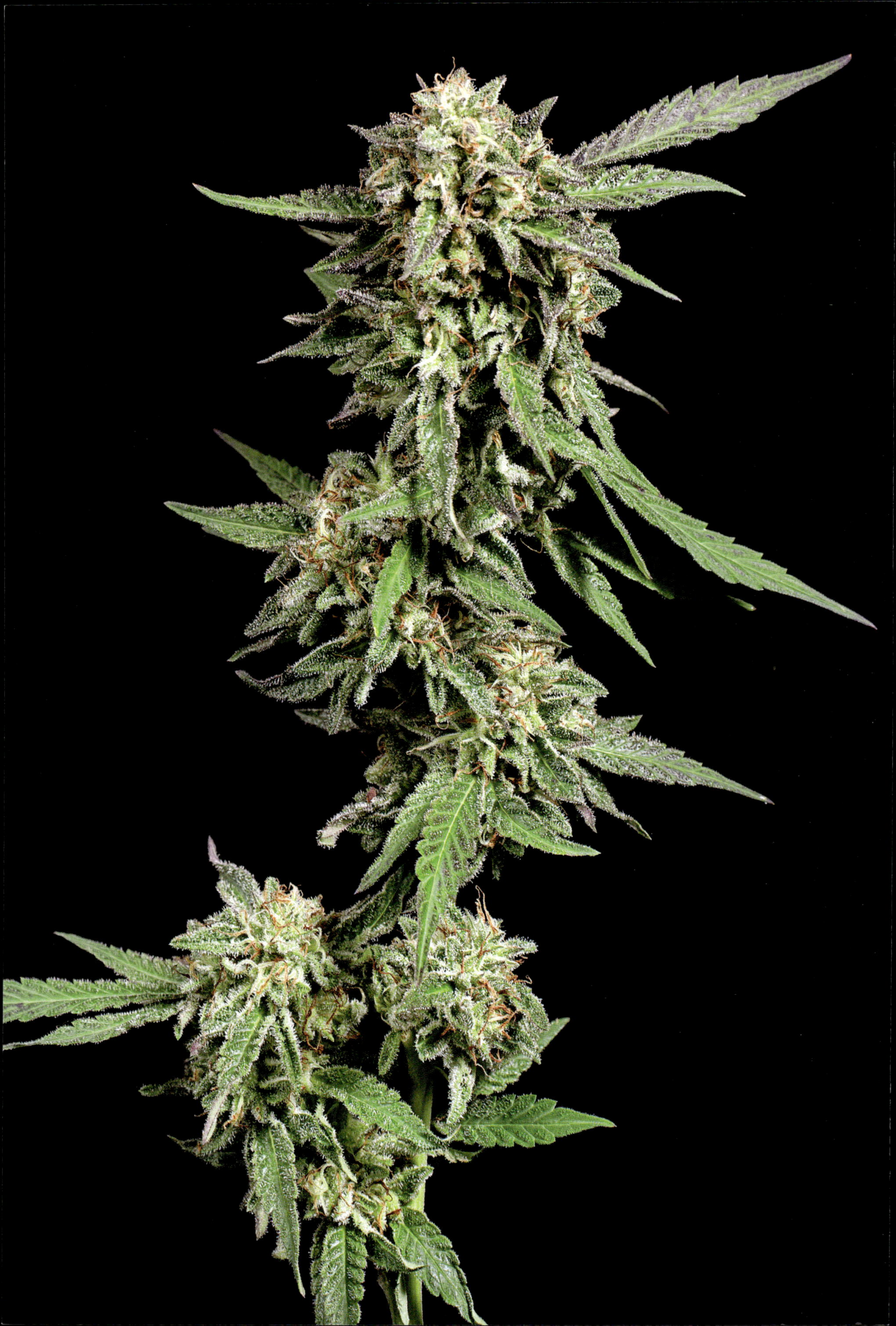

2

The Cannabis Plant

The reason cannabis produces a biochemical response in humans is due to its constant evolution. If human beings didn't have receptors in their brains for cannabis chemistry, the plant would not produce any effect. The cellular responses that create our experiences with cannabis are primarily due to G protein-coupled receptors (GPCRs), which are activated in pathways for signal transduction. Molecules bind to these receptors after entering the human body. The GPCRs for cannabis-related molecules are called cannabinoid receptors. The human body has developed ligands that bind to these cannabinoid receptors. These ligands, *endocannabinoids*, are found in all mammals. Two of the cannabinoid receptors are CB1R and CB2R; the first is known as the "brain receptor," found in the central nervous system and several organs, including kidneys, liver, and lungs. The second is known as the "immune system receptor", found in blood cells inside red bone marrow or in hematopoietic stem cells. We can plot the early evolution of these receptors somewhere around 500 million years ago. The cannabis plant produces cannabinoid molecules that act similarly to endocannabinoids and are capable of binding to CB1R and CB2R. No magic is involved. No mystery. Humans have been using cannabis with their cannabinoid receptors for as long as they've both been around.

Coevolution

Did early humans find a source of cannabinoids in plants, and did natural selection play a role in coevolution? That is an essential question for evolutionary biology. Sufficient scientific evidence indicates that natural selection was part of the adaptive force in the relationship between humans and cannabis. How much have humans influenced this coevolution? Did ancestral primates consume cannabis-type plants? Comparing this relationship to the evolution of cannabis itself is likely to show biochemical changes in humans and plants over significant periods. As we continue to inspect these connections at higher resolutions on the evolutionary tree of life, we can measure the parallel changes between humans and cultivation. For example, mutations have previously occurred to deal with increased starch in our diet, which came

PHOTO: RUSSELL-HOWLAND PHOTOGRAPHY

about by cultivating and breeding crops. Thus, cultivation shapes us. This relationship is known as mutualism; plants thrive when cultivated, and humans benefit from gathering the produce.

How Old Is Cannabis?

To know how long cannabis has existed requires looking at its scientific classification. An angiosperm is a clade of flowering plants that produces seeds, unlike a gymnosperm that produces seeds but doesn't flower. Angiosperms evolved from gymnosperms over 200 million years ago. What existed only 5 million years ago would likely be significantly different from what we see today. Still, as with speciation patterns, we can assume that cannabis-like plants eventually separated, and each population underwent speciation, each with different characteristics until cannabis became the plant we know now.

Cannabis Consumption

Angiosperm provides nutrition to any mammal that consumes it. Seeds and fruits, in addition to being edible themselves, also produce oils, commonly known as "essential oils," such as omega-6 and omega-3. Many mammals, including primates, also eat leaves, stems, piths, and shoots. The gorilla, for example, can eat 66 lbs (30 kg) of plant matter from over 200 species daily. We can only speculate when psychedelic substances began to be used frequently by our evolutionary ancestors. It seems likely that the psychedelic properties were not the original focus of their encounters with plants like ancestral cannabis. Resin glands on the cannabis plant are multipurpose; without human intervention, the functions of resin glands are to protect the plant from being eaten by animals, protect seeds from insects, provide fungal resistance, protect from the elements, and offer some ultraviolet (UV) light resistance. Over long periods, humans began to isolate these chemicals for medical, recreational, and cultural practices.

Cannabis Adaptations

Cannabis is rigorously adaptive. It can grow anywhere if the environment is not consistently cold and has enough sunlight and food for the plant to flourish. To this extent, we can say that the adaptiveness of cannabis is an essential factor in why this particular plant has flourished in many places to which humans have migrated.

In various regions around Mongolia, cannabis plants grow naturally on hillsides and across vast plains, sometimes covering entire hill faces and spreading across the valley below. A massif in Nepal, Dhaulagiri, offers incredible mountain range vistas, but one can't fail to see that cannabis is in such natural abundance as to be treated as a weed. These facts and preliminary evidence seemed to support the hypothesis that the cannabis plant first took root somewhere in the Himalayas. However, an article appeared in the science journal *Science Advances* on July 16, 2021, 7(29), and changed everything. In "Large-scale whole-genome resequencing unravels the domestication history of Cannabis sativa", Ren, Zhang, Li, et al. showed that C. sativa was first domesticated in early Neolithic times in East Asia. All current hemp and drug cultivars diverged from an ancestral gene pool currently represented by feral plants and landraces in China. This research moves the origins of cannabis away from the Himalayas.

Cannabis Paleobotany

Paleobotany is the scientific study of plant fossils and ancient vegetation, while palynology is the scientific study of spores and pollen. Cannabis fossil evidence is accessible in plant fibers, pollen grains, seed remains, trichome remains, and related cannabis compounds found at locations of archaeological interest. Many European sites have recovered an abundance of primordial pollen grains; Asia has seed remains and many cannabis plant impressions on ancient ceramic shards. Africa and Europe have incinerated residue or ash deposits, but these instances are rare. Cannabis trichomes remain the best possible paleobotanical evidence for cannabis history because they do not decompose quickly. Ancient trichome remnants have been analyzed for cannabinoid content and matched with likely cannabis plant populations.

Some evidence suggests that humans have been using cannabis as far back as we have existed. As a common fiber textile, flax is standard, but hemp is also a candidate. The burial shroud of a Celtic chieftain found at Hochdoft (2550–2500 BCE) was possibly made from a cannabis fiber textile. Danish Bronze Age skirt cords were possibly made from cannabis fiber and date back to 3250 BCE.[1] Today, we can use DNA to analyze the origins of cannabis plants and their spread. With the 2021 paper "Large-scale whole-genome resequencing unravels the domestication history of *Cannabis sativa*"[2] we now know cannabis originated in East Asia 12,000 years ago. This is a massive jump in time for us, but only a blink for evolution. The best way to look at what has happened is to look at the new segregation of cannabis based on phylogenetics. It is the same as looking at an evolutionary tree that mimics a cannabis plant with its many branches and stems.

Four Evolutionary Branches

A picture of geographic distribution forms by sampling sites of feral plants, landraces, and cultivars or strains. Genetically, these form four notable groups obtained by phylogenetic analysis (Maximum Likelihood phylogenetic tree based on single-nucleotide polymorphisms (SNPs) at fourfold degenerate sites, using *Humulus lupulus* as an outgroup). The genetic picture that emerges is the spreading of cannabis through pollen dispersal and human intervention. The genetic evidence suggests a new evolutionary origin for *Basal cannabis*, which spread across eastern Asia (China). This is our first branch. Our second branch, called the *hemp type*, spreads across Europe from the East. A third branch, the *drug-type feral*, is found south of China and extends into northern India. The fourth branch is called the *drug type* and is the modern cannabis we mostly encounter in society, located in northern Europe, northern America, and western South America. This perspective gives us more clues as to how cannabis evolved and spread. It is an evolutionary tree showing how cannabis originated from *Humulus lupulus* and branched into four distinct cannabis types in close genetic proximity. Their location on one of the four distinct branches determines how close or far apart they are.

So, we can see that there are four cannabis types in history: *Basel, hemp, drug-type feral*, and *drug-type*. There are three domesticated types: *Cultivar, feral* and *landrace*. The drug-type feral and drug-type can be grouped as one for analysis. 12,000 years ago, early domesticated ancestors of hemp and drug types diverged from Basal cannabis. This indicates that cannabis had already been domesticated by early Neolithic times. Cannabis cord impressions and seed-associated pottery are found in archaeology around this time. Early domesticated cannabis was initially a multipurpose crop until approximately 4000 years BC, when it underwent strong divergent selection for intensified fiber or drug production. Cannabis male pollen has been found in China from more than 5000 years BC. Cannabis strains expanded to later form hemp and drug types around 4000 years BC. Close to this time, multiple fiber artifacts were found in East Asia. The bronze age has archaeological evidence for cannabis spreading west into the Middle East and Europe. Usage would be associated with rituals and medical use to at least 2500 years BC. The first archaeobotanical evidence for cannabis use in India dates back to 3000 years BC and was introduced from China along with other crops. As early as 2000 BC, historical texts from India reveal that the species was only used for drug use. Early European colonists brought *hemp-type cannabis* to the New World during the 17th century, which was later substituted in North America by Chinese hemp landraces by the mid-1800s. Over the centuries after 2000 BC, the *drug-type Cannabis* traveled to various world regions, including Africa (13th century) and Latin America (16th century), progressively reaching North America at the beginning of the 20th century and later, in the 1970s, from the Indian subcontinent. Read the 2021 paper "Large-scale whole-genome resequencing unravels the domestication history of *Cannabis sativa*" to learn more about this content on cannabis paleobotany, and also R. C. Clarke, M. D. Merlin, *Cannabis—Evolution and Ethnobotany* (University of California Press, 2013).

The cannabis plant has managed to travel across the globe without the involvement of humans. The seed has been carried by the wind and bees, in bird droppings, and attached to animals that trek over long distances, thus globally dispersing the plant in an entirely natural way. In more recent times, human intervention has forced the cannabis plant to be grown under more controlled conditions and in areas where the plant would not have previously existed.

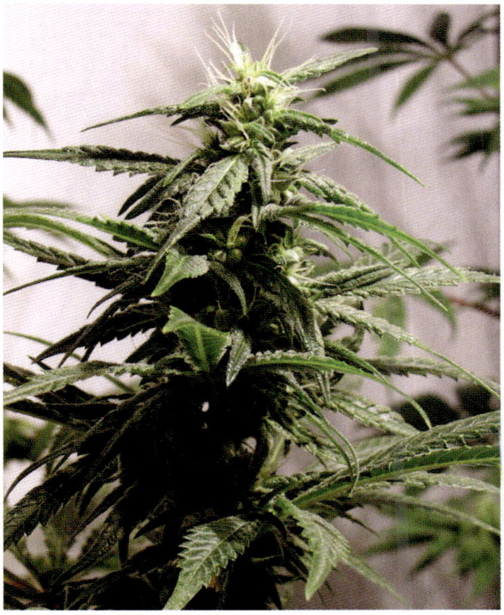

Cannabis indica is short with broad leaves and is known for its body-stone effect.

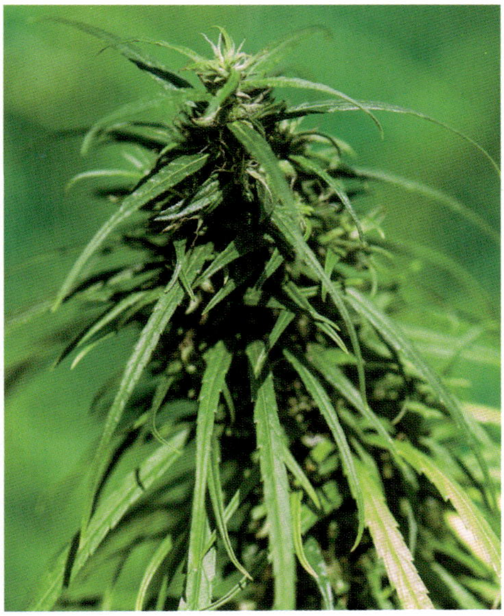

Cannabis sativa is tall with slender leaves and is known for its head-high effect.

PHOTOS: GIBRIDOV (LEFT), DELTA9LABS.COM (RIGHT)

Landrace Cannabis

Landraces, or land races, are defined by J. R. Harlan as:

> ... wild plants having a certain genetic integrity. They are recognizable morphologically; farmers have names for them and different landraces are understood to differ in adaptation to soil type, time of seed, date of maturity, height, nutritive value, use and other properties. Most important, they are genetically diverse. They are balanced populations—variable, in equilibrium with both environment and pathogens and genetically dynamic.[3]

Italian botanical glossarists suggest that landraces are "crop populations in balance with their environment" and "remain relatively stable over a long period of time." Friis-Hansen and Sthapit state that landraces are farmer-developed crop plants that are heterogeneous, adapted to local environmental conditions, and have their local names. In other words, landraces are farmers' varieties, which formal or private breeding programs have not improved. However, farmers can grow modern cultivars which, when self-seeding and selection are practiced over time, can become landrace.

Current Science Association published "Revisit to definitions and need for inventorization or registration of landrace, folk, farmers' and traditional varieties" (2006),[4] in which researchers Saxena and Singh developed a scientific vocabulary, the nomenclature of cultigens, based on the evolutionary process.[5] We expect that the findings of 2021 will influence a revisit to such topics and more. Examples of landraces include the Afghani plant, which has been used by many modern cannabis plant breeders to create improved

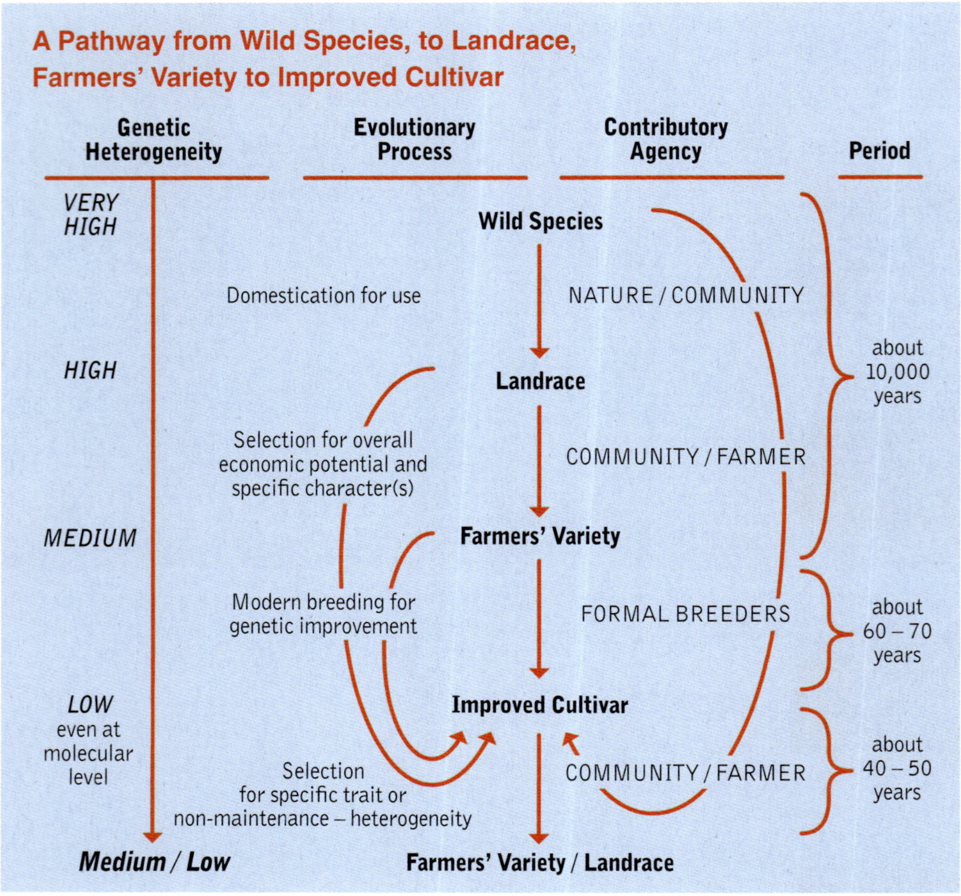

cultivars, as well as Kush, Master Kush, and Hash Plant. As we know definitively, farmers' varieties can make their way back into wild species populations. There are several landrace cannabis strains in Afghanistan and several farmers' varieties. The improved cultivars are mainly bred for modern domestic medical and recreational cultivation.

A popular view of a landrace is that it is a traditional variety, not as consistent as a pedigree breed. Most pedigree breeds have their origins in the landrace. We can say that most modernized cannabis plants come from landraces, but we should adopt the 2021 findings of four distinct cannabis types. An advanced breeder looking to create an entirely new strain could go to landrace origins and start anew, which may be necessary as more patents for cannabis strain genes are granted in the medical industry. Breeders will need to avoid infringing patents, an issue that is bound to occur in the future with the mainstreaming of medical cannabis. Shareholders will treat cannabis no different from any other product that they can patent and control. Medical cannabis genetics, pharmaceutical products, and trademarks can all be covered under laws that protect breeding work.[6]

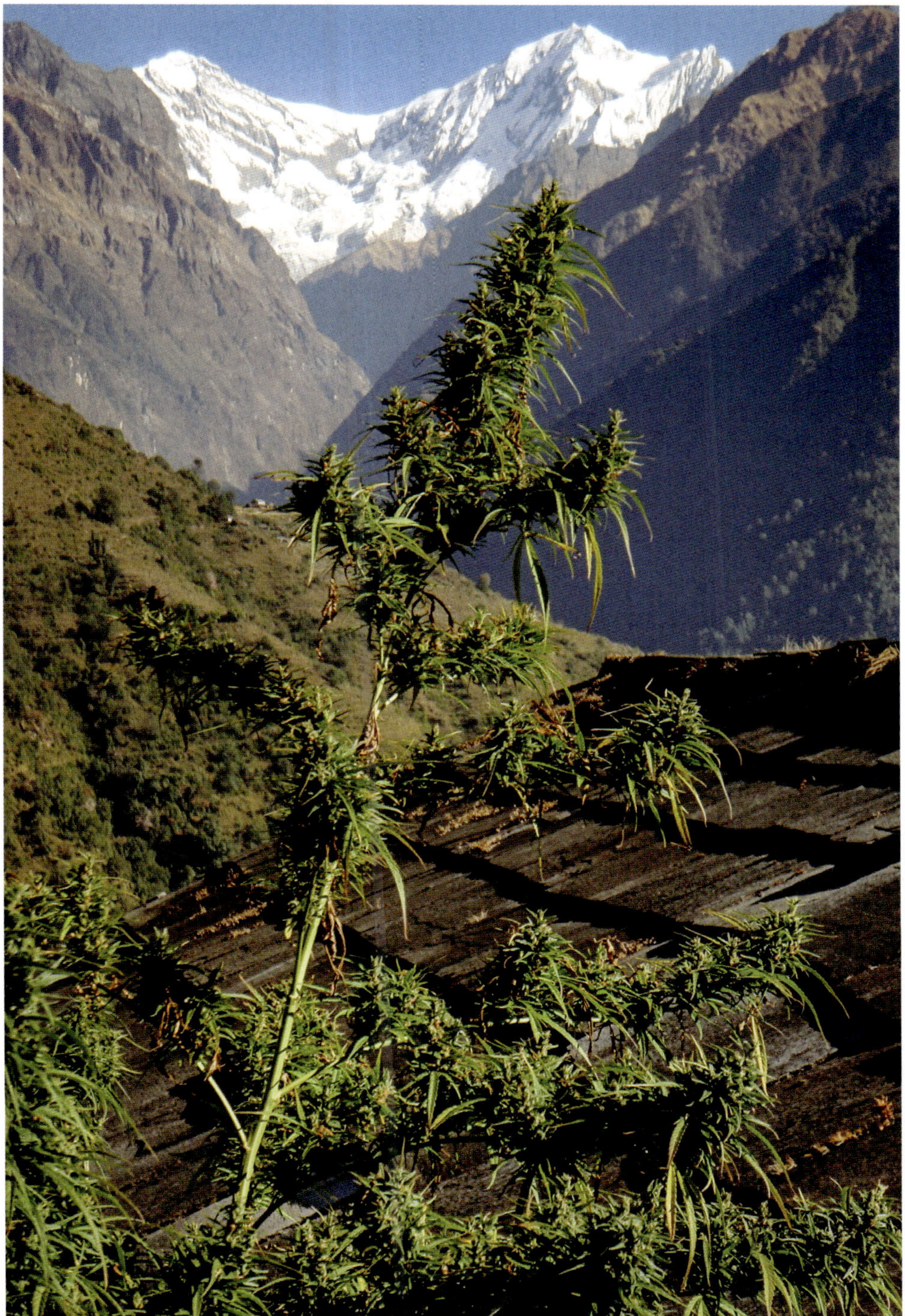

PHOTO: BODHI SEEDS

A Nepalese hash plant outdoors receives light from the sun shining through the clear blue sky and it flowers in darkness at night.

Feral Cannabis

Wild, landrace, and feral cannabis plants are rarer in countries that have tried to eliminate the plant by burning fields and conditioning woodlands. In some countries, cannabis has been identified as a dangerous drug and eradicated by government and law-enforcement officials. As it is highly adaptable, however, the cannabis plant has survived these attempts at eradication in secret indoor and outdoor grow spaces around the world.

Feral cannabis has a slightly more interesting story. Feral cannabis is somewhat connected with landrace. Is it possible that the cannabis local growers have bred has gone from domestication back into the wild? Landrace strains seem more uniform and domesticated than their wild counterparts. Alleged feral cannabis is something that may be more abundant than once thought. In the US, feral hemp may account for over 240 million cannabis plants destroyed by the Drug Enforcement Administration (DEA) in 2003, compared to 3 million cultivated plants. The DEA classed these feral hemp plants as "ditchweed," a type of cannabis that grows wild. The results can be found in the DEA seizures and removals section of the University at Albany sourcebook of criminal justice statistics. If over 240 million cannabis plants grew wild in the US in 2003, feral cannabis might account for most cannabis that grows worldwide; this information isn't from a scientific journal, but the overall picture seems to make sense. It gives us an idea of how humans can influence cannabis dispersal by trekking with seeds. It also ties in with what we know about landrace cannabis strains. Feral cannabis sativa populations have been measured across the Nebraska climate gradient.[7]

Hemp

Some cannabis plants produce very low levels of THC. These plants are mainly bred and used by farmers in countries that permit the growth of cannabis for textiles and birdseed. While this hemp does not produce a high, it can be used as a multipurpose crop. Industrial hemp is a solution to many of the world's problems; a hemp field supports entire ecosystems. Its uses include paper, car panels, and frames from bast fibers; it can be shaped into anything and is robust with high durability. Even though hemp will eventually decay, it will degrade naturally, making it very environmentally-friendly. Hemp products are nearly always significantly better quality than their non-hemp counterparts; in particular, hemp is much stronger than cotton. Despite hemp's usefulness, in the West, the cotton industry was able to topple the hemp industry through legal oppression and media propaganda, such as from the Hearst group. China, Canada, France, and Romania never ceased production of hemp, and China has capitalized extensively from this. After World War II, germplasms bred in America were destroyed by hemp prohibition, so that if the law was changed back, all their essential breeding could never be recovered. A bridge was burned by the prohibition movement so that legalization could never recover quickly. Today, feral hemp can be found in a few parts of the West, but legalization has seen a new wave of outdoor cannabis production

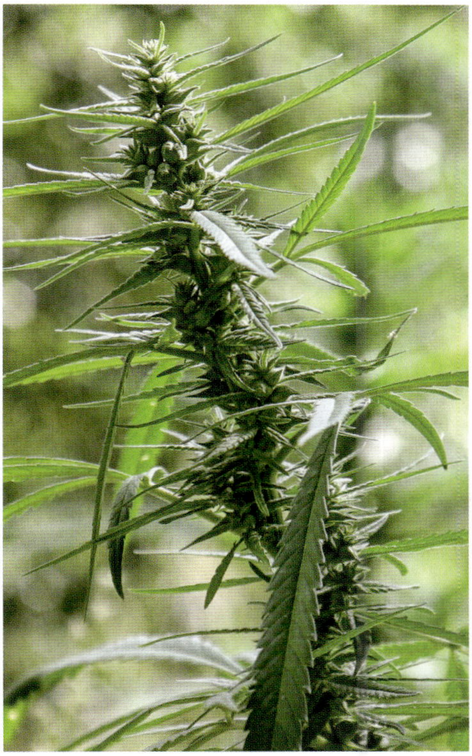

A female hemp plant in the early days of flowering.

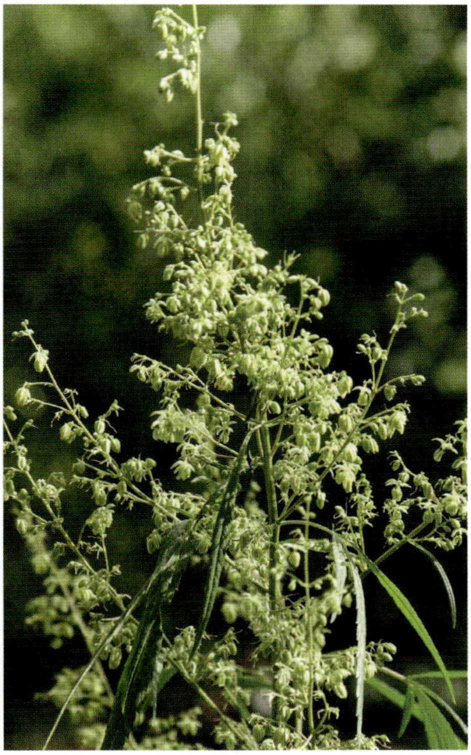

A male hemp plant that is shedding pollen.

PHOTOS: CENTENNIAL SEEDS

of all types. The industry for new hemp breeds is becoming increasingly significant, especially since America passed HR525, the Industrial Hemp Farming Act of 2013. If you can breed cannabis plants with less than 0.3% THC, you have a candidate for hemp production. Whatever your views on genetically-modified plants, the farming of hemp is something every cannabis lover should promote.

Hemp-based cosmetics are now a huge and growing industry. Hemp papermaking is still popular. Biofuels are using hemp. Seeds are found in foods. It is used as an insulator. Livestock feeds include hemp seeds. Hemp is an open industry for breeders to make better strains. The competitiveness focuses on seed, vegetable oil yields, and strains that can grow in conditions further north and south of equatorial zones. Various governments have goals for biomass yields. Seed production can be higher than what it currently is, but climate change may be responsible for lower production. As temperatures rise, breeding will have to compensate for those significant changes. Male flowers are also in higher abundance than they need to be. Breeders, take note: Drug cultivars are not the only cannabis type open to significant breeding. Hemp is an enormous industry and is only going to get bigger. Keep reading and learning about hemp. Members of the cannabis community need to become involved with it.

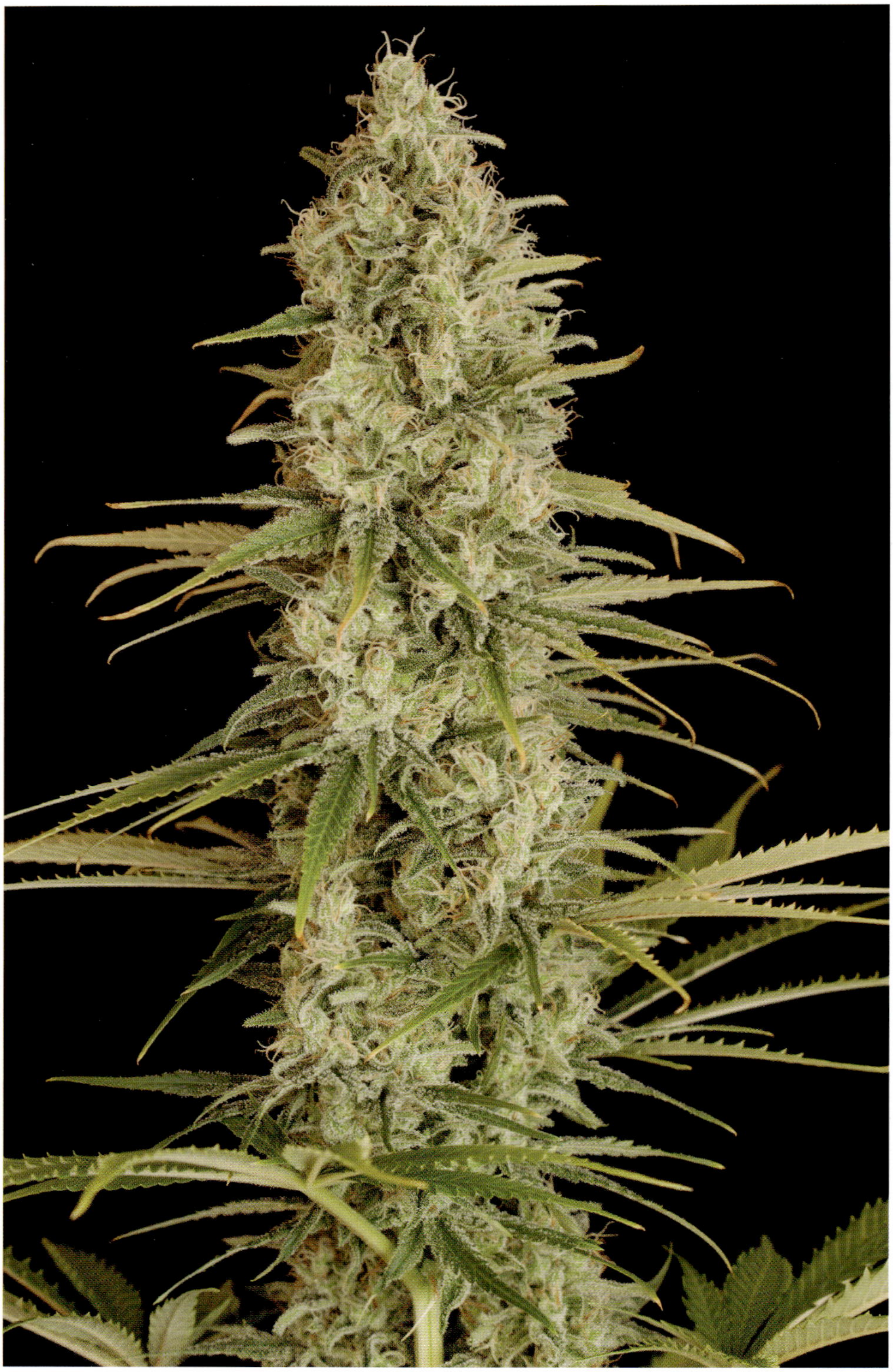

PHOTO: DINAFEM SEEDS

Critical Jack is a popular strain for medical users who are dealing with chronic pain.

Medical Cannabis

The scientific peer-review process has thoroughly debunked any doubts about the medical value of cannabis, though some experts don't believe it despite the science behind it. We are now in the realm of cannabis as therapy, with various treatment types and options, as we understand far more about the biochemical mechanisms involved. Arguments against cannabis prohibition can find an astonishing amount of support from science, which uses the evidence to confirm the case for cannabis as medicine. This book covers a range of methods needed to produce medical cannabis. It is an industry that will keep growing as more cannabinoids are discovered.

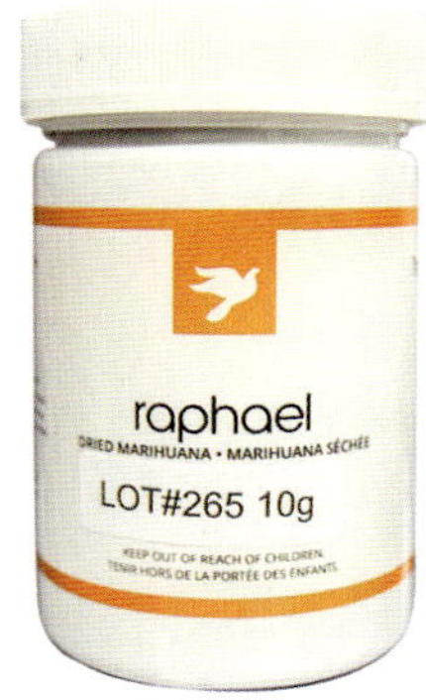

A marijuana dispensary medicine container.

Cannabinoids

Medical cannabis is all about understanding cannabinoids. Cannabinoids change their chemical form and structure, which is how we end up with a group of cannabinoids. For example, the biochemical conversion of cannabigerol (CBG) to cannabidiol (CBD) to cannabichromene (CBC) produces Δ9-THC. In the previous edition of this book, we knew about 85 of these changes. At the time of writing this edition, we know of a lot more.[8] This is all cutting-edge research, and we expect these figures to change. Still, that is an enormous increase. Cannabis is a treasure full of chemistry we have yet to discover.

The main methods of detecting new cannabinoids are gas chromatography, high-performance liquid chromatography, mass spectrometry, and flame ionization detection. There are far too many cannabinoids for this book to cover, and they are not immediately relevant to most growers and breeders. However, we can cover the salient points of cannabinoids and those important to us. The primary cannabinoid compounds are cannabigerol (CBG), cannabichromene (CBC), cannabidiol (CBD), tetrahydrocannabinol (THC), cannabinol (CBN), cannabielsoin (CBE), iso-tetrahydrocannabinol (iso-THC), cannabicyclol (CBL), cannabicitran (CBTC), and tetrahydrocannabivarin (THCV or THV). You will probably be working with them all.

For the benefit of medical growers, we will look at precisely how these work in medicine. The brain receptor CB1 and the immune system receptor CB2 form complexes with cannabinoids.[9] These receptors receive molecular cannabinoids and chemically process them. Agonists cause an action, or produce an increase in some effect. Antagonists block an action, or decrease the effect. However, combinations of cannabinoids can produce different results. THC is an agonist, mainly analgesic (pain relief), with psychoactive effects such as relaxation and a feeling of deeper perspectives concerning the senses. While not overtly psychoactive, CBD can supplement and change the effects of THC when combined with it. Previously it was suggested that CBD didn't interface with CB1 and CB2 but operated on other receptors to alleviate depression, swelling, sickness, unease,

PHOTO: DAVID STRANGE

and seizures.[10] CBD is a CB1 antagonist and indirectly alters the receptors' activity with THC. The affinity of CBD to CB1 and CB2 is extremely low.[11] One hypothesis is that CBD interacts with CB1 by allowing more THC to bind to CB1 receptors.

As THC degrades, it becomes CBN. That is why your stash becomes less potent over time and why you should turn to the sections on curing and storage to learn more.

Degradation of Compounds

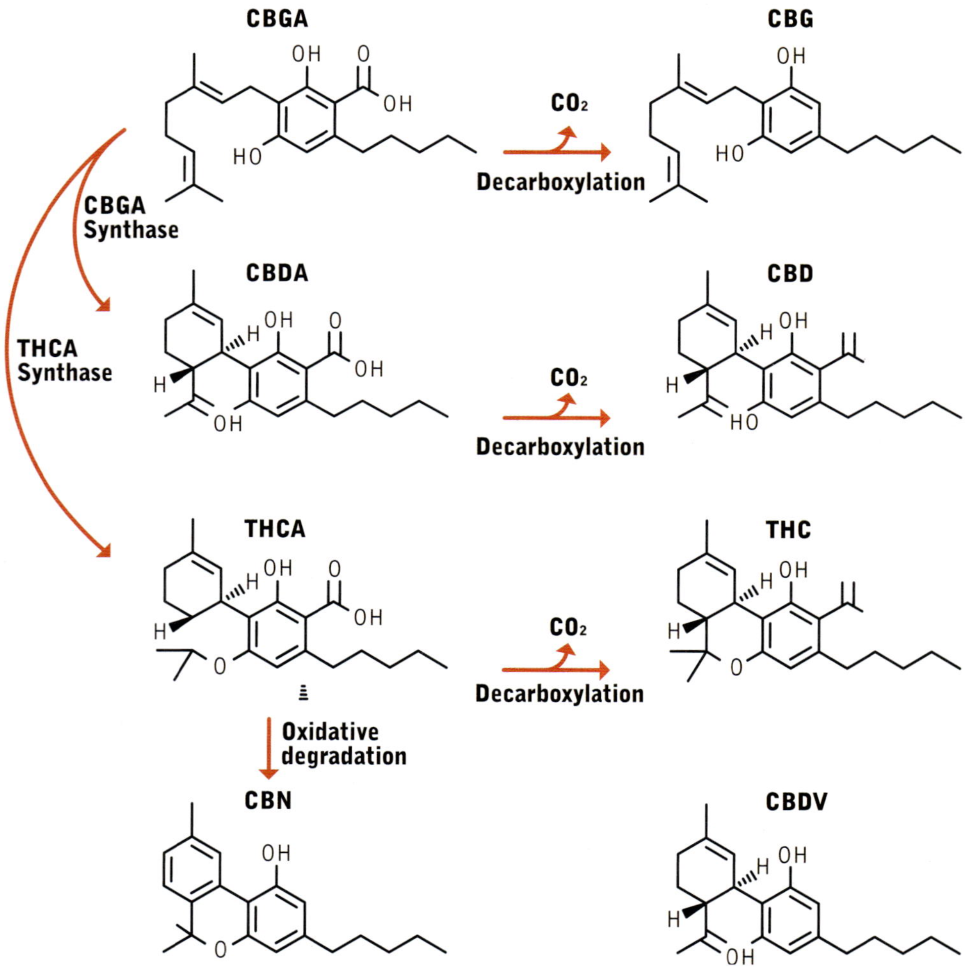

This is the first and only chemical chart you will encounter in this book. After that, all you have to know is how processes like decarboxylation and oxidative degradation can change compounds. The diagram shows the most common cannabinoids and their conversion pathway by decarboxylation because of heat or aging. CBGA can convert to CBDA and THCA by CBDA synthase and THCA synthase, respectively. CBGA: cannabigerolic acid, CBG: cannabigerol, CBDA: cannabidiolic acid, CBD: cannabidiol, THCA: tetrahydrocannabinolic acid, THC: tetrahyrocannabinol, CBN: cannabinol (Fathordoobady et al. 2019).[12]

Avoiding heat, such as from the sun, is the key to retaining THC and other cannabinoids. Cannabis harvesters store their buds in a cool dark place, though lack of heat is more important than lack of light to prevent cannabinoids from transforming into one another. In other words, storing in a cool place is better than storing in a dark, warm place. However, age eventually degrades THC anyway. THCV and THV are non-psychoactive compounds that work like THC in their medical application. Cannabinoid ratios are usually particular to each strain, especially in terms of the cannabinoid variations between sativa and indica strains. Indica strains have lower THC to CBD ratios, and sativa strains have higher THC to CBD ratios. Indica/sativa hybrids offer a way to customize your own medicine.

The G protein-coupled receptor 55 (GPR55) is a cannabinoid receptor, meaning cannabinoids activate it. CBD has been shown to act on it as an antagonist. CBD is also an agonist of another receptor called 5-HT1A, also known as the serotonin receptor. Cannabinoids are terpenophenolic compounds that occur in cannabis plants but can be produced synthetically, even as dangerous full-agonists. The full-agonists never appear in natural cannabis plants, which only contain partial- or half-agonists. That is an important distinction when encountering reports of cannabis-caused deaths, to which synthetic cannabis is a significant contributor. There is no evidence that natural cannabis causes death because the partial-agonist is not powerful enough to do so, and lethal consumption would involve quantities nearly impossible to consume without deliberately force-feeding someone concentrates.

THC and CDB are the two compounds you will come across the most. There are precursor compounds that make them natural homologs. Their precursors are THCA and CBDA.

THC Levels and THC Quantities

Do not confuse levels with quantities (also known as yield). Levels are usually measured as a percentage. THC levels are genetically determined, meaning the grower cannot really influence the potency of the strain. Hemp bred for extremely low potency can't produce highly potent crops. Cannabis bred for higher potency can't produce non-potent crops. THC levels are measured in THC proportion per cannabinoid content per trichome. Let's say the trichomes contain 5% THC along with 95% other cannabinoids. That is a THC level. However, 5% THC doesn't tell you how much you will get in weight—only the percentage per trichome. You could have 1 g of 5% THC or 20 g of 5% THC per plant. That's the quantity in terms of weight. The percentage of THC in a trichome is usually statistically measured from small samples, whereas weight is used to measure the cannabinoid percentage value. In optimal growing conditions, this level is genetically fixed. While there are genetic limits to how much bud volume you can produce, quantities are influenced by the environment. Therefore, a grower who wants stronger THC needs to select a strain with higher THC levels.

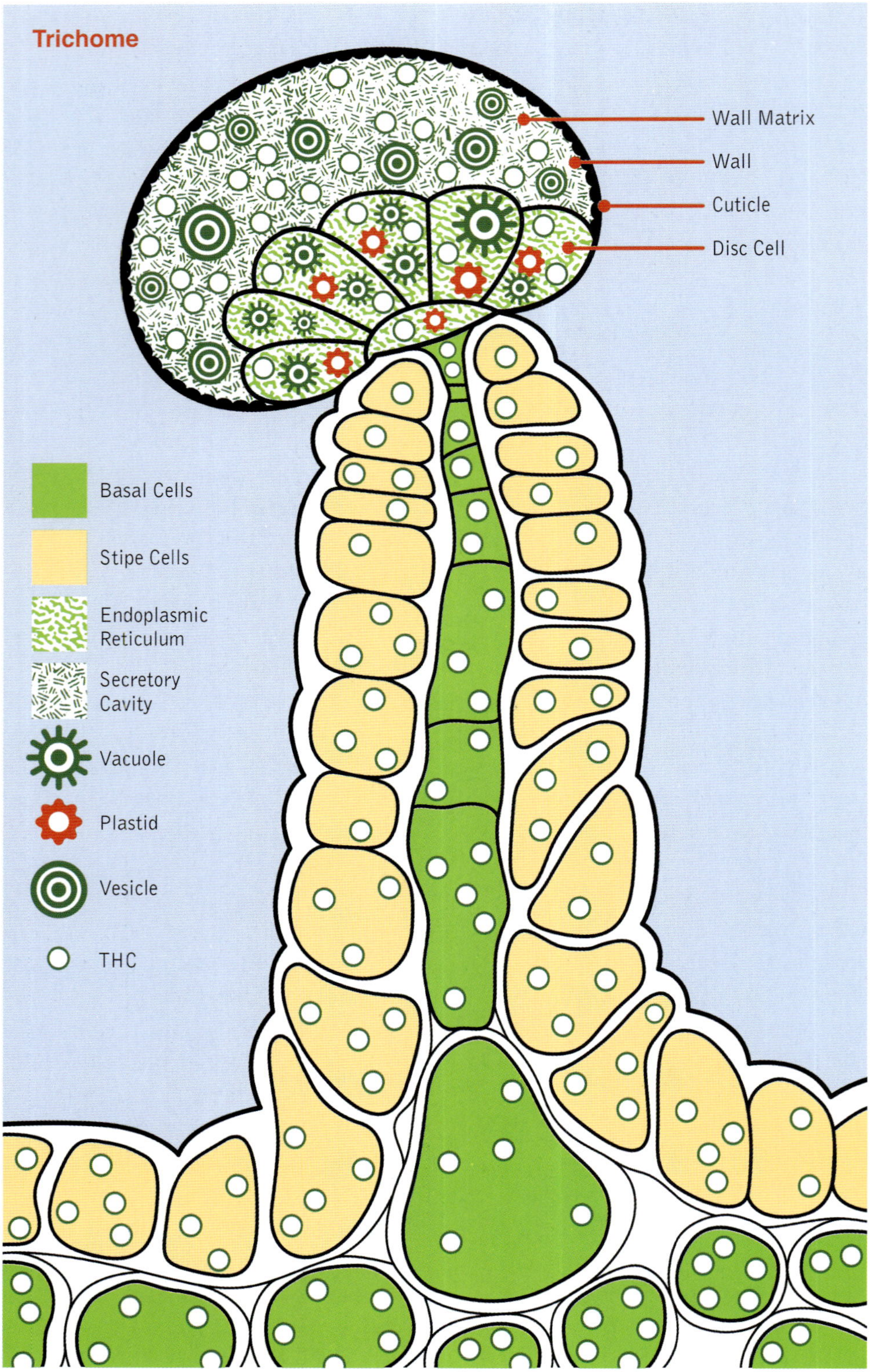
Trichome
Wall Matrix
Wall
Cuticle
Disc Cell
Basal Cells
Stipe Cells
Endoplasmic Reticulum
Secretory Cavity
Vacuole
Plastid
Vesicle
THC

It is possible to process cannabis with extraction techniques so that you can end up with close to 100% THC, a pure sample. Extraction techniques are covered in Chapter 18.

Let's summarize this. Quantities are related to bud mass and how much resin can be collected from that bud mass. For example, the THC level in a single trichome gland was 10%. That plant produced 15 g of resin under average growing conditions. When examining a strain in a seed bank catalog, you can check the THC levels of that plant to understand the potency and quantity. The technical name for quantity is yield; many seed retailers and breeders measure their plants' THC levels and offer accounts of how much THC their plants yield. To know more about the THC level of a specific strain, consult the seed bank or breeder for details or get a THC testing kit. In the past, breeders may have been tempted to embellish the THC levels their plants produce, but because cannabinoid test kits are becoming cheaper and more readily available, it is easier to find out the facts for yourself. As a result, breeders marketing cannabis products need to be aware that, if their ratios differ significantly from expected results under optimal conditions, this will be uncovered quickly by the community. Growers should allow for some variation because of growing conditions, but the strain needs to be in the ballpark of what the breeder describes.

THC Test Kits

The demand for more THC testing has led to a decrease in its cost. Breeders should use a test kit only for general guidance and use a reputable laboratory for actual testing. For growers or users, a test kit is perfect. Most cost $100 to $300, depending on the number of tests you want to do, with prices dropping all the time. More information on using and purchasing THC test kits can be found online.

Advanced quantitative measuring of cannabinoids can also identify the pure compounds we want and undesirable compounds such as microbes, toxins, pesticides, and solvent residues. Heavy metals can also be detected.

CBD Strains

Since the last edition of this book, the surge in the breeding and marketing of high-CBD strains for the medical community has been beyond expectation. Decades ago, CBD was obtained from hemp with lower THC to CBD ratios. The problem was that massive amounts of hemp would have to be gathered because of its low-CBD yield. Many CBD strains also contained some THCL, so if you wanted CBD without THC, you had to perform additional extraction to separate them in the end product. Now cannabis breeders have successfully bred high-CBD level strains without THC.

The CBD market was predicted to be around several billion during the previous decade. It is now predicted to reach over $20 billion over the next decade. That's a mind-blowing amount. There is so much new scientific literature on the subject that even specialists in CBD are having trouble absorbing all the latest data.

CBD strains are not the enemy of drug strain developers; while drug strain producers might aim for the opposite, these are two distinct and separate breeding goals that don't encroach on each other. CBD is also essential for how cannabis naturally synthesizes other cannabinoid compounds through molecular changes in chemical reactions. People still use CBD the same way as many other THC products but without the psychoactive effects.

CBD is only one molecule in the vast cannabinoid molecular library. This book will not detail the biosynthetic pathways of CBD, but, if you learn about cannabis cultivation and processing in this book, much of it can be ported over to CBD. There are similar methods for purity, genetic identity, quantitative analysis, and quality control as well. Exploring the conversion of CBD to THC is cutting-edge cannabis science as it has to do with the sensitivity of CBD to acidic environments. There is no evidence that CBD converts to THC in the human body. To learn more about CBD, read "The Essential Medicinal Chemistry of Cannabidiol (CBD)".[13]

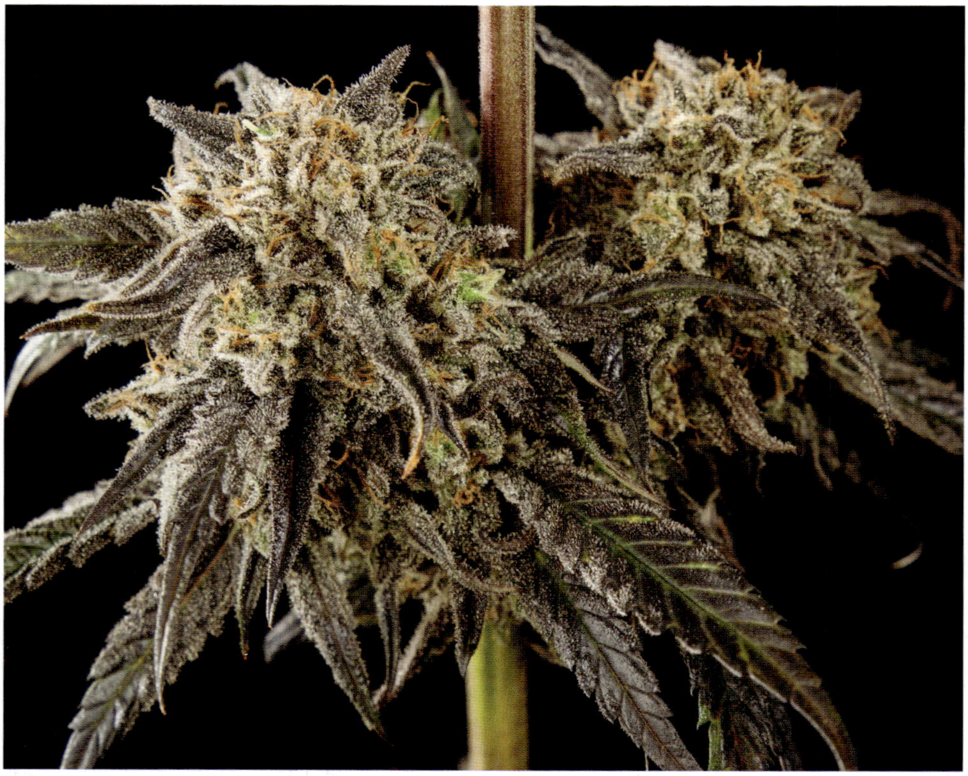

PHOTO: PHILOSOPHER SEEDS

This is a high-CBD strain that is regular and not autoflowering. The sativa-dominant Spicy CBD/SuperJuani: 8% CBD.

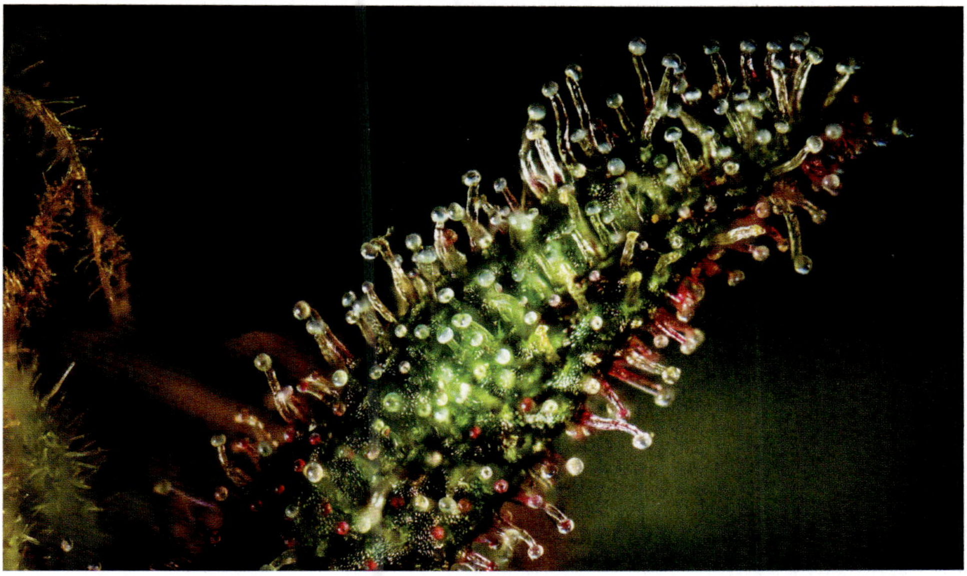

Resin is produced in trichomes and found on pistils and leaves in flowering areas of the cannabis plant.

PHOTO: ERIC PALMER

Resin

Female cannabis plants produce resin glands. Some strains produce resin glands that contain lots of resin that is not very potent. Other strains may have a small amount of resin that is highly potent. More resin glands does not necessarily equal more potency. The market likes to produce strains that look beautiful with lots of resin glands, but these are not necessarily potent buds. The potency of a plant depends on several factors, and the only accurate way to determine potency is to test for it. The topic of resin shouldn't be confused with potency; they are two different topics.

Optimal growing conditions and plant genetics can produce a plant that is both highly potent and produces a high amount of resin—but genes for both have to be present. Some genes produce smaller amounts of resin that are very potent. When it comes to genes and breeding there is a concept known as the 'trade-off'. This has to do with one trait developing more at the expense of other traits. For example, a plant can develop many flowers and a lot of resin, but may lack in other areas; it may have fewer cannabinoids and an unappealing appearance. That mainly has to do with genes that can be linked, and as one trait increases, another trait decreases, much like a see-saw. Some genes have constraints, which is why there are no tree-sized plants producing tons of bud per tree. An additional reason for these links is that plants have limited energy. If a plant puts a lot of energy into bud production, it may not have as much energy for leaf production. However, evolution can and does change those links between genes. Breeding is a way to manage trade-offs so that improvements can occur without significant losses in different plant areas.

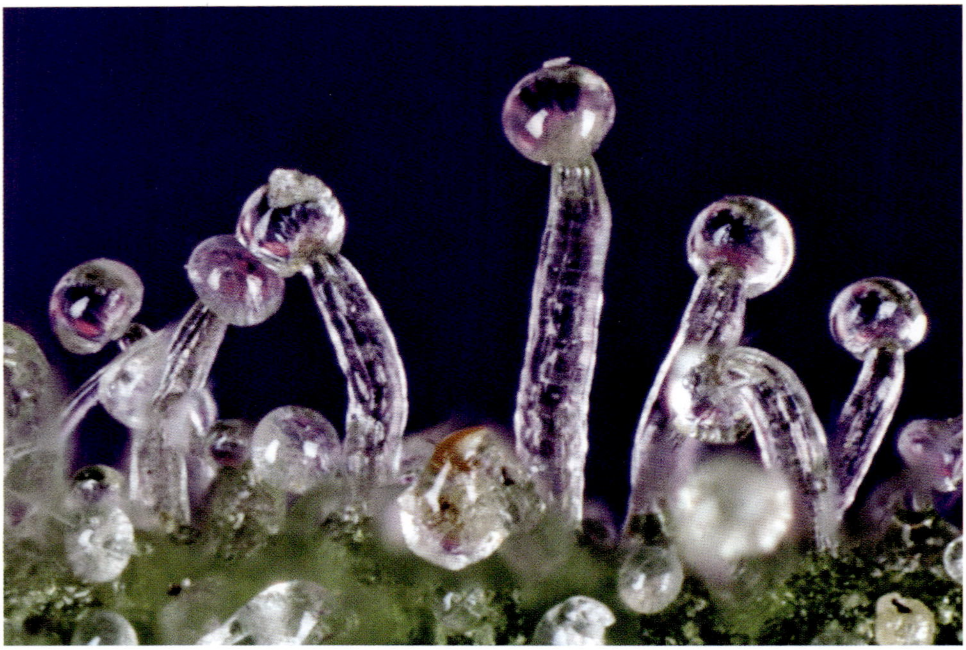

Clear trichomes on a healthy cannabis plant. Several types of trichome are visible here, with the bulbous glandular trichomes clearly visible with their dome tips, and also the more rare cystolith trichomes visible with their pointed, hair-like shape. All are full of cannabinoids like THC and many terpenes, as well.

PHOTO: TRICHOME ART

Resin glands, or trichomes, are produced all over the female flowers and leaves and can be seen clearly with a magnifying aid. You can rub resin off the bud with your fingers and then roll it in your palms to create small balls of hand-rubbed hashish. The main concentration of cannabinoids and THC exists in these glands. When a plant is in full flower, some resin glands may explode or break, dropping resin onto the leaves below, giving these leaves an extra-shiny, potent look during flowering. That is why a leaf that doesn't produce resin glands can still contain a significant cannabinoid amount.

Fan Leaves and Potency

Toward the bottom of the plant are the fan leaves. These are generally large and outstretched to collect light for plant growth. Because they are far from the top of the plant and furthest from the light, they produce the least resin glands and collect the least amount of burst resin from the tops. Therefore, they are not very potent. It is best to separate the fan leaves from the rest of the plant after harvesting, as these leaves will not provide the best high. However, it is essential to keep the fan leaves during cultivation, as these leaves are the primary energy-gathering devices the plant uses in photosynthesis. That is why they are so big. They are the fuel tanks for the rest of the system. Without them, the system has to rely on smaller leaves and whatever is left in its pipes.

Hash

Cannabis can be cured in various forms, including hashish, or hash. Hashish-making can create a product that's of higher quality and is more potent through purification and concentration. The quality of hash has traditionally been judged on the ratio of plant matter to cannabinoids, not potency. Grading hash was once done arbitrarily based on texture and look, producing grades: 00 (Zero Zero), 0, 1, 2, and 3. Zero Zero, the purest form of hashish, involved combining good harvests with an excellent hash-making technique. The other grades were established due to lower quality techniques and crops not as suitable for hashish-making; that is, crops containing a high leaf content. Much of this categorization was done through inspection rather than quantification methods. Likewise, hash was judged by how light or dark it was. Things today aren't clear-cut, as even low-quality hashish can appear light. One older method, the melt test, has become increasingly helpful. The melt test is a visual inspection test that observes how much residue is left after melting hashish. The highest-quality hashish should vaporize without the need for combustion and leave nothing behind that can be observed by the naked eye. Today, we test hashish using lab-based analysis or equipment with much more accurate results than visual inspection.

One way to acquire high-grade hashish is by making it yourself, which will be discussed in Chapter 18. There is no reason why you cannot use part of your first or next harvest to make some hashish. Even if you use a lot to end up with what seems like very little, you may sacrifice quantity for quality and learn a lot.

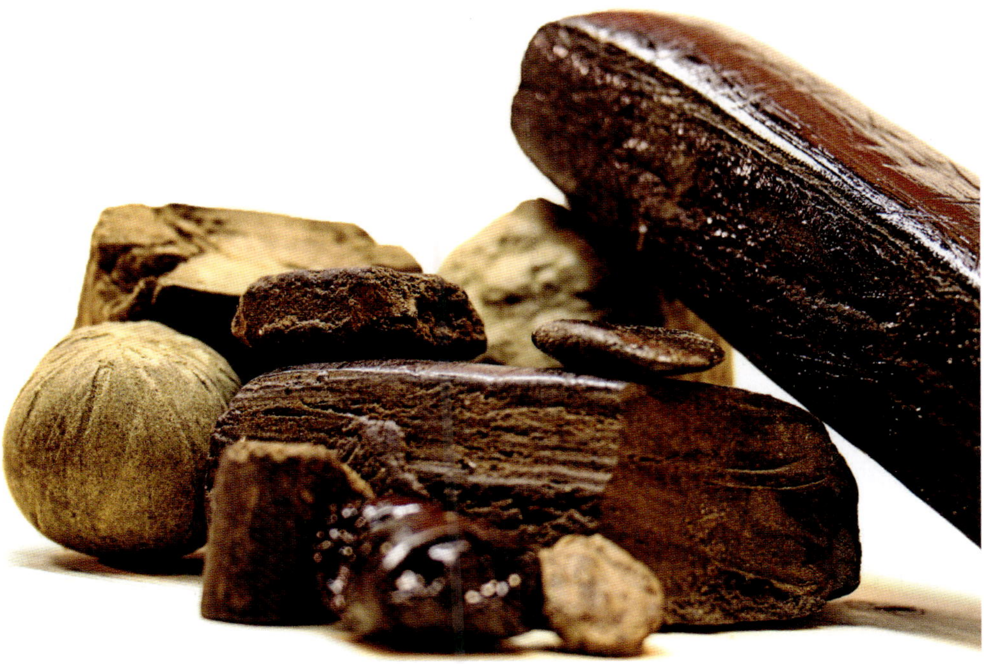

PHOTO: DAVID STRANGE

The wide variations of types and grades of hashish.

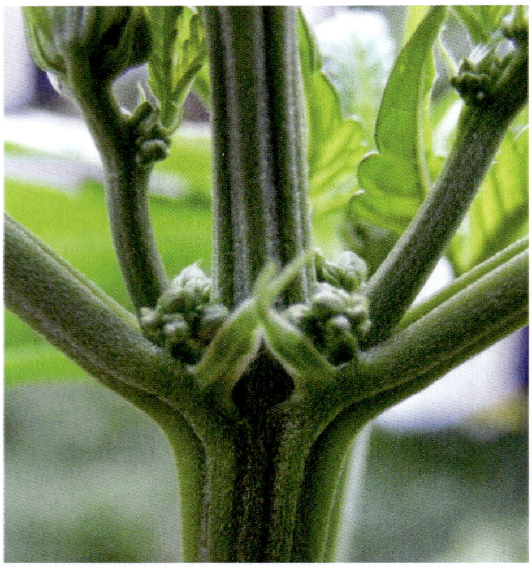

Hermaphrodite combination of both female and male flowers at their early stages.

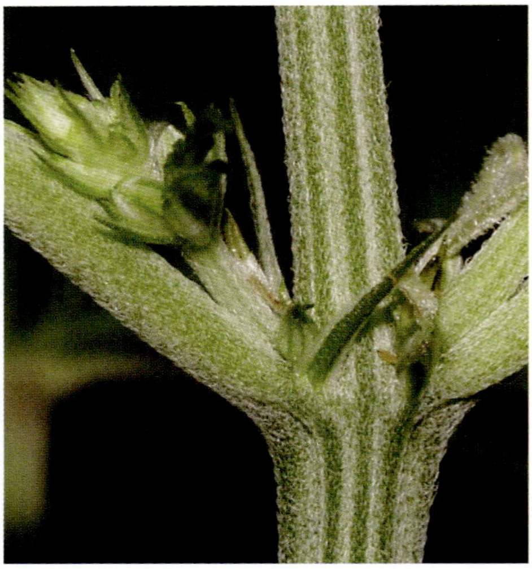

Hermaphrodite male flowers on the left and female pistils on the right at a later stage.

The Plant

The famous serrated cannabis leaf is both a symbol and a powerful cultural image. However, despite the leaf shape being the icon for cannabis, leaves are the least potent part of the plant. The seven sections of the cannabis plant are roots, stem, branches, nodes, leaves, flowers, and main cola. The sexes of cannabis plants are male, female or hermaphrodite (mixed sex).

Males

The male plant contains very low cannabinoid levels, mainly present in the leaf. While it does not taste good, it may provide a low-quality high for new users. Generally, males are not considered potent, and growers and breeders mainly cultivate male plants for pollen to make seeds. Most growers remove male plants as soon as the male sex becomes identifiable. Many breeders will move male plants to a separate grow room to control breeding and avoid randomized pollination, which will occur if the sexes are left together. We will have lots of encounters with male identification in this book.

Females

The female plant, when pollinated, produces THC but also produces seeds, which prevent larger quantities of buds from growing. A seeded female is a natural condition in the wild. Sinsemilla is rare, occurring when few or no males appear in a population, which is statistically unlikely. It can also occur when the males dropping pollen are not synchronized with female flowering, which can happen with new hybrids.

Hermaphrodite plants contain both male and female organs. If the pollen is viable, the plant will automatically pollinate itself, which is called selfing, resulting in a crop

PHOTOS: NMS (LEFT), MANDALA SEEDS (RIGHT)

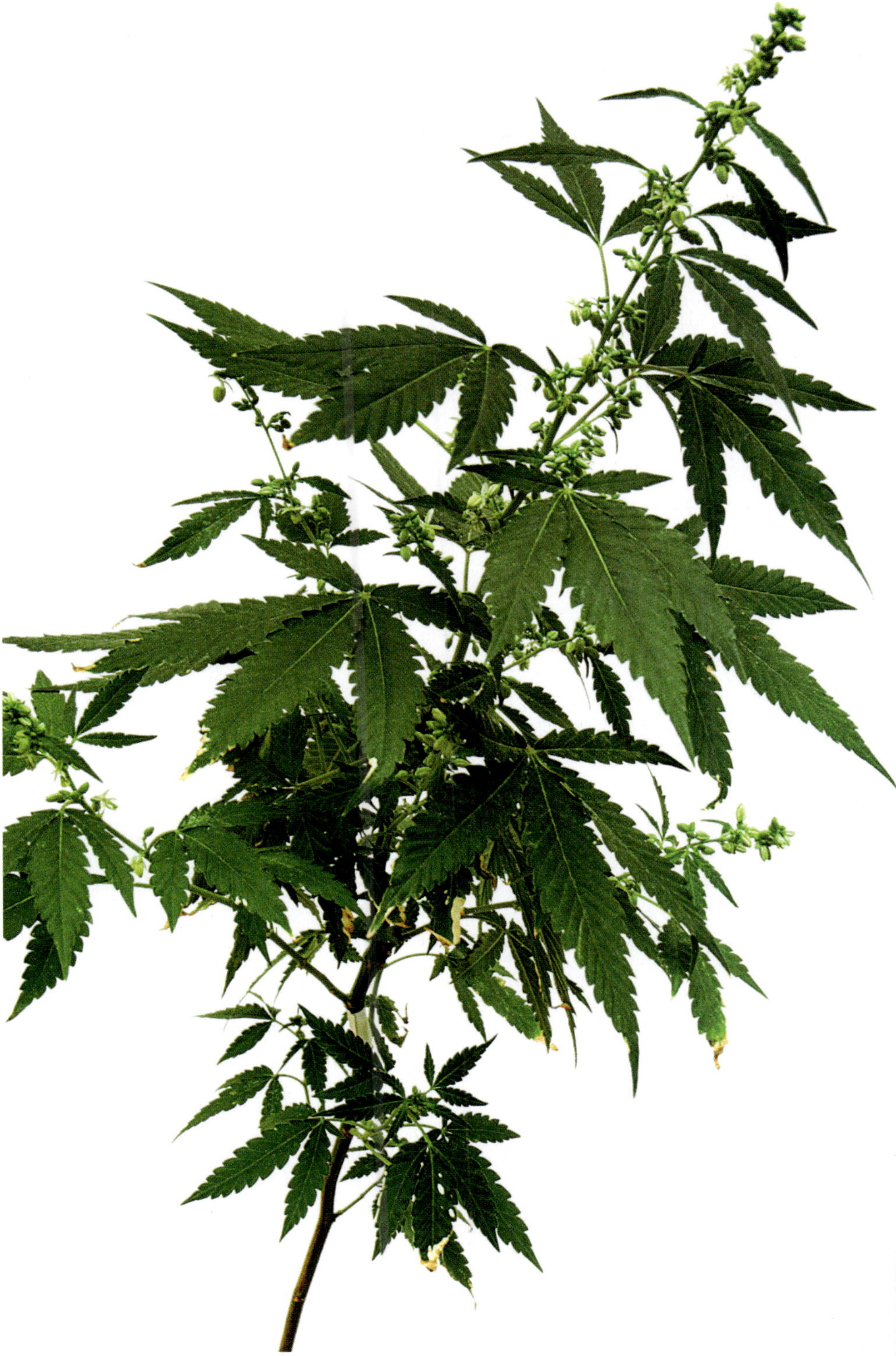

PHOTO: ED BORG

The male plant is mostly only used for breeding seeds.

that can never be sinsemilla. Some strains can become hermaphrodites due to stress under poor growing conditions, while other strains are inherently hermaphroditic. In general, growers avoid hermaphrodites. Optimal growing conditions help reduce this problem, but the genetic selection of a standard strain known to be without these problems is essential.

Sinsemilla Plant

A non-pollinated female, or sinsemilla, (from the Spanish, meaning "without seeds"), will produce more flowering buds and more cannabinoids than the male plant or a seeded female plant of the same strain. The buds produce resin, containing cannabinoids such as THC, that may spread onto the leaves, especially the areas closest to the flowers. Sinsemilla plants are excellent for medicinal use, depending on the grow method, strain, and harvest time. A seedless plant makes processing easier. The goal of a cannabis breeder is to deliver quality seeds and plants. Thus, every cannabis cultivator should aim to grow non-pollinated female plants because these produce the best yield. This book delves into the specific ways growers can achieve these goals.

Cannabis Species

We'll now delve into the history of cannabis species and why you must know about it. However, the existence of multiple cannabis species is disputed in science journal papers. While genetics gives us better insights into the cannabis species problem, it has more to do with an issue of our criteria for taxonomy which is not always precise. In short, taxonomy is flexible to accommodate new findings.

Cannabis Taxonomy for Scientists and Researchers

According to the latest data, reputable government scientific bodies such as the Germplasm Resources Information Network (GRIN) present six potential ways to represent species of cannabis. The first three are from the single-species model, while the latter three are from the multiple-species model. The US National Plant Germplasm System for Species of Cannabis gives six possible names:

Cannabis indica Lam.
Cannabis ruderalis Janisch.
Cannabis sativa L.
Or,
Cannabis sativa L. subsp. indica (Lam.) E. Small & Cronquist
Cannabis sativa L. subsp. sativa
Cannabis spp.

You will come across these names used in the professional literature and can easily see if one fits in the first or latter groups of three. You will generally come across the first three in the commercial sector and the latter in scientific papers. It is all a matter of historical classification, disputes, and modern genetic analysis.

The History of the Scientific Classification of Cannabis

The *Encyclopaedia Britannica* defines Cannabaceae, the hemp family (order Rosales), containing about 11 genera and about 170 species of plants. Its members are distributed nearly worldwide, many occurring throughout temperate parts of the Northern Hemisphere. Older authorities included the two genera *Cannabis* and *Humulus* in the mulberry family (Moraceae), but these and the former hackberry family (Celtidaceae) are now included in Cannabaceae.

The term species is well defined but with some flexible criteria. The biological definition of a species is "in biology, classification comprising related organisms that share common characteristics and are capable of interbreeding."[14] Interbreeding must produce fertile offspring if the parents are the same species. If a cross has infertile offspring, that offspring cannot reproduce, indicating that the parents are not the same species. Species are classifications of a distinct genus into groups that reproduce themselves by breeding within their population groups to produce fertile offspring. Usually, this definition comes with standards that need to be upheld. However, the lines can blur because evolution is often slow. Geography can become a barrier that splits populations off on separate evolutionary paths. Understanding geographical isolation helps us to see how species can evolve. Although considered distinct species, some separated populations can interbreed and produce viable offspring. In this case, what results is known as a "ring species" because of these wider-reaching breeding capabilities. However, some ring species produce infertile offspring. A typical example of a ring species is the Larus gull. In the Northern Hemisphere, these gulls form a ring. Each gull species can breed with the gull next door but not directly across on opposite sides of the ring. That is speciation happening at the level of observation.

Darwin

1859. In *The Origin of Species,* Charles Darwin verified that all organisms had gradually evolved from a common ancestor through natural selection. Imagine a tree; new organisms evolve from the branches, but everything leads back to the common roots. Due to extinction, large segments of this tree vanish from the face of the Earth, while other parts remain. If all biological things in the Earth's history were alive simultaneously, we would have great trouble with the term "species" because the significant changes we expect between populations wouldn't be there; instead there would be minor differences between populations. It might be no more than the difference in hair or fur thickness by a half a millimeter. It certainly does expand the mind to envision such a spectacular zoo. However, Darwin's point was clear: Extinctions allow us to see more significant variation between living things. The concept of species is a human labeling system that gets in the way of seeing biological evolution as a gradual process of biological diversity. If we keep this in mind, but still accept that science has criteria for species, we can make some headway.

Pre-Darwin

Linnaeus

1753. The genus (genera) for cannabis was contested. The father of modern taxonomy, Swedish botanist Carolus Linnaeus (1707–1778), also known as Carl von Linné, invented a scheme of nomenclature classification and published it in his *Systema Naturae*. After observing what he called Cannabis (Hemp), he subsumed all the cannabis varieties he studied under the name *Cannabis sativa*. The genus is called *Cannabis sativa L.*—in the order of Linnaeus. Since we know that all varieties (strains) of cannabis can interbreed and produce fertile offspring, this means that the species *Cannabis sativa L.* satisfies an important criterion for a single-species orientation.

Lamarck

1785. The French biologist Jean-Baptiste Lamarck immediately challenged this single species orientation by classifying a distinctive second species of Cannabis, *C. indica*. Lamarck was very precise about the differences:

> This plant, of which Mr. Sonnerat has sent us some samples which he collected in India, appears to us a species very distinct from the preceding. It is smaller, more branched, with a firmer, nearly cylindrical stem, and it particularly is distinguished in that the leaves are all constantly alternate. The leaflets are very narrow, linear-lanceolate, and very acuminate. Male individuals have five or seven leaflets; but those which are female commonly carry only three on each petiole and the upper leaves themselves are quite simple. The calyces of the female flowers are velvety, the long styles are similarly velvety. This plant grows in the East Indies. Its firm stem and thin bark make it incapable of furnishing similar fibres to the preceding species (*C. sativa L.*) of which so much use is made.[15]

Delile

1849. A.R. Delile named a species found in China as C. *chinensis Delile*. Ind. *Sem. Hort. Monst.* And in 1851, he named another C. *gigantea Delile*. L.

Post-Darwin

Janischevsky

1924. D.E. Janischevsky wrote the paper *Forma konopli na sornykh mestakh v Yugovostochnoi Rossii*. Affiliated with the University of Saratov, in the former Soviet Union, he proposed the species *C. ruderalis Janisch*, or *C. sativa* L. f. *ruderalis (Janisch.)*, or *C. sativa* L *subsp. spontanea Serebr.*

Vavilov

1929. Nikolai Ivanovich Vavilov and D.D. Bukinich wrote the paper *Zemledelcheskii Afghanistan. Trudy po prikladnoi botanike, genetike i selektsii. Prilozhenie* to approve of the use of *C. indica* while naming a wild variety.

Schultes

1974. The botanists Richard E. Schultes and Loran Anderson conducted taxonomic studies of cannabis, concluding that the multiple species model of three species, *C. sativa, C. indica Lam.*, and *C. ruderalis*, should be used appropriately:

> *C. sativa* is tall and laxly branched with relatively narrow leaflets, *Cannabis indica* is shorter, conical in shape, and has relatively wide leaflets, and *Cannabis ruderalis* is short, branchless, and grows wild in central Asia.

Small

1976. Small and Cronquist revised 223 years of taxonomy to conclude that speciation, the creation of a new species by the division of an old one, had not occurred in cannabis. They forwarded the original proposal by Linnaeus for a single species model, *Cannabis sativa L.*, with two subspecies, *C. sativa* L. *subsp. sativa* and *C. sativa* L. *subsp. indica (Lam)*. They classed everything else as just varieties of these two subspecies.

Hillig

2005. K.W. Hillig discovered genetic evidence for speciation in Cannabaceae. A sample population of 157 cannabis accessions of diverse geographic origins was surveyed for allozyme variation at 17 gene loci. The frequencies of 52 alleles were subjected to principal components analysis. A scatter plot revealed two major groups of accessions. The sativa gene pool includes fiber and seed landraces from Europe, Asia Minor, central Asia, and ruderalis populations from Eastern Europe. The indica gene pool includes fiber and seed landraces from eastern Asia, narrow-leafleted drug strains from southern Asia, Africa, and Latin America, wide-leafleted drug strains from Afghanistan and Pakistan, and feral populations from India and Nepal. A third putative gene pool includes ruderalis populations from central Asia. None of the previous taxonomic concepts tested adequately circumscribed the sativa and indica gene pools. He proposed a polytypic (species consists of two or more subspecies) concept of cannabis, which recognizes three species, *C. sativa, C. indica*, and *C. ruderalis*, and seven putative taxa.

Hillig understood that there was a need to know whether speciation had occurred in cannabis. In a follow-up paper, Hillig wrote in the abstract:

> Botanists disagree whether *Cannabis* (Cannabaceae) is a monotypic or polytypic genus.... In summary, the results of this investigation show that a taxonomic revision of cannabis is warranted. However, additional studies of putative wild populations are needed to further substantiate the proposed taxonomic treatment.[16]

Scientific Cannabis Taxonomy

Previously, we discussed the scientific cannabis taxonomy as applied to the GRIN, the USDA Plants Database, and ITIS, which gave us six options divided into two parts. With *breeder terminology*, we select from the first group. For scientific nomenclature, we use the latter.

Conventional scientific nomenclature would appear as follows:

Kingdom	Plantae
Division.	Magnoliophyta
Class	Magnoliopsida
Order.	Rosales
Family.	Cannabaceae
Genus	Cannabis L.
Species	*Cannabis indica Lam.*

The last entry is subject to change. This categorization indicates that this form accepts the three-species model as the single-species model has only sativa. The single-species model would appear as follows:

Kingdom	Plantae
Division.	Magnoliophyta
Class	Magnoliopsida
Order.	Rosales
Family.	Cannabaceae
Genus	Cannabis L.
Species	*Cannabis sativa* L. subsp. *indica*

Which may also appear as:

Genu	Cannabis L.
Species	*Cannabis sativa* L.
Subspecies	*Indica*

These tables all describe the same plant, not three different types of plants. For example, a cannabis plant called indica appears different from sativa but can still be bred with sativa. By definition, sativa cannot be another species, but science holds that tentatively because speciation can be argued due to geographical isolation and other segregating factors.

To sum this up, commercially you will hear of three general types of cannabis plants, and all three can be hybridized to produce viable offspring. They are simply sativa, indica, and ruderalis, which is sometimes called autoflowering. So how do they all combine?

Varieties, Strains, Subspecies, and Hybrids

The most "common" descriptions of cannabis species and hybrids are pure indica (*C. sativa* L. subsp. *indica*), pure sativa (*C. sativa* L.), indica/sativa hybrids (*C. sativa* L. subsp. *indica / C. sativa* L. hybrid), mostly indica (Mostly C. sativa L. subsp. indica hybrid), and mostly sativa (Mostly C. sativa L. hybrid). "Mostly" means greater than 50% content, usually estimated by the breeder. "Mostly indica," for example says that, at one stage, a *C. indica* plant was crossed with a *C. sativa* plant to produce

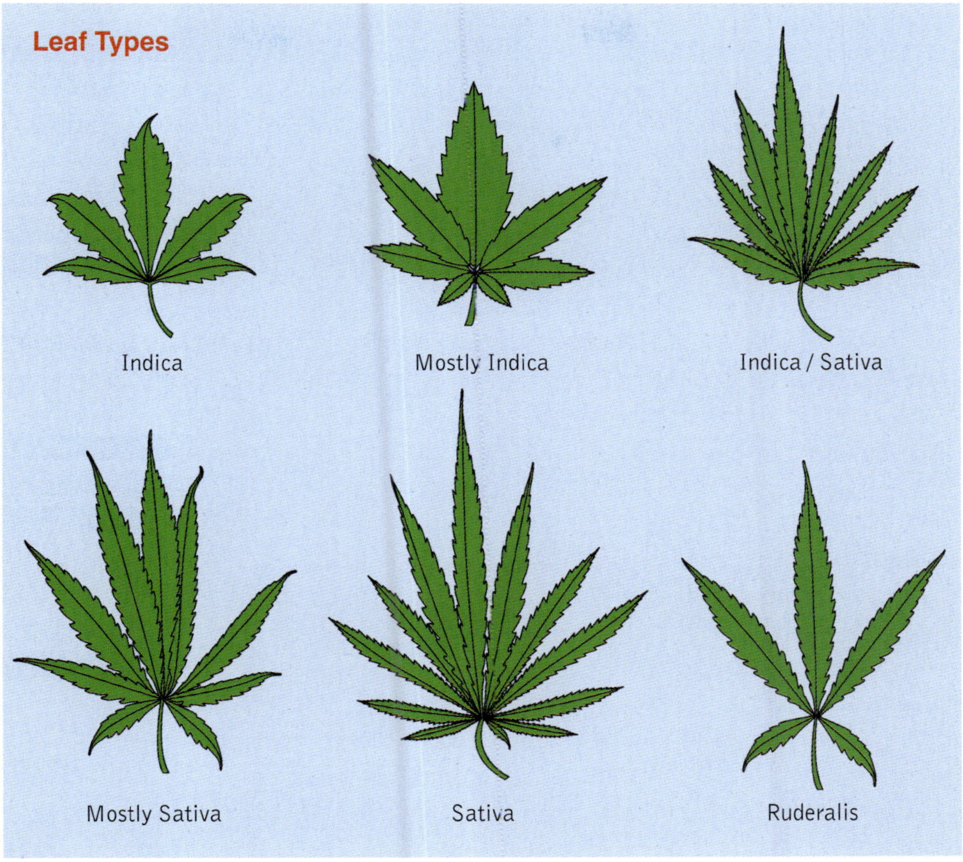

indica/sativa offspring (1:1), and likely that offspring bred with indica to make the strain mostly indica. As a result, the strain will primarily be indica but has some sativa in it.

When researching a strain, you will come across descriptions that fit into these categories. Hopefully, everything you have read up until now about cannabis species explains that layout. We haven't yet discussed ruderalis as it is an autoflowering type of cannabis and needs to be treated differently. Ruderalis is generally a shorter cannabis plant that flowers according to age and not photoperiod as with sativa and indica. It is helpful for locations that need shorter flowering times to finish the plant before late autumn. It is also beneficial if you want shorter plants, though you can also use indica in these situations. We shall discuss ruderalis more later.

Cannabis Reproduction

Genetics suggests the sex of a cannabis plant is set in the embryo. A collection of seeds from one plant will have a roughly balanced mix of males and females. You won't know which are which until the plants mature enough to display their sex. However, the situation is often more complicated than this with cannabis. Genetic studies of cannabis sex chromosomes indicate female plants are homogametic (XX) and males are heterogametic (XY), which is consistent with the science of sex determination but not always consistent with observed results. Growers also observe male organs on female flowering plants, the hermaphrodite condition.

Previous editions discussed how optimal growing conditions could produce a preferable ratio of female to male plants based on the general observations of growers over time. Why do growers see more females from optimal growing conditions if sex is set in the seed? One observation was fewer hermaphrodites in populations growing under optimal, non-stressful conditions. Hermaphrodites may also be weeded out with the males, meaning any that remain in the population would have been female plants if not stressed. To further explain this, we need to look at sex determination systems in cannabis.

Understanding Sex Determination Systems

The sexual systems of cannabis have been widely studied because of observable and repeatable sex-reversal conditions. K. Hirata confirmed the usual expectancy of an XY sex-determination system in 1924.[17] Schaffner disputed this in 1925, when, through sex-reversal studies in hemp, he found that an XA system, an alternative system to XY, was present and highly influenced by environmental conditions.[18] There was doubt concerning how the XY system occurs in cannabis, with statements that the Y chromosome is slightly larger than the X chromosome, thus being difficult to distinguish.[19]

We should be able to say that a plant is male or female by genetic and chromosome analysis. Sex, though, becomes more complicated as we look at more examples in biology. Some organisms, like some wrasse fish, change sex. There are many different types of mating systems in nature.

Cannabis reproduction is botanically similar to that of other flowering plants, which have a structure designed for reproduction in the form of developing imperfect flowers with the male staminate formed separately from the female pistillate, or carpellate. However, in instances where perfect hermaphroditism is observed, staminate form next to or from pistillate with calyx formation.

Understanding sex means identifying female plants, male plants, and hermaphrodites for most growers. Males and hermaphrodites are removed to keep females separate, or the hermaphrodites are removed to make more seeds between males and females. In optimal growing environments with good genetics, you will not see hermaphrodites, but the hermaphrodite condition may express in less than optimal growing environments. How this happens is still an area of research if, as we believe, sex is determined at the gene level. However, there are ways this can be explained.

Dioecious, Monecious, and Hermaphrodites

So how do we describe cannabis in terms of its mating system? Dioecious populations have the male and female reproductive organs borne on loose panicles and racemes on separate individuals of the same species; in other words, there are some plants with male organs and other plants with female organs. Monecious populations have male and female organs found within the same floral cluster, the inflorescence, of the same individual plant. We generally call this the hermaphrodite condition. However, we do find monecious individuals within a dioecious population. So, while cannabis might be mainly dioecious, we must be cautious. Hemp, for example, comes in both monecious and dioecious forms.

Sexually, we can describe any cannabis member as:

Dioecious	Only dioecious plants.
Monecious	Only monecious plants.
Hermaphrodite	Only hermaphrodite plants.
Gynodioecious	Both female and hermaphrodite plants present.
Androdioecious	Both male and hermaphrodite plants present.
Trioecious/Subdioecious	Male, female, and hermaphrodite plants in the same population.

All dense clusters of female flowers produced by cannabis are loosely referred to as "bud," which generally should be without seeds. They contain no seeds because they never came into contact with pollen. All unfertilized female flowers are called sinsemilla. While seeded bud is generally regarded as low in quality, this is not because of genetic potency factors (as long as the pistils have time to mature to optimal potency, it is fine), but because it is harder to work with seeded bud. The plant has devoted more energy to seed production than pistil growth and cannabinoid production. As a result, the cannabinoid levels and ratios shouldn't alter too much, but the final yields will be lower. Post-harvest manicuring techniques become more complex and often involve sieving at large production scales to shake the seeds out. Seeds are made by breeding programs and usually only with healthy dioecious parents.

What could explain the presence of more females in optimal grow rooms? Sex is predetermined, but several factors can influence maleness in plants. Sex-determining genes, sex chromosomes, epigenetic control by DNA methylation, microRNAs, and physiological regulation with phytohormones influence sex expression (Galoch, 1978;[20] Dellaporta & Calderon-Urrea, 1993;[21] Hall et al., 2012;[22] Punja & Holmes, 2020[23]). The most recent paper on evidence for altering these factors comes from Flajšman et al. They wrote that the phenomena of alteration of cannabis sexual reproduction can be influenced chemically in their article "Production of feminized seeds of high-CBD *Cannabis sativa* L. by manipulation of sex expression and its application to breeding".[24] They also identified over 10,500 differentially expressed genes, of which around 200 are potentially responsible for male flower development in female plants in "Comparative RNA-Seq analysis reveals genes associated with masculinization in female *Cannabis sativa*" in *Planta* 253 (17) 2021.[25]

So today, we can say that while sex is determined at the gene's level, that gene's expression will go through various regulated pathways that will influence the final expression of sex in the cannabis plant.

Advanced Sinsemilla Facts

Sinsemilla is a type of cannabis, and the terminology was first used by the American Spanish-speaking cannabis cultivation community. It occurs in cultivation where male plants are removed from the population, leaving only the female plants to promote optimal yields and results. However, fertilization can still occur because the technique produces stress-related sexual change where some dioecious females will express gynodioecious sexuality by bearing male organs. We don't know all the reasons stress can cause hermaphrodites. Still, we know cannabis sexual expression involves complex pathways.

For this reason, growers must take great care in choosing a mother plant for a perpetual clone sinsemilla system that will maximize the female's pistil gland production without male flowers showing. A grower will typically manually remove any male reproductive organs in a gynodioecious occurrence, though sometimes it is better to remove a mostly female plant with a few male flowers to avoid the risk of pollinating the other sinsemilla females. If the hermaphrodite condition is too profuse, the grower will usually not grow that strain again and must find a more suitable candidate. Over the decades, breeders have been trying to make their females hermaphrodite-free. Good sinsemilla needs to start with good genetics. While some sustainable evidence supports a case for more psychoactive cannabinoids in the sinsemilla product, there is little evidence to support the claim that sinsemilla glands themselves have higher cannabinoid levels. Sinsemilla simply produce more of these glands, making the cannabinoid quantity of the whole plant higher.

In previous editions, there was insufficient evidence to note a substantial increase in average potency, but the past ten years have provided us with more data. The US Federal Potency Monitoring Project noted in 1985 that the average THC content of commercial-grade cannabis was 2.84%, and the average for high-grade sinsemilla was 7.17%. In 1995, the potency of commercial-grade cannabis averaged 3.73%, while that of sinsemilla averaged 7.51%. In 2001, commercial-grade cannabis averaged 4.72% THC, and the sinsemilla averaged 9.03%.

Around 14,000 samples of herbal cannabis were analyzed between 2009 and 2019 to determine potency increases in the US. Mean Δ9-THC concentration increased from 9.75% in 2009 to 14.88% in 2018 and 13.88% in 2019. The mean Δ9-THC:CBD ratio rose substantially from 24.81 in 2009 to 103.48 in 2017. A decrease in THC:CBD ratio was recorded in the last two years, 54.39 in 2018 and 24.58 in 2019, indicating a trend in producing more high-CBD-containing products. So, there has been a potency increase of 10% in 2009 to about 14% in 2019, according to ElSohly *et al.*'s study "A Comprehensive Review of Cannabis Potency in the United States in the Last Decade" *Biol Psychiatry Cogn Neurosci Neuroimaging* 2021 Jun 6(6):603–6.

Breeding for Desirable Traits

The creation of a large-volume, high-yielding, resinous, potent dioecious population of female-only sinsemilla plants, with high calyx-to-leaf ratio and high trichome production, has led to an increase in well-refined strains available to the cultivator. Tried and tested clones are ideal for those who want to start growing immediately. For this reason, most growers are concerned with obtaining hermaphrodite-resistant clones that meet the standards the grower wants from the genetic material.

The average grower, certainly beginner growers, will probably not be concerned with breeding cannabis seeds. The indoor grower is usually interested in C. indica species or subspecies indica/sativa hybrids; they will most likely exclude pure sativa because it is an expert plant to work with and suitable for only a very sizable growing area with longer flowering times. Even a mostly sativa strain can grow tall. Always check what heights the breeder claims. Growers generally avoid autoflowering ruderalis in favor of photoperiod-controlled sinsemilla results. However, they may select outdoor ruderalis or indica hybrids if they have a short flowering season. Breeders work to deliver strains with the traits you need.

General Cannabis Morphology

Sativa

Height: Tall, averaging 4 to 15 feet
Nodes: Long internodes between branches, 3 to 6 inches
Leaves: Thin, long, and pointy leaves with no markings or patterns
Blades: Usually 6 to 12 blades per leaf

Indica

Height: Small, averaging 6 inches to 4 feet
Nodes: Short internodes between branches, 3 inches or less
Leaves: Wide, short, and rounded leaves with marble-like patterns
Blades: Usually 3 to 5 blades per leaf

Ruderalis

Height: Small, averaging 6 inches to 4 feet
Nodes: Very short internodes without much branching
Leaves: Small and thick
Blades: Usually 4 to 6 blades per leaf

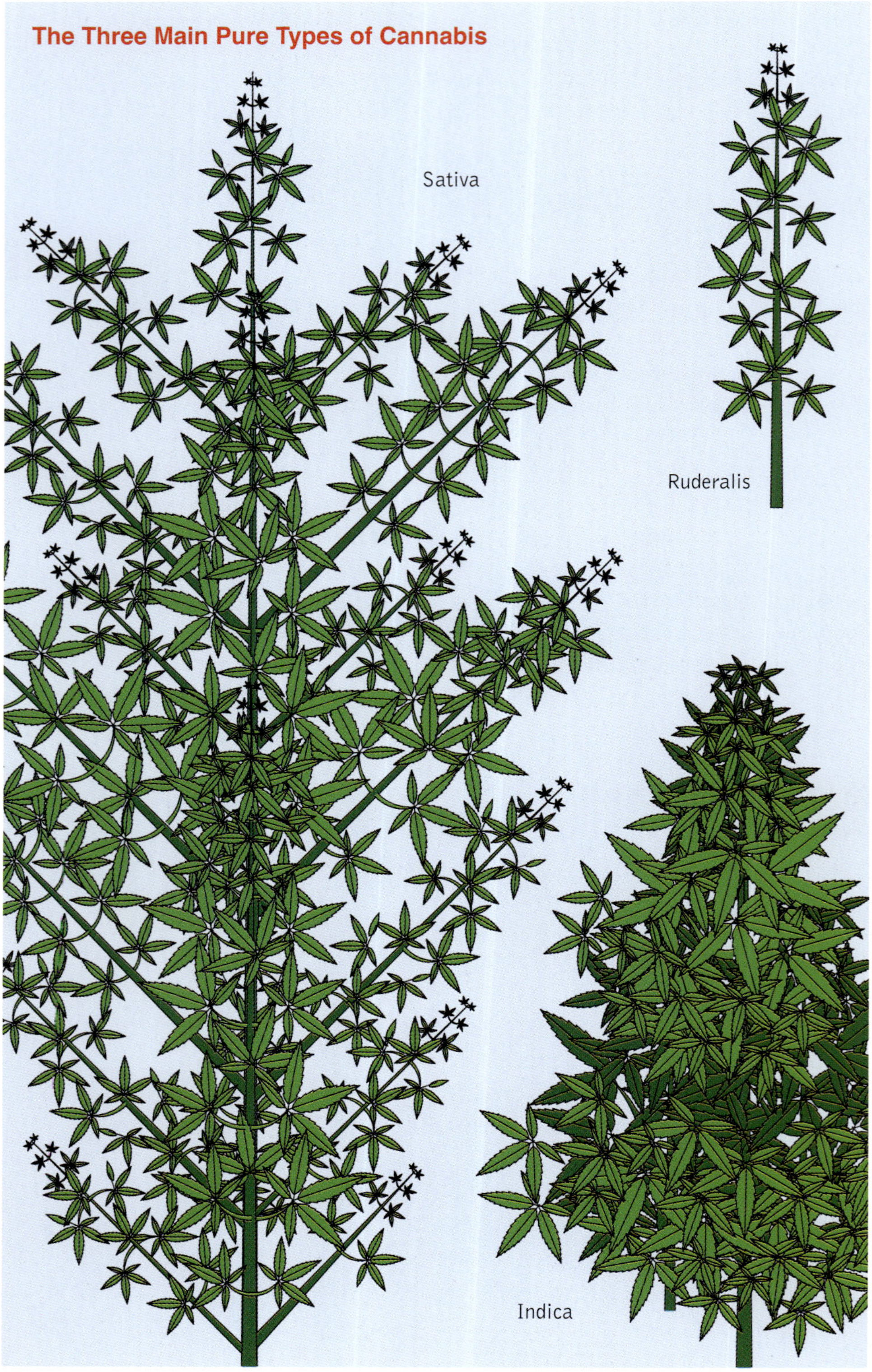
The Three Main Pure Types of Cannabis
Sativa
Ruderalis
Indica

The Life Cycle of the Cannabis Plant

The cannabis plant grows in three main stages: Germination, vegetative growth, and flowering, and three additional sub-stages.

Germination

Developmental biology deals with the embryology of the organism. A plant starts its life as a single cell. As the embryo develops as a seed, it eventually breaks through its shell. Germination is the initial growth stage, when the seed's embryo breaks through the shell, or the testa, and the seedling produces its first initial root, the plumule. This root fixes itself into the germination medium and pushes the developing seedling up and over the surface. Following surface contact, two embryonic leaves, the cotyledons, open outward to receive sunlight, pushing the empty testa away from the seedling. It takes 12 hours to three weeks for seeds to germinate. In nature, the wind helps to shake the shell away. Since artificial wind is not initially used in the germination environment, some seedlings find it harder to shed their shell. If the shell obstructs the seedling's growth, you can remove it by hand, being careful not to damage the seedling.

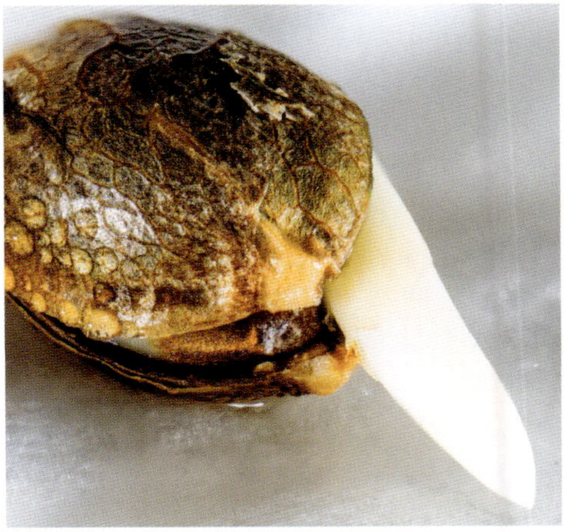

Embryo breaking the testa and producing its first initial root, the plumule.

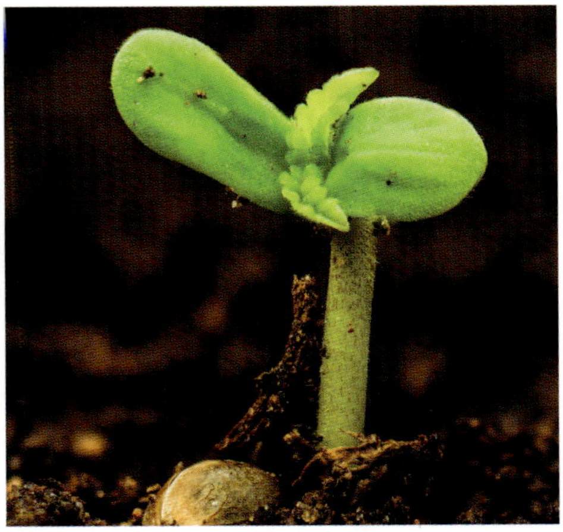

Two embryonic leaves, the cotyledons, push the testa away from the seedling.

Seedling

After the first pair of embryonic leaves receive light, the plant produces another small set of new true leaves, which may have more noticeable cannabis characteristics, such as the three rounded, finger-shaped points. As the seedling grows, more of these leaves are formed and bush upward along with the stem. Some stems are fragile at this sub-stage and need the support of a stake tied to the seedling with some fine thread. The seedling sub-stage can last one to three weeks. At the end of the seedling sub-stage, the plant has four to eight new leaves, while some of the original bottom leaves and cotyledons may have dropped off. Remove any support strings when you feel the seedling is independently stable enough.

PHOTOS: ERIC PALMER

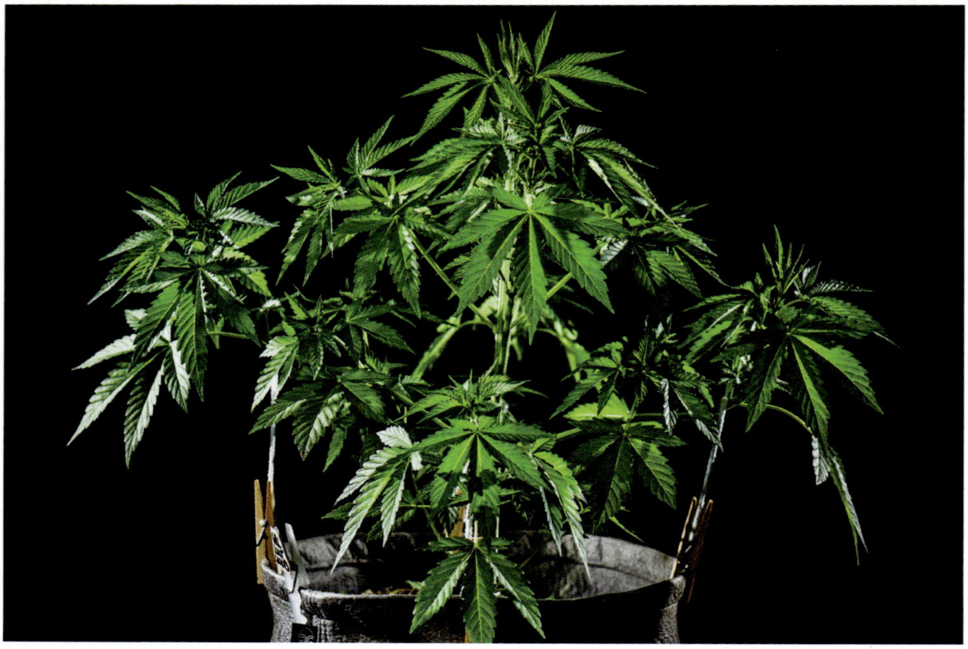

Vegetative growth occurs over weeks, growing leaves for energy-intensive flowering later.

Vegetative Growth

The plant begins to grow at the rate its leaves can produce energy. At this stage, the plant needs all the light and food it can use. It continues to grow upward, produce new leaves, and develop a thicker stem, thicker branches, and its maximum number of blades on the leaves. When mature, the plant shows its sex. The vegetative growth stage is approximately five weeks, depending on the strain, with some sativa able to go longer, over six weeks, all before flowering. Cannabis takes eight to 12 weeks for a cycle, so subtract the vegetative stage to get your flowering time estimates.

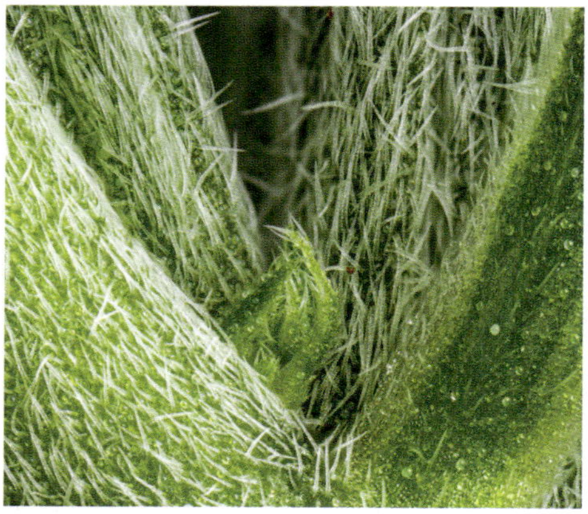

Calyx development signals the pre-flowering phase.

PHOTOS: ERIC PALMER (TOP), ROB BRAMHILL (BOTTOM)

Pre-Flowering

At this sub-stage, the plant's upward growth slows, and it produces more branches and nodes. The plant fills out and shows a calyx where the branches meet the stem at the nodes. This calyx is the ultimate indicator that the plant is in the pre-flowering growth phase and is mature enough to flower. The plant starts to exhibit signs of its sex, and more calyx development takes place at other node points. Pre-flowering can last one day to two weeks.

Flowering

The plant continues to fill out. Its sex is now clearly evident. The male plant produces a collection of creamy yellow banana-shaped flowers clustered together that dispense pollen when they open. The female plant produces tiny white pistils that look like curly oily tentacles coming out of a pod. Both males and females have a green hue in the initial development days. After that, each plant continues to fill out its floral traits. Depending on the strain, it can take four to six weeks to develop its flowers fully, but some sativa can go much longer: Two weeks of pre-flowers max and then four weeks to six weeks. Consult breeder's terminology.

Seed Production

In the wild, male plants release pollen only when females have developed their flowers. Natural selection ensures that synchronization occurs as only plants that sync will contribute to future offspring through seeds. Indoor breeding operations involve pollen gathering and application to females in a sealed-off growing environment, changing how hybrids, even out of sync, can be pollinated.

The female plant produces seeds if she has received viable pollen from a male plant. The seeds grow in the female bud, taking two to 16 weeks to mature fully. The female pistils may change color before finally bursting the seedpods, sending them to the soil below. Breeders like to collect seeds before the seedpods burst.

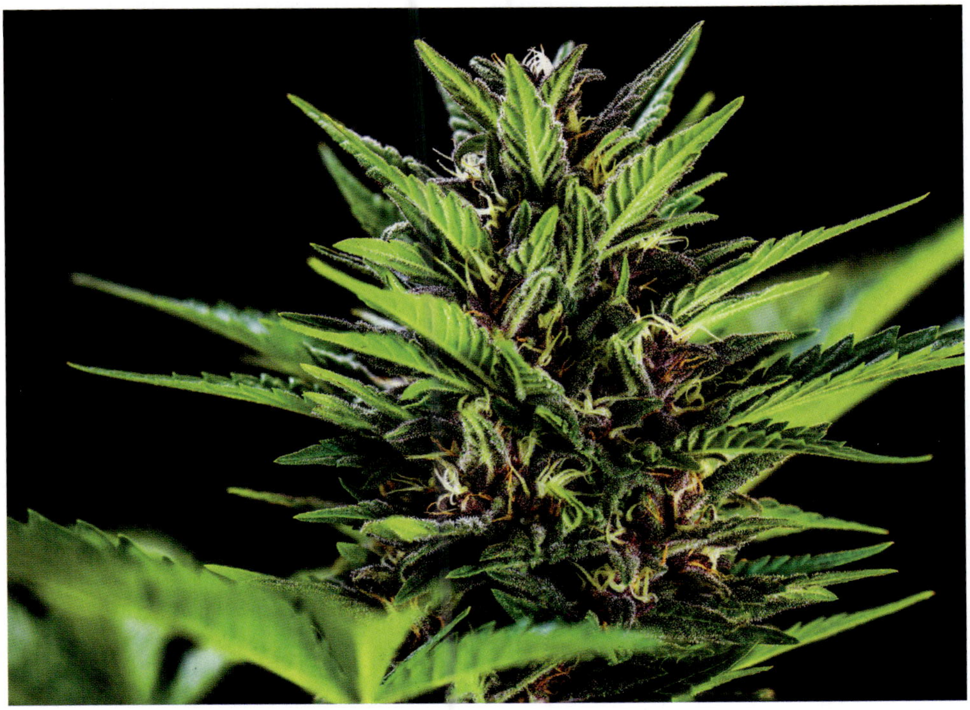

PHOTO: ERIC PALMER

Cannabis flowers can dramatically shift in color values throughout the flowering period, especially around harvest week.

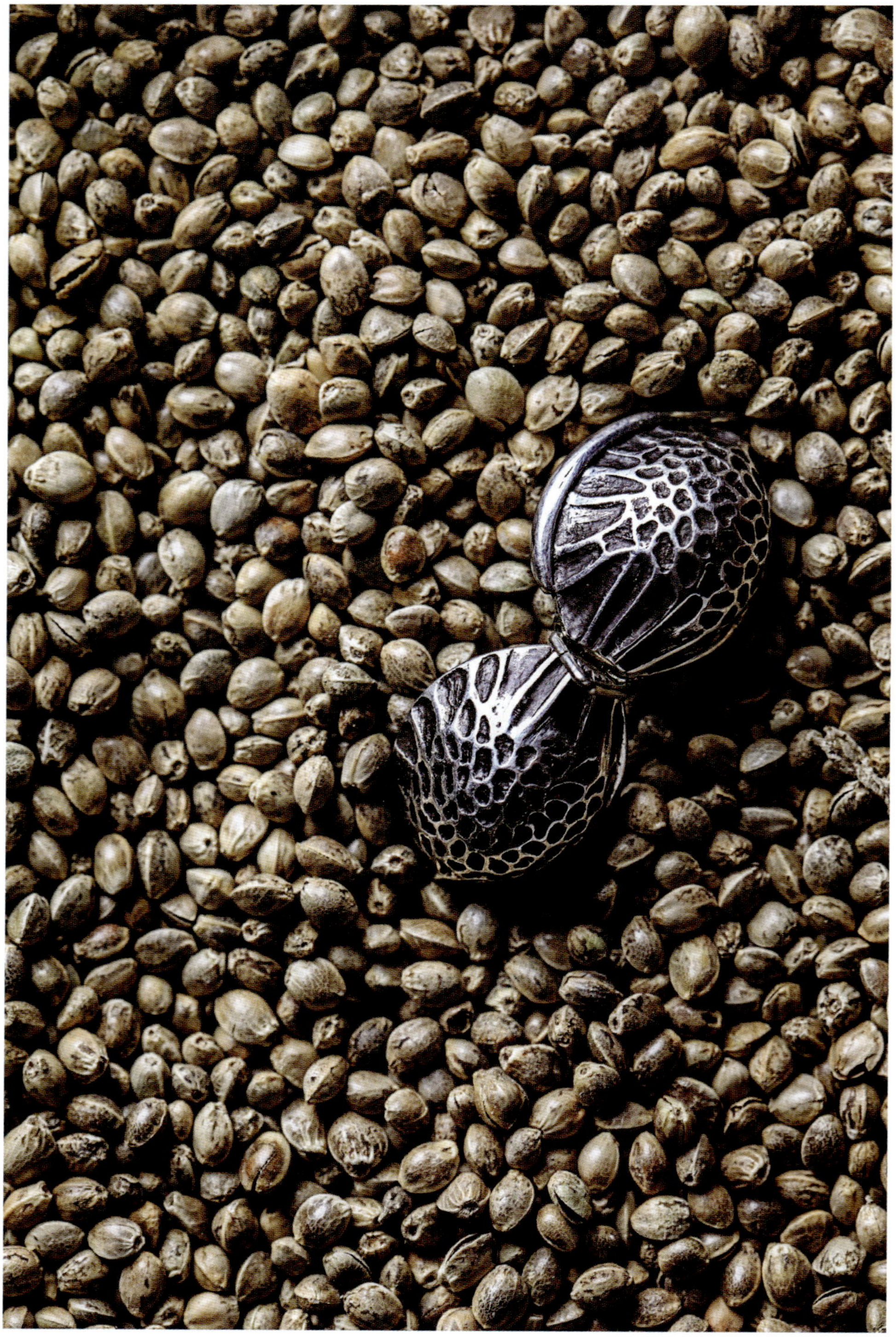

PHOTO: KAYA

A large selection of seeds ready to be packaged. Each seed has its own unique pattern, ranging from no pattern at all to deep brown markings.

If no males are present to pollinate the female plants during the flowering stage, the buds grow larger and develop more resin glands. The resin may drop down onto the leaves, making the plant very sticky. The pistils on the buds begin to thicken and cluster more. The high increase in bud growth indicates that the female plant is trying its best to attract male pollen. This is the sinsemilla condition. Toward the last days of flowering, the pistils may change color, indicating that the plant is ready for harvest.

Cycle Times

Growing from a seed to a fully matured plant can take anywhere from 10 to 36 weeks, most commonly falling between 13 to 17 weeks. Timing depends on the strain you select. Pure sativa can take six to nine months. Indica can flower in six weeks. A sativa/indica hybrid plant falls into the two- to four-month flowering period. Hybrid cycle times vary the most.

Keeping Notes

It's important to take notes. Record-keeping enables you to measure the flowering times and backtrack over plant growth to see areas where you could have made improvements or encountered problems. You can also highlight the parts of this text that you want to remember. Recording soil, nutrients, feeding regime, temperatures, humidity levels, pH levels, and harvest times can improve your cultivation techniques. Undoubtedly, the best growers keep some notes and even write articles about their experiences. Labeling is a must. You don't have to label a plant "Skunk #1" directly; you can give it an ID tag such as "1789" and have this correspond to SK1 or something similar in a spreadsheet. Not using notes usually has negative consequences and limits opportunities for optimization.

Strain Name	Age	Stage of Growth	Watering Times and Amounts	Nutrients Times and Amounts	Estimated Harvest Times	Growing Mediums	General tasks (pruning, tying, etc.)

You can use software for cultivation; some are for managing medical communities, but private grow apps are on the rise. Remember that you are tracking your progress and that the information is sensitive. Most of the premium software packages are encrypted. This software's objective is to store information on grow rooms and the setup in each room. It allows you to print tags and labels. You can measure and plot the height of your plants. Daily reminders can be entered. Costs may be included.

You can create your own spreadsheets with these columns: Strain name, age, stage of growth, watering times and amounts, nutrients times and amounts, estimated harvest times, growing mediums, general tasks (pruning, tying, etc.).

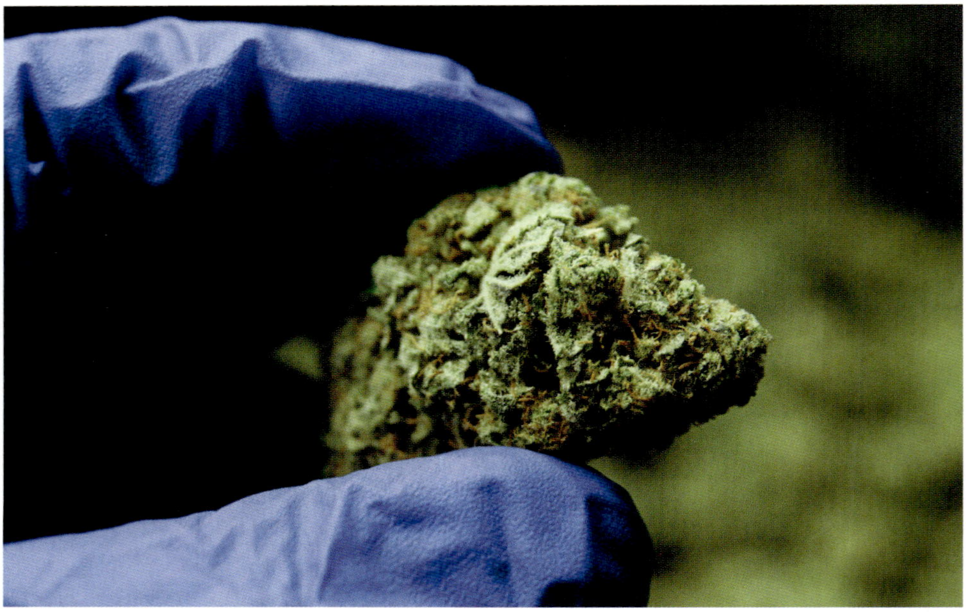

Freshly-harvested and manicured marijuana bud. If you are harvesting a large amount, you should wear gloves to prevent a contact high and any skin irritation from the plant matter, especially if you need to use the washroom or touch any sensitive body parts.

By keeping notes, you can plan successive grows better. It is impossible to remember everything about that crop you had a few years ago that you want to try again. You will not remember everything you had to deal with or what you can improve upon with that strain. You cut your research time down if you have notes and know what to expect. Note-keeping can make the difference between average and excellent results. If you grew a strain with great success, the second round with experience grows even better. This will help you improve as a cannabis grower.

Considerations Before You Start Growing

There are several things to consider before you start to grow cannabis. Better to think of these now rather than halfway through your grow when you learn that the smell is too strong to continue or you're growing the wrong strain.

- What do you hope to achieve? High potency, high yield, one or many plants?
- Which species/strain best meets your needs?
- Are you willing to spend over $100 for 10 seeds?
- Will you grow indoors or outdoors?
- How do the people you live with feel about this?
- Do you have time to take care of your plants?
- Do you have someone you trust to care for your plants in your absence?
- How secure is your grow area?

PHOTO: DAVID STRANGE

- Are people going to walk past your grow site?
- Can you hide the smell when the plants start to flower?
- Do you have the patience to wait a few months before sampling what you produce?
- Are you prepared to spend money on lights and other grow items?
- Are you prepared to pay the costs of a higher electricity bill?
- Are you aware of the legal risks for the amount you plan to grow?
- Can you afford a good attorney if you think there could be legal consequences to your grow?
- Do you have any previous convictions that could be used as a legal prejudice against you if you are charged with growing cannabis?
- Do you know what your legal rights are?
- Can gun ownership be used against you if you are caught growing cannabis?
- Can other drug possession in your home be used against you if you are caught growing cannabis?
- Can your children be taken from you and put into social care if you are caught growing cannabis?
- Is your home safe to grow in?
- Are there any pets that can damage your crop or start an electrical fire by knocking over things?
- Can you deal with a fire?
- Are you a tight-lipped person?
- Do you want to be another dull cash-cropper who wastes their life just selling cannabis, or do you want to be a new-wave frontier grower who grows to rid themselves of the connection to the black market to enjoy their favorite herb?
- Do you want to grow?

When you feel confident that you have addressed these questions, start roughly outlining your plan. You need a general idea of what to look for in a plant to produce a high-quality product. Medicinal cannabis growers aim for a high cannabinoid ratio. Connoisseur growers aim for taste, color, visual appeal, and yield. These goals may be different for average growers. The everyday gardener is looking for non-pollinated female plants that produce lots of bud with resin glands containing high levels and quantities of THC. They are also looking for flowers that have been well-cured and processed to sample the plant's full flavor, smell, and potency. Some people prefer plants that provide an effect that does not cause drowsiness, where the body becomes less responsive to stimuli, or they may prefer more of a sativa cerebral effect to the indica one. Both effects can be found in hybrids. These effects are to do with strain type and harvesting times. Variations in cannabinoid ratios are something that medical users pay attention to as it guides them toward similar strains. Growing your product ensures that you have natural and unadulterated cannabis.

Let's get growing.

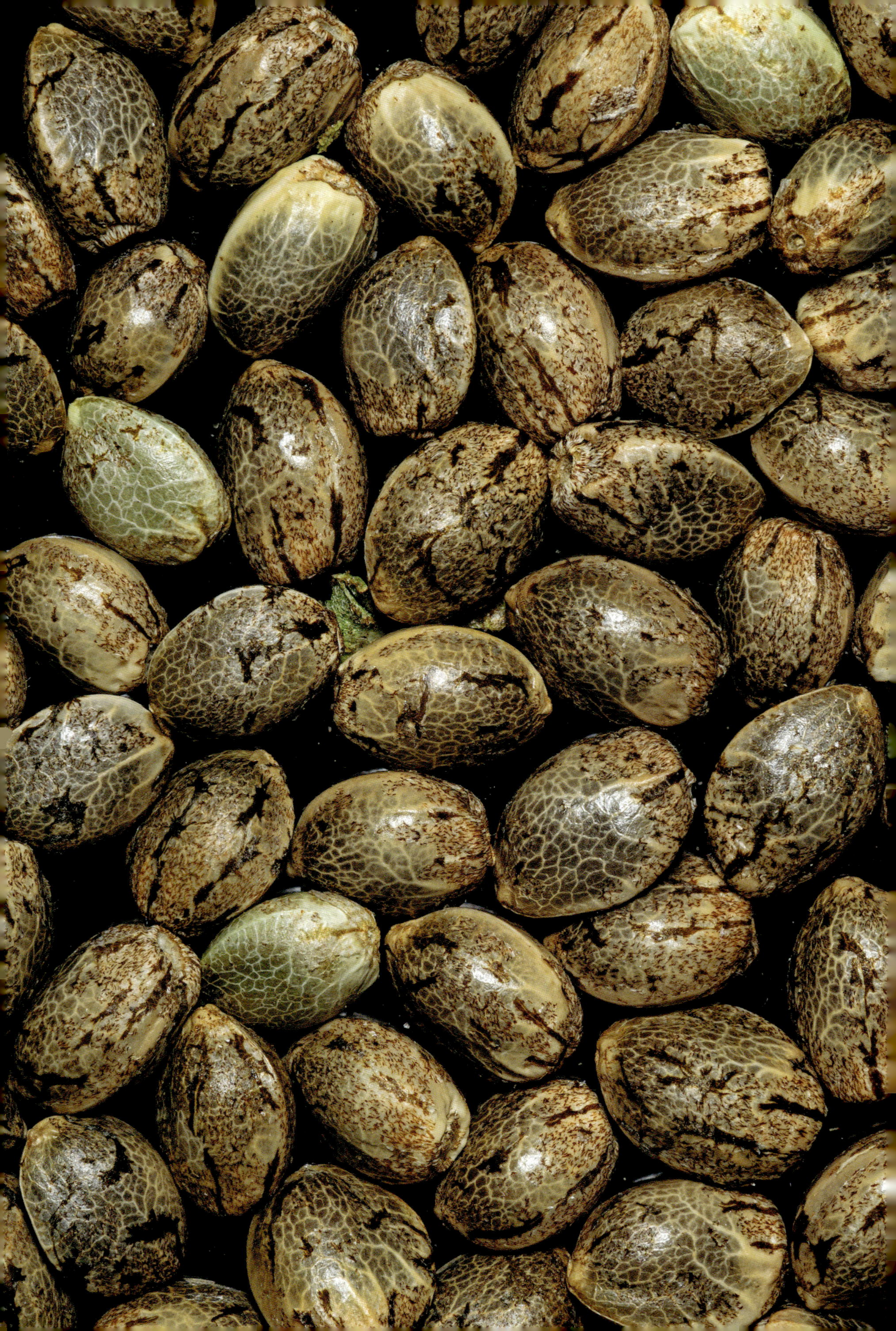

3

Seeds: Selection, Banks, and Storage

This chapter provides all the information you need to select the right strain for you. As you become more familiar with your cultivation style and the characteristics you desire in your final product, you'll find numerous strains to choose from, and become better at picking those that suit your grow setup and style.

How Many Strains Exist?

By 1999, there were about 450 cannabis seed varieties available on the market. Of these, growers suggested that 200 were worth considering, but only about 50 were outstanding. The first decade of the 21st century witnessed an enormous increase in the number of breeders and strains available, making it a daunting task to keep track of them. Still, you can follow cannabis-related social media accounts and read articles in online cannabis magazines to stay informed about the latest developments in the cannabis industry. One great online resource is seedfinder.eu. It's always a good idea to fully research before spending your money.

What's a Hybrid?

A hybrid is the offspring of two animals or plants that belong to different breeds, varieties, species, or genera. In the context of cultivation, it primarily refers to plants that have been intentionally bred to exhibit specific genetic characteristics. Cultivators often create these "strains" by carefully selecting parent stock lines with desirable traits. The term "breed" is also used in describing plants. Academic journal articles use both terms to describe plant populations, including those of cannabis.

Stable strains exhibit consistent genetic traits, ensuring that their offspring will closely resemble one another. Stabilizing hybrids is crucial for several aspects of cultivation,

PHOTO: ROB BRAMHILL

including preventing competition for light between shorter and taller plants, which can lead to excessive internode lengthening. While variations between populations of different strains are expected, even desirable, stable strains should exhibit minimal variation within their own population.

New hybrids tend to be highly unstable, or variable, and genetically unpredictable. There are often substantial variations among their offspring, including differences in scent, taste, appearance, cannabinoid ratios, and disease resistance. If a strain is labeled as "mostly sativa," and its offspring produce a range of plants displaying traits from sativa-dominant to indica-dominant, then it is an unstable hybrid and not recommended for novice growers. Experienced cultivators typically use these hybrid seeds to identify and maintain a suitable "mother" plant for cloning.

You can obtain a stabilized hybrid from most breeders. Over time, a stabilized hybrid can evolve into a stable strain.

Most new hybrids are not immediately commercially available, usually being limited to breeders experimenting with plant genetics. However, new hybrids can offer advantages to cultivators who use clones for their "hybrid vigor." In a large hybrid population created by crossing two genetically distinct strains, one or more plants may possess all the desirable traits from both parents. Instead of breeding a stable line that consistently exhibits these traits, a grower may select one of these plants as a mother donor for cloning. The grower can later use male pollen from the same plant to replicate its genetic makeup in the female plants of the population.

Hybrid vigor thrives in large populations. The more plants you cultivate, the greater the chance of finding an exceptional mother donor. The key to discovering an outstanding mother plant lies in large sample sizes and a touch of serendipity. Conversely, obtaining seeds from a breeder who has already stabilized a hybrid's traits will yield more consistent results.

Some strains can be obtained only in clone form because no male counterpart exists.[1] Working with clones requires knowledge on how to maintain them. Ultimately, what suits your preferences as a grower is what matters most.

Seed producers typically categorize their strains into these groups:
- Pure sativa
- Sativa (mostly sativa species with some indica)
- Pure indica
- Indica (mostly indica species with some sativa)
- Indica/sativa (a 50/50 cross between indica and sativa species)
- Ruderalis

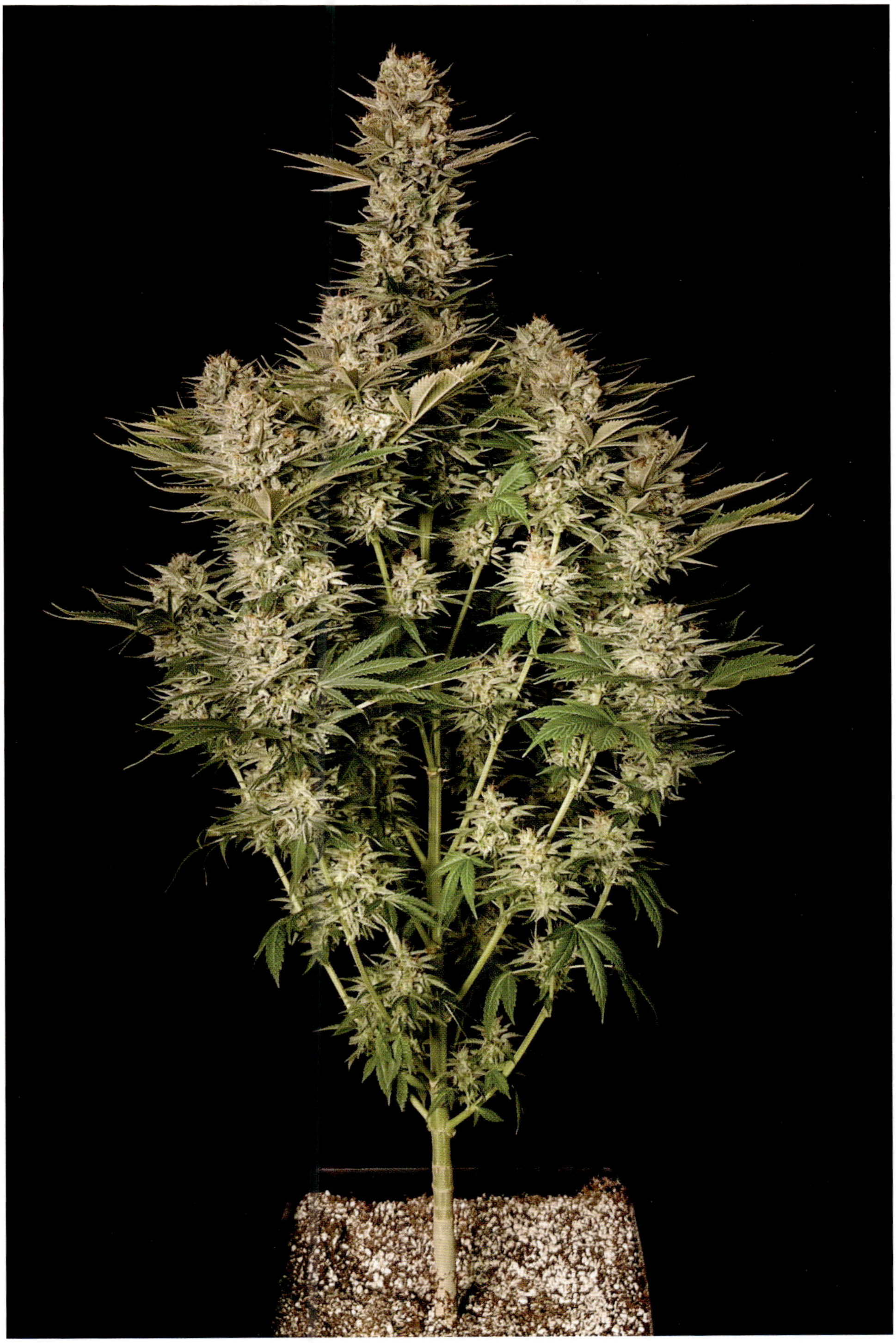

Autoflowering plants are a great choice for many growers who do not want to depend on a photoperiod for flowering. These plants automatically flower when they reach a certain age.

PHOTO: DOCTORSCHOICE.FARM

What is Ruderalis?

Ruderalis, while posing challenges for new growers, has its niche in hybridizing with outdoor strains in regions with less-than-ideal climates. This plant does not yield large quantities of flowers, nor does it boast a high THC content. Growers often regard ruderalis as subpar because it flowers based on its age, rather than responding to changes in photoperiod. A ruderalis plant will enter the flowering stage when it reaches a certain level of maturity, and this process is beyond the grower's control.

Ruderalis is commonly found in regions with cold climates, such as Russia, Eastern Europe, and Alaska, where it thrives in the wild. It is an exceptionally robust plant for outdoor cultivation. However, its autoflowering nature makes it challenging to manage. Attempting to clone a ruderalis plant can be difficult since maintaining the clone in the vegetative growth stage of the plant's cycle is a complex task. Traditional photoperiod manipulation, a fundamental aspect of cannabis cultivation, does not apply to ruderalis plants. Photoperiod will be discussed in more detail in later chapters.

The compact size and rapid maturity of ruderalis hybrids make them an excellent option for growers who need their plants to complete flowering before the first frost of the season, or where photoperiod is otherwise of no concern. Ruderalis has been hybridized by outdoor growers to create award-winning outdoor cannabis strains; however, these hybrids often exhibit a reduction in cannabinoid content and bud yield.

Novice growers should begin with regular strains and only consider experimenting with ruderalis plants once they've gained some experience in cannabis cultivation.

Indica or Sativa?

There are several factors to consider when choosing a strain for cultivation. The most fundamental is whether to go with an indica or sativa strain. A pure sativa strain typically delivers a predominantly cerebral high, while a pure indica strain tends to produce a more physical effect, often referred to as a body-stone or couch-lock sensation. Hybrids, on the other hand, blend elements of both sativa and indica strains. A 50/50 hybrid, for instance, offers a balance of head-high and body-stone. Breeders have the ability to adjust this ratio through their selections. For example, if a breeder crosses a pure indica with an indica-sativa hybrid, the resulting plant might be about 75% indica and 25% sativa. Though these ratios can vary, strains are commonly described as "mostly" indica, "mostly" sativa, "indica-dominant," or "sativa-dominant."

The next consideration is whether to cultivate your chosen strain indoors or outdoors. In theory, any strain can be grown in either environment, but doing so may not yield optimal results. Generally, indica strains are preferred for indoor cultivation, while sativas tend to thrive outdoors. Your decision should hinge on what is most important regarding your cultivation goals, such as the medicinal properties of the strain or the

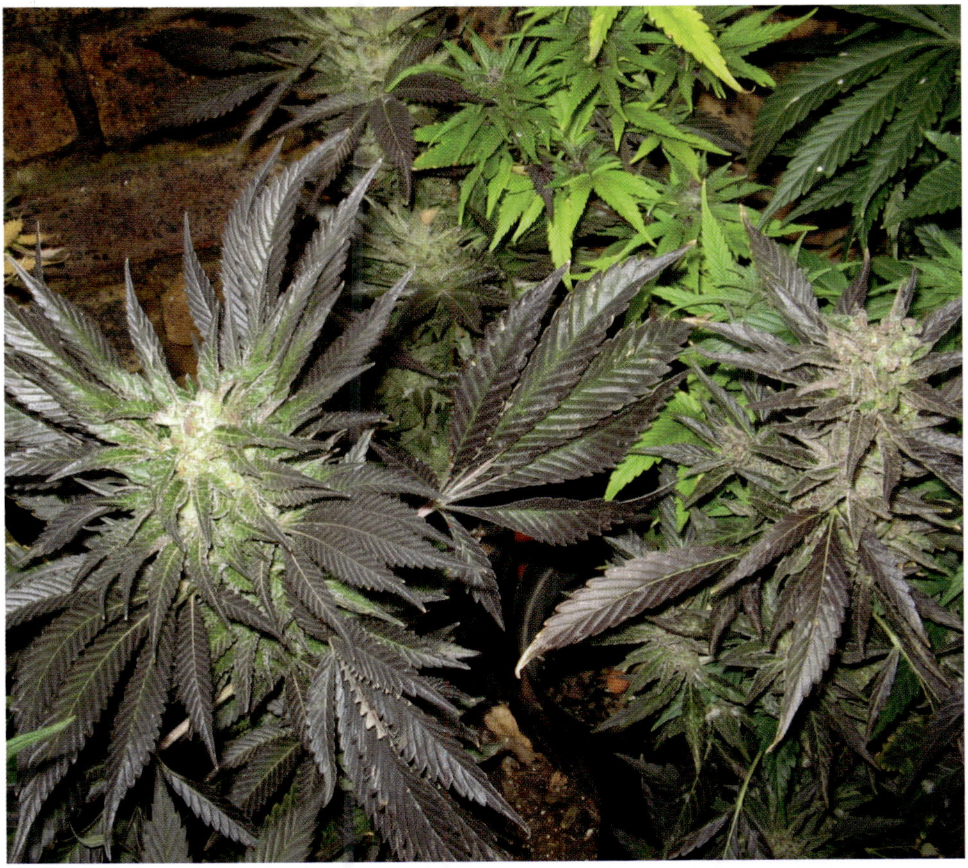

Fantastic frost on this Lebanese landrace pure sativa from the Bekka Valley, grown in South Africa. A combination of natural and human selection generates great plants for cultivation.

PHOTO: WEED.CO.ZA

environment in which you intend to grow. In certain climates, particularly in northern and southern regions of the world that have shorter flowering seasons, indica strains are more suitable for outdoor cultivation than sativas.

Now you can select a strain that aligns with your requirements in terms of plant height, potency, and the desired type of high, often referred to as its "medicinal value." Your choice of seeds should depend not only on whether you plan to grow indoors or outdoors but also on the other characteristics of your growing space. For example, attempting to cultivate an 8-foot-tall sativa indoors would be impractical if your indoor space lacks the necessary height. Similarly, a 2-foot indica plant may struggle to survive outdoors if it has to compete with other plants and weeds for light. You can trim and shape a larger plant through pruning, but it is impossible to double a smaller plant's height if its genetic makeup restricts it to a growth range of 2 to 3 feet, even if you attempt to extend internode lengths through light manipulation. Later chapters discuss indoor and outdoor growing spaces in greater detail.

Selecting Good Strains

There's no one-size-fits-all chart to determine the best strains because what's considered "good" is highly subjective. People's preferences and reasons for using cannabis can vary greatly, and such characteristics as the type of high, plant type, potency, and flavor can influence what each person considers "good." However, we can evaluate what a particular strain excels at or is suitable for.

While some strains are versatile and well-rounded, a strain is unlikely to excel in every trait. For example, the highest-yielding strains often aren't the most potent, and strains that are easy to grow may not yield a substantial harvest. If you choose a strain for its high potency and exceptional taste, you might have to accept lower yields and a less visually appealing final product. These trade-offs are inherent to genetics, and there's no single "ultimate" cannabis plant. Instead, you must make wise choices based on your specific goals as a grower and/or consumer.

All cannabis seeds can be cultivated both indoors and outdoors. However, it's advisable to consider what the breeder intended for the best results. If the breeder designed

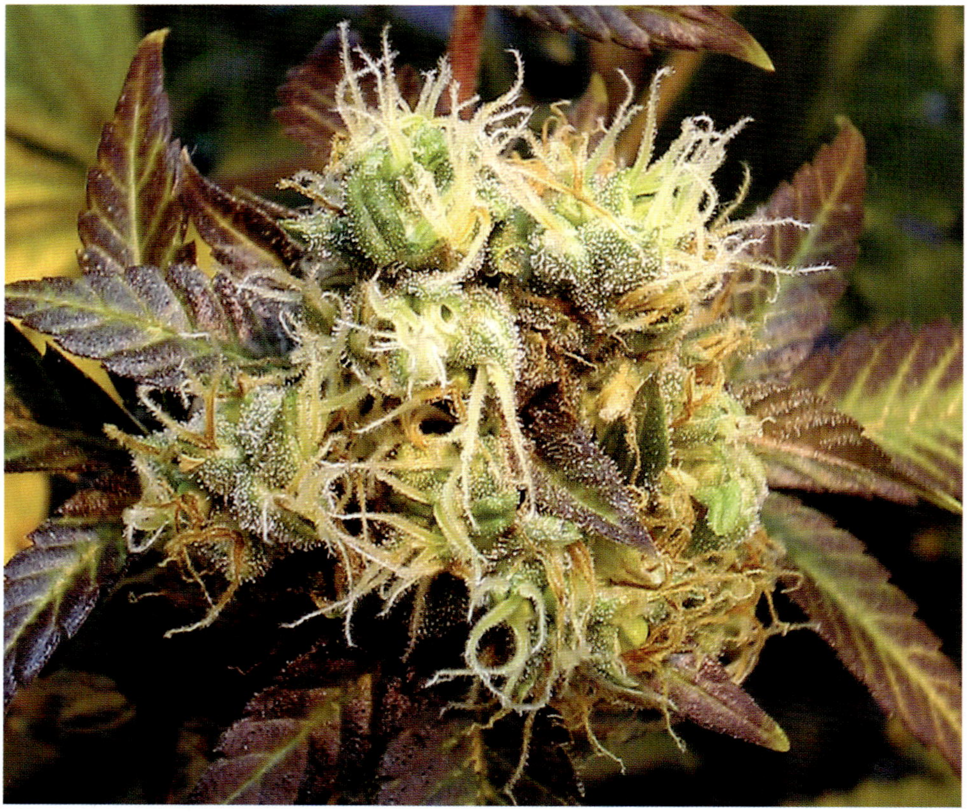

PHOTO: ORIGINAL SEEDS

This pure indica is highly resinous and perfect for hash making. This "Hindu Kush" is very close to its landrace Afghanistan parentage and was imported to the West in the 1980s.

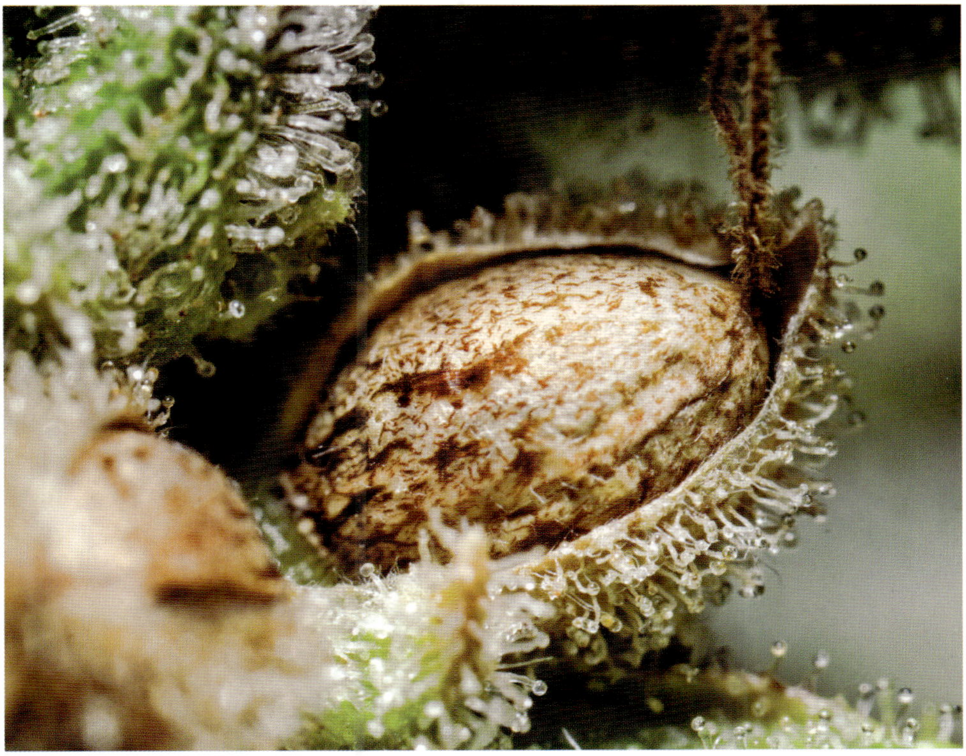

At the end of flowering, the mature seed will cause the calyx of the pollinated females to split open. Gravity, wind, and animals will naturally carry that seed away from the plant.

a strain for indoor cultivation, grow those seeds indoors. If you decide to grow the plant outdoors, it may not perform well. Of course, there's room for experimentation, and some growers have achieved excellent results by going against breeder suggestions. But if you're new to growing, it's wise to follow the breeder's advice.

When selecting seeds, evaluate the strain's characteristics. Most seed sellers provide this information along with the seed type on the packaging. Try to anticipate which characteristics the plants are likely to display, keeping in mind the ongoing species debate. For example, some sativa plants may be shorter due to their indica genetics, while some indica plants may grow taller because of their sativa genetics. In later chapters, we'll delve into how breeders can control specific features of the plant, such as its appearance, growth pattern, and height.

Growers can also influence the plant's medicinal qualities by harvesting it at specific times. Harvesting the plant later in its growth cycle enhances its body-stone effect, while harvesting just before peak growth induces a more cerebral high. Harvest timing can thus be used to enhance these properties when working with strains intended for either cerebral or body-stone effects.

PHOTO: DINAFEM SEEDS

Harvesting Seeds

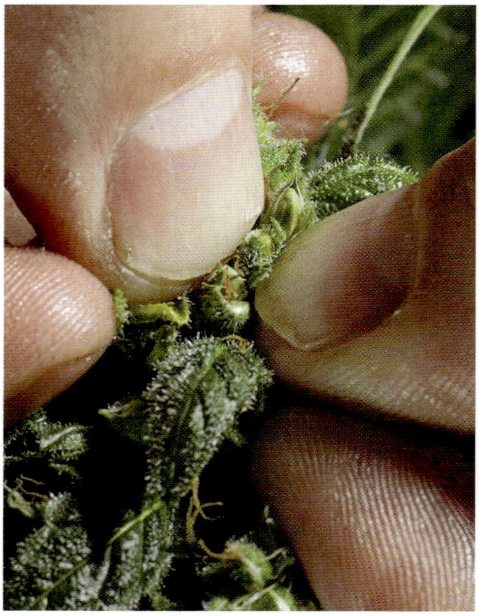

Teasing a seed from the bud. Here, a calyx containing a seed is being lightly squeezed between the thumbs at its base so as to not damage the seed.

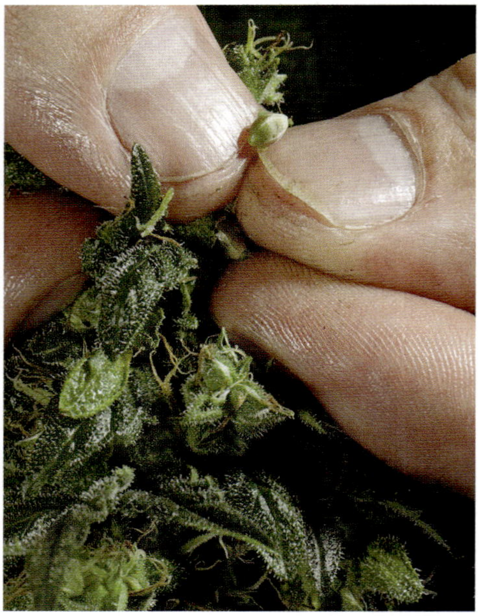

The calyx opens and the seed comes out. Do this carefully. It is easy to lose the seed by dropping it or having it fly out.

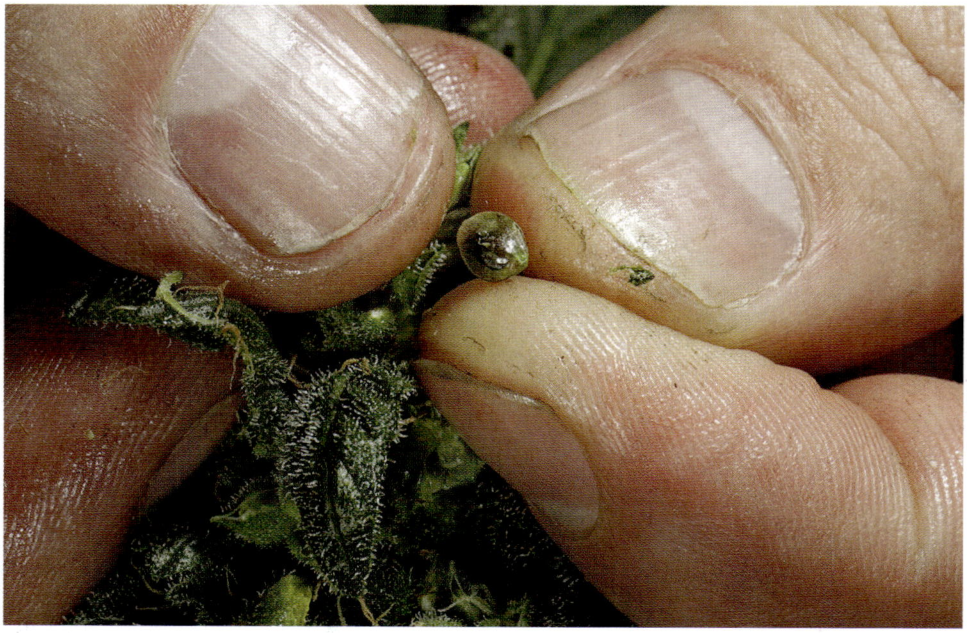

This is the seed. It is not pale and so is likely viable. However, some pale seeds can be viable, depending on the strain.

PHOTOS: MG IMAGING

Medical Equivalents of High Types

The terms "cerebral" and "body-stone" are often used by the general public to provide a broad description of the effects of using cannabis. These terms typically correlate with the medical usage of cannabis. Sativa strains, which tend to produce more cerebral effects, are primarily used in treating psychological issues, such as depression and withdrawal, but they can also help alleviate physical pain. On the other hand, indica strains, known for their body-high or couch-lock effects, are primarily used to address physical pain conditions, including those associated with ailments like cancer and HIV/AIDS. In the last decade, CBD-rich strains have expanded medical choices, delivering therapeutic benefits without strong psychoactive effects.

Within the cannabis community, there are alternatives to smoking cannabis. It's been suggested that one of the healthier methods of lung inhalation is through the use of high-quality vaporizers, which do not involve combustion and thus harmful carbon monoxide. Vaporizers achieve this by maintaining temperatures below combustion thresholds, ensuring that only the desired cannabinoids are converted into vapor. However, much more research is needed to confirm whether vapes are healthier than smoking. Cannabis can also be consumed in the form of oil droplets, or tinctures, or as an ingredient in cooking.

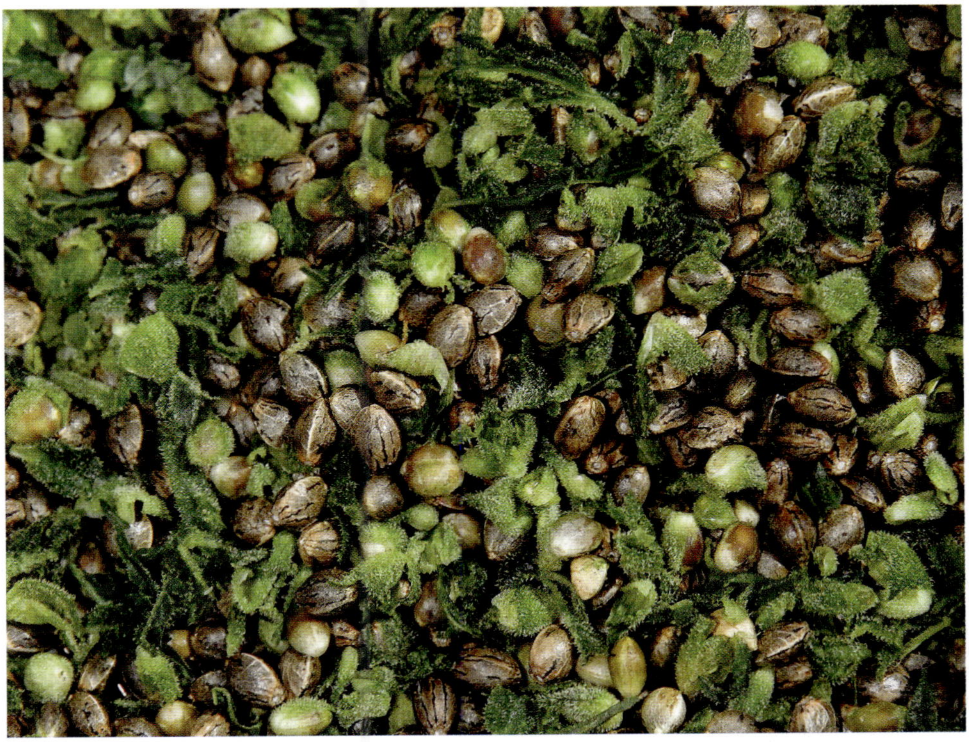

PHOTO: DINAFEM SEEDS

Freshly harvested seeds teased out from the calyx parts, which appear as green matter surrounding the seeds.

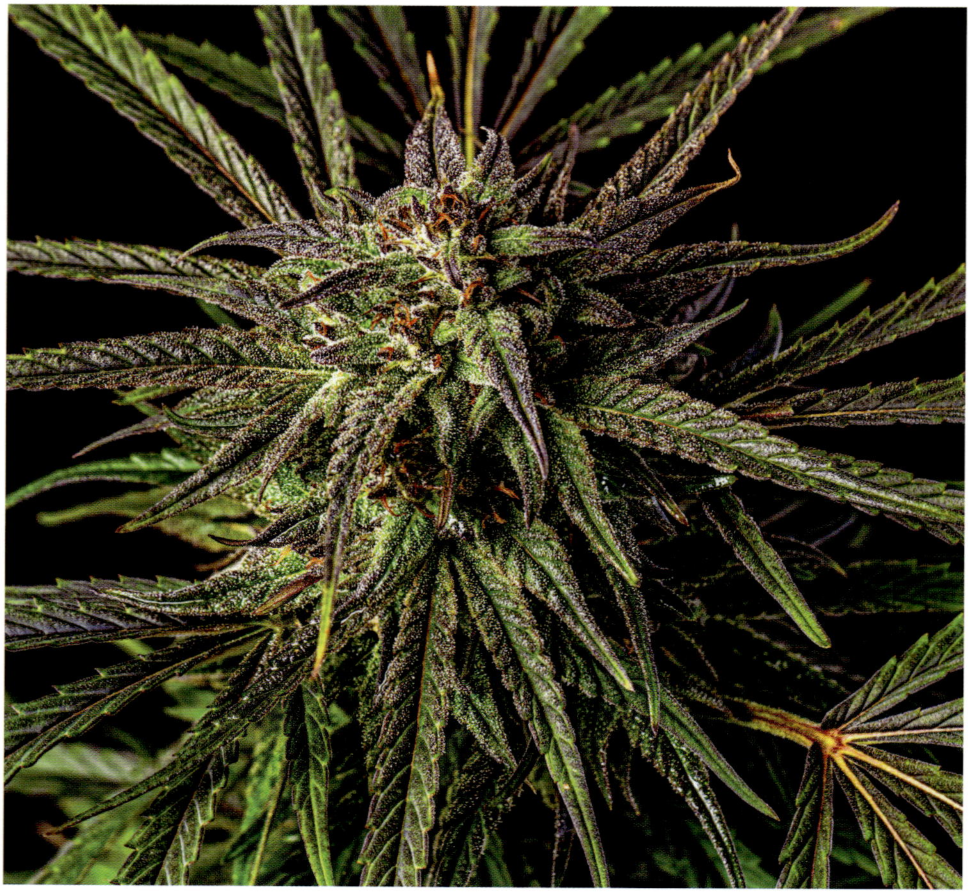

This Purple Orange by Dinafem Seeds is a wonderful option for anyone needing to medicate throughout the day to control pain, inflammation, anxiety, or other chronic conditions.

PHOTO: ROB BRAMHILL

Consuming an oil extraction of a cannabis plant may yield different effects than vaporizing the herb of the same strain. Some strains are particularly well-suited for producing hashish or oils, and breeders may recommend specific strains for this purpose. Therefore, when selecting a strain that suits your needs, consider such factors as cultivation, intended use, and delivery method.

Seeds and Flowering Periods (Photoperiod)

When selecting a strain, you must consider its flowering period, which can vary significantly from one strain to another. You'll want to time your harvest towards the end of the flowering phase. For example, if a seed bank states "flowering time seven to nine weeks," you can estimate when your plant will be ready for harvest. In this case, it will be about seven to nine weeks from the moment your plant begins to flower. In the harvesting section of this book, we delve into how to pinpoint the exact day for harvesting by examining trichome colors.

Acquiring Seeds

One of the most reliable methods of obtaining quality seeds is from another experienced grower who has successfully developed a plant you enjoy. This approach offers several advantages, including acquiring seeds without cost and obtaining firsthand knowledge of the medicinal value and effects of the strain by sampling it. However, a potential drawback to obtaining seeds from another grower is that you might experience some inconsistency if that particular strain hasn't been fully stabilized, though the grower can often assist you since they are well-acquainted with that strain. By the time you've completely read this book, you'll likely be prepared to provide seeds to newcomers.

Given environmental factors like temperature and sunlight duration, some outdoor strains may be better suited to thrive in your specific location than others. As such, outdoor growers might benefit most from swapping seeds with other growers. New growers may spend many years experimenting to find the ideal outdoor strain for their particular environment. By connecting with a local outdoor breeder and selecting seeds that have thrived in your region, you can bypass much of this trial and error. Obtaining seeds from a local outdoor grower ensures that those seeds are well-suited to your environment. These environmental adaptations are more prominent along longitude lines rather than latitude lines, so new strains often need to be bred to suit varying longitudes.

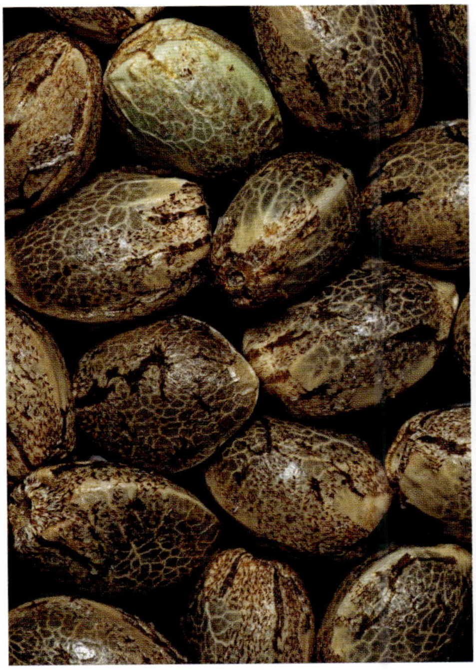

Cannabis seeds generally look like brown pods with dark and light markings.

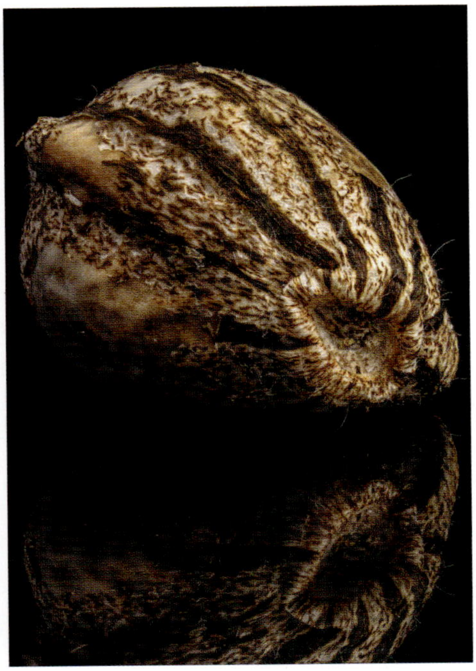

The seed's integument shell may be patterned. Dark stripes are most common but some seeds have none.

PHOTOS: ROB BRAMHILL

Indoor growers don't face this geographical challenge. If indoor grow rooms are replicated to consistent specifications and conditions, the same strain should grow consistently, regardless of the location. In this sense, indoor growers have more flexibility when purchasing seeds because they have full control over the growing environment.

At some point, almost everyone requires a seed bank. The internet is teeming with seed banks eager to sell you their products, but there are certain risks. First, some of these seed banks may not be reputable and rip you off. Second, not all seed banks ship worldwide, making their products inaccessible to you. Third, some seed banks may misrepresent their stock, although this issue is not unique to the cannabis community but rather a consequence of the vast scale of online commerce. Some scammers exploit a customer's need for privacy and believe they can get away with incomplete or erroneous orders. The next section provides comprehensive guidance on finding a reputable seed bank.

Because of the costs associated with buying seeds, be aware of the risks when purchasing seeds online and conduct thorough research before making a purchase. A pack of 10 to 16 seeds can range from around $85 to as much as $300, with an average price of about $150. Although many seed banks will now sell seeds in custom numbers, anywhere from one to 100 seeds.

Choosing a Good Seed Bank

Identifying a reputable seed bank can require some effort. Medical dispensaries can often offer recommendations on seed banks, usually on their websites. In previous editions of this book, we mentioned that search engines and seed review websites were becoming less reliable, and the shift towards social media was inevitable. It may seem counterintuitive for individuals with security concerns, but social media has a thriving cannabis community. If privacy is a concern, you can use a VPN to maintain your anonymity and avoid tracking cookies. On platforms such as YouTube, Instagram, and TikTok, where influencers often share valuable insights, you can read and watch content without the need to post anything. As long as you refrain from sharing personal information, social media can be an effective way to stay informed about the community and research seed banks discreetly.

You can verify if a seed bank is still operating by examining the latest grow pictures shared online. Many individuals on platforms like Instagram post images of their plants, along with the strain and seed bank information. This allows you to read about what people are growing, view photographs, and gain a general understanding of the available options and what fellow growers are achieving with their seeds.

Once you've located a seed bank, verify that the place you intend to buy from has a registered URL, such as one ending with ".com" or country-specific domain. Avoid seed banks that use free website services, as most of them disappear overnight. Reputable

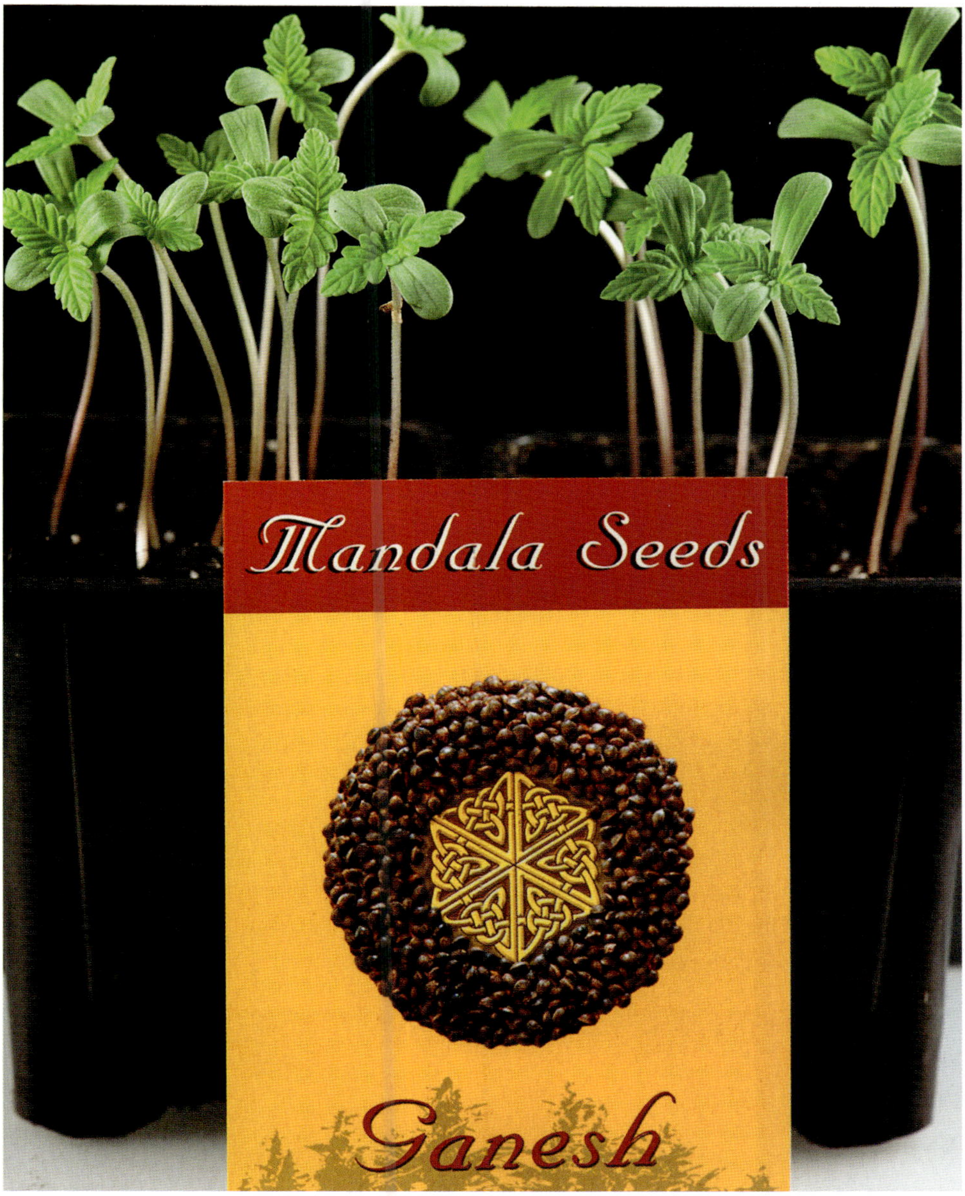

An example of seed bank stock of a breeder's strain being germinated.

PHOTO: MANDALA SEEDS

seed banks should also encourage customer feedback and provide a means of contact. Contacting the seed bank before making a purchase is strongly recommended. In your email, be sure to ask about the following points.

Delivery Times

Ensure that the seed bank offers quick delivery. Ideally, it should take no more than 30 days for the seeds to reach you. Some seed banks have introduced back orders that can take over two to three months to clear; for instance, seed orders placed around Christmas might not arrive until the following March. If you place an order without inquiring about these specifics, you may end up receiving "similar" seeds instead of the ones you ordered, with the explanation that the ordered seeds were "out of stock." It's crucial to reach out to the seed bank via email to confirm seed availability. While it is normal for a breeder to take some time to generate a batch of seeds, extended delays can be indicative of counterfeit products. Waiting three months for a seed order is excessive. You should be willing to wait only for high-quality genetics that are rare, recent, and worth the delay, such as new cup-winning hybrids with sudden high demand.[2] Sometimes, a breeder may not produce viable stock for that season, but a good seed bank will inform you about this issue before you make a payment. The general rule is to steer clear of seed banks with extended delivery times. You want a prompt service, and standard delivery within 30 days. Some seed banks even have a one-to-two-day shipping policy, and these are typically favored by growers. Clarify all these details in writing before placing an order.

Deals

Some seed banks offer deals on seeds, and prices can vary from one bank to another. Strains that win awards or become trendy may see price increases. Nonetheless, keep an eye out for special deals, as many seed banks provide discounts, price reductions, or buy-one-get-one-free offers, just like any other retail business. Even if these offers are not visibly displayed on their website, you can inquire about them in your email.

Shipping and Protective Packaging

Before making any purchase, inquire about the seed bank's services, delivery options, postage, packaging, and security measures. Unforeseen issues can arise during transit. Seeds can become non-viable due to accidental damage during shipping, like a

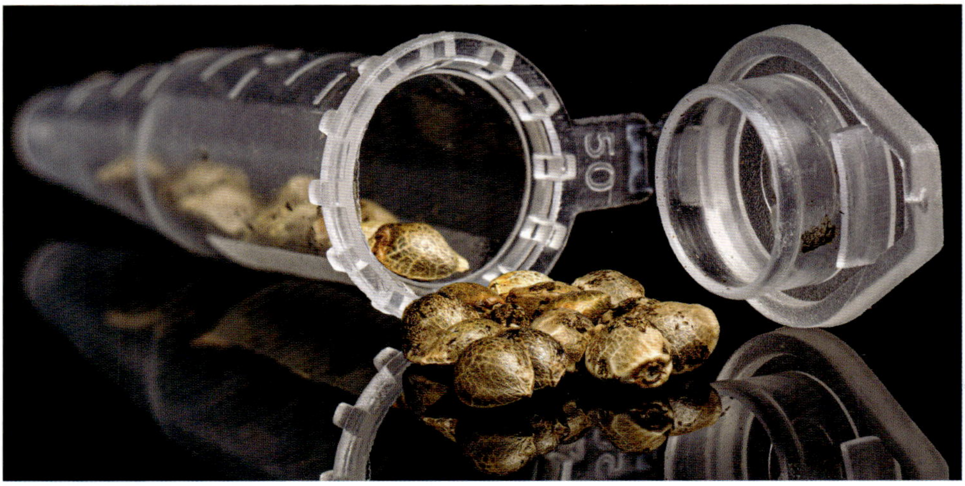

PHOTO: ROB BRAMHILL

Small ampules make perfect containers for seeds. They prevent the seeds from being crushed.

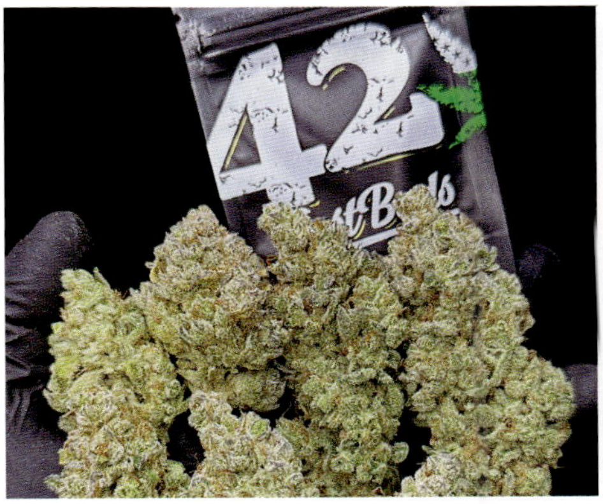

Strawberry Banana Auto, autoflower with sweet and fruity terpenes.

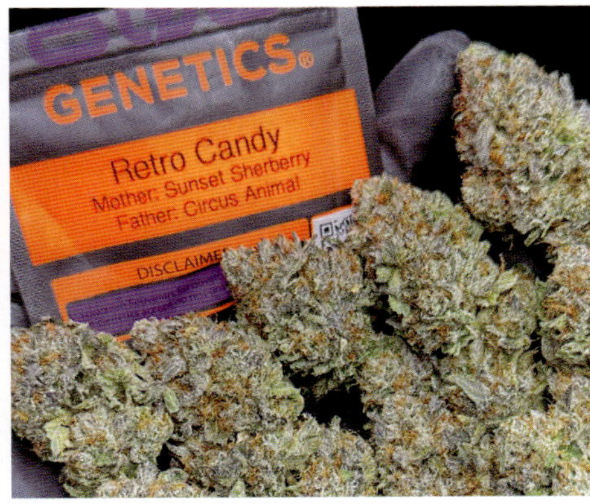

Retro Candy, a hybrid that really brings the gas.

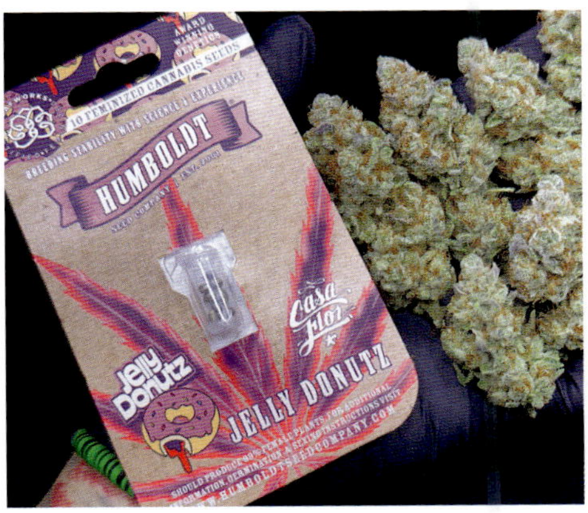

Jelly Donutz, very candy-like with terpes like a delicious dessert.

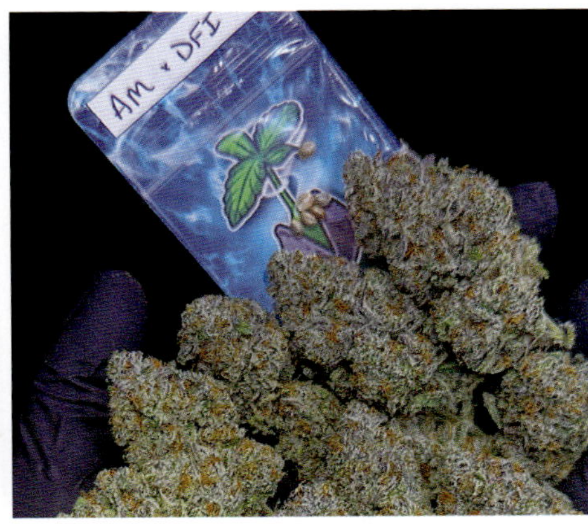

AM x DFI, wonderful earthy, minty flavor, a beautiful strain.

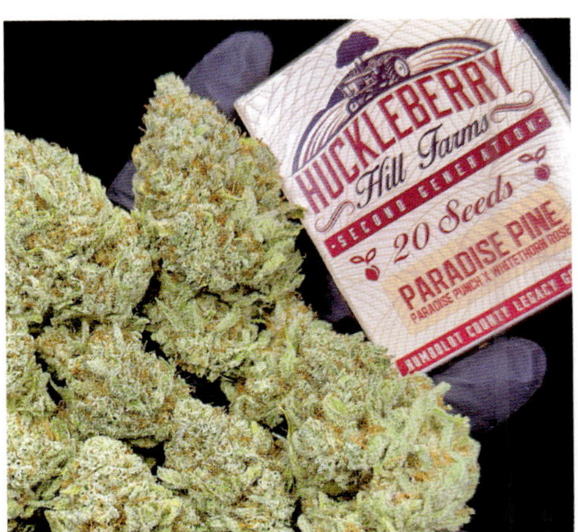

Paradise Pine, beautiful neon green buds that smell earthy and fruity.

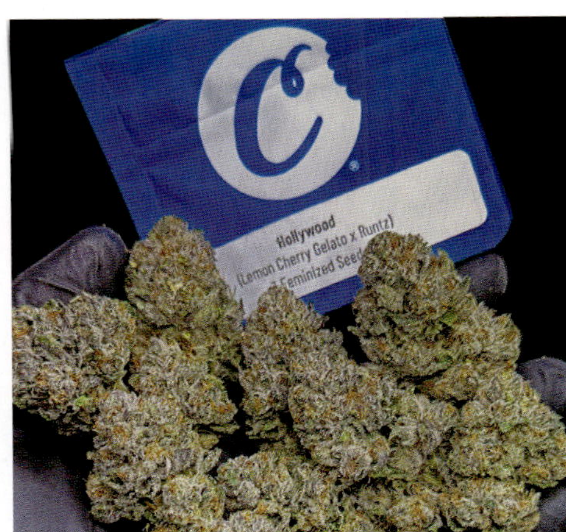

Hollywood is a great strain with an earthy, sweet candy, zesty fruit aroma, and a hint of gas.

PHOTOS: SHOPFREEGROW8.COM

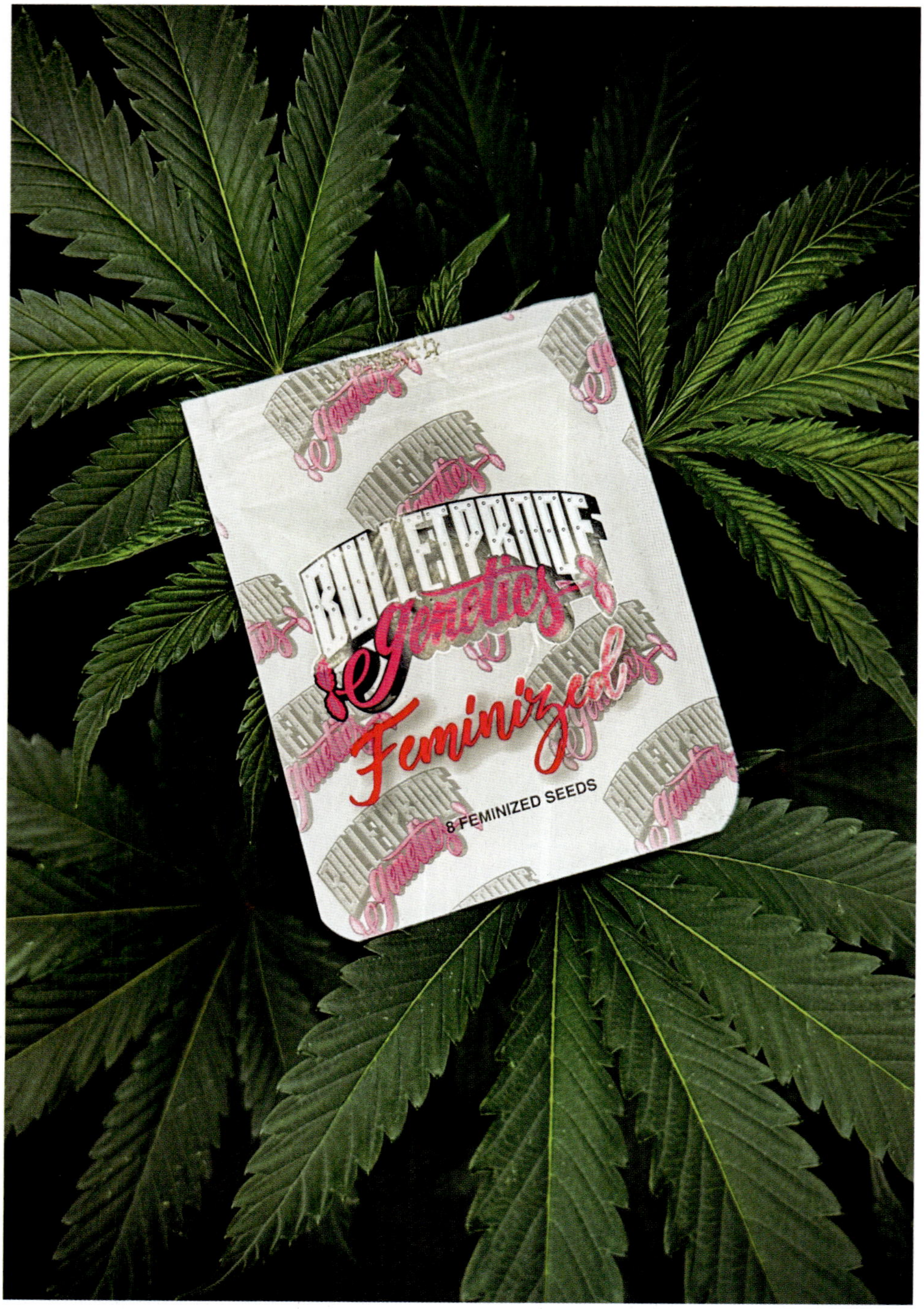

PHOTO: SHOPFREEGROW8.COM

Each edition of this book is marked by the loss of many cannabis greats. Regrettably, Eddie Ray, the founder and breeder at Bulletproof Genetics, passed away in late 2023. He was genuinely passionate about the art of cultivation, and his breeding efforts will perpetuate his legacy. Rest in peace, Eddie.

misstep at the postal office. To prevent damage to the seeds, high-quality seed banks use robust protective packaging. In your email, inquire whether they use such packaging. If they fail to respond, it's best to avoid using that particular seed bank. If your seeds do not arrive within a reasonable time frame, contact the seed bank and inquire about the delay. Initiating contact will also foster better communication with the seed bank in your future seed purchases.

Always communicate with the seed bank about your chosen strain. They may even provide suggestions that better suit your requirements. You will likely have various delivery options to choose from, and many seed banks sell their seeds in batches of 10 to 20.

Below is an example email to a seed bank:

> Subject line: Interest in your seeds
>
> Dear [seed bank company],
>
> I have reviewed your catalog and have a few questions about purchasing some seeds.
>
> Do you currently have [strain] in stock? What are your delivery options, and how long will it take for you to send the seeds to me? Do you provide protective packaging?
>
> I am also concerned about data privacy. How long do you retain my information on file?
>
> Additionally, are there any special deals or offers I should be aware of when I place my order?
>
> Best regards,
> [Your name]

This email comprehensively addresses the essential points. In the reply, you should learn when to expect to receive your seeds in good condition, and you'll know that your personal information won't be retained. Furthermore, if issues arise with the delivery of your seeds, it is helpful to already be in contact with the seed bank. A simple photo attached to the email can explain a lot, especially in cases where issues like crushed or damaged seeds arise.

Transporting Seeds

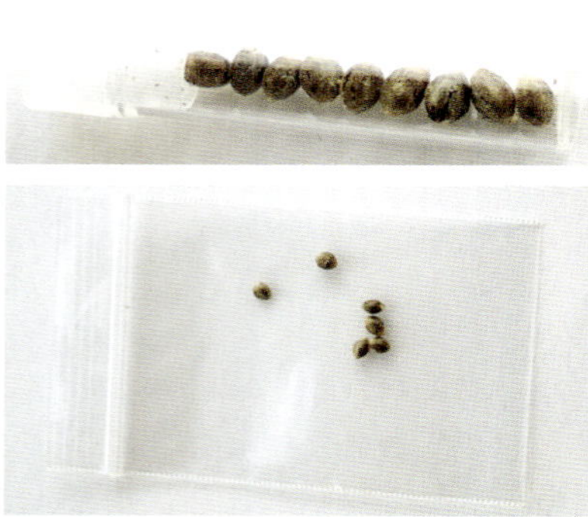

Step 1: Get your seeds ready.

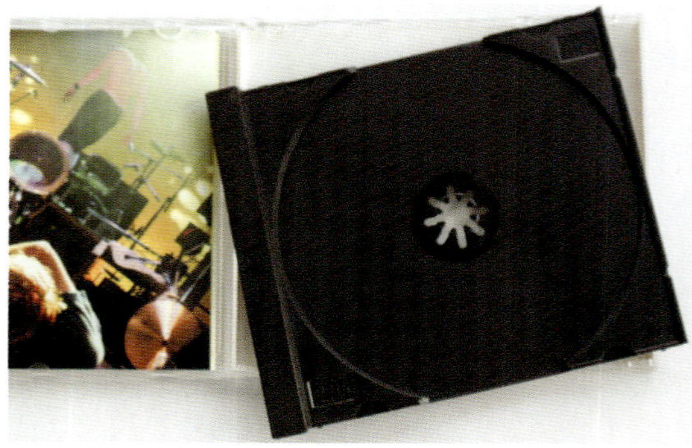

Step 2: Take the CD case apart and flip the base over.

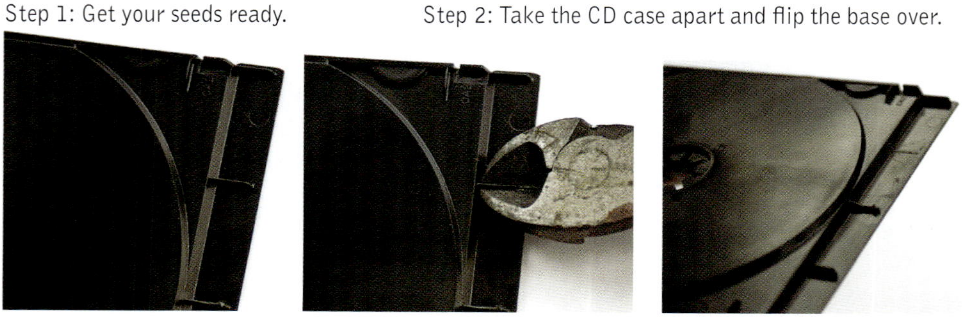

Step 3: Use pliers to break the back side of the case here.

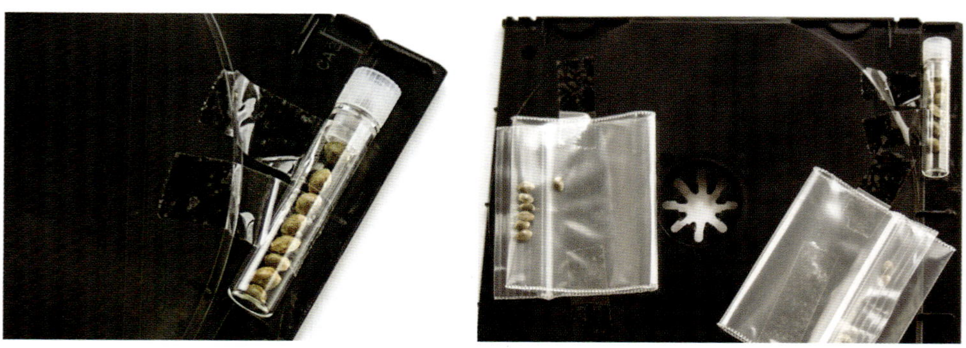

Step 4: Carefully tape the seeds inside.

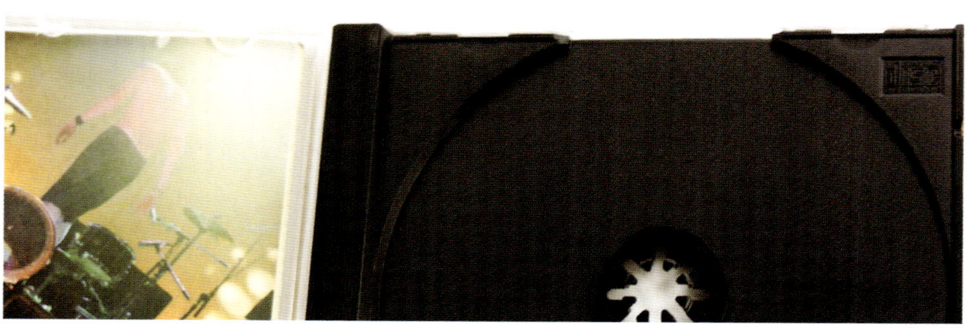

Step 5: Put it back together.

PHOTOS: WEADO

Storing Seeds

Seeds should be stored on a dry surface due to their permeability. Despite their seemingly solid shell, they have microscopic openings, including an area called the micropyle at the seed's point. Water triggers germination, so ensure you work with seeds with dry hands in a dry environment. If moisture comes into contact with the embryo inside the seed shell, germination is definite and no longer a matter of "if."

If the seeds appear to be in good condition, remove them from the bag and place them in a small, clean, and thoroughly dry container, such as old camera film canister, a similar container sold by the seed shop, or a dark, non-transparent plastic vitamin or medicine container. Seal the container and be diligent in labeling and dating it. Labeling is essential to prevent forgetting the seed type and storage duration.

The dark canister serves as a short-term solution for seed storage, preventing seeds from being exposed to light, bacteria, moisture, and air. For longer-term storage, especially if you plan to store seeds for over a year, you should use an airtight container and place it in the freezer.

Long-Term Storage

For long-term seed storage, include a desiccant packet containing either silica or clay in a vacuum-sealed storage medium. Moisture barrier bags with desiccant packets provide

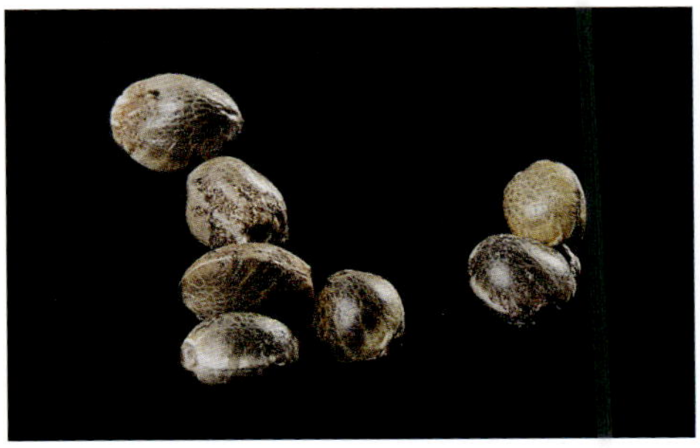

Healthy, viable, non-crushed seeds.

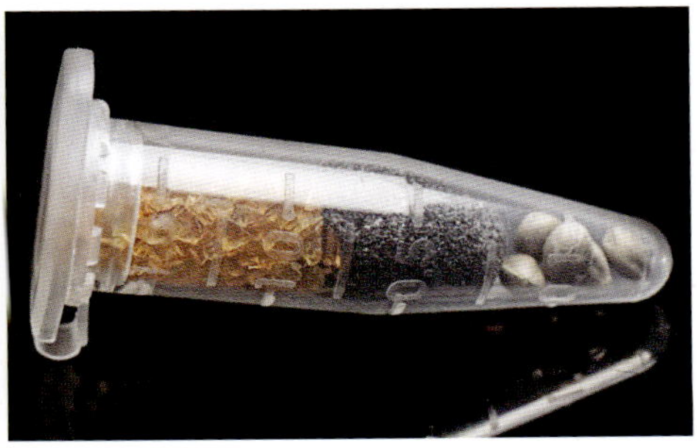

Pearls of silica gel absorb moisture, ensuring the seeds stay dry.

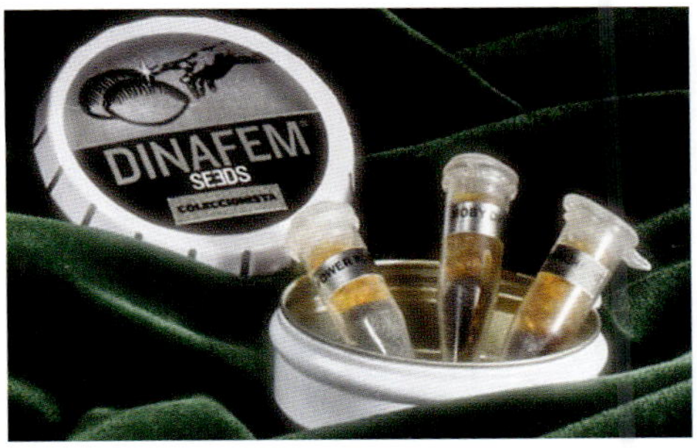

A micro-conical tube offers protection but should be kept out of the light.

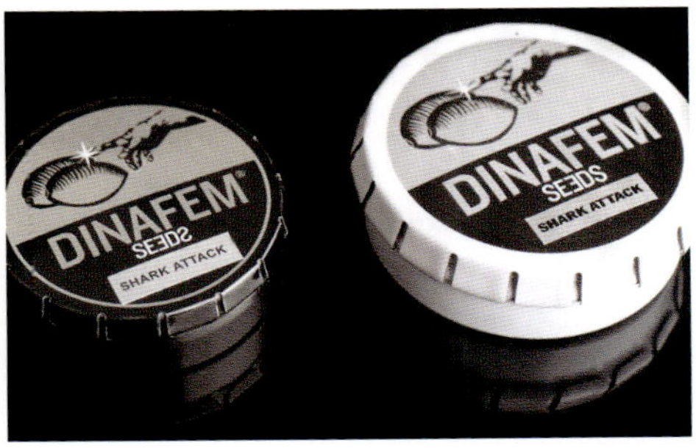

Stash tins can be used to store seeds.

PHOTOS: DINAFEM SEEDS

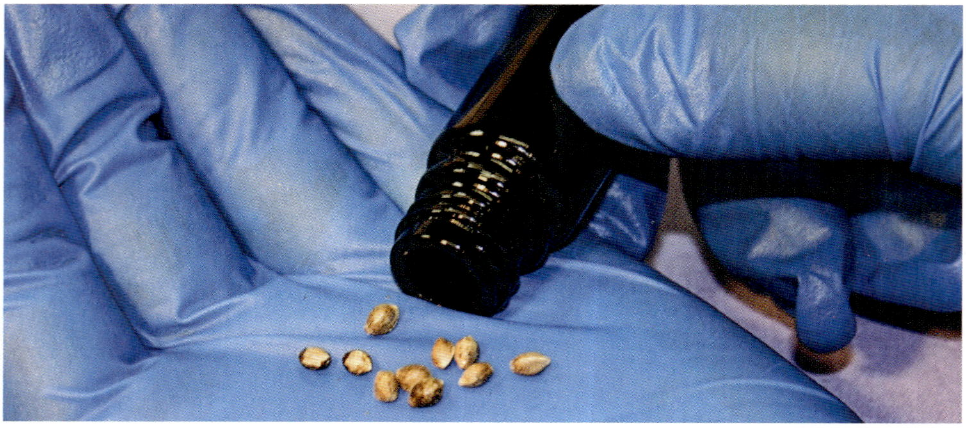

Seeds stay viable in these short-term storage solutions. Dark containers keep light out.

the most robust protection against seed degradation. Similar to the static-shielded bags used for electronics, like computer memory cards, they feature an aluminum foil shield and additional layers, such as nylon, making them resistant to puncturing. These bags are designed to minimize humidity and moisture contamination of their contents. To monitor humidity, add a humidity indicator card to the bags. If it changes color, it indicates an increase in humidity, and the potential spoilage of seeds.

Vacuum-sealed bags are an affordable solution and also have various applications in the kitchen, such as packing items for the freezer or preserving food as they are usually equipped with an additional heat seal.

The longevity of frozen seeds varies based on several factors, and many variables can affect seed viability. Seeds can typically be stored for up to 10 years without a freezer and up to 20 years in one. However, some seeds may deteriorate much faster, while a few might remain viable for more than 20 years. To prevent long-term degradation, most growers and breeders cycle their seed stock using the "first in, first out" method, using the oldest stored seeds before adding new ones to the collection. Store seeds for an extended period only when you are faced with difficulties in cultivation. If you are regularly growing crops, you can use your seed stores every few years, ensuring that they remain fresh and suitable for germination. In this way, you can avoid wasting time and effort on seeds that become unusable due to age. Remember, time passes quickly, so get on with growing the seeds you have.

In plant science, the term "germplasm" typically refers to seeds stored for future use. However, germplasm can encompass any genetic material from which an organism can grow. Breeding facilities, as well as individual breeders who maintain seeds in storage, have their own germplasm lines. As a grower, you can establish your very own private germplasm line.

PHOTO: GCP

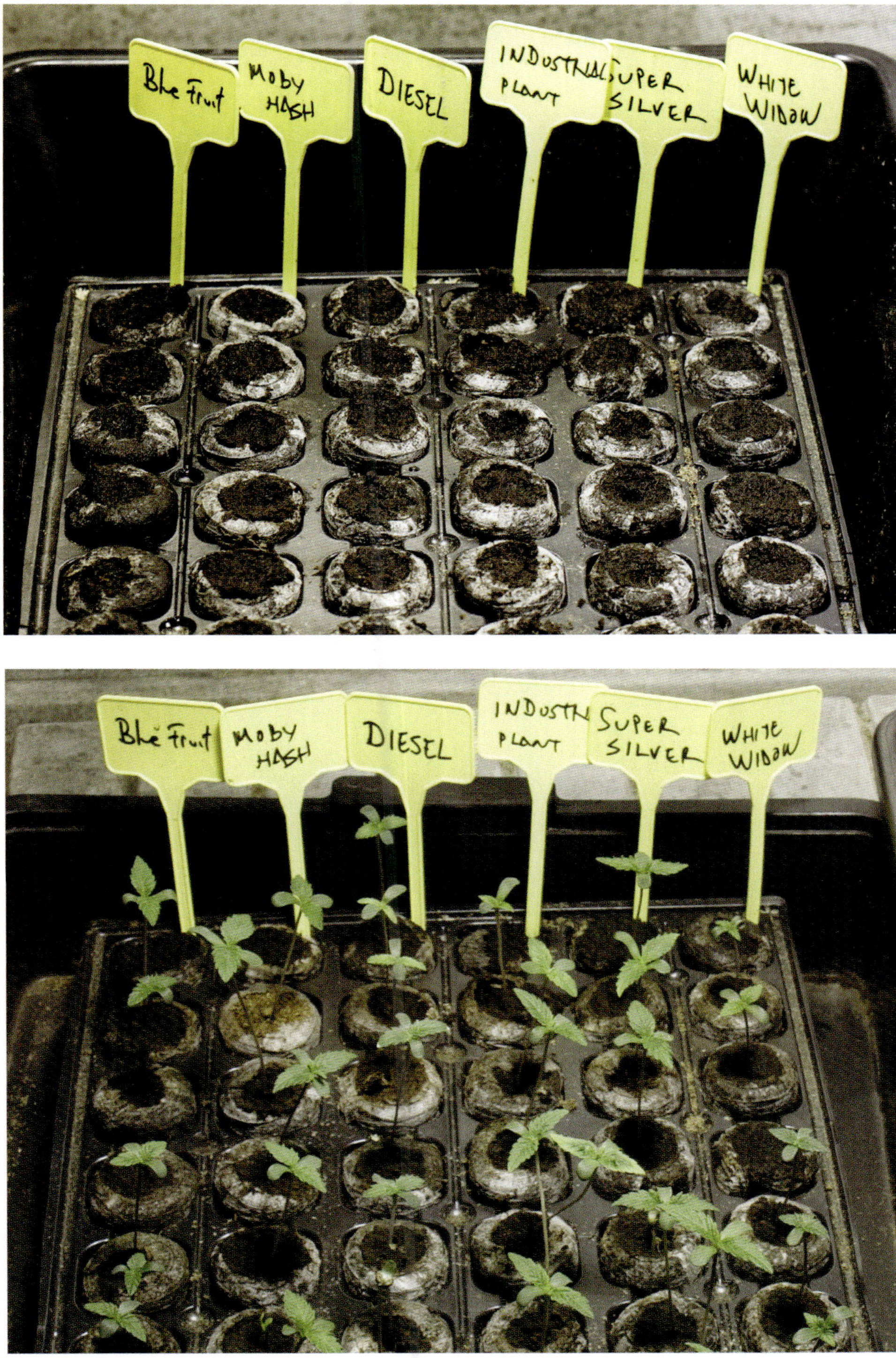

The importance of labeling should not be underestimated. It is very easy to mix up strains, especially in these beginning stages. Introduce good labeling practices from the start.

PHOTOS: DINAFEM SEEDS

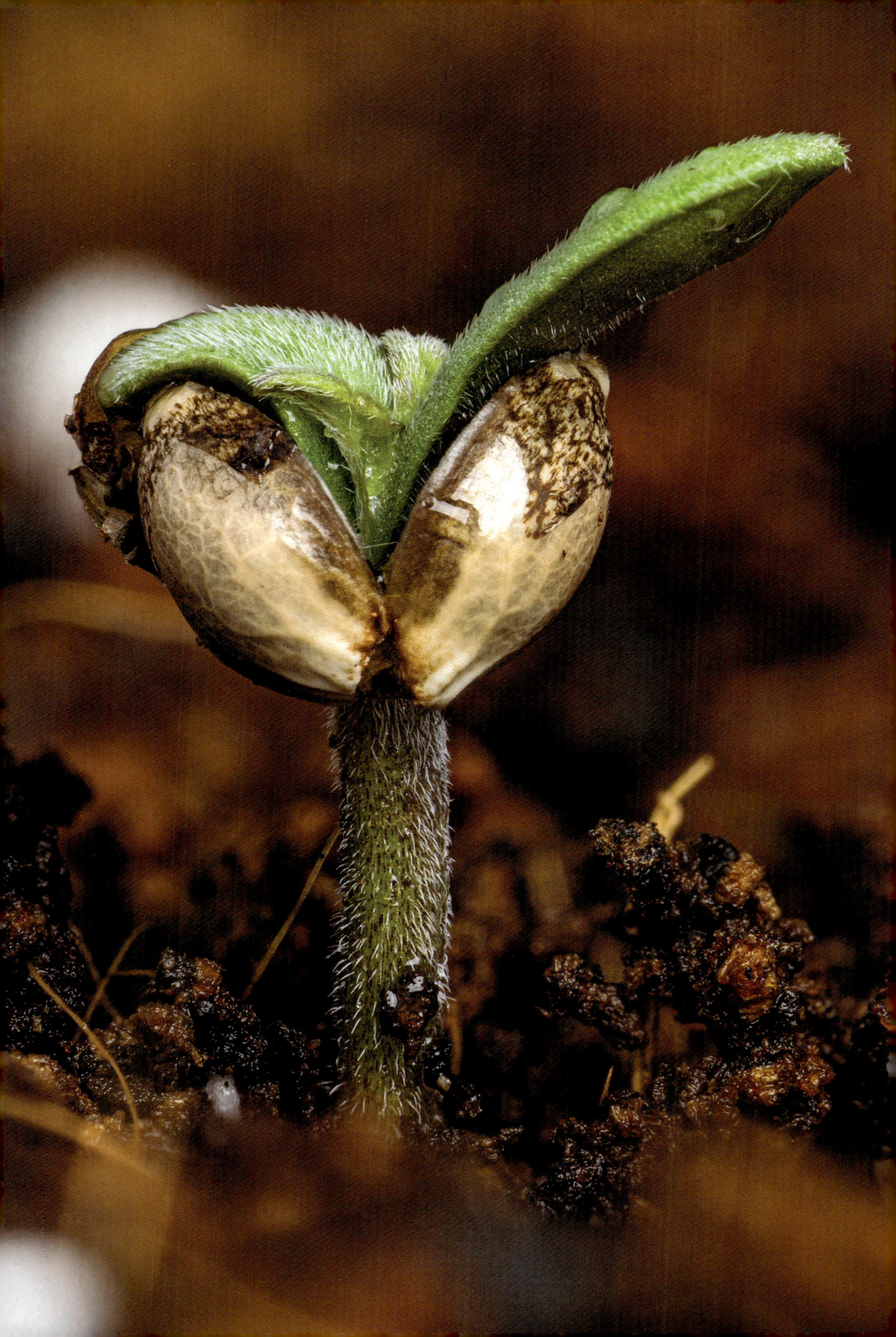

4

Germination and Propagation

Starting off on the right foot is crucial for a successful cultivation journey. Germination often appears intimidating to new growers, but it doesn't have to be. You may have invested a considerable sum in acquiring 10 tiny seeds, and the prospect of failure might seem daunting. However, even in failure, there's an opportunity to learn and improve. If you're new to working with seeds, plenty of stable, high-quality genetics are available at affordable prices. Strains like Skunk, Afghani, and Kush won't break the bank, and if things don't go as planned, you can always try again. This chapter will guide you towards success. It will save you both time and money when germinating seeds. If you prefer, you can opt for clones instead of seeds, but starting from seeds shouldn't be an issue, especially if you have prior experience with cloning.

Cannabis Seed Morphology

Cannabaceae, or the hemp family, are members of the angiosperm phylogeny group.[1] Cannabis is a member of that family.

A seed, also known as an achene, is the result of the fertilization of a plant, specifically the ripe ovules of female flowers in angiosperms, as well as gymnosperms. Seeds are essentially small embryonic plants enclosed in a protective seed coat and that typically contain nutrients for nourishment. A fully formed seed signifies the culmination of a plant's reproductive process, which starts with the development of flowers, pollination, and the formation of seeds within plant's fruits.

In the initial stage, angiosperms are fertilized twice, with the fusion of egg and sperm nuclei forming a zygote. The second sperm cell nucleus combines with polar nuclei to create a primary endosperm, which eventually becomes a source of nutrition. This source is depleted after the formation of the root and stem. In contrast, gymnosperms have two sperm cells transferred from pollen, with only one fertilizing the egg. A seed consists of the embryo and some parental plant tissue that surrounds it.

PHOTO: ROB BRAMHILL

Parts of a Seedling

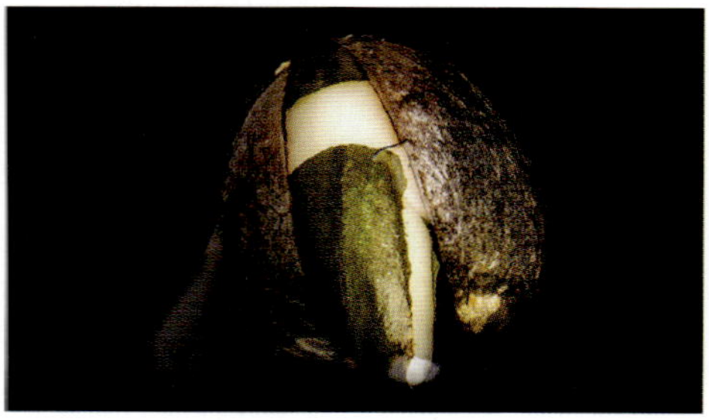

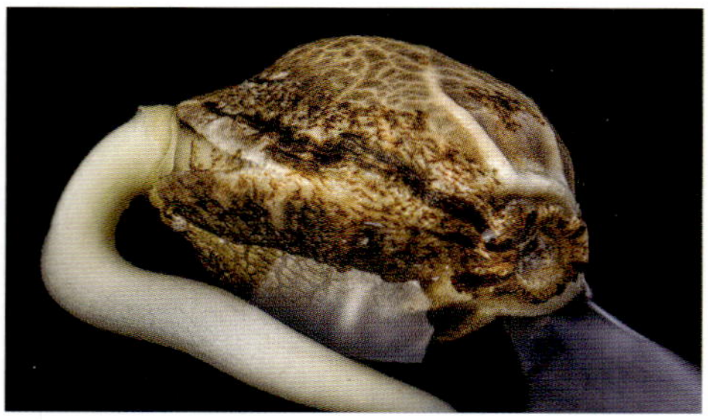

The seed absorbs water, causing it to swell and break its outer shell, or integument, with the radicle, an embryonic root, being the first part to emerge from the splitting shell.

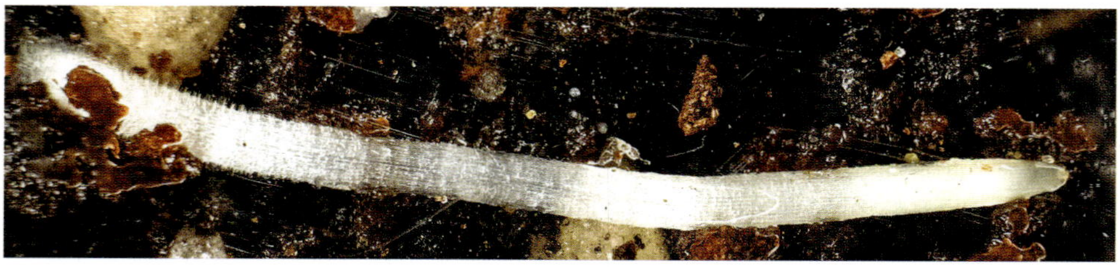

Radicle elongation supports the vulnerable seedling and absorbs nutrients.

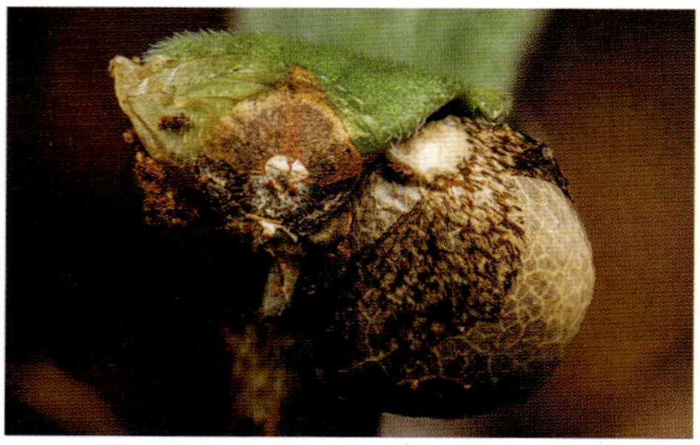

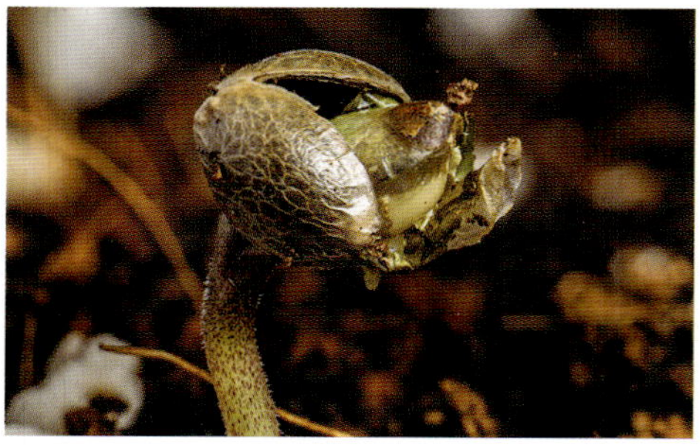

Next, the plumule, the embryonic stem, emerges, and as it develops, the integument is pushed off, falling to the ground.

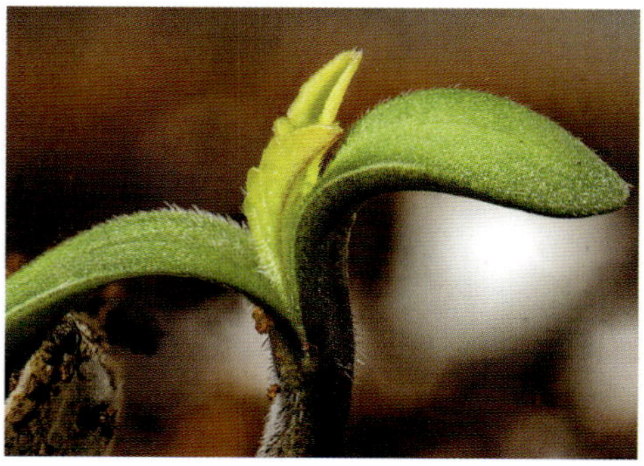

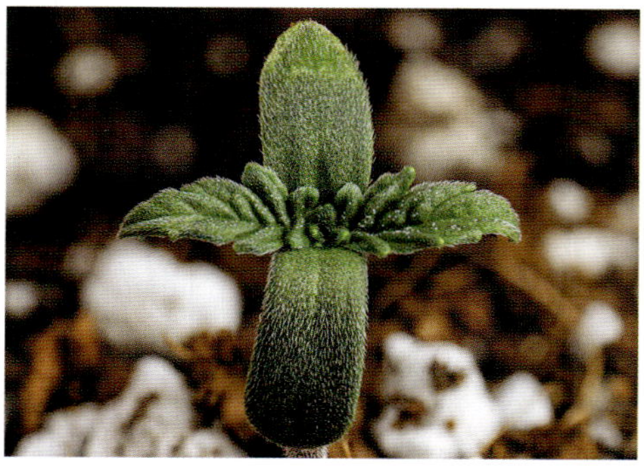

Two cotyledons unfurl like green tongues, with the first true leaves emerging between them, signaling the plant's readiness for light.

PHOTOS: ROB BRAMHILL

In simpler terms, a seed is a biological entity that is sown to propagate a plant. However, seeds aren't the only method of plant reproduction. Ferns, for example, reproduce via spores and possess an intermediate plant stage known as the gametophyte.[2] Nonetheless, seeds are the primary means by which plants spread and establish themselves in various environments.

Seed shape and structure can vary significantly among different plant species, and even within cannabis varieties. For instance, cannabis seeds may exhibit stripes, blotches, or a solid dark color, with some being brighter than others.

The cannabis plant embryo typically features two cotyledons (dicotyledons) and seed leaves.[3] These cotyledons anchor themselves through the radicle, the embryonic root, found at either end of the plumule, the embryonic plant shoot. Above the attachment point of the cotyledons lies the epicotyl, while below it is the hypocotyl.

In cannabis seeds, the food reserves are located in the endosperm, containing oils, proteins, and starches produced during seed reproduction. Cannabis seeds are albuminous, meaning they consisting of simple, water-soluble proteins that can coagulate when exposed to heat, similar to egg whites. The outer layer of the seed, or integument, is a hard tissue that covers the ovule.

Understanding Propagation

Propagation is the process of reproducing and multiplying plants through natural methods, including procreation, generation, and reproduction. Some growers use the term to mean those activities that occur between planting seeds and transplanting the resulting seedlings into the main growing environment. However, we'll consider propagation as the entire cultivation process, from seed to harvest. It's important to remember that propagation is an ongoing process that occurs in stages. This chapter focuses on the initial phase—germination.

Cannabis Seed Anatomy

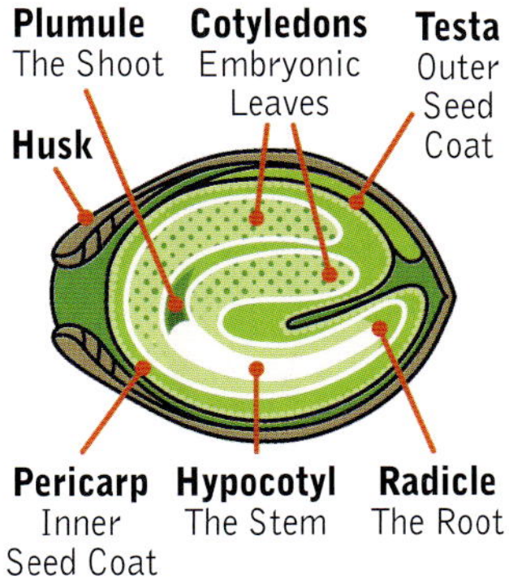

Managing Propagation Logistics

What's your plan? Will you purchase a batch of 10 seeds and grow them all at once? Do you intend to eliminate the male plants and cultivate only the females? Or do you want to keep the males to generate more seeds from the females? How many seeds can a female plant produce, and what steps can you take to ensure all your seeds germinate successfully? These questions are where propagation logistics come into play, and the answers largely depend on the size of your growing area, your budget, and how much time you can invest in your grow.

Let's assume you have a budget of $100 to $300 for seeds. With an expensive strain that may be all the rage on social media, you have the potential to grow the hybrid and generate additional seeds. Depending on plant size and growing conditions, you could potentially yield hundreds or even thousands of seeds. If you produce a substantial number of seeds in one season, you might never need to repurchase seeds for this strain. But make sure they are stored correctly, especially for those in long-term storage.

However, if you want to produce seeds and pollinate the females during your plants' growth AND want to cultivate sinsemilla—seedless female plants—you'll need two separate growing areas. One area would be dedicated to growing all your female plants as sinsemilla, while the other would be used for growing one or more females alongside the males for pollination. This arrangement will depend on the size of your grow space and budget constraints. Your pollination room should be physically separated from your all-female sinsemilla grow room, as pollen can be transported through the air. Bees and other insects, as well as you, can spread pollen. Always wash your hands and face after handling male plants to prevent pollen from reaching females you intend to keep seedless.

If you plan to make seeds after experimenting with various strains, it's wise to select your favorite strains for seed production. New growers should initially aim for sinsemilla cultivation.

Cloning can also eliminate the need to repurchase seeds. Cloning involves growing numerous plants initially and selecting a high-quality plant, typically a female in cannabis cultivation. You take cuttings from the chosen plant's branches and cultivate them into new plants. Clones inherit the same sex and vigor as the mother plant, allowing you to create a garden of cloned plants that can last indefinitely from a single mother plant. Cloning is discussed in detail in Chapter 13.

It's perfectly acceptable to split a seed pack and germinate only a portion of the seeds. For example, newcomers with 10 seeds could choose to germinate just three at first, then three more a little later, then the final four seeds, providing three opportunities for success. Any mistakes made during the first attempt can be corrected in subsequent tries; any successes replicated for the remaining seeds. The waiting period between attempts depends on the success rates of each method. If germination occurs in the first batch, proceed with the next three seeds, and so on. This approach allows for error correction while preserving seeds.

For experienced growers who have previously germinated seeds, it's advisable to begin with five seeds, followed by another five the following week. Long-time growers with ample experience can germinate all the seeds at once. Even under optimal conditions, failure may occur. Nonetheless, there are ways to minimize these failures.

Germination

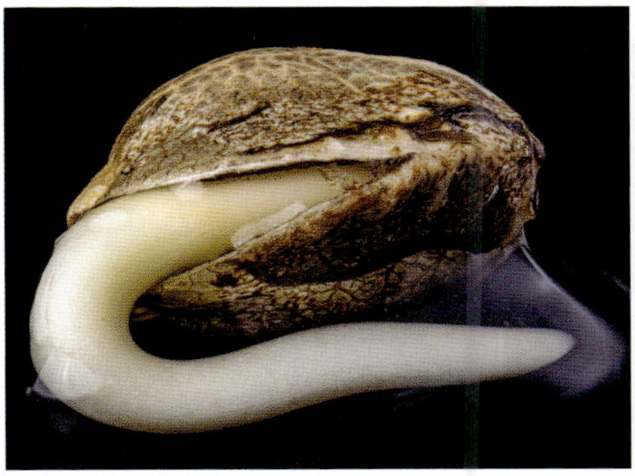
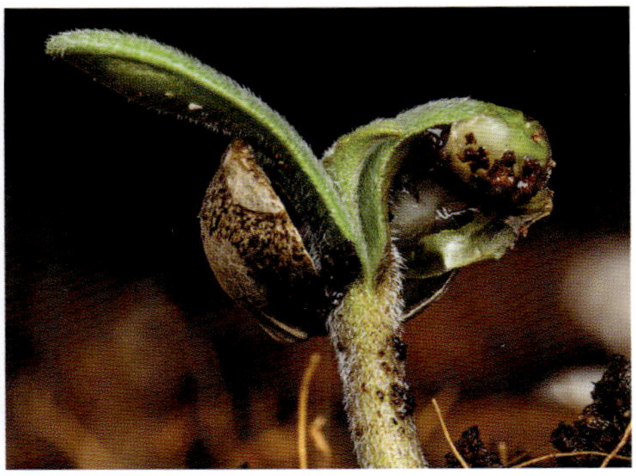

Stored starch and proteins fuel the germination of seedlings, while cellular expansion contributes to the elongation of the seedling.

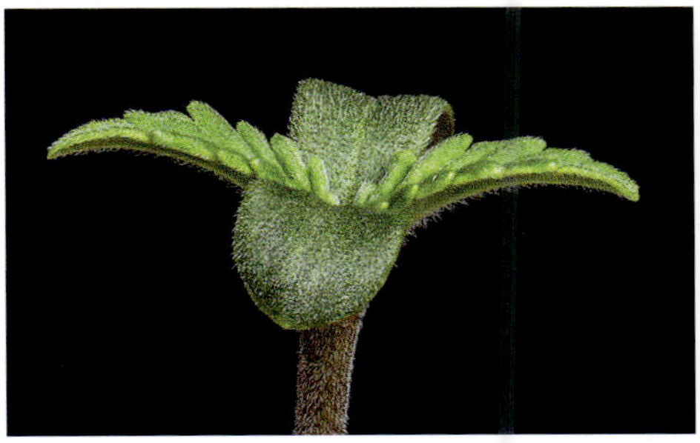
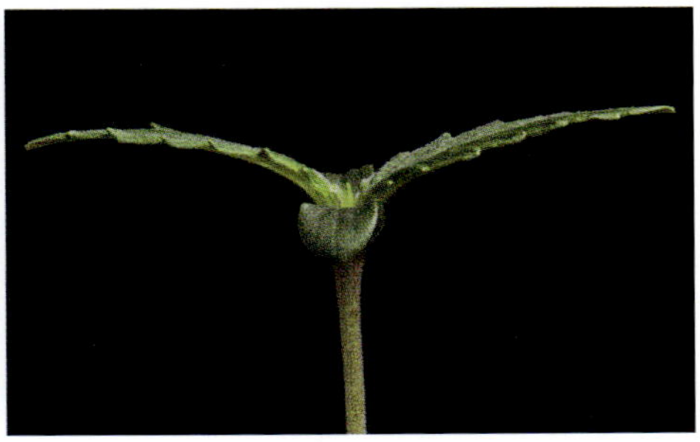

The initial set of primary true leaves specializes in photosynthesis, with vascular tissue absorbing nutrients to support the utilization of light by the true leaves.

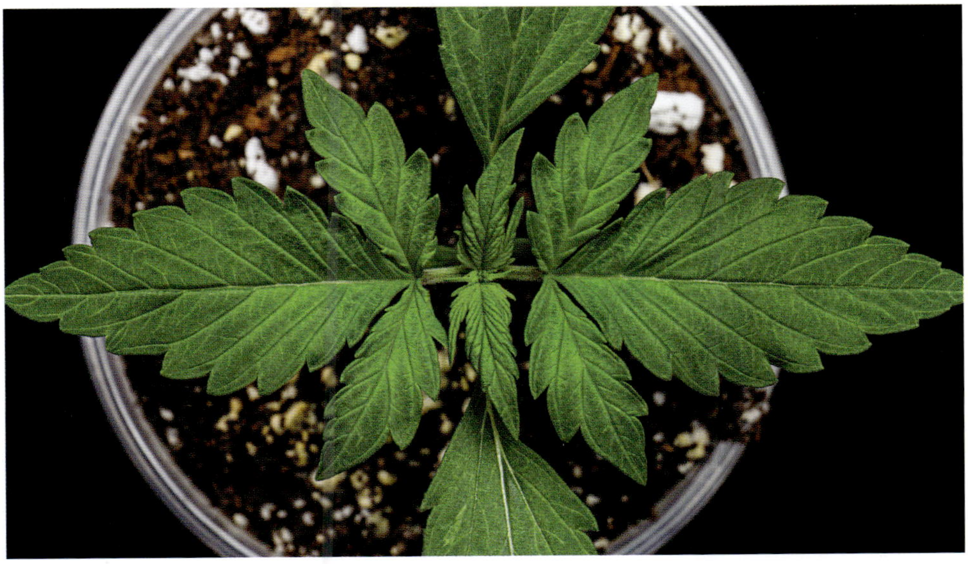

Leaf morphogenesis influences the shape of the cannabis leaf. All leaves after the primary true leaves are called secondary leaves.

PHOTOS: ROB BRAMHILL

Water

In most cases, tap water is suitable for growing, and does not negatively affect plants. Maintaining a neutral pH level is crucial, as is ensuring the water is at room temperature. There's no need to boil or use distilled water unless your tap water is unsafe for consumption, in which case you should find a different water source. You can easily obtain pH test strips for water testing. We will discuss water pH throughout this guide.

Germination Techniques

Seeds can be germinated in various ways, with some methods proving more successful than others. The highly effective Rockwool SBS propagation tray method, which involves using small germination cubes to initiate seedlings, boasts a near 100% success rate and will be discussed in detail in the Propagation Cubes, Trays, and Domes section later in this chapter.

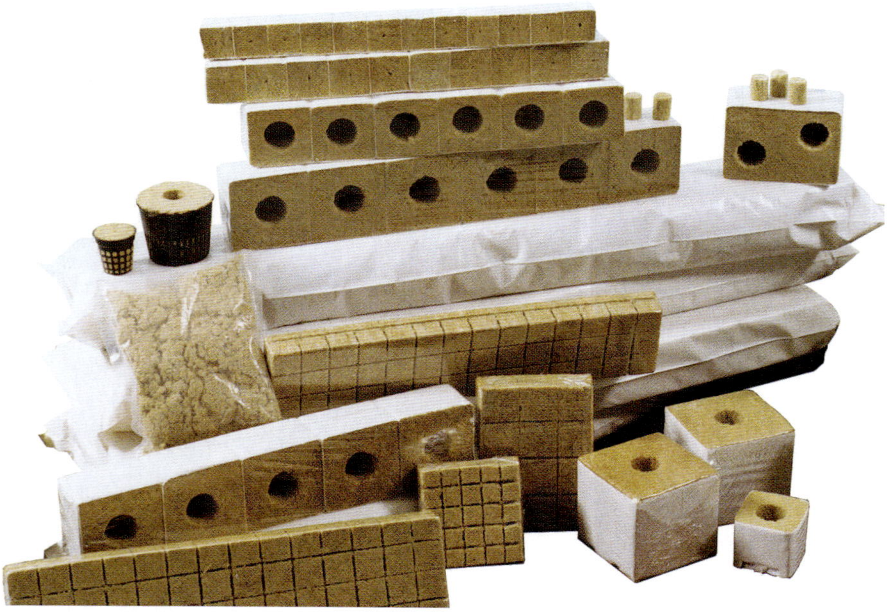

Rockwool comes in all shapes and sizes including slabs and mats. Some net pots are prefitted with shaped Rockwool.

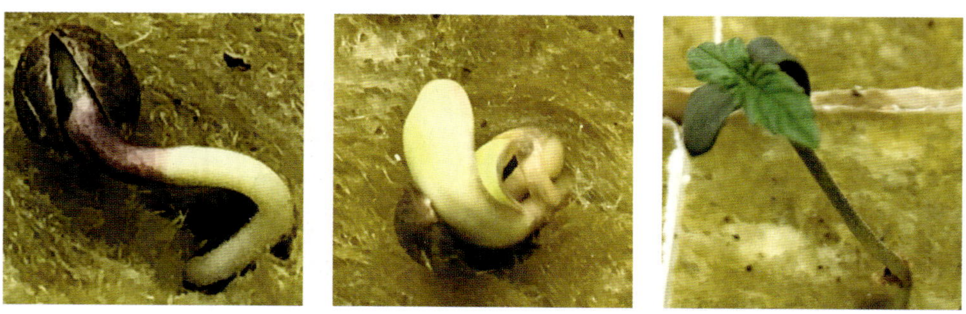

Rockwool germination is a great substitute for soil germination as it is easier to transport.

PHOTOS: HYDROFARM.COM (TOP), GRUBBYCUP STASH (BOTTOM ROW)

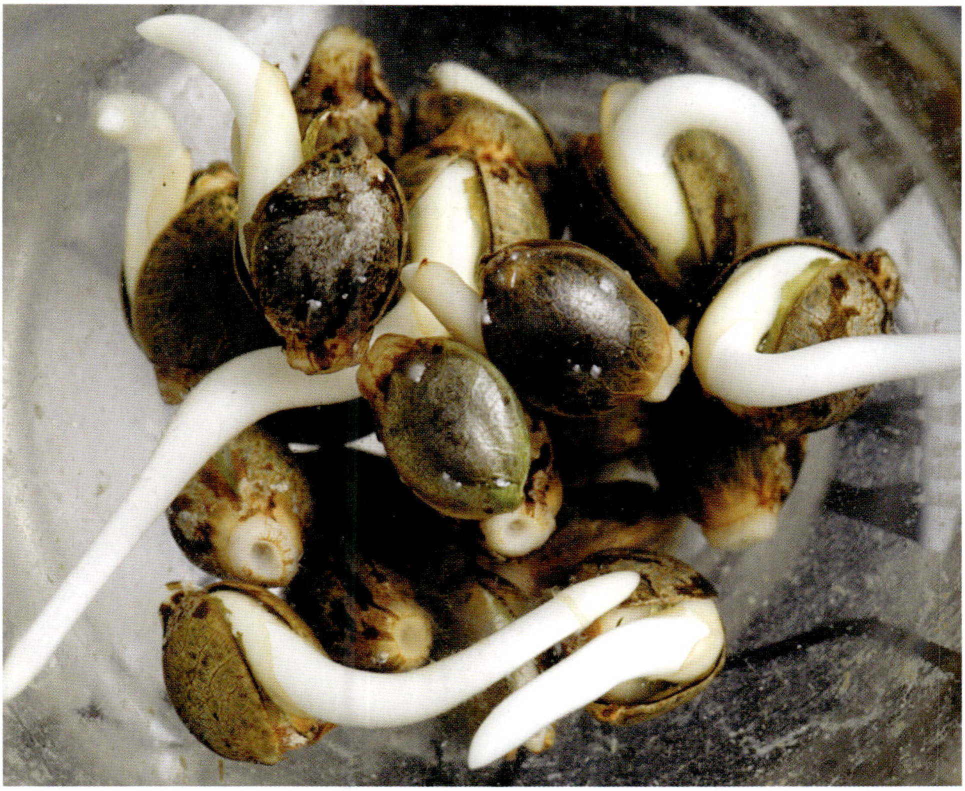

Water germination allows you to see the radicle protruding, signaling it is time to transplant.

Water Germination

Germinating seeds in a container of room-temperature water is a viable method. It involves using maximum moisture, which also softens the seed shells. As soon as germination starts, you must transplant the seedling into a growing medium by carefully removing it from the water with tweezers. If you're dealing with many seeds, you can empty the container onto cheesecloth to facilitate water drainage. You can put any seeds that haven't germinated back into fresh water at room temperature. This method offers the advantage of allowing you to observe germination, but it necessitates transplanting as soon as germination begins. Prolonged exposure to water can hinder a germinating seed's access to the air it requires. If other methods fail, this water-soaking approach can be attempted.

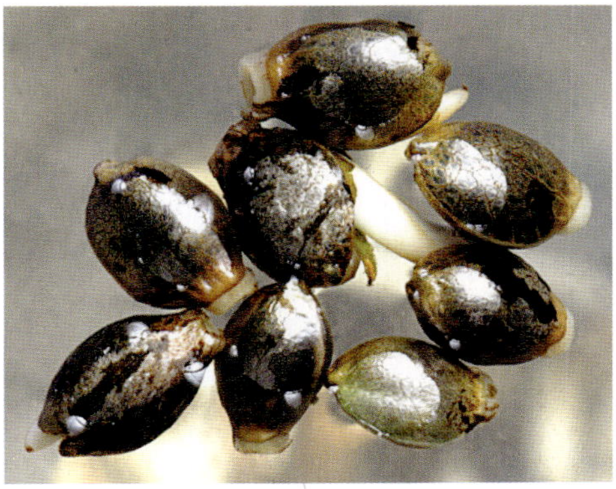

Water germination should be somewhat synchronous with healthy seeds from the same batch.

PHOTOS: ED BORG

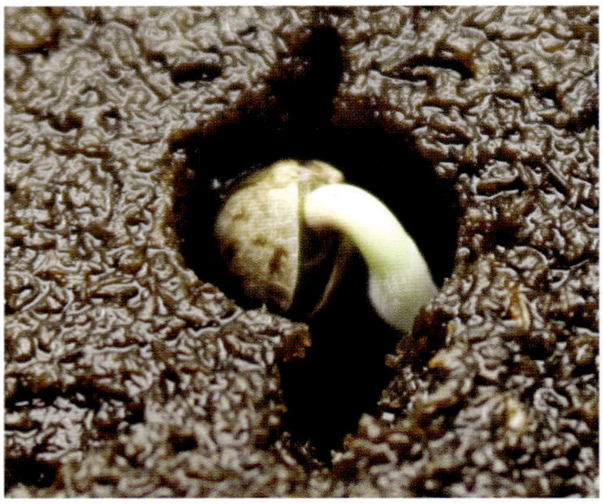

Seedlings will automatically lift the shell out from the medium.

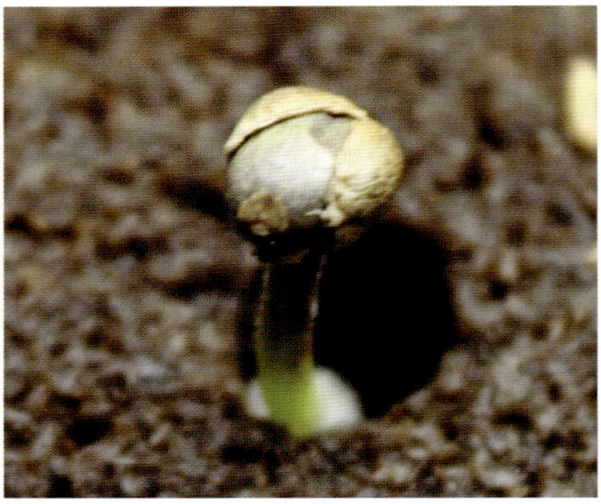

The hypocotyl, or seedling stem, elongates, lifting the shell out of the medium.

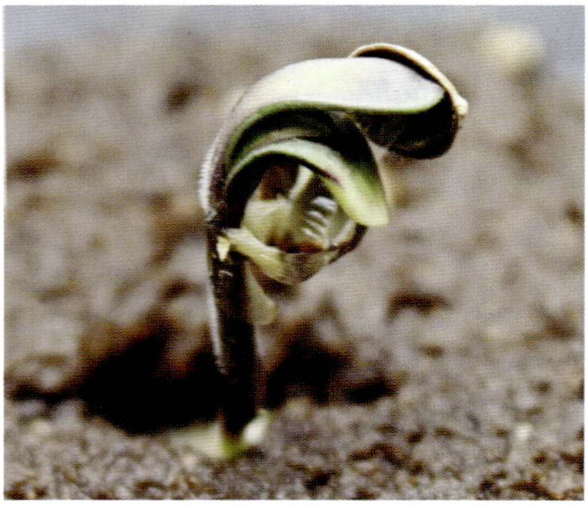

Cotyledons open, forcing the shell away.

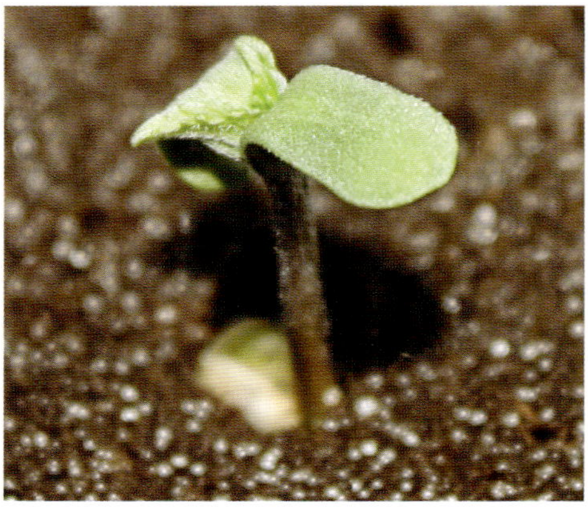

Shell is shed and cotyledons are open to receive light.

Seed in Soil Propagation

With this method, you place seeds into moist soil, about 3 mm below the surface, roughly the length of the seed. Keep the soil moist but not saturated by sprinkling water over it once daily. Direct-to-soil germination has a moderate success rate, with about seven to eight out of 10 seeds expected to germinate.

Germination Soil

Several soils are marketed specifically as germination soils. These are similar to regular soils but contain lower-level micronutrient blends suitable for seedlings and are sifted and free from contaminants and compost. These soils promote root development and are often labeled as organic and bio. They may be referred to as potting mix, seed starter, rooting soil, or cutting soil. Germination soils are used in conjunction with the seed soil propagation method and typically yield higher success rates compared to untreated outdoor soil.

PHOTOS: GRUBBYCUP STASH

Growers more commonly use regular loam soil with a pH level of 7 and an NPK (nitrogen, phosphorus, potassium) ratio with levels of N equal to or higher than P and K. NPK ratios like 5:1:1 or 8:4:4 work well. Ensuring that N is equal to or higher than both P and K is key.[4] Lower NPK ratios are preferable, as seedlings require minimal nutrients. Since you may transplant seedlings,[5] loam offers a slightly lower success rate than germination soil but performs better than untreated soil.

Seed Towel Propagation

Towel propagation, when executed correctly, is a highly successful germination method. Place seeds on a damp paper towel or piece of cheesecloth or damp cotton balls. Then cover them with additional damp material. It's crucial to keep the material moist, as drying out can damage the seeds. Check daily to monitor root development. When roots appear, promptly transfer the seedlings to a growing medium, such as soil, using tweezers. Be careful not to touch the delicate roots, as this can harm your seedlings. This method exhibits a moderate-to-high success rate, with eight or nine out of 10 seeds often germinating. One advantage of towel propagation is your ability to visually confirm seed germination and detect any failures early, without disturbing potential late-developing roots.

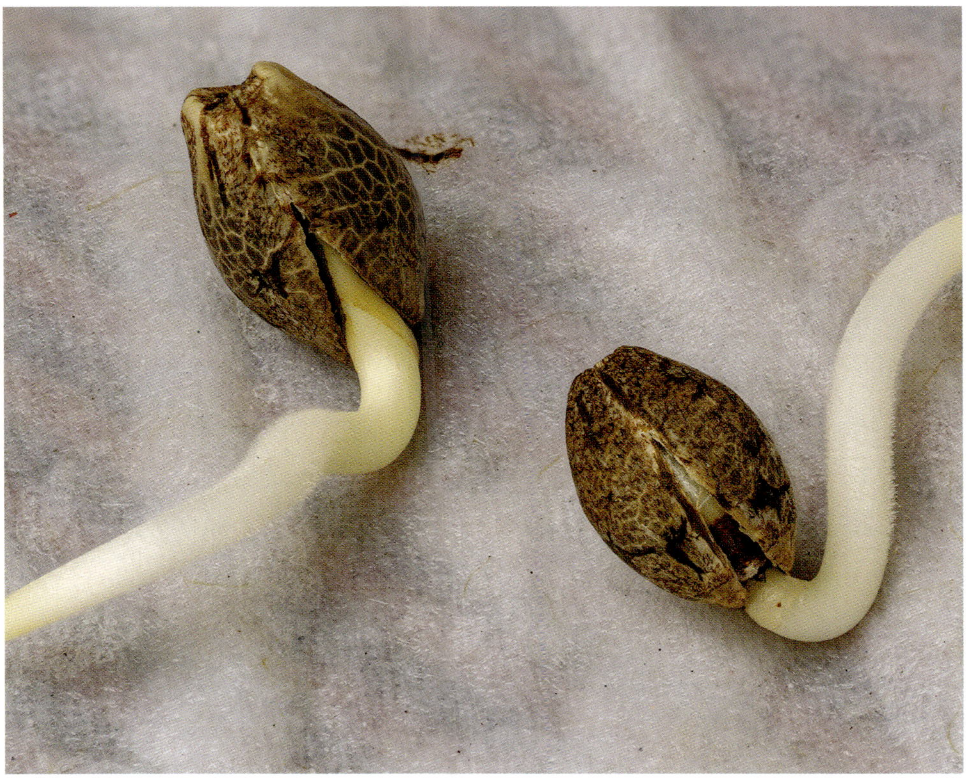

PHOTO: ROB BRAMHILL

Germination can also be observed when using the towel method. This is 48 hours after the radicle shows.

Seed Towel Propagation

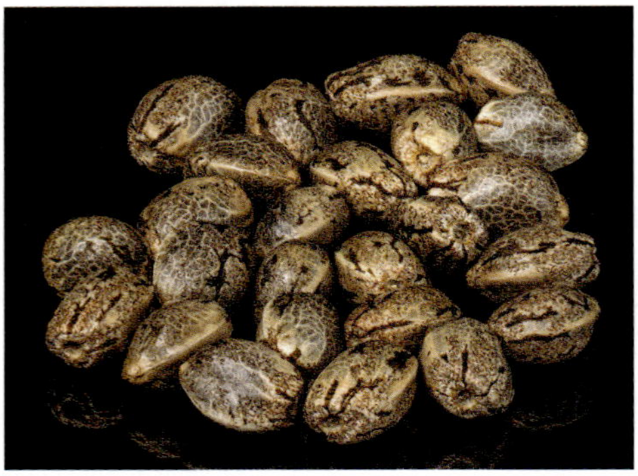

Seeds of the same batch should be high quality, healthy, and show no damage.

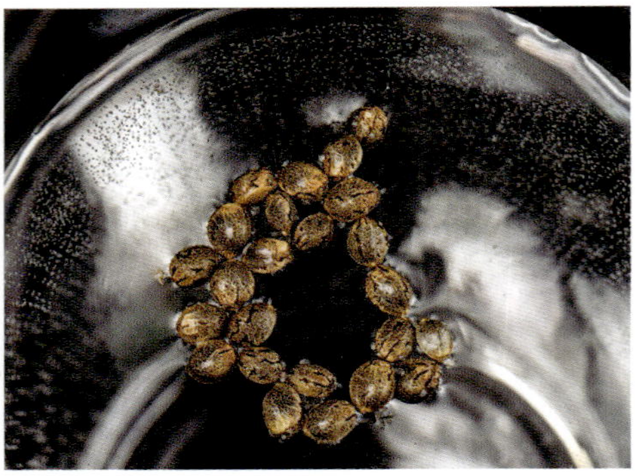

You can start the seeds in water or on a damp towel.

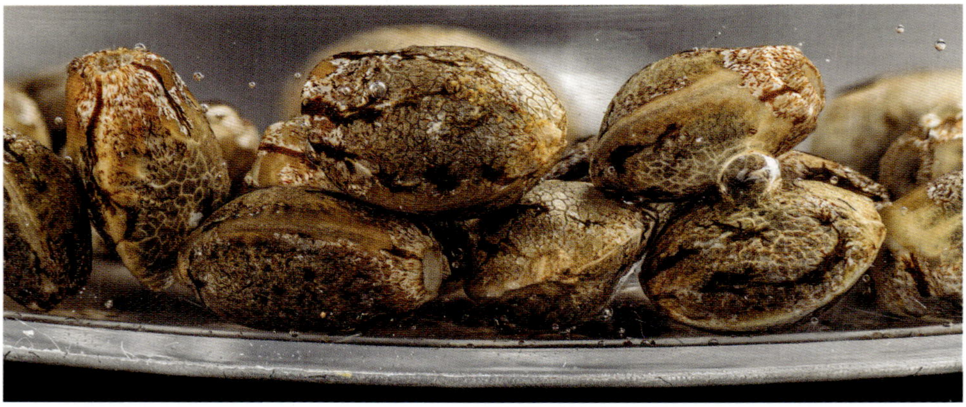

Total submersion ensures water completely envelopes the seed for imbibing. The embryo starts to swell and split in response.

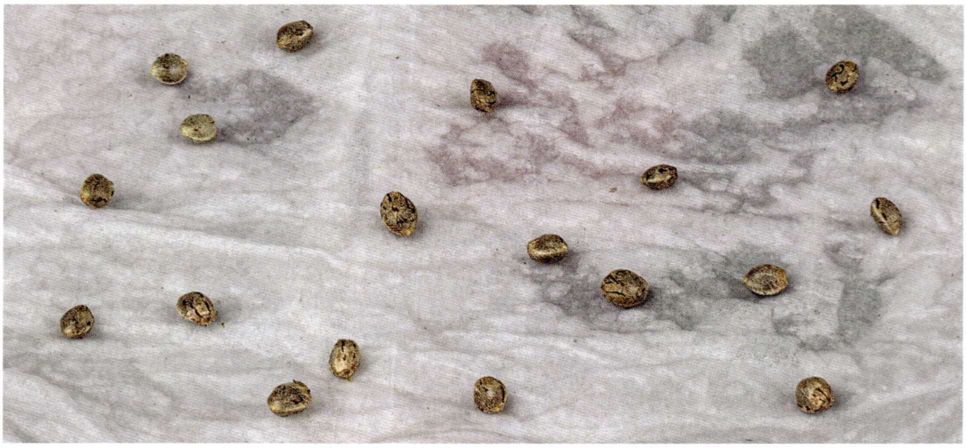

As soon as initial radicle growth shows, move seeds to a damp towel. Using a dish can make for an easier transportation.

PHOTOS: ROB BRAMHILL

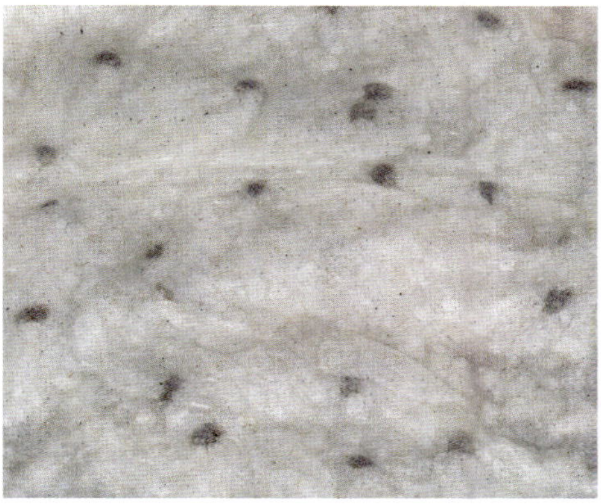

Cover the damp towel with another damp towel.

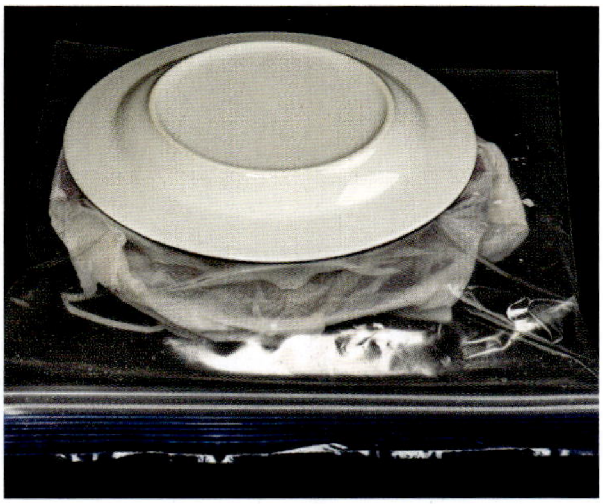

Place the towel in a ziploc bag and a dish on top so it doesn't dry out too quickly.

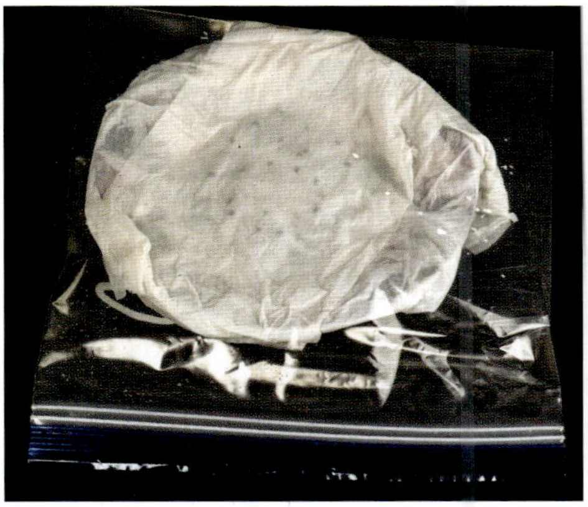

Check your towel regularly to ensure it is kept damp.

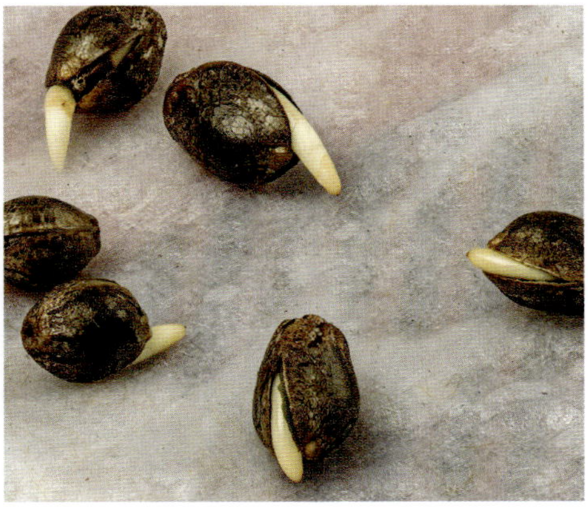

Radicle growth after 24 hours.

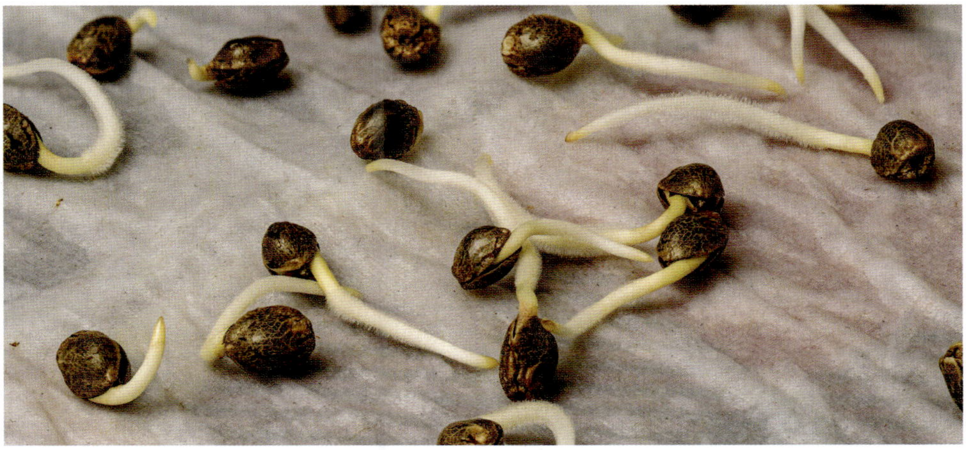

48 hours later, these seedlings are ready to transplant. Germination is the most rapid phase of cannabis growth.

Propagation Cubes, Trays, and Domes

Batch seed propagation is typically done on trays under LED lights in designated germination rooms with controlled environments. In such conditions, these trays are often lidless. However, many home growers prefer using kits to maintain environmental control. These kits typically consist of a tray with a transparent dome with air slots to exchange fresh air.

Propagation trays often come with a humidity dome. Opting for the dome is beneficial, for both humidity control and protecting your seedlings. At the tray's bottom is a small area where water or germination hormones can be added. Rockwool cubes, known as the single block system (SBS), are placed into slots within the tray, which automatically immerses the Rockwool in the solution. Seeds are then planted into small holes in the cubes, and the holes are filled with Rockwool particles to shield the seeds from direct air exposure. Finally, the dome is placed over the tray with the air slots left open to facilitate fresh air circulation.

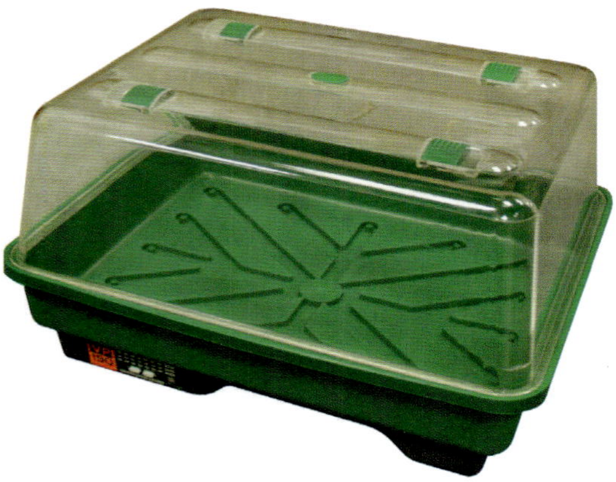

Propagation tray used mainly for the single block system (SBS).

Some propagation kits are heated and resemble miniature greenhouses. A typical kit includes about 24 Rockwool cubes, 50 ml of Clonex, 100 ml of Formulex, and

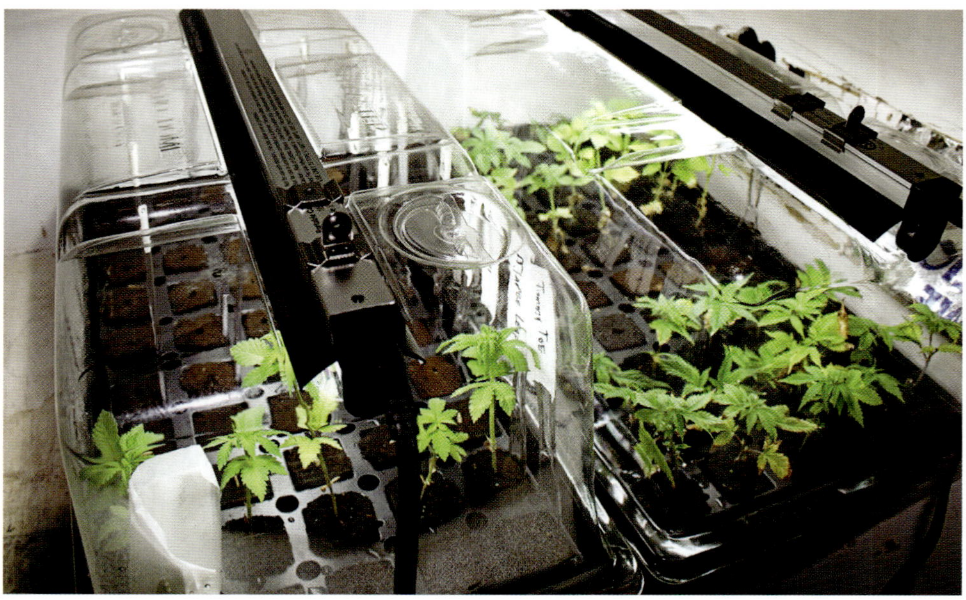

Domes create humidity by trapping air moisture, creating perfect conditions for seedling growth.

PHOTOS: HYDROFARM.COM (TOP), GRUBBYCUP STASH (BOTTOM)

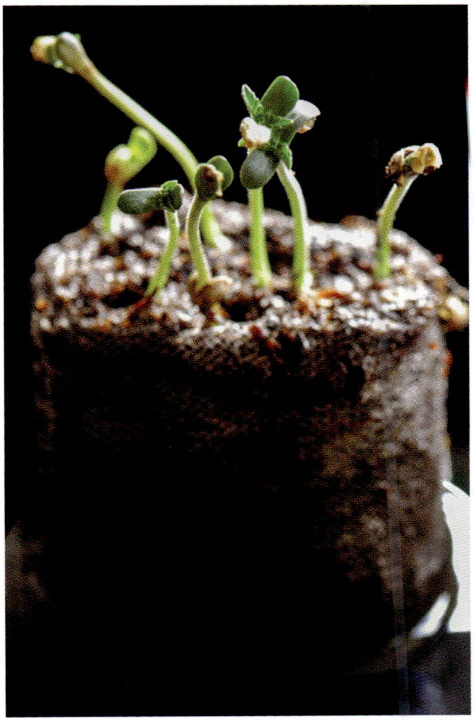

Jiffy peat cubes are like miniature grow bags for seedlings and cuttings.

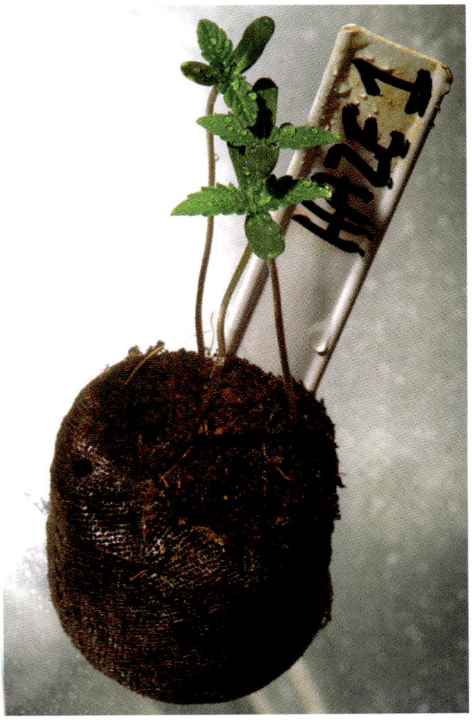

Cut the side to unpack one with several started seedings ready for transplanting.

possibly some cutting tools. Such kits can also be used for cloning cuttings, as Clonex and Formulex encourage root growth. For seed germination, the use of fertilizers or growth hormones is generally not recommended unless you have prior experience. Even slight overfeeding can harm seeds or seedlings, so rely solely on water for seed germination. To date, no cannabis strain needs growth hormones or fertilizers for successful germination.

Managing water content in the Rockwool cubes is essential. If the cubes become too dry, the growing roots can push the seedling out. Conversely, excessive moisture can oversaturate the cubes, making it challenging for seedlings to emerge. Various cube types, such as Jiffy, pellet cubes, and coconut substrates, retain water differently. Experiment with water retention for the cube type you have. Learning the moisture level and drying time for your specific cubes will allow you to establish a germination watering schedule before planting seeds.

Tray prices range from $10 to $50, depending on size. Slabs of 50 to 100 small (1″ × 1″) Rockwool cubes cost around $20, while a six-pack of larger cubes (4″ × 4″) ranges from $10 to $20. As discussed above, fertilizers for seed starting are generally unnecessary, but if you do choose to go that route, small bottles are available for around $5. If you've invested significantly in quality seeds, you can assemble a small

PHOTOS: ED BORG

kit like this to increase your chances of achieving a 100% germination rate. Alternatively, consider investing a bit more in a quality kit that adds the advantage of rooting your clones.[6] Don't miss out on this opportunity.

If you're planning to root numerous cuttings but lack the suitable kit, you can use a transparent covering placed over a container for cloning. The transparent cover allows light penetration while trapping humidity, creating a propagation-kit-like environment. Typically, these containers are placed outdoors in warm conditions and opened once or twice a week for fresh air exchange. If you do it properly, you will see signs of moisture accumulation within the container. If moisture levels are insufficient, add more water to the medium. Always clean up any plastic materials after use. This method provides an excellent way to work with outdoor propagation and should not be overlooked.

Scaling Up

If you plan to increase the number of seeds you germinate and transplant, consider using a seedling cloche or a portable cold frame. Always ensure there's adequate air circulation in these setups, just as with your propagation kits. Proper maintenance, including regular cleaning, is crucial to maintain the right temperatures and prevent unwanted pests and the growth of bacteria and mold. The main purpose of these tools is to help you create a controlled microclimate on a larger scale. For large-scale germination, tray frames on coasters equipped with LED lights on each shelf are commonly used. These trays are sometimes used to transport germinated seedlings over long distances for transplantation elsewhere.

Cannabis Germination Mechanisms

"Imbibing" is the absorption of water by the seed, eventually causing the seed coat to split open. The hardness of the seed coat can vary among cannabis seeds. Ripe seeds

Root Growth from Seed to Seedling

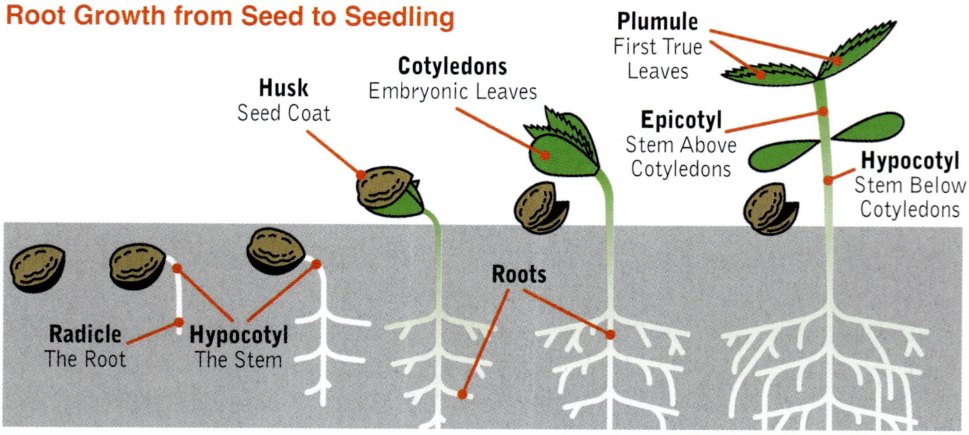

The radicle and hypocotyl allow the seedling to grow in opposite directions, below and above the surface. The shell is raised by the hypocotyl and falls off when the cotyledons and plumule open out.

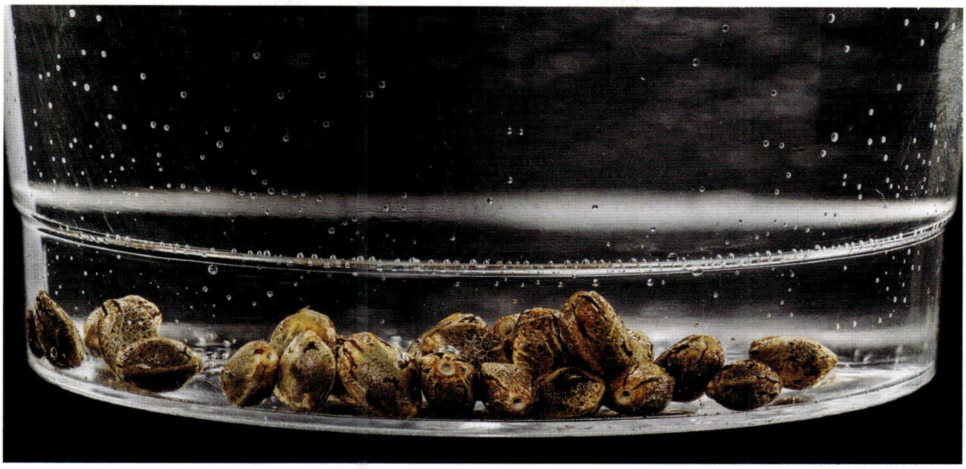

Water germination allows you to move the seeds around so you can see every part of them. They are not fixed in soil or rockwool.

should germinate, but immature seeds are often nonviable. Immature cannabis seeds usually have a soft, whitish appearance, though some strains naturally exhibit this characteristic. If in doubt about maturity, consult the breeder. Another issue can arise from excessively hard seed coats, preventing water absorption, requiring intervention by the grower or natural processes for germination. Both the water or towel methods of germination allow for visual inspection of the seed and are useful for identifying this problem. Using soil and growing cubes necessitate digging up the seed to check for failure.[7]

Cannabis seeds don't require light for germination, unlike some other plant species. Water and temperature are the primary factors influencing germination. However, once the seedling emerges from the soil, it requires light for proper growth, otherwise it won't establish roots and may die. While cannabis seeds possess a relatively permeable seed coat that allows some light to penetrate, exposing them to direct sunlight for extended periods may hinder germination success due to potential damage from UV light. Several factors can inhibit germination, including seed immaturity, unsuitable soil types, excessive exposure to environmental elements, incorrect planting depth, weeds, high nutrient content, physical damage from animals or environmental factors, and fungi.

Cold drafts can also impede germination, so it's crucial to keep germinating seeds away from open windows or fans and ensure that the room maintains a warm temperature[8] during the germination and transplantation phases, when the plants are most vulnerable.

By following proper germination methods, you can mitigate these inhibitors and potential issues. However, if problems do arise, it's essential to identify their causes and take corrective measures.

PHOTO: ROB BRAMHILL

Germination Timing

The time required for germination can range from 12 hours to 10 days, depending on seed structure and germination conditions. In most cases, healthy seeds and optimal conditions should result in germination within a few days.

It's essential to exercise patience and avoid unnecessary disturbance during this phase. While you may be tempted to check on your seedlings frequently, touching them or shifting them can damage young roots. It's crucial to refrain from interfering with your growth process; intervene only when necessary. If you want to observe the process, use the previously mentioned cheesecloth method as it provides a clearer view of the germination process.

Cannabis Seedling Nutrition

The primary requirements for seedlings are water and light. Keep the soil or growing medium consistently moist but not waterlogged. Overwatering can lead to damping-off disease and root rot, which are common issues in young cannabis plants, so ensure that your seedlings receive adequate but not excessive moisture.

Fertilizing Cannabis Seedlings

Cannabis seeds contain enough nutrients for the cotyledons, the initial seed leaves, to support the seedling during its first couple of weeks of life. Fertilizing is unnecessary and, in fact, providing too many nutrients too early can harm the delicate seedlings. However, once the cotyledons start to yellow and wither, indicating that the seedling needs additional nutrients for healthy growth, and the seedlings develop their first set of true leaves, it's time to introduce a mild nutrient solution.

When it's time to start fertilizing your cannabis seedlings, use a balanced, water-soluble fertilizer with a formulation designed for seedlings or young plants. These fertilizers typically have a lower concentration of nutrients to avoid overwhelming the delicate roots of young seedlings. Follow the manufacturer's recommendations for dilution and application frequency and start with a weaker solution to prevent over-fertilization.

When applying fertilizer, it's essential to water your seedlings thoroughly with the diluted nutrient solution, ensuring even distribution throughout the growing medium. Be cautious not to splash fertilizer on the leaves, as this can lead to nutrient burn or leaf damage. Only use foliar spray feeding for plants in the vegetative growth stage. Misting the seedlings with water is fine, just be sure not to overwater them.

Carefully monitor your seedlings for any signs of nutrient deficiencies or excesses, including yellowing or browning of leaves, stunted growth, or unusual discoloration. Identifying and addressing these issues promptly is crucial for fostering healthy and robust plant development.

Healthy Root Growth

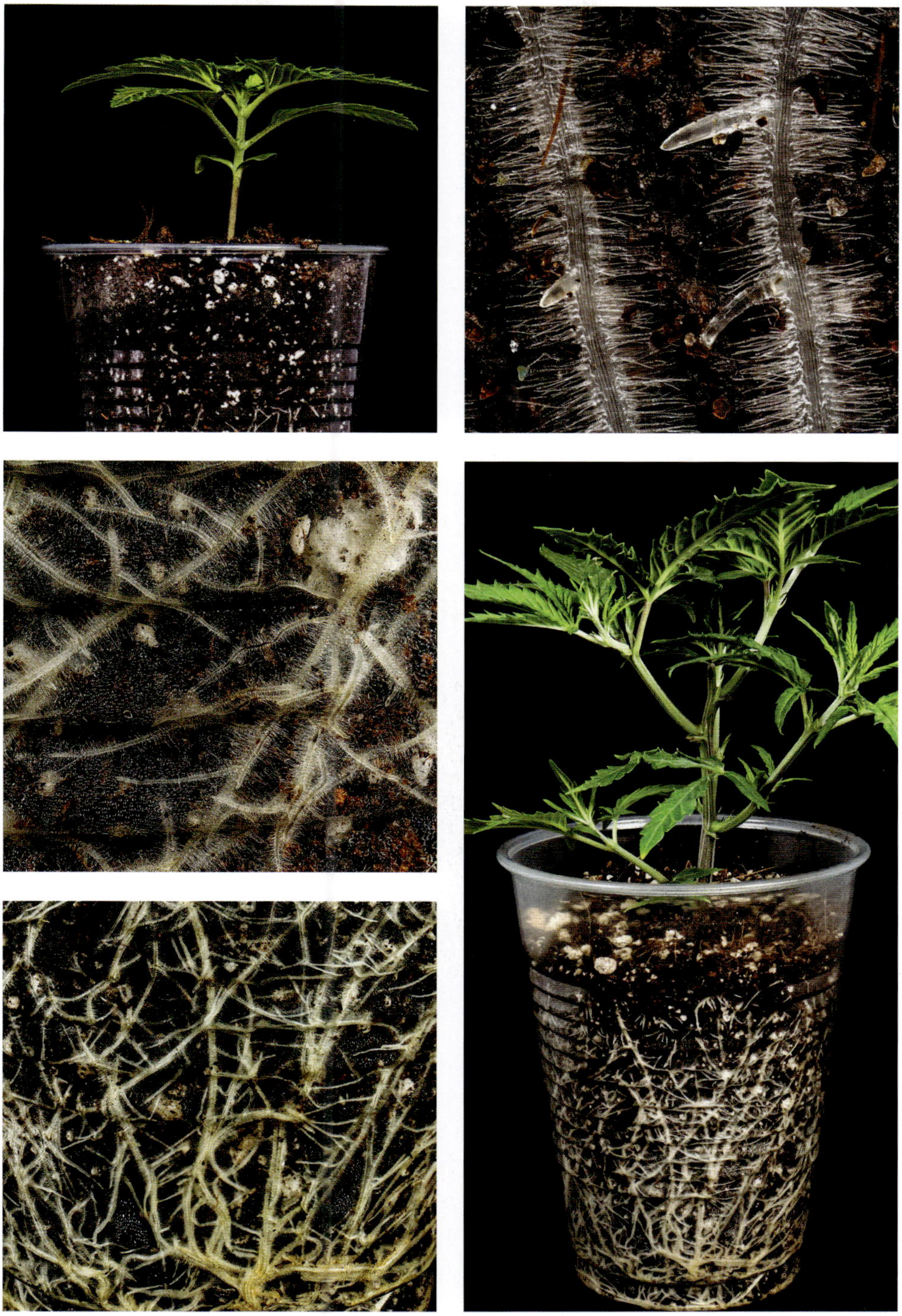

PHOTOS: ROB BRAMHILL

Lateral roots grow from the primary root, and microsized root hairs absorb nutrients and water. Roots will grow into any area with nutrients and water, including traveling back upwards again.

As your cannabis seedlings continue to grow and transition into the vegetative stage, you can gradually increase the strength and frequency of your fertilizer applications to meet their increasing nutrient demands. However, avoid over-fertilization, which can harm your plants.

Cannabis Seed Functions

Cannabis seeds play a dual role in the life cycle of the cannabis plant, serving as both its inception and its culmination. From a seed, a new plant emerges, eventually giving rise to more seeds. As the seeds are released, the plant can persist until a drop in temperature halts its metabolic processes, leading to the plant's demise. This marks the start of a new cycle. The nutrients within the seeds facilitate the proliferation of embryo cells, driving growth. Cannabis seeds tend to be relatively heavy, limiting their dispersal by wind. Animals, primarily birds, are the natural agents responsible for distributing cannabis seeds over long distances.[9]

Cannabis flowers yield both seeds and resin, enabling seeds to adhere to almost any surface when the opportunity arises. They can latch onto animal fur or get transported through digestive systems, occasionally stored as a future food source by these animals. For the survival and establishment of a new population, all that is required are a male and a female plant to endure the journey.

We should not exclude humans from the natural dispersal of cannabis seeds. Throughout history, people have used these seeds for various purposes, even today, extracting essential oils from them. Human cultivation and harvesting have long served as methods for the dispersal of cannabis seeds. Today, the postal system and over-the-counter seed purchases have become the most prevalent means of cannabis seed distribution. Looking ahead, the future might usher in drone-based transport for these seeds. Such a development would have been unimaginable even a century ago when considering the fate of cannabis.

Overstretching

Some cannabis strains produce seedlings with weak stems, leading to seedlings that may lean to one side. This stretching is often indicative of issues with seed-to-light distances, especially when using natural light, causing seedlings to reach for light sources and resulting in longer stems than desired during this early stage. It's essential to understand internode lengths and their significance in plant growth; we will learn more on why this matters in Chapter 7. To address overstretching, consider using LED grow lights, which help keep seedlings more compact. In the past, people commonly used fluorescents or low-wattage HID lights for seedlings, both of which generate more heat than LEDs.

To deal with stretched seedlings that need support, use small sticks to gently brace them. Attach the stem to the stick using a piece of thread. Avoid tying the thread above a growing shoot, as this can lead to damage. Over time, you can replace the

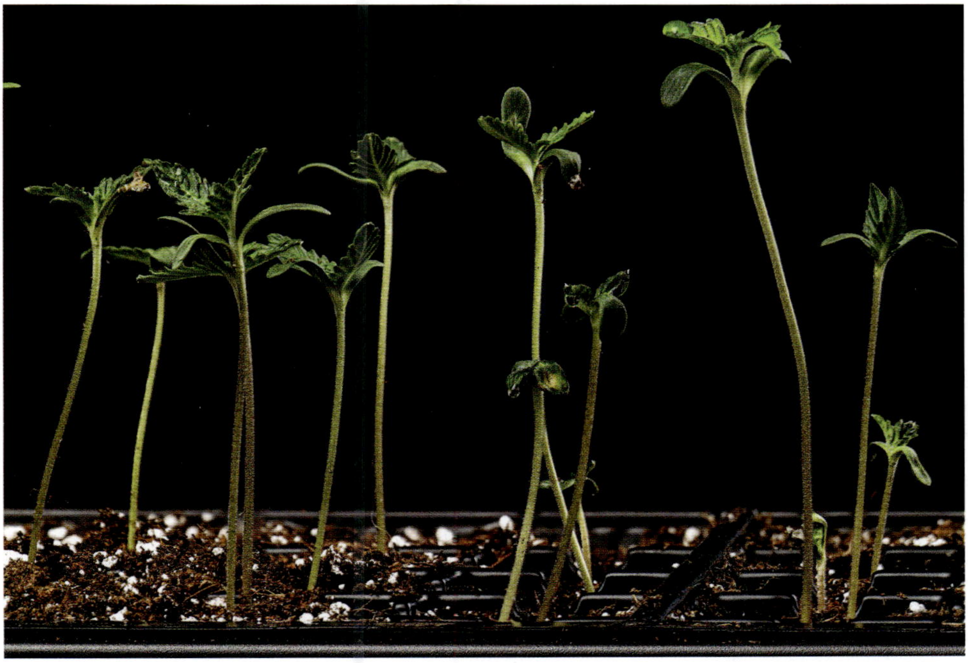

If you do not keep the light close, seedlings can stretch. These seedlings should not be allowed to stretch any more than they have. A closer light should ensure this.

stick with a stake to support your plant's growth—although this shouldn't be necessary, as even weaker seedlings tend to develop into sturdy vegetative plants. Avoid bringing support sticks from the outdoors to an indoor grow space, as they may harbor pests like spider mites in their incubation nests inside the wood. Consider using LED lights earlier in the growth process to prevent seedling stretching in the first place.

As seedlings grow and transition into vegetative plants, particularly if they have weak stems, it's beneficial to gently shake the base of the stem every morning and evening. This mimics the effects of wind, promoting the development of a more robust stem. Outdoor plants tend to be sturdier due to natural wind exposure, while indoor plants require the assistance of indoor fans to stimulate wind-induced stem strength.

Transplanting Seedlings

Transplanting seedlings is a necessary step in their growth journey, especially when they outgrow their initial containers or need more space. The transplanting process is similar regardless of the propagation method used, with the exception of outdoor plot sowing.

Transplanting should be done during the transition phase between the seedling and vegetative growth stages. However, it's crucial to ensure that the seedlings have developed sufficient roots to support the transplant. Visual and timing cues can help determine when it's the right time to transplant.

PHOTO: ROB BRAMHILL

Transplanting a Plant

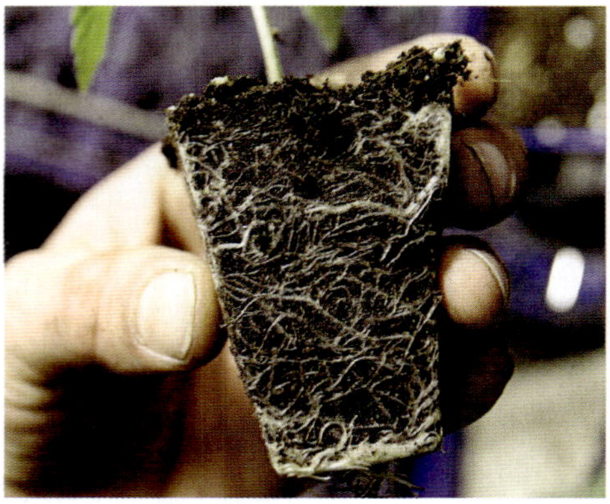

You must dry out the soil medium. Cubes should not be moved when wet.

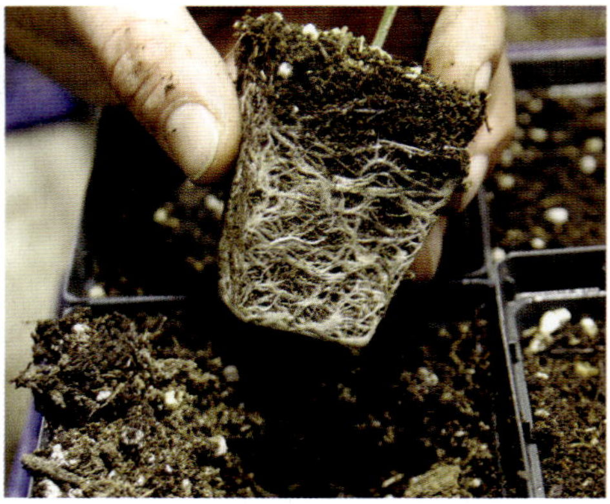

A dry medium will stay together and not crumble when moved.

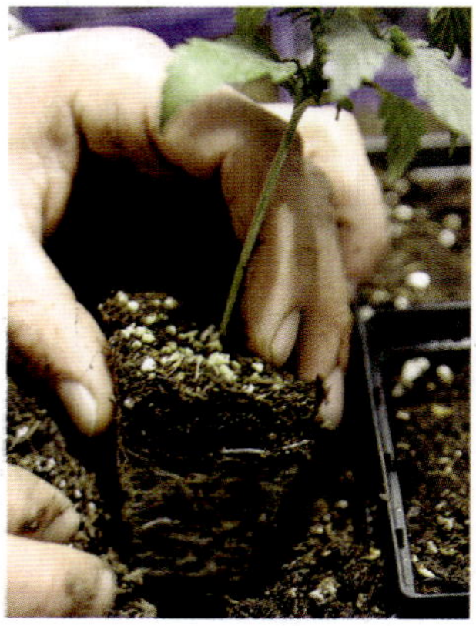

Pre-dig your hole before you move the plant.

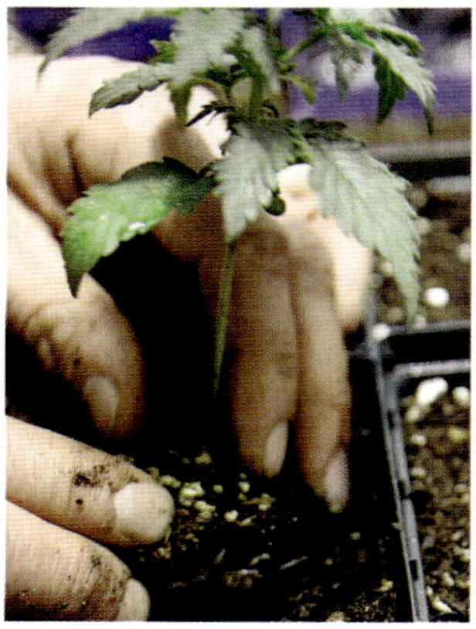

The hole needs to be deep and wide enough.

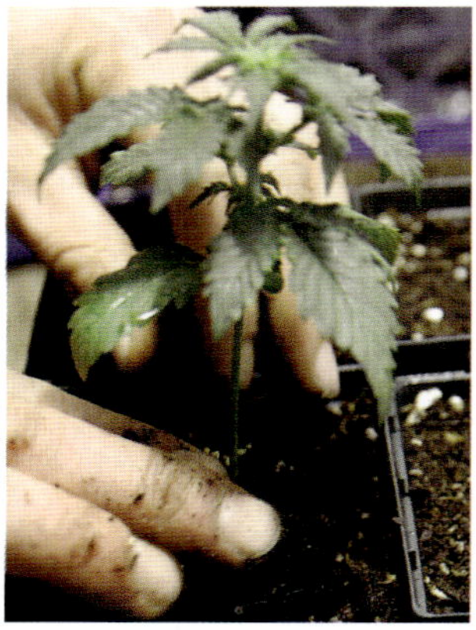

Position the plant and hold it vertical as you fill in the sides.

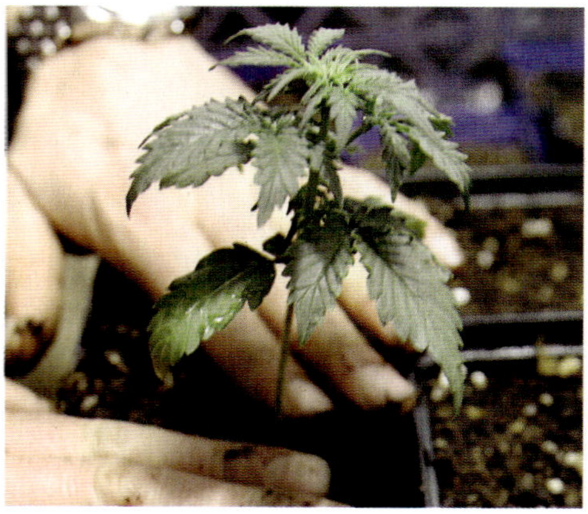

Use some extra soil to fill in around the plant.

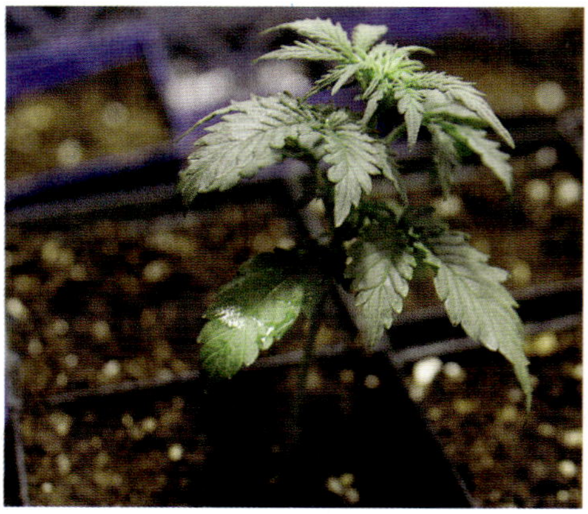

Do not feed transplanted plants. Allow them time to recover.

PHOTOS: DAVID STRANGE

For example, if you're using growing cubes, you may notice roots penetrating the sides of the cubes. In pots with drainage holes, roots may start growing externally. The visual cue from the plant itself is when your seedling begins to resemble a typical cannabis plant, with branching and leaf patterns that resemble the classic cannabis shape. The plant should remain relatively short, with the root mass and medium no larger than what can be comfortably cupped with one hand when dry between waterings. Smaller plants are easier to transplant successfully.

When the seedlings are ready for transplanting, gently lift them from the propagation tray, along with their cube if applicable, and place them into the new growing medium. If you're using a larger cube, insert the smaller cube into a slot cut through the other. Alternatively, you can transplant directly into soil in a pot or a hydroponic or aeroponic setup.

To ensure a smooth process, maintain a plan and work out the steps before transplanting. The cube won't interfere with your plant's growth in any medium and provides additional support as the plant adapts to its new environment.

Even if you started your seedlings in soi , transplanting them into larger pots doesn't have to be complicated. The key is to handle the plant and soil carefully to minimize disturbance. Wait for the soil to dry. Gradually lift the plant out, keeping the root ball as intact as possible. Avoid moving the soil around too much, as disturbing the roots can stress the plant. If you must transplant from one type of growing medium to another, it's best to choose options that are easy to manage and minimize the risk of root damage.

Several methods can be used to transplant seedlings.

Upside-Down Technique

If the soil is compact and stable, you can turn the pot upside down and gently tap it to release the entire root ball as a solid mass. This method requires practice and works best with dry soil. Hold the stem between your fingers to ensure it doesn't get damaged during the process.

Pot-in-pot method

This involves leaving the plant in a perforated pot for the transplant—for example, a smaller pot goes into a bigger pct, or outdoors, the pot goes into the ground. Look up pots for the pot-in-pot method if you want a removable base. Grow bags are more popular because the base can be sliced open easily and placed on top of a larger grow bag. Bags and pots can be used together—a small grow bag in a big plant pot or a small plant pot in a grow bag. These ways, you avoid having to cut any plastic up.

Germination and Transplanting

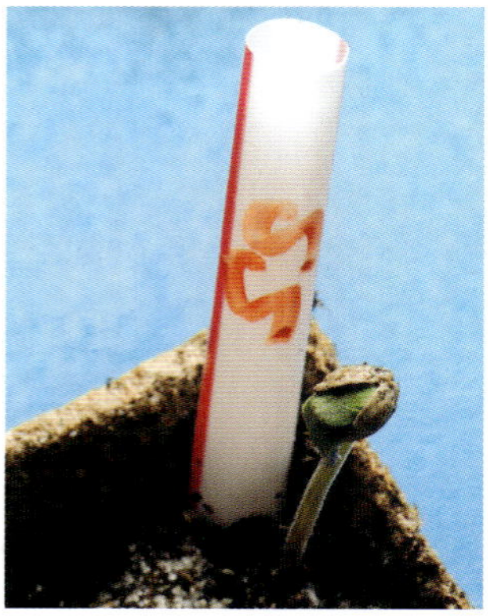

When seedlings germinate, they grow quickly.

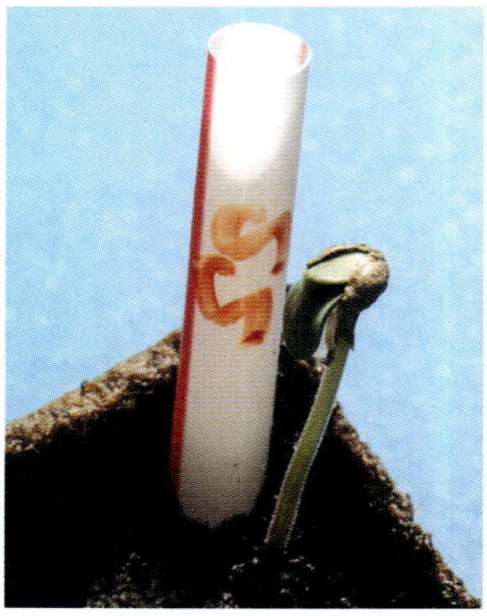

The seedling shows more growth after only a few hours.

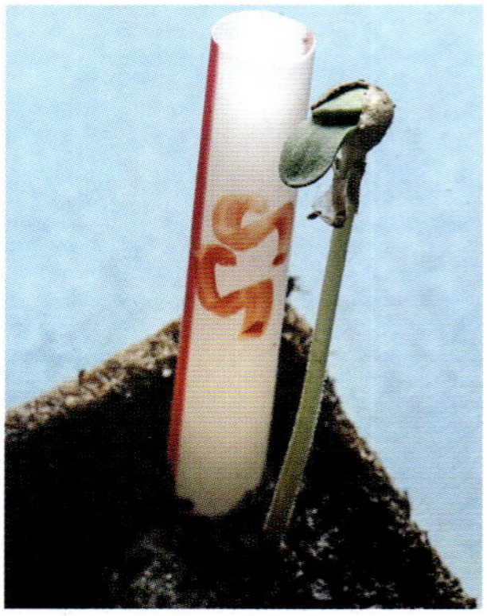

Within a few days the shell will naturally fall off.

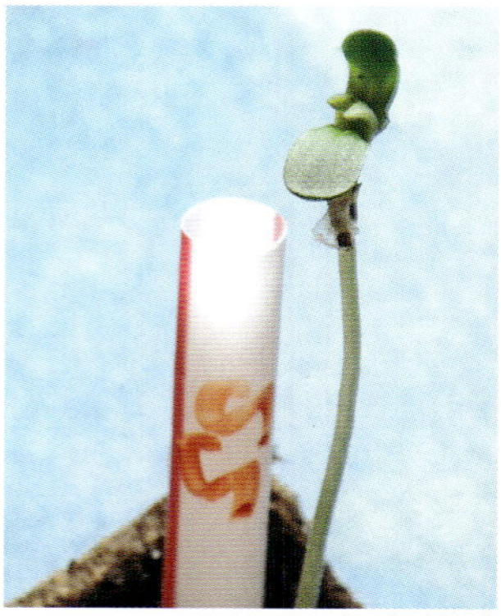

When the cotyledons are open you need to give them light.

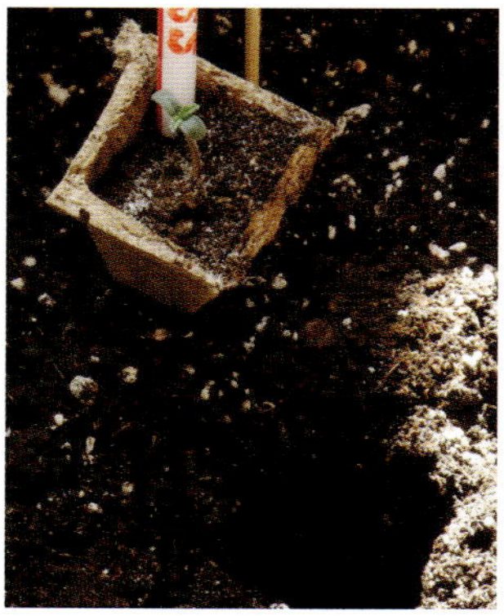

Biodegradable cubes and pots can be placed in the soil.

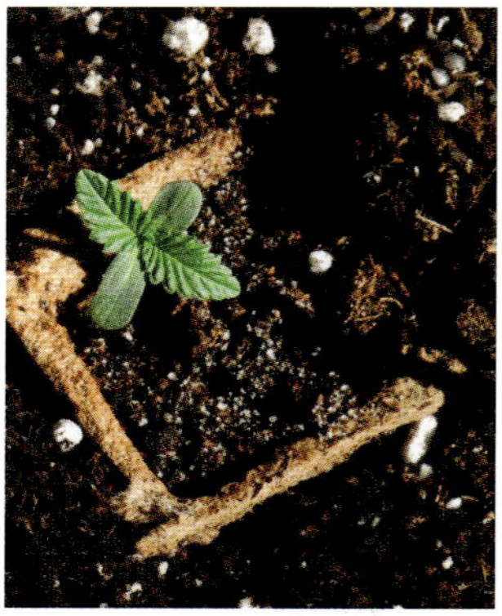

Make sure some of the stem stays above the surface.

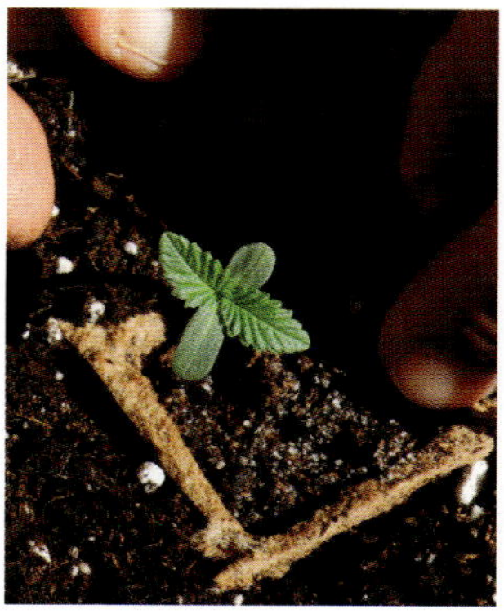

Fill in the sides to cover the biodegrable starting medium completely.

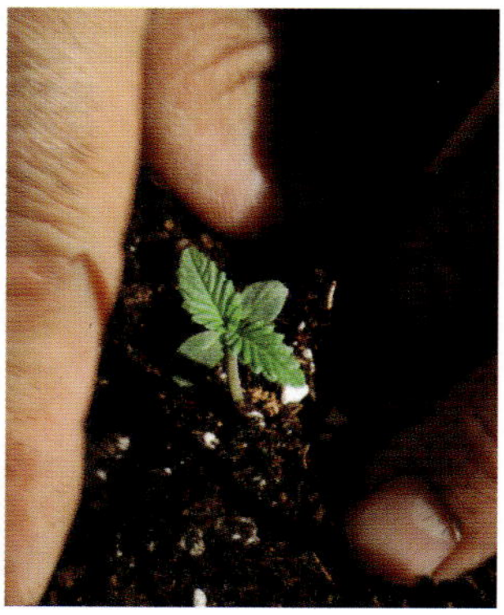

A slight mound is good because watering will level it out.

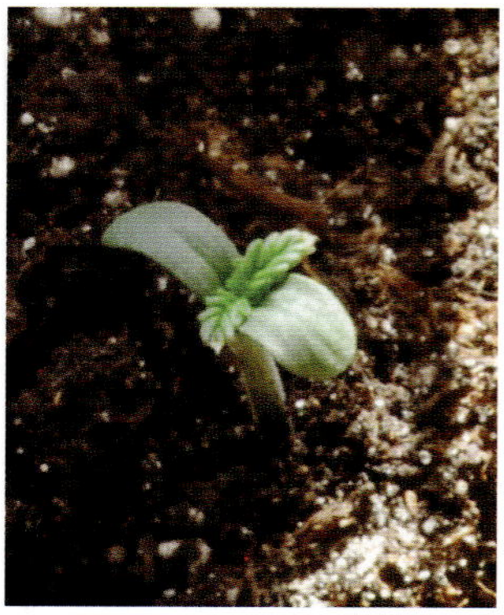

After watering, the surface should be even and flat, not dipping. If dipping, use more surface soil.

PHOTOS: ED BORG

Pulling Method

This last resort should be used only when the soil is extremely dry and the plant is in a contracted state due to dehydration. By delaying watering and letting the soil become stiff, you can attempt the upside-down method first. If it fails, use a clean knife to carefully cut around the inside edge of the pot, then gently lift the plant and soil out. Some soil may break away, but this should not significantly harm the plant. Place it immediately in the new growing medium and water thoroughly to help it adjust.

Whichever transplanting method you choose, your goal is to minimize stress on the seedling and ensure a smooth transition to its new home. Always handle the plant gently and take precautions to protect the delicate roots during the process.

Transplanting from Indoors to Outdoors

Before transplanting your cannabis seedlings into an outdoor location, they must be hardened off in a gradual acclimatization to prepare them for the outdoor environment and reduce the risk of transplant shock.

Hardening Off Cannabis Seedlings

1. Start the hardening-off process about one to two weeks before you plan to transplant your seedlings.
2. Choose a sheltered, partially shaded outdoor location, such as a covered porch or a spot with dappled sunlight, where your seedlings will be protected from strong winds and direct sunlight.

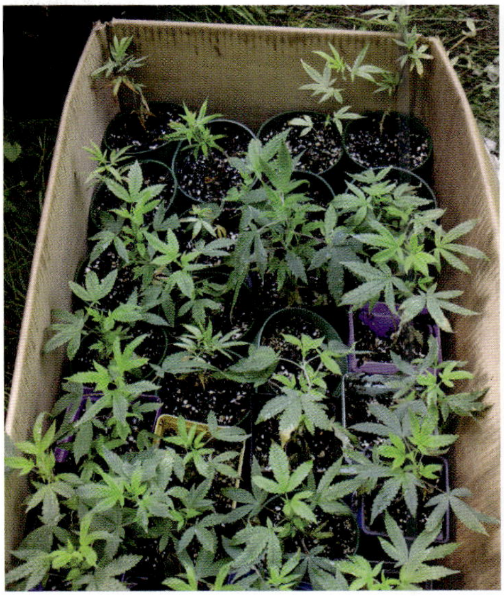

A box of 30 mature seedlings after hardening up outdoors for a week. Ready for transplanting.

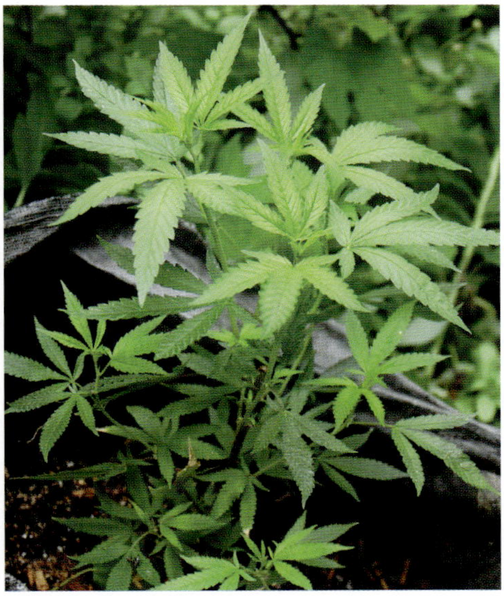

Outdoor environmental factors and stressors influence the plants to grow more robust and sturdy.

PHOTOS: DAVID STRANGE

3. Place your seedlings outdoors for a few hours on the first day. Gradually increase the amount of time they spend outside each day.
4. Over one to two weeks, expose your seedlings to increasing amounts of direct sunlight and outdoor conditions. This will help them adjust to the changes in temperature, humidity, and light intensity.
5. Keep a close eye on your seedlings during the hardening-off process. If you notice any signs of stress, such as wilting or leaf damage, reduce their exposure to outdoor conditions and provide more shelter.
6. Once your seedlings have been outside for several hours each day and show no signs of stress, they should be ready for transplanting into their final outdoor location.

Hardening off is critical to ensure the success of your outdoor cannabis plants. It helps prevent shock and stress that can occur when moving seedlings from a controlled indoor environment to the unpredictable outdoor conditions. By gradually acclimatizing your seedlings to their new surroundings, you increase their chances of thriving in their outdoor home.

Transplanting Cannabis Seedlings Outdoors

Transplanting cannabis seedlings from an indoor environment to an outdoor grow requires careful planning and execution. Follow these steps to successfully transplant your seedlings into their final outdoor spot.

1. Choose a suitable outdoor location for your cannabis plants by carefully evaluating the area. Consider such factors as sunlight exposure, soil quality, drainage, and proximity to water sources. Ensure that the chosen spot receives ample, consistent sunlight throughout the entire day.
2. Prepare the soil. Prepare the planting holes by loosening the soil and amending it with organic matter if necessary. Ensure that the soil has good drainage to prevent waterlogging.
3. Choose the timing. Wait until the risk of frost has passed in your region and the weather is consistently warm. Cannabis plants are sensitive to cold temperatures and can be damaged by frost.
4. Dig holes. Make holes in the prepared planting area that are large enough to accommodate the root ball of each seedling. Space the holes according to the recommended distance for your cannabis strain.
5. Transplant seedlings. Gently remove each seedling from its container, taking care not to damage the roots. Place them in the prepared holes and fill in the soil around them, ensuring they are at the same depth as they were in their containers. Tamp down the soil gently to eliminate air pockets.
6. Water the newly transplanted seedlings immediately after planting to help settle the soil and provide moisture to the roots. Use a gentle stream of water to avoid disturbing the soil around the seedlings.

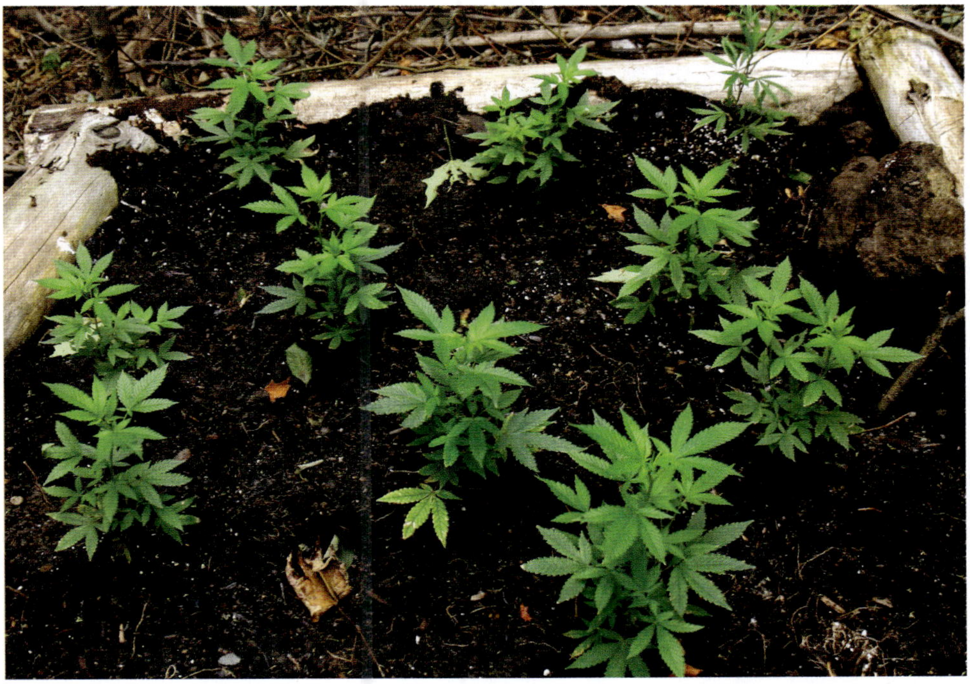

Squared off with logs to retain moisture, the spacing between these plants will fill with vegetative growth.

PHOTO: DAVID STRANGE

7. Add mulch. Apply a layer of organic mulch, such as straw or wood chips, around the base of each plant. Mulch helps retain soil moisture, suppress weeds, and regulate soil temperature.
8. Provide support. If your cannabis plants are expected to grow tall and bushy, consider providing support in the form of stakes or cages to prevent them from falling over as they mature.
9. Monitor and care for them. Keep a close eye on your newly transplanted seedlings over the coming weeks. Ensure that they receive adequate water, monitor for pests and diseases, and provide any necessary nutrients based on soil tests or plant symptoms.
10. Expose to sun gradually. If your seedlings have been growing indoors or in a greenhouse, gradually expose them to increasing amounts of sunlight over the first few days to prevent sunburn.

Advanced Transplanting

Transplanting involves moving a plant from one location to another, regardless of the distance. Your primary concern is plant health, with the aim of minimizing damage by keeping the plant and its root mass intact. Transplanting can range from simply moving a germinated seedling from its incubation cube to soil in a swift "pick up and bury" manner to relocating multiple fully grown plants over long distances. Transplanting

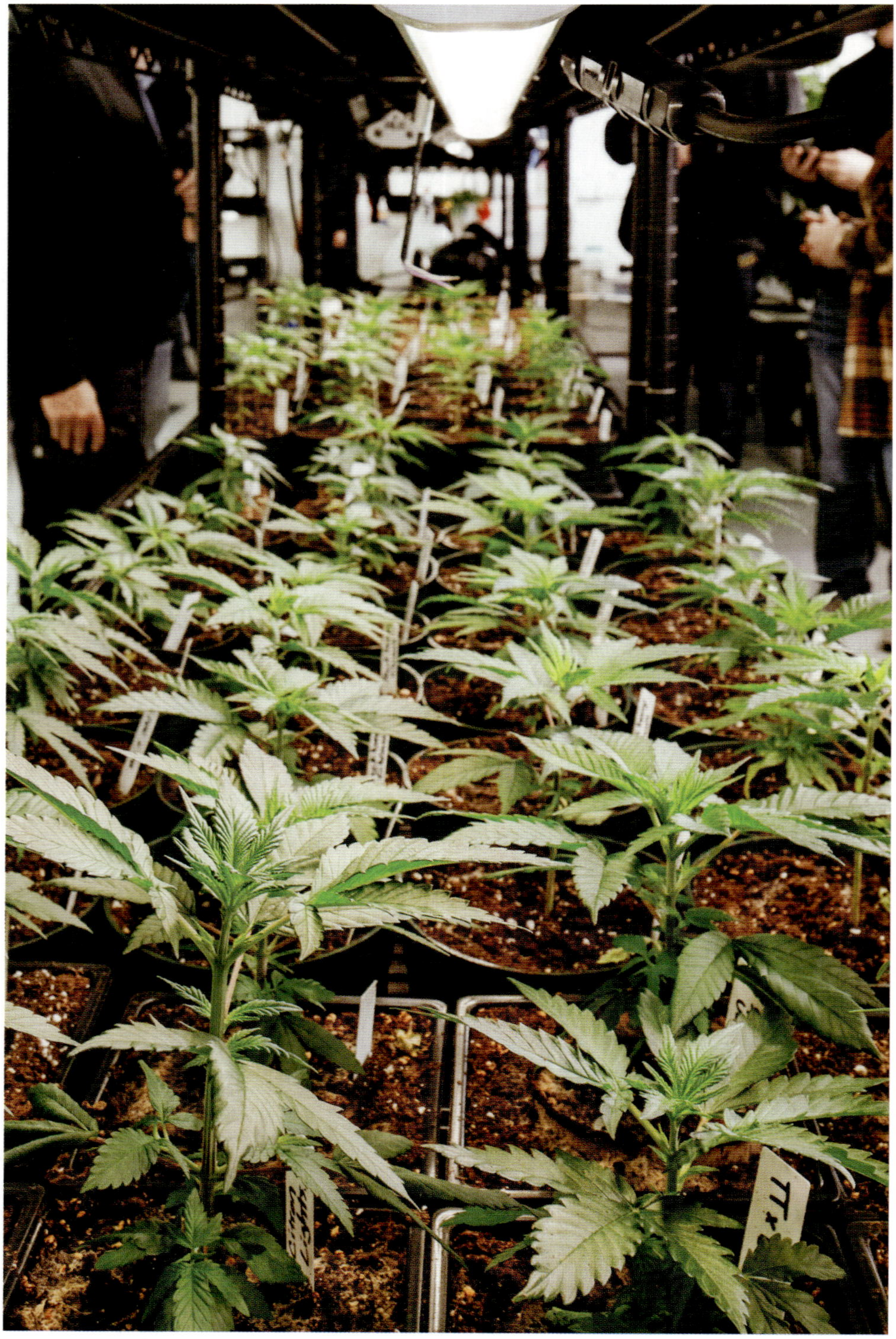

PHOTO: HORTICULTURE LIGHTING GROUP, HLG.COM

Cannabis is a cottage industry. These racks support rows of plants ready to be bought and transplanted to their new home for vegetative and flowering.

requires thorough planning and meticulous execution. While it can be challenging, experience will make it easier and boost your confidence in achieving a high success rate. If you have a choice, vigorous plants are generally better suited for transplanting.

Ensure your tools and containers are clean. For small plants, use a hand-held trowel with a pointed, scooped metal blade to prepare the soil. Specialized transplanting trowels are available at plant nurseries for those involved in high-volume work. It's crucial to prepare the new medium before proceeding with the transplant. Dealing with damaged or plants in need of emergency transplanting often reduces the success rate. If you are transplanting outdoors, consider weather conditions. Try to avoid transplanting on a cold, windy day. Plants moved from one environment to another, especially into worse conditions, are more susceptible to problems than those placed in similar or better conditions. The more you learn about these factors through this guide, the better you'll understand what matters for success.

Estimating the size of the root ball comes with experience; the size can vary based on strain and growing conditions. Hydroponic growers can often see the root mass and do not need to dig, but they should be cautious as these early roots, grown in water, can be more fragile than those developed in soil, where plants must develop stronger roots to push through the medium.

A pot-bound plant may develop a wall of roots around the inner rim of the container, choking its roots and causing stress. Transplanting it to a larger medium can alleviate this issue. Always mentally plan out your transplant and prepare the transplant medium in advance. The choice of transplant medium is up to you.

Plants nearing maturity with thick stems may require two people to support both the root mass and the plant itself during transportation. A canvas spread can serve as a stretcher to carry the plant, and will also come in handy during harvesting. Transplanting at later stages is less common due to the risk of transplant shock, which can produce suboptimal results. However, with proper preparation and care, transplants can be successful regardless of plant size and distance.

Transplant shock can occur for various reasons, the most common being root damage, plant damage, and overexposure of roots to the upper environment. Plants can also pick up pests and diseases if they come into contact with contaminants during the transplant. When transplanting multiple plants near each other, take care not to crowd their roots over each other. Proper spacing is essential to avoid undue stress and transplant shock. The wrong or low-quality growing medium can also contribute to transplant shock, as the plant needs time to adapt to the new medium before feeding can resume. Dealing with transplant shock will be discussed in more detail later in this chapter.

Transplanting with BudCups™

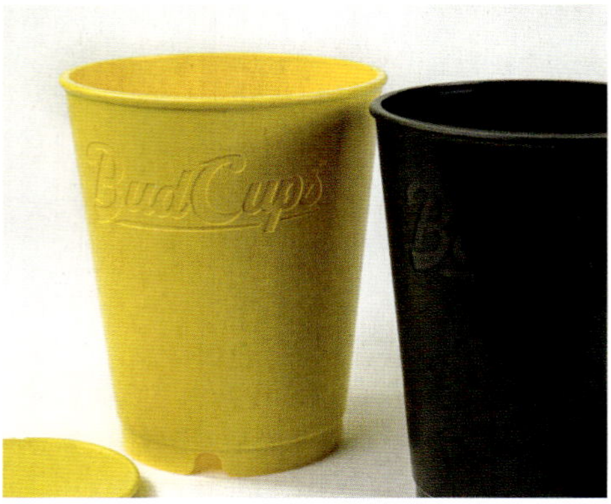

The BudCups are self-draining, easy-to-transplant pots that provide maximum rootzone growth.

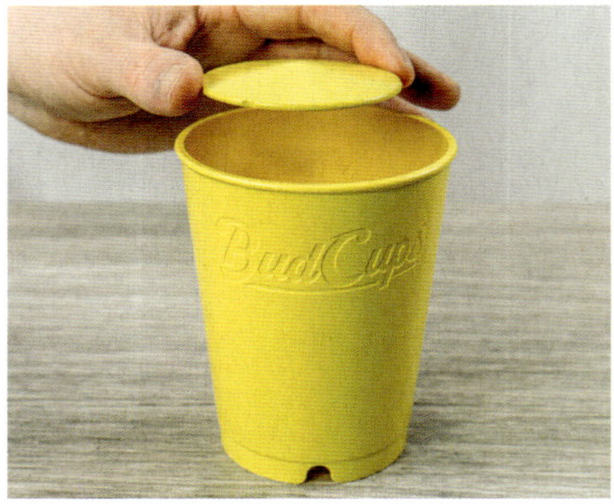

The first step is to insert the BudCups' bottom plate with the pointy side facing up.

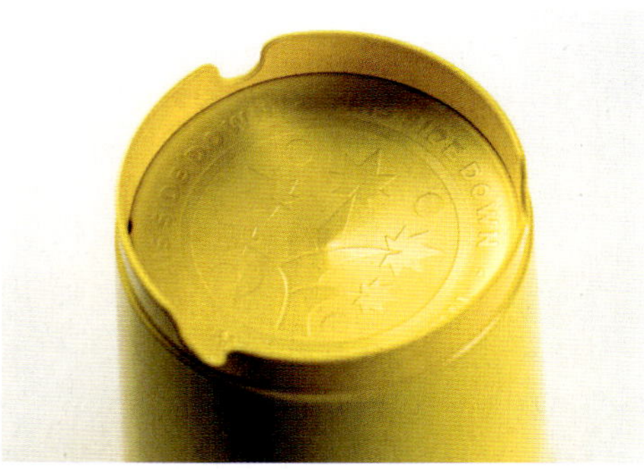

The BudCups' Triple Drainage mechanism allows for fast drybacks while preventing root rot.

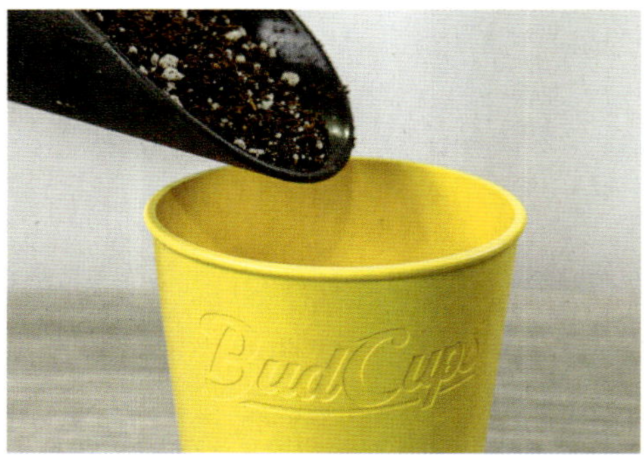

The second step is to add your media to fill the BudCups, about 16 oz in total.

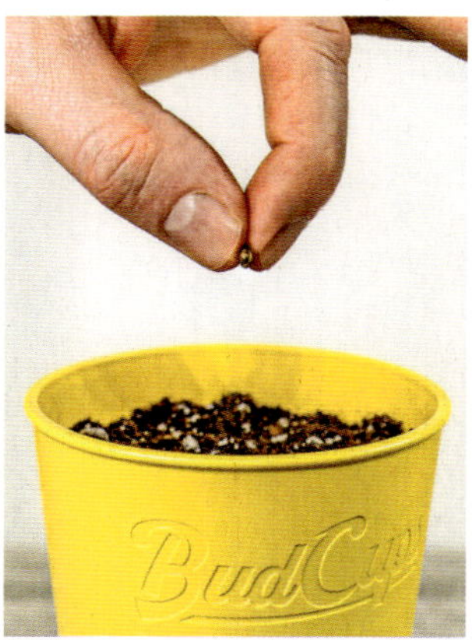

Plant your seed ¼ inch in and cover with media. Don't push or shake the soil down.

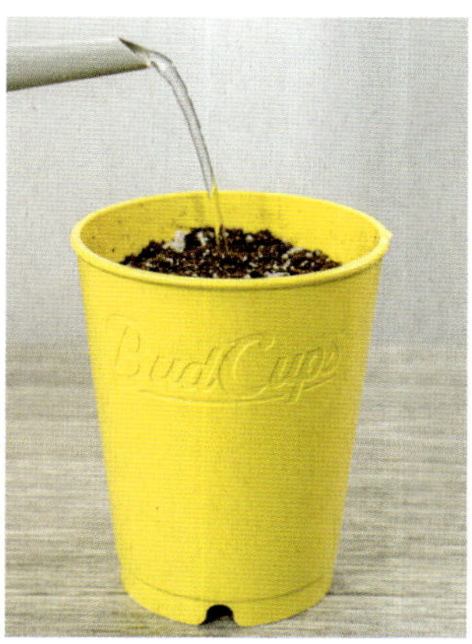

Water over 30 seconds until you see runoff. If needed, recover seed with media.

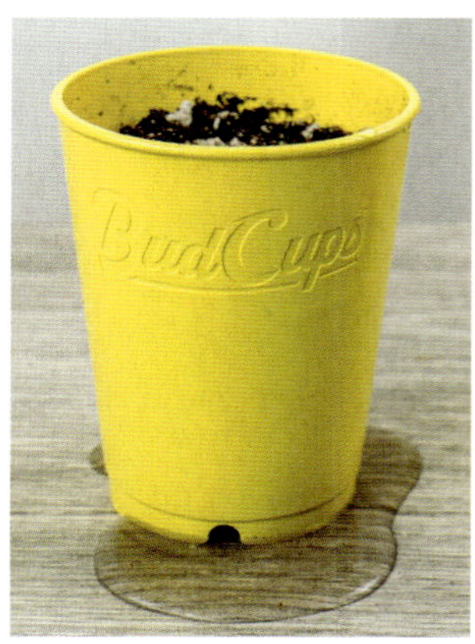

The BudCups' Triple Drainage mechanism prevents roots from sitting in runoff water.

PHOTOS: BUDTRAINER.COM

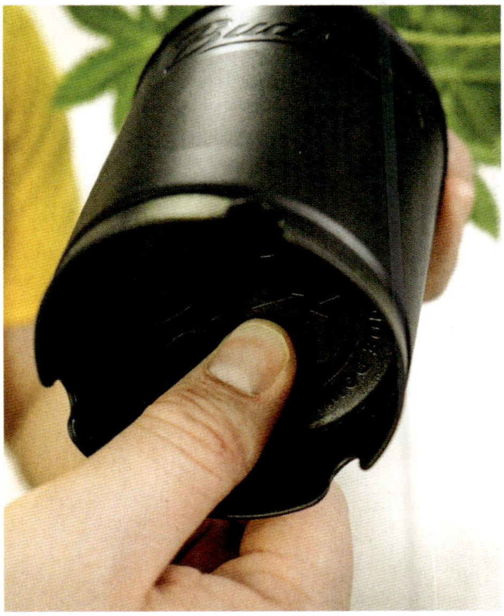

Once your seedling has grown 3 to 4 nodes (3 to 4 weeks), push the bottom plate of the BudCups to check the size of your roots.

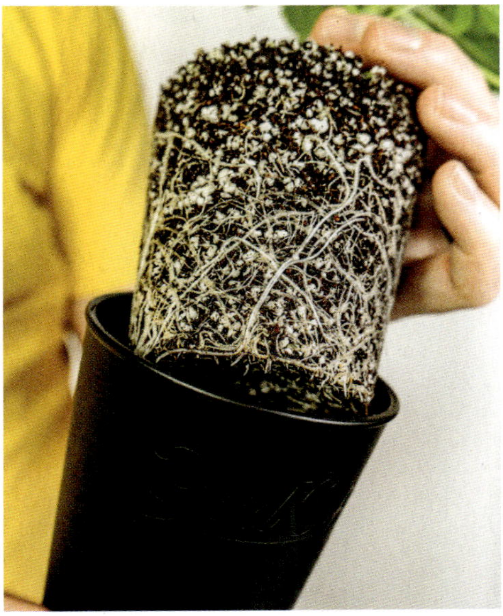

If your roots are well developed and touching the sides of the media, it is time to transplant your seedling into its new, bigger pot.

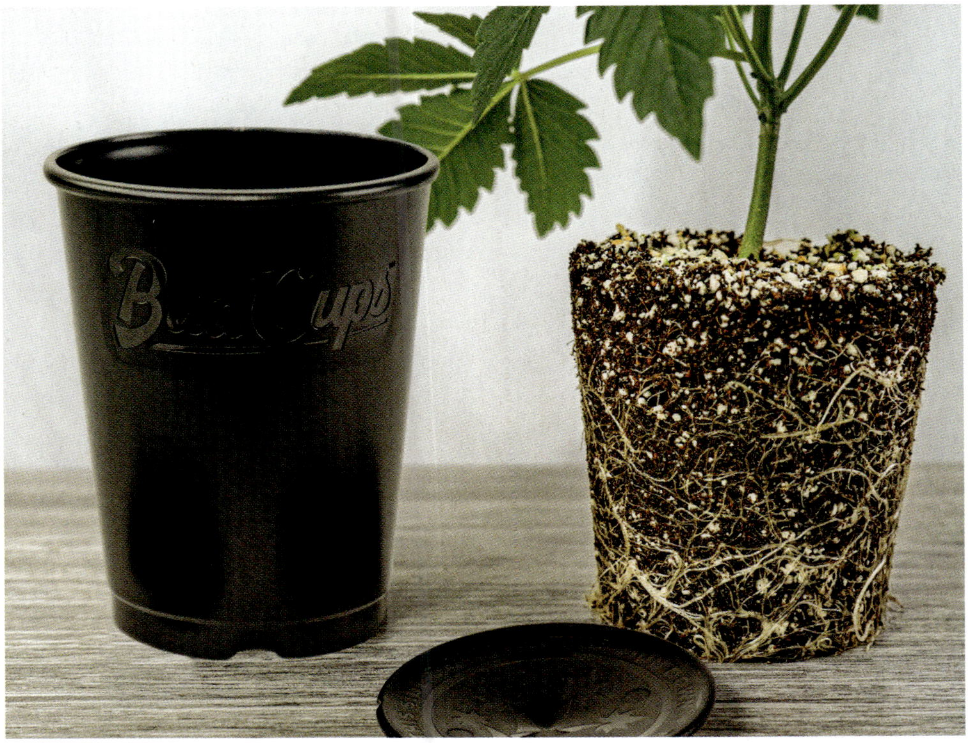

The BudCups allow your plants to be transplanted with no root stress, promoting a seamless transition into their new medium.

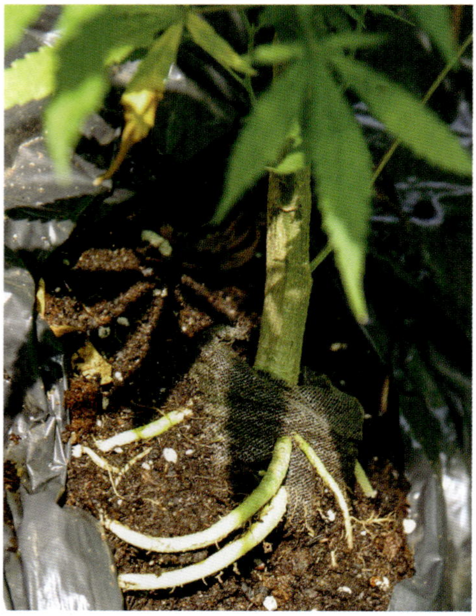

After harvest, you can see how easily the roots grow from a Jiffy or Rockwool cube. They spread fast and thick.

PHOTO: DAVID STRANGE

Under optimal conditions, cannabis tends to develop an extensive root system during the vegetative growth phase. If you observe the plant from above, the root system will approximately cover the same surface area. The lateral spread is similar, so the longest side branch serves as a measure of where the root tips will be. The depth will be around the same, and this area contains the mass of the root ball. Use a trowel to cut around the estimated root ball size. Be cautious and slow in this process, using your hands to gently part the soil and check for roots. If you encounter roots on both sides or slice roots, widen the cut accordingly. Roots can grow unevenly, so avoid damaging them as much as possible.

Once you've cut through the medium, you can lift the root ball out. Remove any roots attached to objects that could obstruct a clean uprooting. Plants with intertwined roots due to crowded conditions may pose this issue. If you can't loosen the roots gently, you can either cut down halfway or preserve one plant's roots by cutting away more roots from the other. After taking these steps, you're prepared for the actual lifting.

Depending on the root ball size, you may need two people to lift the plant, stabilizing the root ball with one hand and the stem with the other. Larger root masses moving over longer distances can benefit from being placed on canvas for transport. Transporting the plant sideways on the canvas is acceptable if the root mass is properly bagged.

The topic of root pruning before transplanting is a cause of debate amongst growers. Some believe the roots should be untouched; others that they should be cleaned and pruned to fit the transplant medium. While pruning may be necessary in cases of restricted transplant space, it's best to avoid it for now. Plant into the new medium and clean your tools afterwards. You can experiment with root pruning when you have the necessary resources and time.

Some growers prefer cleaning roots before transplanting, although this may not suit cannabis unless the root mass is small and undemanding. Cleaning cannabis roots can result in root damage, stunted growth, and even plant death. Root care is crucial for successful transplantation.

Transplant Shock

Even if a transplant is performed cleanly and quickly, cannabis plants may experience transplant shock. Healthy plants should recover; neglected ones may struggle. Transplant shock leads to delayed or slowed growth due to root damage or disturbance. To avoid it, maintain a firm hold on the soil during transplanting. Refrain from feeding plants suffering from transplant shock for at least one week, as shocked plants struggle to use fresh nutrients properly. The uptake mechanisms aren't functioning correctly, making them susceptible to nutrient burns even with low-strength nutrients. Feeding is different from using transplant and rooting formulas. Various effective transplant-feeding products are available, such as Superthrive, which contains the auxin NAA (Naphthaleneacetic acid), a proven growth regulator, and the vitamin B1, for plant health. Most transplant additives promote root growth. Some are in powder form, others are gels. While not essential, they can be beneficial for strains that don't transplant well. When using these products, always follow the directions and wear gloves.

Room Temperature Water

Cold water can shock transplants by rapidly reducing the soil's temperature. Always let tap water reach room temperature before using it on your plants. Similarly, when feeding your plants, prepare mixtures in advance to allow them to reach room temperature. Get into the habit of using only room-temperature liquids.

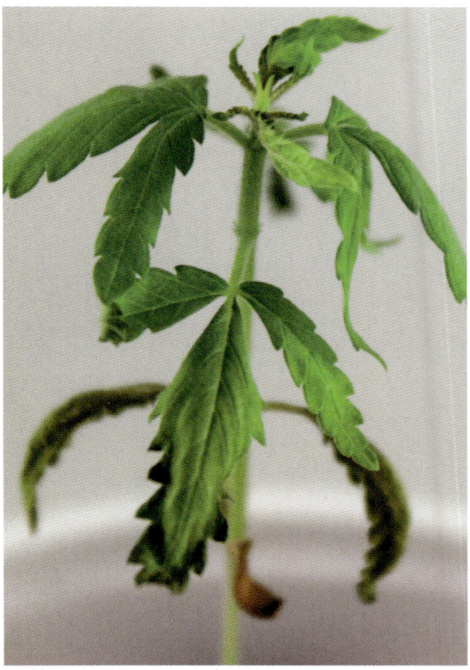

Leaf wilting during light times is a sign of underwatering or overwatering. Underwatering will show a spreading dryness at the leaf tips.

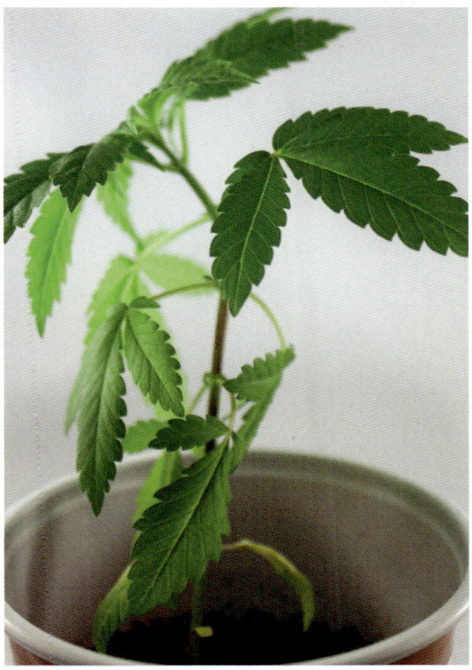

Overwatering will not show signs of dryness at the leaf tips but will show a similar droopiness and collapse.

PHOTOS: GCP

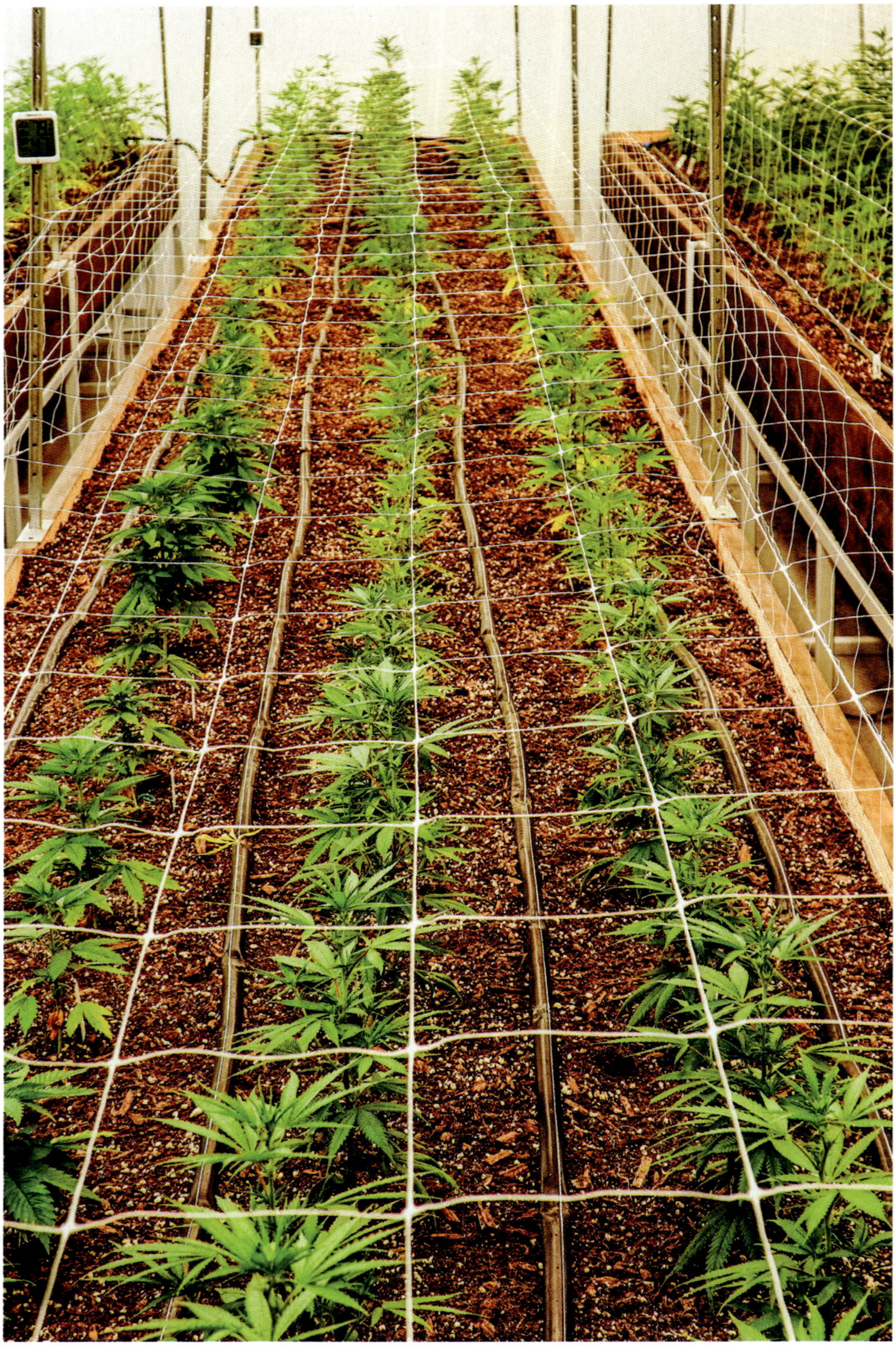

PHOTO: HORTICULTURE LIGHTING GROUP, HLG.COM

Note the irrigation system. Experience with your strain allows you to calculate the exact spacing between plants for maximum efficiency.

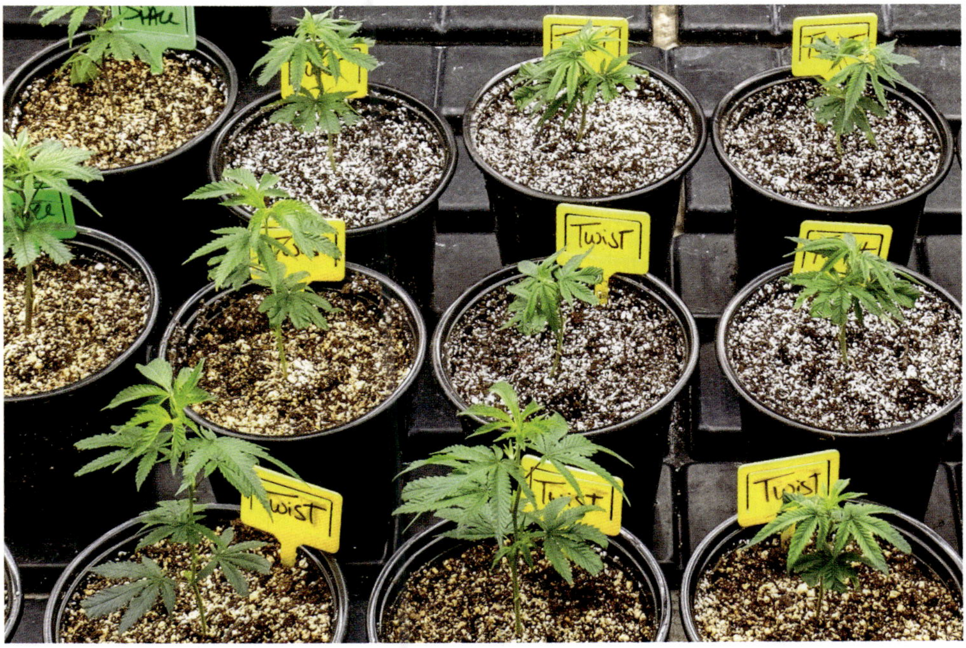

During the early phase of vegetative growth, plants can be bunched more closely because they are not very wide. However, this may change considerably depending on the strain and growth time.

Air

Plants require fresh air throughout their life cycle, even during germination. Stale air can change gas ratios and accumulate new gases. Avoid overwatering, as it can also interfere with air circulation. Roots rely on gases in small air pockets within all growing mediums.

Substrate Misting

Misting the medium to make it moist is a safe alternative if you tend to overwater. Misting is easier than watering to maintain moisture. If overwatering is an issue, consider adding perlite or vermiculite to containers to absorb excess liquid.

pH

A pH below or above 7 can cause problems. Test your medium's pH before planting seeds or transplanting. If you have a pH issue, it's best to replace the medium with something neutral (pH 7). If you can't replace it, pH-up and pH-down products can be used to adjust the pH. We will discuss pH testing and adjustments in Chapter 8.

So far, we have covered the history of cannabis, species, seed banks, and germinating genetics. Now, we reach a point where we must choose between two different growing methods—indoors or outdoors. Each method requires a distinct approach, and the decision will significantly influence your cultivation journey.

PHOTO: BONSAIBUDSRI.COM

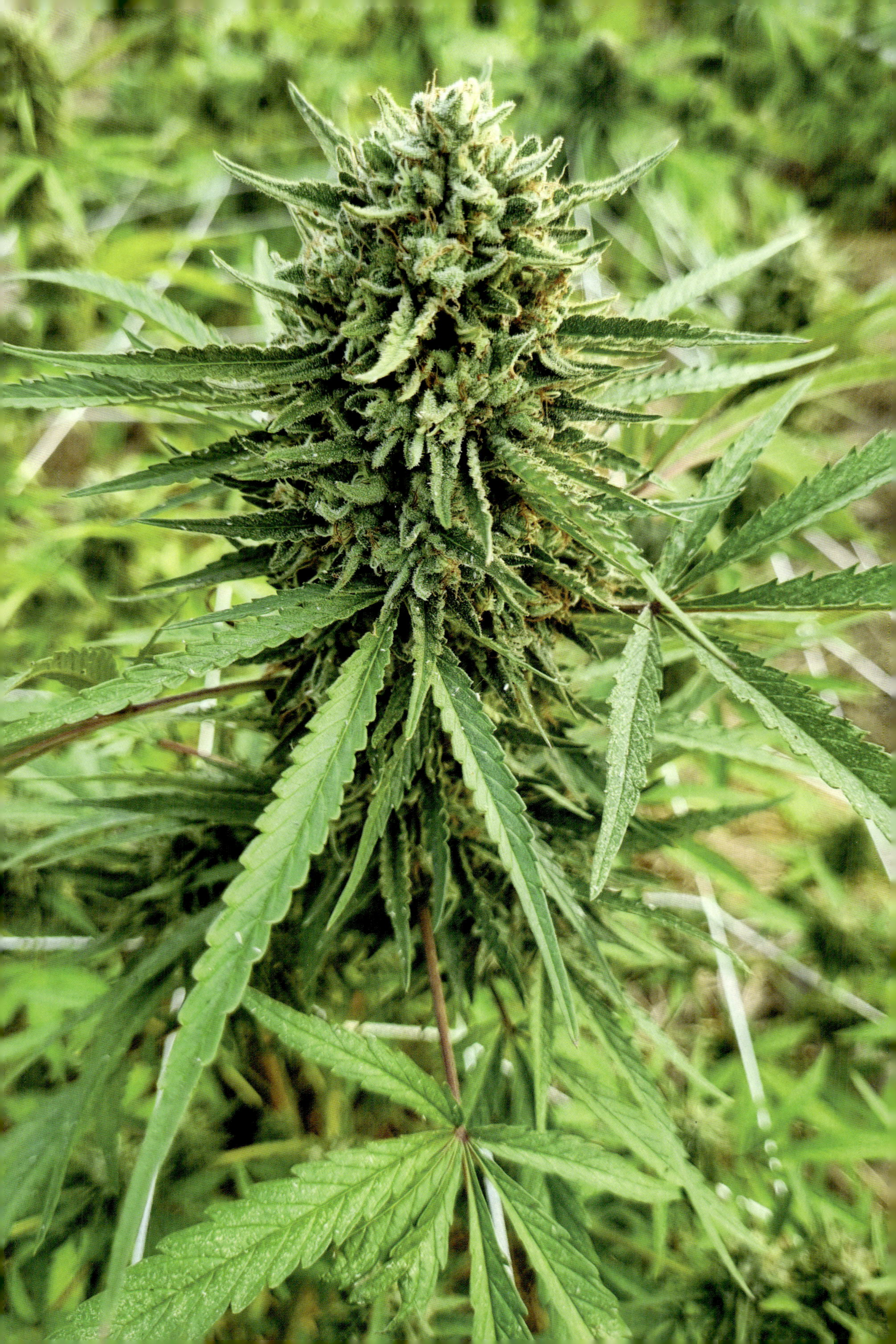

5

The Great Divide: Indoors or Outdoors

We have now reached a critical juncture in our marijuana cultivation process: The choice between indoor and outdoor growing. Even if you plan to grow outdoors, you should read the sections about indoor cultivation, as indoor growing encompasses a wealth of theoretical and practical knowledge that also applies to outdoor growing. In this chapter, we will explore the similarities and differences between the two approaches.

Sunlight

Next to selecting the right strain, light is one of the most critical factors to consider when growing cannabis. Cannabis plants have high light requirements. The intensity of sunlight varies, depending on the atmospheric conditions, time of day, and seasons. Light, which is covered in detail in Chapter 7, is measured in lux. Lux is defined as one lumen, or the total quantity of light over time, per square meter, and is typically used as a measure of light intensity. Light from the sun takes about 8.3 minutes to reach Earth and has an approximate value of 98,000 lux without atmospheric conditions. A clear day in North America or Northern Europe can get about 20,000 lux, while equatorial regions receive higher lux values. The amount of natural light is also affected by altitude, pollution, ozone layer conditions, global mean surface temperature (GMST), and volcanic aerosols. You can easily find mean temperature and weather data for your region online when planning your grow.

Sunlight and Glass

Success depends on the amount of sunlight your plants receive. Sunlight can penetrate a clear glass window, and your plants should thrive. However, it's essential to ensure the glass isn't tinted or stained, which can alter color of the sunlight.

Initially, it might appear that indoor plants under grow lights outperform those near

PHOTO: ED BORG

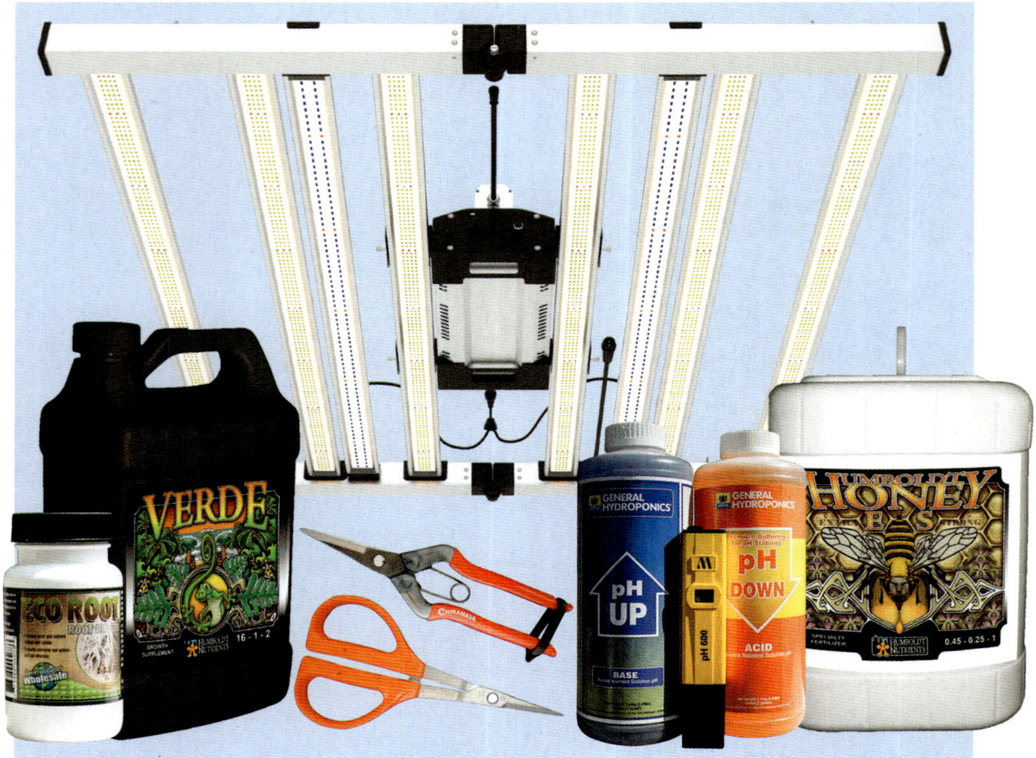

Lighting systems, nutrient bottles, pH meters, and pruning scissors are standard items in many grow rooms. Your plants depend on these items throughout their growth, so do your research and choose them carefully.

PHOTOS: HORTICULTURE LIGHTING GROUP, HLG.COM, HUMBOLDTNUTRIENTS.COM, STONED ROSIE, CHIKAMASA

Cultivation Tools

Here is a list of essential items that growers will need for successful cannabis cultivation. You will likely accumulate these tools as you gain experience in cannabis cultivation, so you don't need to acquire all of them immediately.

- cloning gel
- fertilizers
- gardening gloves
- good LED lighting system for indoors
- nutrients
- organic pest control
- pH test kit
- pH-up/down
- pots
- propagation trays
- Rockwool cubes (Oasis or Jiffy cubes are just as good)
- rubbing alcohol (to clean resin from tools)
- scissors
- sharp knife
- small shovel or trowel
- soil/medium
- support stakes
- thread
- water source and delivery system

This list covers only the fundamental tools you'll need. You'll discover that growers often acquire additional items to achieve larger yields.

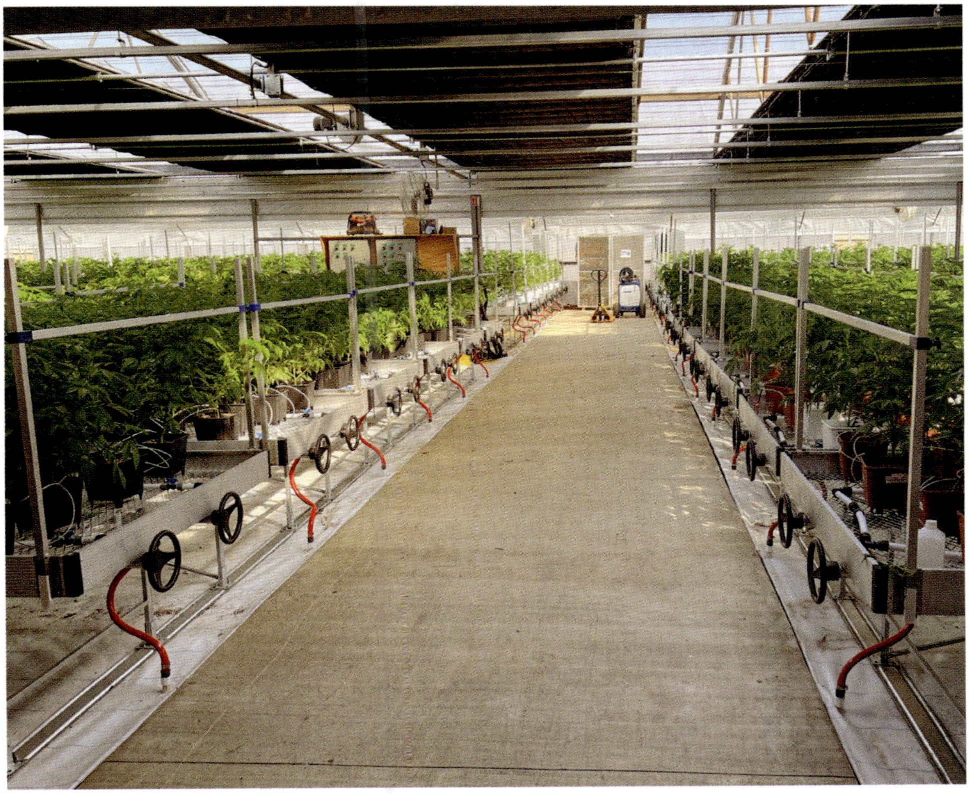

If the plants are from the same strain, the lighting, nutrients, and pH maintenance requirements will be the same for all the plants. Large grows are duplicated from smaller ones. This ebb and flow hydroponic system is an example of this duplication.

PHOTO: GREENHOUSE BY ISSAC PABST AND HENRI VAN DEN BOS

windows. This depends on the sun's light intensity at a given time. Growers in the Northern and Southern Hemispheres often find that the farther they are from the equator, the less likely it is that window cultivation will yield optimal results. However, if you have access to areas with abundant natural light, then window grows and glasshouse extensions can support successful growth.

However, most places rarely receive a consistent 12 hours of intense sunlight throughout the day, making artificial lighting more reliable. Grow lights can create an environment that closely matches the optimal light cannabis requires, leading to better flowering and increased bud production compared to plants relying on natural light through clear glass.

If you choose a window grow, try to position your plant near the window that receives the most sunlight during the day. Keep in mind that you'll want your plant to receive most of its light during the flowering phase. Estimate when you'll have the best weather conditions and coordinate this with the flowering times recommended by the breeder.

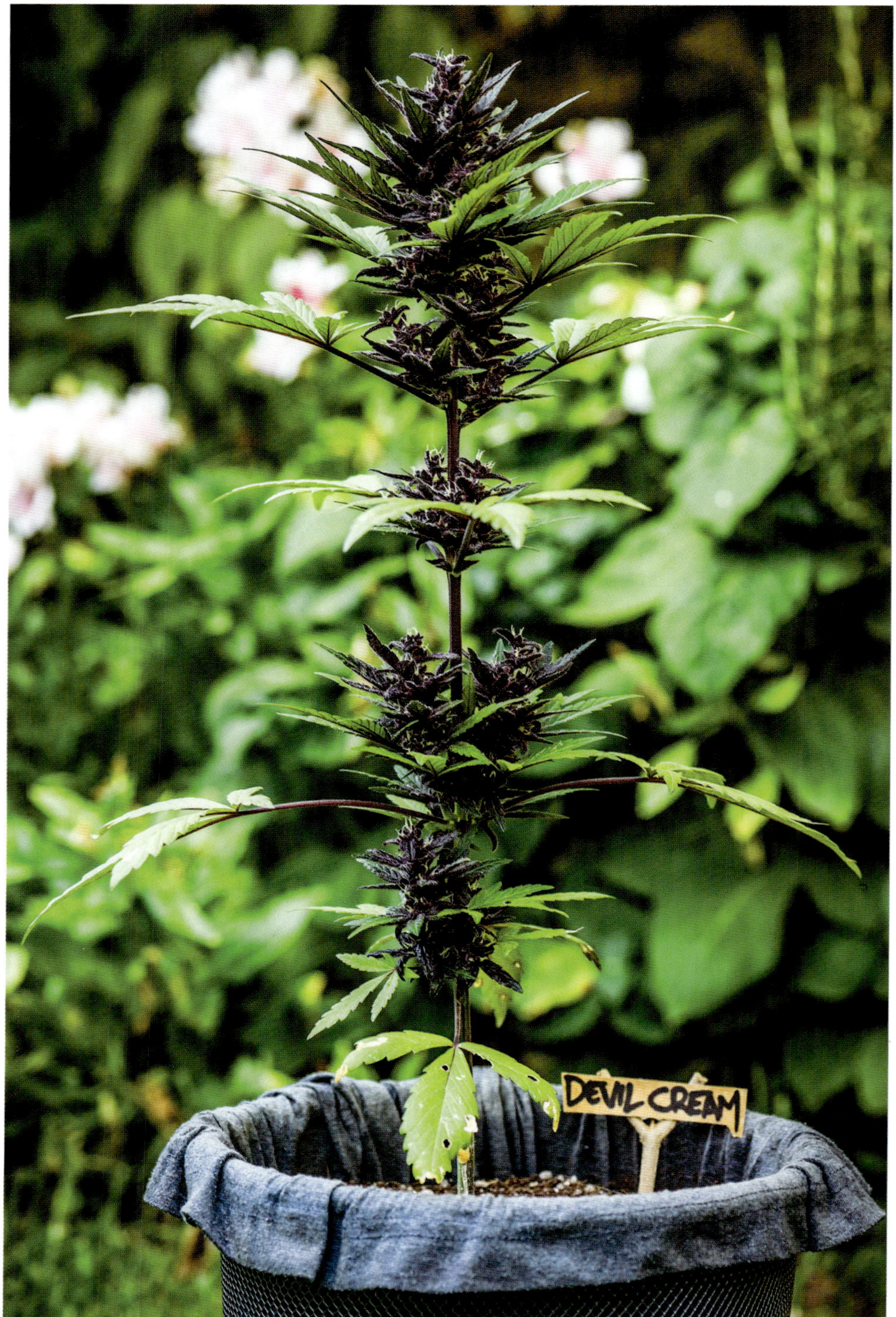

PHOTO: ERIC PALMER

Some autoflowering plants can reach three feet in height in just two months from seed germination. This hybrid comes from crossing Dark Devil Auto and Black Cream Auto.

If, for example, July offers the best sunlight, consider germinating your seedlings in April or May, or even as early as March. Outdoor growers also need to consider these factors while taking into account the 12/12 photoperiod recommended for flowering.

Indoor growers have control over their lighting systems. However, note that, while natural light is free, electricity is not, and some grow lights can be expensive to purchase and operate, especially in larger setups. Also consider privacy and security. People may notice your plant if it's growing near a window, particularly if it's a sativa plant that can grow large and conspicuous. Furthermore, while window growing can result in limited success, the results often fall short of a cannabis plant's true potential. You should weigh all these factors when deciding between growing in natural sunlight indoors and artificial lighting.

Some growers grow on a balcony, so the plant spends the day outdoors and is brought indoors at night. This isn't classified as window growing because the plant receives direct natural sunlight outdoors. Greenhouses are similar, as they provide an outdoor growing environment protected from the elements by glass panes. If you're growing indoors, you might dedicate a room to cultivation—an attic, closet, basement, or spare bathroom—which will require artificial lighting. We will discuss in detail in Chapter 10 various ways to set up an indoor grow room.

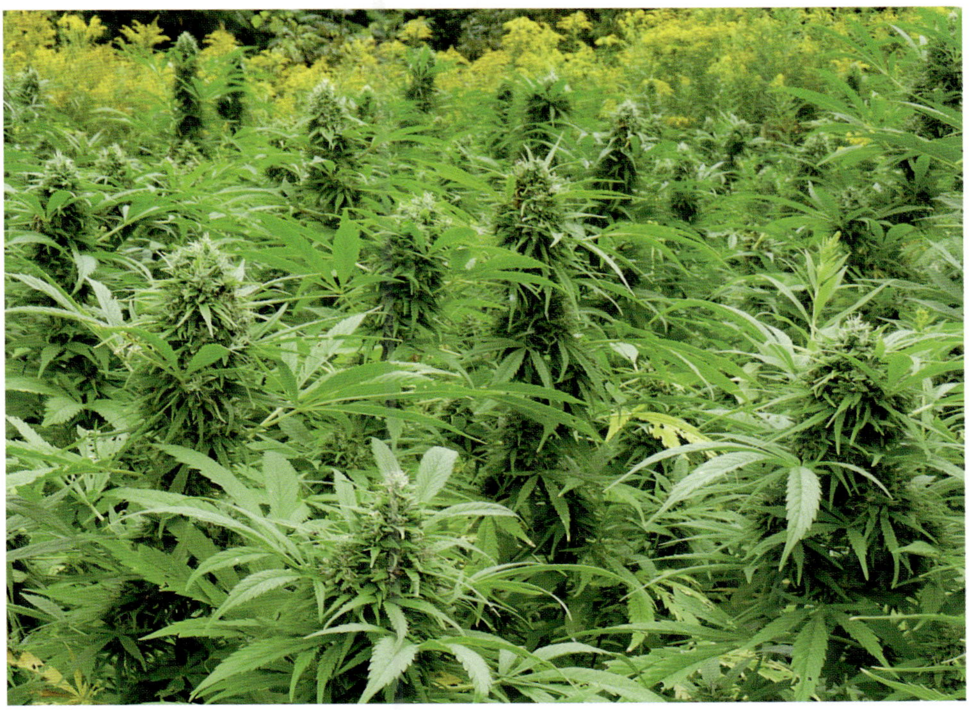

Outdoor plants get big fast and need sunlight and space to grow. Some side branches can appear as if they are the top cola. With all the extensive side branching, the grow may appear to have 20 plants when in reality, it only consists of 10 or even five plants.

PHOTO: DRGREENTHUMB.COM

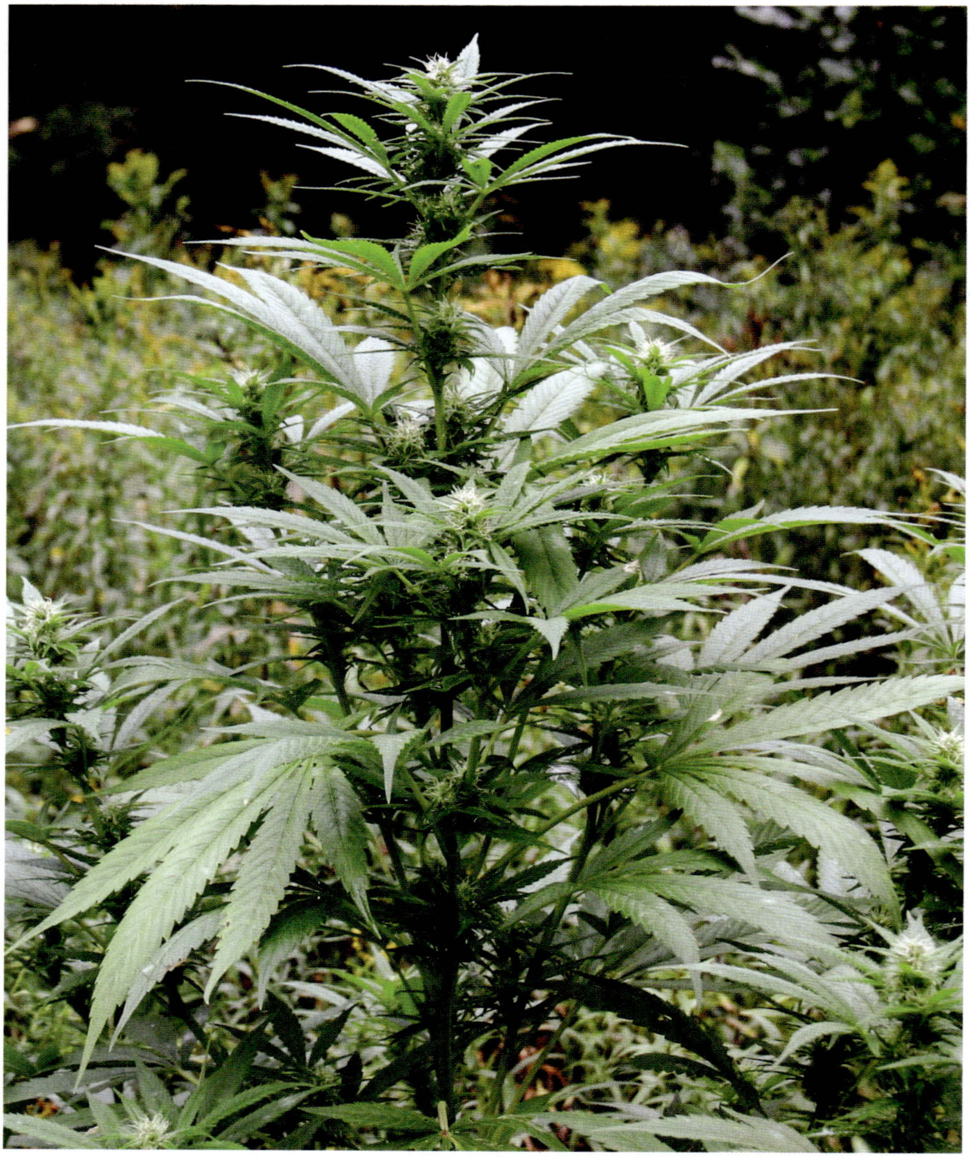

A single plant growing outdoors in a remote natural area can blend in well with its surroundings. This particular flowering plant demonstrates significant healthy growth

PHOTO: DAVID STRANGE

Outdoor Growing

There are two types of outdoor growing: Growing on your own property and guerrilla farming away from your property, such as in public areas. Regardless of whether you're growing on your own property or in a more discreet location, your grow patch requires careful preparation and regular maintenance. Simply planting seeds in the soil and returning months later is unlikely to yield favorable results. To begin the process, you have two essential tasks to do on your grow patch: Weeding and digging.

Planning for Outdoor Growing and Guerrilla Farming

Security is the primary concern when it comes to outdoor growing, as your grow area must remain discreet and secure to protect from thieves and prying eyes. Some experienced thieves may even target your grow for their supply.

One effective cost-efficient and low-profile method to conceal an outdoor garden is to intersperse cannabis plants with other types of plants that can act as camouflage. If you live in a remote area, you can also consider growing your cannabis plants within a brick enclosure with glass sheets on top. This setup resembles a greenhouse, though without glass walls, and can be designed to look like a small shed. However, it allows light to reach only the canopy of the plants, resulting in limited bud production beneath. If you opt for a greenhouse, it's advisable to paint the sides white to prevent prying eyes. The white exterior helps reflect sunlight internally, promoting growth on lower leaves and bud areas, but reflects light away from the outside.

Guerrilla Farming

Guerrilla growing is challenging and carries a higher risk of theft. Finding the right location is key to its success. By planting in forests or on someone else's property, you avoid the risk of having cannabis plants on your own property. However, you put that person's property at risk, which is unethical and reflects poorly on the cannabis cultivation community. Instead, look for a secluded public area like a forest or hill slope that receives adequate sunlight. A spot near a river is ideal as it provides easy access to water, which can help your crop survive during dry periods. You'll need to balance security with accessibility, as a less accessible location is generally more secure. Take your time finding the perfect spot. Once you do, it's like striking gold. Finding the right strain is also important. Ruderalis hybrids have become more popular with guerrilla grows due to their autoflowering properties.

Transporting your plants for guerrilla farming often requires moving quickly. Many guerrilla farmers use grow bags for transplanting. You can use plastic wrap to tighten up any bundles when transporting them to their new location. Larger grow cubes are also an option, allowing the seedlings to develop further during the vegetative growth stage before they are transported to the patch. This approach improves their chances of survival. It's crucial not to let the plants develop too far beyond the early vegetative growth stage, as this makes transplanting more complicated and may hinder success.

Once you have a successful transplant, you need to worry only about secondary factors, such as light, security, and pests.

Security

Keeping your cannabis cultivation activities discreet is of the utmost importance. Avoiding discussions about your cultivation reduces the chances of security issues arising, but does not eliminate all risk. You can inadvertently reveal your growing operation in phone messages; acquiring equipment, seeds, or clones; and by the presence of strong-smelling plants. While it may be challenging to commit to complete secrecy, about 99.9% of security-related issues can be attributed to talking about your operation with others. The remaining 0.1% is due to inadequate preparation and insufficient concealment efforts. If you plan to share your crop with friends, consider methods that maintain secrecy.

Security is a concern whether you are growing cannabis outdoors or indoors. It's crucial to prepare for any potential security breaches to protect your cultivation area, especially in jurisdictions where cannabis prohibition is enforced. Some covert

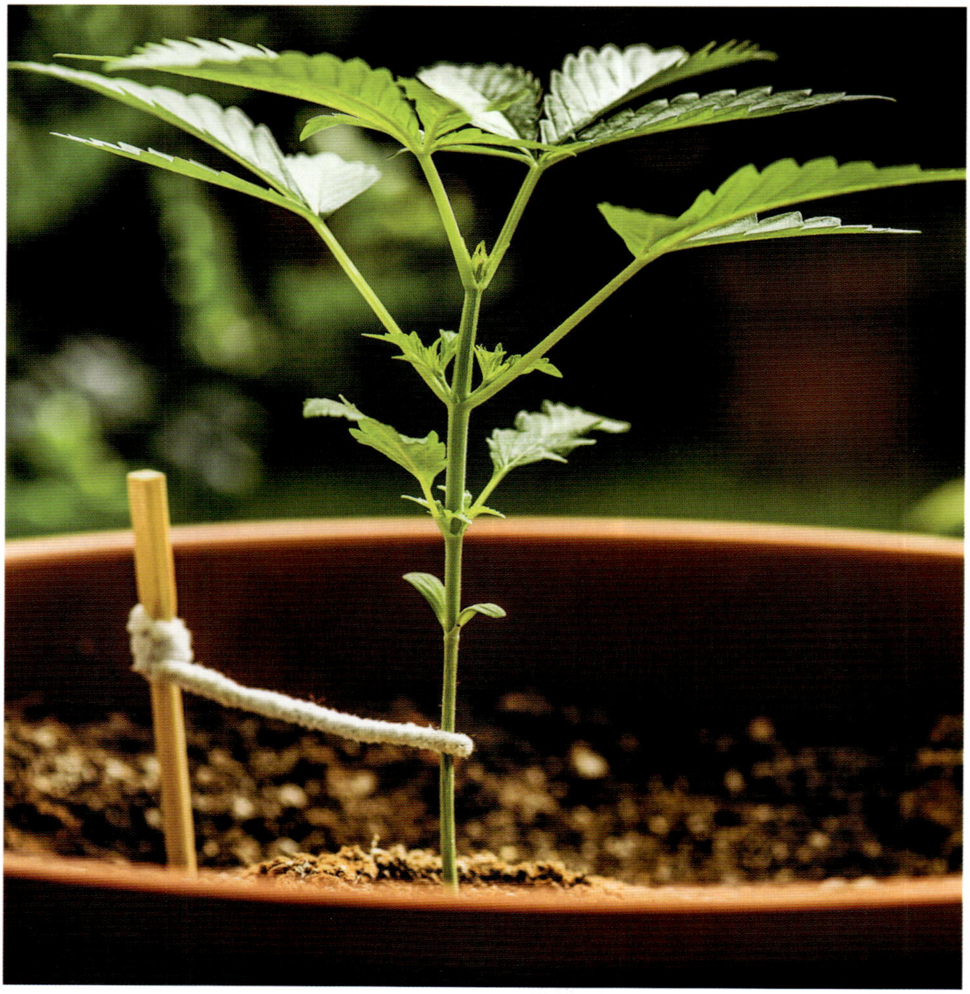

PHOTO: ERIC PALMER

Mini plant stakes and pipe cleaners are a great way to give seedlings the initial support they may need to stay upright. If you find your seedling bending to one side, this is a solution, in addition to bringing your light lower.

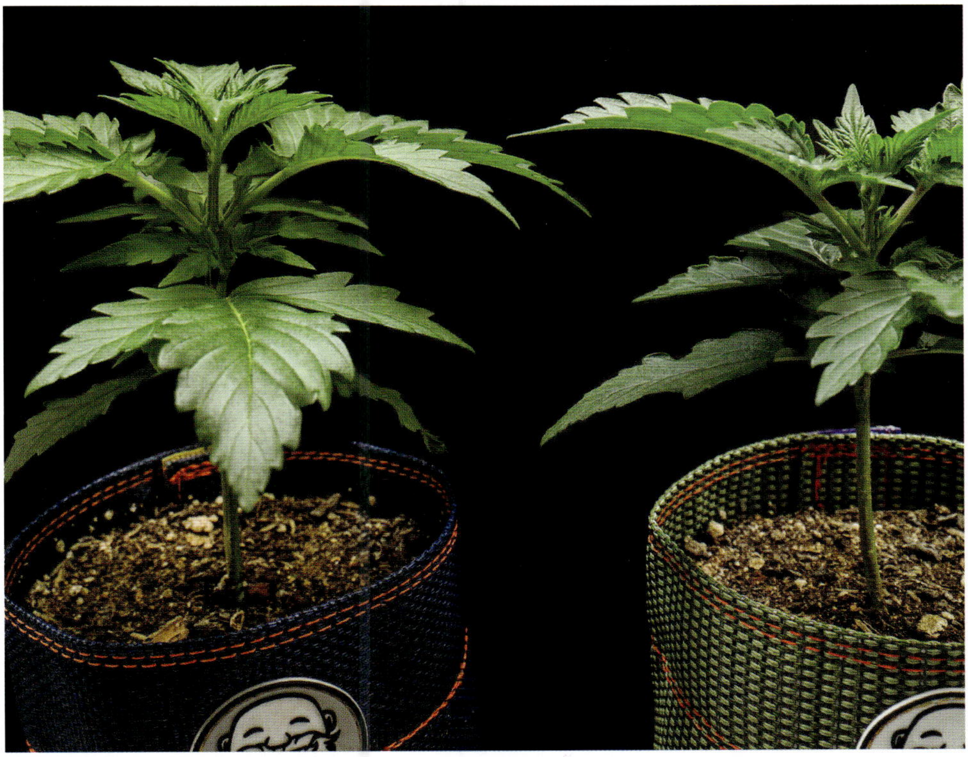

This is an example of seedlings kept squat because of their optimal distance to light. Stretching towards the light causes internode lengths to become overextended.

PHOTO: JOE'S CANNA GROWS

methods can lead to your detection as a grower. For example, a sudden and significant increase in your electricity bill may attract unwanted attention from authorities. Modern heat sensors can detect unusually hot attics, so it's important to ensure that your grow room doesn't become excessively warm. Another covert technique used to identify growers involves tracking purchase orders. While online tracking typically requires special court orders, in many jurisdictions law enforcement agencies can obtain these orders and uncover any suspicious purchases made using the same credit card or accounts. Unfortunately, many growers have been apprehended this way. To avoid this risk, try to make purchases with cash where possible.

Some agencies also track seed bank mail, specifically looking for incoming mail with specific stamps and envelope headers. Most seed banks have adapted by not marking their mail in this way to avoid detection and employ effective stealth techniques to ensure safe delivery. If a seed bank you're considering still uses identifiable mail, choose a different one. Maximum security precautions entail purchasing all your growing tools and equipment using cash and obtaining your seeds from a reputable seed bank that prioritizes discreet and secure shipping methods. Most importantly, never have seeds sent directly to your grow area.

No one can be completely immune from security concerns until cannabis is decriminalized worldwide. Cannabis is just a plant, and growers shouldn't have to resort to growing it in remote, snake-infested areas to enjoy its benefits. Until that day arrives, let's continue to exercise caution and be mindful of the potential risks.

Indoor Security

In smaller indoor growing setups, it's possible to move a small number of plants if needed. When cultivating cannabis indoors, be aware of short-term security issues, such as visits from service personnel. Experienced growers typically have a well-organized grow room that can be quickly cleaned and secured. In the event of unexpected visitors, they may have a nearby security closet where they can relocate their plants.

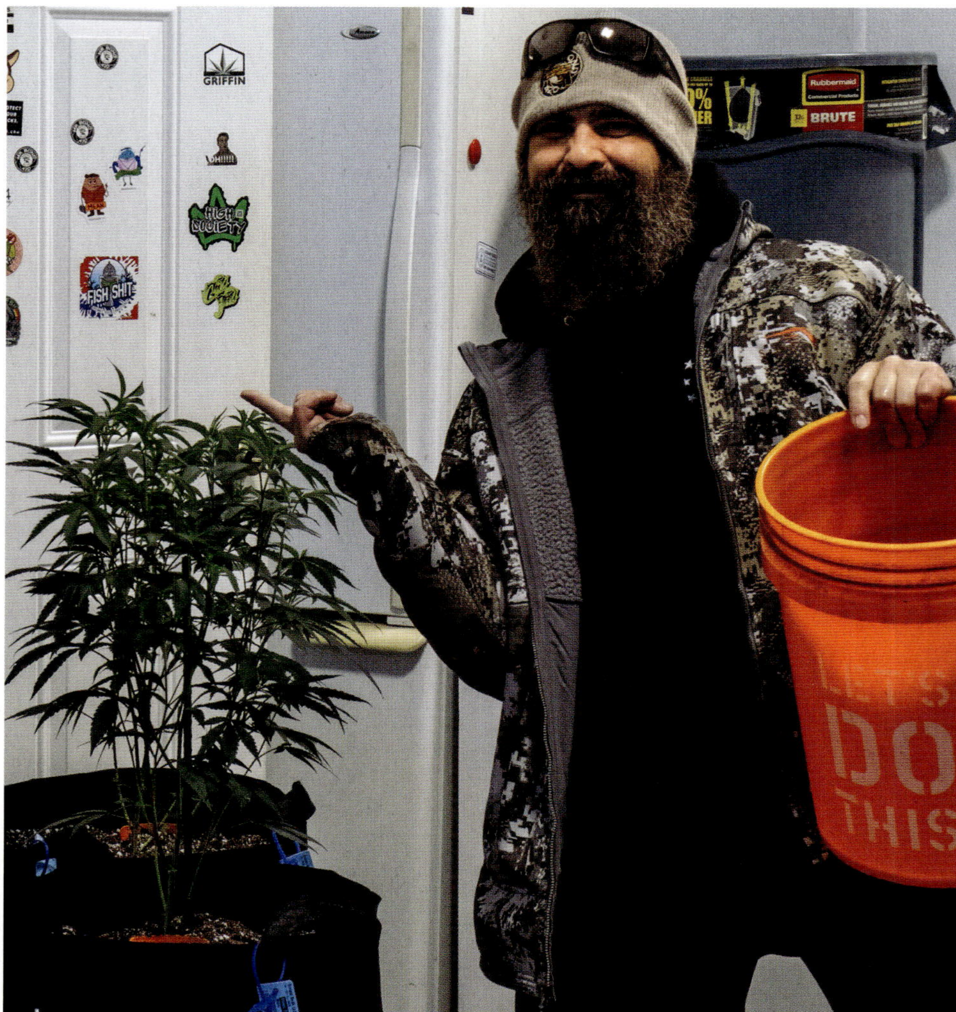

PHOTO: BONSAIBUDSRI.COM

Grow bags with handles make it easy to shift plants quickly. Here, they are moved inside a home for a fun photo op. These plants are in vegetative growth.

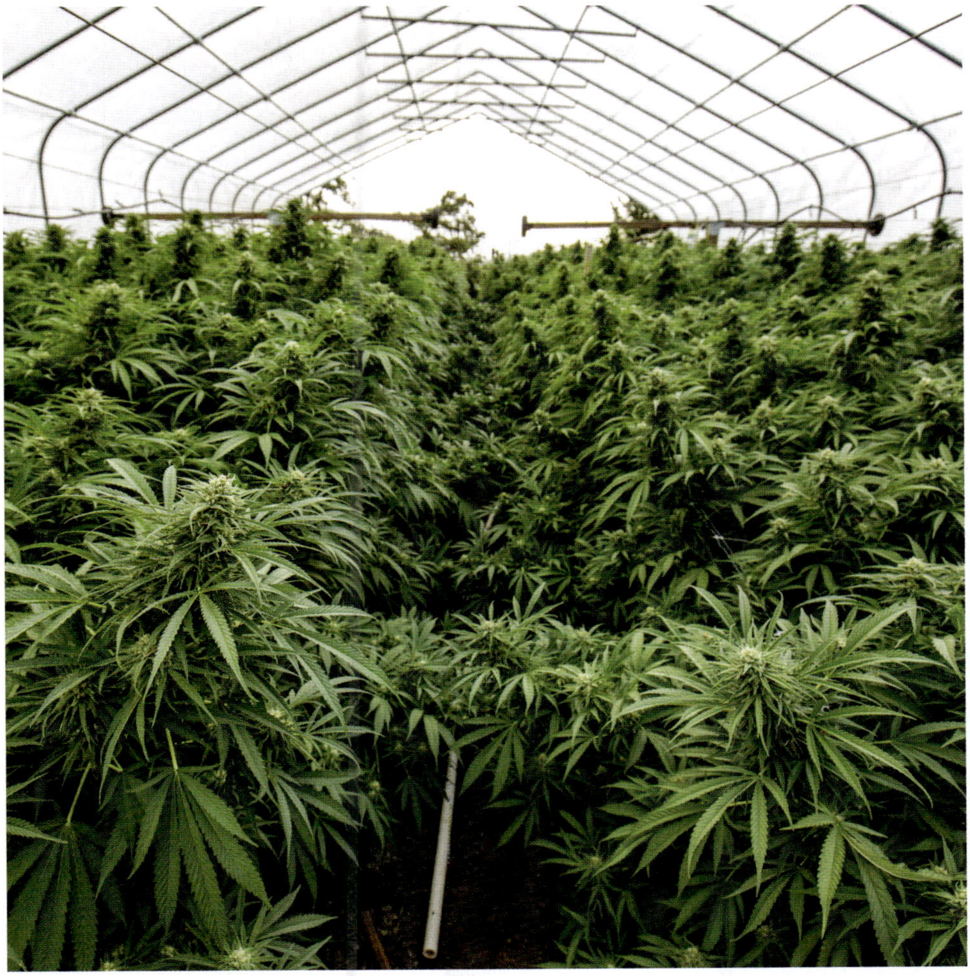

Some outdoor strains get so big so fast that a greenhouse grower must factor in their large size if they want to grow the plants without pruning.

PHOTO: DINAFEM SEEDS

It's advisable to keep your security closet close to your grow area to facilitate swift action. Using a bathroom as an alternative security area is not recommended unless you have another bathroom accessible to guests. For larger-scale operations, securing the entire setup away from prying eyes may be necessary.

Accidental walk-ins can happen when people mistakenly open doors and take the wrong turn. To maintain security, do not leave any grow-related items outside the grow area. Items like nutrient bottles, soil bags, or plant matter left lying around can arouse suspicion. It should not be evident that you are cultivating cannabis. If possible, load and unload items from your car in a closed garage rather than on the curb. Whenever and wherever possible, items should be locked securely. It's a simple step that can make all the difference in ensuring a secure environment.

Flushing Plants at the End of Flowering

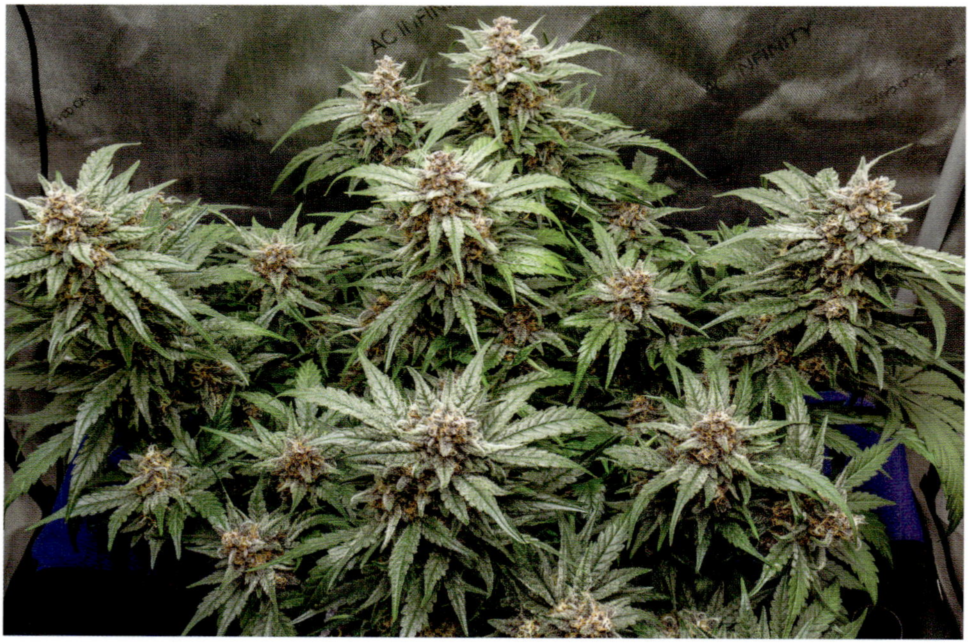

Flushing plants encourages the plant to use its internal sources of nutrients instead of absorbing more from the medium.

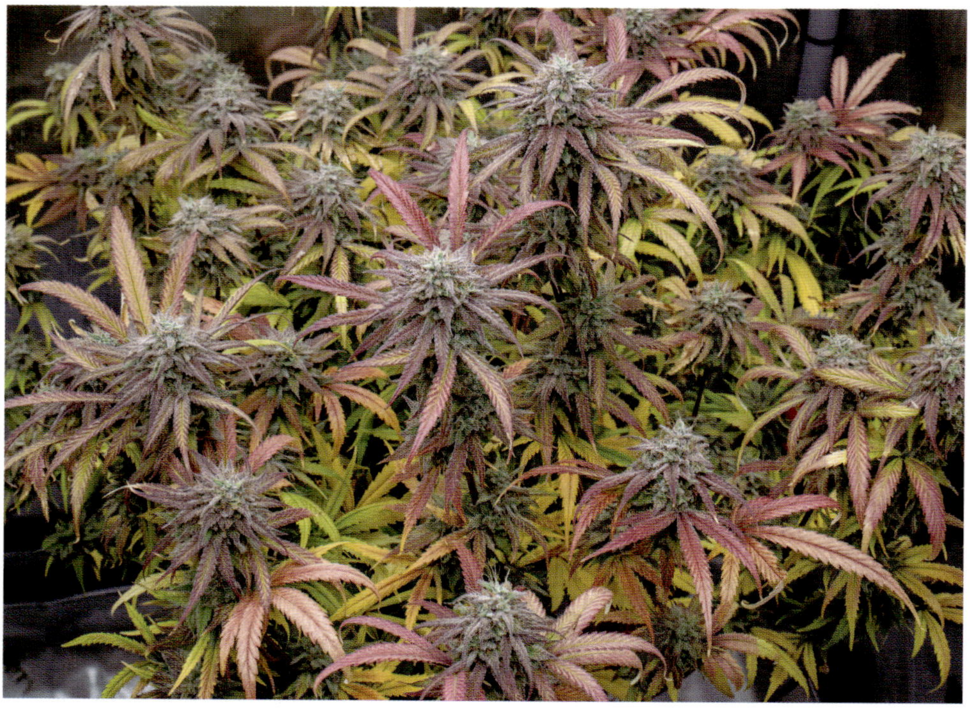

PHOTOS: JOE'S CANNA GROWS

Some plants will show colorful changes as they use up all their internal stores after flushing.

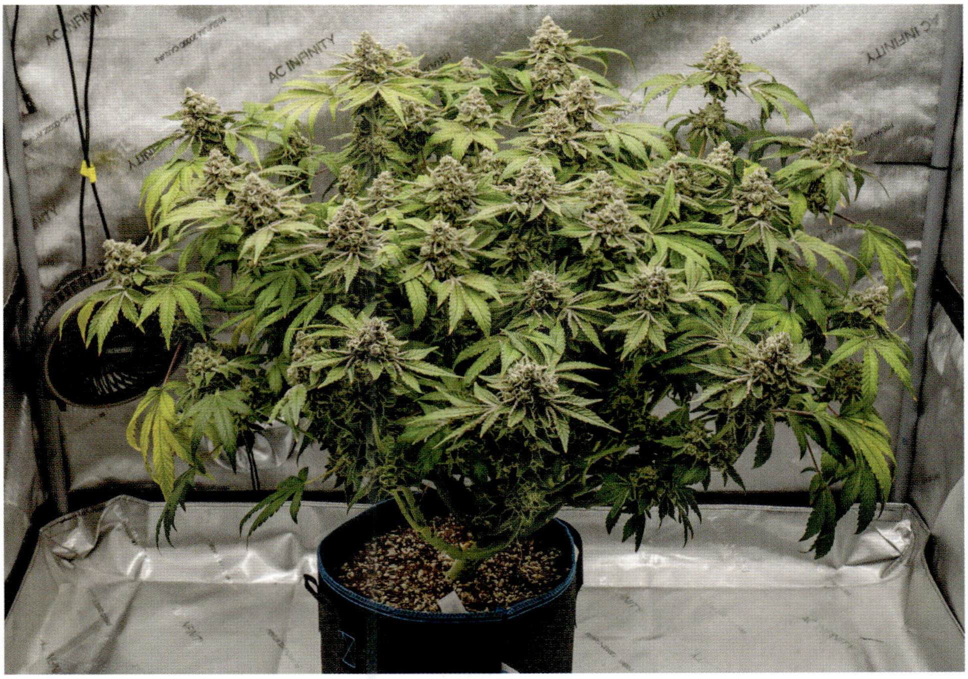

Some growers choose not to flush their plants and let the plant finish with all their chlorophyll.

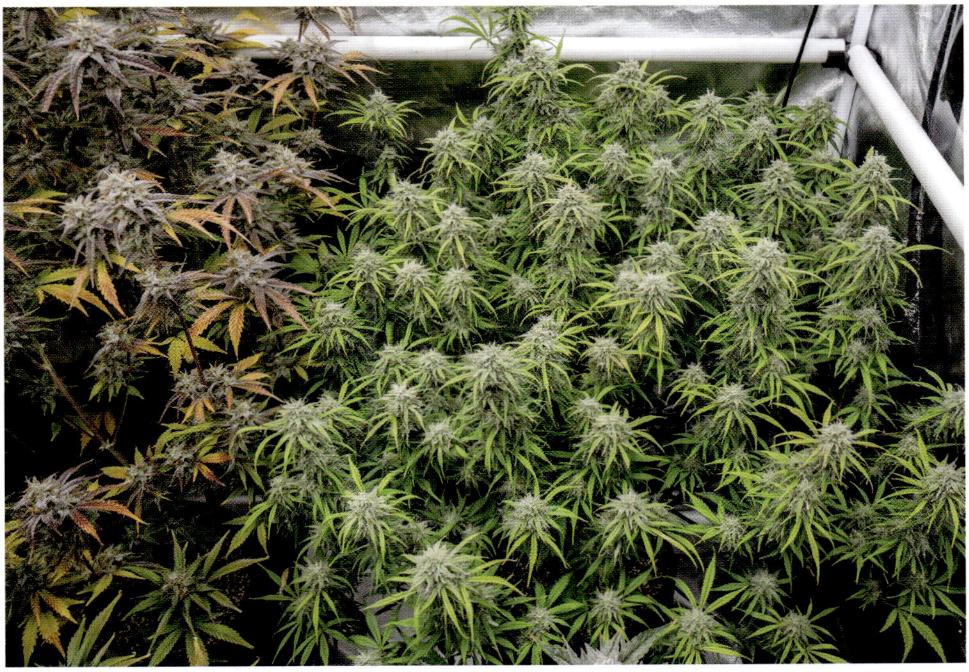

A side-by-side comparison of a flushed plant and one that hasn't been flushed. You will still need to cure the buds from both.

Never use butane extraction or similar explosive methods near your grow area, as accidents can compromise your grow operation. Safer and more efficient extraction methods, such as subcritical fluid extraction, are recommended. No one has the right to enter your property without a warrant and probable cause. You are not obligated to open your door to anyone without a warrant, and you have the right to remain silent until you consult with a lawyer. Authorities may cite the smell as probable cause, but you still have the right to take the necessary steps and seek legal counsel before allowing entry. These rights apply to everyone.

Effective odor control is important for indoor security. Some cannabis strains, such as Skunk, emit strong odors, especially during the flowering stage. In certain indoor setups, fans can help remove unwanted odors from corridors and high-traffic areas. Air can be directed through a window or a filter, typically a carbon filter, to another area where the odor won't be noticeable. Fans can also provide fresh air and simulate natural airflow for the plants. If you live in an apartment complex, it can be challenging to conceal the smell unless you have proper odor control measures in place, such as an extraction fan and possibly an ozone generator, which is available at most grow shops. We will discuss these odor control systems in more detail in Chapter 8.

Fires

Fires pose a significant security risk for growers, particularly for those cultivating indoors. Electrical fires are among the most dangerous. Subpar lights or fixtures can pose a genuine fire hazard. Get a fire extinguisher specifically designated for electrical fires, usually called Class C fire extinguishers. Note that before using a fire extinguisher on an electrical fire, you should shut off the electricity at the junction box. Preventing electrical fires hinges on using electricity safely and correctly. Never take shortcuts with lighting and electrical systems, as that can result in suboptimal results at least, and at worst, it can destroy your home and everything in it. Proper lighting systems, including budget-friendly options, will be discussed in Chapter 7. Moreover, your grow room should not be excessively hot. By following the correct procedures, you can ensure that the temperature remains within the optimal range for your plants while keeping your space safe.

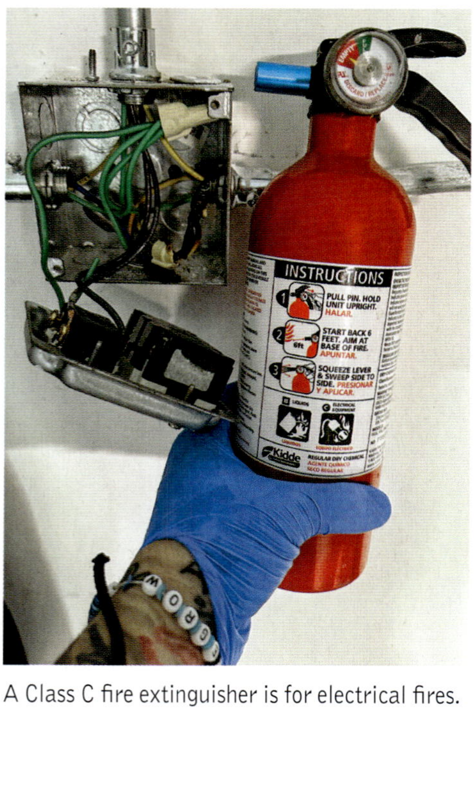

PHOTO: SHOPFREEGROW8.COM

A Class C fire extinguisher is for electrical fires.

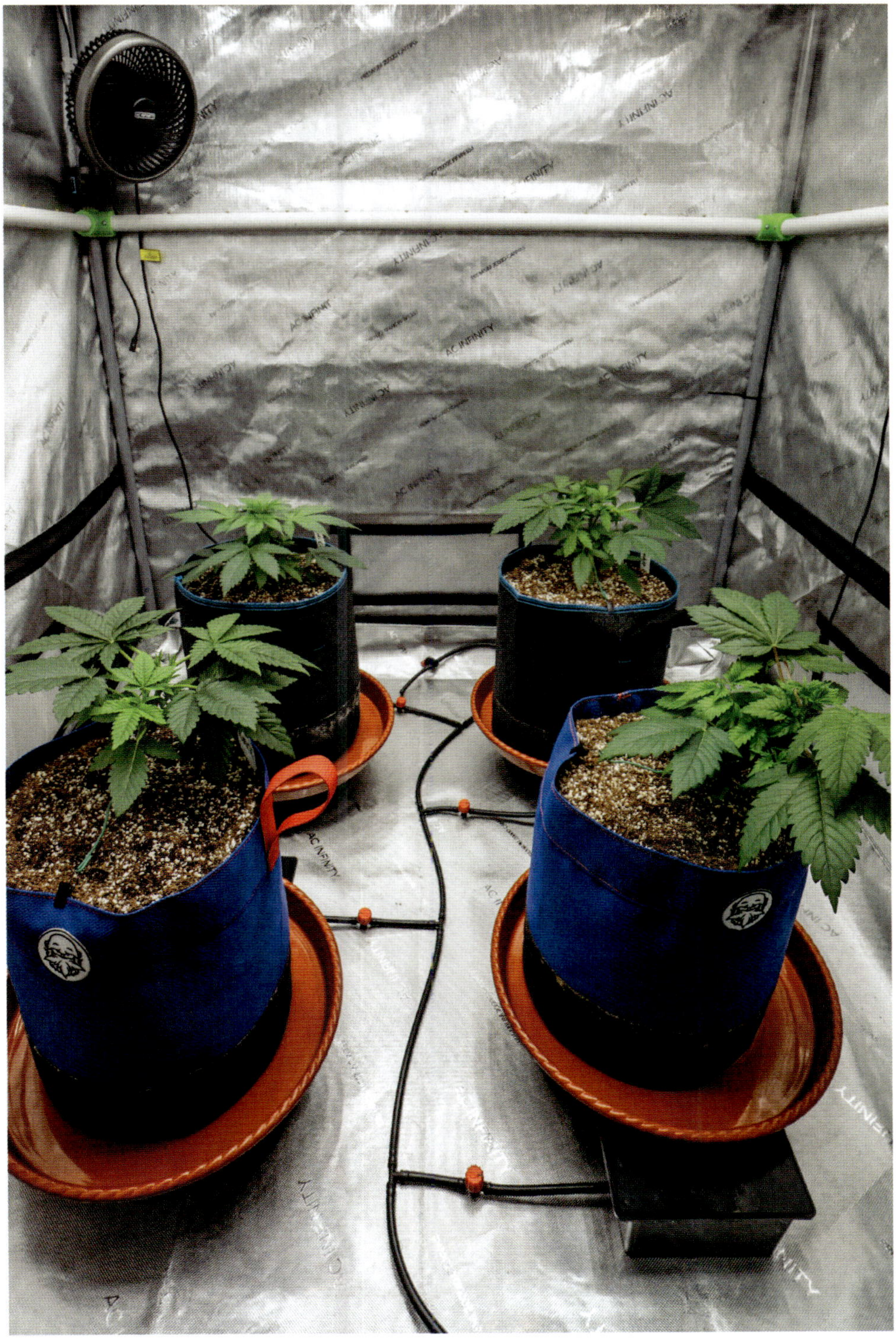

A fan in the grow room creates an internal breeze that encourages the plants to harden up and prevents excessive bending during flowering.

PHOTOS: JOE'S CANNA GROWS

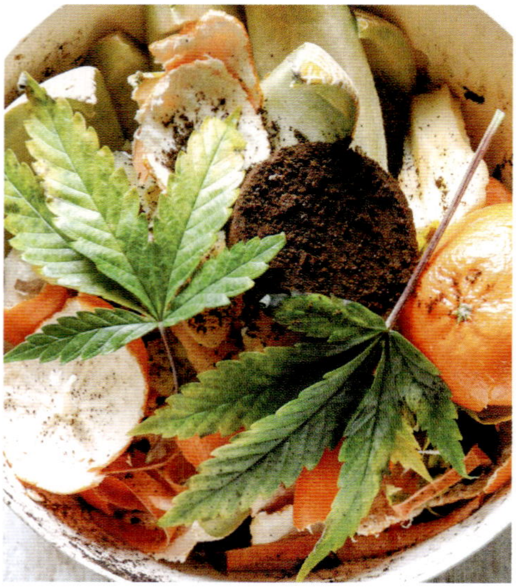

You can use many leftover items for compost, from foods to leaves.

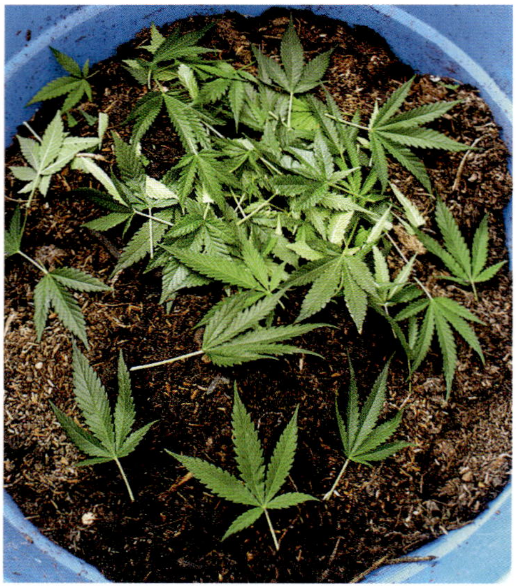

Even the cannabis leaf itself can be used for composting. Read the organics chapter.

Other Issues

When disposing of leaves and branches, place them in a compost container rather than your regular garbage can. This practice is not only more secure but also environmentally-friendly.

Maintaining computer security is essential. As the number of plants you grow increases, the risks also escalate. Never discuss your cultivation activities on your phone, whether through a call, text, email, tweet, or internet communication. While it may be tempting to share on social media, it's best not to. Because phones can be traced and triangulated, take extra precautions with your phone when visiting your grow operation, such as by using a VPN. If you have concerns about advanced detection methods used to identify cannabis cultivation, you can review various surveillance reports that lawmakers have made public online. The less attention you attract, the better. Thus, if you are growing in or near your home, it's important to be a considerate neighbor. Keep a low profile, maintain your lawn and garden, avoid anything unsightly or antisocial, and be polite and friendly with your neighbors.

Outdoor Security

The best way to secure your outdoor garden is by using a shelter. During flowering, cannabis plants emit a noticeable odor, which can travel a short distance depending on wind conditions and climate. To address this issue, many growers opt for cannabis strains with minimal odor. When contacting your seed bank, inquire about these strains. They should be able to recommend options with less pronounced odors, though all cannabis plants produce some level of smell during flowering.

PHOTOS: ED BORG

Another aspect to consider is how to harvest your crop quickly and discreetly. Standing under a small shelter and placing cannabis cuttings into large black garbage bags is not the most secure method. Using plastic bags is also ill-advised as they can easily tear and accumulate resin on the inside. A more professional approach is to use canvas bags. Growers typically bring a canvas bag to their garden, drop it over the plant, and then lift the entire plant, ensuring the crop remains hidden from view. It is advisable to use dark colored canvas bags, such as dark green bags, and avoid bright colors. Some growers choose to harvest at night, but using a flashlight in the dark can attract unwanted attention. Daytime harvesting offers better visibility of your surroundings and is generally a wiser choice unless there is a specific reason to do it at night, such as reduced activity in your area during those hours. The details of this process will be covered in Chapter 16.

If you are growing your plants outdoors without shelter and away from the general public, consider creating a protective enclosure for your plants. A chicken wire pen can be effective in deterring unwanted predators like deer. Predators are a significant concern for outdoor growers and will be further discussed in the chapter on dealing with pests.

Guerrilla Growing Security

Tracks left behind from your trips to and from your guerrilla grow area are a significant security concern. Hikers often explore woods and trails, and an obvious path may pique their curiosity. To maintain secrecy, avoid creating a visible trail when accessing your grow area. Even revisiting the same spot once every two weeks can leave a noticeable trail. Instead, aim to access your grow site via multiple routes and save the most apparent one for your final visit during harvest.

Struggling through dense brambles or overly sparse areas to reach your grow site can also leave a trace. When selecting a location, look for an area that strikes a balance between dense and sparse vegetation.

Some guerrilla farmers grow cannabis in baskets suspended from trees hidden from public view. If well camouflaged, these baskets can be used discreetly. However, growing in hanging baskets requires prior experience. Creating them is relatively straightforward. You'll need a 3-gallon wire hanging basket, a plastic garbage bag or grow bag that fits inside the basket, and some wire. After lining the basket with these bags, lightly perforate the bottom of both the basket and the bag to allow for drainage. If possible, use biodegradable bags and ensure the bag is entirely covered by soil. Fill the basket with soil, transplant your seedling, and hang this basket high on a tree branch. Hanging baskets are best used with slow-release fertilizers, such as granular foods, which store nutrients in the soil throughout the plant's growth cycle and allow for less frequent feeding. You should rely on rain for watering where possible to minimize the need for bringing the baskets down. Balancing workload versus output is essential, as infrequent

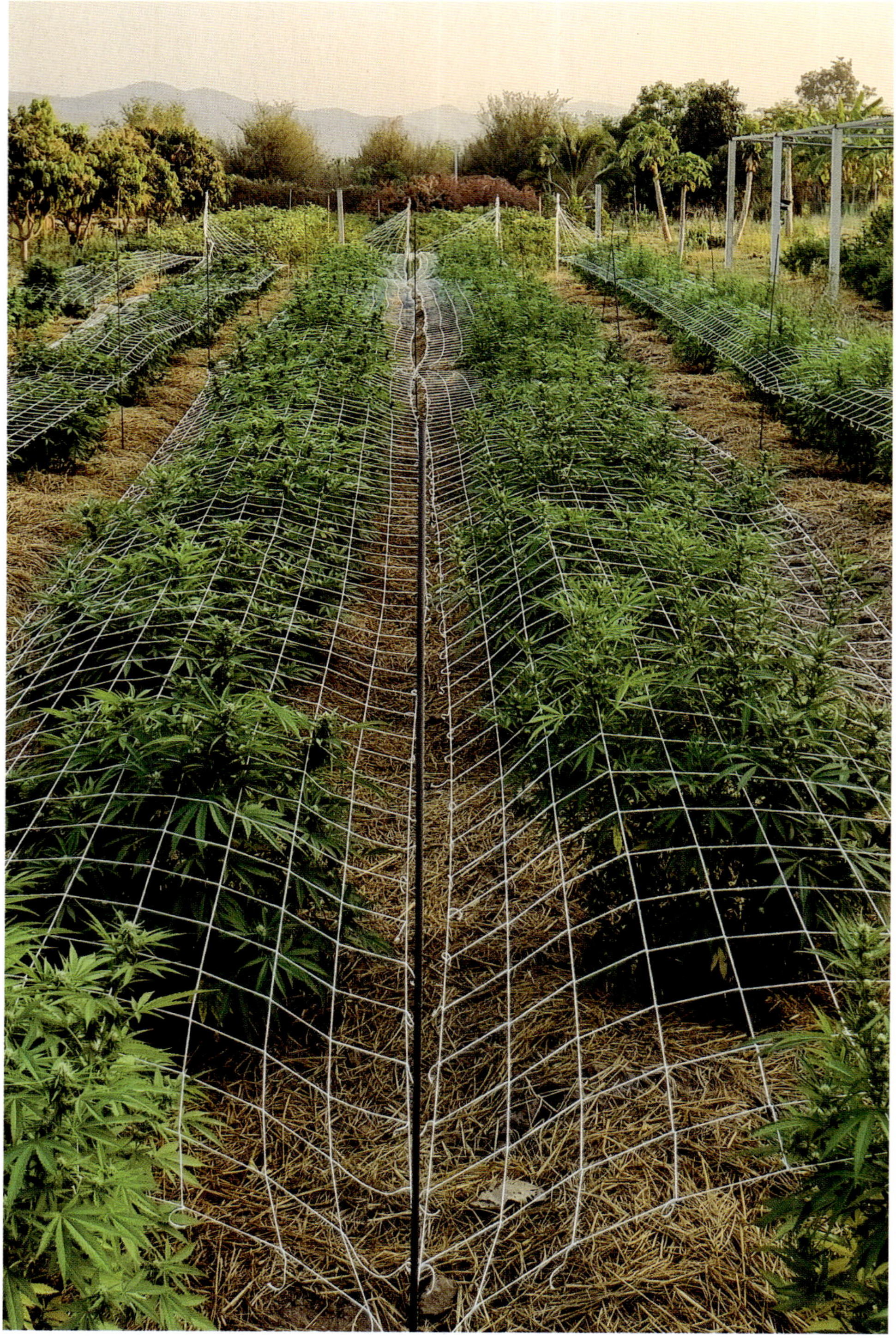

PHOTO: ED BORG

Some netting is essential to keep larger plants from curving over too much during flowering. The net is placed on top during vegetative growth.

visits may yield suboptimal results, but more effort may lead to better results. Once you establish a system that works, you can continue using it year after year.

Vigilance and careful planning are crucial for maintaining security. Wearing gloves when handling your grow and tools is essential. Be mindful not to leave fingerprints on nearby buckets or equipment. Carrying fishing gear or birdwatching binoculars can give you a plausible excuse for being in your grow area. Keep an eye out for any suspicious individuals in the vicinity of your grow site. Generally, guerrilla growing is best suited for remote locations accessible to few people.

The riskiest time for any guerrilla grower is during the harvest, when you must transport your yield from the grow area to your home or another location. Always conduct this operation in the morning, as early as possible, and thoroughly inspect the area for any suspicious individuals. Pack your buds and plants into a canvas bag and place this inside a backpack. Before approaching your vehicle, discreetly leave your bag near a bush, cover it, and carefully survey the area once more. You may even want to drive for about five minutes to watch for any signs of surveillance or followers. If everything appears normal, retrieve your bag and hide it in your vehicle, in the trunk if possible, and drive home cautiously. Chapter 12 will provide additional guidance on treating your outdoor grow patch.

While some individuals engage in large-scale guerrilla farming, this is a commercial endeavor on a risky scale, usually occurring in regions where cannabis is prohibited. Growers in such cases often reside deep in remote forests, miles away from the nearest town, dedicating several months to cultivating large quantities of cannabis. This practice has become increasingly competitive and hazardous in some regions due to its prevalence. Remember that not all individuals involved in guerrilla growing are friendly, and some may pose risks to your security. Check local news sources for information on guerrilla grow seizures and any incidents involving armed individuals. Though this issue is gradually being addressed through decriminalization, it remains a significant concern associated with cannabis prohibition. Cannabis cultivators should never feel compelled to arm themselves because they are involved in cultivation, as this goes against the ethics of the cannabis community.

We do not recommend guerrilla growing for most of our readers, as it is suitable only for individuals living in remote areas with infrequently visited land. However, if you have the right environment and can execute it without stress, it can complement your indoor or outdoor cultivation plans. Furthermore, even if you don't use cannabis personally, reintroducing cannabis to the wild can be a valuable contribution and can provide birds and other organisms with seeds and a source of sustenance for generations to come.

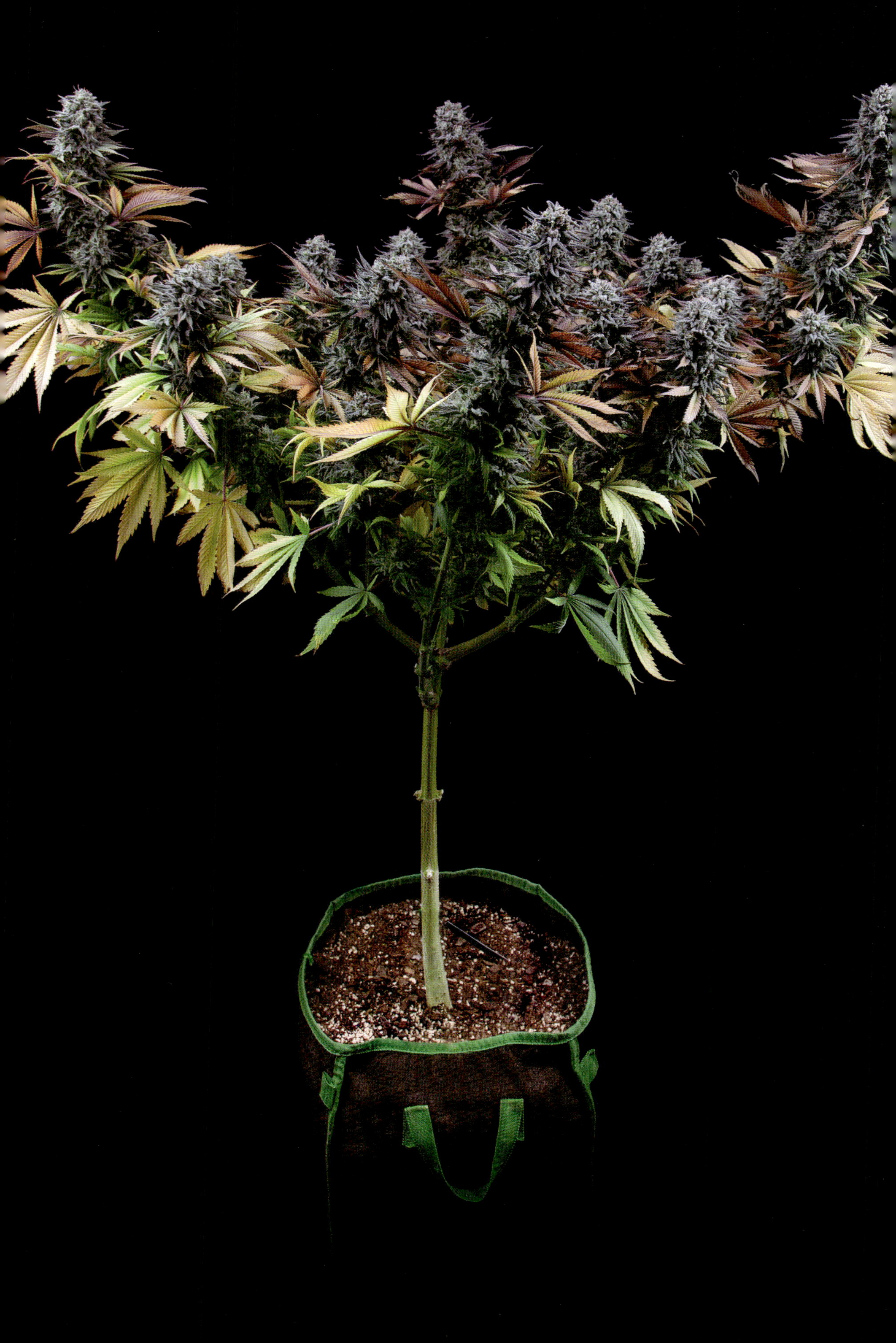

6

Nutrients and Soil

This chapter covers a wide range of topics on growing indoors, including basic setups, environmental control, plant care throughout the life cycle, and advanced techniques. This information can help you enhance plant health and growth in various growing environments. Knowledge gained in one area can often be applied to another, so read the outdoor and indoor growing sections regardless of where you plan to grow. In this section, we focus primarily on soil or semi-solid media, with a dedicated hydroponics chapter to follow.

The Basic Setups

Many large-scale, professional indoor grow rooms use one light per plant. A 1:1 ratio of female plants to lights is ideal for strains that can efficiently use most of the light, but unused light results in excess illumination, which is wasteful. Introducing more plants can help harness that surplus light, but risks overcrowding, leading to plants overlapping and obstructing each other's access to light. Consequently, indoor cultivators have devised methods to maximize light and space, balancing the number of plants and their growing style.

Indoor gardens can range from basic to advanced setups. The most common basic indoor setups are soil or substrate grows, which use any semi-solid mixture as the medium, and hydroponic or aeroponic grows, which use a liquid-only medium.

The most popular indoor setup styles include the following, and each can be paired with soil/substrate or hydroponic/aeroponic styles:

- Sea of Green (SOG)
- Screen of Green (ScrOG)
- Cabinets
- Indoor tents

There are variations of these setups, but most indoor cannabis cultivation can be categorized into at least one of them. Some combinations may also work—for example,

PHOTO: RUSSELL-HOWLAND PHOTOGRAPHY

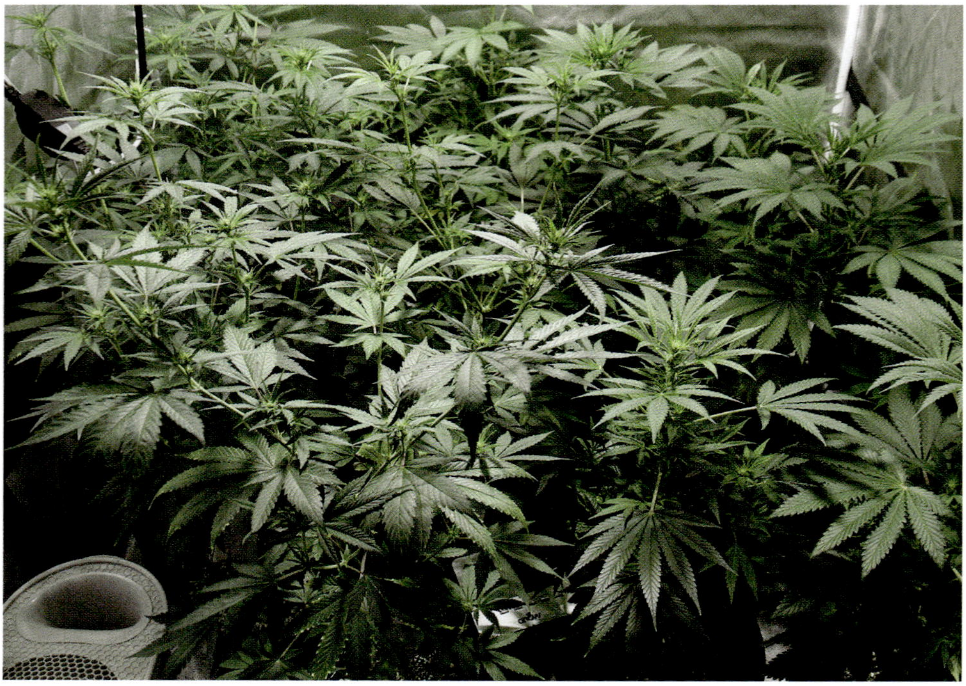

Sea of Green (SOG) requires plants of the same strain, preferably clones, to maintain a uniform canopy across the top without additional aids like mesh screens.

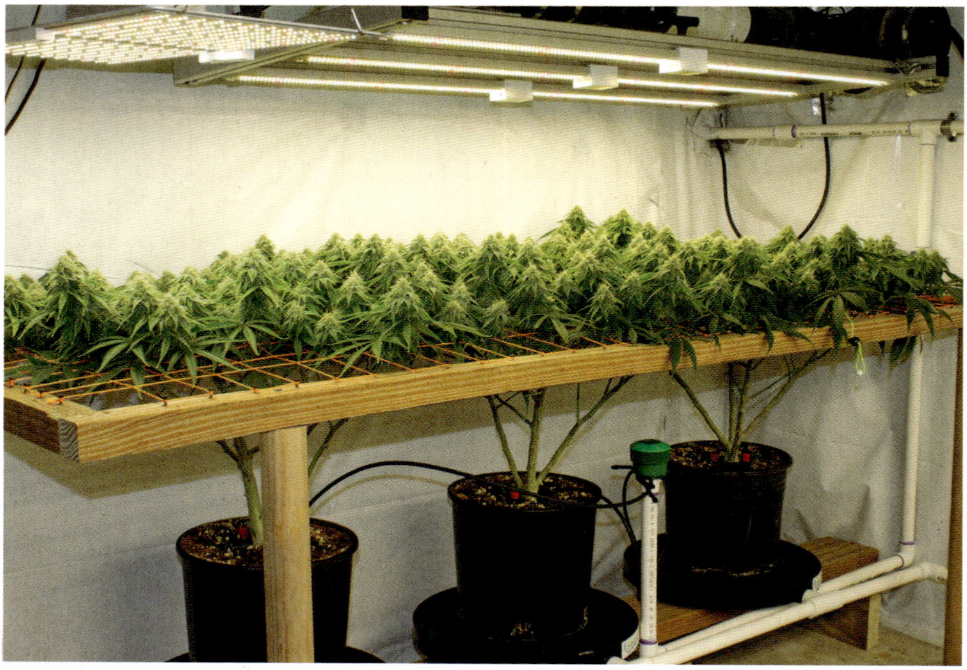

Screen of Green (ScrOG) requires a mesh screen and plants of the same strain, from seeds or clones, to maintain a uniform canopy across the top.

PHOTOS: DAVID STRANGE (TOP), TRAVIS HOELLERER @SOFAKINGHIGH (BOTTOM)

a tent with a ScrOG. By learning about these styles and media, you'll gain a solid understanding of the vast spectrum of indoor cannabis cultivation methods available. Chapters 10 and 11 will detail more advanced indoor setups.

Environmental Controls: The Vegetative Photoperiod

Cannabis is a light-demanding plant. During the vegetative photoperiod, growers keep the light on their plants for 24 hours a day. When grown under optimal conditions with a 24/0 photoperiod, plants flourish and do not require a period of darkness to rest. These plants form more nodes, create additional branches, and produce more leaves.

Some growers choose to use an 18/6 photoperiod, which involves 18 hours of light and 6 hours of darkness, for vegetative growth to reduce electrical costs, but this may result in a lower final yield. The plant will grow naturally, but not as vigorously as with the 24/0 photoperiod because it receives only 75% of the light. While this doesn't necessarily mean the plant will produce 25% fewer leaves, branches, and nodes, it does highlight the strong correlation between light and cannabis growth. Some growers have attributed cannabis sexual dysfunction (the hermaphrodite condition) to the 18/6 photoperiod, but these issues are more likely related to genetics and stress factors.

In summary, the 18/6 option is more cost-effective, prolongs the lifespan of the light, and is still able to provide good results, though in most cases, the yield will be less than that of the 24/0 photoperiod.

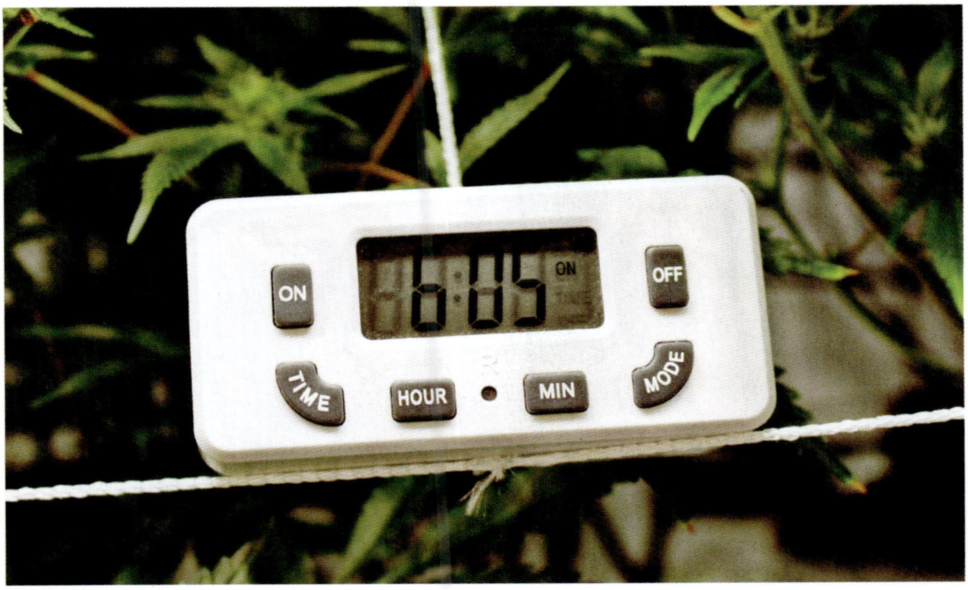

PHOTO: TEE ROBERTS

Timers can be used to control the photoperiod automatically and are especially useful for flowering in a 12/12 photoperiod.

Indoor Soil Garden

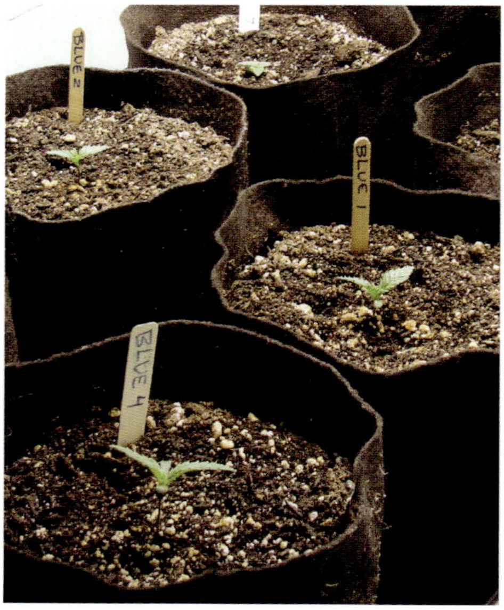

Note the use of labels. These are not optional, but essential to make life easier for you.

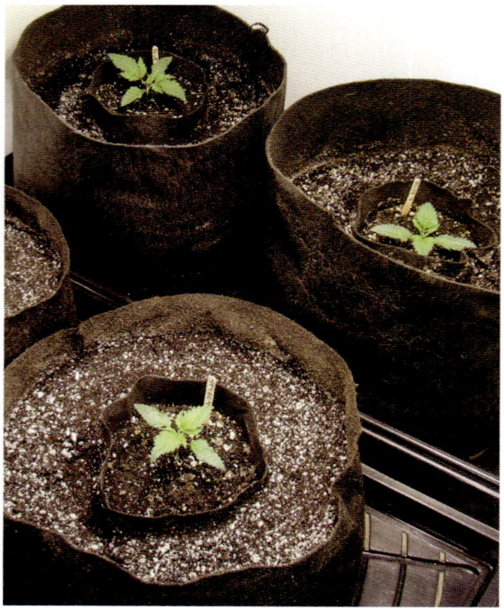

Seedlings transplanted from small grow bags into big grow bags. Notice the labels and relative size.

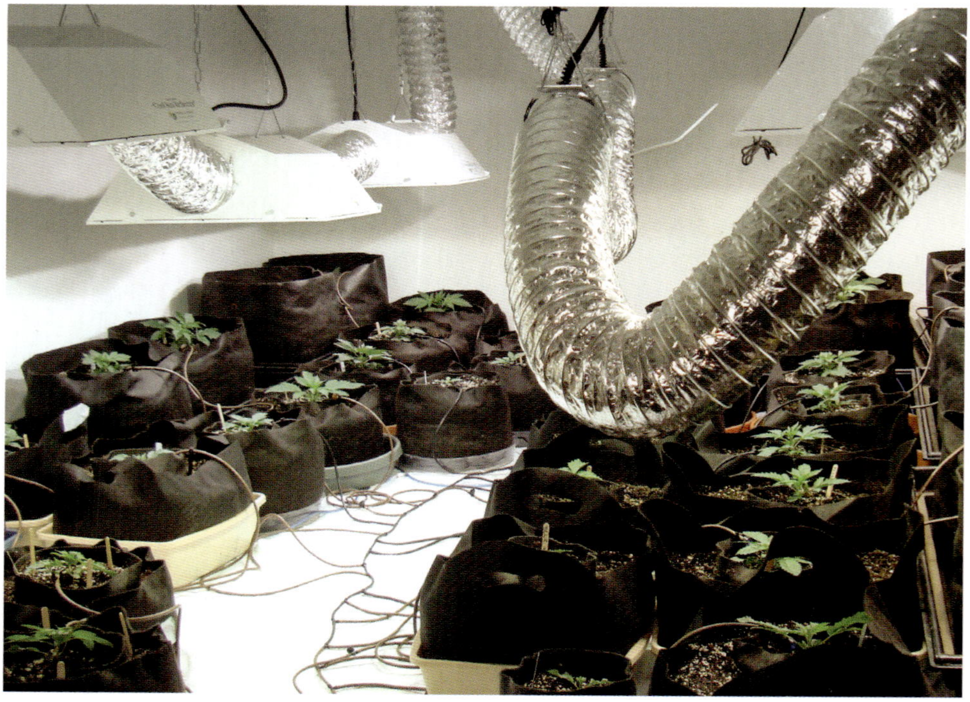

The grow room has four white walls and a white floor for maximum reflectivity. Even the HID lights are white.

PHOTOS: MAX BORTNICK

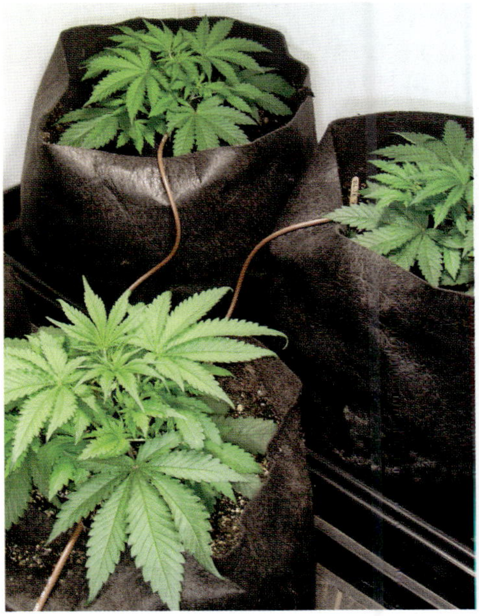

The diameter of the grow bag is a good indicator of how wide your plants will get.

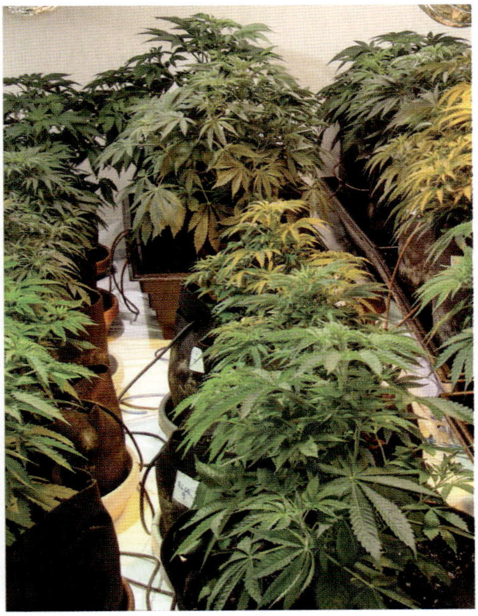

The uniformity of your grown plants is dependent on the stability and uniformity of the seed's genetics.

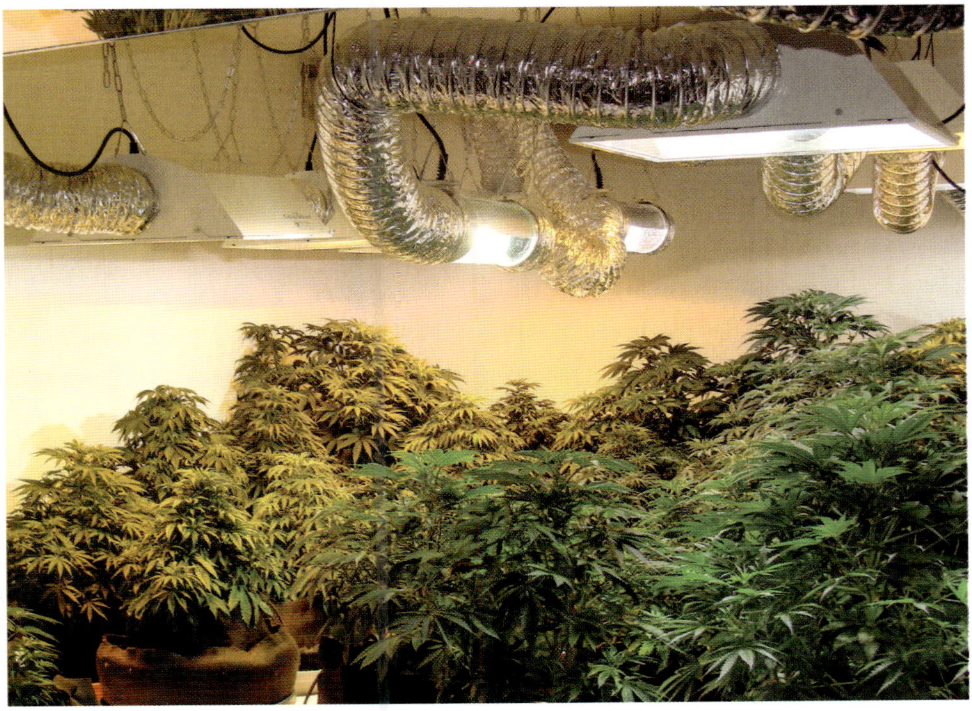

An uneven canopy is not uncommon when growing new hybrids. Future breeding makes them more uniform.

continues...

Indoor Soil Garden *continued*

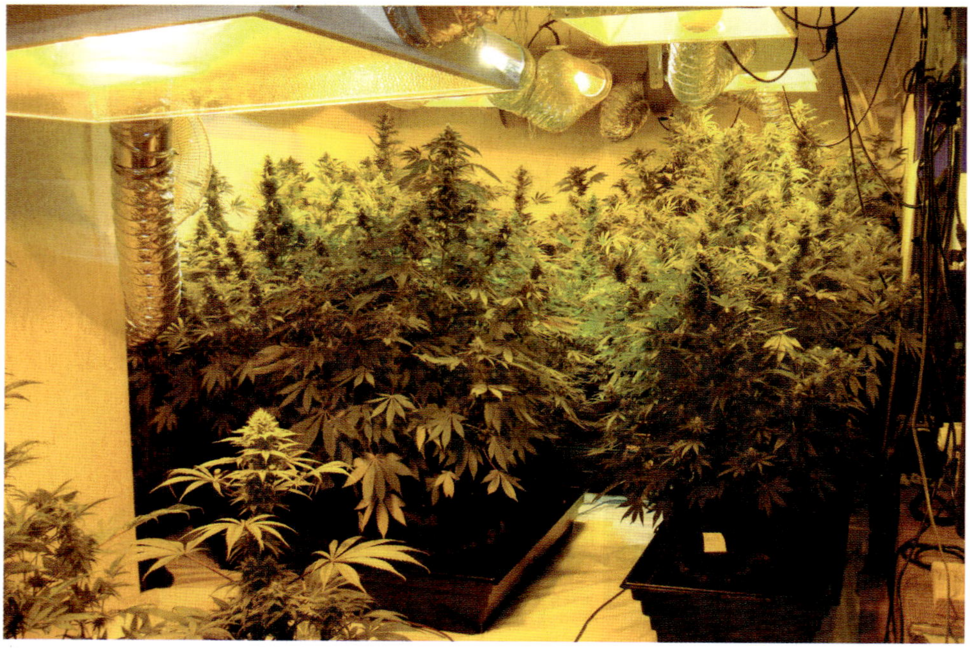

You may have to create a gap between plants to get to the plants in the back for watering and feeding.

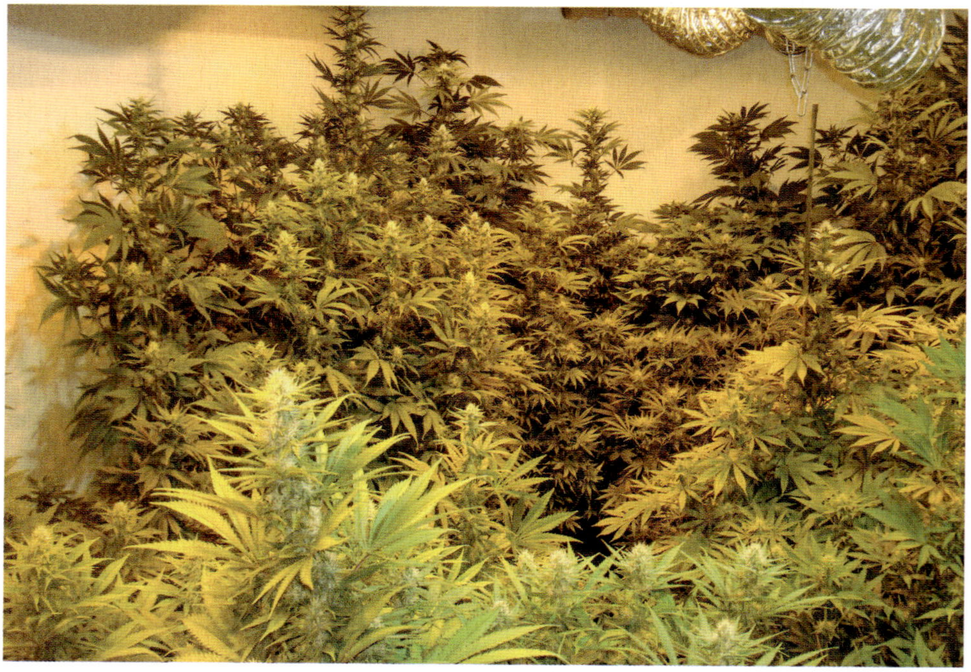

PHOTOS: MAX BORTNICK

The canopy is uneven but there are a lot of flowers here. Next time, you can estimate how to use more space.

Maintaining the Photoperiods

Both 24/0 and 18/6 photoperiods share the same issue: Once you initiate a photoperiod, it's crucial to maintain it, especially as the plants approach the pre-flowering phase. An irregular photoperiod can induce stress and, when combined with genetic factors, may lead to underwhelming results. Whether you choose 24/0 or 18/6 as your vegetative photoperiod, strive to keep that consistent until your plants enter the flowering stage. Indoor grows that don't maintain fixed vegetative and flowering photoperiods often yield suboptimal results.

Soil

Soil comes in various types and varieties. This section discusses natural soils as opposed to synthetic media, primarily focusing on soil types without delving into nutrient ratio or the functions of individual nutrients. As you gain experience in growing, you'll learn to enhance plant growth by creating your custom soil mix with different ingredients. Cannabis plants develop long, winding roots, which delve into the soil to absorb water and essential minerals for growth. Roots also require some access to air. During dry periods when you're not watering your plant or when the plant has taken up most of the water, air can infiltrate the spaces between soil particles, allowing the roots to breathe. You should NEVER introduce natural outdoor soil into an indoor grow space because it can contain bugs and pests that may jeopardize your grow. Always purchase your soil from a gardening shop. Soil will be the least expensive component of your grow, but do not underrate its significance.

When selecting suitable soil, consider three main factors: Composition, pH, and nutrient content. Soil growers typically use a loam mix.

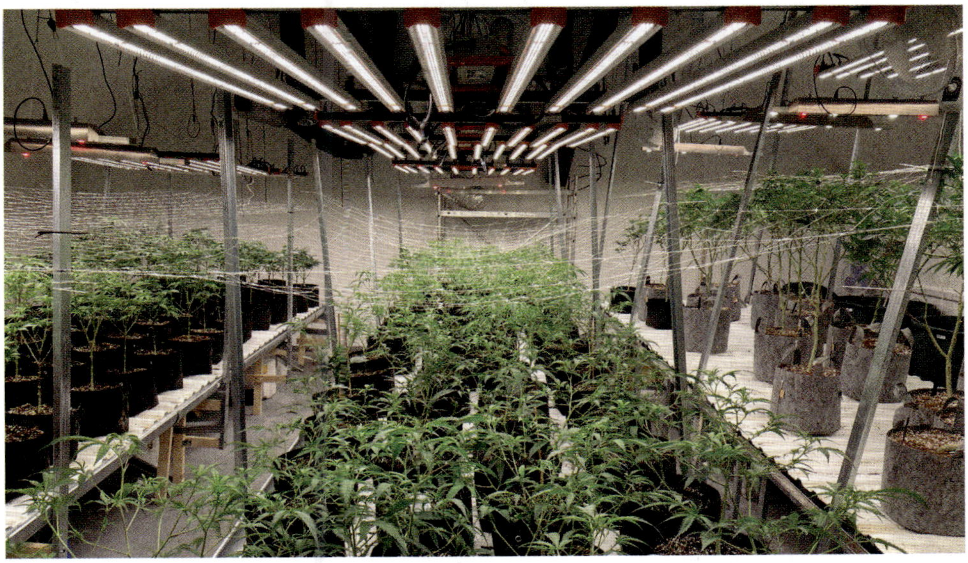

Preparing the ScrOG involves estimating the height at which the plants will be trained.

PHOTO: SPIDER-FARMER.COM

Composition

Ideally, your soil should have a balanced consistency, not overly wet or dry, which allows the roots to access the right amount of water and oxygen. Many brands offer loam with differing moisture levels, though they all have similar nutrient values. Aim for a compromise between wet and dry soils; the packaging should indicate whether the soil is wet, dry, or balanced. If no balanced option is available, purchase both wet and dry soils and mix them. Try to mix soils with the same NPK ratio listed on the bags; otherwise, you'll need to calculate the difference in nutrient ratio. Wet soil can sometimes harm plants by obstructing airflow to the roots, while dry soil can quickly dehydrate and deprive the roots of moisture. Look for a loose soil mix that feels fine but slightly heavy. Avoid purchasing anything excessively hard and bulky, or overly soft and weightless. Instead, aim for a balanced composition using a mix of soil types, or loam. Due to its composition, loam is usually the ideal type of soil for growing cannabis. The following are the most common types of soil media available.

Clay

Clay is a dense, fine-grained soil composed of hydrated aluminosilicates, which become pliable when moistened. Marijuana roots don't favor clay soil on its own, so clay is usually mixed with other soil types to create a suitable medium for cannabis growth.

Humus

Humus is the organic component of soil formed through the decomposition of plant materials. It can be purchased in bags from local gardening stores. These products usually claim to be free of bugs and other living matter, but you may occasionally find small organisms in the package. Humus makes up the organic matter added to the mixture of manure and loam soil known as "compost." When mixed with clay, sand, and silts, humus is a more natural soil option.

Sand and Silts

While sand and silt are not commonly used alone, they are important for soil mixes. Sandy soils may be pure sand or a sand-soil mixture. Sand drains water and minerals too quickly and is unsuitable for cannabis growth on its own. Silts, which have a consistency similar to clay though are darker in color, hold nutrients well but don't retain water effectively. These soils are also typically mixed with other types to create loam.

Loam

Loam is a balanced mix of various soil types and is highly fertile. In most cases, store-bought soil already contains a mix of humus, sand, silt, and clay; the composition should be indicated on the bag. You can mix your loam soils using the soil types mentioned for precise control over ratios.

Perlite and Vermiculite

Artificial media can be mixed with soil in soil growing. These media are typically not used on their own to support the plant as they lack the necessary composition, drain too quickly, and require intensive monitoring if used in higher ratios than other soil types. However, they retain nutrients exceptionally well when mixed with soil. Some other media involve processing.

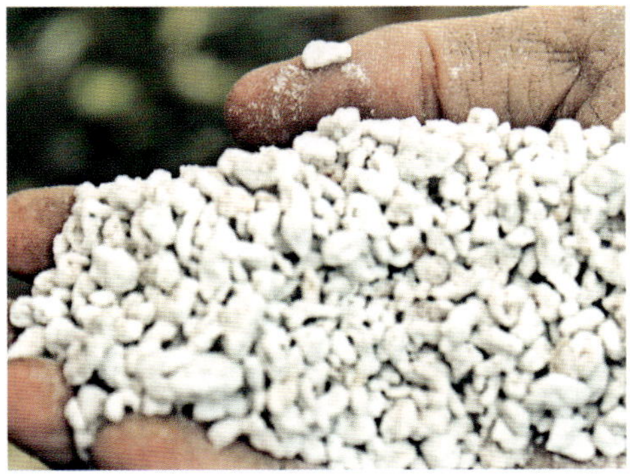

Perlite. When heating volcanic glass, you get this expanded lightweight medium.

Though perlite is technically not artificial, the raw form needs processing before it can be used in agriculture. Perlite originates from the hydration of obsidian, a natural amorphous volcanic glass. It serves as a suitable medium but lacks nutrients, so perlite is often mixed with other soil types to create an optimal growing environment.

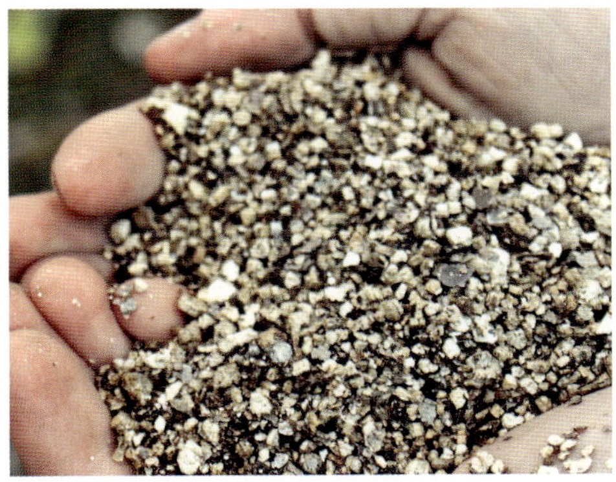

Vermiculite. Heated mica produces this water- and nutrient-absorbing medium.

Vermiculite is similar to perlite, belonging to the phyllosilicate category of hydrous minerals, often referred to as mica. There is a debate regarding how 'organic' these products are. Some growers refer to them as semi-organic, which may not align with the preferences of organic growers. While both are naturally occurring minerals, they undergo treatment by heating to become lighter and more porous. However, the process of heating soil to sterilize it does not necessarily make it any less organic. In this sense, we can consider these minerals as having natural origins, even though they are partially processed. Due to the mining process and the use of energy-intensive heating methods, they are not entirely environmentally-friendly. Therefore, it's essential to evaluate each source and decide if you are comfortable using it. This applies not only to substrate choice but also to anything used by pure organic growers for cannabis cultivation.

Both perlite and vermiculite are considered "inert" soils because they lack nutrients. If you're using them for the first time, mix them thoroughly with soil. You can start with a ratio of one part substrate to four parts soil. As you gain experience, you can adjust the mixture ratio, aiming for 1:1. Remember that pure vermiculite or perlite mixtures do not retain moisture effectively, and are typically only used in their pure form as substrate support for hydroponic systems, which we will explain in Chapter 11.

PHOTOS: STONED ROSIE

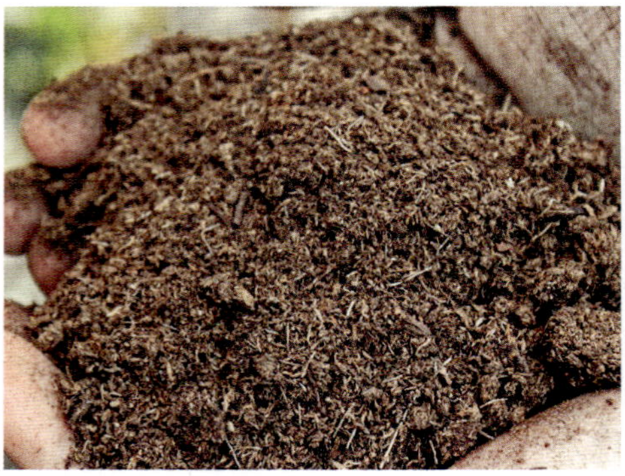

Peat moss is an alternative to soil or can be mixed with soil. Peat moss is very fine.

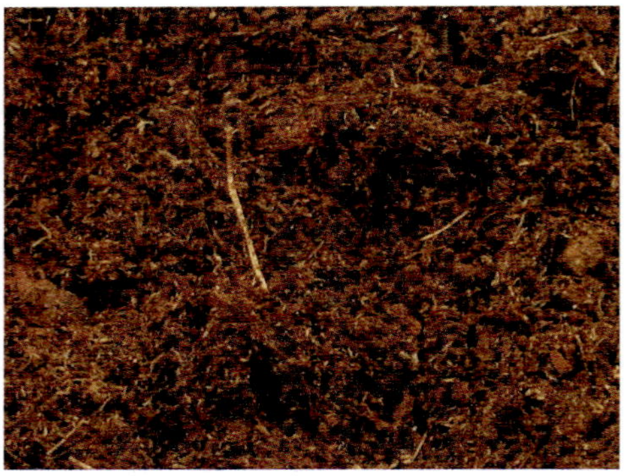

Coco coir is even finer and is sold in blocks that expand in a bucket of warm water.

Moss and Coir Brick Blocks

Sphagnum and peat moss are the two most common types of moss-like substrates on the market. These mosses are collected from bogs, dried, processed, and dyed, usually colors like green, gray, brown, and black. They are then compressed into blocks and used widely as substrates by gardeners due to their excellent capacity to absorb and retain nutrients. However, moss tends to decompose quickly after repeated watering, potentially necessitating the addition of more to your mix before the end of the growing cycle.

Moss blocks can be expanded by soaking them in warm water, similar to coconut coir, which also comes in block form. Adding warm water to the moss block causes it to expand, creating a semi-solid growing medium that can be blended into your soil mix. Allow it to cool down before incorporating it into your soil. Coir blocks are also an excellent choice for introducing a neutral substrate to your mix, offering advantages in water retention, nutrient absorption, and overall composition when combined with high-quality loam soil.

pH

pH measures levels of acidity and alkalinity in the soil. It's crucial to understand because different chemicals react differently in various pH environments. The pH scale ranges from 0 to 14, with 7 being neutral, 0 representing strong acidity, and 14 indicating high alkalinity. Cannabis typically thrives in an environment that leans toward a neutral pH of around 7, although this can vary depending on the growing method. When selecting your soil, aim for a pH level of 7, which should be indicated

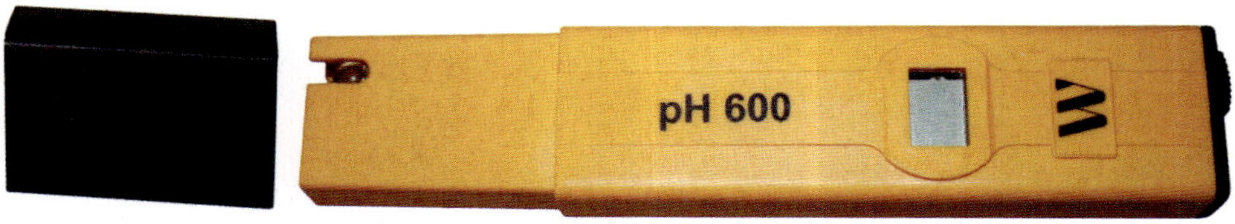

A pH test pen. The reading will be on the screen, from 1 to 14, with 7 being neutral, 1 very acidic, and 14 very alkaline.

PHOTOS: STONED ROSIE (TOP LEFT), HYDROFARM.COM (TOP RIGHT), STONED ROSIE (BOTTOM)

on the bag. Although cannabis can tolerate pH levels ranging from 6 to 8, deviating by one pH unit above or below this mark can lead to problems in your plant's growth. Some organic systems perform best at a slightly lower pH, just below 7. However, when the pH exceeds 7, it may slow down the uptake of phosphorus.

You can purchase pH readers, ranging from affordable liquid test kits to more expensive digital readers, from most gardening shops to measure and monitor the pH of your soil and water. We cover how to adjust the pH in various sections throughout the book. A low-effort way to make necessary pH adjustments is using pH-up and pH-down liquid products.

Nutrients

The three most crucial nutrients for soil-grown plants, known as macronutrients, are nitrogen (N), phosphorus (P), and potassium (K). NPK can be provided in two forms: Either pre-mixed into the soil or as stand-alone fertilizers, usually in liquid or granular form. The percentage of each nutrient should be clearly indicated on the packaging, typically as a ratio. For example, 20:20:20 signifies 20% nitrogen, 20% phosphorus, and 20% potassium, with the remaining 40% consisting of other essential elements found in the soil. Keep in mind that the NPK ratio may vary among different nutrient and soil brands, so it's crucial to understand the nutrient requirements of cannabis and the appropriate amounts needed during different stages of its life cycle.

During the vegetative growth stage, cannabis plants thrive with a soil or fertilizer

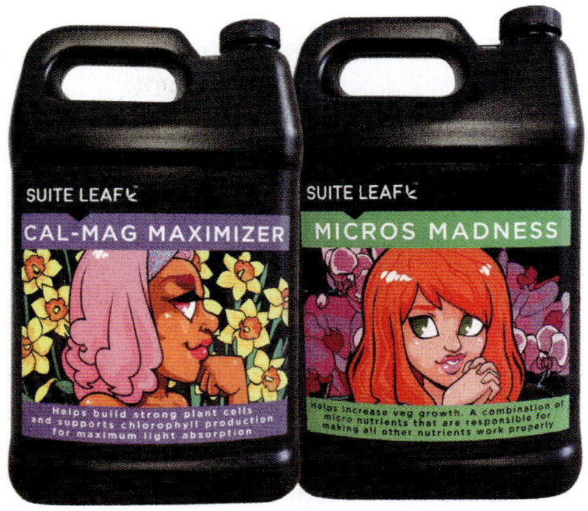

Calcium/Magnesium suggests a secondary supplement. Micro suggests micronutrients that you also need.

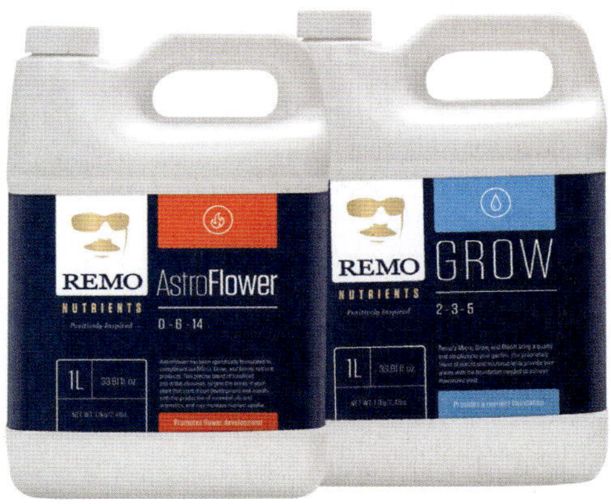

Flowering nutrients with no nitrogen, medium phosphorus, heavy potassium. Vegetative nutrients with nitrogen, medium phosphorus, medium potassium.

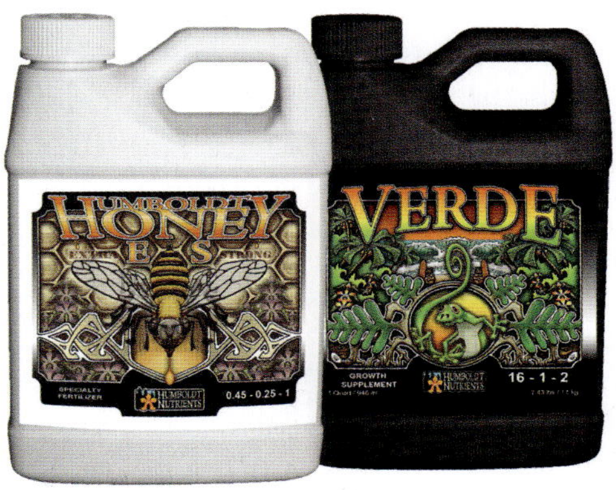

Honey ES, high in potassium, contains cane molasses, seaweed, and Quillaja Saponaria.

PHOTOS: SUITELEAF.COM (TOP), REMONUTRIENTS.COM (MIDDLE), HUMBOLDTNUTRIENTS.COM (BOTTOM)

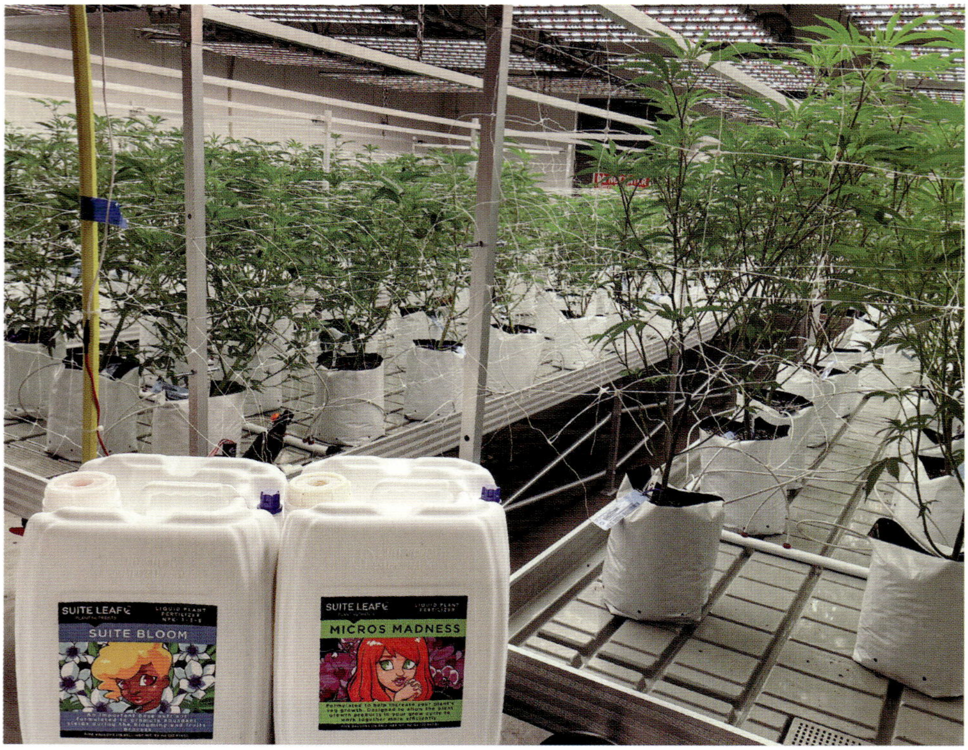

This is an example of several feeds that are combined to ensure these plants get a full complement of primary, secondary, and micronutrients.

PHOTO: SUITELEAF.COM / EXCELSIOR EXTRACTS

mixture that provides high levels of nitrogen and moderate levels of phosphorus and potassium. When selecting a soil or fertilizer, look for a balanced combination of these nutrients, with phosphorus and potassium levels equal to or lower than the nitrogen value. Suitable combinations include 12:12:12, 20:20:20, 12:6:6, or 18:4:5, with the first two being the best choices.

As cannabis transitions to the flowering stage, it requires a higher level of phosphorus. Therefore, carefully choose your soil or fertilizers to meet this increased phosphorus demand. Since cannabis plants are typically not transplanted between the vegetative and flowering stages, planning to adjust nutrient levels for flowering by adding appropriate nutrients is crucial.

Mixing Soils

There's no one-size-fits-all soil mix for cannabis plants because different strains have different nutrient requirements. Some strains thrive with abundant nutrients, while others are more sensitive and can easily suffer from nutrient burn. Therefore, choose a soil mixture that aligns with your specific strain's needs. These loam soil mixes are designed to cater to different plant requirements.

For Strains That Require High Levels of Nutrients:

1. NPK loam soil (20:20:20)
2. Moss

Combine the soil and moss in a 3:1 ratio. This mixture features loam soil with a high NPK ratio combined with moss, providing robust nutrient retention.

For Strains That Require Average Levels of Nutrients:

1. NPK loam soil (10:10:10)
2. Perlite or vermiculite

Mix the soil and perlite or vermiculite at a 4:1 ratio. This blend combines loam soil with a moderate NPK ratio with perlite or vermiculite for excellent nutrient retention.

For Strains That Require Low Levels of Nutrients:

1. NPK loam soil (5:5:5)
2. Sand
3. Perlite or vermiculite

Mix the soil, sand, and perlite or vermiculite at a 1:1:1 ratio. This soil mix doesn't retain minerals or water as effectively, making it suitable for plants with lower nutrient needs. Keep in mind that lighter mixtures like this will require more frequent watering.

These examples demonstrate the versatility of soil and substrate combinations to meet your plant's specific needs. You can always adjust these soil mixtures to tailor them to your plants. Do not rely solely on these soil mixtures to nourish your plants throughout their life cycle unless you are using slow-release organics, which will be covered in Chapter 14. To maintain a balanced nutrient profile over time, you'll need to supplement your mix with additional nutrients.

Understanding the NPK Ratio

To gain a deeper understanding of the NPK ratio, consider this example of a soil mixture:

NPK loam soil (20:10:10) and vermiculite.

We chose 20:10:10 because we need additional nitrogen. In this case, you would mix four parts loam soil with one part vermiculite to create a medium suitable for a plant that requires slightly above-average nutrient levels. Here, 20:10:10 represents 20% nitrogen, 10% phosphorus, and 10% potassium. Unless otherwise specified on the packaging, you can assume the remaining 60% is composed of soil particles or, in the case of bottled nutrients, water. When we transition into the flowering stage, we'll adjust our nutrient mix to include higher phosphorus values, such as 10:20:10 or 5:10:5, to meet the specific needs of the plants during that phase.

As we progress through this book, especially in the hydroponics sections, we'll delve deeper into nutrient management, which can also be applied to soil cultivation.

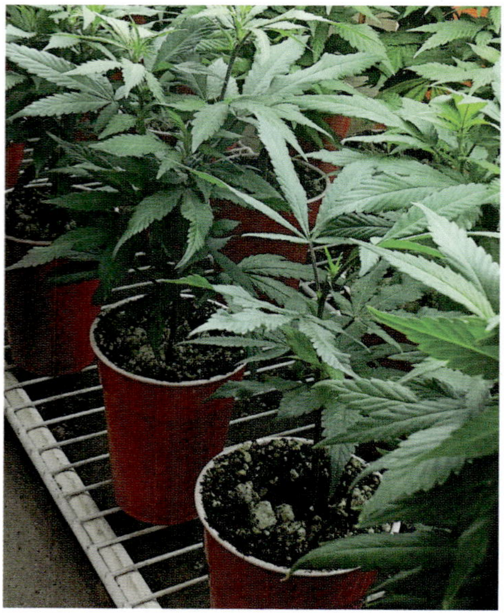

Narrow pots allow for compacting many plants together, like in a SOG grow.

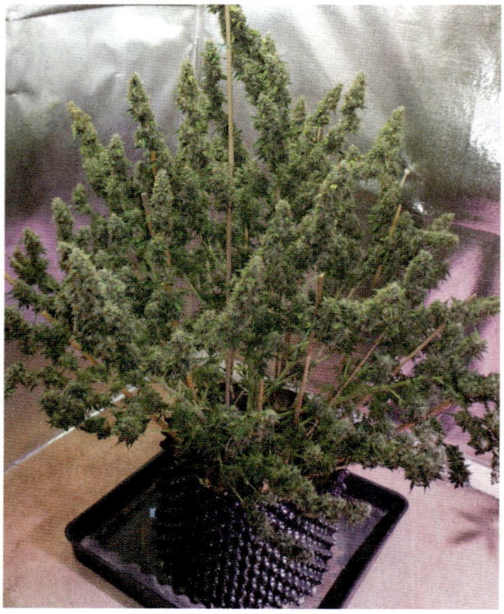

One big pot and one high-yielding strain under a single lamp. Pruning helps to establish many branching parts.

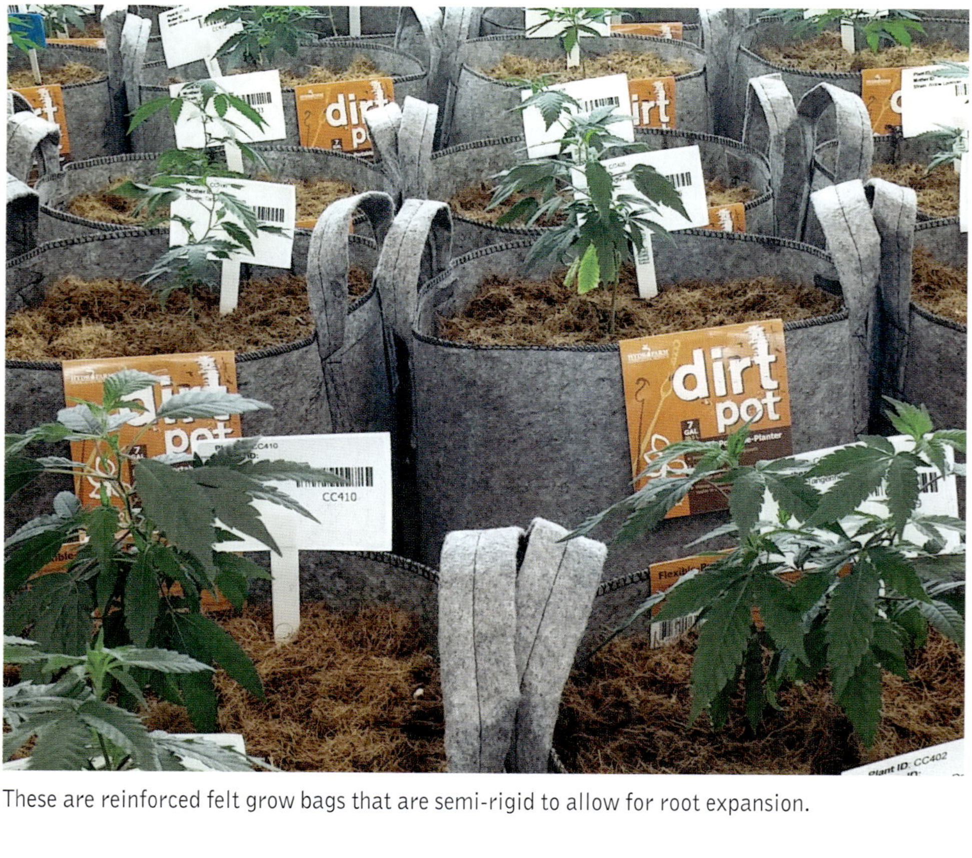

These are reinforced felt grow bags that are semi-rigid to allow for root expansion.

PHOTOS: MONICA GRIFFIN (TOP LEFT), DUTCH PASSION (TOP RIGHT), MONICA GRIFFIN (BOTTOM)

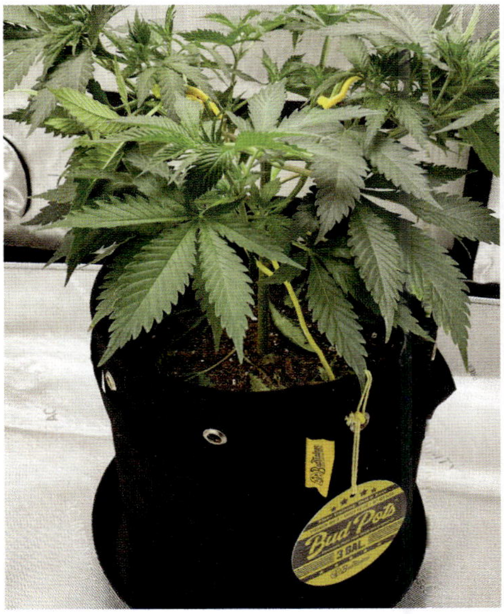

Eco-friendly fabric bud pot with peat moss in the medium.

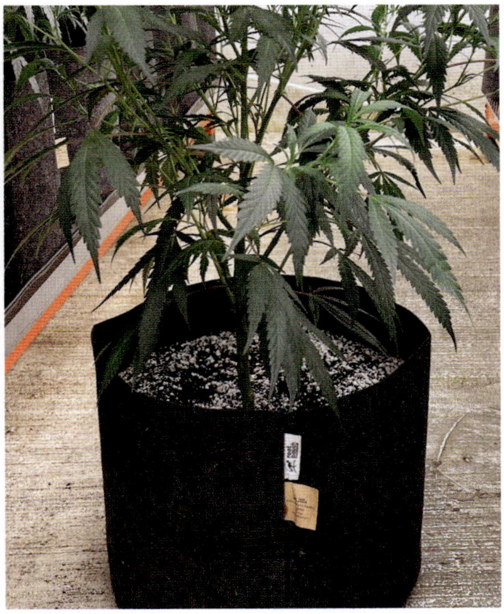
Eco-friendly fabric bud pot with coco coir and perlite in the medium.

Pots, Dishes, and Trays

Pots come in a variety of shapes and sizes. Cannabis plants do best in larger pots, ideally 1.5 to 3 gallons in size, as they develop extensive root systems, and larger pots provide ample space for root growth. When selecting pots, choose ones with holes in the bottom, and place them inside dishes, which are typically available where you purchase your pots.

When you water your plants, some of the excess water will drain through the soil and exit through the holes into the dishes. It's important to periodically empty these dishes to prevent water spills. Remember that water on the floor can pose an electrical hazard, which is why it's crucial to have a system in place to capture drained fluids.

Alternatively, you can opt for trays instead of dishes. Trays can be used for more than one plant, and are usually deeper, to hold more reserve water that may be absorbed by the roots later. However, they can be a bit more challenging to empty if you accidentally spill water. While holes in pots help prevent overwatering, water can leach out some of the nutrients in your soil. Overwatering can lead to wasted nutrients and time, and, in severe cases, can harm your plants. Advanced growers may opt for pots without holes because they know how to avoid overwatering or overfeeding. As you gain expertise, you can consider transitioning to non-perforated pots if you prefer.

Before introducing a pot into your grow space, it's essential to thoroughly clean it to remove any unwanted chemicals or dust that may have accumulated during production or storage. It's most practical to use one pot per plant so that, if any issues arise

PHOTOS: PHOTOS: BUDTRAINER.COM (LEFT), ROOTPOUCH.COM (RIGHT)

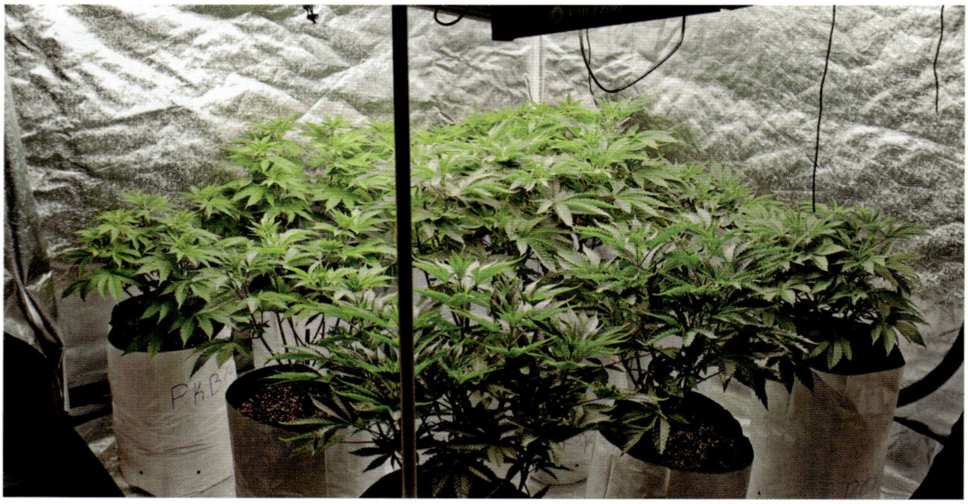

Using grow bags in a tent is a fantastic way to maximize your space and control over your plant.

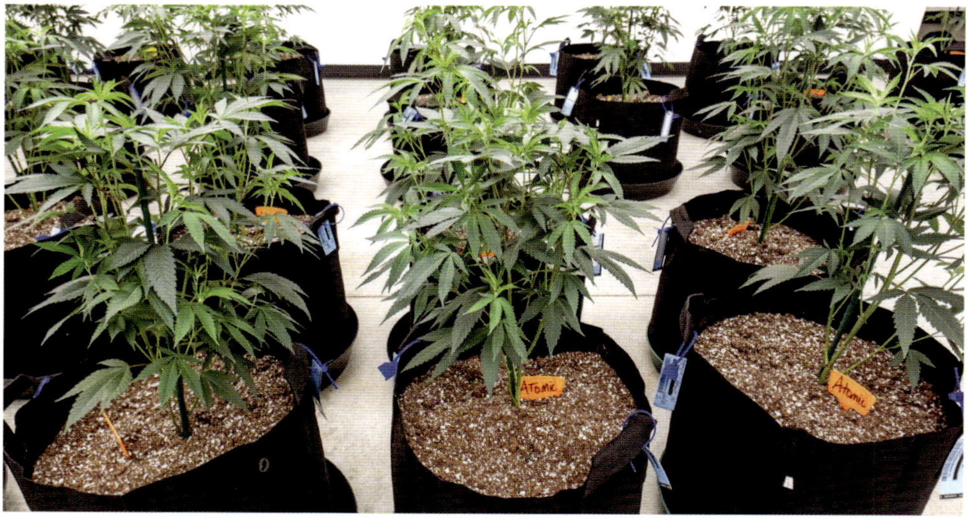

During the middle to later phases of vegetative growth, plants often need more spacing as they expand laterally. A wider grow bag accommodates this increased lateral growth.

PHOTOS: TEE ROBERTS (TOP), BONSAIBUDSRI.COM (BOTTOM)

related to the soil, watering, or nutrients, only one plant will be affected. Larger, wider pots are beneficial as they allow for more extensive plant growth by enabling the roots to stretch out further. This increased root support promotes lateral growth, which is particularly desirable for vegetative plants. Encouraging as many natural branches as possible to form before flowering is vital, as each node has the potential to become a bud site. Wider pots play a significant role in achieving this goal.

These fundamentals cover the basic requirements for indoor cannabis cultivation. In Chapter 7, we will delve into artificial lighting.

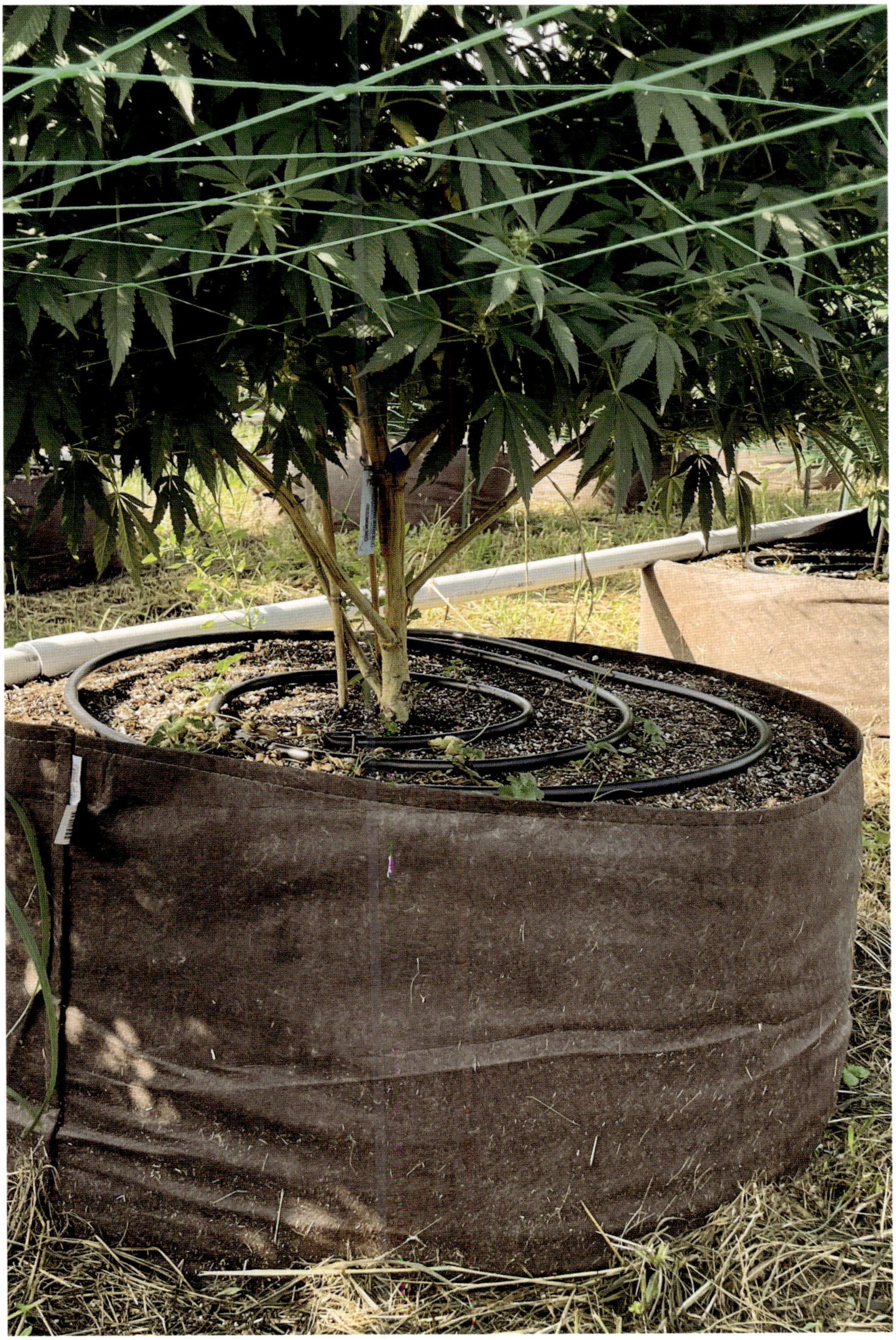

PHOTO: ROOTPOUCH.COM

You can clearly see how the width of the grow bag determines the plant's width. The plant's genes are allowed optimal performance in that area.

Cleaning Your Pots After a Grow

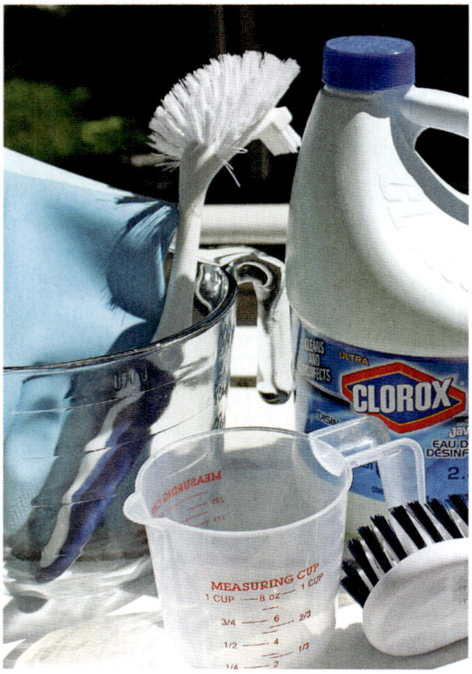

Prepare sterilizing tools and use rubber gloves.

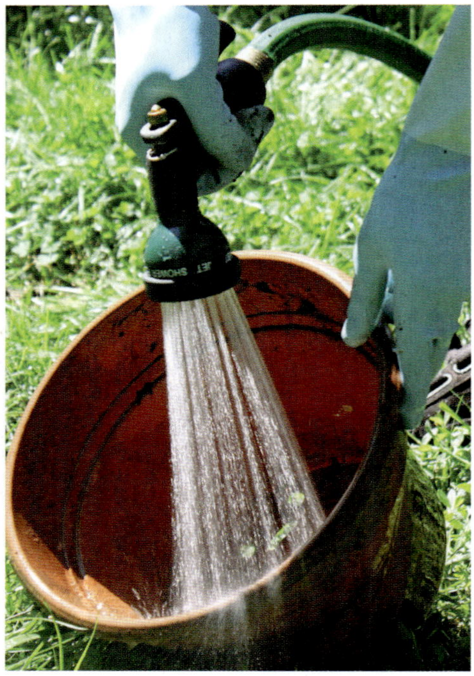

Put on rubber gloves and wash off excess dirt.

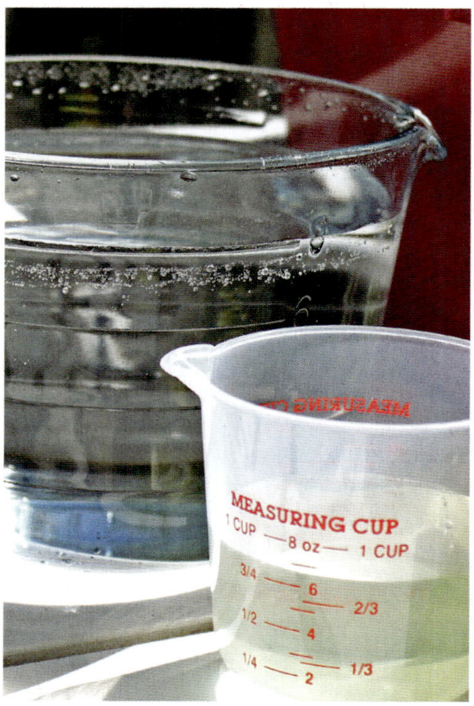

Follow bleach instructions to mix with water.

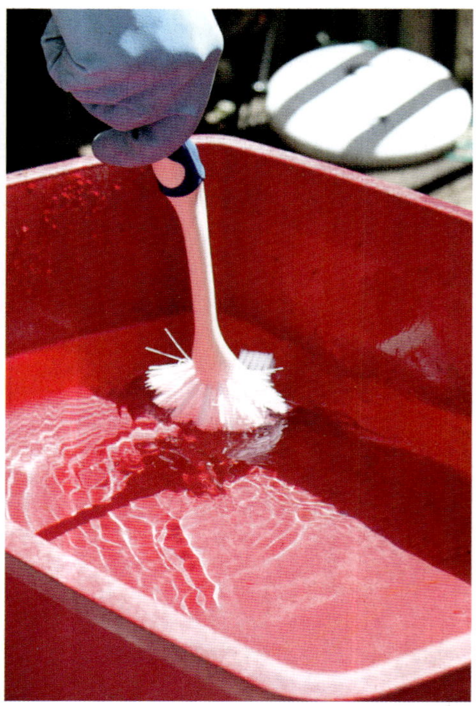

Thoroughly mix beach and water in a basin.

PHOTOS: STONED ROSIE

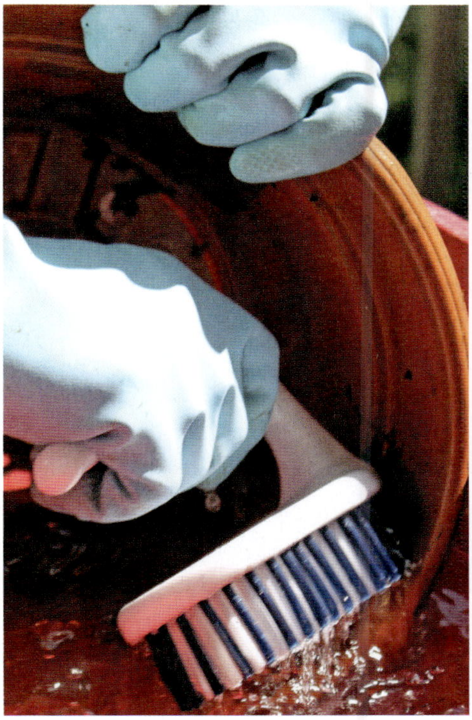

Scrub pots in bleach-water solution.

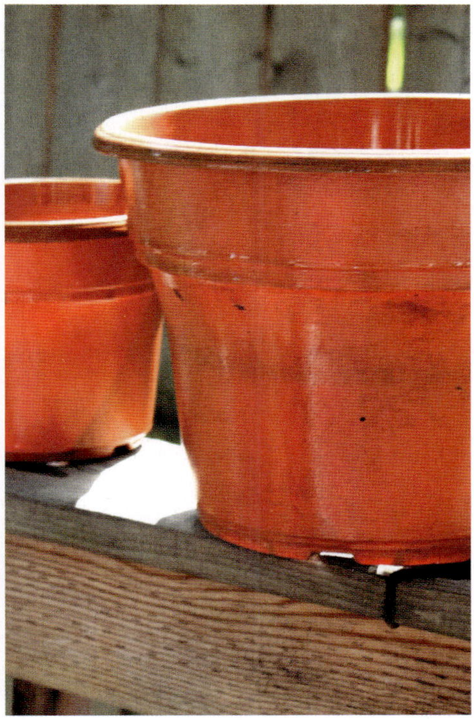

Let pots air dry.

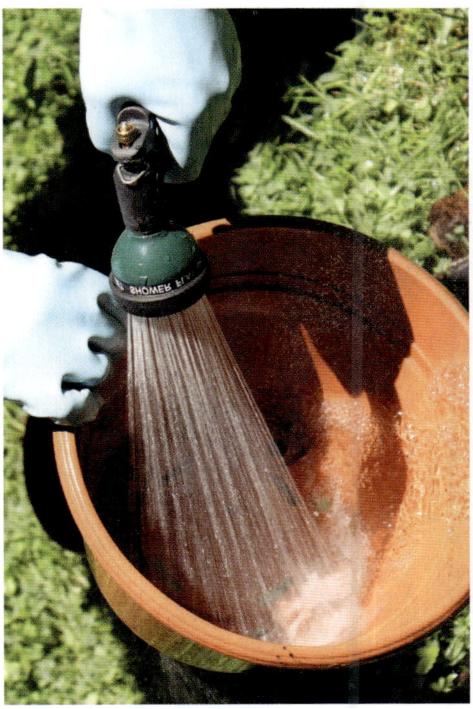

Rinse again with fresh water.

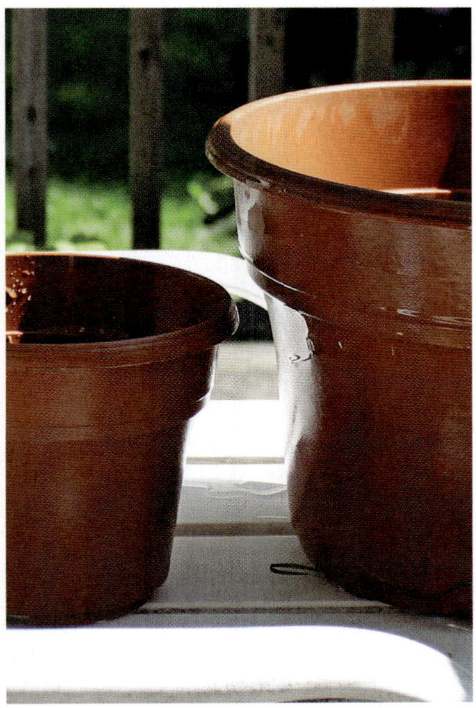

Your pots are ready!

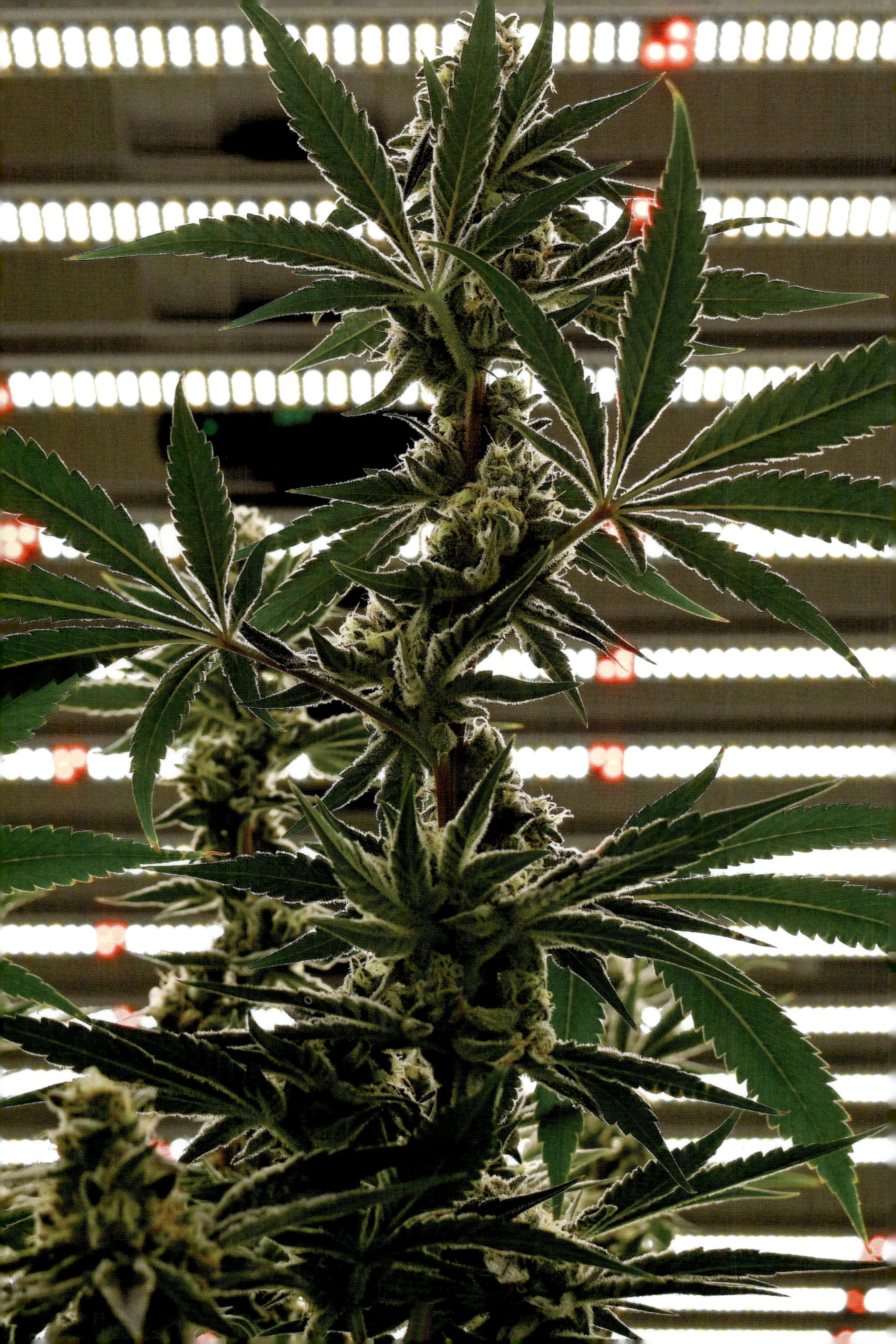

7

Grow Lights

A significant technological advance of this century, with implications for growers, is the light emitting diode, or LED, as it can be used in grow lights. Embracing LED technology opens up entirely new possibilities for cultivation, despite the fact it was once considered the realm of science fiction. However, transitioning to LEDs requires some adjustments and a bit of understanding. In this section, we explore light systems before and after LEDs, making the topic more comprehensive.

Voltage Differences in Different Countries

Before purchasing a grow light kit, it's crucial to know its voltage compatibility, since this varies between countries. A light kit with a power supply intended for European use is incompatible with electrical systems in the US. For a US light kit you wish to use in Europe, you might have to invest in a voltage converter or risk damaging your ballast and potentially the entire light system, including bulbs/LEDs. Make sure the kit is designed for your local power systems. Most reputable kits are, but when buying from platforms like eBay, global options are prevalent. Some units may include a voltage switch, so ensure you select the correct setting for your country.

Electricity and Water

Remember that plants require water, and lights consume electricity. Mixing these two elements can be deadly, so exercise safety and caution. Keep your plants and liquids away from all electrical outlets. Consider mounting your power supply strips on the wall, as those on the floor can be a problem when water accumulates on the ground. LED light systems are mostly internally powered, offering an advantage over high-intensity discharge (HID) lights, which typically require a separate ballast box for power.

Protective Film and Packaging

Pay attention to the protective film and packaging of your grow lights, which can be incredibly subtle. LEDs generate some heat, leaving protective film on some areas can pose a hazard or, at least, reduce the efficiency of your lighting system. Examine the edges of new products to see if any film needs to be peeled away. Reflectors often have protective films both inside and outside, which should be removed for optimal performance.

PHOTO: MIAMIMANGOCA.COM

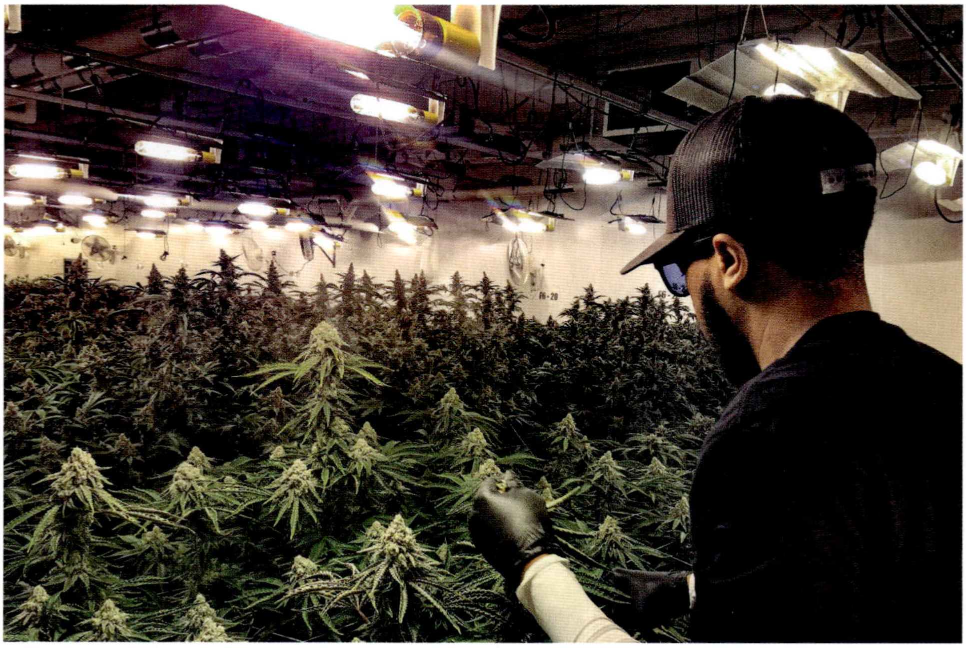

HID lights are evident in their oblong shape under reflectors that bounce the light onto the plants below. Here, you can see some huge top colas.

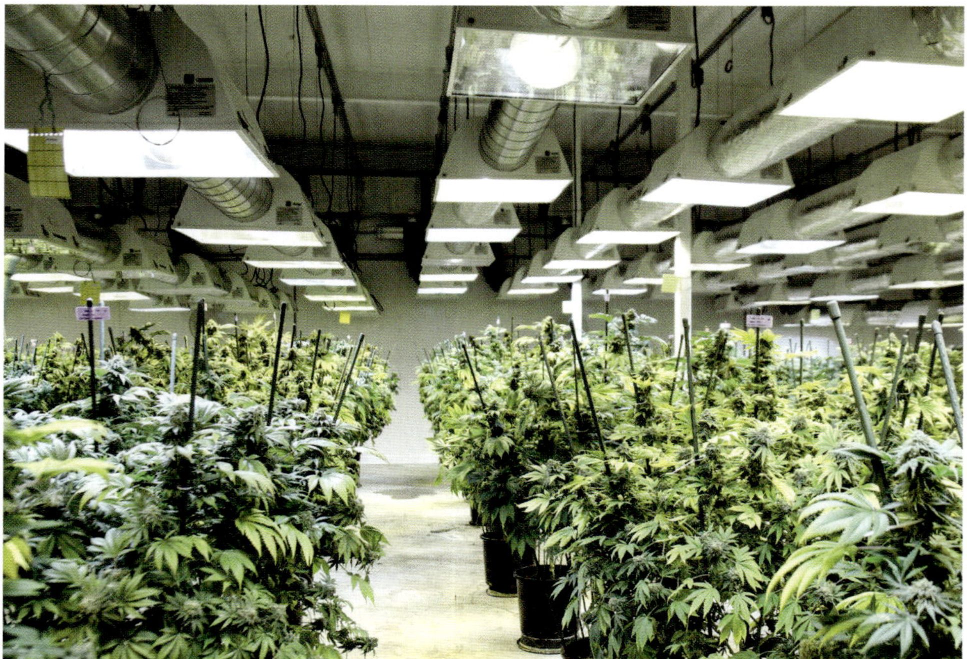

Air-cooled hoods for HID lights. Each hood can channel the bulb's hot air through a fan-driven outtake exhaust.

PHOTOS: HIP2THECROP (TOP), DAVID STRANGE (BOTTOM)

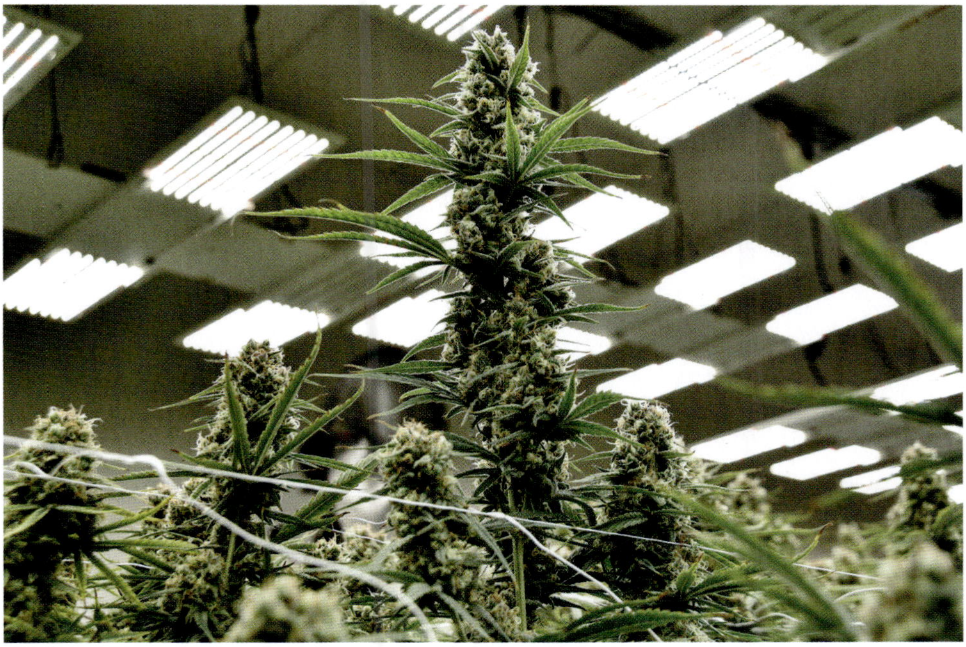

LED lighting is replacing HID lighting worldwide due to its affordability, ease of use, and range of options.

PHOTO: HORTICULTURE LIGHTING GROUP, HLG.COM

Learning About Grow Lights

Approaching the topic of lighting can be quite daunting, but I've found a method that works well for almost everyone, blending a bit of science with information about the gear commonly used by growers. The journey of learning about grow lights takes us through various stages, starting with light calculations, understanding the importance of selecting lights with the correct color bands, and gaining a basic grasp of photosynthesis. From there, we discuss different types of lights, focusing on HID and LED lighting systems, which are essential to understand for cannabis cultivation. Then we explore which type of light is best suited for different growth stages and delve deeper into the LED revolution before touching on advanced light systems. While it may require some effort, by the time you've completed this journey, you'll have acquired the same knowledge that expert growers possess on this subject, which ranks as the second most crucial aspect of cannabis cultivation right after genetics.

Indoor Lights

When we're growing plants indoors, understanding the concept of lighting is crucial. While the sun provides about 98,000 lux of light on Earth, the intensity of light can vary as we move from the equator to the Northern and Southern Hemispheres. Lux is a common unit of measurement for light intensity, but when it comes to plants, we use more specialized units, including photosynthetic active radiation (PAR), photosynthetic photon flux (PPF), photosynthetic photon flux density (PPFD), and the Daily

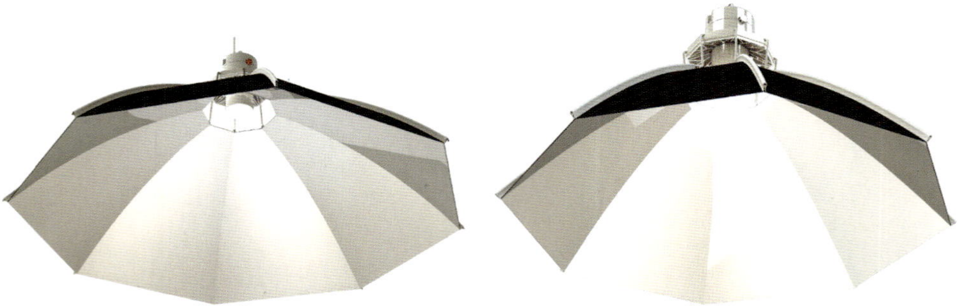

Reflectors come in all kinds of shapes, including octagonal.

Light Integral (DLI) which assess the efficiency of light sources for plant photosynthesis. These measurements play a significant role in optimizing grow room setups, and you'll often find them in the specifications of grow lights. To understand these values, how they relate to each other, and why they are important, we first need to cover some basics about light intensity and distribution.

To grasp the idea of grow lights, think of a sphere. Imagine the sphere's center is a hot, deep red that gradually transitions to yellow as you move toward the surface. This is like the sun, which radiates light in all directions from its spherical surface. However, for indoor plant cultivation, we need to focus all that light on our plants. To achieve this, we use reflectors.

Reflectors are essential components in grow light systems because they direct the light downward onto the plant canopy. The beauty of reflectors is that they can be adjusted to various angles, allowing for precise control of light distribution. Virtually all grow lights come equipped with reflectors, but they can also be purchased separately.

The relationship between the distance from the bulb and the light's color is noteworthy. As you get closer to the bulb, the light appears redder; as you move away from the bulb, the light takes on a more yellowish hue. The distance between the plant and the bulb dictates what temperature of light it will receive. We use a fundamental equation to calculate the intensity of light.

$$\text{Intensity of Light (lumens)} = \text{Light Output} / (\text{Distance (ft)})^2$$

For example, if your light output is 1000 lumens (lm), that equates to 1000 lm for every one square foot (1 ft^2). At two feet away, you'll have 2 ft^2, resulting in $1/4$ of the lumens, or 250 lm. Moving another foot away, you'll be at 3 ft^2, which is $1/9$ of the lumens, about 111 lm. At 4 ft^2, you're down to $1/16$, or roughly 62.5 lm.

While the lumen output of indoor grow bulbs is typically much higher than in this example, the formula remains the same.

PHOTOS: SECRETJARDIN.COM

Grow lights come in a range of shapes and sizes, boasting different wattages and lumen outputs. In the market, you'll find both LED kits and HID kits, and here's what you should know about them.

In a complete HID indoor lighting kit, you should expect to find these essential components: A bulb, a reflector, an internal or external ballast, a timer, and electrical inputs/outputs. It's important to note that the transition from gas-based tube lights to LEDs has already occurred, but you might still encounter HID light systems.

HID lighting kits are often designed in an open style, meaning they lack a glass cover or hood to shield the bulb. Instead, the bulb is securely fixed into a socket positioned inside the reflector. This horizontal positioning aligns with how many grow bulbs are tested, and it's the configuration you should maintain, even if you have the flexibility to hang it in different ways in practice, such as placing bulbs to the sides of your plants. The bulb socket is connected to an internal or external ballast. With an external ballast, a cord usually links it to the bulb's socket. The ballast may be directly attached to the bulb socket, and it might even support the reflector if it's an internal ballast.[1] Some ballasts come with built-in timers. The ballast then plugs into a standard domestic light socket. This whole system is what we refer to as the lighting system.

Exponential Decay of Light Intensity

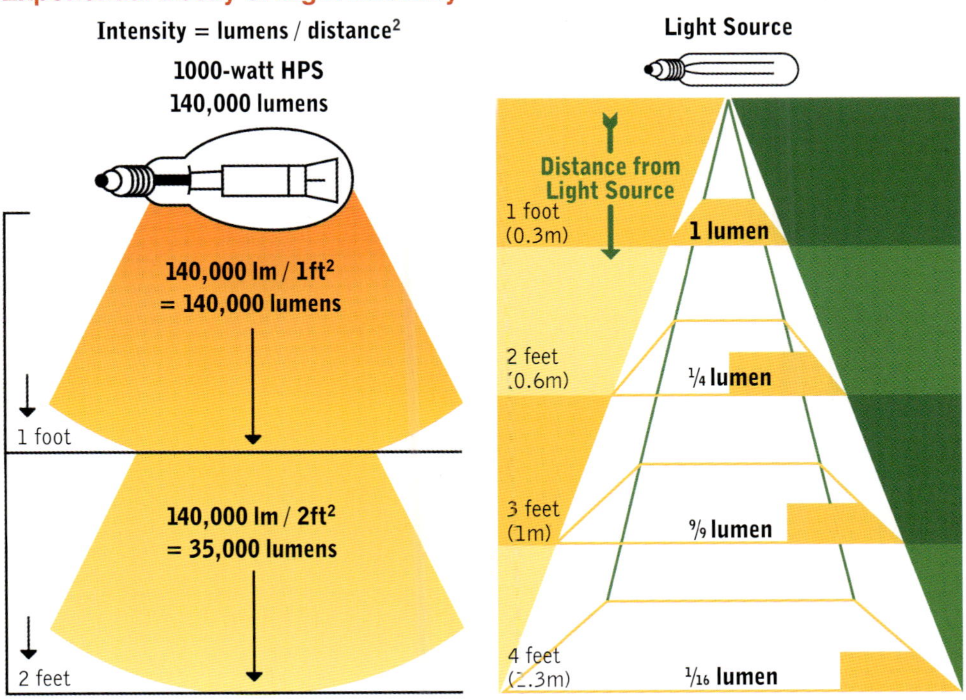

These are just theoretical amounts. Actual light intensity is found in the lamp's specifications or by using a Quantum Sensor PAR Meter Full-Spectrum PPFD Tester.

Radiant Hydrofarm HID Lights

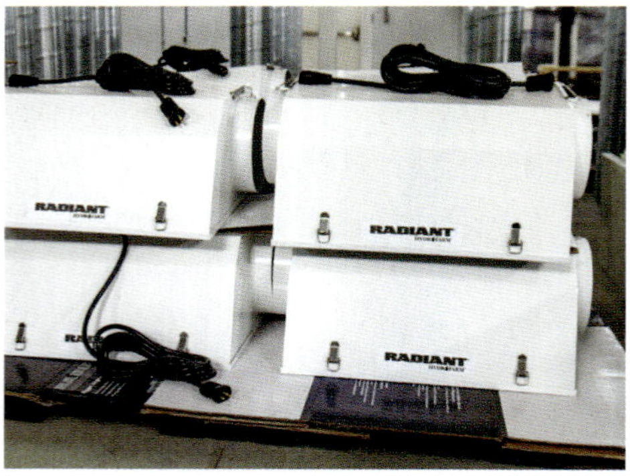

Air-cooled hoods allow for direct airflow through the light, reducing heat.

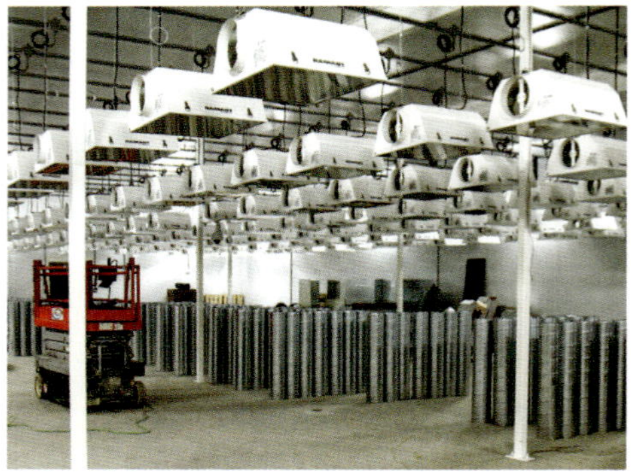

Air-cooled hoods aligned and prepared for ducting.

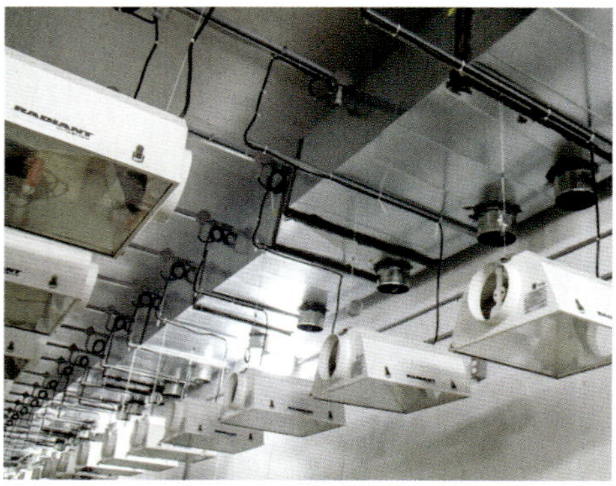

Air ducting will be fitted between hoods and eventually attached to an outtake system like this metal vent shaft.

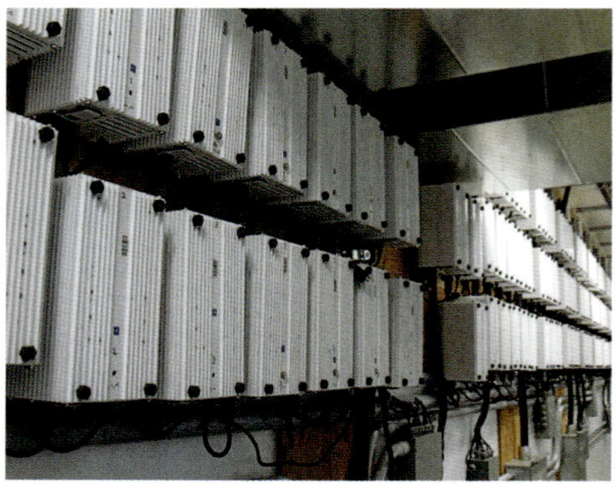

External ballasts separate power source and the bulb. Here they are maintained in another room.

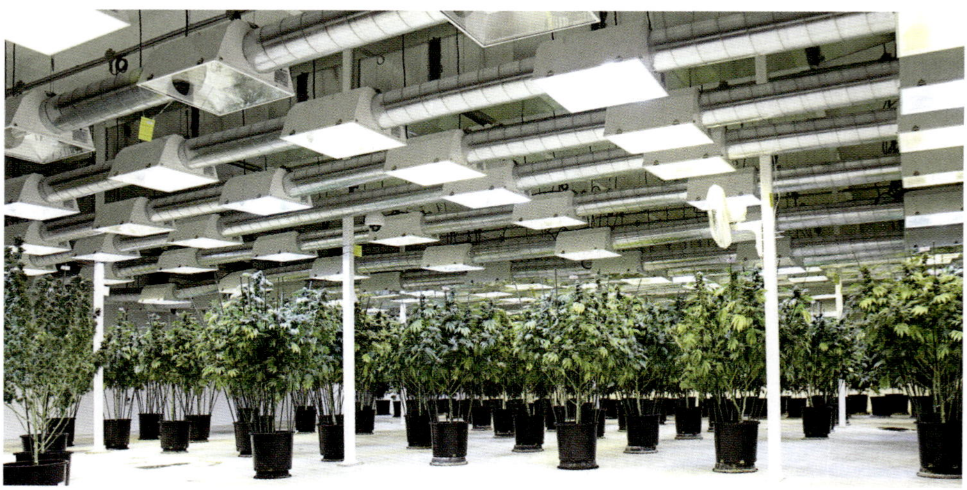

A finished air-cooled grow room. Cables connect up each light to the adjacent room's ballast farm.

PHOTOS: DAVID STRANGE

LED grow lights are typically available as complete light kits. Everything you need, including the reflector and power unit, is integrated into a single unit. Some LED systems are modular, allowing you to upgrade the reflector or add more LEDs. However, for the most part, you can find LED systems tailored to your specific grow space requirements, such as tent-sized kits or multiple LED systems for larger spaces.

When you decide to purchase a lighting system, look for a comprehensive package and consider buying an extra bulb, especially if you're working with HID lighting. Ensure that the lighting system adheres to safety regulations and provides guarantees. With LED systems, it's advisable to have a spare system on hand. If you ever need to replace your main LED light, you don't want your flowering plants to go without light, as it would negatively affect your harvest. Having a backup light source is more cost-effective than missing out on a quality harvest. You can always use the extra light for seedlings and clones; it doesn't need to be identical to your main LED system, just of lower wattage, to prevent photoperiod interruptions.

Color Bands and Plant Growth

When light is dispersed through a prism or diffraction grating, it gives rise to various color bands, representing the colors of the rainbow: Red, orange, yellow, green, blue, indigo, and violet. Color temperature, typically measured in degrees kelvin (K), correlates with the colors produced in a blackbody radiation experiment at different temperatures. These colors correspond to the frequencies emitted by a heated light source and can also be measured in nanometers (nm).

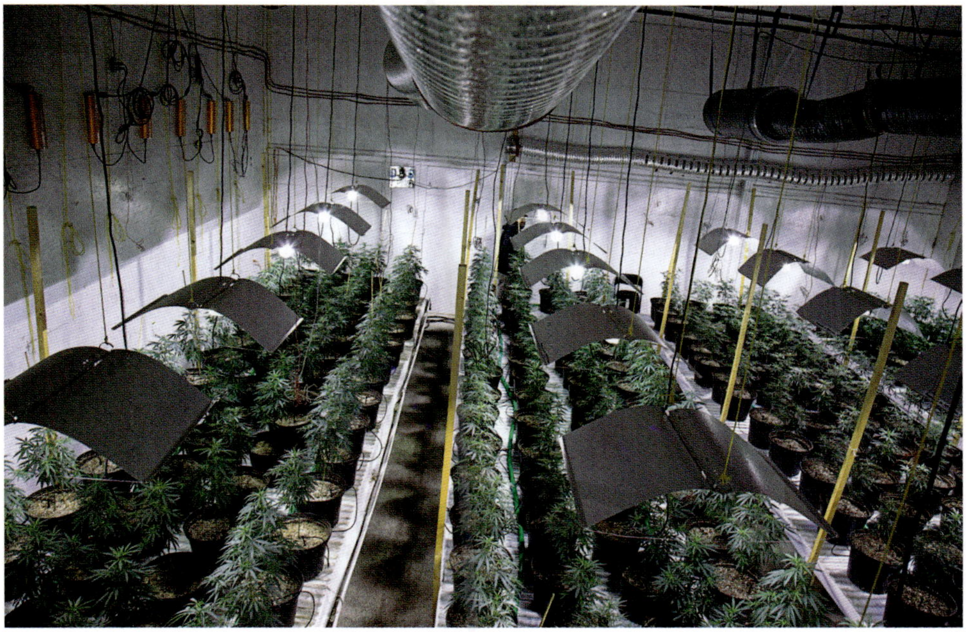

PHOTO: BUBBLEMAN

The blue tint of these metal halide bulbs simulates the sun during the vegetative phase of growth.

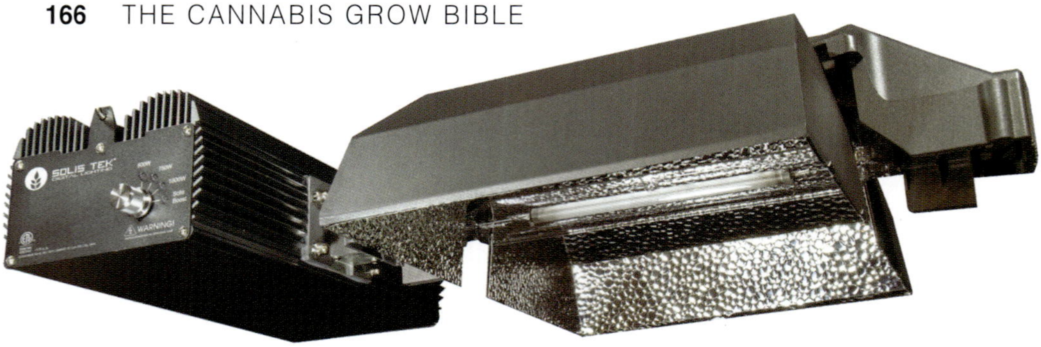

A DE (Double Ended) lamp. Notice how it has two sockets? These are becoming more popular compared to the standard single socket HIDs you see in this book.

PHOTO: SOILIS TEK

The electromagnetic spectrum describes the distribution of electromagnetic radiation based on its energy. The table below provides approximate values for wavelengths, frequencies, and energies in various regions of the spectrum, which you may find useful for assessing your light bulb's qualities. Information about your bulb can usually be found on the bulb's packaging, including wavelengths and frequencies ranging from the infrared to the ultraviolet regions, although manufacturers may have varying specifications regarding a bulb's ability to emit artificial light.

Spectrum of Electromagnetic Radiation

Region	Wavelength (Angstroms)	Wavelength (Centimeters)	Frequency (Hz)	Energy (EV)
Radio	109	>10	<3 x 109	<10-5
Microwave	109-106	10-0.01	3 x 109-3 x 1012	10-5-0.01
Infrared	106-7000	0.01-7 x 10-5	3 x 1012-4.3 x 1014	0.01-2
Visible	7000-4000	7 x 10-5-4 x 10-5	4.3 x 1014-7.5 x 1014	2-3
Ultraviolet	4000-10	4 x 10-5-10-7	7.5 x 1014-3 x 1017	3-103
X-rays	10-0.1	10-7-10-9	3 x 1017-3 x 1019	103-105
Gamma Rays	0.1	<10-9	>3 x 1019	>105

Notably, many new grow lights extend slightly beyond the visible region (400–700 nm). In this range, 400 nm represents the blue end and 700 nm the red end of the spectrum. Research suggests that ultraviolet light (10–400 nm) can enhance a plant's resistance to diseases. Wavelengths beyond 700 nm influence plant competition for light. Nevertheless, the visible light range (400–700 nm) remains the most critical for plant growth.

The color of light produced depends on the mechanisms of the light source. Artificial grow lights are engineered to emit a strong, clean, white light that adheres to specific color and temperature criteria, classifying the bulb as a "grow bulb." This pure white light can be adjusted with various gases to achieve a blue or orange hue. When dealing with HID grow lights, you'll come across two main categories of hue: Cool colors, ranging from whites to blues, and warm colors, spanning from yellow to red.

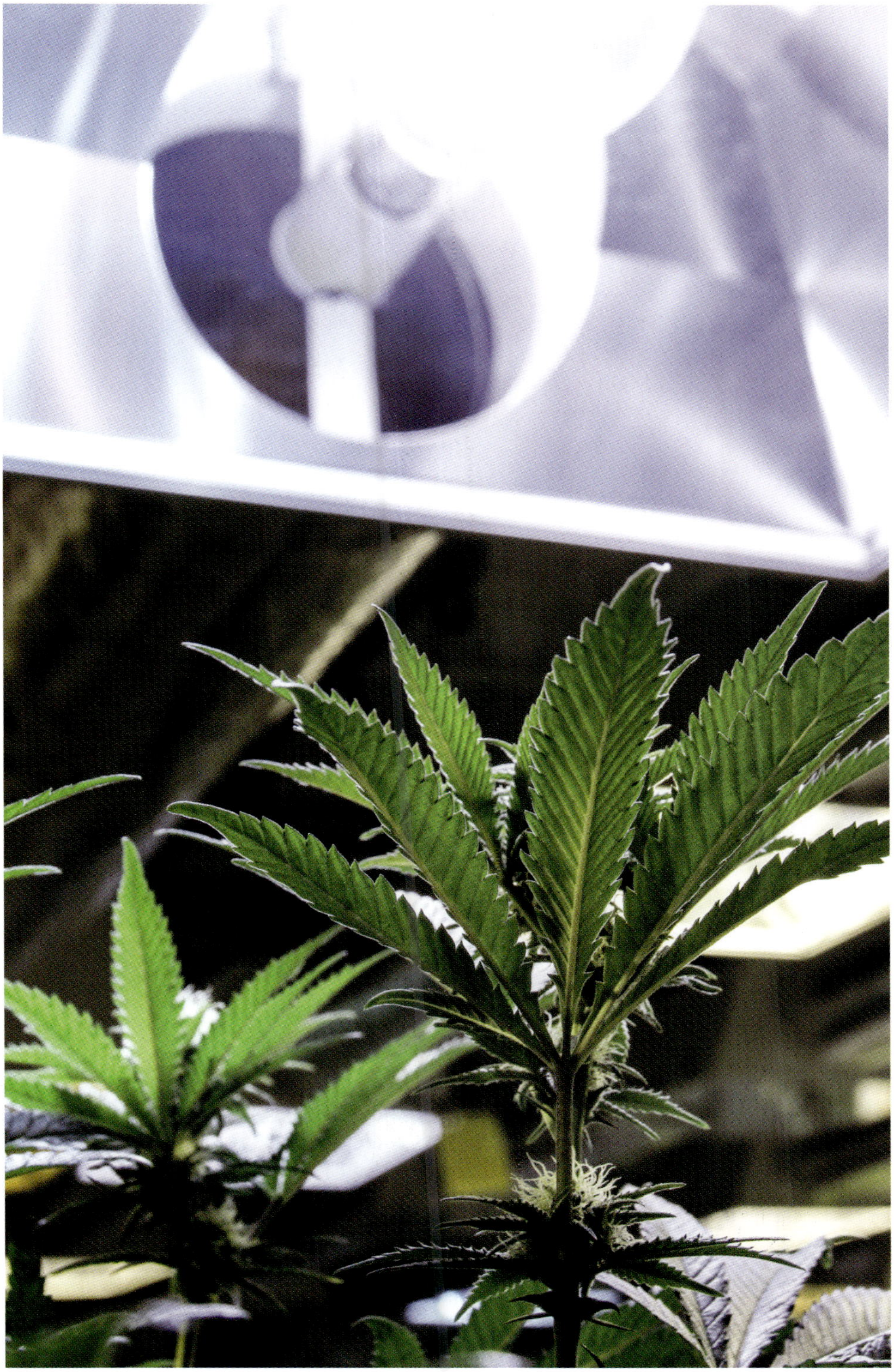

PHOTO: DAVID STRANGE

Leaves lying flat to receive light, on branches angled upwards, are a good sign of a healthy plant.

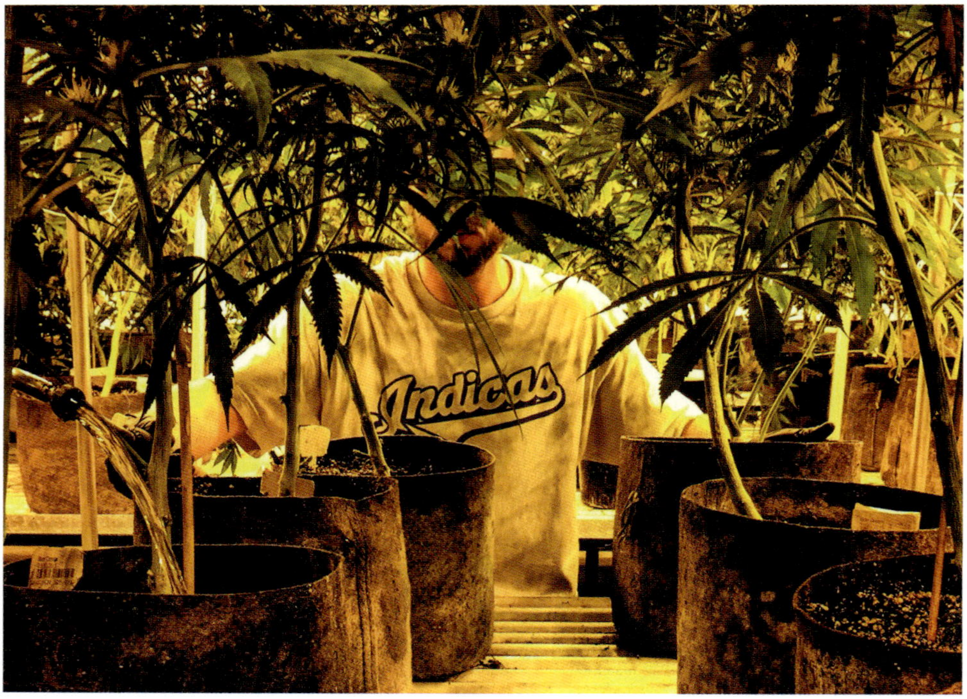

Orange glow means HPS lights. The pot at the left is being watered.

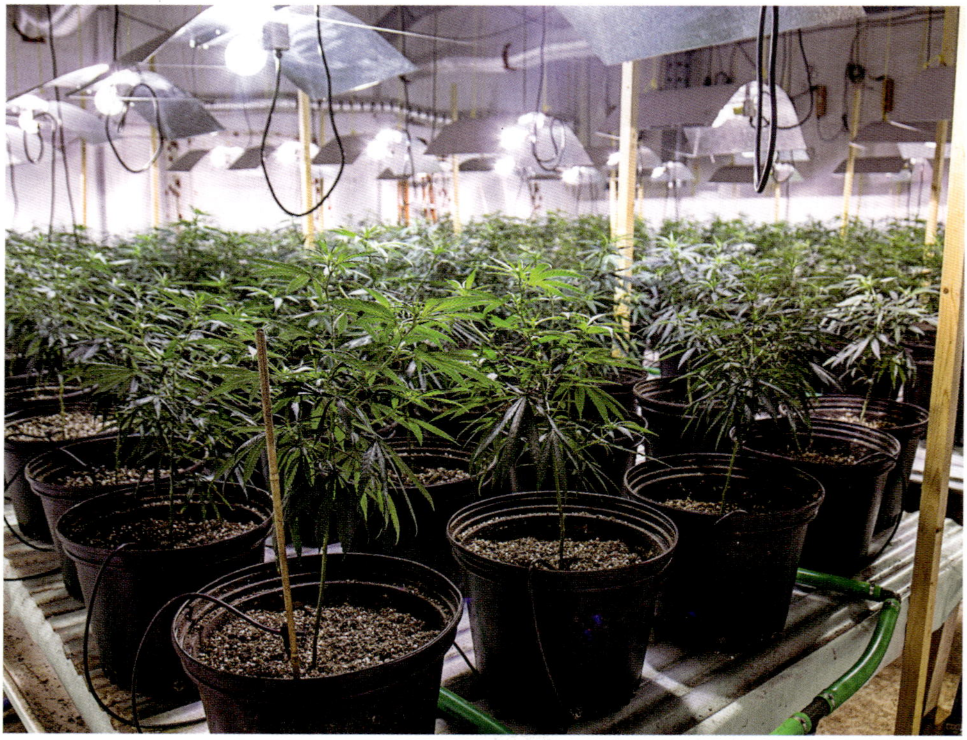
Blue tint expected from vegetative plants under MH HID lights.

PHOTOS: HIP2THECROP (TOP), BUBBLEMAN (BOTTOM)

For example, metal halide (MH) bulbs with a color temperature of 5,500 K appear blue. A fluorescent cool white tube, at approximately 4,200 K, emits light in the blue to white spectrum. Clear MH bulbs with a color temperature of 4,000 K produce white light. Warm MH bulbs at 3,200 K emit light ranging from white to yellow. High-pressure sodium (HPS) bulbs with a color temperature of 2,200 K cast an orange hue. LEDs are capable of emulating these color temperatures but use a distinct mechanism involving semiconductors to produce an electroluminescence. We will go into more detail on LEDs in this chapter.

Correlated Color Temperature (CCT)

The correlated color temperature (CCT), expressed in degrees kelvin, signifies the thermal temperature of a light source. The source emits light when the bulb's components and gas compounds are heated. As these elements heat up, their color changes within a specific range, ultimately peaking when the bulb reaches its maximum temperature. This peak color is the bulb's CCT rating. A bulb with a CCT rating of 3,000 K is referred to as "warm," one with a CCT rating of 4,000 K is categorized as "neutral," and one with a 6,000 K CCT rating is labeled as "cool." The bulb's CCT is a result of the diverse colors emitted by the bulb's hot elements or the LED mechanism.

Color Rendering Index (CRI)

While CCT reveals the bulb's color temperature, it does not indicate how effectively each color band is represented. To evaluate color distribution quality, we refer to the lamp's color rendering index (CRI).

CRI is determined in a controlled laboratory setting by comparing the bulb's CCT with a reference material under the same CCT. In the horticultural community, there is a general consensus that a higher CRI rating indicates better color distribution quality. Therefore, by considering both CCT and CRI values, we can identify the most suitable bulb for our specific needs.

For most growers, natural daylight during the daytime hours measures around 5,500 K. The table below provides an overview of the colors typically encountered when using artificial light sources and their impact on cannabis plant growth.

Kelvin Color Temperature Scale

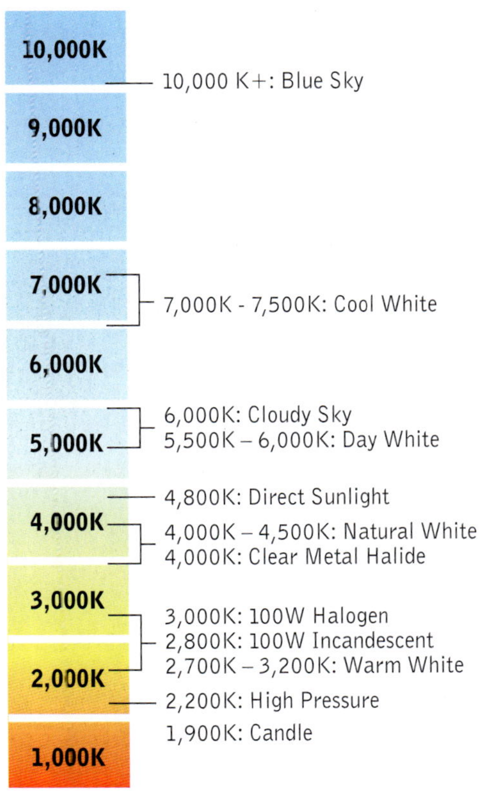

Impact of Light Color on Plant Growth

CCT in Kelvin (K)	Light Color	Effect
5000 to 8000	Deep blue	Encourages excellent leaf and stem growth
4000 to 5000	Light blue	Encourages good leaf and stem growth
4000	Neutral white	Promotes normal growth
3700 to 4000	Warm neutral	Promotes rapid growth
3000 to 3700	Warmer yellow neutral	Highly active photosynthesis for all stages of growth
1500 to 3000	Hot orange or red	Promotes flowering

Ultraviolet, Visible, and Far-Red Light

Plants appear green because they reflect green light, which is not extensively used for photosynthesis in cannabis and most other plants. This phenomenon is related to the plant pigment chlorophyll. Despite reflecting green light, plants still use some green in the visible light spectrum (ranging from 400 to 700 nm) for photosynthesis. This means that grow lights do not need to minimize green light, which occupies a central position in the visible light spectrum, in their design. Therefore, any grow light you consider should encompass the entire visible spectrum, even if it leans more towards the blue or red end. Avoid any gimmicks aimed at reducing green light. When selecting a light, check if the manufacturer has provided a spectrograph, allowing you to review the color data.

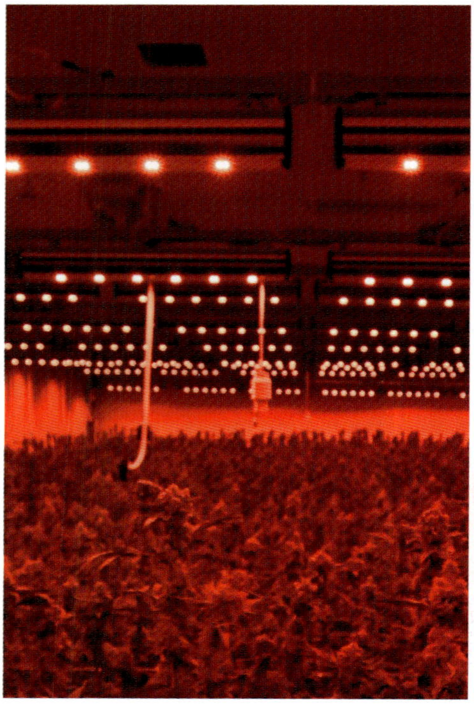

Far-red light experimentation to see how it may impact final results.

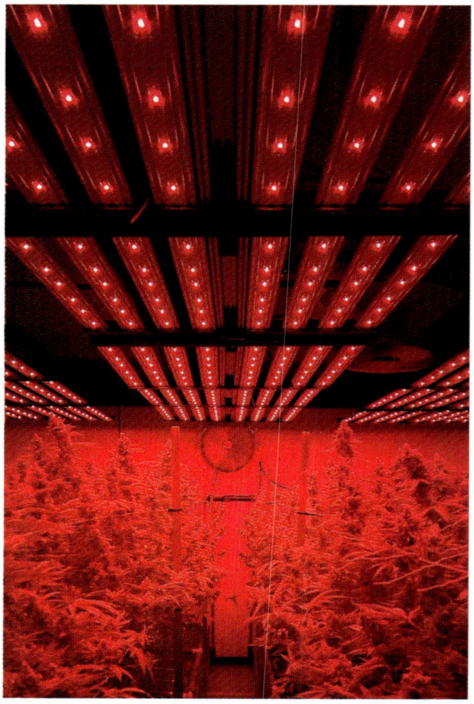

Far-red light is very noticeable due to the intense red coloration of the grow room.

PHOTOS: MIAMIMANGOCA.COM (LEFT), GRANDMASTERLEDS.COM (RIGHT)

Ultraviolet light on the left side of the visible band appears to influence a plant's defense mechanisms against pathogens and potentially some forms of cannabinoid synthesis. On the far-red side of the visible spectrum, plant structure is affected. The examined UV region spans from 350 to 450 nm, while far-red light ranges from 700 to 750 nm. However, the significance of UV and far-red light for cannabis plants is not as established as the visible light spectrum (400 to 700 nm) and requires further research to determine their specific roles. UV light has the downside of destroying DNA bonds.

These are the basics of light mechanisms and the associated measurements and values found on bulb packaging. Now we discuss how plants use light, which will lead us to a deeper exploration of lighting in the context of plant growth.

Understanding the Fundamentals of Photosynthesis

To grasp the essence of cannabis plant energy systems, it's essential to understand the basics of photosynthesis. With the exception of some algae and bacteria, plants are the only organisms naturally capable of converting simple substances into complex food materials. Most other organisms lack the ability to synthesize their own sustenance and instead seek complex foods, whether in the form of other organisms or plants.

Chlorophyll

Plants inherently produce chlorophyll, the green pigment responsible for their characteristic coloration. Chlorophyll constitutes a group of green pigments containing magnesium, which serve as a light energy absorber for specific wavelengths. The plant harnesses this absorbed light energy and converts it into chemical energy.

The Process of Photosynthesis

The term "photosynthesis" literally means "combining with light." It represents a "reactant-product" process that takes place wherever chlorophyll is present in the plant, primarily in the leaves. The symbolic equation for photosynthesis is:

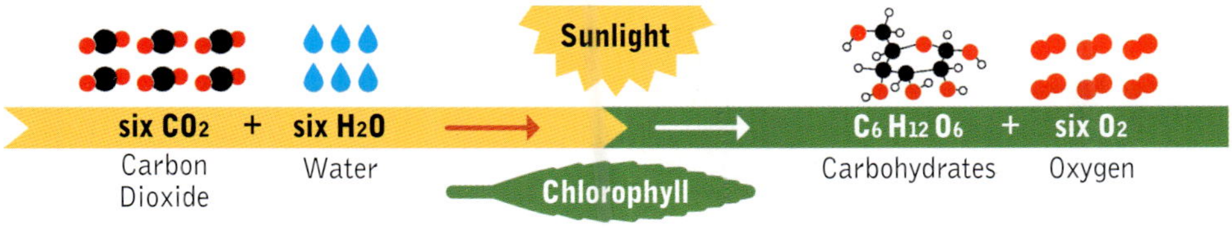

This equation illustrates that six atoms of carbon dioxide ($6CO_2$) and six molecules of water ($6H_2O$), exposed to sunlight (or artificial grow lights) and chlorophyll in plants yield a sugar molecule, typically glucose ($C_6H_{12}O_6$), and release six oxygen molecules ($6O_2$). Photosynthesis requires light. Therefore, during the night or when grow lights are off, photosynthesis comes to a halt.

Temperature plays a critical role in photosynthesis, as all chemical processes in living organisms operate within a specific temperature range. Consequently, photosynthesis may slow down or even cease if temperatures deviate significantly from the optimal range for the particular plant species. Sufficient nutrient availability is another fundamental aspect, as a shortage of nutrients leads to a halt in chlorophyll production and, subsequently, photosynthesis.

The above equation encapsulates the entire process. The basic components for plant growth are synthesized internally by the plant, using gases, sunlight or artificial light, and nutrients drawn from the growing medium. The sugars generated, particularly glucose ($C_6H_{12}O_6$), combined with the essential nutrients, shape every aspect of a plant's physiology.

Notably, plants have evolved to adapt to the natural variations in sunlight throughout the seasons. Therefore, it's crucial to adjust lighting in indoor environments to simulate natural changes in light. This is achieved by using different types of lighting at various growth stages.

Lighting for Different Growth Stages

Seedling Lighting

During the initial stages of germinating seeds, there's no need for light until the first leaves, the cotyledons, emerge. While window light can suffice, it's not ideal, as it may cause seedlings to elongate or "stretch." To maintain short internode lengths, low-wattage LEDs are a suitable choice. Traditional fluorescent lights are gradually being replaced by LEDs whose better performance and reduced heat production make them a favorable option. HID lighting is too intense for seedlings.

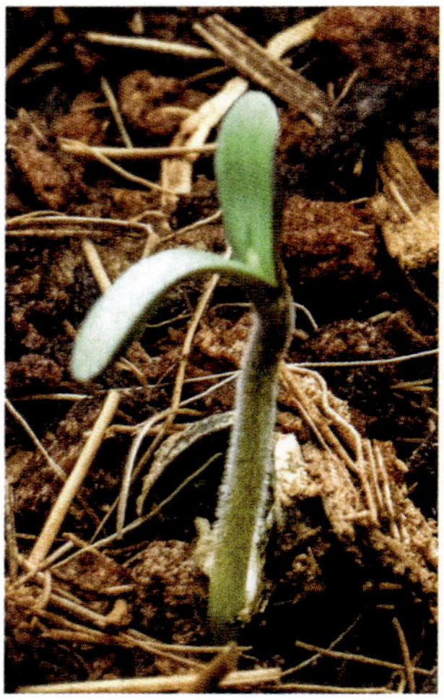

It is essential to keep the seedling short.

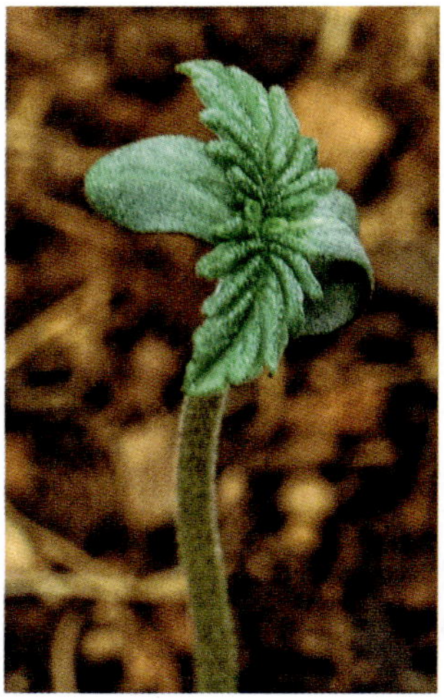

Soon, this germinating seed will seek light.

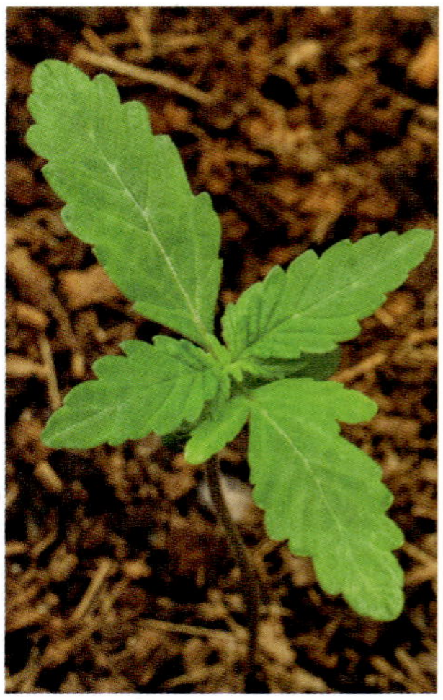

Seedlings tend to chase light quite early on.

PHOTOS: JOE'S CANNA GROWS

Clone and Small Plant Lighting

When preparing to take cuttings for cloning, or if you plan to prune your plants, you'll need a light source to support healthy growth. Natural sunlight and window light can lead to extended internode lengths. To encourage compact and sturdy growth, opt for LEDs. While higher-wattage fluorescents or low-wattage HIDs have been used in the past, you'll find LEDs more convenient and effective.

Vegetative Plant and Clone Mother Plant Lighting

Plants that have grown more than four leaves, not counting cotyledons, are ready for vegetative or clone mother plant maintenance. To stimulate vigorous growth, it's crucial to provide adequate lighting. Natural sunlight and window light can result in elongated internode lengths. To maintain a more compact plant structure, high-output LEDs and high-wattage HIDs are preferred. Outdoor growers may tolerate longer internode lengths, but for indoor vegetative growth, HID cultivators use MH lights.

Flowering Plant Lighting

Mature plants that have undergone preflowering calyx development are ready for the flowering stage. To induce flowering, you must adjust the photoperiod to a 12/12 light-dark cycle. Although natural sunlight and window light can initiate flowering in mature plants, a consistent 12/12 photoperiod is required. For indoor flowering, high-quality results can be achieved with LEDs. HID users commonly opt for HPS HID lighting, which meets their needs successfully.

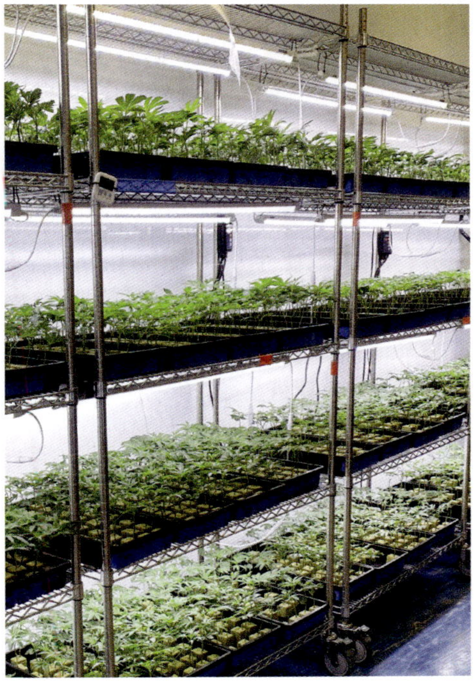

Some fluorescent-type grow lights are popular for shelf growing.

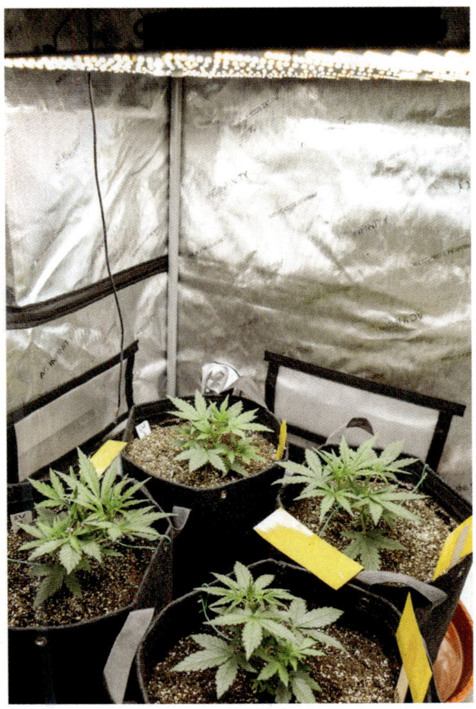

LED lights are very popular for tent growing.

PHOTOS: HIP2THECROP (TOP), JOE'S CANNA GROWS (BOTTOM)

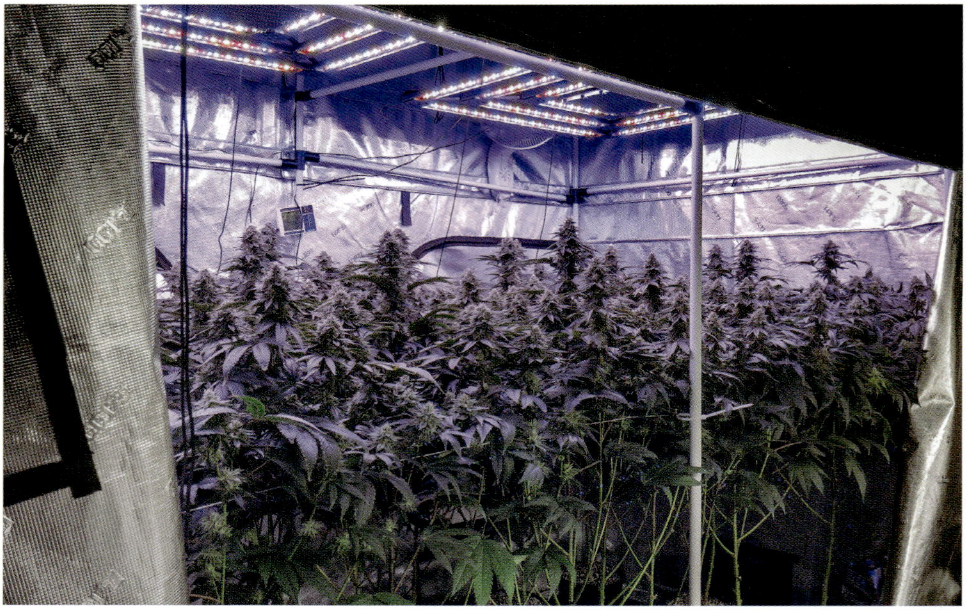

LEDs for tents are much easier to install and use than HIDs. The larger the tent, the more LED arrays you might need.

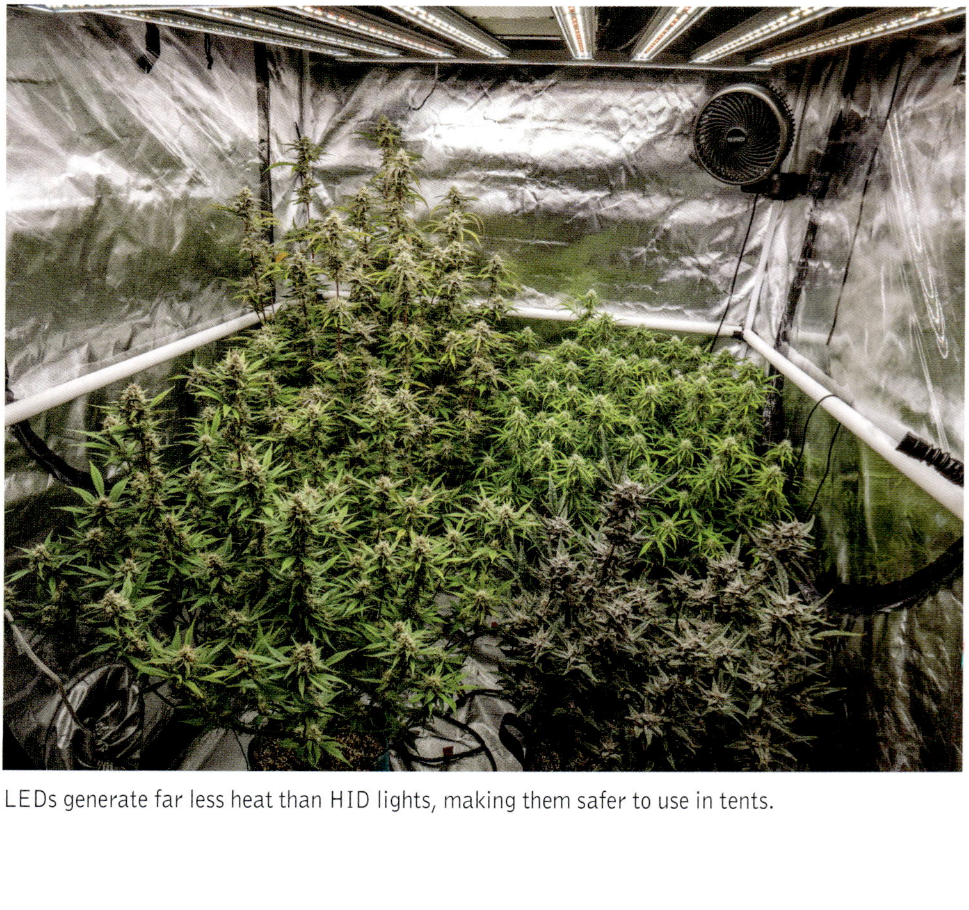

PHOTOS: KINDLEDGROWLIGHTS.COM (TOP), JOE'S CANNA GROWS (BOTTOM)

LEDs generate far less heat than HID lights, making them safer to use in tents.

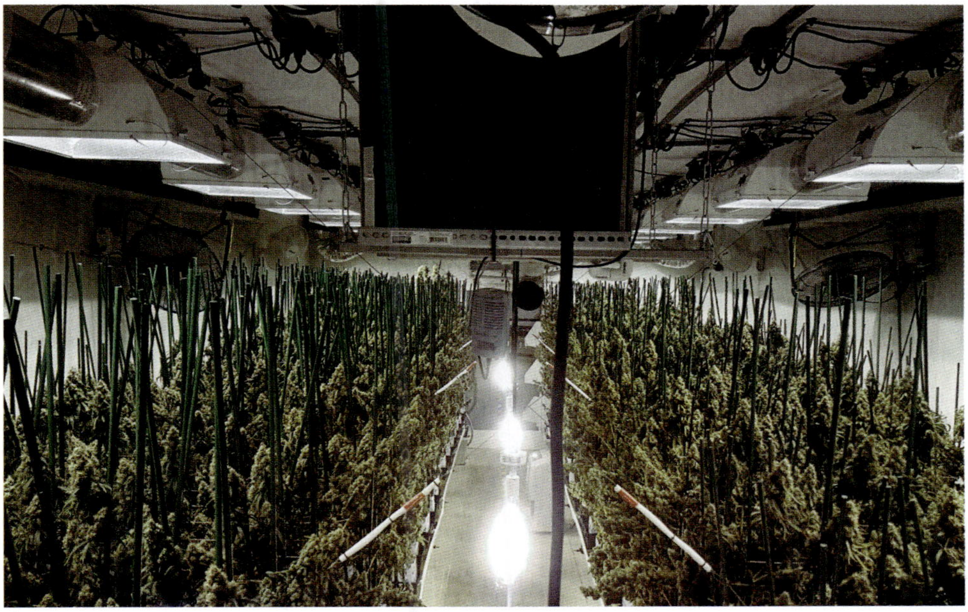

HIDs with air-cooled hoods and ducting, suspended over staked flowering plants.

HPS HID lights are suitable if you use HIDs and can't afford two separate bulbs. However, transitioning to MH bulbs for vegetative growth is recommended if feasible. This transition helps adjust the light spectrum according to the plant's adaptation to the natural color bands, which change outdoors over the course of the months.

To understand how to use each of these lighting options, consider your entire setup rather than focusing on light strength and color bands. The choice of lighting should align with the specific requirements of your setup. Keep in mind that the lighting needs for tents, cabinets, and full-scale grow rooms can vary significantly.

Many cultivators gradually expand their setups from small to large over time and with greater experience. Starting small and gradually progressing has advantages, including the ability to recoup a substantial portion of the equipment cost when selling, as horticultural items tend to hold their value. Smaller systems can also serve for nurturing seedlings and clones when you transition to a larger setup.

Even if you don't plan to use HID lights, it's valuable to learn about them, as they serve as a benchmark for comparing LED systems. For instance, you may come across claims that certain LED systems can match the performance of a 600-watt HPS light. However, these comparisons may not make much sense unless you have a basic understanding of what HID lights and specifically 600-watt HPS lights actually do.

Now, let's dive deeper into the characteristics of different lighting types.

PHOTO: ALEX

Bulbs

When purchasing a lighting system, it is recommended that you look for a complete system and buy an extra bulb. Check to make sure that the lighting system meets safety regulations and has some sort of guarantee or warranty.

1000-watt DE (double ended) HPS light. DE lights are becoming more popular.

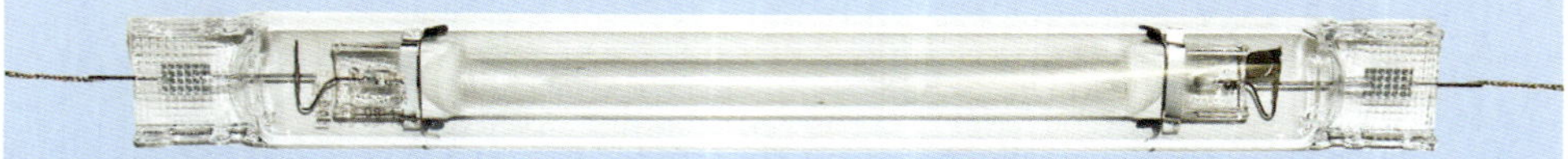

1000-watt DE MH light. DE requires you have a DE socket/reflector.

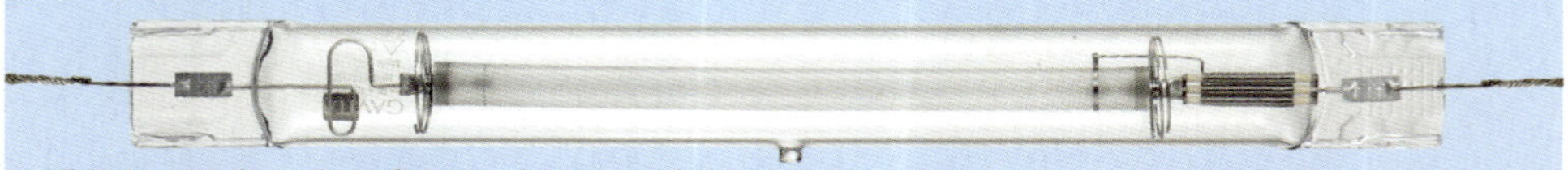

This is a high-end professional DE, combining high optical quality with a high photosynthetic photon flux (ppf).

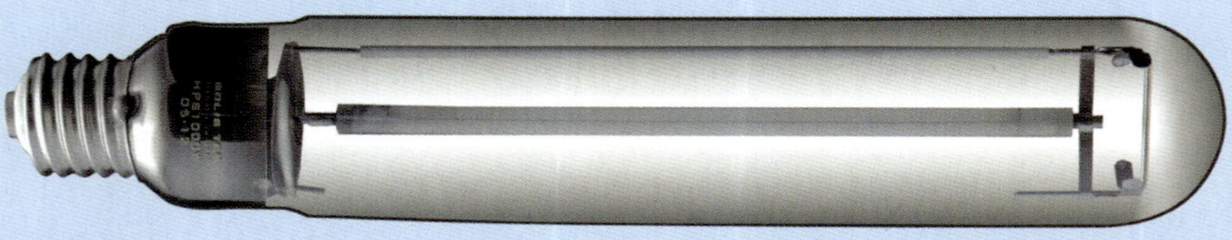

1000-watt HPS. This is a regular 1K HPS light that uses a standard single HID socket.

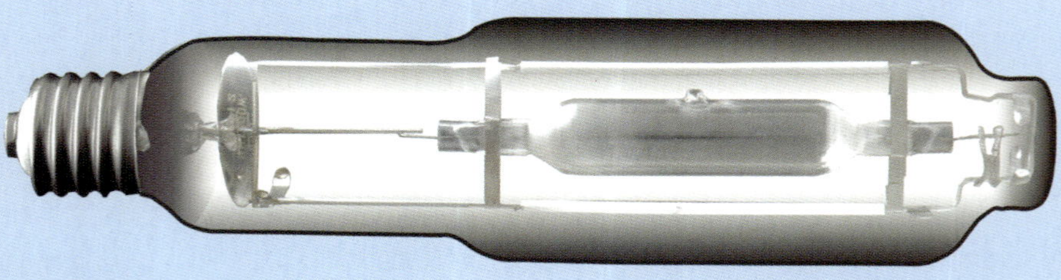

1000-watt MH. Also regular but MH. It's important to get the right socket/ballast for all these bulb types.

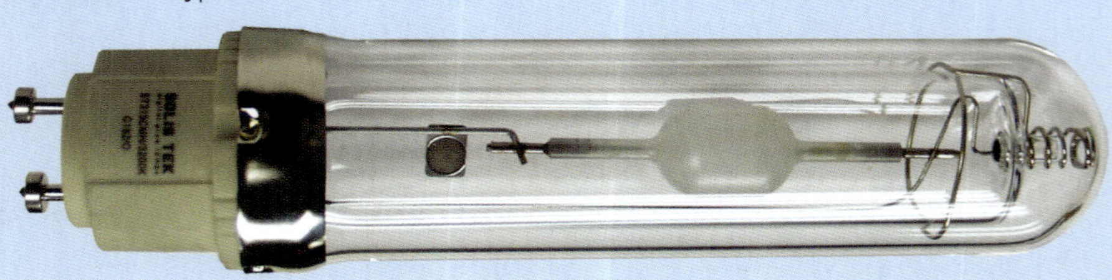

Energy-efficient CMH (Ceramic Metal Halide). This is a new HID technology for increased efficiency. They often have unique wattages. A bulb may be 315-watt, for example.

PHOTOS: SOILIS TEK (TOP FIVE), GAVITA (BOTTOM)

Common Lighting Types

Incandescent Bulbs

Formerly known as domestic bulbs, incandescent bulbs were commonly used in households but have mostly been replaced by LEDs. They are available in various sizes and typically range from 15 to 150 watts. However, they are unsuitable for growing due to their low light intensity and poor CRI rating. Standard domestic incandescent bulbs have a CCT rating of about 2,700 K.

Halogen Lights

Halogen lights, although small and often used for night-time floodlighting, have been largely replaced by LED bulbs. They can range from 75 to 4,000 watts. However, halogen lights generate excessive heat, making them unsuitable and potentially dangerous for indoor cannabis cultivation. They also have a low CRI rating. Halogens have a CCT rating of about 3,000 K.

Fluorescent Tube Lights

These long, tube-shaped lights, once common in industrial and commercial settings, have been largely replaced by LEDs. They come in various lengths and sizes, with bulbs between 2 and 10 feet long being the most common, and they range from 10 to 300 watts. While these lights are acceptable for growing, they provide lower light intensity and can be challenging to set up correctly. Moreover, their light spectrum may not be ideal for cannabis growth due to their poor CRI ratings.[2] However, some fluorescent white lights are designed for plant growth.

Fluorescent White Tube Lights

Unlike standard fluorescent lights, white tube lights have a higher CRI rating and were recommended as cost-effective grow lights. They were particularly useful for rooting clones and starting seeds. Fluorescent white tube lights are typically available in 10, 30, 60, and 100 watts. Lights of 30 watts or higher are suitable for inducing floral development, while those with less than 30 watts are sufficient for rooting cuttings and starting seedlings. Cool white fluorescents have a CCT rating of about 4,200 K. LEDs can effectively replace fluorescent lights.

Horticultural Lights

Professional horticultural HID lights are specifically designed for promoting indoor plant growth. These lights are typically available in kits, which include a bulb, reflector, ballast, and timer. They come in various wattage levels, shapes, and sizes. HID high-powered grow bulbs can deliver light intensities comparable to the natural sunlight on Earth without harming the plants when proper ventilation and control are in place. These bulbs are available in four major wattage options: 1000, 600, 400, and 250 watts. In addition, there are two less common wattage levels: 150 and 430 watts.

HID lights can be categorized into three distinct subtypes: Metal halide (MH), mercury vapor (MV), and high-pressure sodium (HPS).

MH and HPS are the most widely used HIDs. MH lights are typically used for the vegetative growth stages of plants, as they emit cooler-toned light. While MH lights can also be used for flowering, HPS lights are more suitable for this stage. They are available in various shapes and sizes, and range from 75 to 4,000 watts. MH lights tend to produce light in the blue spectrum, earning them the cool designation. Daylight MH lights typically have a CCT rating of around 5,500 K, while standard clear MH lights have a CCT rating of about 4,000 K. Warm MH lights with a CCT rating of about 3,200 K are also available, but it is generally recommended to opt for daylight halide as it provides the best MH light for cannabis. When choosing between MH and MV, MH is generally preferred as MV lights tend to emit light that is slightly out of the optimal spectrum range, appearing too blue.

HPS lights have long been the preferred choice among cannabis cultivators. These are available in various sizes, ranging from 75 to 4,000 watts. They emit light in the ideal spectrum for growing cannabis and are particularly recommended for the flowering stage of the plant's life cycle. HPS lights tend to produce an orange hue, indicating that they belong to the warm category. HPS bulbs typically have a CCT rating of about 2,200 K.

HID kits are generally designed to accommodate specific bulb wattages and types. For instance, if you have a 600-watt HPS system, you should use 600-watt HPS bulbs, not MH bulbs. However, some lighting kits include a switchable ballast, allowing you to use both MH and HPS lights with the same system.

Note that more power is not always better. A 4,000-watt HID is excessive for a typical grow room and can generate too much heat. One 4,000-watt bulb or four 1,000-watt bulbs, when placed too closely, can scorch and bleach cannabis plants. There's an optimal point of light saturation for plant growth, and exceeding it can lead to photoinhibition, potentially reducing production. As a rule of thumb, 1,000 watts is the maximum recommended for an average-sized space, as we will explain further using the illumination-to-space formula. For larger spaces, you can use multiple bulbs to provide adequate light coverage.

The LED Revolution

Between 1999 and 2009, LED manufacturers were in the midst of fundamental research aimed at bringing about better, brighter, and more cost-effective systems for the grow-lights market. In the years that followed, lower-wattage HID lights and low-wattage fluorescents were phased out, with growers increasingly favoring 400-watt and then 600-watt options. Today, LEDs have not only caught up with but also surpassed 1000-watt HIDs. LEDs are particularly well-suited for the close proximity

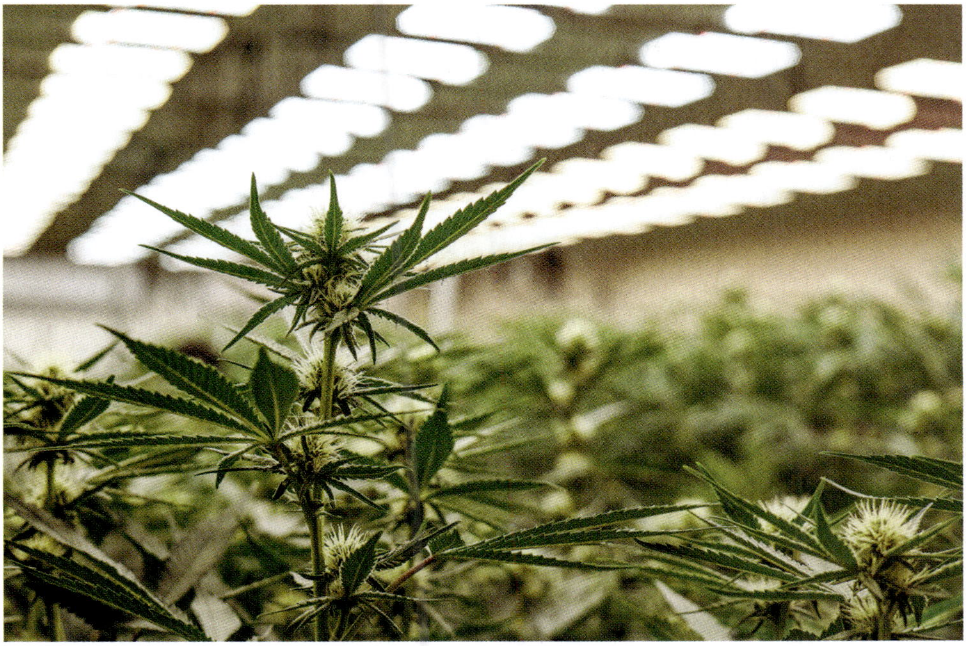

Leaves outstretched, flat, and receiving light are signs of a healthy plant.

PHOTO: HORTICULTURE LIGHTING GROUP, HLG.COM

required for seedlings, clones, and the initial vegetative growth stages. There's little reason to use an HID in these scenarios. However, HID systems are still viable for the flowering stage, particularly with 600-watt and 1000-watt HPS HIDs. LED systems can also compete effectively in this context.

Adopting LEDs in the grow-light sector involved not only altering lighting setups but also embracing a different approach to cultivation. This shift in methods led to distinct indoor growing practices, and these have become the dominant approach, with systems increasingly transitioning to LEDs, especially in grow tents. HID lights produce heat, which can contribute to elevated temperatures in the growing space. LEDs, on the other hand, operate at cooler temperatures, with some making very minimal contributions to overall heat. Consequently, some LED grow spaces may require heating rather than cooling.

Research efforts for both LED and HID technologies aim to achieve these objectives:

1. Reduce the amount of electricity required to operate the lights, thereby lowering operational costs.
2. Minimize heat generation by lighting systems to mitigate heat stress issues.
3. Replicate the light colors and lumens of natural sunlight for optimal plant growth.
4. Demonstrate environmental sustainability in both construction and usage.
5. Provide accurate and transparent product specifications.

LEDs have the advantage in many of these aspects.

LED and Arrays

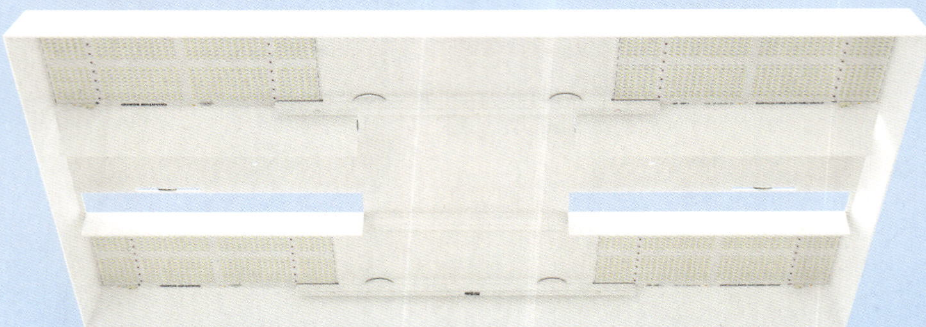

There are many shapes of LED array out there, such as this rectangular one.

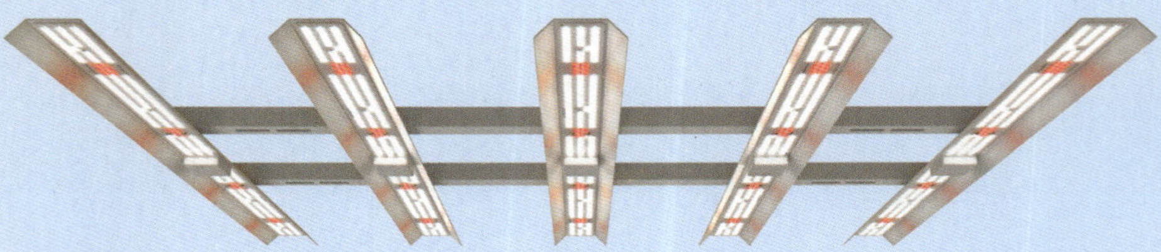

Some LED arrays are borderless and more like a satellite array.

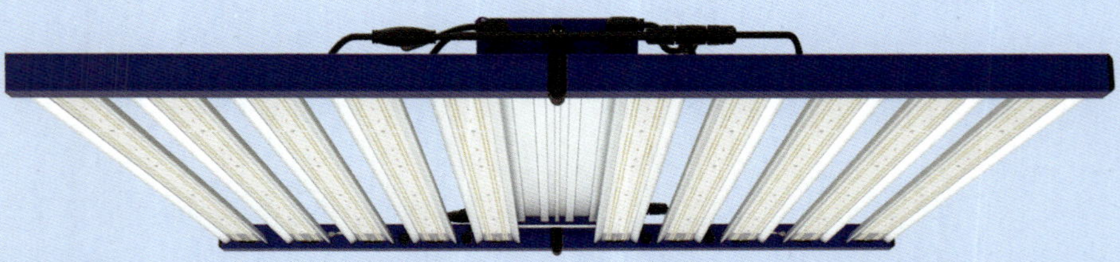

Other LED arrays have borders on two sides with the lights close together.

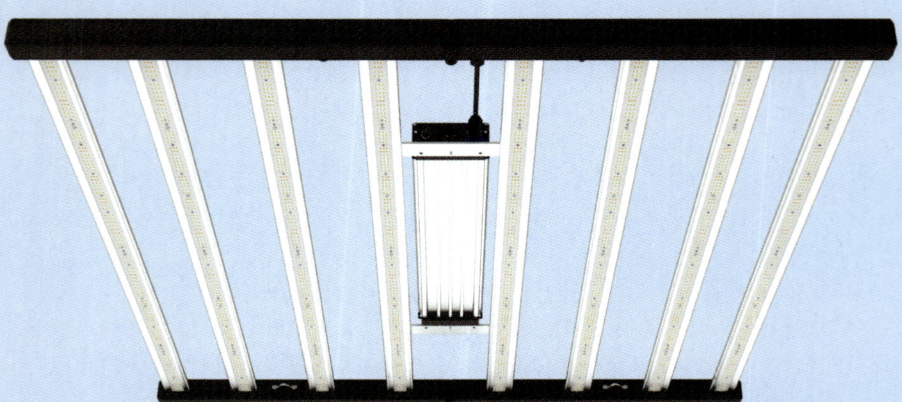

LEDs with a central cluster in the array are also available.

PHOTOS: HORTICULTURE LIGHTING GROUP, HLG.COM (TOP TWO), GRANDMASTERLEDS.COM (BOTTOM TWO)

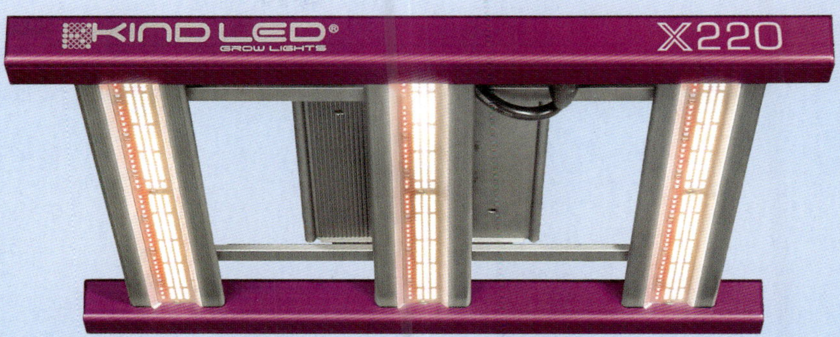

It is not uncommon to find that professional LED systems come in a series of different intensities.

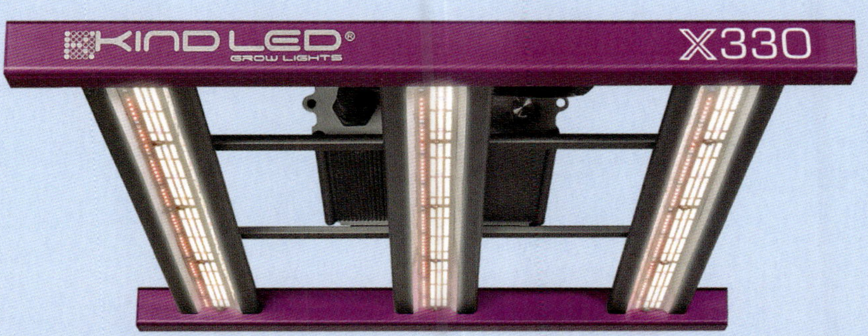

The more advanced units try to increase their PPF by a factor of a few hundred with each model.

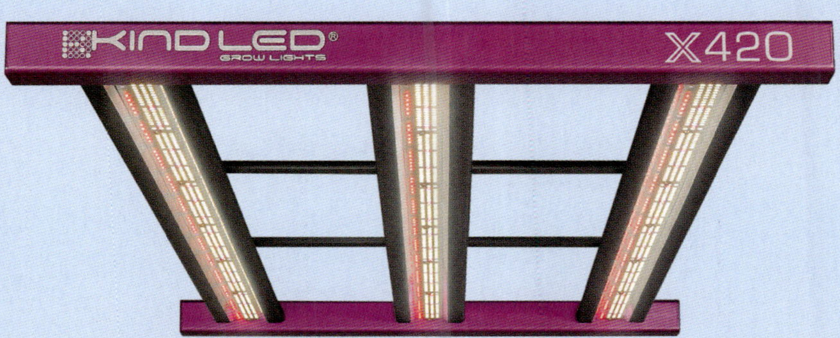

This X420 model of KindLEDs puts out around 1000 PPF.

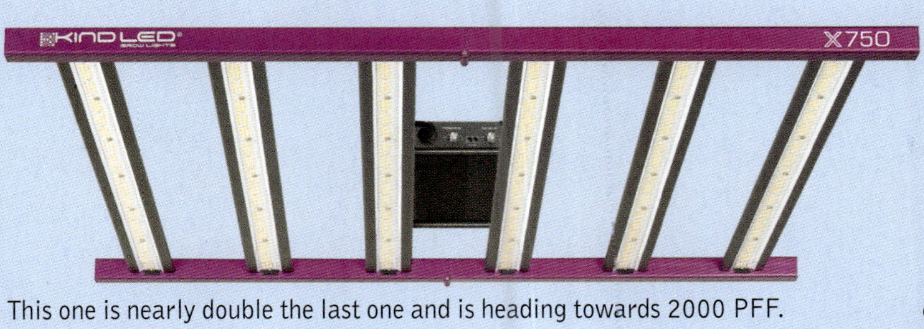

This one is nearly double the last one and is heading towards 2000 PFF.

continues...

PHOTOS: KINDLEDGROWLIGHTS.COM

LED and Arrays *continued*

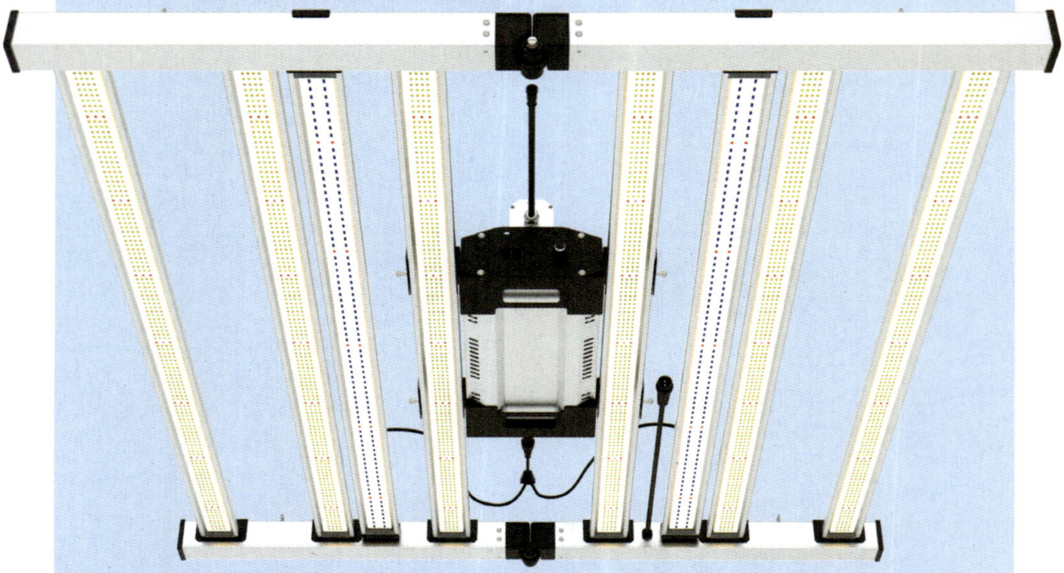

Industrial-sized arrays are available for the most intense growing operations.

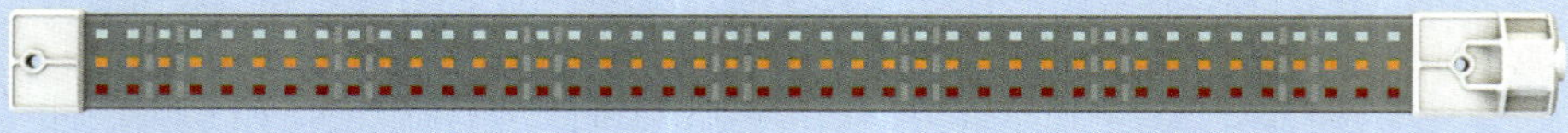

Diodes can be seen aligning the inside of the array unit holder.

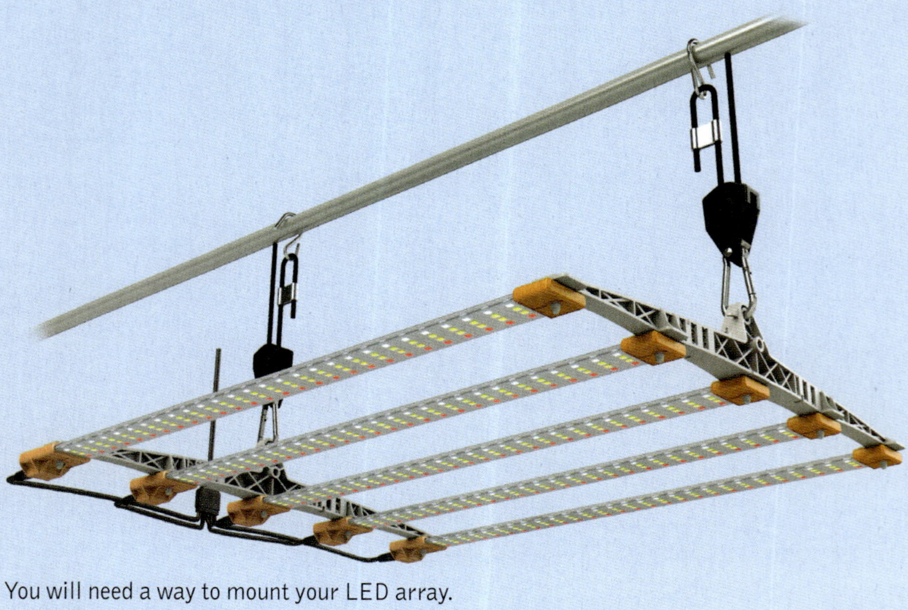

You will need a way to mount your LED array.

PHOTOS: MAMMOTHLIGHTING.COM (TOP), SECRETJARDIN.COM (MIDDLE AND BOTTOM)

LED Power

LED grow bulbs have successfully reduced the operational cost of lighting. Consequently, even though LEDs might initially cost more than HIDs, the long-term use of LED systems over HIDs results in reduced electricity consumption and lower overall costs. The numbers included in an LED brand's name, such as 100, 400, 600, or 1000, can be misleading; they are essentially arbitrary labels. To make an informed choice, you need to delve into the LED's specifications and description.

HID lights differ in that their numbers typically correspond to wattage. If you know any two values among watts, amps, and volts, you can calculate the third using this formula: watts = amps × volts. However, remember that light intensity represents just one facet of the equation; the light must also encompass appropriate color bands. The wattage indicated on LED bulbs may exhibit slight variations around the average, meaning that the actual wattage they consume may be slightly more or less than what's stated, depending on their energy efficiency.

LED Advantages over HID

LED systems offer several advantages over HID lights. HID bulbs are comparatively less robust due to their glass and gas components. While it's not advisable to subject LED systems to physical stress, they are inherently more rugged. High-quality and well-maintained LED systems also can achieve lifespans with double or even triple the duration of HID bulbs. Unlike HIDs, LEDs require no warm-up time. When you turn them on, they are instantly ready for operation. However, LEDs may take a few minutes to reach a stable temperature, particularly when equipped with plate fin heatsinks. It's advisable to check the LED temperature after it has been running for at least 10 minutes.

LED Heatsinks

The advancement in LED cooling technology involves the use of heatsinks, similar to the cooling methods used for computer graphics cards or processors, incorporating fans, cooling pastes, and thermal-resistant components. In contrast, HID lights, with either an external or an internal ballast, tend to be heavy and generate substantial heat.

Two types of heatsinks are commonly used: Pin heatsinks and fin heatsinks. Each type has its own thermal resistance (Rth), indicating its capacity to dissipate heat. Pin heatsinks can sometimes outperform fin heatsinks in cooling, but the addition of airflow to a grow environment can bring the cooling efficiency of fin heatsinks to a level comparable to that of pin heatsinks. In practical operation, the two types offer similar performance. To customize your LED systems, it's possible to acquire replacement LED heatsinks. However, it's essential to select a heatsink that is compatible with your system. The heat reduction achieved with heatsinked LEDs represents a significant improvement from HID lighting. Many LEDs remain cool to the touch or become just mildly warm. This makes LEDs a safer choice for growers concerned about the risk of fire.

Additive and Subtractive Mixing of the Primary Colors

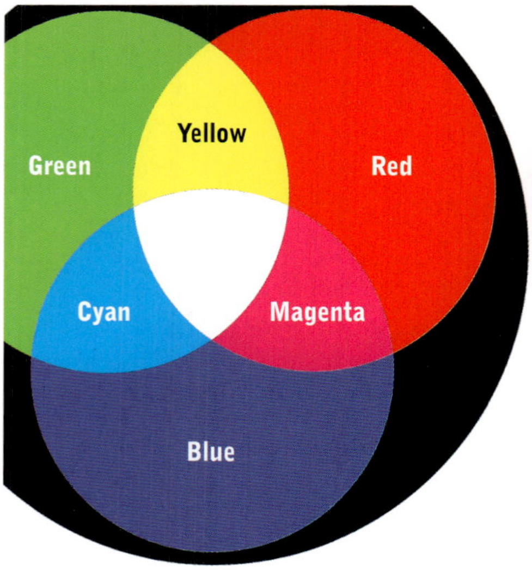

ADDITIVE
combining light

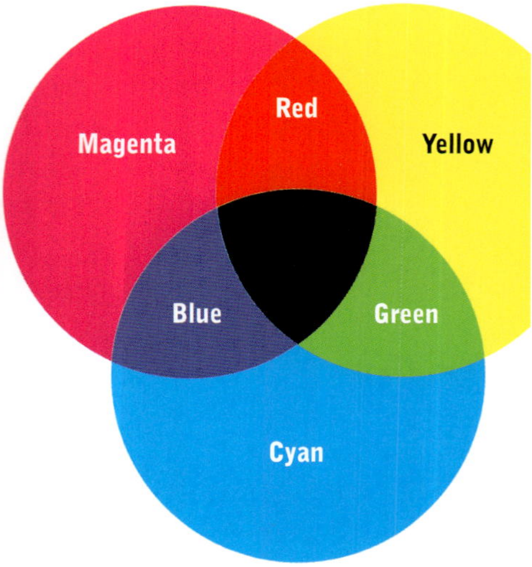

SUBTRACTIVE
mixing paints or inks

Diodes

Diodes are tiny semiconductors that can be precisely engineered to cover specific parts of the electromagnetic spectrum. They are capable of emitting extremely bright light, making them competitive in the 1000-watt HID market. The science of electroluminescence is based on the spacing between semiconductors within a diode. Different spacings generate different wavelengths of light. Therefore, to create light within a specific range, an array of diodes is needed.

You might be familiar with the scientific RGB model, which consists of three intersecting circles: Red and blue combine to produce magenta, blue and green create cyan, green and red yield yellow, and the mixture of magenta, yellow, and cyan results in white light at the center. White light cannot be achieved with just two primary colors. A light that leans toward a blueish tint is suitable for vegetative growth, while one with an orange tint is ideal for flowering, as seen in HIDs. However, you require white light for optimal results.

A single diode can emit primary colors. Some LEDs are known as multicolor white LEDs, while others are RGB LEDs. The primary consideration with grow LEDs is that they be categorized as white LEDs. The method of producing white LEDs varies, leading to variations in product descriptions. In a single LED system, one LED produces all the primary colors, which blend to create white light. These are known as multicolor LEDs or RGB LEDs, which can be configured to emit a balanced grow light spectrum. In a phosphor LED system, phosphors in the LED convert different light sources, such as blue and UV light, into white light.

In addition to housing quality and electrical components, a superior LED system provides extensive information on the specific spectral color bands it can produce. The higher quality the LED, the broader the range of spectral color bands it covers. Understanding the concept of white light LEDs and the color spectrum they generate will enable you to choose a suitable LED system. The next question is how to match the LED wattage to achieve results comparable to those of higher-wattage HIDs.

Replacing HID with LED

Before switching from HID to LED lighting, it's essential to understand how HID lighting works. HID bulbs aim to mimic the sun's natural spectrum of light. The sun is essentially a giant ball of burning gases, and HID lights recreate this spectrum by burning specific gases in a sealed tube. In contrast, LEDs model this spectrum through electrical means. High-quality LEDs focus on providing specific parts of the light spectrum, while the best LEDs aim to replicate a fuller spectrum, closely resembling HID lights.

Concerning HID lighting, there's an ongoing debate about which bulb is the best. In theory, a linear progression suggests that doubling the wattage of a bulb should double the yield, forming a straight line on a graph from lower wattage on the left to higher wattage on the right. However, experienced growers have noticed that there isn't a direct linear correlation between bulb wattage and yield. While upgrading from a 250-watt to a 400-watt bulb might nearly double the yield, transitioning from a 400-watt to a 600-watt bulb results in almost double the yield. Nevertheless, a 600-watt bulb produces about 75 to 80 percent of what a 1,000-watt bulb can yield with most strains.

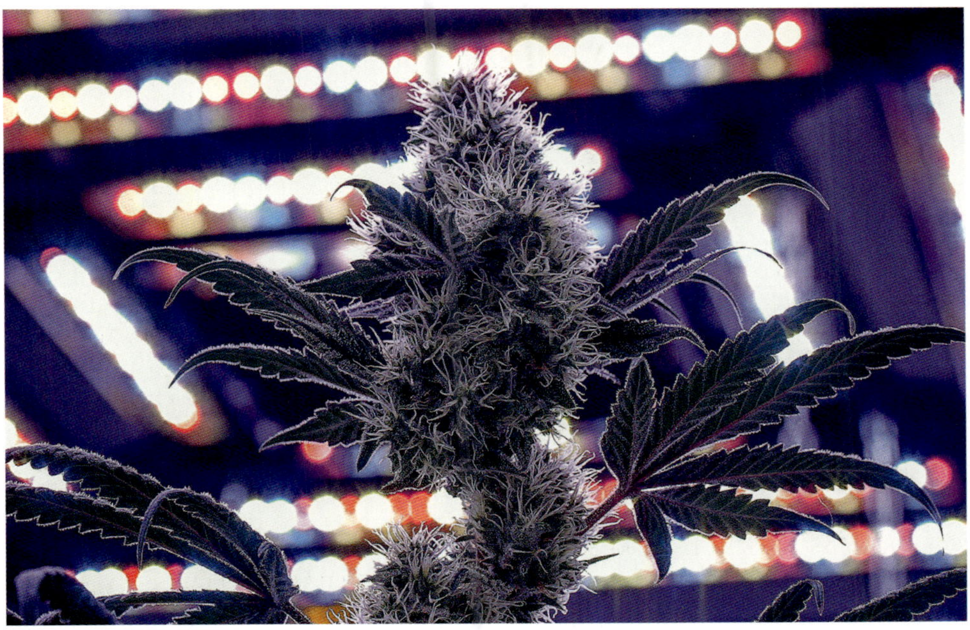

PHOTO: KINDLEDGROWLIGHTS.COM

Some LED kits allow you to change which way they lean in the color spectrum, such as blue or orange.

Scaling Up for Industrial Cannabis Production

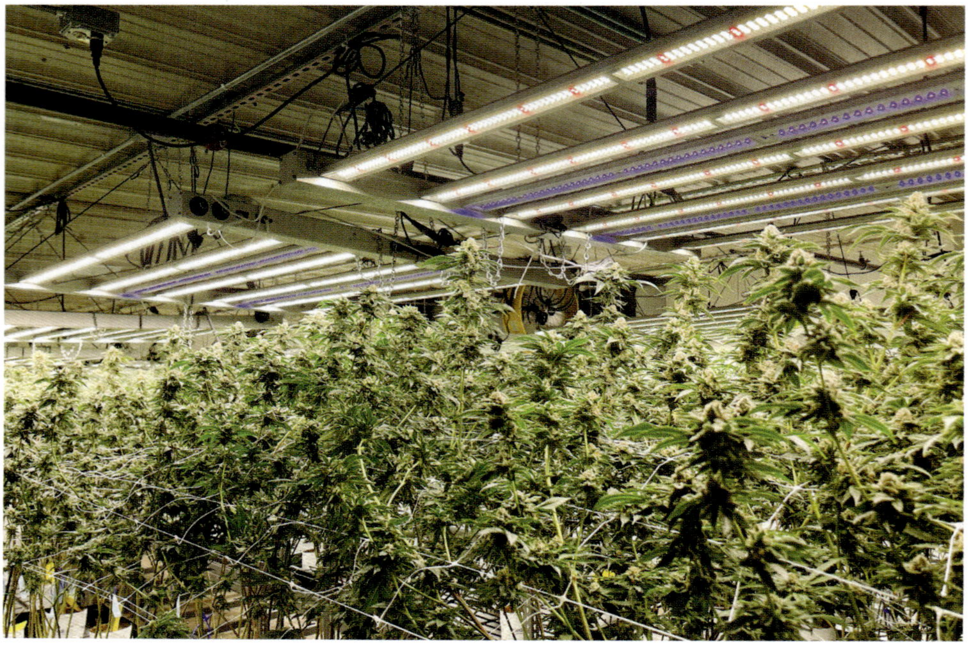

There is no longer any doubt about how well modern LEDs can grow cannabis, as we can see from this bountiful crop.

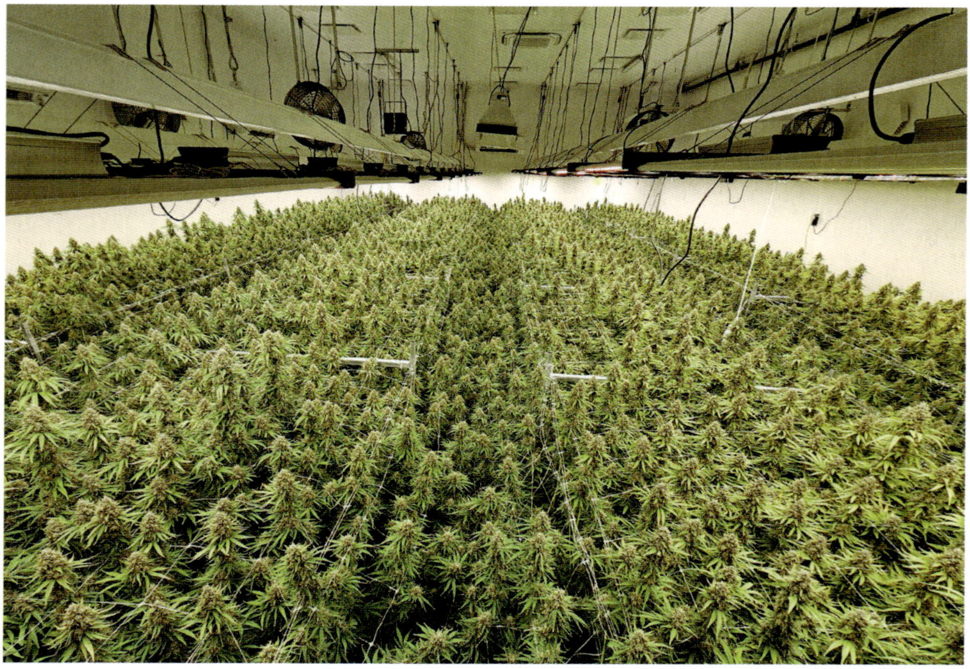

If you thought the previous photo was a big bounty, look at the size of this LED crop. LEDs are more than capable of competing with HID lights.

PHOTOS: MAMMOTHLIGHTING.COM (TOP), GRANDMASTERLEDS.COM (BOTTOM)

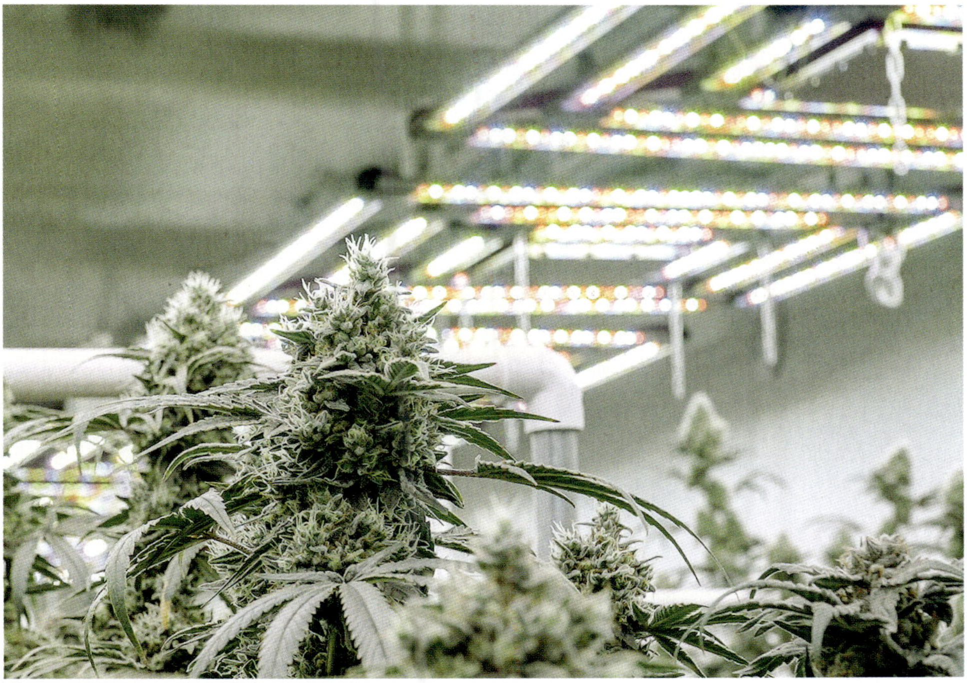

The double-blind test determining if bud comes from LEDs or HIDs shows that nobody can tell the difference. This one is under LEDs.

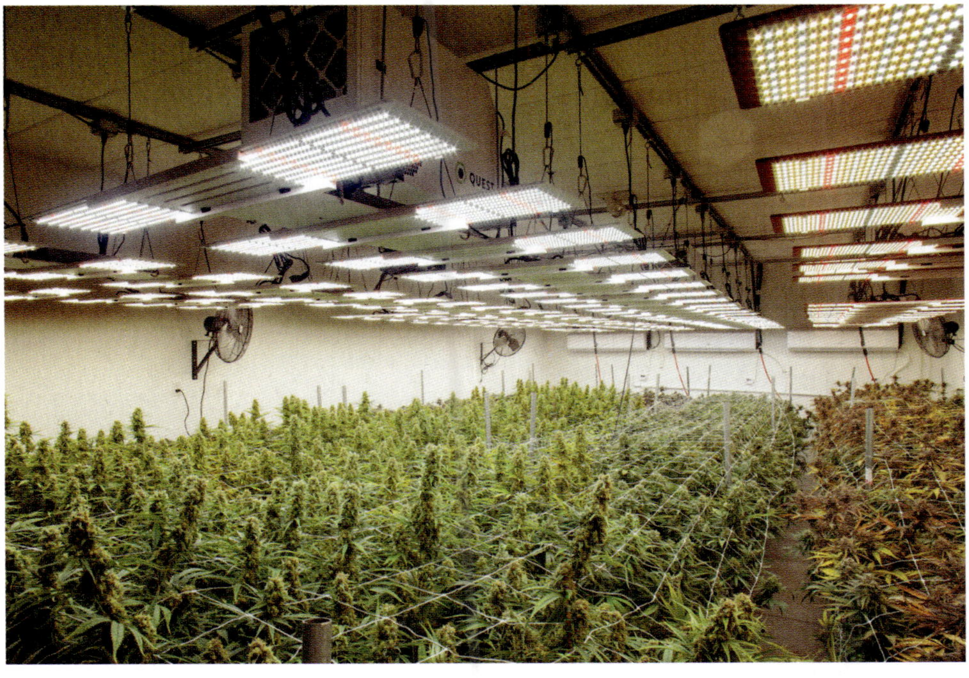

Horticulture lighting can replicate the outdoor environment. Here, LEDs again rule the show with their efficiency.

PHOTOS: KINDLEDGROWLIGHTS.COM (TOP), HORTICULTURE LIGHTING GROUP, HLG.COM (BOTTOM)

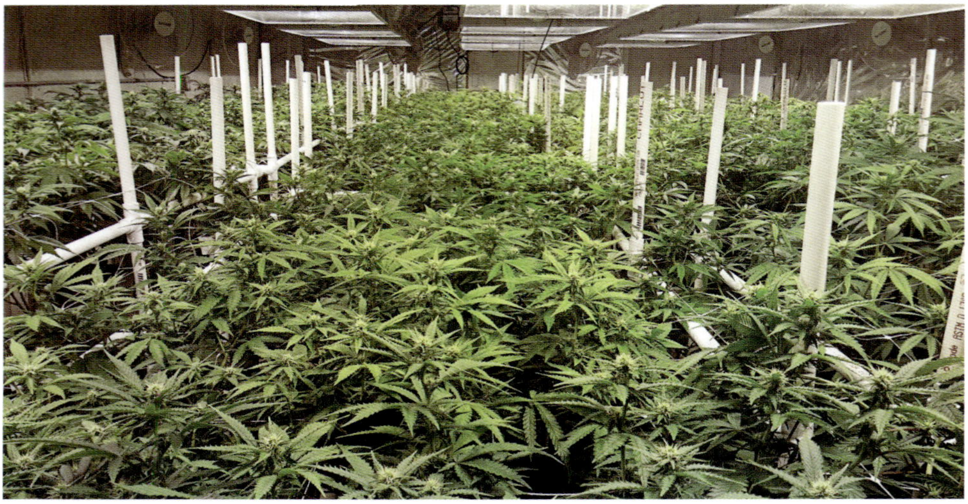

An even canopy is an important goal. This is done by using enough light to avoid significant competitive growth between plants for light.

Sometimes, a 1,000-watt bulb doesn't significantly outperform a 600-watt bulb because the strain's optimal growth falls between these two wattages. This means that in certain cases, a 1000-watt bulb exceeds what the plant actually requires.

For this reason, many growers experiment with both 1000-watt and 600-watt bulbs for different strains. While there may be some improvement under the former, it's essential to weigh whether the added expense and energy consumption are justified. Often, it's more effective to allocate the 1000-watt bulb to a strain that fully uses it.

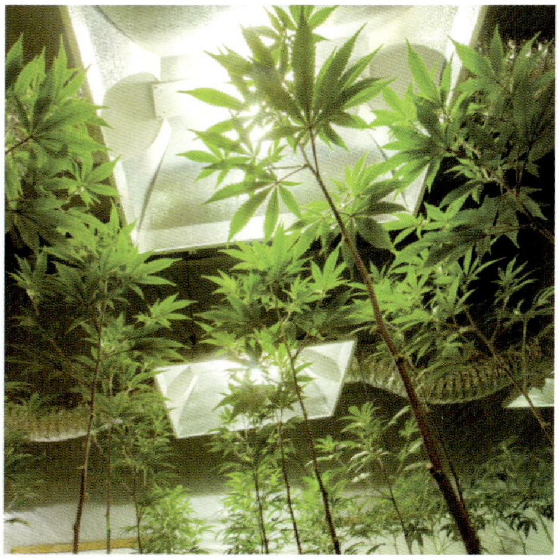

This is an example of significantly long internode lengths, caused by the plants stretching towards a light that's too far away.

PHOTOS: MONICA GRIFFIN (TOP), HIP2THECROP (BOTTOM)

In comparing LED and HID lights, the discussion often revolves around 1000-watt and 600-watt HIDs compared to LEDs. It's crucial to emphasize that not all LEDs are of equal quality. Optimal LED setups usually consist of rectangular or square arrays of LED chips. It's also possible to customize your own LED configuration.

How HID Works

HID systems are regulated by a ballast, which can be either internal or external. The ballast transforms and delivers electrical power to the HID lamp. The ballast efficacy factor (BEF) measures the light output relative to the power input, with the system's efficiency rated in lumens per watt (LPW). The ballast factor (BF) is a ratio that compares the output of various ballasts using the same lamp. High BFs typically reduce bulb life compared to average BFs, but low BFs also lead to a reduced bulb lifespan. The three primary types of ballast are electronic, hybrid, and magnetic.

HID lamps are designed to create an electrical arc discharge within an arc tube made from fused quartz or fused alumina, which contains a gas. The ballast electrically regulates this arc discharge. Essentially, the HID lamp consists of two tungsten electrodes between which an electrical arc ignites. Some HID lamps have a single glass tube, while others include an inner glass tube. The glass tube, usually made of the translucent aluminum oxide alumina, is filled with gas that ignites the lamp. When the metal electrodes heat up, they produce a specific band of light, vaporize, and transform into glowing plasma. Common types of HID systems include HPS (CRI 22–75), low-pressure sodium (LPS; CRI 0), mercury vapor (MV; CRI 15–55), and MH (CRI 65–90).

HID lamps receive continuous AC power from the ballast. These lamps produce light through mercury sodium emission. The most prominent emission in HID lights is the D-line emission, which is primarily due to sodium. When HID lights become damaged but remain functional, they can lead to such issues as sunburn or eye damage. To mitigate this risk, it's advisable to use self-extinguishing HID lamps that turn off instantly or within 15 minutes if they break. If you encounter a broken bulb in a socket, it's essential to turn the light off and unplug it, including from the ballast, which may retain a residual charge. Understanding how to safely remove the broken bulb is crucial, and it typically involves counter-clockwise rotation. In some cases, using long-nosed pliers or a cloth wrapping will make removal safe.

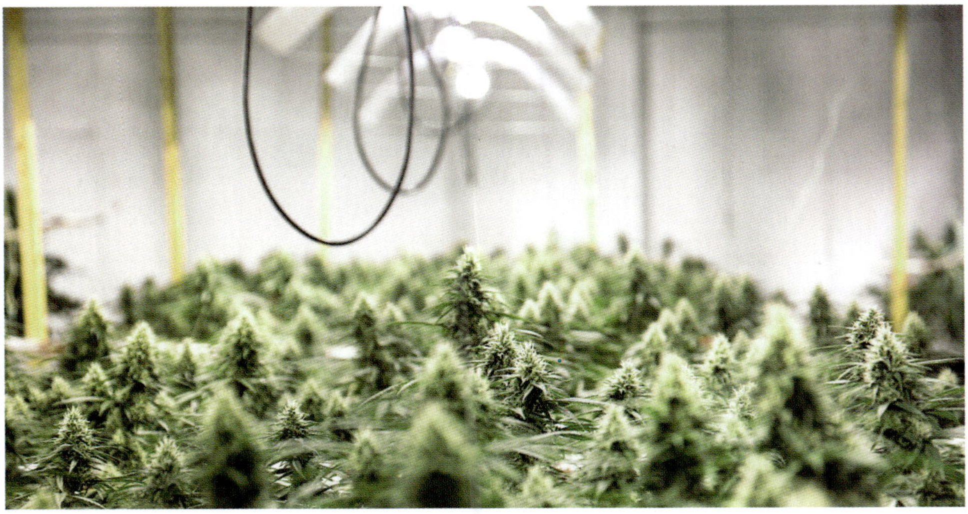

PHOTO: BUBBLEMAN

If plants are not putting energy into competitive growth then more energy is available for flowering production. Even canopies are a good sign of lack of competition.

Approximate to Light

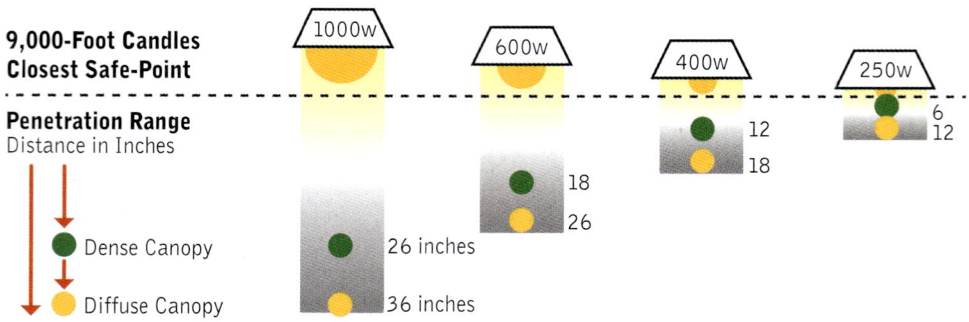

How HPS Works

HPS lamps do not eliminate mercury entirely. HPS lamps contain mercury, sodium, and xenon gas for ignition, which initially emit a white-blue or faint pink light. As the lamp's heat increases, this light transitions into an orange hue. The variation in color is due to the different heating rates of the gases, which ultimately produce a consistent light spectrum.

An amalgam of sodium and mercury, created when mercury is mixed with an alloy, is used to produce the vapor that sustains the electrical arc in HPS lamps. The temperature of the amalgam is determined by the power supplied which then influences the pressure inside the lamp. This process results in stable lamp operation.

The HPS lamp remains operational as long as there is electrical power. If the vapor in the lamp is depleted and the amalgam evaporates, the light intensity decreases, and the lamp eventually extinguishes. If excessive power is used, it can cause the lamp to fail due to the rapid increase in current and the decrease in the lamp's resistance. To avoid this, it's crucial to use lamps specified for particular kits. A functional circuit breaker board and power conditioners are also essential to protect the bulbs and ballasts from electrical surges.

Lumens and Cannabis Cultivation

The light output of a bulb per square foot is measured in lumens. Although lumens and wattage are related, their relationship can vary significantly between different lighting systems. This metric is not solely dependent on wattage but also on the light's design. A high-quality lighting kit emits more lumens.

How many lumens you need to grow cannabis depends on three factors:

1. Budget: How much you're willing to invest in your lighting setup.
2. Number of Plants: The quantity of cannabis plants you plan to grow.
3. Grow Area Size: The dimensions of your cultivation space.

Installing HID Lights

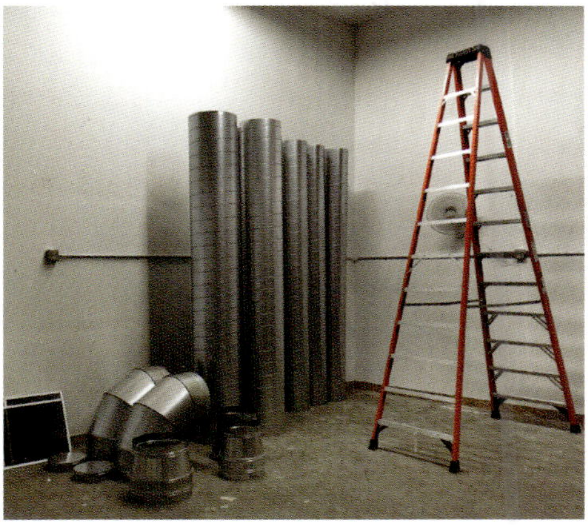

Elevated lights and ducting are a must.

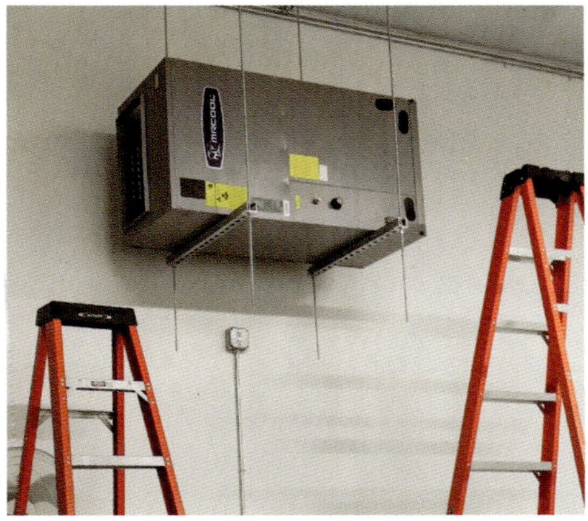

The ventilation goes in first.

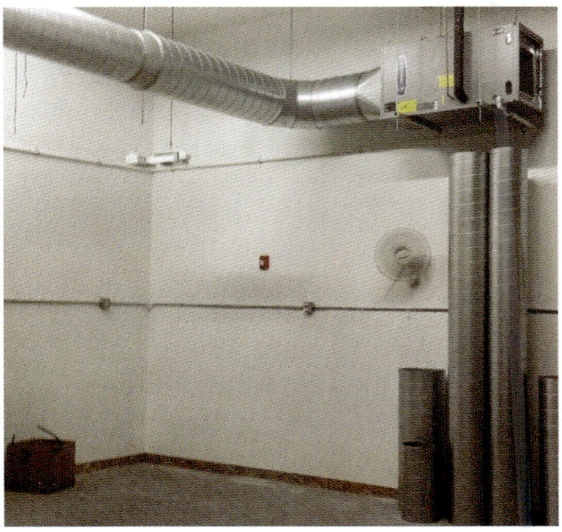

Followed by ducting.

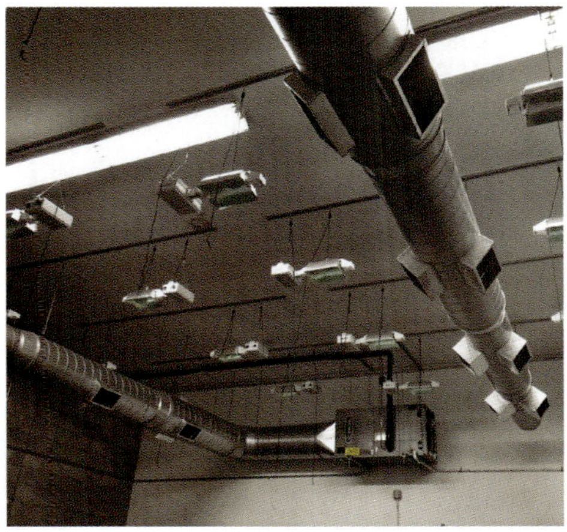

Followed by the lighting.

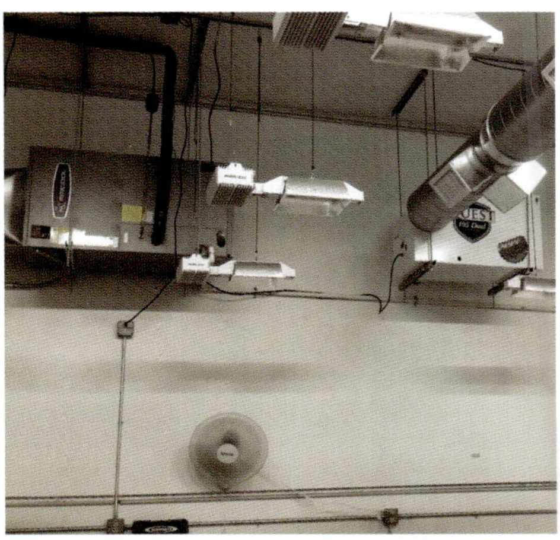

Everything is then hooked up electrically.

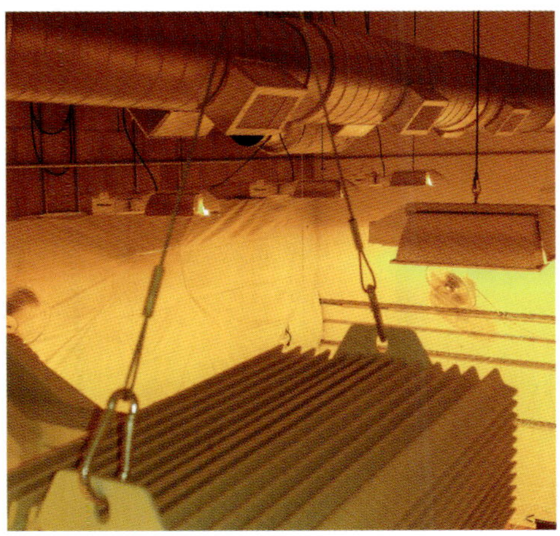

Finally, the whole setup can be turned on.

PHOTOS: @BEAM401 / CH9 FEMALE SEEDS

Never use less than 2,500 lumens, even for a single cannabis plant. One light source emitting around 45,000 lumens is generally sufficient for a grow space of about 3 feet × 3 feet. We'll discuss depth considerations shortly. A 3 × 3-foot area is a common size, accommodating anywhere from one to 12 indica plants, depending on the strain's growth characteristics. Keep in mind that a single large sativa plant can rapidly cover a nine-square-foot grow space, while shorter indica plants behave differently.

A 45,000-lumen output is typically associated with a high-end 400-watt HID system. Cannabis can use more light, so upgrading to a 600-watt HID system can boost your available light to around 60,000 lumens. For larger grow spaces, you might require two or more 600-watt HID lights to achieve this level of illumination. Although 1,000-watt HIDs are costly, they often deliver the best yields.[3]

The HID Illumination Formula

We have a simplified formula for HID wattage[4] based on the grow area. Aim for about 50 watts of HID light per square foot of your grow area, using this formula:

250-watt HID = 22 foot area
400-watt HID = 32 foot area
600-watt HID = 32 foot area
1000-watt HID = 42 foot area

This straightforward watts-per-square-foot calculation assumes that each square foot of space receives the same number of lumens. In practice, however, bulbs don't distribute lumens evenly across the entire area; you also must consider the depth of your grow space. As light travels away from its source, its intensity diminishes by one quarter each time the distance it covers doubles. Using a 1,000-watt HID light on a few plants is acceptable, and they will likely flourish under the intense light. But it's essential to select strains that can fully use the available light. "Lighting overkill" occurs when a powerful HID light is used to grow a genetically low-yielding plant. Most strains from reputable breeders yield generously, so using a 1,000-watt light can lead to significant yields, with growers sometimes harvesting two pounds or more of buds from a single plant.

We've now covered the topic of HID lighting in relation to cannabis yields and can proceed to explore how LEDs compare, introducing PPFD values to our LED area formula.

Measuring LED Light Intensity

In today's market, numerous new LED manufacturers are emerging, and their claims about their products may not always align with the output you observe. Fortunately, reliable tools are available to gauge LED light intensity with measurements in PPFD. LED light meter apps can be found in online stores and are budget-friendly. If you want to assess the light intensity in your grow space accurately, check out what is

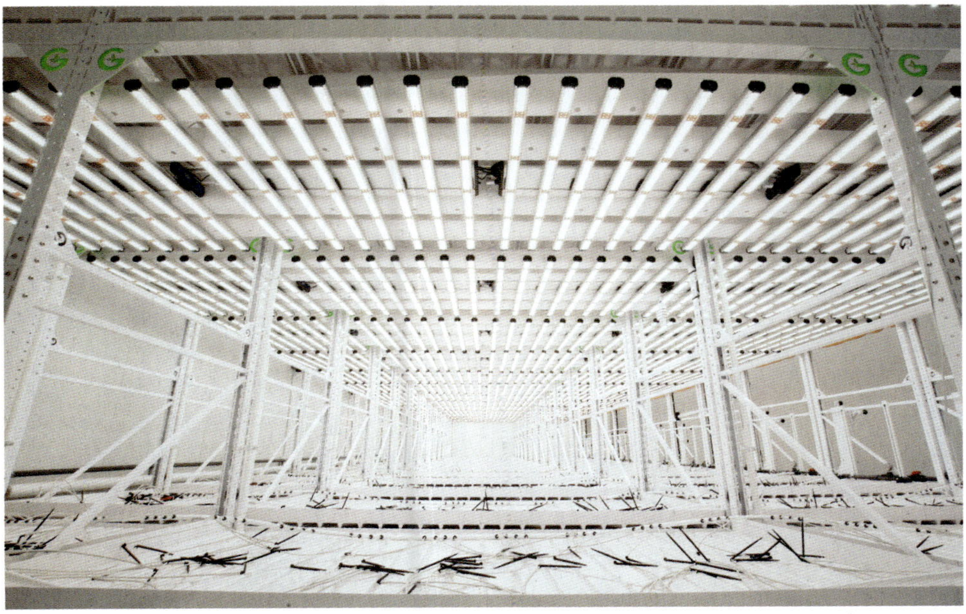

Racks and carriages can be multiplatform units designed for different types of grow trays. LEDs work well with this box-type modular grow rack.

currently considered the best app and try that. You may be impressed to find they are just as good as equipment such as light meters, costing three figures. You will use your results to compare with the manufacturer's specifications to see if there are any disparities. In addition to PPFD and lux readings, some devices provide micromole measurements. For scientifically precise measurements, you may opt for photon sensors, which are known for their accuracy but are more expensive.

Ambient room lighting is typically of low intensity and will yield low readings. When you move to measure the light intensity under an LED grow light, you should observe a significant increase. However, it's important to note that different LED grow lights will exhibit varying intensity levels. The readings you obtain will depend on factors such as the LED manufacturer and the distance between your light source and the light meter.

Investing in a reliable light meter or photon sensor can ensure that your plants receive the appropriate amount of light for their growth. By accurately measuring light intensity, you can fine-tune your cultivation environment to optimize the growth of your cannabis plants.

Understanding PPF, PPFD and DLI

In our exploration of lighting for plant growth, we've briefly mentioned various key measurements, including PAR, PPF, and PPFD, all of which relate to light intensity and its correlation with photosynthesis, the process essential for plant growth.

PHOTO: MIAMIMANGOCA.COM

Cannabis, having evolved in high-altitude regions exposed to intense sunlight, falls into the category of plants that can thrive under high light levels. This characteristic sets cannabis apart from many other plant species, especially common edible vegetables that typically require far less light for optimal growth. It's crucial to understand this distinction, particularly if you intend to cultivate various plant species in your lifetime. Cannabis has adapted to flourish under the intensity of natural sunlight, making this level of light its preferred threshold. Below a certain light threshold, plants cannot thrive, and insufficient light can result in plant death.

So far, we have considered measurements that give us a snapshot of an illuminated grow space. The Photosynthetic Photon Flux (PPF) is specified in micromoles per second (μmol/s). The value is limited to a duration of one second of light and doesn't tell us about the area. PPFD (Photosynthetic photon flux density), tells us about area coverage because the unit of measurement is micromoles per square meter ($\mu mol/m^2/s$).

PPFD can describe the specific light intensity measured at a point on the canopy. That makes PPFD useful for immediate measurements. It is often the value given on light specifications. However, in horticulture, plants are exposed to light for more than one second. 24 hours is a typical period of plant growth measurement, so the daily light integral (DLI) calculation is the total light energy available for photosynthesis per day. If you were to take PAR (photosynthetically active photons) readings at intervals during the day and plot these on a graph, the DLI would be all the area under the plots. DLI units are given as moles of photons per square meter per day ($mol/m^2/day$), also expressed as micromoles of photons per square meter per day ($\mu mol/m^2/day$). This DLI value is simply the quantity of photosynthetically active radiation delivered to a specific area over 24 hours for healthy growth.

It's a common misconception that doubling DLI (or light wattage as an easier example) equates to a proportionate increase in crop size; in reality, there's a point of diminishing returns. Increasing light intensity or wattage will lead to more substantial yields, but the returns will start to decline once you reach the optimal light conditions a plant can use efficiently. Finding the "Goldilocks zone" involves achieving the most economical means of obtaining the highest yield with the least investment in lighting and electricity.[5] This DLI value is useful for planning and achieving long-term optimization goals. In addition to PPFD, some lighting systems offer DLI charts as part of their specifications. They help you find the ideal balance, which considers cost-effectiveness, as spending large sums on lighting and electricity for incremental gains may not be the most efficient approach.

PPF falls between 500 and 700 PPFD, which roughly equates to 65 μmol PPF per square foot. Cannabis can potentially benefit from even higher levels, possibly reaching around 1000 PPFD. The DLI for cannabis is approximately 45 ($\pm$5) DLI.

Both HID and LED lighting systems have their merits, with HID lights being more cost-effective initially but generating more heat and having shorter lifespans, while LEDs are more expensive upfront but offer a more energy-efficient, longer-lasting, and heat-reducing solution.

Understanding LED RGB Ratios and Spectra

The rapid development of LED technology has created an ever-evolving landscape for cannabis growers. The contents of this book may become outdated as LED manufacturers continue to make advancements, which is why it's essential to stay up to date with the latest market trends through personal research.

In the world of LED grow lights, "full spectrum" is the buzzword, indicating that these lights are equipped with phosphor-coated diodes. These coatings enhance the number and diversity of color bands emitted, ultimately producing a white light spectrum. While the inclusion of phosphor coatings may slightly diminish the intensity and efficiency of LEDs, high-intensity LED grow lights tend to compensate for this effectively. LED manufacturers have been working to extend their spectrum coverage to include UV and far-red areas. However, it's important to bear in mind that, for the stages of vegetative growth and flowering in cannabis, we are primarily interested in the visible part of the light spectrum.

LED manufacturers typically provide detailed specifications, including RGB values, as well as percentages of UV and far-red. These values give growers insights into the spectral characteristics of the LEDs.

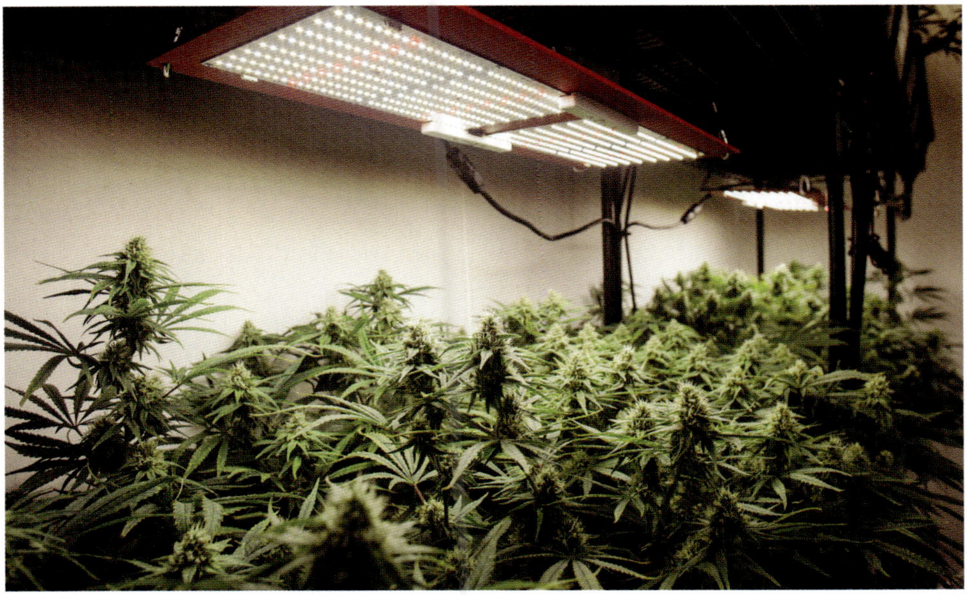

PHOTO: HORTICULTURE LIGHTING GROUP, HLG.COM

A rack system using LEDs to flower these cannabis plants.

HID lighting systems, such as MH and HPS, have distinctive spectral properties. MH lights predominantly emit blue light, while HPS lights offer a higher proportion of red light. LED lighting seeks to replicate this.

Certain LED types have higher percentages of red light, indicating their suitability for the flowering stage. Meanwhile, other types might incorporate more blue light but still contain significant amounts of red. This implies that the "blue" LEDs are designed for vegetative growth, whereas the "red" ones are intended for flowering. It is advisable not to draw conclusions based on cross-comparisons between different manufacturers, as this may lead to the misconception that a broader spectrum presentation is inherently superior to a narrower one. These distinctions are often rooted in marketing strategies.

The best approach is to focus on examining the LED systems within each brand's product range. By doing so, you can gain a more comprehensive understanding of how manufacturers describe their LED products in terms of RGB ratios and color spectra. Ultimately, this research will help you identify which manufacturers are more transparent and capable of delivering the expected results.

As a word of caution to LED manufacturers, it's important to acknowledge that a growing number of cultivators are investing in light quantum sensors, which are becoming more affordable. These sensors enable growers to independently verify the spectral claims of LED products, reinforcing the need for honesty and accuracy in product descriptions. This evolution in technology highlights the importance of providing accurate information and adhering to the standards set by the industry.

Blue, Red and Full-Spectrum LEDs

The influence of light spectra on plant development varies across different species. Some plants thrive better under continuous exposure to blue-type light throughout their growth cycle. Cannabis is unique in its preference for a specific light spectrum, particularly during the flowering phase. Many LED manufacturers use blue diodes alongside a substantial number of red, and vice versa. In most cases, LEDs lean toward producing a redder spectrum, but this is far from a groundbreaking revelation. In response to the varied needs of cultivators, LED manufacturers are focusing on offering full-spectrum LED systems. These lights aim to provide an evenly balanced blend of blue and red light, with additional emphasis on the other essential parts of the spectrum.

In the ever-evolving LED lighting market, it's clear that the trend is shifting towards full-spectrum solutions that strike a harmonious balance between blue and red wavelengths. To make the best choice for your specific cultivation needs, you may need to delve deeper into the available information and resources provided by LED manufacturers to find a light system that aligns with your plant variety and growth objectives. In an era of transparency, accurate information and research will be your allies in selecting the most suitable LED grow light for your unique cultivation requirements.

Shade Avoidance

Phytochrome, the plant's main chemical compound, is used to detect changes in light falling on the plant. When a plant shades another, phytochrome is inactivated in the shaded plant, producing a response that compels the plant to find light. Auxins are released for cell elongation, and this is part of the physical phototrophic response that causes the plant to move away from the shade and toward the light. Hence, shade avoidance is a response. It is important to note that here again, we encounter how and why internode lengths can stretch because of lack of light.

As you research plant responses to artificial light, you will encounter cutting-edge technologies that often explore poorly understood phenomena to see if they can benefit crops. The far-red area of the light spectrum is where some of this exploratory research is, and this research includes you, the grower, because these units are now commercially available. In many cases, the far-red part of LED technology is controllable, meaning you can experiment with the levels. The experiment is to see what using some far-red will do.

The standard monochromatic light for photosynthesis drops away at approximately 685 nm. The far-red light region peaks at 735 nm and is the more extreme red end of the visible spectrum. It is barely visible to our eyes. After this comes infrared light (invisible to our eyes).

Some LEDs come with far-red claims to improve results in some way. The improvement could be yield or rooting success, for example. At the time of writing, the far-red may improve rooting success rates. However, it will likely also increase internode lengths; this is to be expected because far-red light inactivates phytochrome, so auxins are released for cell elongation.

The hypothesis is that cell elongation is advantageous for rooting but may not be for yields, because instead of flowering development, the plant expends this energy on cell elongations, meaning internode length increases at the expense of yield. Plant height should increase and yield decrease. However, the ratio of monochromatic light to far-red light may shift these values, and it is here in these ratios that the experiment resides. The point is that the blue part of the spectrum may not be as crucial as the red part for rooting. That does not mean that the blue part of the spectrum is not essential. It still is, for regular plant growth. Some possible negatives from using too much far-red light could be leaf senescence, meaning you may observe parts of a leaf appearing to die similarly to aging. Whatever happens, make sure to record your data. You will adjust your experimental values according to your findings.

Lighting Spectrum with Miami Mango

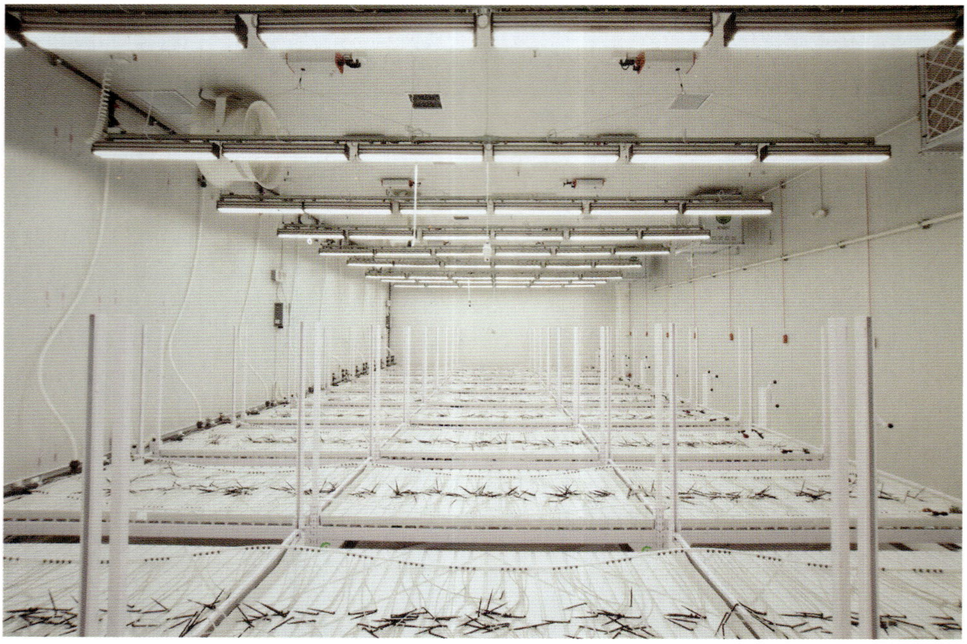

Modular racks and carriages can sometimes remove the tops to allow room LEDs to take over the role of light.

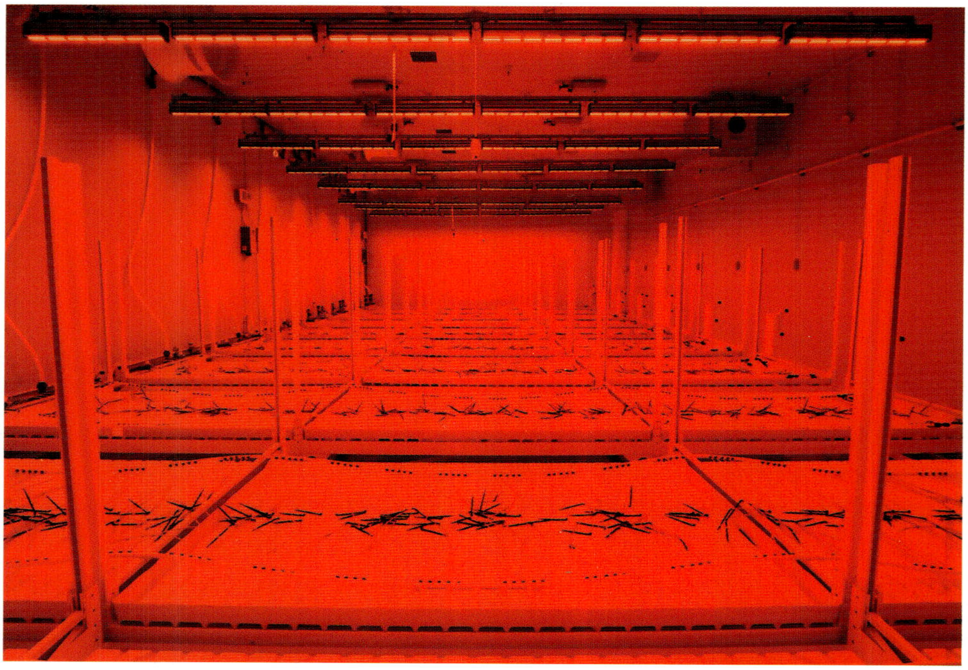

Many professional LED systems allow you to switch to and from UV, blue, far-red, and deep-red light. These can also be used with a modular system.

PHOTOS: MIAMIMANGOCA.COM

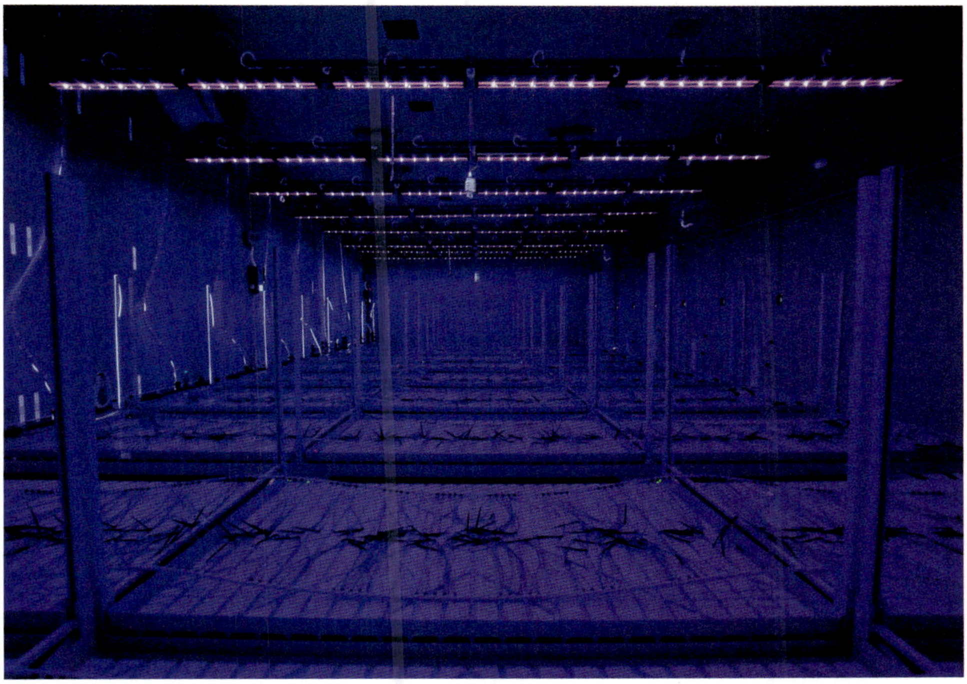

This system applies UV light intermittently for a few hours each day at the end of the harvest. It enhances trichome production, boosts potency, and improves terpene profiles.

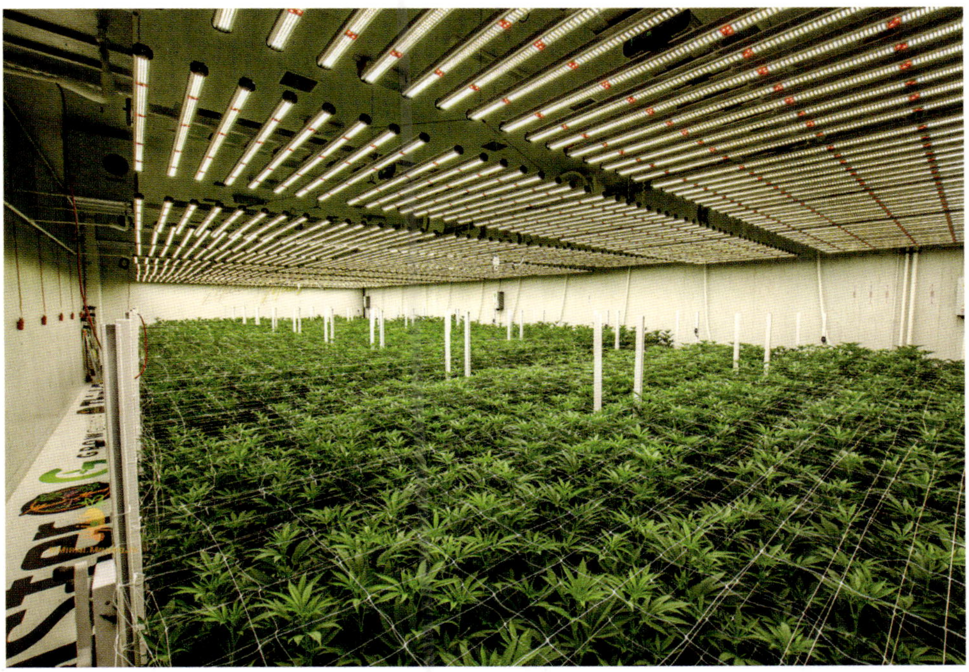

The flat, outstretched leaves on these plants clearly show that they are receiving LED light efficiently and benefiting from optimal light conditions.

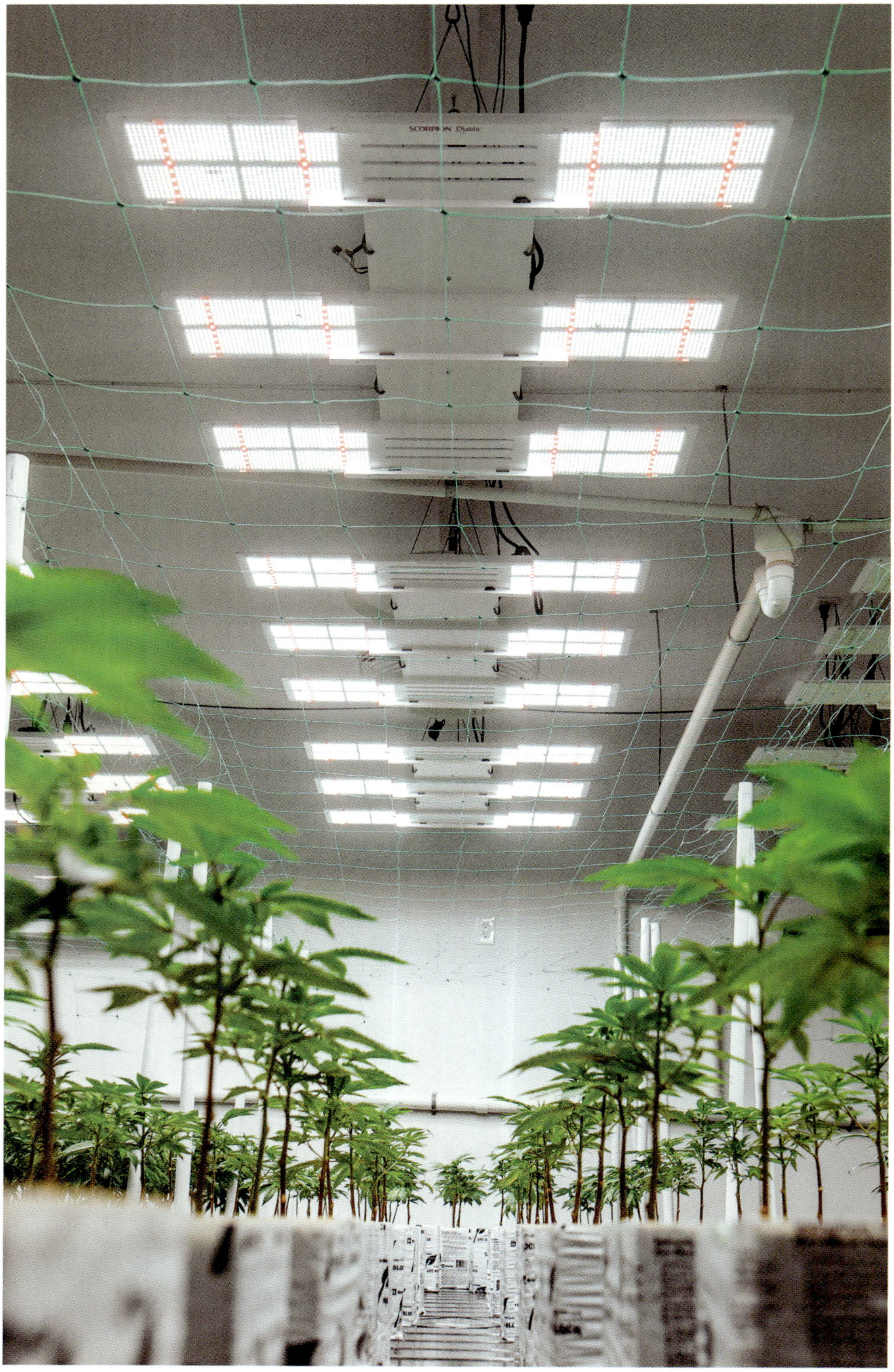

PHOTO: HORTICULTURE LIGHTING GROUP, HLG.COM

These young plants in vegetative growth enjoy the rays from the LEDs onto their open leaves.

LED Illumination Estimations

As we mentioned, PPFD units are given as μmol/m^2/s and are found on most LED specifications. This provides valuable information about the area that can be covered by light. You may also see the PPF (Photosynthetic photon flux) measurement in μmol/s, although a measurement of time, is often converted into PPFD for area μmol/m^2.

You may also come across another metric: μmol/J. This value is the Photosynthetic Photon Efficacy (PPE) and it is calculated by dividing the total PPF output of a light source (PPF in μmol/s) by power use (in watts).

It's possible to encounter a 100-watt LED system that delivers more light intensity than a 200-watt system, especially when dealing with older LED models. Developers aim to get the most output per watt. Understanding PPFD and the related metrics is crucial for evaluating these systems, and LED manufacturers should make this information readily available.

Not all areas of an LED panel provide uniform PPFD. PPFD measurements vary with the distance from the light source to the plant. LED manufacturers often provide a PPFD chart of their LED system, illustrating values that decrease from the central LEDs to those on the edges of the panel. These numbers offer insights into the coverage you can expect, with each dot representing a PPFD measurement.

PPFD values can be improved by upgrading to a better light system or by reducing the coverage area using a reflector. When you decrease the spread of the light, PPFD increases, resulting in a higher yield.

PPFD Chart in a 4x4-Foot Grow Tent

Height: 8 inches (20 cm) (4 feet × 4 feet; axes 0–3.5)

1190	1350	1401	1480	1487	1405	1354	1197
1272	1481	1501	1550	1558	1506	1480	1282
1310	1500	1550	1631	1630	1560	1510	1320
1340	1540	1590	1671	1675	1596	1546	1343
1341	1541	1591	1665	1672	1590	1540	1340
1320	1511	1560	1631	1630	1550	1510	1330
1280	1475	1506	1558	1555	1506	1480	1282
1195	1354	1405	1487	1481	1400	1350	1190

Height: 12 inches (30 cm) (4 feet × 4 feet; axes 0–3.5)

1110	1300	1350	1410	1420	1353	1307	1113
1181	1371	1410	1470	1480	1410	1370	1186
1222	1411	1451	1510	1520	1459	1410	1226
1250	1450	1460	1540	1549	1470	1455	1254
1254	1452	1470	1541	1542	1460	1451	1251
1226	1400	1455	1520	1510	1459	1410	1225
1186	1362	1411	1480	1470	1410	1370	1181
1111	1301	1353	1424	1420	1350	1300	1110

PPFD value valid only at specified distance on chart; changing distance changes PPFD value.

Many growers are happy to choose a reputable brand, rely on the PPF or PPFD specifications, and follow the manufacturer's recommended coverage area. Once you understand what a specific brand and model can achieve, you can determine the number of panels needed for your growing space or opt for a grow tent of suitable size. This is a common approach, with growers selecting their lights first and then matching the tent accordingly. If you're using multiple panels, you can either add more tents or choose a larger tent to accommodate them.

As mentioned previously, the ideal range for cannabis lighting in terms of PPF falls between 500 and 700 PPFD, which roughly equates to 65 μmol PPF per square foot. Cannabis can potentially benefit from even higher levels, possibly reaching around 1000 PPFD. Additionally, the DLI should ideally be 45 ($\pm$5) DLI.

Keep in mind that PPF values can vary between different LED systems, but here are some general guidelines:

260 PPF is suitable for a 2^2-foot area
585 PPF is appropriate for a 3^2-foot area
796 PPF can cover a 3.5^2-foot area effectively
1,040 PPF is sufficient for 4^2-foot area
1,625 PPF is ideal for a 5^2-foot area

Large cannabis plants can handle PPFD levels in the range of 1000 to 1500 effectively, but exceeding 2000 PPFD might lead to photoinhibition. Going below 500 PPFD is not advisable if you aim for more than just low yields. The optimal zone lies somewhere in between these extremes.

PPFD values can be influenced by various environmental factors. For instance, the PPFD measurements are under optimal conditions, which may include the addition of supplemental CO_2 to the grow area. Therefore, if you're not achieving the desired results with a good light system, it may not be the light that's the issue, but rather your growing environment, choice of strain, and/or CO_2 levels.

Make sure to familiarize yourself with these measurements and their values, and understand how recommended guidelines are calculated for you. Once you grasp these concepts, it's all about selecting the right LED system that aligns with your specific needs.

After acquiring the suitable system, you'll generally follow the recommended surface area for the desired PPFD during the vegetative growth phase before transitioning to a 12/12 light cycle for flowering. Keep in mind that PPFD values can change when you use different light regimes. LEDs are straightforward to use once you've made the right prepurchase considerations, and this preparation phase is half the battle.

Hagstone under an HLG-600H Quantum Board

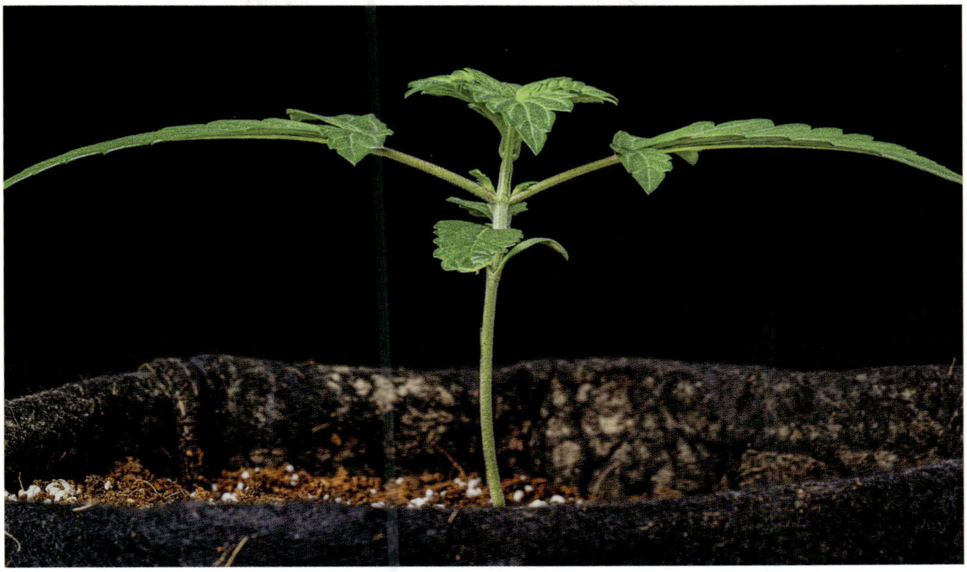

Seedlings enjoy LED light because it discharges less heat than HIDs. Heat stress is dangerous for young seedlings.

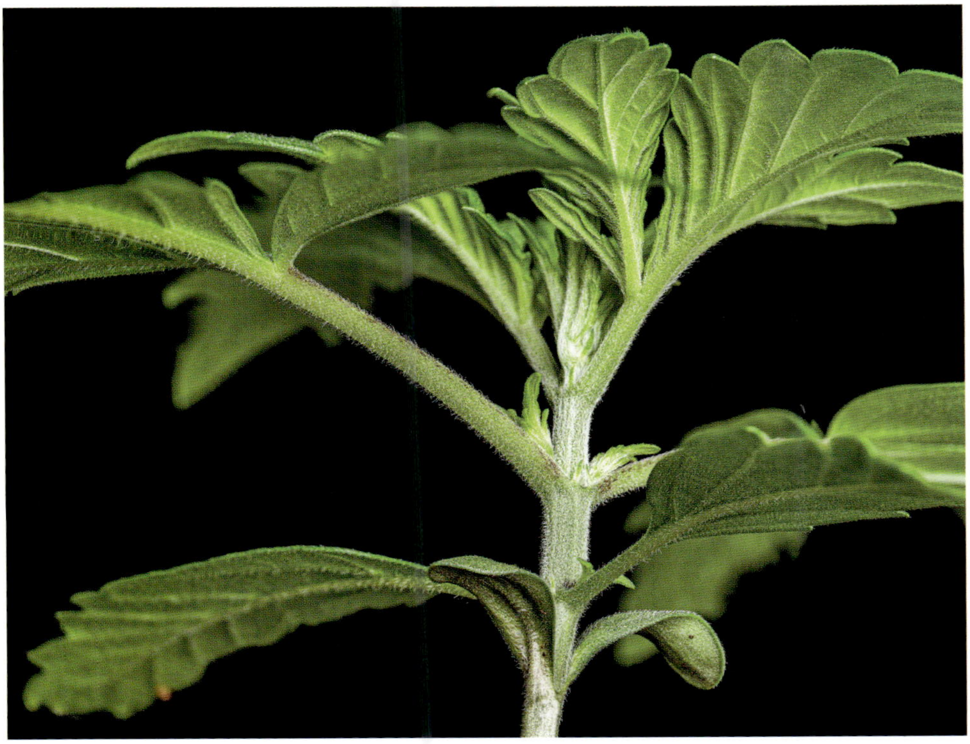

PHOTOS: ROB BRAMHILL

Healthy seedlings should show new growth under gocd growing conditions and LEDs can provide that environment.

continues...

Hagstone under an HLG-600H Quantum Board *continued*

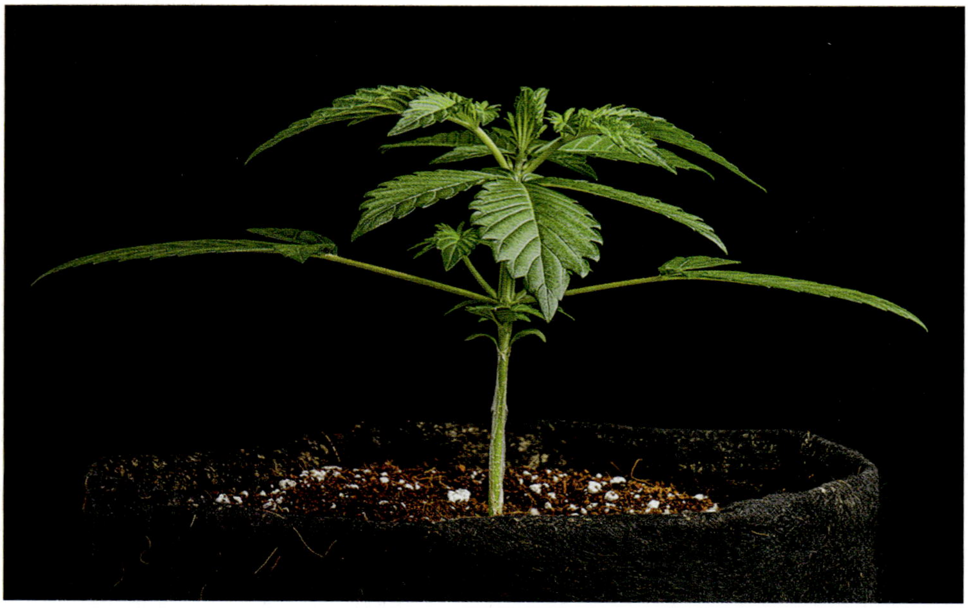

This plant has been kept short by keeping a light down close to the developing plant. This keeps internode lengths to their genetic minimum.

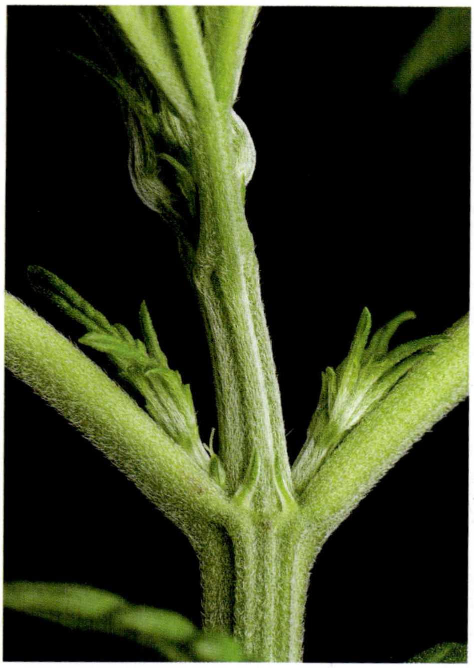

We can find a bract and stigma at this internode, but there is also the emergence of female pre-flowering calyx development.

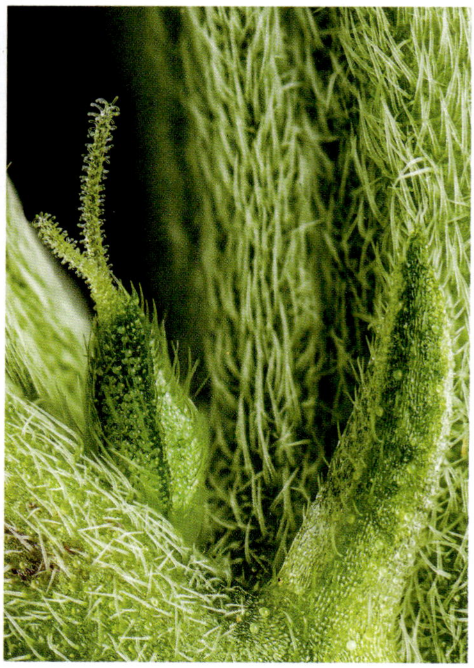

A closer inspection of the pre-flowering calyx development reveals two pistils and the presence of trichomes on them.

PHOTOS: ROB BRAMHILL

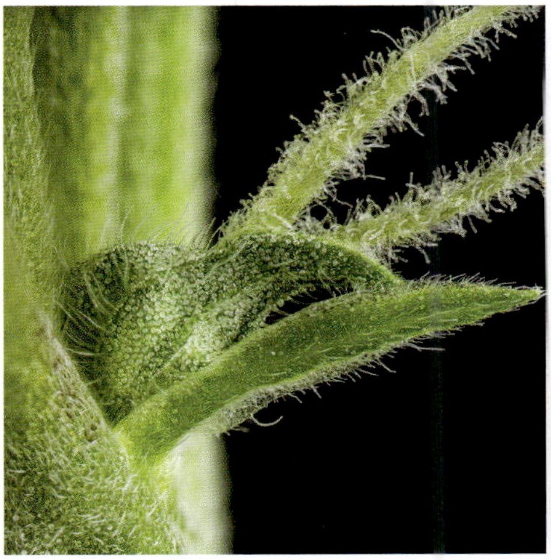

Over the coming days, the pistils will grow in length as pre-flowering development covers most node regions.

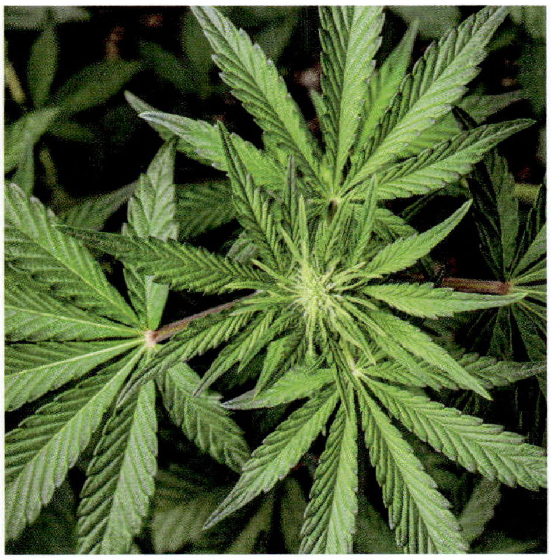

The top of the plant has an apical or terminal bud site, which will start to show flowering.

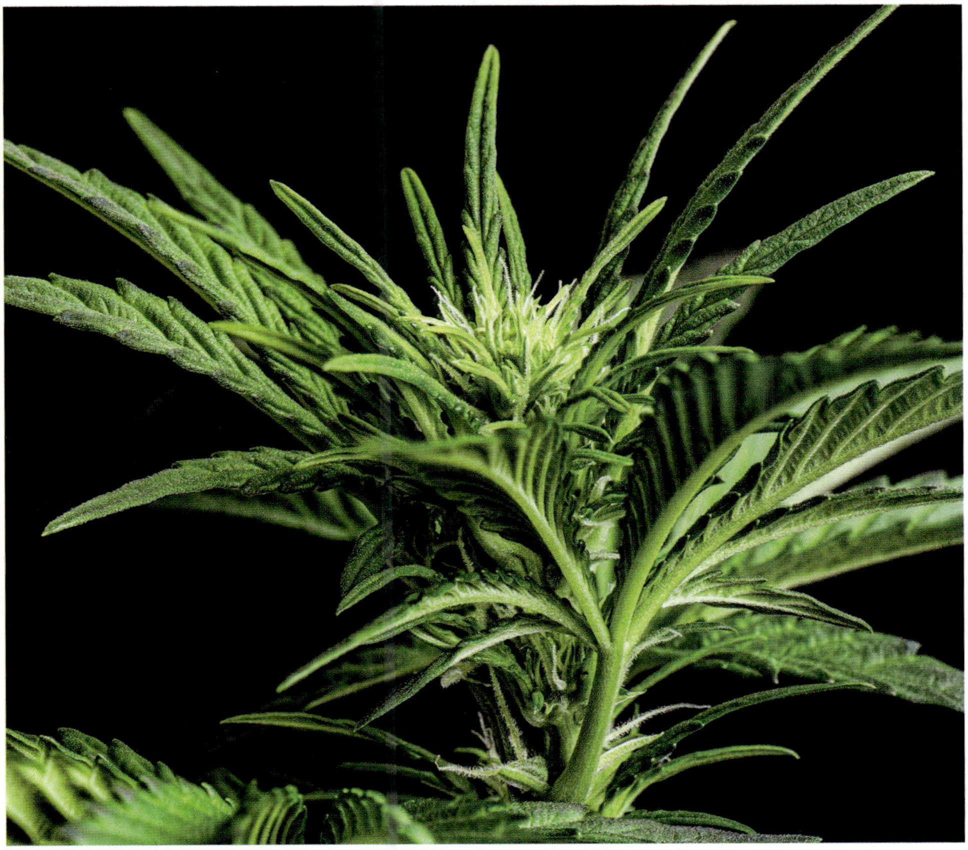

As more pistils are produced, they will eventually become colas thick with flowers and the internode lengths will elongate.

continues...

Hagstone under an HLG-600H Quantum Board *continued*

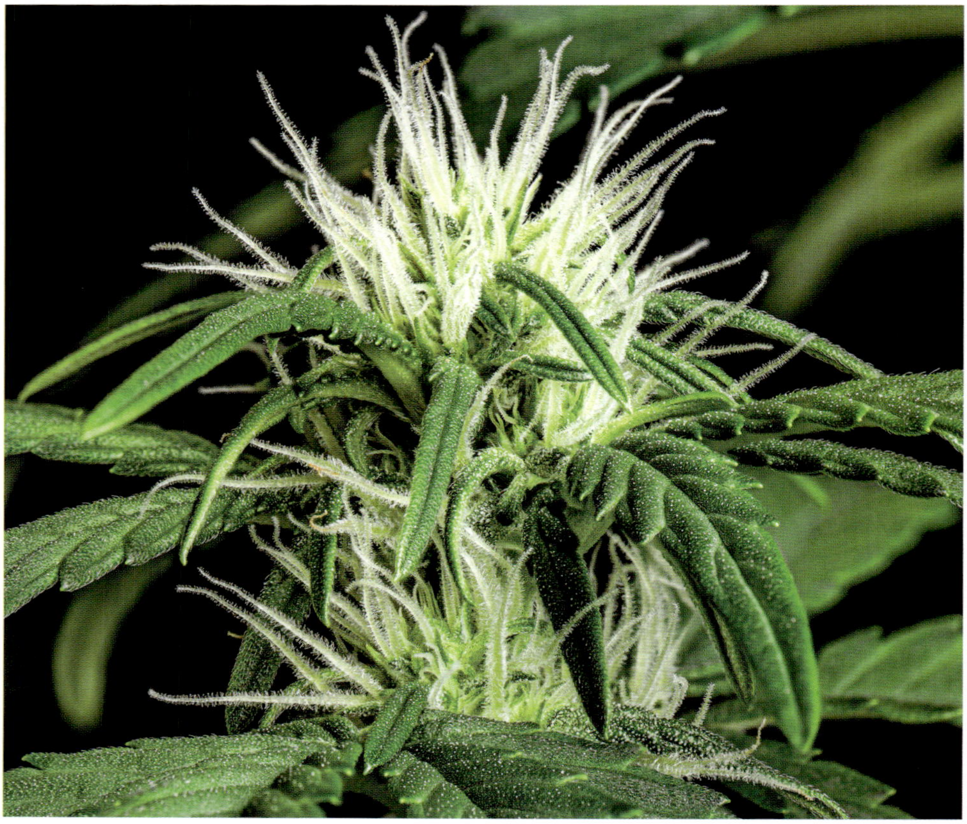

The tops of branches will also develop their own colas, but these are not expected to be as big as the main top cola.

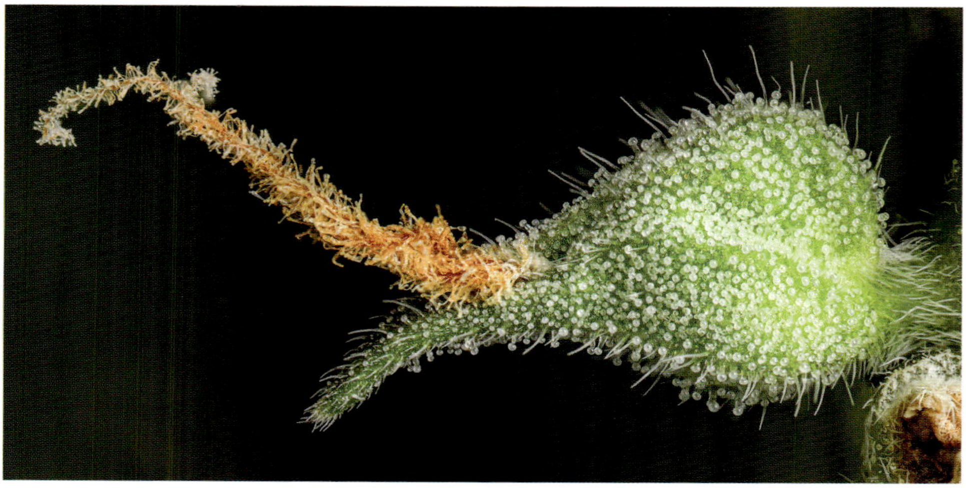

It is not uncommon for pistils to produce a range of colors. Also, notice that the pre-flowering calyx has trichomes.

PHOTOS: ROB BRAMHILL

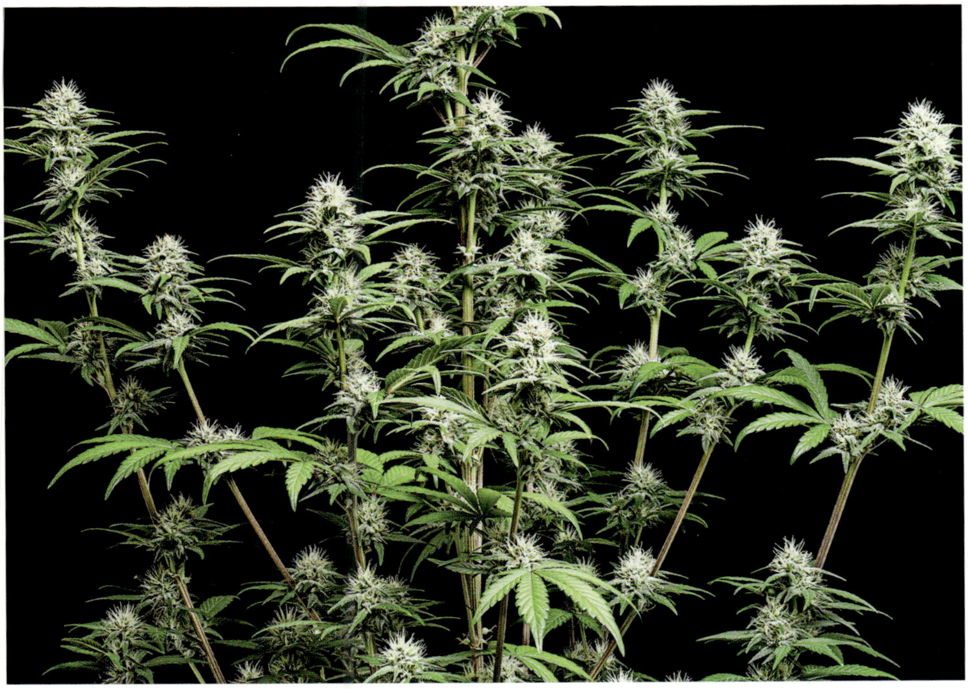

This plant is around 40 days from the start of flowering. Every node region is showing considerable flowering growth.

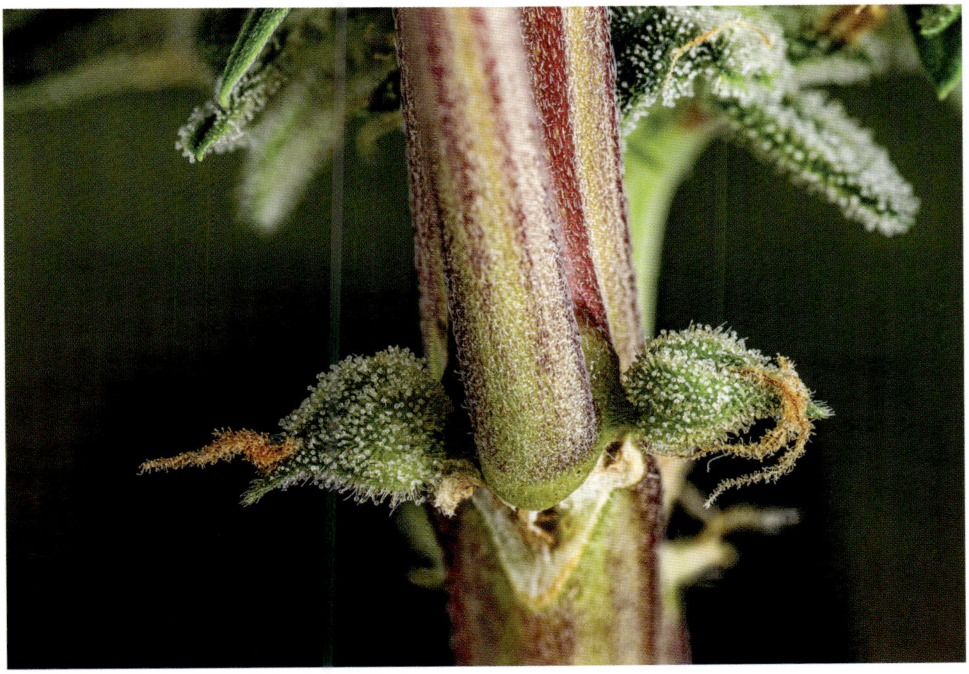

Calyx trichome development will continue along with the shorter leaves near the trichome-filled flowers.

continues...

Hagstone under an HLG-600H Quantum Board *continued*

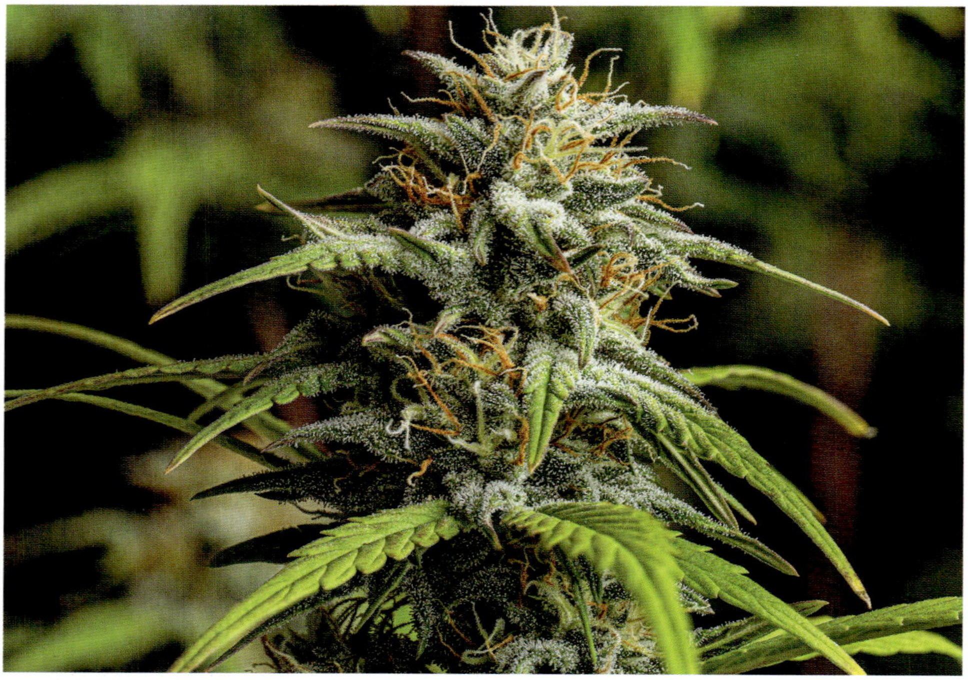

This plant is around 50 days into flowering, and trichomes are abundant on the leaves growing with the flowers.

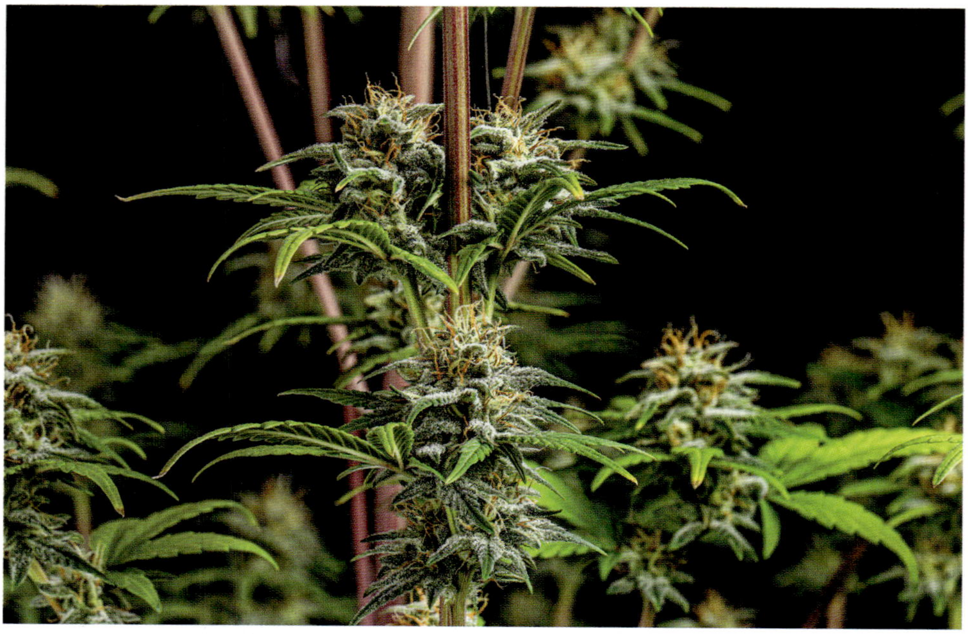

At 50 days into flowering, internode gaps should fill with growing buds. Leaves may start to show some discoloration as the plant uses its stored nutrients.

PHOTOS: ROB BRAMHILL

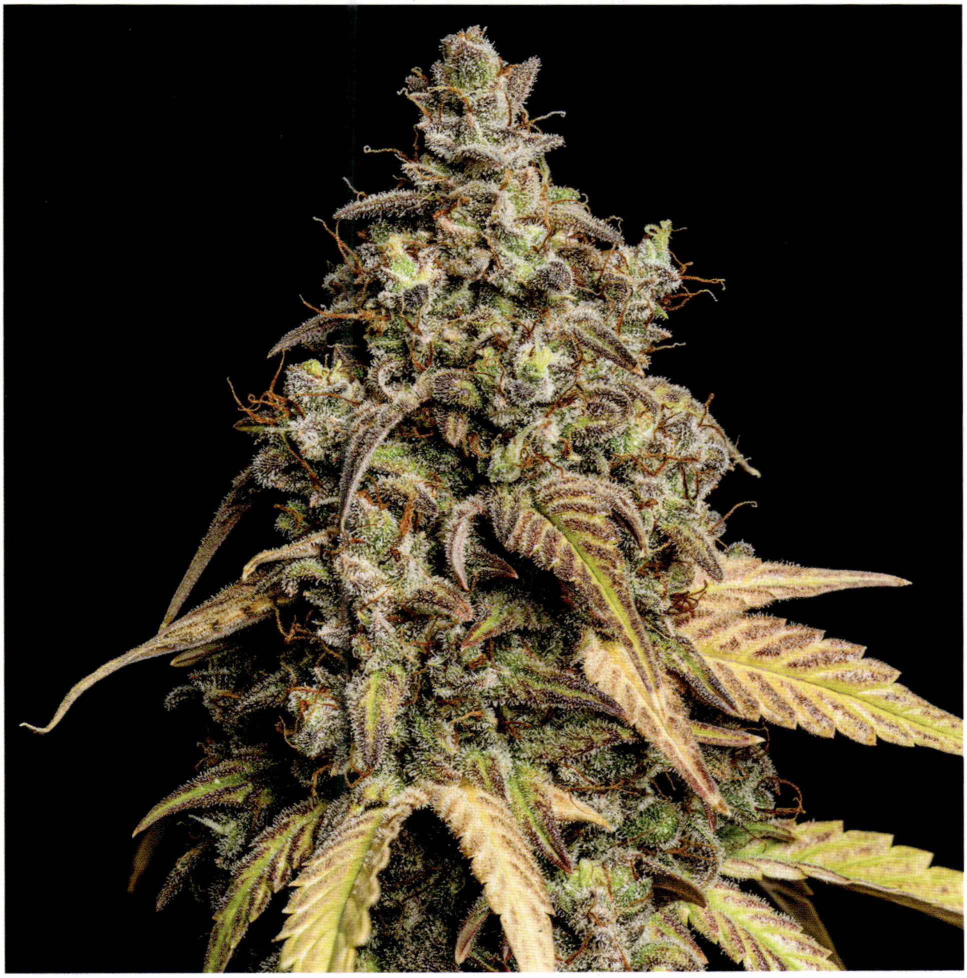

Day 80 of flowering shows a pistil-filled anc trichome-covered top cola with many color changes, including the leaves.

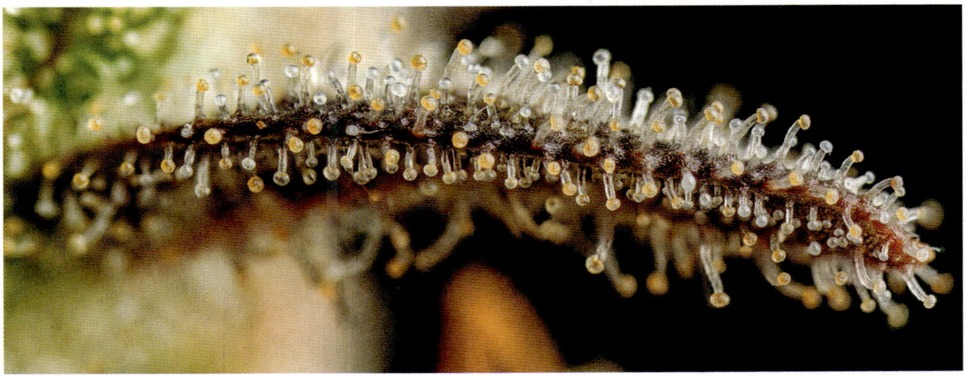

Even the trichomes themselves may change in color in their heads compared to their stalks and each other.

Understanding Electrical Costs for Indoor Growing

Electricity prices are variable, subject to the ever-evolving landscape of green and clean energy. Economic fluctuations worldwide can also lead to unpredictable surges in energy costs. Therefore, the question often arises as to how much it costs to operate a grow light system for a small number of plants. When growers embark on indoor cultivation using artificial lighting, their concerns are often about their resulting electricity bill and whether it's justifiable. HID lights will consistently be more expensive in terms of electricity consumption than LEDs, which are renowned for their energy efficiency and thus cost-effectiveness. It is possible to calculate the anticipated costs, based on the rate your electricity provider charges per watt or unit of electricity consumed. Additionally, it's important to recognize that electricity rates can vary throughout the day, with peak and off-peak hours leading to fluctuations in costs.

Calculating the Cost of Power

Typically, one unit of electricity equates to about 1,000 watts per hour and this translates into a measurable monetary value. To determine your specific costs, check your electricity bill and locate the applicable price per unit. Once you have this figure, you can plug it into the following formula to calculate the expenses:

1 kW × 24 hours = 1 kW × [price per unit] × 24 = daily cost = weekly cost (multiplied by 7) or monthly cost (derived from the weekly figure, multiplied by 4).

For instance, if the price is 10 cents per unit:

1 kW × 24 hours = 1 kW × 0.10 × 24 = $2.40 per day = $16.00 per week or $67.20 per month.

Therefore, running a 1,000-watt grow light for four months could incur expenses of up to $268.00.

While the cost of electricity may appear high, the returns generated by the cultivation effort more than justify this expenditure. Depending on factors like quality and market demand, a dispensary can price an ounce of cannabis anywhere from $100 to $350. In light of this, it becomes evident that even a small portion of your yield can cover all your expenses. Cannabis, as it turns out, possesses remarkable economic resilience, often immune to the effects of inflation. LEDs, with their energy-efficient operation, further lighten the financial burden, ensuring a cost-effective approach to cultivation.

Adjusting Your Lights

Many reflectors and grow light kits come equipped with chains and hooks, making it easy to adjust the height of your lights to accommodate plants at various growth stages. All you need is a hook in your ceiling or tent frame, or you can also use rails

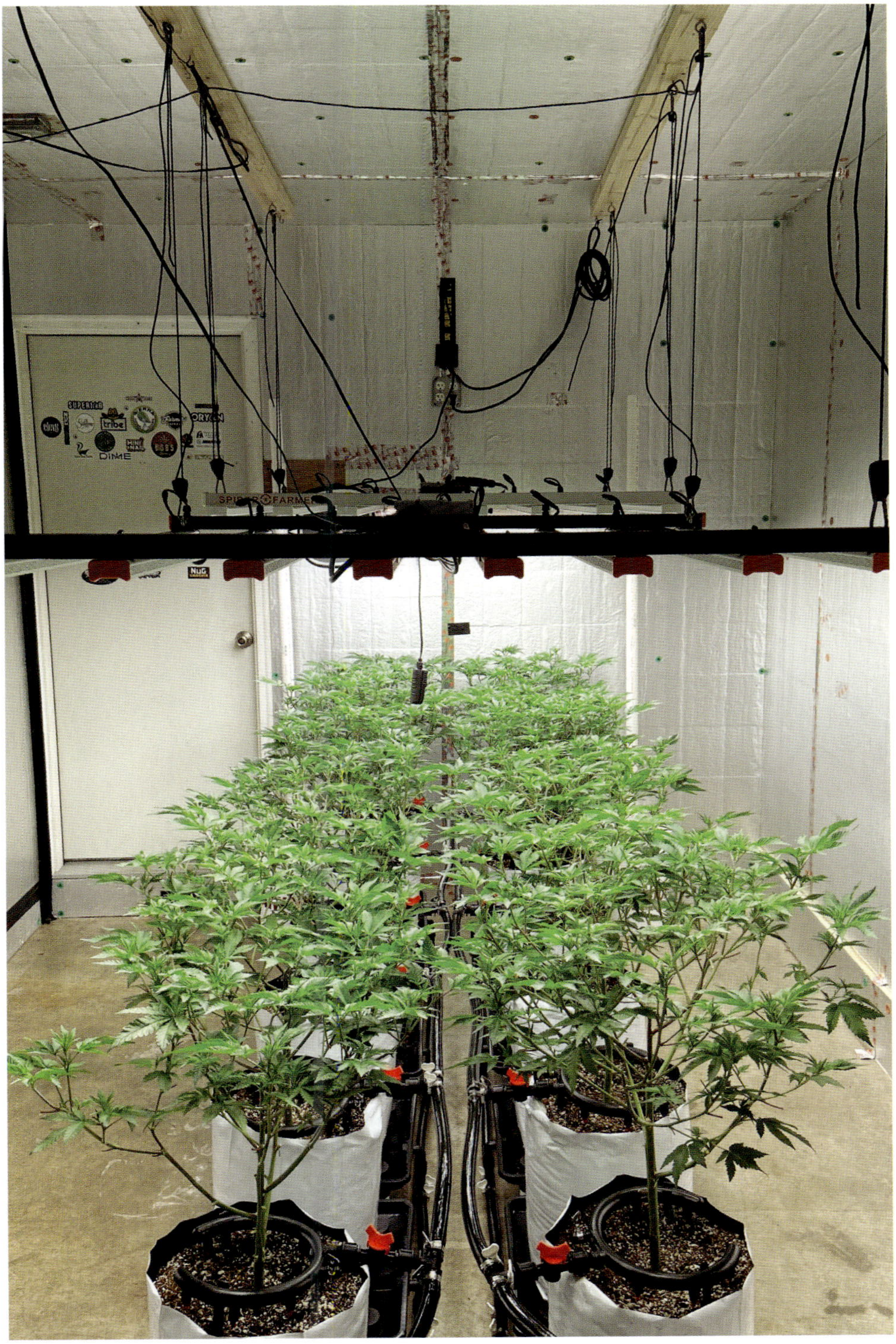

PHOTO: SPIDER-FARMER.COM

Keeping an array down close to these pruned plants has helped maintain an even canopy which will be beneficial for the flowering phase.

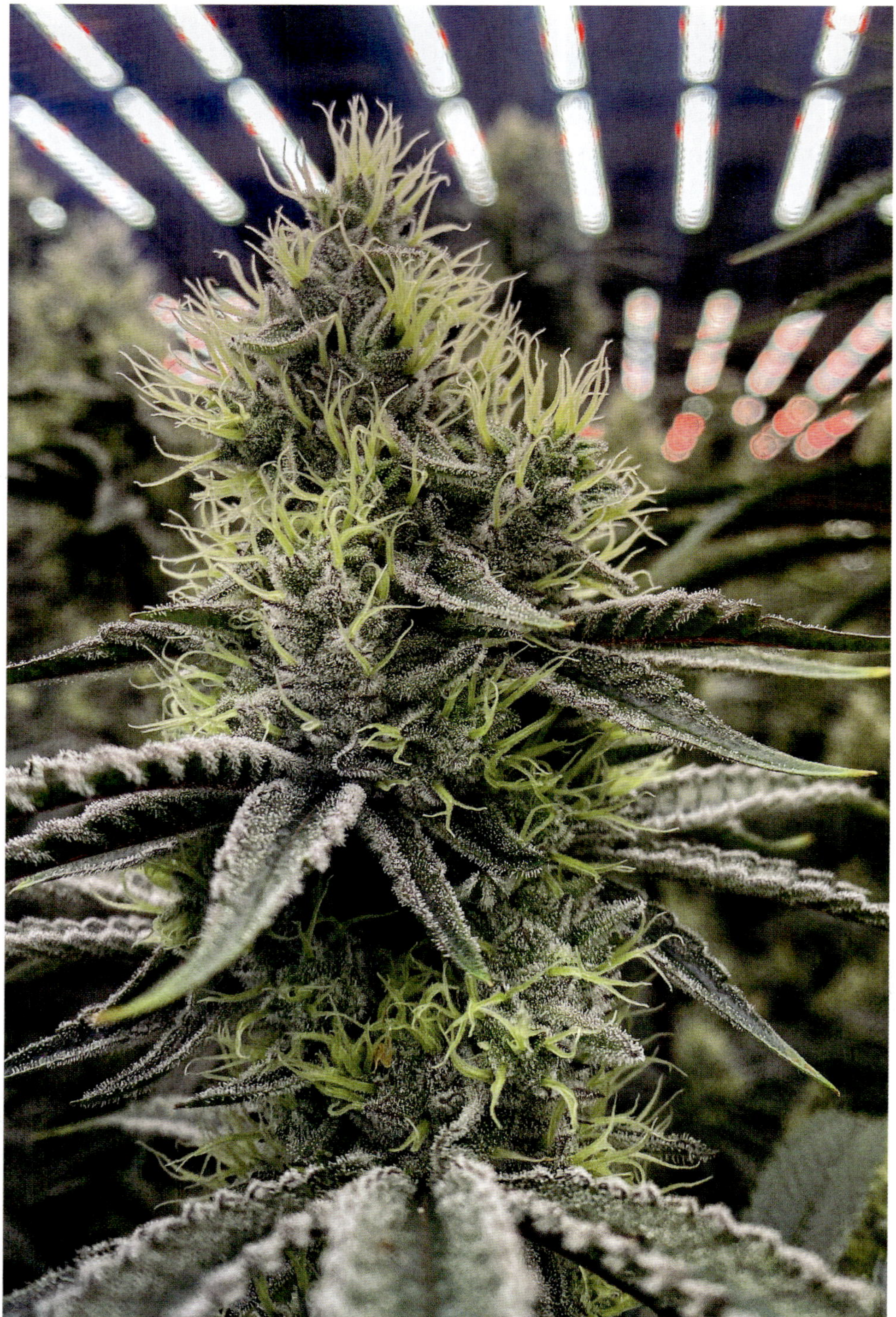

PHOTO: HIP2THECROP

Pistil growth and trichome production are pretty much the same for LEDs as they have been for HIDs. Is it possible to tell the difference between them? Probably not in blind tests.

for advanced systems that enable light movement. Grow stores usually carry the necessary accessories, but if you're having trouble finding them, TV mounts designed for ceiling mounting can also serve the purpose. In grow tents, the frame often features a light mount in the ceiling piping. Be sure to review the specifications to ensure the mount can support the weight of your lighting system.

Always remember that light intensity increases the closer the lighting is to the plants. However, placing the lights too close to your plants can lead to leaf burn. Follow this simple rule of thumb to determine the appropriate distance: If you can hold your hand under the light without discomfort, your plants should also be okay. Use common sense and adjust your lights accordingly to achieve optimal light intensity without causing harm to your plants.

Maintaining Ideal Temperatures

Chapter 8 discusses the temperature range suitable for cannabis cultivation, taking into account atmospheric CO_2 levels. In general, it's essential to maintain a temperature range of 75–85°F (24–29°C) to ensure your cannabis plants thrive. This means you may need to reduce heat, possibly with extraction fans, or increase heat with heaters if the temperature falls below the desired range.

You should now be familiar with setting up your grow area and addressing security concerns. Your lighting kit should be properly suspended over your grow area, and you should have installed some form of light reflection to optimize light conservation and direction around your plants. You should have already acquired seeds, initiated the germination process, and prepared for transplanting the seedlings into larger pots. These larger pots will accommodate your plants throughout their entire life cycle. During this period, you will provide the most suitable growing medium for your plants to flourish. In the upcoming chapters, we will explore how to fine-tune various aspects of the indoor environment to maximize your yield and achieve the best results from your cannabis plants.

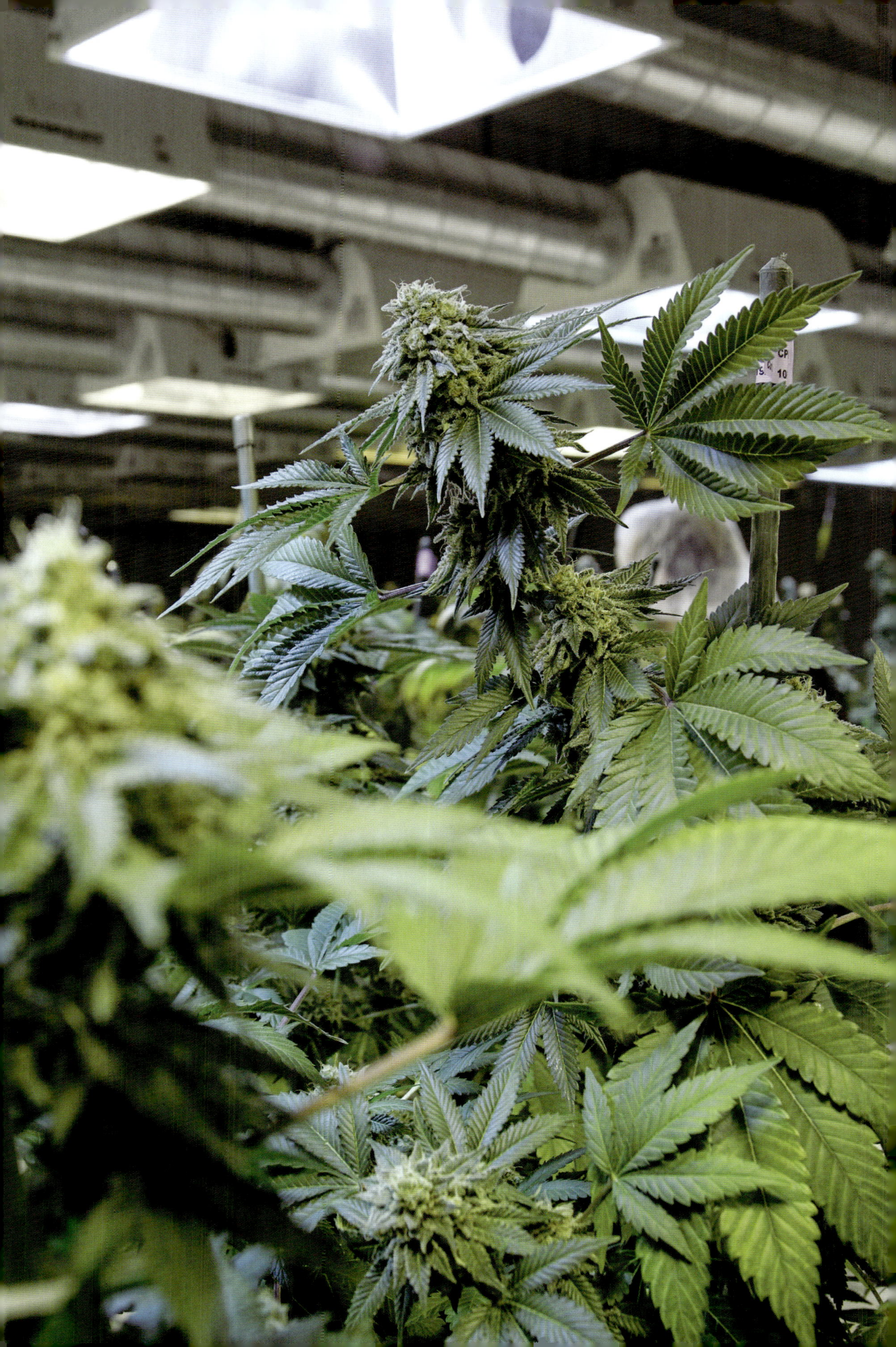

8

Indoor Environment Control

Previous chapters have shown you how to establish an indoor environment to replicate weather conditions for your cannabis plants. As the grower, you wield complete control over this environment and must make sure that it meets your plant's requirements. A breeder who develops a strain suitable for a specific indoor environment can distribute it anywhere that same environment and setup can be replicated. Most indoor environments can replicate standard cannabis grow rooms. However, if you attempt to cultivate an outdoor strain indoors, you will need to adapt the strain through pruning and training to maintain a more compact size.

This chapter addresses the control of four crucial environmental factors for plant growth: Nutrients, soil, water, and air. These, alongside genetics and lighting, the main considerations, constitute all the plant's essential needs to flourish. Each component contributes to the others in a chain of optimization that ultimately leads to the best outcomes. A chain is only as strong as its weakest link, so, even if everything else is in order, if something crucial is lacking, the results won't be optimal. Your plants will thrive when each area receives the right care.

One of your grow's crucial components is soil. Some growers choose a medium that doesn't involve soil, such as hydroponics. We will delve into these systems later, but the same principles for soil apply to other mediums.

PHOTO: PEACE NATURALS / PHOTOGRAPHED BY DAVID STRANGE

Nutrient Control

Before addressing nutrient problems, always check the pH level of your growing medium. You can find instructions on how to do this in later sections of this chapter and others. pH alterations can affect nutrient activity, potentially rendering them inactive, so you won't be able to accurately predict how nutrients behave in your

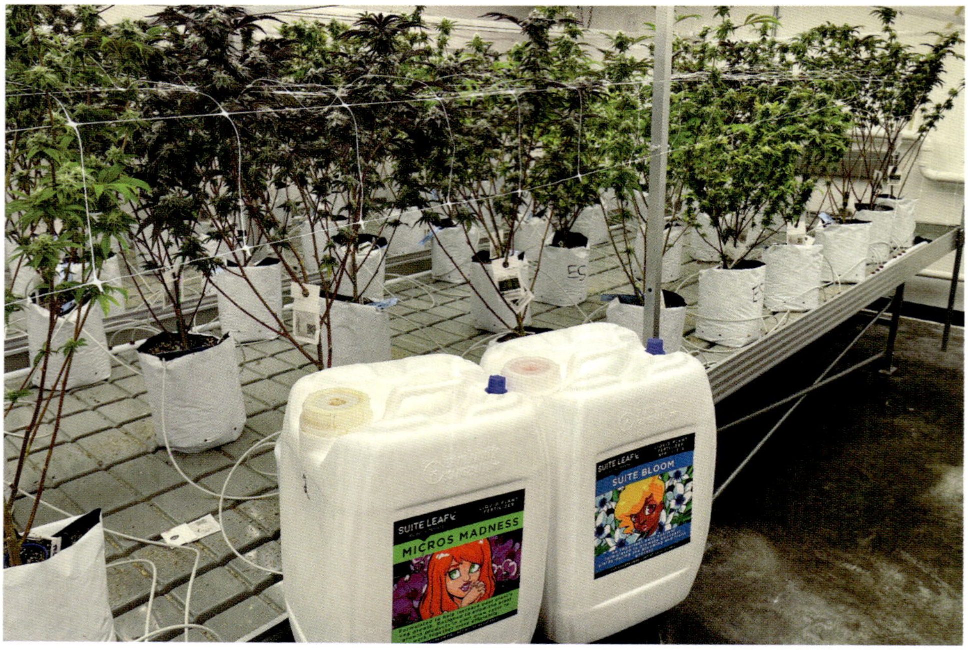

Growers often mix up their plant food with segregated macro and micronutrients.

PHOTO: SUITELEAF.COM / EXCELSIOR EXTRACTS

medium without knowing your pH level. Cannabis thrives in a pH-neutral range of around 7. We'll explore this further after covering nutrients.

In Chapters 6, we encountered the macronutrients nitrogen, phosphorus, and potassium (NPK), the primary nutrients essential for the health of a cannabis crop, whether grown in soil or another medium.

The secondary nutrients calcium (Ca), magnesium (Mg), and sulfur (S), collectively abbreviated as CaMgS, are generally present in soil, though their levels might not always be sufficient, they are vital to the metabolic cycles necessary for robust plant growth.

Eight additional plant micronutrients—iron (Fe), boron (B), chlorine (Cl), manganese (Mn), copper (Cu), zinc (Zn), cobalt (Co), and molybdenum (Mo)—also contribute to metabolic processes in plants and are essential for overall health, though they are less critical than NPK or CaMgS. Check the labels on your soil bags and feeding products to determine if they contain micronutrients. If they are present in the medium, they're usually sufficient for the entire growth cycle. However, you will still require primary and secondary nutrient sources, and non-soil mediums will likely need additional micronutrients.

You can use electronic or manual nutrient testers to monitor the nutrient content and levels in your soil. Digital testers are quite affordable and provide the most accurate measurement of primary nutrients in your growing medium. An NPK meter, for example, can deliver precise readings. Digital meters often include pH, total dissolved solids (TDS) for parts per million (PPM) and electrical conductivity (EC) readings. Take measurements at intervals to see changes over time and to aid against overfeeding. If you're on a budget, start with rapid soil test kits that use strips. Growers successfully nurtured plants long before electronic readers were invented, so don't worry if digital readers are not readily available to you. The key to nutrient control lies in having a well-planned feeding regimen.

As you gain experience with each strain you cultivate, you'll likely develop a specific nutrient mixture and feeding schedule for the vegetative growth phase and another for flowering.

Most nutrient products cater to a broad spectrum of plants. These nutrient concentrations often require some dilution based on the breed and cultivation methods. A limited number of nutrient products specifically tailored for cannabis may also require dilution. Undiluted products may be the same price or less expensive than diluted products.

While there is no one-size-fits-all formula for nutrients, and no single nutrient product suits every strain, the method outlined in this guide has proven effective for me for over 20 years. It focuses on understanding macronutrients and micronutrients, their ratio, strengths, growth phases, and timing. Cannabis is a nutrient-demanding plant. It may require lower-strength additions than other plants but more frequent applications.

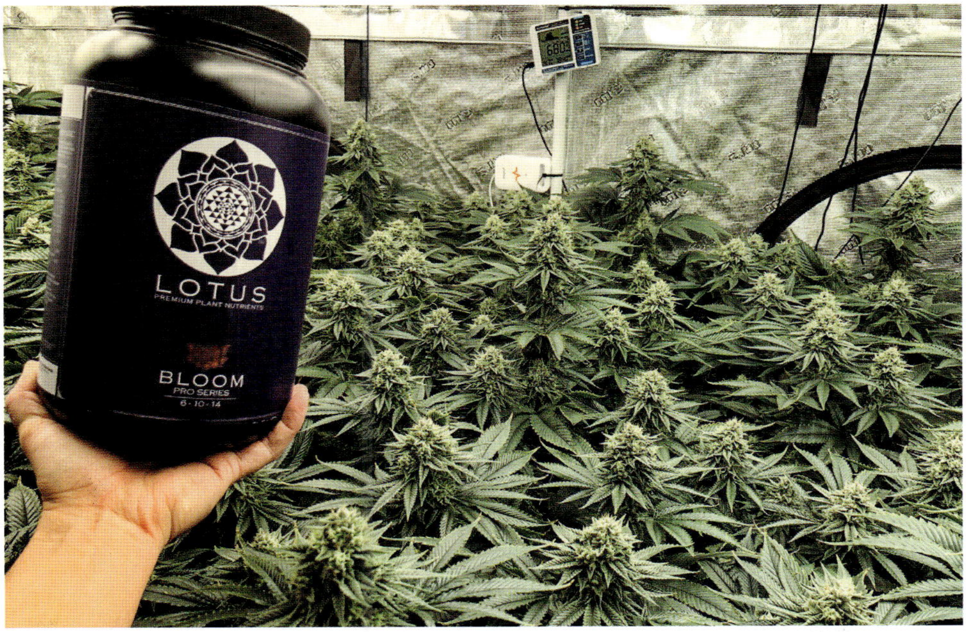

Macronutrients for flowering plants contain less nitrogen than phosphorus and potassium. Higher phosphorus and potassium promote flowering growth, as seen with this abundance of cannabis.

PHOTO: LOTUSNUTRIENTS.COM

Soil Cannabis Feeding Schedule

DWC / recirculating; teaspoons per gallon

		EC (mS/cm)	PPM (500 scale)	Grow Powder	CAL/MAG Powder	Bloom Powder	Boost Powder	Carboflush Powder
Well-Rooted Clones / Seedlings	Week I	0.9EC	430 ppm	0.75 tsp 3.6g				
	Week 2	0.9EC	430 ppm	0.75 tsp 3.6g				
Vegetative Stage	Week I	1.8EC	900 ppm	1.5 tsp 7.5g				
	Week 2	1.8EC	900 ppm	1.5 tsp 7.5g				
	Week 3	2.2EC	1100 ppm	1.75 tsp 9.0g				
	Week 4*	2.4EC	1200 ppm	2.0 tsp 9.5g	0.5 tsp 1.8g			
Flower Stage	Week I	2.3EC	1150 ppm	0.75 tsp 3.5g	0.5 tsp 1.8g	1.0 tsp 4.5g		
	Week 2	2.6EC	1300 ppm		0.5 tsp 1.8g	1.25 tsp 5.0g	0.5 tsp 3.5g	
	Week 3	2.6EC	1300 ppm		0.5 tsp 1.8g	1.5 tsp 5.0g	0.5 tsp 3.5g	
	Week 4	2.8EC	1400 ppm			1.5 tsp 7.5g	0.5 tsp 3.5g	
	Week 5	2.8EC	1400 ppm			1.5 tsp 7.5g	0.5 tsp 3.5g	
	Week 6	2.8EC	1400 ppm			1.5 tsp 7.5g	0.5 tsp 3.5g	
	Week 7	2.1EC	1050 ppm			1.5 tsp 7.5g		0.75 tsp 2.3g
	Week 8**	0.3EC	140 ppm					0.75 tsp 2.3g

Parts per million (ppm) values are calculated on base water treated with a reverse osmosis filter at 0ppm.

*For extended VEG cycles, repeat week 4 of VEG table.

**For extended Flower cycles, repeat week 6 of the Flower chart for any additional weeks added, making sure to follow week 7 and 8 the final two weeks of Flower.

NOTE: For light feeding plants/gardens with lower light intensity/no CO_2—adjust down as much as 30%. For heavy feeding plants/high light intensity rooms/high CO_2—adjust up as much as 20%

SOURCE: LOTUSNUTRIENTS.COM

Basic Feeding Plan

Most growers begin a new strain with a basic feeding plan. Unless you have prior experience with a strain similar to the one you're cultivating, you'll find yourself navigating through a trial-and-error process.

Seedlings

Do not feed seedlings. For seedlings in soil, it's better to use soil with a low NPK ratio, such as 5:5:5 or 1:1:1. Avoid adding extra nutrients. Seedlings can be sensitive to nutrient-rich environments, and soils with a high NPK ratio can burn them. When the plants remain in the seedling stage for an extended period, nutrients should be used sparingly, not exceeding 12.5% of the recommended strength, and should be diluted thoroughly.

Post-Germination

Refrain from feeding plants in the initial three weeks after germination, unless the seedlings display signs of yellowing. Once they develop a second set of leaves after the cotyledons, marking the start of the first week of vegetative growth, introduce them to the vegetative growth environment. For younger, smaller plants, provide them with an even NPK ratio (1:1:1), or one with higher nitrogen (2:1:1), at 25% the recommended strength for the first week. Stronger nutrient ratios, like 10:10:10 or 20:10:10, can also be used at 25% strength. Your aim is to determine the plant's needs gradually, as it's easier to recover from a deficiency than from nutrient burn. Use 100% strength only with cannabis-specific mixtures that are already diluted, as indicated on the label.

Vegetative Growth

Primary Nutrients

You can determine the dilution ratio that growers use for cannabis with your chosen brand of primary nutrients by looking it up online.

Any yellowing on your plants is a sign that they need more nutrients. As soon as you identify the yellowing, feed again; this may resolve the issue immediately. You'll need to increase the strength of your feeding solution until the yellowing stops. Since nutrients are already present in the system, you might wonder how much more you need. This is where nutrient meters can be handy.

Imagine a leaf transitioning from yellow to green to brown. Yellow indicates that the plants require more nutrients, while green means they're getting the right amount. If the leaf tips start turning brown, it's a sign of overfeeding. Your goal is to find the ideal balance, where the leaves are a happy, healthy green.

Some growers suggest beginning with a 33% strength solution to address yellowing,

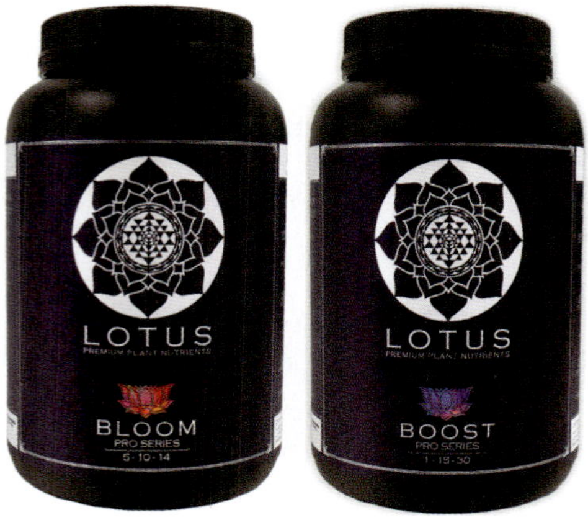

Bloom is 5:10:14, and Boost is 1:15:30. For flowering.

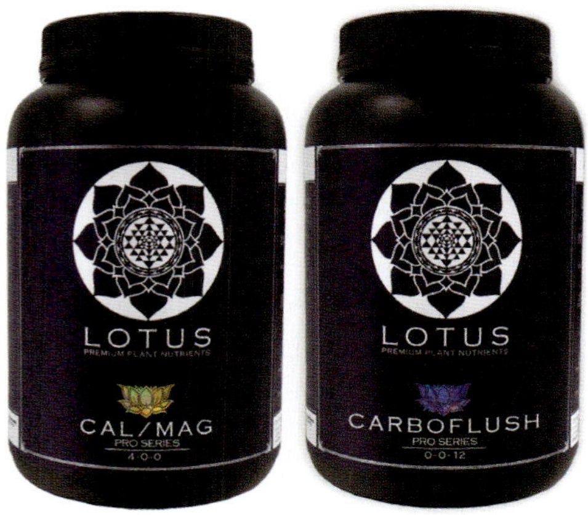

Secondary feeds calcium and magnesium. Also, a flushing agent to help finish flowering plants.

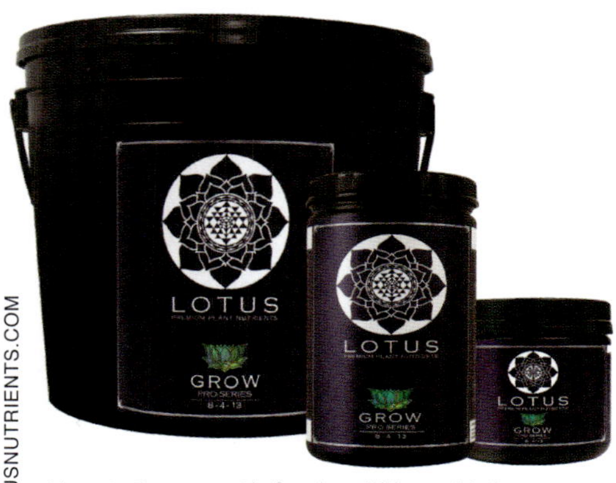

Vegetative growth foods will have higher nitrogen to phosphorus ratios. Although they come in different quantities, the ratios are the same.

PHOTOS: LOTUSNUTRIENTS.COM

which raises the nutrient content to about 50%, depending on the plant's uptake and response time. Plants typically respond to treatment within a few days, so you should start to see the yellowing subside, replaced by healthy green leaves. However, this approach can lead to burns due to overshooting the strength. If burning is severe, it may be necessary to flush the medium, which will be discussed later.

Other growers recommend adding another 8% dilution to the initial 25%. While you won't burn your plants, you may be undershooting your target. You may need to repeat the process by adding more nutrients or reverting to the 33% strength approach, as nutrient uptake might be vigorous. Persistent yellowing indicates suboptimal vegetative growth.

Which approach is better—undershooting or overshooting? Even professionals can get it wrong when switching to a new strain, even with a nutrient reader. Because strains vary in their requirements, all you can do is research the strain and learn from others' experiences. Undershooting may be advantageous because, if you don't observe improvement within a few days of adding more nutrients, you can top up again, taking only a week or a few days to figure out the ratio. In overshooting, if you burn your plants, you'll still need to determine the correct strength and address the nutrient burn.

With this information in mind, you should be better equipped to get it right. It's normal to adjust when dealing with new strains. The key is to avoid losing control early and resorting to emergency flushing. The less you interfere with your plants, the better. Try your best to start out on the right foot.

If your plant's health doesn't improve, refer to Chapter 15 on troubleshooting nutrient deficiencies. Find the appropriate regimen for vegetative growth with your specific strain and nutrients, and be diligent about keeping notes.

Secondary Nutrients

During the second week of vegetative growth, introduce secondary nutrients to your plants. Mix them at 25% of the strength recommended on the label. Incorporate secondary nutrients once every other week. Follow the same trial-and-response approach as you did with the primary nutrients during vegetative growth.

Micronutrients

Every other week, add micronutrients to your plant's feeding regimen at 25% of the recommended strength. Apply the same trial-and-correction approach. While micronutrients are not as critical as primary and secondary nutrients, they play essential roles in various parts of the plant's metabolism. Without them, optimal growth cannot be achieved.

Continued Vegetative Growth

During this phase, your goal is to foster lush, green foliage with sharp, pointed cannabis leaf tips, ensuring they spread out and appear healthy under the grow lights. This book contains numerous images illustrating this stage.

Nutrients are typically added once a week. You can address nutrient deficiencies by not increasing the nutrient strength but rather by adjusting the feeding frequency. For example, you can shift from weekly feedings to feeding every five days. However, shorter feeding intervals can suffocate the roots. Plant roots require oxygen, and the soil needs to partially dry out to become adequately aerated, so if you feed daily, this doesn't leave enough time for it to dry. You don't want to create a swamp-like environment. If you want to feed daily, consider aeroponics. Wilting leaves during the light period indicate that your plants might be dry, and you should water them.

To cultivate a bushy plant, maintain light on a 24/7 cycle once the plant reaches maturity but before it begins flowering. This forces the plant to remain in a vegetative state, diverting its energy into growing branches and increasing in size. The plant's potential for growth is still constrained by genetics, pruning techniques, and growing conditions. The choices you make—from your seed purchases to the grow setup to the way you train or prune your plant—will either help them to express their full growth potential or strategically restrict it. Recognizing maturity is relatively straightforward and is usually followed by triggering the flowering stage with a 12/12 photoperiod.

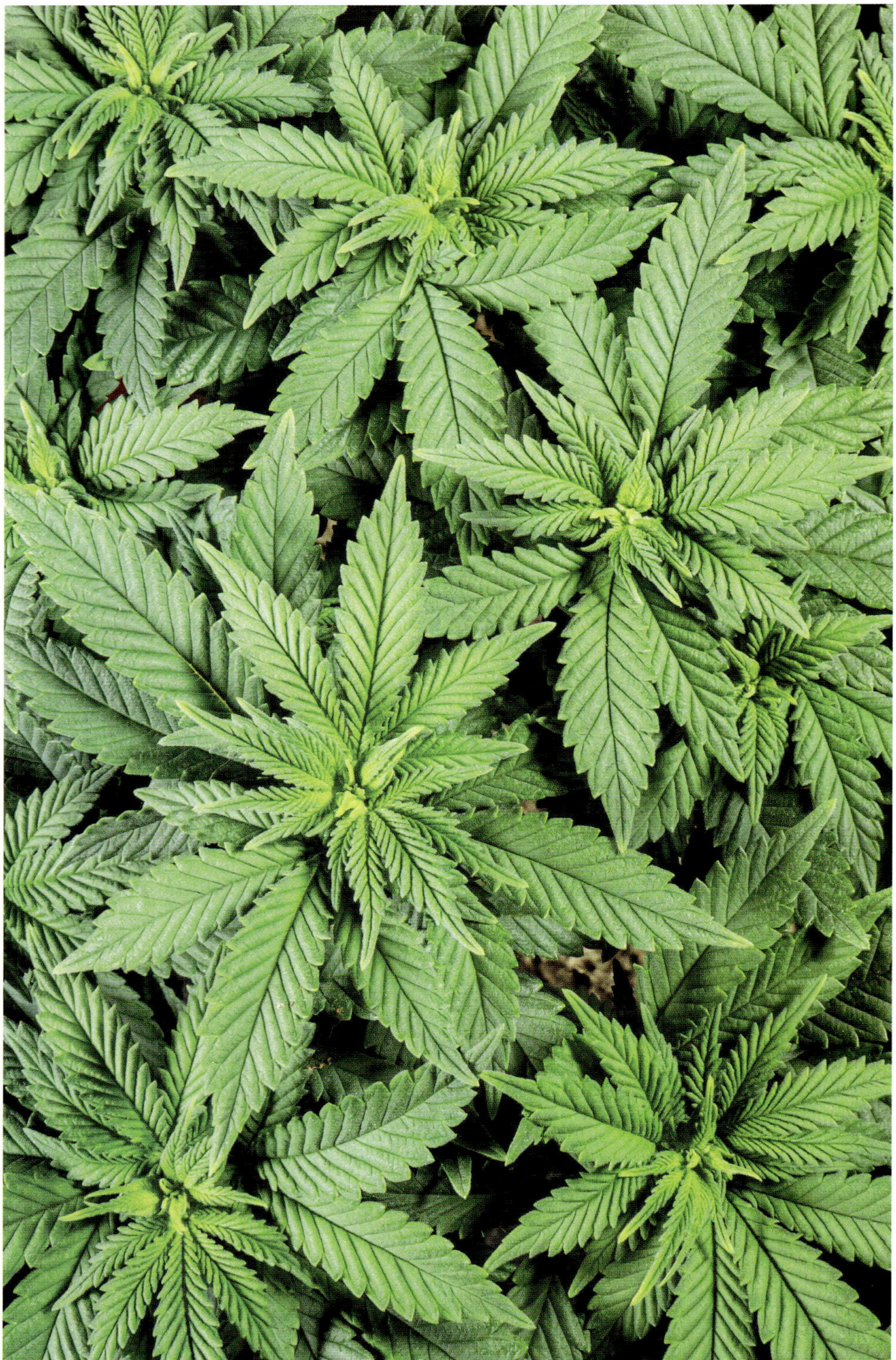

PHOTO: ROB BRAMHILL

Frequent low-intensity feedings have resulted in a healthy, even canopy.

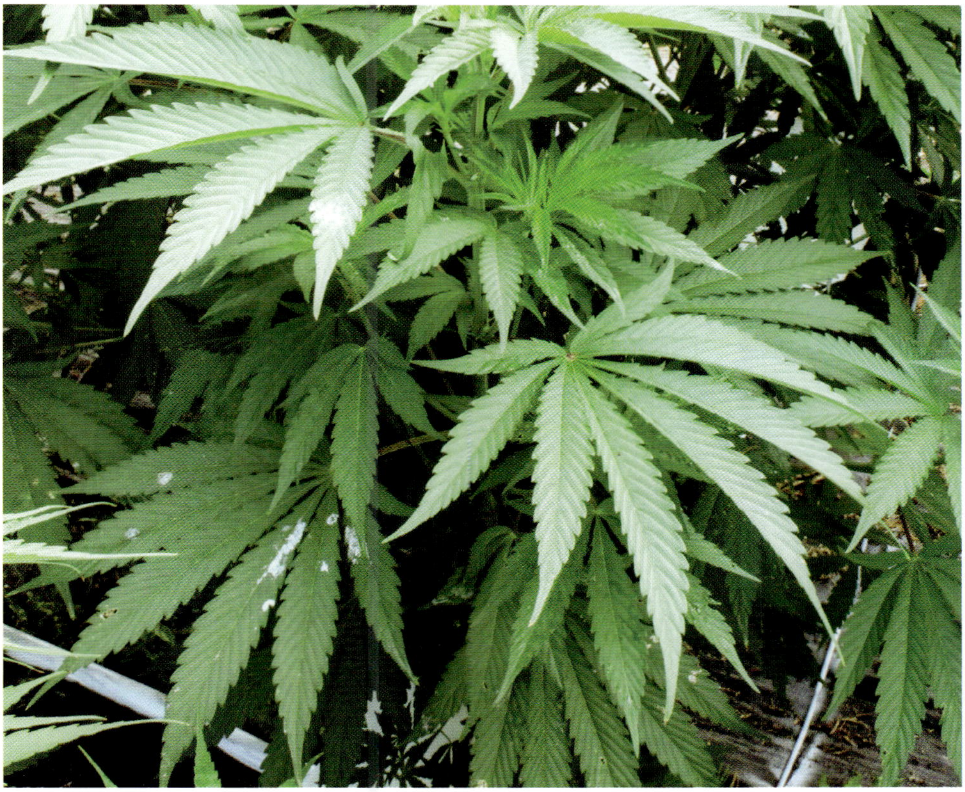

A healthy bush outdoors not only catches the light but also bird droppings from time to time. Rain will wash these away.

PHOTO: STONED ROSIE

Pre-Flowering Maturity and Flowering

Once you observe the development of ca yxes, transition to a nutrient solution with a phosphorus content higher than nitrogen and potassium, such as a 10:20:10 ratio. Maintaining the regular feeding schedule for your plants, replace the vegetative nutrient solution with the flowering formula. Use the same tests and techniques as those during the vegetative growth phase to determine the appropriate feeding regimen for your plants.

Balanced or Unbalanced Nutrients?

Some plants require higher doses of certain nutrients than others. While the feeding frequency and nutrient strengths required may vary between different strains, the nutrients themselves remain relatively consistent. Your plants rely on NPK as the fundamental components of their diet. Some soils and growing mediums deplete nutrients more rapidly than others, depending on their composition and how they hold water. When choosing a soil type, look for one with a balanced NPK ratio. A ratio like 10:10:10 is considered balanced, while 20:10:10 is unbalanced. However, both are suitable for the vegetative growth phase of cannabis.

If you're growing a new strain for the first time, starting with a balanced ratio is important. However, if you discover that your strain benefits from more nitrogen, say, consider using an NPK ratio like 20:10:10. Maintaining a balanced NPK ratio during vegetative growth is generally easier, so you might find that a ratio like 20:10:10 is too much; you'll require a 0:10:10 mixture to rebalance. It's unlikely that the nutrient ratio of a well-balanced soil composition will be significantly altered during vegetative growth. Nutrient meters can help make this process much more manageable.

Consider this scenario. You've accidentally used a soil or nutrient type with a ratio like 10:20:10 for vegetative growth. High phosphorus levels can be detrimental to the plant, outcompeting other essential nutrients, like nitrogen, preventing the plant from accessing them. This condition, nutrient lockout, can be caused by an unbalanced nutrient ratio. To address this issue, simply add a 10:0:10 mixture to the soil during the next feeding. Nutrient packages typically provide you with the flexibility to adjust and mix different ratio. You can also add separate bottles of nitrogen and potassium to achieve this balance. If all else fails, you may have to flush the medium and transplant the plant into a properly balanced mixture.

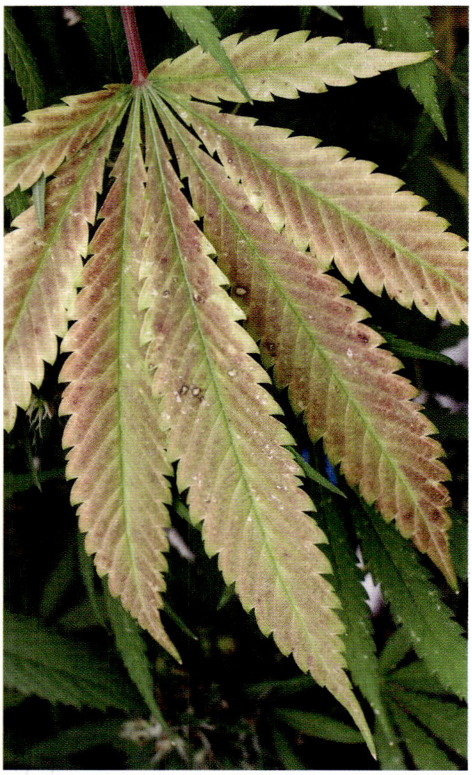

The most common nutrient deficiency during flowering growth: Lack of phosphorus.

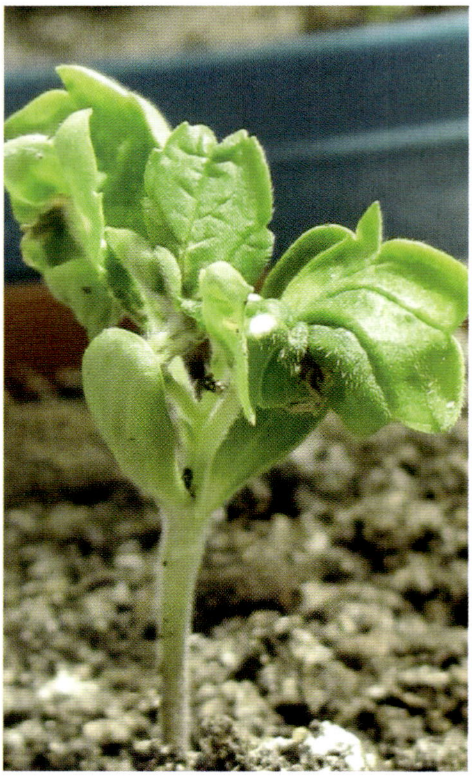

This seedling was fed nutrients prematurely.

PHOTOS: HANNA BLISS (LEFT), STONED ROSIE (RIGHT)

Classic Nutrient Types

Growers typically have access to four main types of nutrients: Primary vegetative nutrients, primary flowering nutrients, secondary nutrients, and micronutrients. These are the classic nutrient types you'll come across:

Most Common

1. NPK 10:10:10—a balanced vegetative primary nutrient pack.
2. NPK 10:20:10—a flowering primary nutrient pack.
3. CaMgS 1:1:1—a balanced secondary nutrient blend.
4. CaMgS 2:3:4—a secondary nutrient blend.

Less Common

5. NPK 0:20:10—a flowering nutrient without nitrogen.
6. NPK 10:0:10—a vegetative nutrient without phosphorus.

Pure Supplements

7. NPK 10:0:0—a pure nitrogen supplement.
8. NPK 0:10:0—a pure phosphorus supplement.

Mixed Supplements

9. NPK with CaMgS 10:10:10:1:1:1—a nutrient solution that contains both primary and secondary nutrients.

Micronutrient contents are sometimes presented as a ratio, but it's more common to find them listed individually in a comprehensive nutrient mix. A micronutrient brand used by many growers is Formulex.

Avoid this nutrient solution unless you're balancing a low phosphorus and potassium system:

NPK 10:20:20, a flowering nutrient that isn't suitable for cannabis due to its equal phosphorus and potassium values but lower nitrogen values.

Secondary Nutrient Deficiencies

Secondary nutrient deficiencies, though less common than primary nutrient problems, can be challenging to identify, so include secondary nutrients in your soil mix or feeding routine. Adding too much of the wrong secondary nutrient can harm your plants. Once again, an electronic nutrient reader is useful.

Some secondary nutrient deficiencies are more subtle and harder to detect than primary nutrient disorders. For instance, a calcium (Ca) deficiency primarily stunts growth without displaying the usual signs associated with nutrient disorders, such as leaf discoloration, rusting, blotching, leaf curling, or other chlorotic conditions.

Therefore, focus on prevention rather than cure and incorporate a secondary nutrient plan into your feeding routine.

Professional growers often obtain separate packs of nitrogen, phosphorus, and potassium for complete control over their primary macronutrient ratio. With these, they create custom nutrient blends for vegetative growth and flowering, such as mixtures of pure nitrogen, pure phosphorus, or pure potassium. With a custom nutrient blend, you can also adjust the ratio as needed. However, these separate packs are more expensive because they require additional processing to maintain purity (or stay close to it). Identifying the problematic nutrient or nutrients for a specific strain is the first step before finding the right feeding product. You might start with a balanced mix but switch to a ratio that aligns with what you've discovered through trial and error.

Breeding Specialization

The occurrence of problematic deficiencies has increased with the advancement of stabilized plant breeding. As breeders develop strains with specific characteristics such as flowering times, potency, yield, or color, they may unintentionally influence other traits, affecting nutrient requirements, smell, or taste. Some breeders provide guidance on the nutrient needs of their strains, such as more potassium or magnesium, which is valuable information when selecting a strain and its feeding products.

Image and Deficiency

Breeders might suggest reducing the dosage of specific nutrients or nutrient ranges to achieve colorful floral and leaf displays. For example, a potassium deficiency can result in reddish hues across your plant and may even turn the buds purple. While nutrient deficiencies can enhance the visual appeal of your plants, you may be sacrificing yield and potency by not allowing the plant to thrive under optimal conditions.

Nutrient Disorders

Macronutrients, vital throughout the cannabis plant's growth, are used extensively. However, it requires most micronutrients in such small quantities that their role in plant functionality is limited. Most loam soils already contain sufficient micronutrients, so you don't need to add much. However, skilled growers always add a small dose of micronutrients because prevention is more effective than cure. Always ensure that you have established correct NPK values before addressing secondary nutrient concerns. By making these adjustments, you should prevent this issue from recurring, and sustain your plant's optimal health.

This guide will help you understand how various nutrients function and how to identify nutrient disorders in your grow.

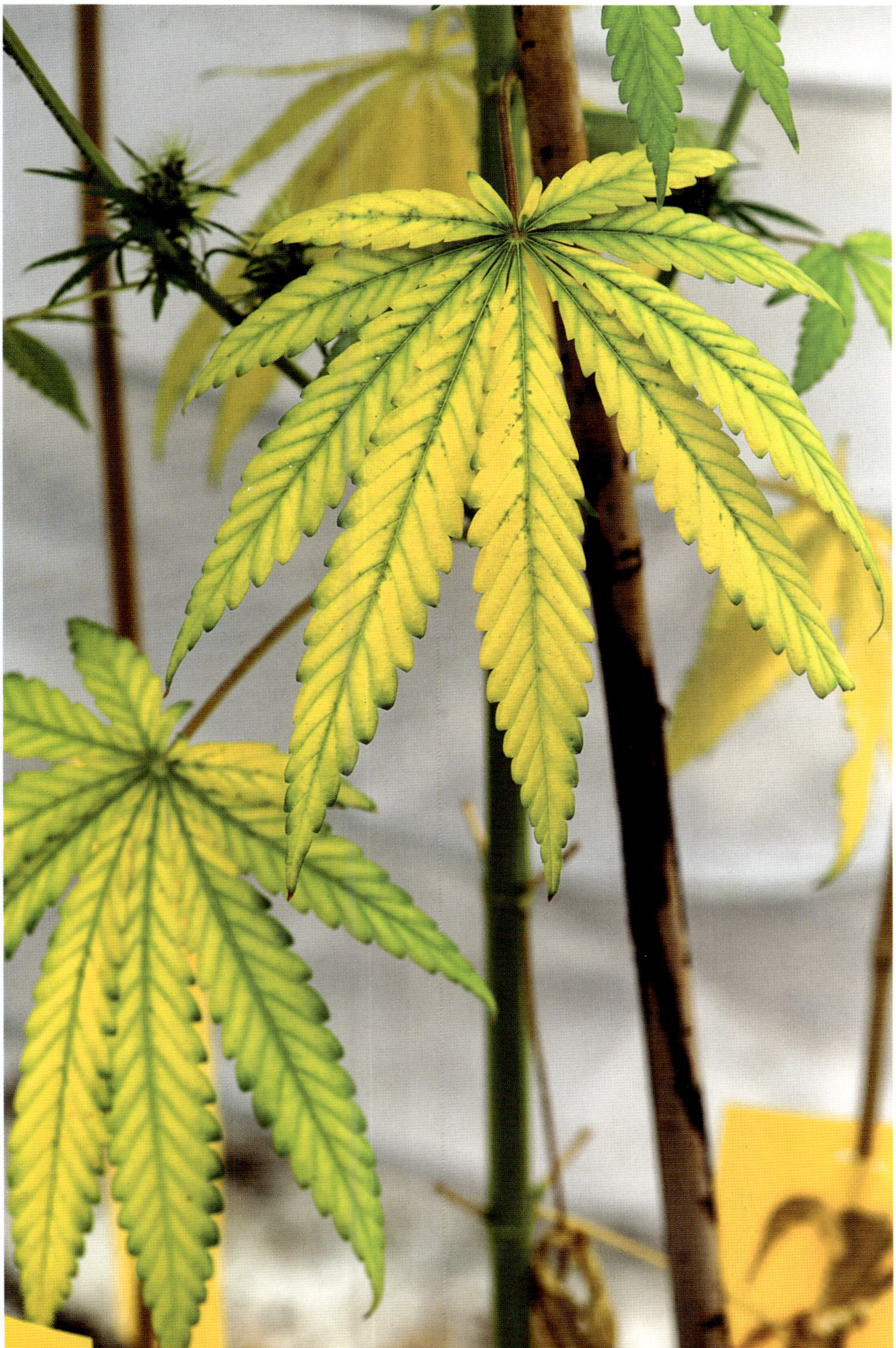

The most common nutrient deficiency during vegetative growth: Lack of nitrogen.

PHOTO: HANNA BLISS

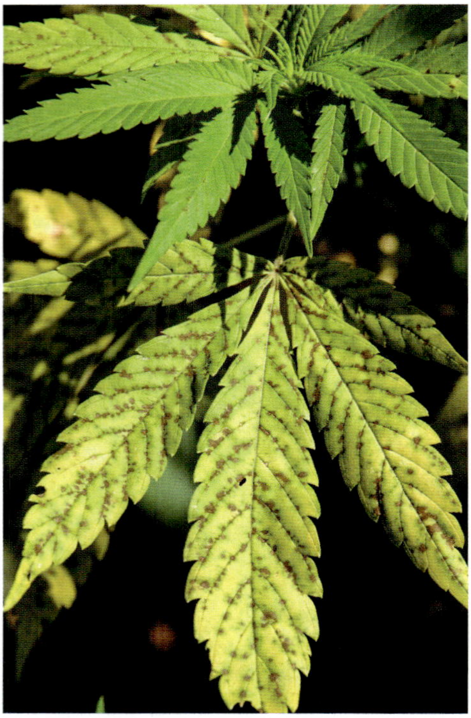

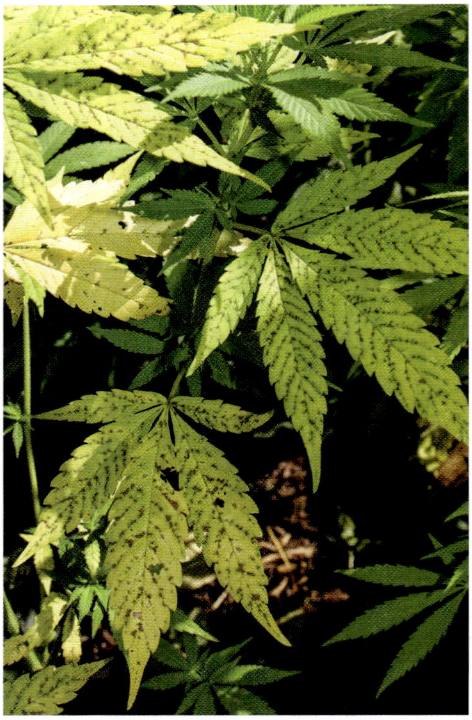

Leaves yellowing from the bottom up during vegetative growth indicates a lack of nitrogen. The deficiency is resolved by feeding the plant more nitrogen than phosphorus and potassium.

Nitrogen (N)

Yellowing during the vegetative growth stage is likely due to a nitrogen deficiency. Cannabis, like most plants, requires more nitrogen than any other nutrient during the vegetative growth phase. Nitrogen plays a direct role in chlorophyll production and is essential for photosynthesis and energy generation in plant cells. Inadequate nitrogen levels lead to cannabis plants turning pale yellow-green, starting with lower leaves and progressing upward. Eventually, affected leaves wither and drop off. Increasing nitrogen levels will resolve this issue.

Nitrogen Deficiency

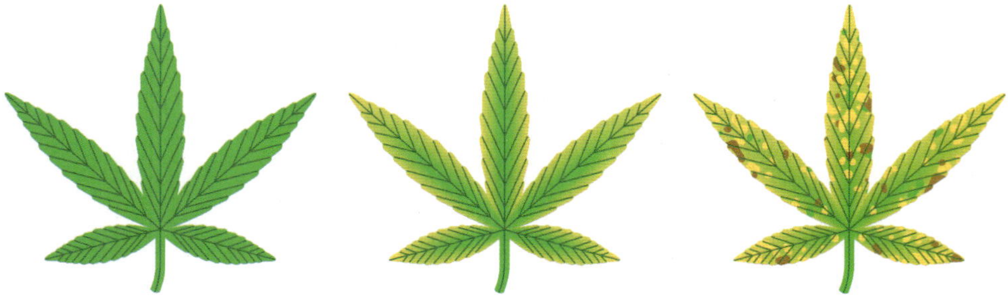

PHOTOS: DAVID STRANGE

Phosphorus (P)

Phosphorus should be present in your vegetative nutrient mix, most critically during the flowering stage. Like most plants, cannabis uses phosphorus in photosynthesis to create essential compounds, especially during floral development. A phosphorus deficiency causes the veins on plant leaves to turn red and inhibits plant growth. To address this, supplement with additional phosphorus if you suspect your plant isn't thriving. However, keep in mind that genetics can sometimes play a role in this.

Phosphorus Deficiency

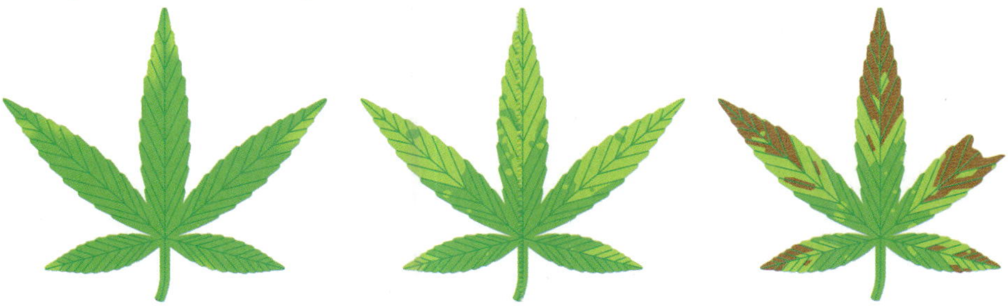

Early stage | Middle stage | Late stage

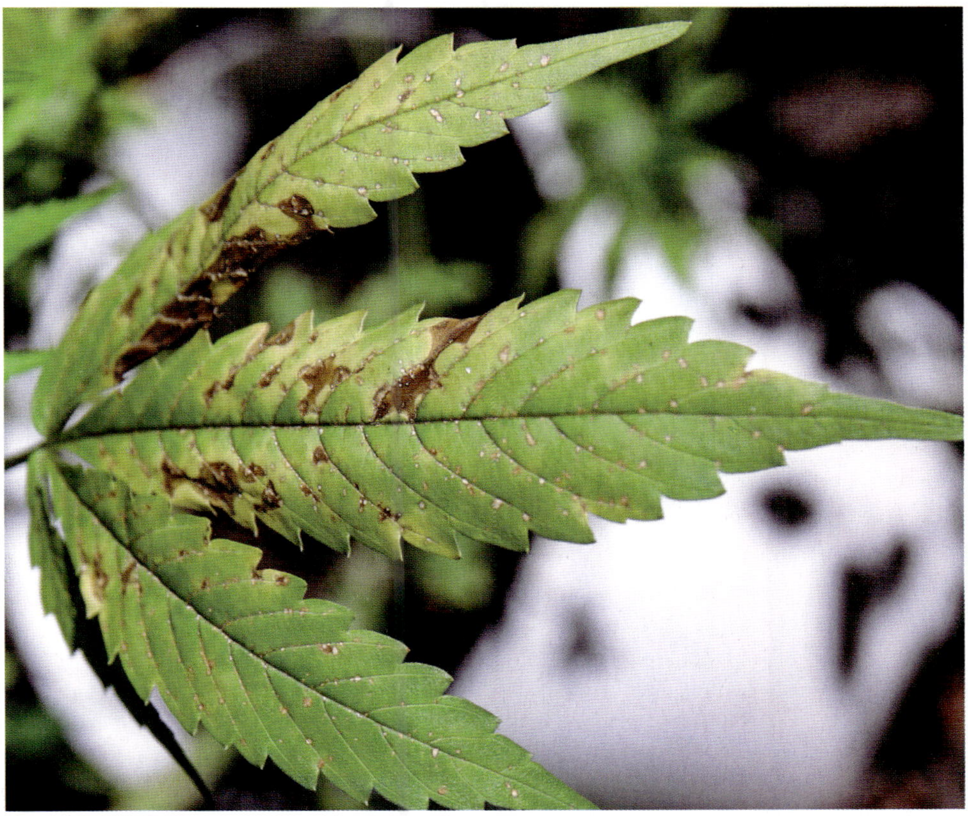

PHOTO: DAVID STRANGE

A phosphorus deficiency appears to cut into the leaf's veins, turning them red and necrotic.

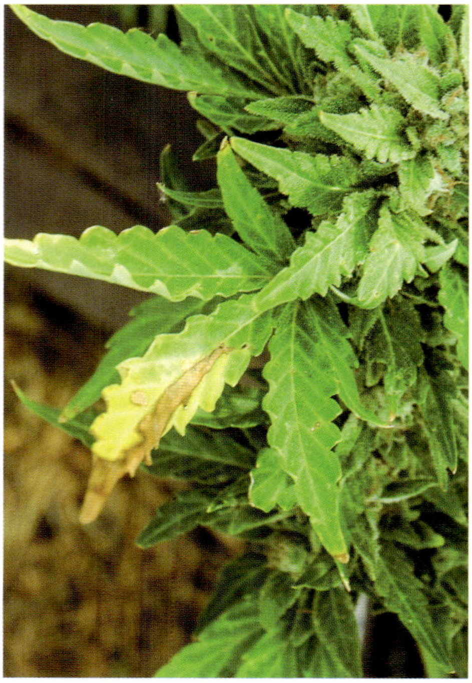

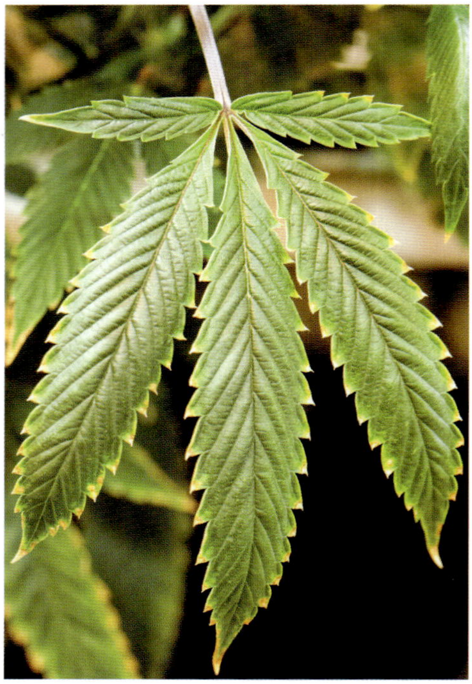

A potassium problem causes leaves to become weak and brittle. Stems may turn red.

Potassium (K)

Potassium supports various chemical synthesis processes and overall plant metabolism. Some processes contribute to disease resistance, so a potassium deficiency can make your plant susceptible to mold, fungi, and wilting. Potassium also aids in seed and stem development. Without enough, stems and branches become weak and prone to breaking. Symptoms of potassium deficiency include necrotic patches on leaf tips at the base of the plant and blotchy patterns in the middle of leaves. While red stems can indicate a potassium problem, they can also be a result of cold temperatures or a genetic trait in some plants, especially equatorial strains. Avoid misdiagnosing these symptoms as a potassium deficiency and overfeeding your plant.

Potassium Deficiency

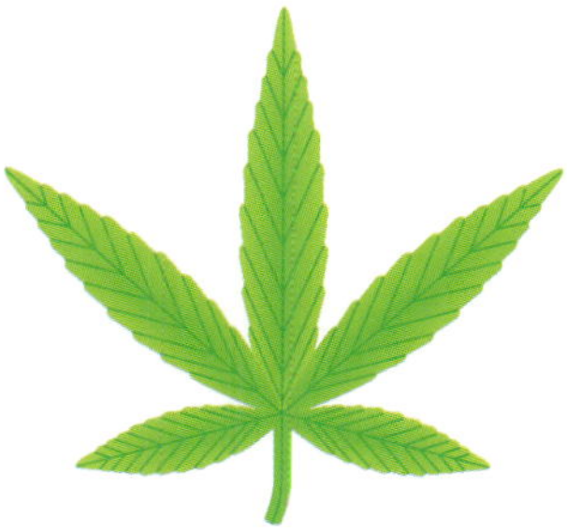

Early stage

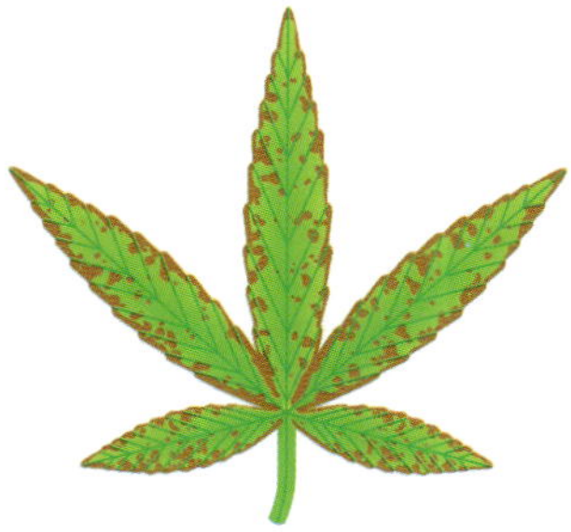

Middle stage

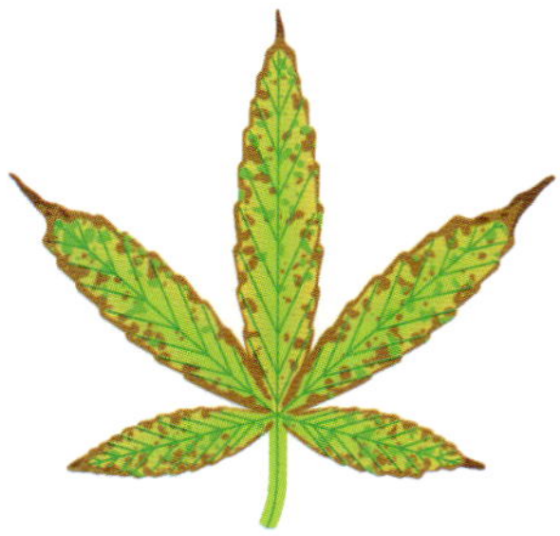

Late stage

PHOTOS: STONED ROSIE

Calcium (Ca)

Plant cells require calcium for development and storage. Calcium deficiencies are rare in cannabis, and their symptoms are often subtle. However, they can stunt growth and lead to wilting. If your plants exhibit slow growth without displaying symptoms associated with another nutrient disorder, consider adjusting the calcium content in your feeding plan. Take notes to help ascertain whether this change is helping the issue.

Stunting

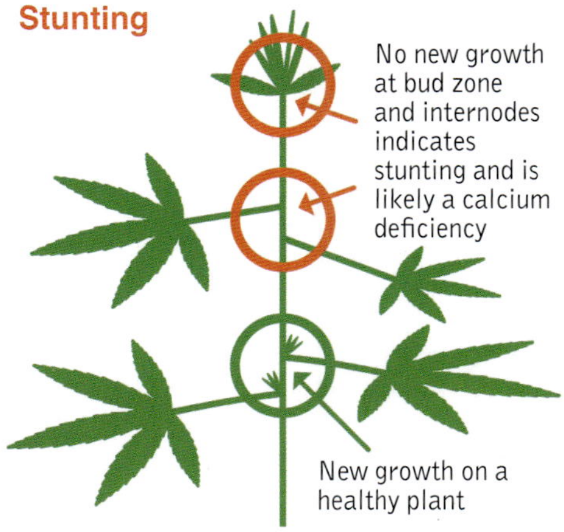

Calcium Deficiency

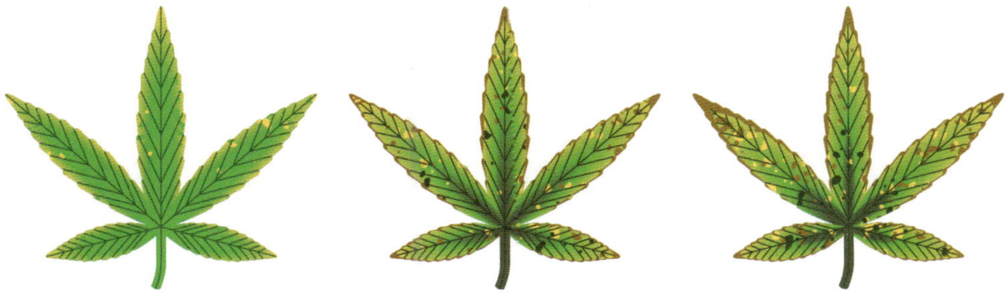

Sulfur (S)

Sulfur contributes to chemical synthesis and metabolic processes in the plant and is also involved in the formation of amino acids and proteins. In the absence of sulfur, the plant will appear yellow and pale. Detecting sulfur and nitrogen deficiencies early is crucial, as they can become challenging to distinguish from each other as they progress. Nitrogen disorders typically start from the bottom of the plant and move upward, while sulfur issues begin with new growth and spread from there.

Sulfur Deficiency

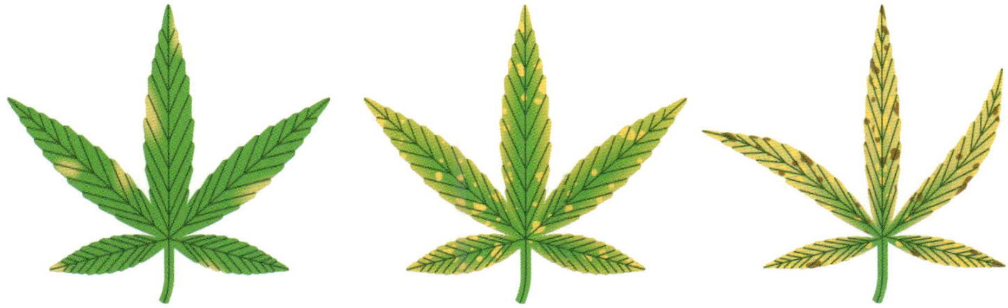

PHOTO: HANNA BLISS

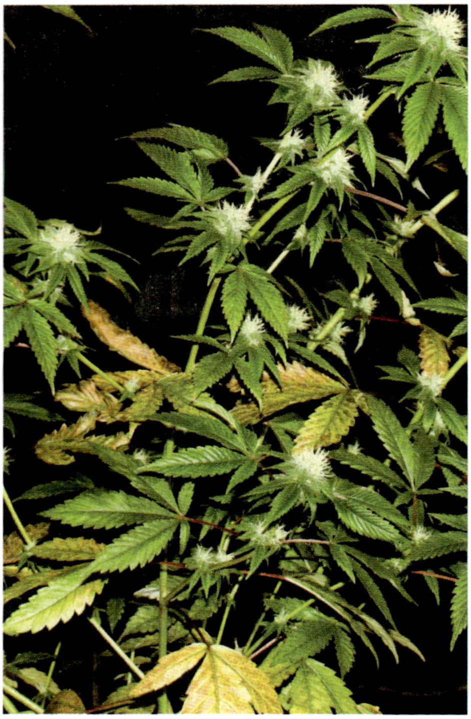

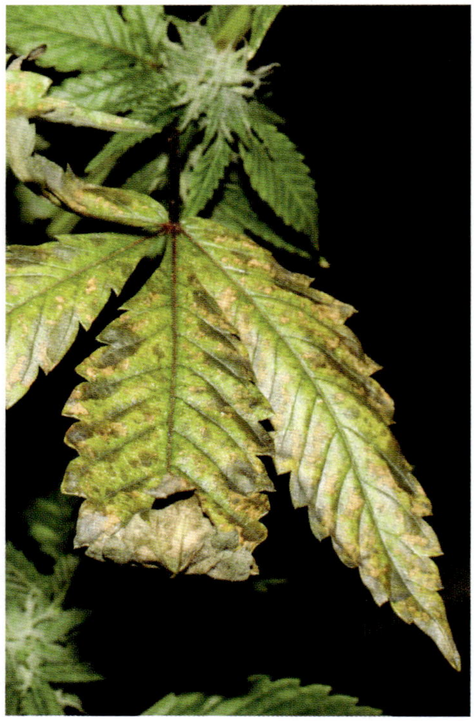

The edges of this midway leaf are curling up as if praying for Mg. Treat with Epsom salts or a secondary nutrient feed.

Magnesium (Mg)

Magnesium deficiencies are among the most common secondary nutrient disorders you may encounter, especially if you have already balanced the NPK ratio correctly. Many strains are more susceptible to magnesium nutrient disorders if they are also deficient in another secondary nutrient. You may need to introduce pure magnesium or a secondary nutrient-feeding product, preferably one with a higher magnesium to calcium and sulfur ratio. However, any balanced secondary nutrient product containing magnesium is better than none.

Magnesium Deficiency

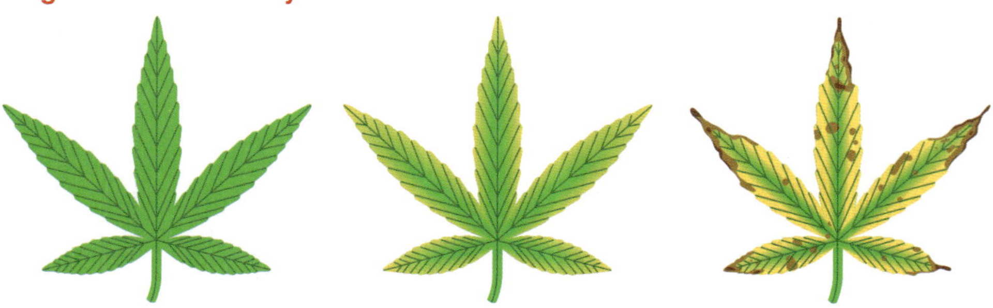

Early stage Middle stage Late stage

PHOTOS: ALPINE SEEDS

Magnesium is contained in chlorophyll, which imparts the characteristic green color to foliage, facilitates photosynthesis, and plays a central role in chlorophyll production. As such, it is vital for photosynthesis. Therefore, plants with magnesium problems often display such symptoms as yellowing and leaf curl, particularly in leaves that curl upward at the base of the plant, thus the saying "the plant is praying for magnesium."

To address magnesium deficiencies, feed your plant one teaspoon of Epsom salts per three gallons of water every three to four weeks. Epsom salts specifically designed for plant use are available at grow shops, and dissolve more effectively in water and offer better value than regular Epsom salts. You can also opt for a medium with higher magnesium content.

Secondary nutrient products are available in liquid, powder, or granular forms at your local grow shop. Avoid using granules for immediate magnesium deficiency correction, as they take longer to break down in the soil and are considered slow-release products. For immediate solutions, opt for liquids such as Formulex.

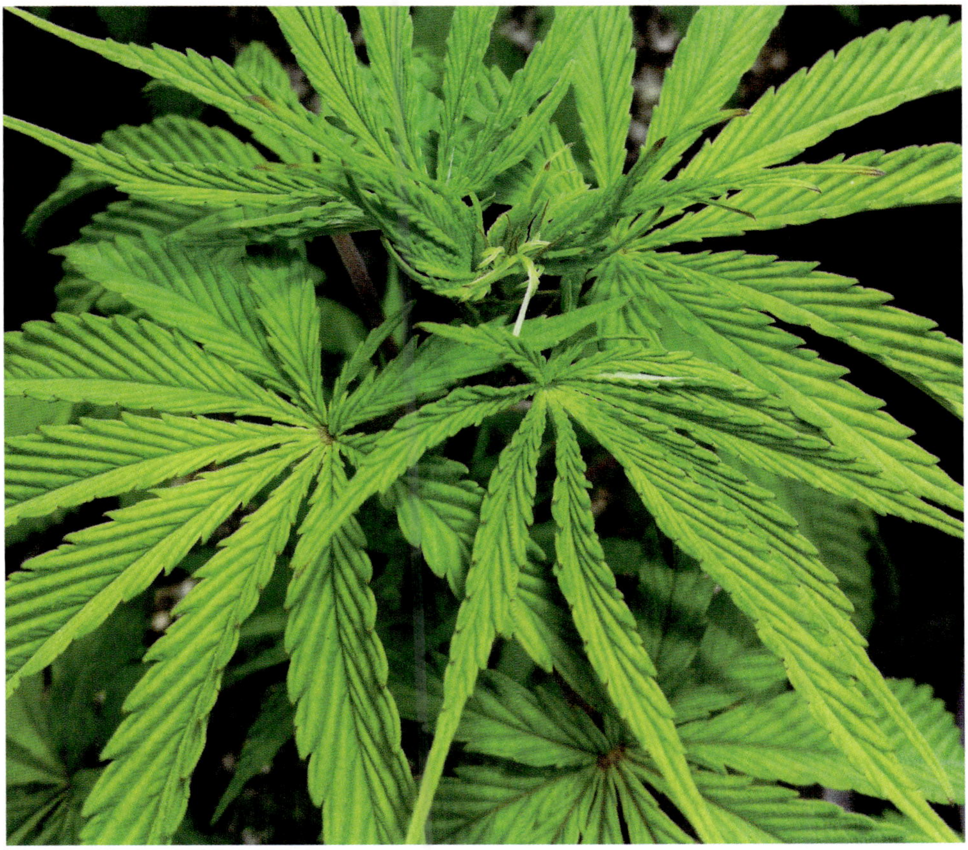

PHOTO: TYLER J. MARKWART AND DANIELLE HALLE

Plants start to look pale and unhealthy when they become unable to take up nutrients because of toxins and pH problems.

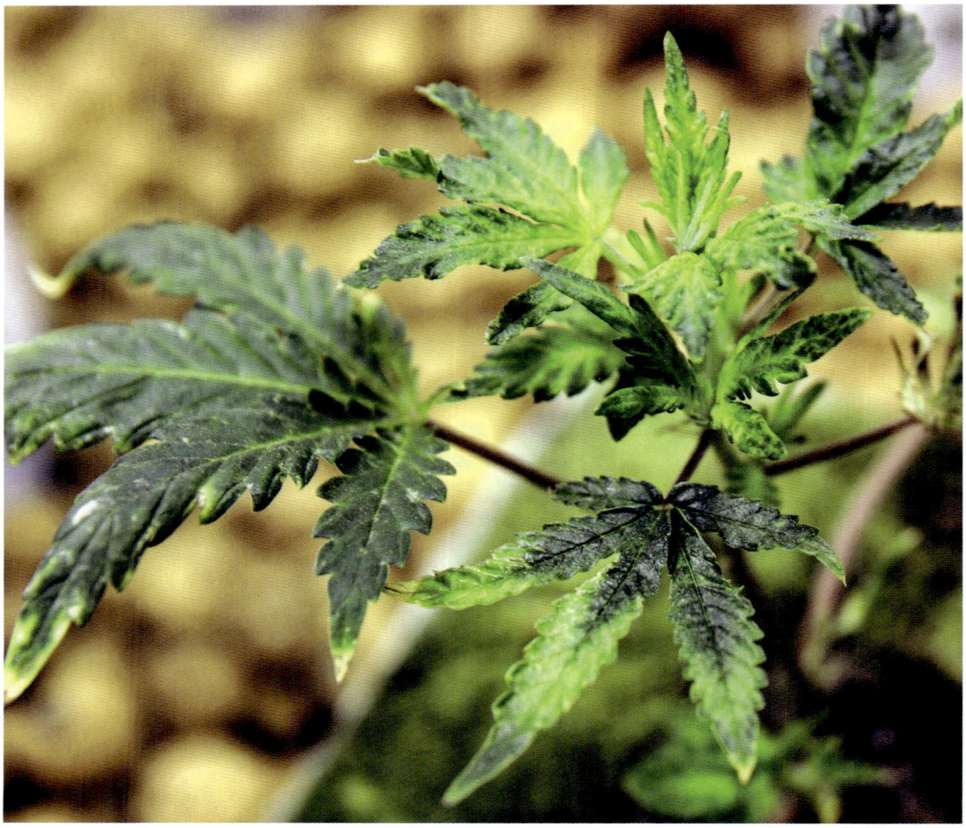

Manganese or zinc problems occur in the upper portion of the plant and indicate the need for micronutrients.

Lockout

Micronutrient problems are rare unless lockout occurs. This is a chemical reaction in which nutrients combine to form new compounds that the plant cannot use, typically resulting from an excessive amount of one nutrient or the introduction of salt into your mixture. This transformation turns a dissolved substance into an insoluble solid from a super-saturated solution. Using expired nutrient formulas past their shelf life can also lead to a lockout.

You can use different brands for primary, secondary, and micronutrients. However, many growers prefer using the same brand for all nutrients to prevent potential lockout issues, as mixing brands can sometimes lead to unintended chemical reactions within the medium. Though NPK and CaMgS represent pure substances, some nutrient products may have impurities or contain additives to enhance their effectiveness. The brand's formulation specifications will say if it can be mixed with another. However, in most cases, it should not be problematic. You can experiment with the combination of two brands, but exercise caution.

PHOTO: DAVID STRANGE

If you do use different brands, space out their use, with several days to a week between applications rather than adding them together or on consecutive days. For example, if you run out of brand A for NPK and switch to brand B, avoid mixing the remaining brand A with brand B.

This practice is recommended because lockout can be challenging to detect. Even after exploring various deficiency possibilities, solutions, and pH correction, you may still encounter lockout as the underlying cause. In such cases, you will need to flush your soil, a process we will describe later. It is perfectly normal to learn through mistakes as part of the process of optimizing your results.

Avoid relying on the actual bottle caps for measurements when using nutrient products. Use a proper measuring flask to prevent issues with cap precipitation and the inadvertent addition of unwanted chemical compounds to your plants. Refer to the product instructions to determine what constitutes a capful, measure it out in a flask, and keep a record of the measurement. Be sure to clean your flasks, segregate them for primary, secondary, and micronutrients, and designate specific flasks for mixing as trace amounts of residual nutrients can accumulate in them over time.

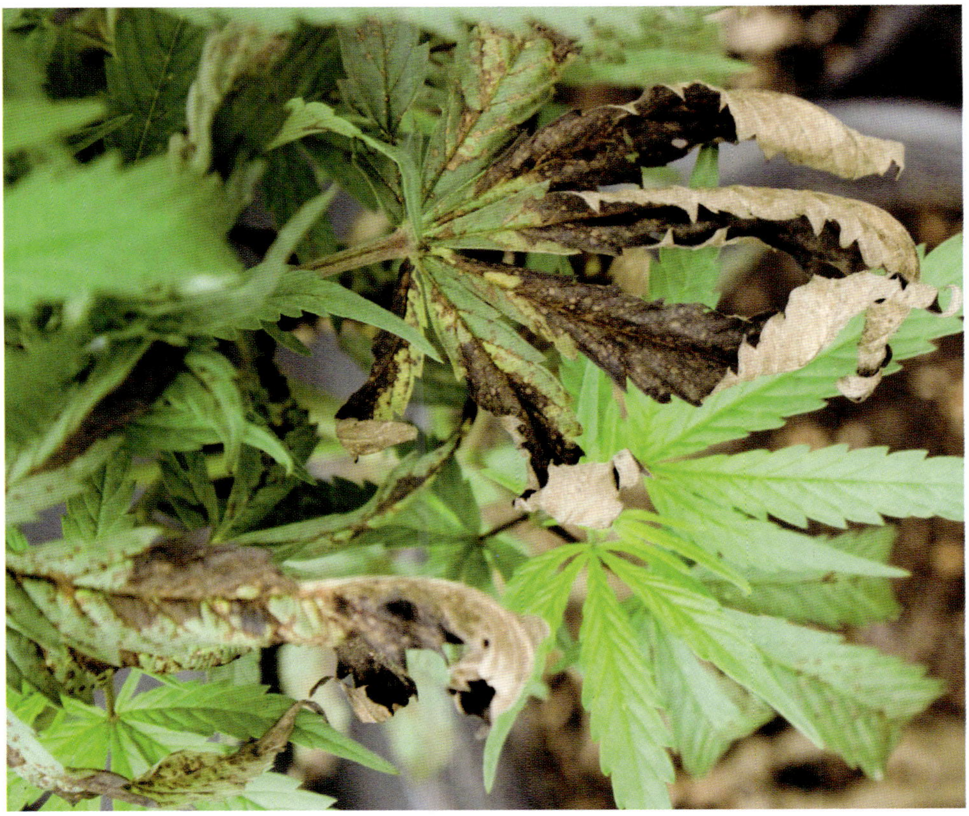

PHOTO: DAVID STRANGE

This plant has been burnt from overfeeding, meaning a transplant is needed.

Nutrient Experiments and Testing

You can experiment with nutrient solutions by preparing mixtures in an open flask, allowing them to settle, and returning after a few days to observe any precipitation and to gain valuable insights into potential issues with your nutrient mixture. You are specifically looking for significant clumping in the solution. The fluid content of the mixture should not change significantly when exposed to air in this manner, though you may encounter clumping around the rims of nutrient bottle caps where the remaining liquid has been exposed to air. This clumping can resemble a powder or a residue and may lead to nutrient lockout.

Using this method along with a preliminary test can help you avoid nutrient adjustment errors. While having a nutrient reader can be beneficial, these devices can be relatively expensive. However, you can opt for more affordable nutrient testing strips, which can also be used for pH testing. Even if your testing results are not precise, they will still bring you closer to optimization. Over time, you can refine your testing methods.

To conduct a nutrient test, extract a sample from the medium you intend to adjust, whether that's soil, a nutrient reservoir, or a substrate mix, and place it in a jar. Typically, you won't require more than a few spoons of soil. For hydroponic reservoirs, you can fill a jar with the nutrient solution. Begin by taking a nutrient reading and then proceed to prepare your nutrient adjustment. After mixing, test the solution once more. Repeat this process until you determine the necessary nutrient adjustment. Once you've identified the correct adjustment, you can apply it directly to your actual grow in a single step, without the need for further testing on your plants.

Additional Notes on Feeding Strengths

Feeding your plants replenishes nutrients that have been depleted from your growing medium. You will need four different feeding solutions throughout your plant's growth cycle, two for primary nutrients and two for secondary and micronutrients. The first is used during vegetative growth, the second during flowering. Plant food comes in various forms, including solids, liquids, sprays, powders, and granules. Liquid form is the most common, available in bottles or larger containers.

Solutions with nutrient values below 5% must be mixed at a higher ratio for certain plants. For example, if you have a nutrient mix with an NPK value of 5:5:5, it means that 15% of the solution contains nutrients, while the remaining 85% is primarily water. If you are flowering large nutrient-demanding strains, you may have to provide a higher-strength mixture, particularly one with more phosphorus.

Large outdoor hybrid strains can consume significant amounts of water and nutrients daily. In some regions, hybrid sativa strains can grow to almost tree-like proportions. Even if you ensure that the soil around the plant is rich in nutrients, you may need to

Step-by-Step: Watering with Nutrients

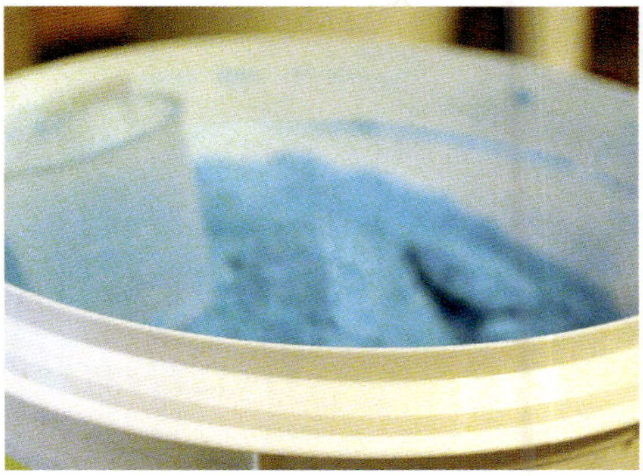

Measure out fertilizer.

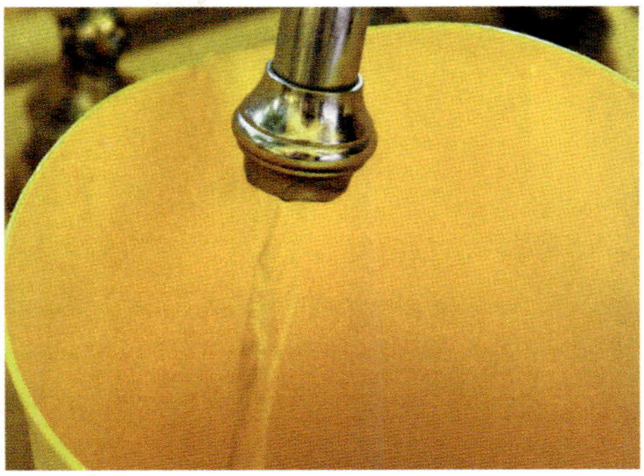

Add water slowly.

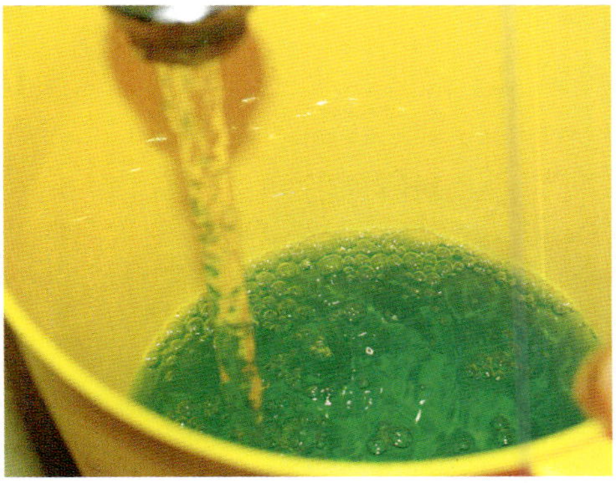

Mix carefully.

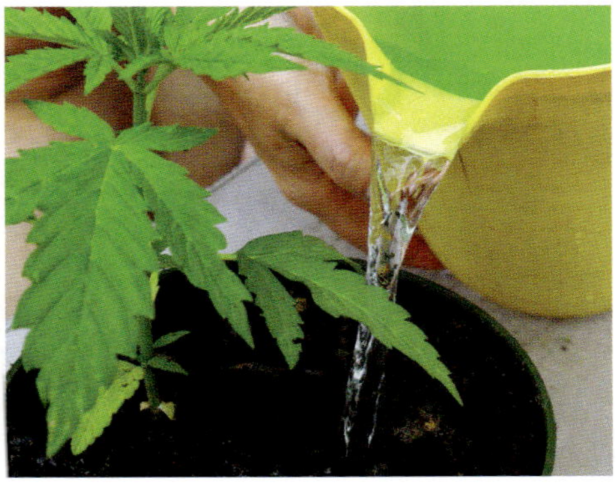

Add to soil.

increase the frequency of feeding with a high-strength bloom mix to promote robust bud growth. A 100% strength solution can be beneficial for large outdoor plants, as long as you ensure even distribution around the base. Water in a circular pattern, starting from the plant's base and moving outward, ensuring uniform distribution of the strong solution to the surrounding area. The soil absorbs these concentrated minerals at full strength, and, as the roots extend, they can access these nutrients.

Never introduce nutrients directly from the bottle into your plant's soil, as this may harm or even kill your plant. Instead, mix nutrients with water first. In the case of accidental spills, emergency soil flushing may become necessary.

pH Control

Chemical reactions are influenced by ions, electrically charged atoms or molecules. The pH scale, ranging from 0 to 14, measures the presence of hydrogen ions in a substance. Any substance that contains or lacks hydrogen ions affects pH. The fact that water contains hydrogen bonded to oxygen holds significant importance for growers. Neutral is represented at the midpoint, which is a pH of 7. Values below 7 are considered acidic,

PHOTOS: GCP

while values above 7 are alkaline, or basic. The further away from 7 a substance's pH is, the more extreme the conditions become, potentially inhibiting or promoting chemical reactions. Cannabis thrives at a neutral pH of 7, although cannabis in hydroponic systems can tolerate a slightly lower pH of around 6. Most grow shop products, including soil, nutrients, and other growing media, typically have a pH of 7. However, some products may disrupt this pH balance, with tap water being a common culprit.

Some industrial acidic substances have a pH of 0. Lemon juice is between pH 2 and 3, coffee measures at pH 5, milk is just under pH 7, baking soda is pH 9, and lye is between pH 13 and 14. As a cannabis plant grows, it absorbs minerals from the soil and deposits waste materials, which can lead to fluctuations in pH levels. Maintaining the proper pH is crucial for enabling normal chemical reactions and preventing nutrient lockout.

Check the pH of your medium at least once a week and, more importantly, a day or two after feeding. You can buy a pH test kit, the most accurate way to testing a mixture's pH, at most grow shops, or you can also use affordable pH paper strips for testing. If you are growing hydroponically or organically, consider investing in a quality digital pH meter, which has a greater tolerance for pH variation. If your soil's pH deviates from the 6 to 8 range, it is essential to adjust it to the optimal level of 7.

Acids and Bases

pH-adjustment products often contain water in addition to components that influence acidic or alkaline properties.

pH-down products, or pH-down acids, often contain trace amounts of phosphoric acid, citric acid, and mono-ammonium phosphate, which collectively create an acidic solution.

pH-up products, or pH-up bases, often include substances like potassium hydroxide and potassium carbonate, which together form an alkaline solution.

Ensure that you use pH-adjustment products exclusively designed for horticulture and avoid using other chemical products, such as those meant for aquariums. Some pH products can be phytotoxic, meaning they can harm or kill plants.

When handling more concentrated pH-adjustment products, exercise caution and wear gloves, as they can be corrosive to the skin and pose risks if ingested. In case of contact with eyes or skin, immediately rinse with water. Another method to adjust the pH of your soil, typically reserved for extreme circumstances, such as severe pH fluctuations or chemical burns, is soil flushing. A detailed explanation of this is given later in this chapter.

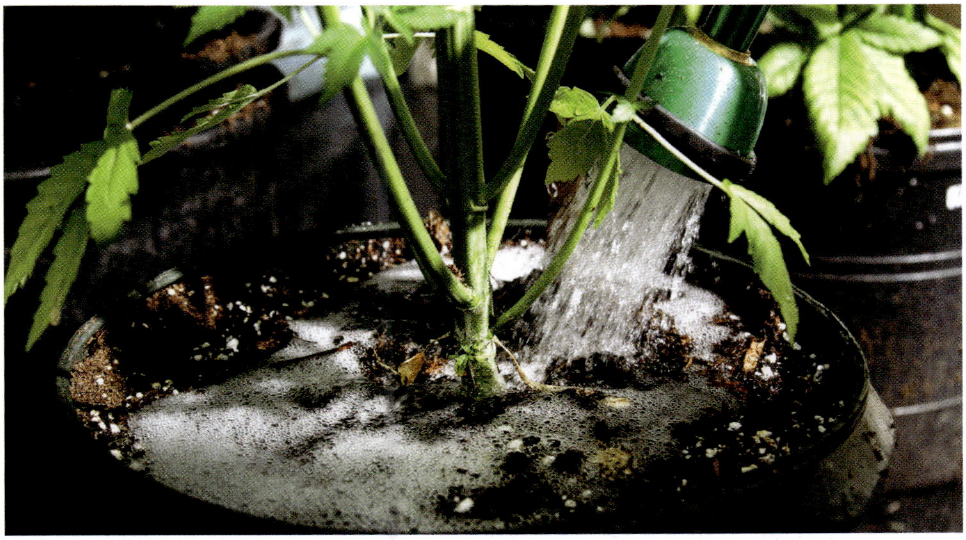

Watering: Besides light it's the next most important thing the cannabis plant needs to grow.

Water pH

Always check the pH of your water, because it can affect your pH adjustment calculations. Adjusting the pH of your growing medium without considering that of the water used can lead to inaccurate results. Measuring the pH of both will enable you to determine the precise pH adjustment needed.

For example, your growing medium has a pH of 6, and you aim to raise it to 7 by adding a pH-up product. You apply the product, assuming that the resulting pH will be 7. However, you overlooked the pH of the water you mixed it with, and it turns out that the water has a pH of 6. Consequently, your overall pH remains at 6.

If your water has a pH of 5 and your growing medium has a pH of 4, you will need to increase the pH of the water by 2 to reach 7 and raise the pH of the medium by 3 to attain a pH of 7. In total, you need a pH adjustment of 5 to achieve the desired pH level. When making such substantial adjustments, do it incrementally using pH-up and pH-down products rather than attempting to make the full adjustment in one step. For minor adjustments of about 1 pH in either direction, you can make a direct correction by following the instructions on the liquid pH-up or -down product.

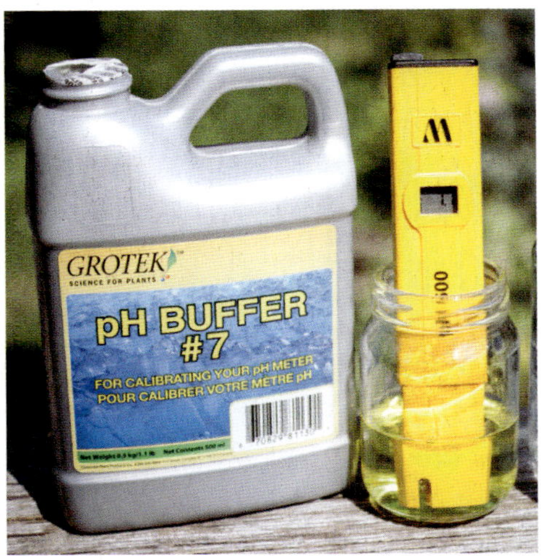

A pH test buffer solution to calibrate your reader.

PHOTOS: DAVID STRANGE (TOP), STONED ROSIE (BOTTOM)

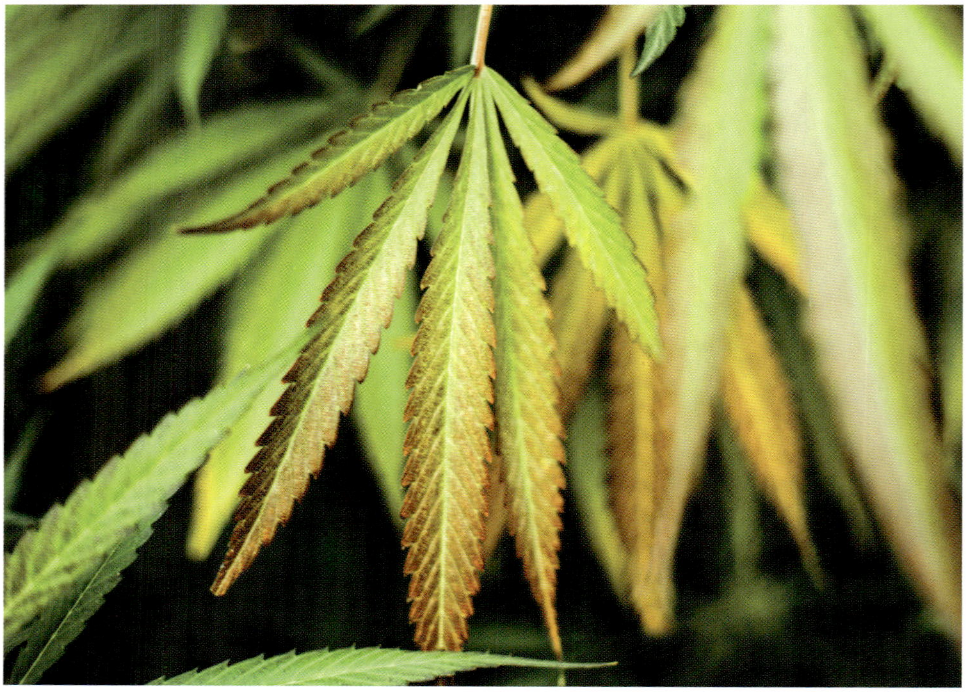

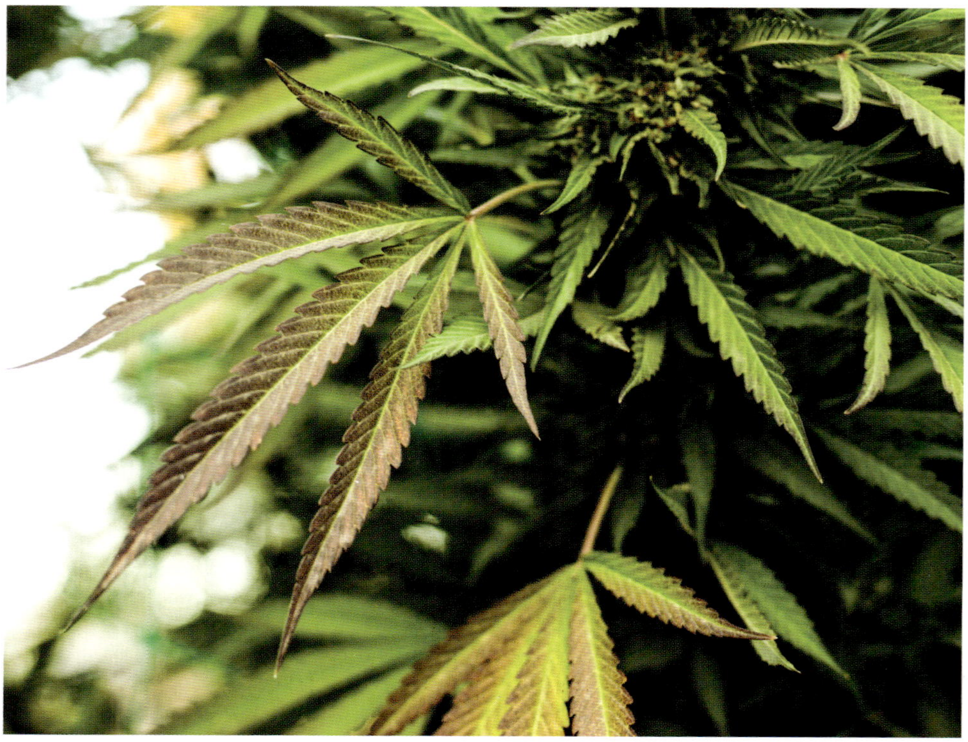

PHOTOS: TRICHOME ART

Acidic soils (pH less than 6) can reduce the availability of molybdenum (Mo). Mo becomes more soluble and available in neutral to slightly alkaline soils.

You can conduct tests on your growing medium and pH adjustments in a controlled environment, such as a flask, before applying them to your plants. This helps ensure that your adjustments are accurate and will not negatively affect your plants.

pH Adjustment: Restoring Soil to Neutral from an Acidic State

If your soil's pH becomes excessively acidic, you'll need to restore it to a neutral level of 7. You can use lime, alkaline calcium oxide, which is a brittle white caustic solid obtained by heating limestone. It is readily available in small containers from reputable grow shops. Add only a small amount to your soil when watering your plant and then test the pH the following day to assess the impact. If necessary, repeat the process. With some experimentation, you'll determine the quantity required. Experienced growers fine-tune the amount of lime through trial and error to effectively raise the pH of acidic soil. As a starting point, try adding two tablespoons of lime per gallon of soil. Some limes contain secondary nutrients. One is dolomite lime, which contains calcium and magnesium and is commonly used in organic gardening. Ensure you choose gardening lime, as not all types work effectively for this purpose.

pH Adjustment: Restoring Soil to Neutral from an Alkaline State

When the pH of your soil becomes too alkaline, you'll need to bring it to the neutral level of 7. This can be achieved by adding small amounts of any of these acidic substances: Liquid humic acid, cottonseed meal, lemon peels, coffee grounds, or high-acidity fertilizer. Always introduce them gradually, monitor the pH level the next day, and make necessary adjustments as required. Most growers find pH-down products to be more efficient due to their quicker action. Some substances may take longer to break down and correct pH imbalances, sometimes over several weeks, making them more suitable for organic growing methods.

Advanced pH Testing

To avoid errors when adjusting pH, first conduct experiments in a flask. Extract a few spoonfuls of the medium you intend to adjust, whether that's soil, a nutrient reservoir, or a substrate mix, and place it in a container. If you are growing in a hydroponic system, you can use a flask to test a sample of your intended nutrient solutions. Take a pH reading of the sample, then prepare your pH-adjustment solution. Add a small, precisely measured amount of the pH-adjustment mixture to the sample, let

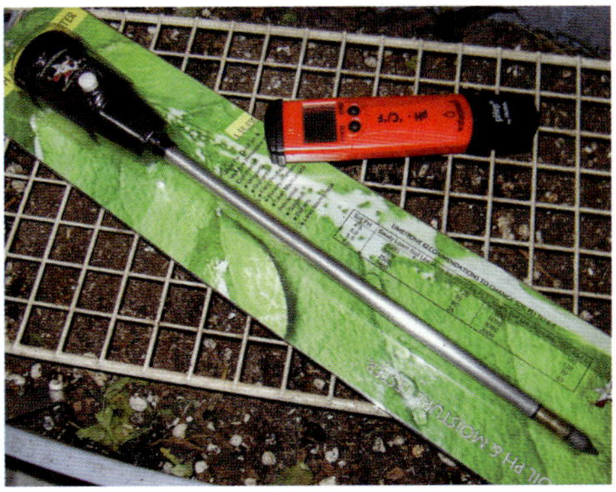

pH meters can come in different lengths for deeper measurements.

PHOTO: THE REV

it settle for an hour, and then retest the pH. Repeat this process until you determine the required pH adjustment and the time it takes to achieve the desired pH level. This approach minimizes the number of attempts required and increases accuracy.

pH Bouncing

Some growers encounter challenges with maintaining pH levels, especially when using organic methods. Fertilizers can be highly alkaline, making it difficult to keep the pH below 7. Certain nutrient solutions may cause pH fluctuations, bouncing below and above 7. Reverse osmosis (RO) or deionization (DI) filter systems are recommended for improving water quality, as better water quality can mitigate many of these problems. Another solution is the use of liquid humic acid in conjunction with pH-down products. Humic acid can be obtained from various sources, such as ground leonardite, coal, or potassium humates, with further processing to reduce unwanted heavy metal content. The quality of liquid humic acid depends on the fineness of the screening process and the water used.

pH Buffering

Buffers—substances that help maintain a stable pH—are typically used for calibrating equipment. When using buffers, avoid placing measuring tools directly into the buffer bottle to prevent contamination and maintain accuracy. Instead, use a clean flask for preparing and using buffer calibration solutions. Handle these concentrates with care, as they can be corrosive. Some pH-up and pH-down products may also contain buffering agents, which help stabilize pH levels and prevent rapid fluctuations. These products can maintain the desired pH for an extended period, although the duration will depend on the specific formulation and its buffering capacity.

pH-Up / pH-Down Measurements

When measuring pH-up or pH-down solutions, use a clean syringe, beaker, or plastic measuring jug. Always follow the provided instructions. Generally, about 0.5 ml of pH-up or -down solution will adjust the pH by +/– 0.1 pH per three gallons of water. A standard-sized syringe dispenses 0.1–0.5 ml.

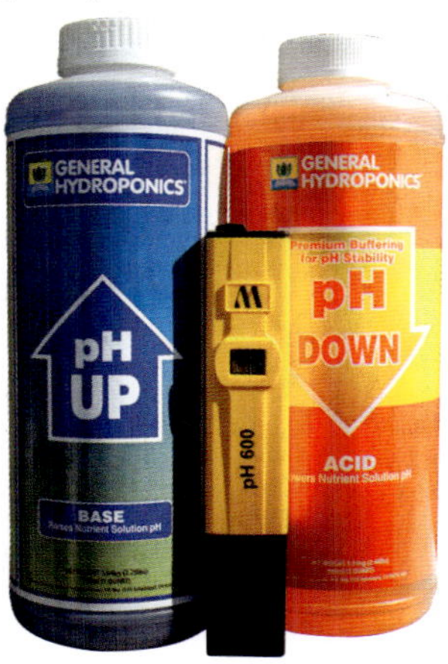

PHOTO: STONED ROSIE

pH-up and -down solutions.

For example, if your soil tests at a pH level of 5.6, and you aim to increase it to a stable 7 by using pH-up and a three-gallon pot:

1. Fill a watering can with three gallons of water and measure its pH with a pH meter.
2. If the water's pH is 7, proceed. If it is lower than that, adjust it to 7 by adding the required amount of pH-up.
3. Apply a total adjustment of +1.4 pH to raise the soil mixture from 5.6 to 7.
4. Add the necessary pH-treated water to the soil.

You may spread this application over several days while testing the medium daily to monitor the pH change. This process should gradually raise the pH to a balanced 7. Always follow the product instructions for the recommended quantities of pH-up or -down.

Other pH Considerations

Before addressing any nutrient-related issues, assess the pH levels of the medium and the nutrient formula. You can use a pH meter to check a sample in a flask. If you need to balance the nutrient pH, do not add the adjustment directly to the nutrient bottle; instead, incorporate it into your mixtures. Many nutrient brands strive to maintain a balanced pH between 6 and 7 in their products.

While a pH of 7 is generally preferred, cannabis can thrive within a pH range of about 5.5 to 8. Severe pH irregularities in cannabis cultivation occur when the pH falls outside these parameters. However, in hydroponics, optimal cannabis growth has been observed at pH levels as low as 5.5 and, in some cases, above 7. This variation is attributed to how pH levels influence chemical interactions, making some systems work more effectively in slightly acidic conditions. Strain-specific preferences and adaptability to varying pH ranges further influence the ideal pH range for cannabis.

Water Control

In cannabis cultivation, finding the right balance in water management is crucial. Begin by watering your plant every second or third day, and adjust this schedule based on your observations. Avoid allowing the soil to dry out completely for extended periods. This watering schedule works well with three-gallon pots:

Day 1: Water
Day 2: Allow to dry
Day 3: Allow to dry
Day 4: Check the soil and water if necessary

Watering frequency depends on the pot size and substrate type. You can compare the weight of the pot when dry and when it has been watered to help you develop a knack for determining when your pots require watering. Repeat this process at different stages of plant growth to account for variations in plant weight.

Two Types of Wilting

Wilting can be a sign of both underwatering and overwatering. Closely observe your plants' leaves. Do they point outward to receive more light, or do they wilt downward? Wilting downward during the light period signals water imbalance. Next, examine when the wilting started and how your plant responded for two to three days after watering. Probe the soil's dampness by inserting a wooden craft stick, letting it sit for a few minutes, pulling it out, and checking the dampness. If the stick is not damp, the soil is dry throughout, indicating more water is needed. Additional factors

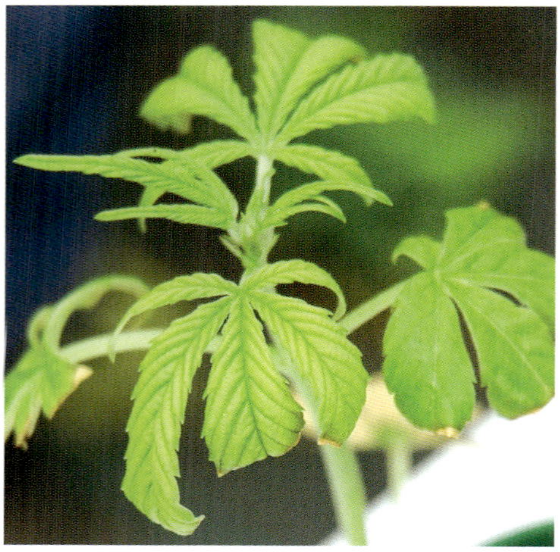

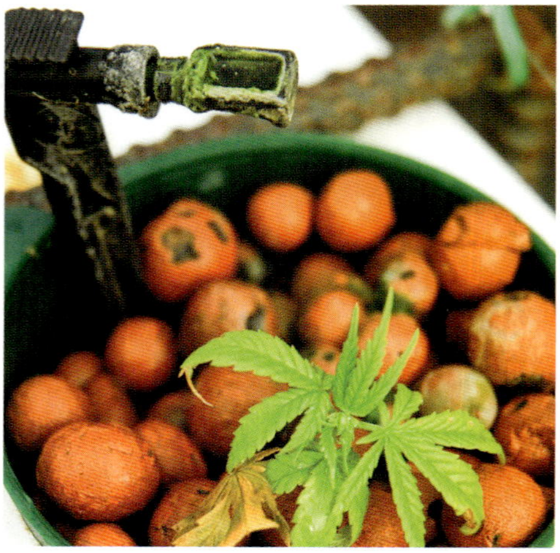

Wilting during the light hours suggests overwatering, so the medium must dry out. This can be done by placing fans near the overwatered plant.

like high temperatures or quick-draining soil may necessitate daily watering. If the soil is wet, allow it to dry out before watering again once the leaves show signs of improvement. Overwatering can be detrimental to your plants; if it occurs, just let the soil dry out. Using a fan near the soil's surface can help address mild overwatering issues. Be cautious when transplanting overwatered plants, as the wet soil can break apart easily.

Air Control

When considering the atmosphere around your cannabis plants, remember that it's not just about oxygen and CO_2. Air varies in temperature, cleanliness, and speed of movement, all of which can impact plant development. Hydroponic nutrient reservoirs are often aerated to provide oxygen. Dust can affect air quality, highlighting the importance of air filtration.

In nature, open air allows plants to thrive optimally. When you grow indoors, assume that all air can be improved through filtration. In particular, areas that are isolated from a fresh air source, such as grow tents, cabinets, small rooms, attics, basements, and internal compartments, may require air treatment. Air can carry pathogens and spores, and poorly ventilated areas can become stale. That said, the advantage of compartmentalization is the ability to control the air, which is not possible outdoors without a greenhouse.

Opening windows for air exchange is better than having no exchange at all, but it may not fully address odor issues. If possible, exchange air directly from the outdoors to your growing area using filters and fans. If direct outdoor ventilation is not feasible, you may need air ducting to channel fresh air into the growing area.

PHOTOS: STONED ROSIE

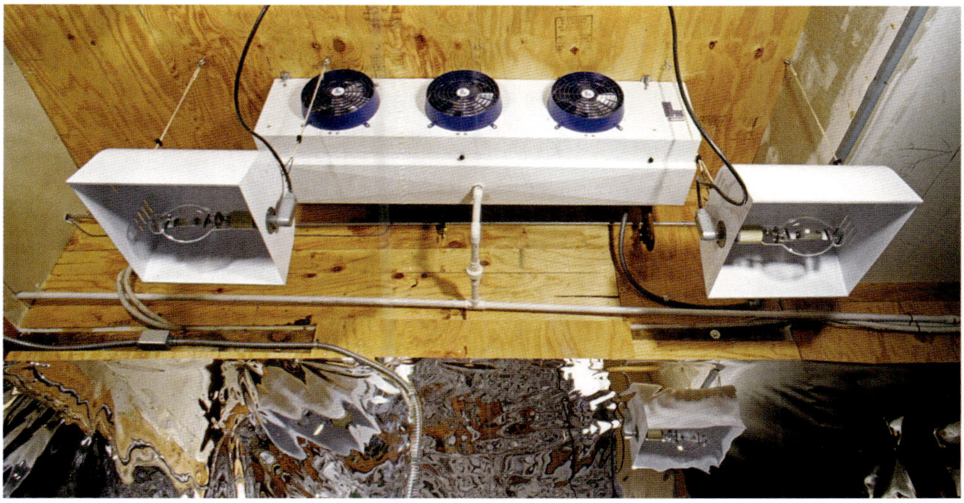

Hot air rises. Having extraction at the top or near the lights is the best way to get rid of the heat.

PHOTO: ANDRE GROSSMAN

Fresh Air

During the vegetative growth and flowering stages, cannabis plants benefit from a supply of fresh air. Its composition, of about 78% nitrogen, 21% oxygen, 0.05% carbon dioxide, and other gases, is relatively consistent across fresh air samples, though poorly ventilated areas can experience fluctuations, as well as the introduction or removal of other gases. Plant productivity can sometimes be enhanced through manipulating gas conditions, such as with CO_2 manipulation.

Windows

In warm weather, you can open windows as long as there are no security concerns. Add screens to prevent unwanted pests from entering. In winter, keep windows closed, except for brief 15 to 20-minute air-refreshing intervals, as cold temperatures may hinder plant growth.

Even when you use an extraction or intake fan, open windows can facilitate the input of fresh air and the output of used air. To help this, you can use air ducting and vents, a topic we'll explore later.

Odor Control

You may need to consider other aspects of air control, such as managing odors, especially when ensuring discretion during cannabis cultivation. Cannabis strains possess varying scent profiles due to the recombination of genetic material through natural selection and breeding. During the vegetative growth stage, cannabis emits a distinctive, easily detectable odor, which typically becomes noticeable around the first week of vegetative growth. This scent, unique to the cannabis plant, is a sharp, pleasantly pungent aroma akin to freshly cut grass, with a hint of spice. Cannabis scents can

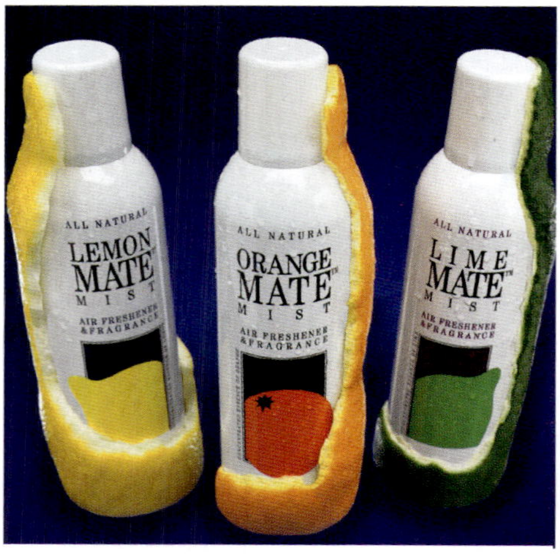

From basic air fresheners...

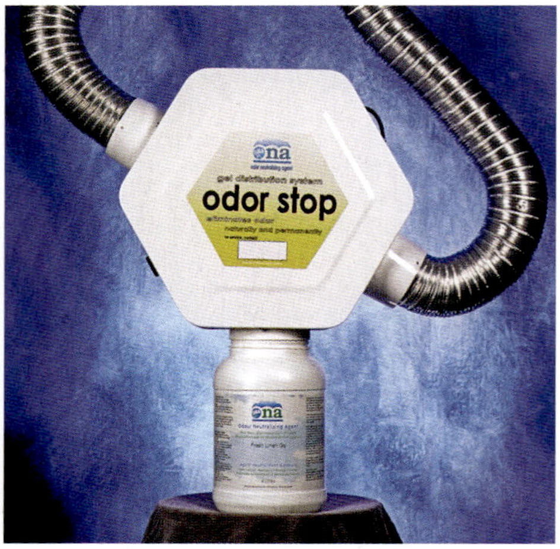

...to automated odor stop dispensers.

carry quite a distance, and this poses security concerns. The flowering stage intensifies the release of aromatic molecules into the air, resulting in a more potent odor profile, ranging from freshly cut grass to fruity, forest-like, hashish, and even strong skunk odors. It's crucial to appreciate the strength of these odors, even in strains considered less aromatic.

Growers use three main methods to control cannabis odors within the grow room before they escape.

Ionizing

Ionizers are air purification systems designed to manage odors, smoke, mold, bacteria, chemical gases, mildew, pollen, dust, and static electricity. They emit negatively charged ions into the environment, which neutralize odor molecules in the air, causing these and other particles to become charged, and to fall onto surfaces. However, using ionizers may require thorough cleaning of the grow area. Furthermore, extended exposure to ionizers has been linked to minor respiratory distress as they are believed to produce ozone. Ionizers are most suitable for smaller growing operations with up to six medium-sized plants, as there are more effective odor control options for larger-scale growers. For home cultivators in particular, ionizers can be a helpful tool in reducing odors.

Ozone Generating

Ozone molecules, which are activated oxygen, contain three oxygen atoms, one more than in the air we breathe (O_2). Ozone, which can be naturally occurring or generated, acts as a potent sterilizer; however, it has a relatively short lifespan of about 30 minutes. When ozone (O_3) encounters an odorous molecule, one of its atoms separates and attaches to it, oxidizing its cell walls and eventually breaking them down and leaving only oxygen behind. Exercise caution with ozone, as excessive exposure can be

PHOTOS: HYDROFARM.COM (LEFT), ANDRE GROSSMAN (RIGHT)

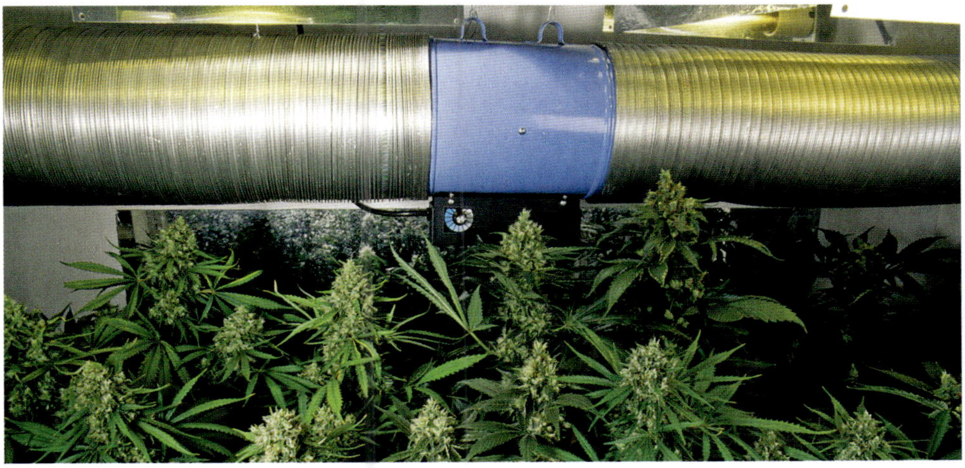

Ozone Generators are another way of removing odors from the grow room.

harmful to both plants and humans. Most ozone generators designed for horticultural use produce minimal ozone exposure, typically around 0.05 ppm over a timed interval, well below the legal exposure limit for humans of about 0.1 ppm for eight hours. Ozone generators are more effective than ionizers at controlling cannabis odors.

Carbon Filtering

Using activated charcoal is the safest and most effective choice for managing cannabis odors. When charcoal, a form of carbon, undergoes a treatment process with oxygen, countless tiny pores are opened in its atoms. This activated charcoal is often broken into pellets to serve as the primary ingredient in carbon filters and air filtration systems. The unique quality of activated charcoal lies in its capacity to chemically attract and absorb odorous molecules.

The activated charcoal is contained in a metal tube with filters that screen the air passing through it. This entire activated carbon filter requires specific ducting attachments for proper venting.

Not all activated carbon filters exclusively use charcoal. Some use other materials that function similarly, such as coconut husks. To continue effectively filtering out odorous molecules, you must replace the carbon material every couple of months. Activated carbon is readily available at most reputable filter supply stores. Select only activated carbon pellets as crushed activated carbon is less effective.

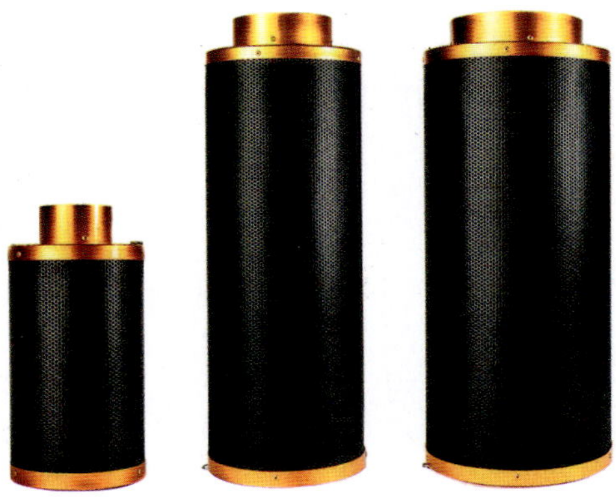

Carbon filters come in various sizes.

PHOTOS: ANDRE GROSSMAN (TOP), GORILLAGROWTENT.COM (BOTTOM)

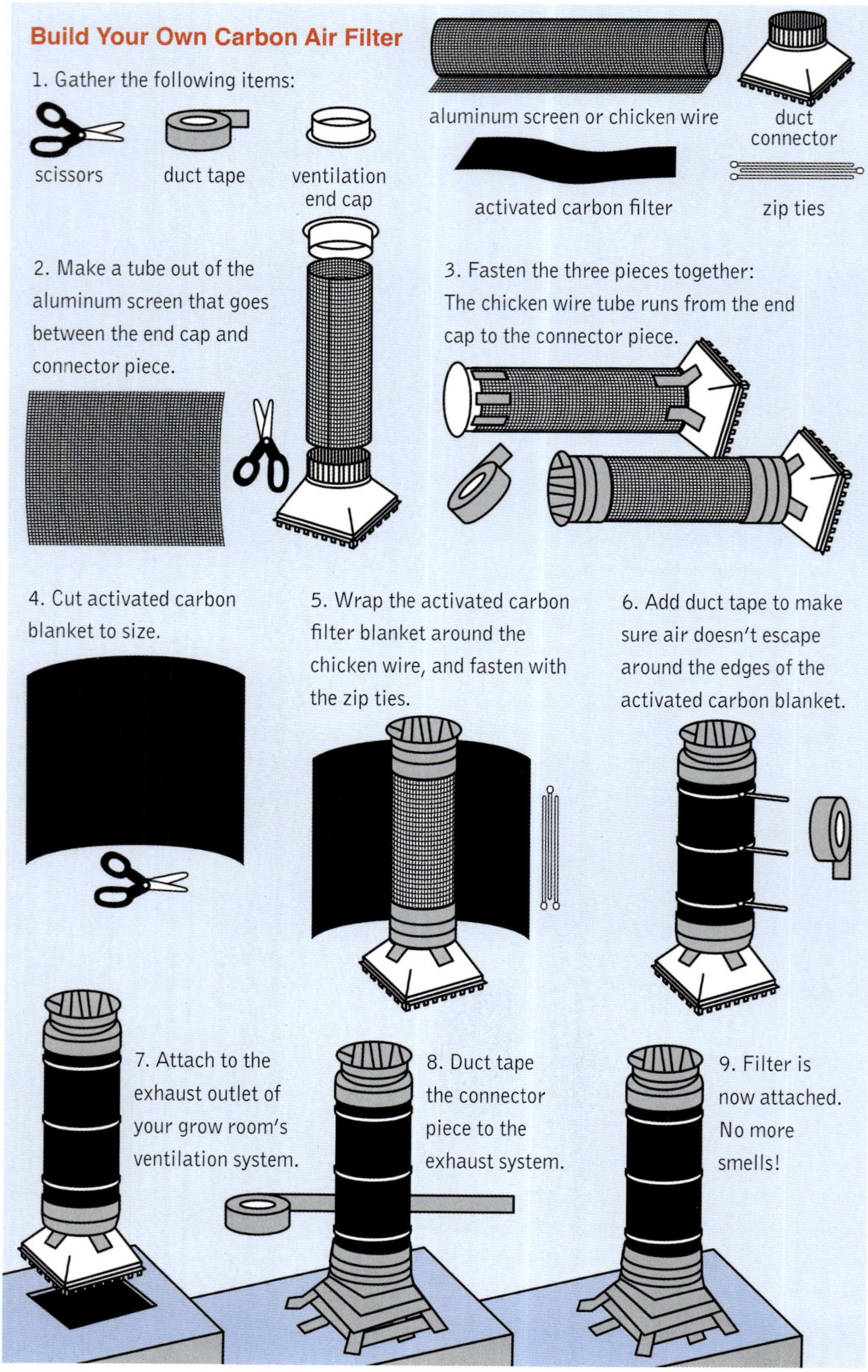
Build Your Own Carbon Air Filter
1. Gather the following items:
scissors
duct tape
ventilation end cap
aluminum screen or chicken wire
duct connector
activated carbon filter
zip ties
2. Make a tube out of the aluminum screen that goes between the end cap and connector piece.
3. Fasten the three pieces together: The chicken wire tube runs from the end cap to the connector piece.
4. Cut activated carbon blanket to size.
5. Wrap the activated carbon filter blanket around the chicken wire, and fasten with the zip ties.
6. Add duct tape to make sure air doesn't escape around the edges of the activated carbon blanket.
7. Attach to the exhaust outlet of your grow room's ventilation system.
8. Duct tape the connector piece to the exhaust system.
9. Filter is now attached. No more smells!

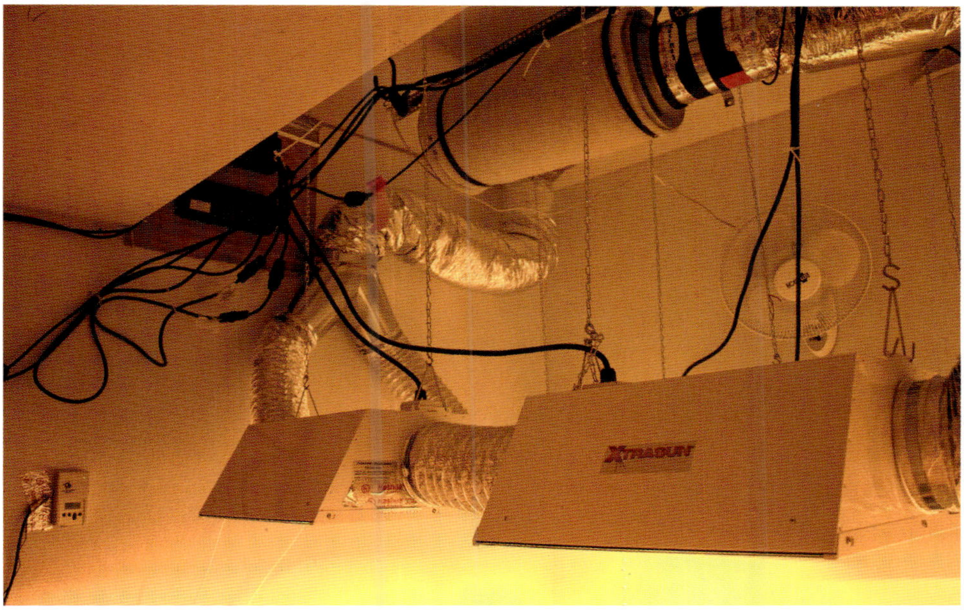

HID lights with air-cooled hoods connected to the carbon filter above them at the outtake fan.

Activated carbon filters have become standard equipment in all types of grow rooms, including those used for large-scale medical cannabis cultivation. Most do not come equipped with an active fan, though some models may include one. Air circulation within the filter is typically facilitated by venting, a topic we'll delve into.

Size Considerations

Sizing of filters commonly causes confusion. Measurements of filter dimensions often indicate the filter's width but not its length. Furthermore, the filter's size corresponds to the opening at each end rather than the total diameter of the tube.

For example, a carbon filter listed as 8 inches (20 cm) has openings of that size at each end; the measurement given is not its total length. To determine the filter's full specifications, consult the complete length measurement. For example, an industrial-sized filter suitable for horticultural use may be over 24 inches (60 cm) long, more than 8 inches (20 cm) wide, and weigh upwards of 20 lbs (9 kg). Yet, the same filter is often still referred to as an "8-inch carbon filter."

Thus, the actual size and weight of a filter can differ significantly from what you might expect based solely on the nominal width. Particularly for smaller grow areas, 6-inch and 4-inch filters may be recommended, but these measurements pertain to the width, not the diameter. A 6-inch (15-cm) wide carbon filter, for example, may measure 18 inches (45 cm) in length and weigh about 11 lbs (5 kg), while a 4-inch (10 cm) wide carbon filter might be 6 inches (15 cm) long and weigh around 6 lbs (2.5 kg).

PHOTO: PURE BRED GROWERS

Placement and Mounting

Carbon filters are often suspended near the top of the grow room, typically above the LED or HID lights. Many come equipped with mounting holes designed for attaching lighting systems underneath them. Before setting up a filter system, take into consideration the combined weight and the capacity of the mounting unit and supporting chains.

Filter systems involve the movement of air in terms of both volume and speed, typically measured in cubic feet per minute (CFM). It is not always necessary to calculate this number, as even a small amount of activated carbon can suffice for multiple grow rooms. However, here is a basic method to calculate the required CFM of activated charcoal based on your grow area's volume:

1. Measure the length, height, and width of the grow area in feet, and then multiply the three measurements together to calculate the volume of the space in cubic feet.
2. If you aim to replace all the air in your grow area in one minute, the necessary CFM will be equal to the grow area's volume.
3. If you prefer air replacement to occur over five minutes, divide the grow area's volume by five to determine the CFM required for that duration.

Growers generally opt for air replacement once per minute, although some choose longer intervals to retain CO_2. Activated carbon filters will specify their CFM rating, which should guide your selection.

CFM filter measurements are typically determined under optimal conditions, and the type of ducting used can affect these calculations. If it is not installed in a straight path, ducting may reduce the CFM by a small percentage while longer ducting lengths can result in more significant reductions. Some growers opt for filters with a slightly higher CFM rating to compensate for potential ducting-related losses. Avoid sharp bends in the ducting; instead cut it to the necessary length. Temperature is another important factor to consider, as excessive heat inside the grow area may require the removal of hot air through proper ventilation.

Before purchasing your filter, continue reading and consider the factors discussed here and in the following sections. These will play a crucial role in ensuring the optimal performance of your activated carbon filter and, in turn, contribute to effective odor control and air quality in your grow room.

Ventilation

Ventilation is essential for maintaining the indoor environment of a grow room. Not to be confused with the mere use of fans, ventilation encompasses methods for replacing air within a space through intakes, vents, and ducting. Before setting up your grow room,

Odor control devices, such as activated carbon or charcoal filters, are often attached to or positioned near the active vent to help manage and eliminate unwanted odors effectively, ensuring that the air leaving the grow room is clean and odor-free.

Solve False Intakes

The motion of air as it is drawn out of the room by the ventilation system creates a vacuum effect, which requires fresh air to enter the grow room through any available path. Vulnerable spots in your grow room, such as improperly sealed tents, gaps in cabinet frames, or even keyholes, can serve as unintended air intake routes. Deal with these false air intakes promptly since controlling airflow is essential for an efficient system.

To mitigate false intakes, take these steps:

1. Seal vulnerable spots: Identify any areas in your grow room where air can infiltrate from unintended sources. Use sealing materials, such as the reflective material Mylar, to seal these openings effectively.
2. Control light leaks: Maintaining a controlled light environment is also essential for successful cultivation, especially when transitioning to a 12/12 light cycle during the flowering stage. This transition requires you to block all potential sources of light leaks, including vents that could potentially allow light to escape.
3. Implement ducting: In many cases, using ducting can help prevent both false intakes and light leaks. Properly installed ducting can channel air in a controlled manner, ensuring it passes through your ventilation system without allowing uncontrolled air exchange through unintended openings.

By addressing these issues, you can significantly enhance the efficiency of your grow room, leading to improved yields and better environmental control.

Passive Intake

Passive intakes, equipped with screens and ducting to prevent the ingress of dust and light, operate without the need for power. Typically installed at a lower position in the grow room, they allow fresh air to flow over and through the plants, assisting in temperature regulation and facilitating airflow between the grow lights and the top of the plants.

While passive intakes do not require fans for operation, some growers opt to use them as a means of regulating the volume of incoming air. Filters are often incorporated to further enhance their effectiveness, serving to block out dust particles. However, the mesh micron size of standard filters may not be adequate for preventing the entry of pathogens, such as fungal spores or mold.

Where stringent pathogen control is necessary, higher-quality filters, such as HEPA filters, can provide the level of filtration required to maintain a clean and pathogen-free growing environment.

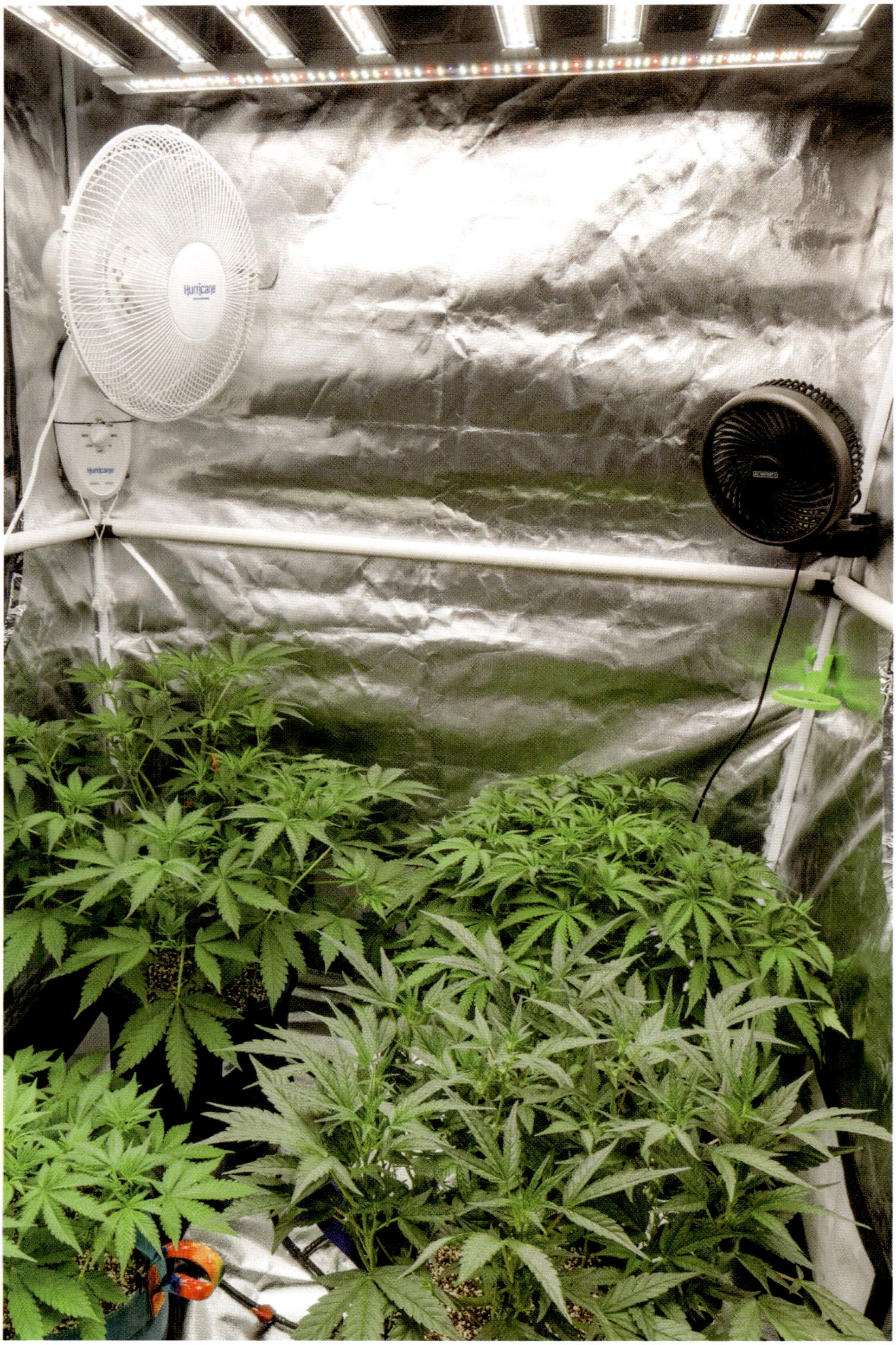

PHOTO: JOE'S CANNA GROWS

Active fans for breezes are not the same as passive intakes and active outtake fans. These fans strengthen cannabis plants. Intakes and outtakes control airflow.

Fans

Fans circulate air to provide a cooling effect, playing a crucial role in enhancing cannabis productivity. However, they should not be used as a substitute for a proper ventilation system.

You can use standard domestic oscillating fans to ensure that all areas of the grow room receive an adequate supply of fresh air. They create a gentle breeze that helps plants develop sturdy stems and branches, emulating the conditions they'd encounter in their natural outdoor environment. Though these fans can be positioned relatively close to mature marijuana plants, exercise common sense when using them. The speed of the fan should be based on the degree of movement that the plants require; while plants benefit from gentle movement, excessive force can lead to uprooting or falling over.

The same calculations you use for carbon filters can be used to determine CFM rating and specifications for fans.

Ventilation Calculations

To ensure effective ventilation, aim to replace the air in your grow room at least once every minute. If your room becomes too hot, you may need to increase the frequency to as much as five times per minute. Most growers opt for a ventilation system capable of cycling the room's air volume three times a single minute.

The rate at which you choose to remove air from your grow room depends on the internal temperature of the room, the external temperature of the incoming air, and whether you are using CO_2 supplementation.

Let's consider a grow room with dimensions of 2 × 5 × 5 feet, or a total volume of 50 cubic feet. For an air exchange rate of three times per minute, select a fan with a capacity of 150–250-CFM for your grow room. A 150-CFM fan can effectively circulate all the air in the grow room three times per minute, while a 250-CFM fan accomplishes this task five times per minute. The CFM rating is usually displayed on the fan's side.

Squirrel-cage fans are strongly recommended. However, before finalizing your decision, gather more information and consider additional factors related to air management in your environment.

Humidity

Cannabis plants thrive in an environment with a relative humidity (RH) of 40% to 80%. The most effective way to regulate humidity levels is by introducing fresh air into the environment. If you have implemented a robust air circulation system, you

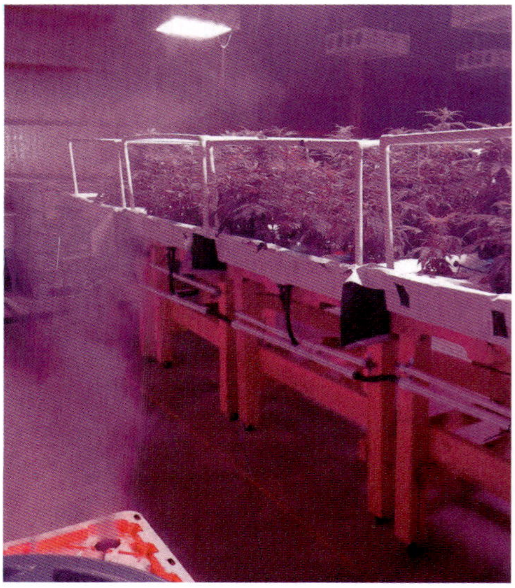

Humidity can also be raised by using mist makers.

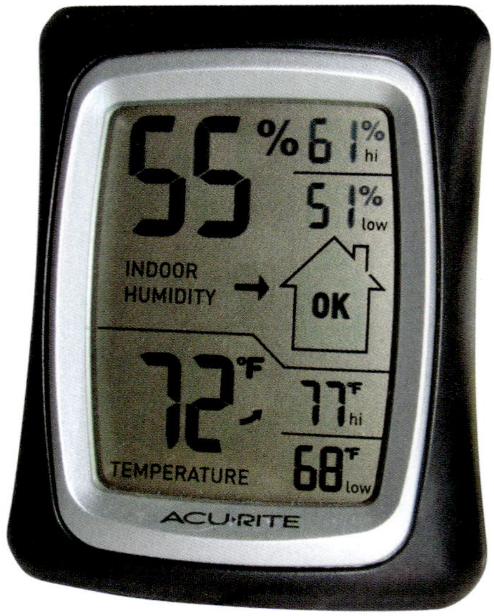

Thermometer and humidity gauge combo monitor.

should maintain suitable humidity levels in your grow room. However, if the air in your space becomes excessively humid, a dehumidifier will bring the RH down to an acceptable level.

A dehumidifier cools the air as it passes through the unit, leading to condensation, the removal of water vapor, and a reduction in RH. Some dehumidifiers have built-in RH meters, or hygrometers, which can measure the humidity levels in the room. These devices are relatively affordable and often available as part of a digital temperature reader combo. Many can be connected as smart devices for remote monitoring and control.

By using an RH measuring kit, you can gauge the amount of fresh air required to maintain the optimal 60% RH level for cannabis growth. Cannabis cultivators typically aim to avoid the need for a dehumidifier by establishing an effective air circulation system from the start. Always prioritize ventilation as the initial solution for addressing RH issues, turning to a dehumidifier only when no other viable options remain.

Temperature

Cannabis plants thrive in a temperature range that is also comfortable for people. If you find your grow room too cold, your plants will likely feel the same way. Likewise, if it's too hot for you, it's too hot for your plants. Room temperature can typically be regulated with a thermostat. However, in a grow space, temperature fluctuations can be influenced by lighting, particularly during the 12/12 flowering phase, when lights cycle on and off.

PHOTOS: THEHOUSEOFHYDHO.COM (LEFT), THE REV (RIGHT)

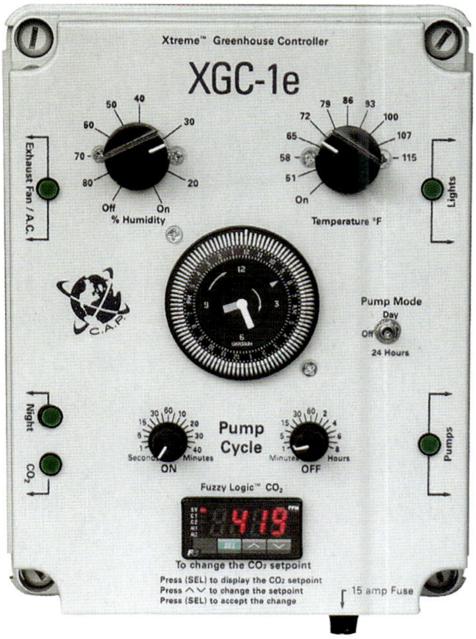

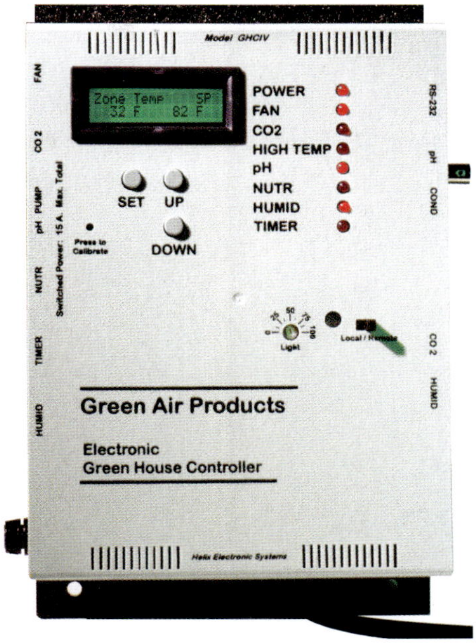

All-in-one controllers can automate a lot of different tasks. Some are partially analog and others fully digital.

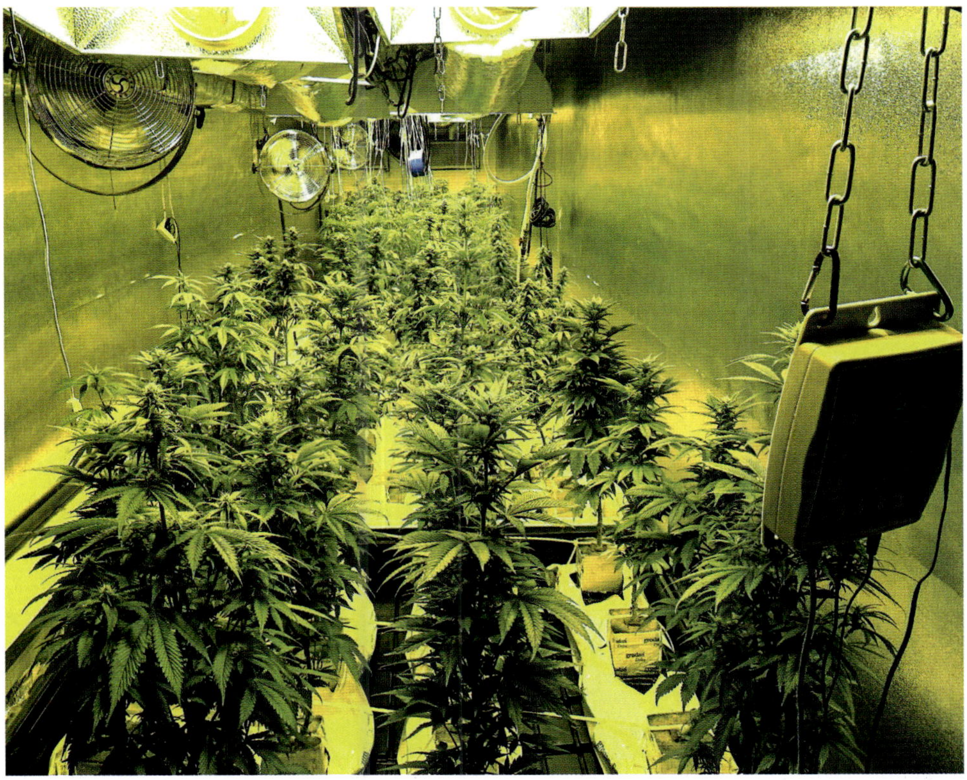

Controlling power, lights, humidity, temperature, fans, and more all from one box.

PHOTOS: CAP (TOP LEFT), ANDRE GROSSMAN (TOP RIGHT), RIOT SEEDS (BOTTOM)

The ideal temperature is around 75°F (24°C), although slightly warmer temperatures may encourage plants to finish their growth cycle a bit earlier. To monitor temperature variations accurately, use multiple thermometers, fixed in place, or moved as needed, at different locations in your room. Warm air rises, so the temperature above a thermometer will typically be higher than the air beneath it. The area closest to the grow lights will be the warmest, while the floor of your grow space will be the coolest. Temperature fluctuates, though it is crucial for it to stay within the ideal range throughout your grow room.

Learn the temperature ranges in your room, such as at the root, light, or canopy levels. Do not let the temperature exceed 85°F (30°C), as higher temperatures can lead to heat stress and hinder plant growth. Going above 125°F (51°C) will likely result in the death of most cannabis plants, although some equatorial strains have adapted to thrive in such heat. You can cool your room with the ventilation methods previously discussed.

If cold temperatures are a concern, you may need to incorporate a heater into your setup and adjust it to maintain the desired temperature.

In the flowering phase of the cannabis life cycle, when you switch to a 12/12 photoperiod, the temperature drops when the lights are off. This is normal, and cannabis plants can tolerate temperatures as low as 55°F (13°C) during this phase. If it drops significantly below this threshold, it can slow down growth and lead to stunting, where development is halted. If the temperature falls below 30°F (–1°C), it can cause cold damage to the plant.

24/7 Ventilation

Plants in the dark phase don't undergo photosynthesis, which requires light. Instead, they undergo the dark reaction, which is responsible for creating the carbon-based building blocks necessary for growth. While photosynthesis is a light-dependent reaction, the dark reaction is an ongoing metabolic process that operates 24/7 within the cell organelles. While the dark reaction is continually active, it doesn't seem to be directly influenced by ventilation during the dark period. Nevertheless, 24/7 ventilation should be maintained.

Why is 24/7 ventilation preferred? While you could opt to turn off air circulation for 12 hours during the dark phase, doing so can lead to RH issues. Ventilation plays a crucial role in preventing mold growth on your flowers. Additionally, by keeping the ventilation running continuously, you ensure that fresh air is readily available when the lights come back on. Pausing ventilation for 12 hours may not yield the best results and could potentially introduce problems, so it is likely not worth it for whatever savings you may make in utility bills (if that is your concern).

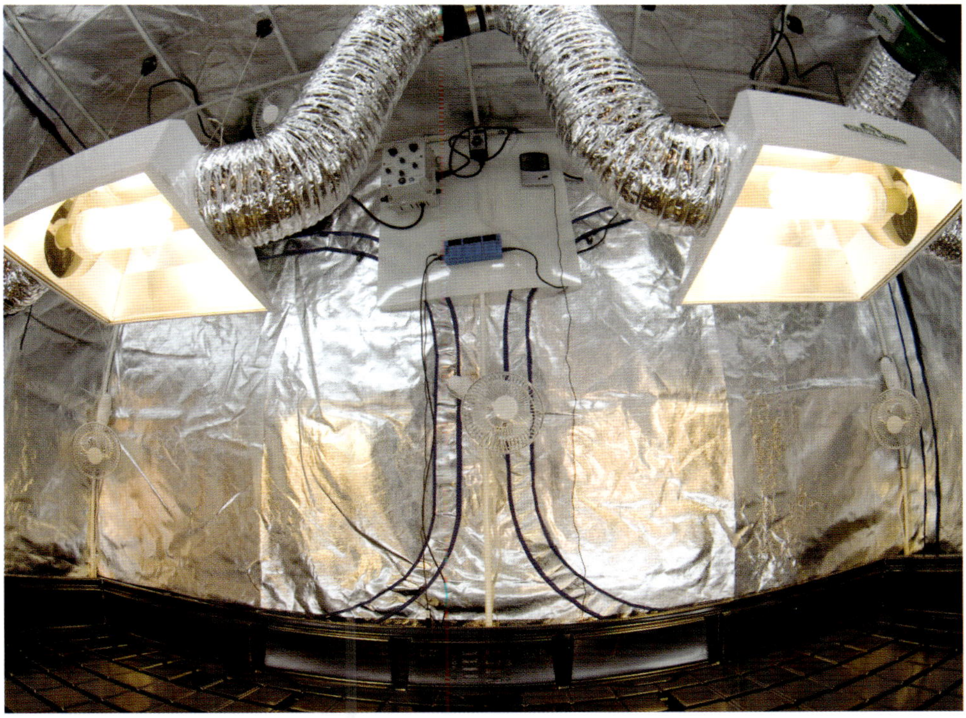

S-bends in air ducting add more distance, which helps cool the air passing through HID air-cooled hoods.

In summary, address temperature concerns without compromising ventilation. As you design your grow room, conduct temperature tests, and even simulate a 12/12 light cycle without plants to assess the temperature range you can achieve.

Timers

Timers are essential for automating tasks and eliminating the need for constant manual intervention in your grow room. They are indispensable for controlling the timing of lights, heaters, fans, and other electrical devices. If your lighting kit, ballasts, and fans do not come equipped with built-in timers, you can easily adapt any electrical appliance to work with one. Setting up and using timers is straightforward. Plug your device into the timer, plug the timer into your electrical outlet, and set it to turn on when you want the device to activate and to turn off at the desired shutdown time.

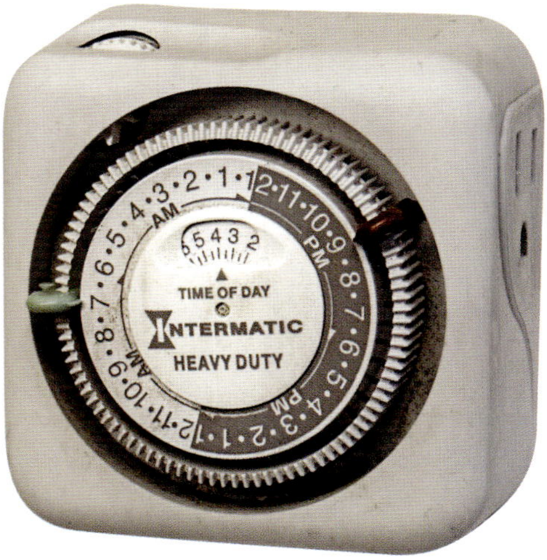

The indispensable timer, perfect for 12/12 flowering.

PHOTOS: HYDROFARM.COM (TOP), JUSTINCANNABIS.COM (BOTTOM)

Most timers come in digital and analog displays. Automated timing is generally more precise and reliable than manual adjustments.

It may be necessary to use multiple timers in your grow room to avoid overloading them. Familiarize yourself with your timer's specifications and consult its manual for guidance. Attempting to run multiple appliances on a single timer can lead to power overloads, tripped circuits, and even electrical fire hazards. Climate controllers, devices capable of managing multiple devices simultaneously, might better meet your needs if you require multiple timers. These controllers, which will be covered in a later section, can also regulate CO_2 levels.

Never place timers or any electrical appliances directly on the grow room floor, which can become wet. Instead, mount them securely to prevent damage or accidents.

Carbon Dioxide (CO_2)

CO_2 plays a vital role in promoting plant growth, especially during the flowering phase. About 0.03% of the Earth's atmosphere by volume consists of CO_2, a gas that is natural and not inherently harmful. Plants absorb CO_2 from the air and use it for photosynthesis. When the supply of CO_2 is insufficient, photosynthesis is hindered. Thus, increasing the supply of CO_2 can optimize the process of photosynthesis.

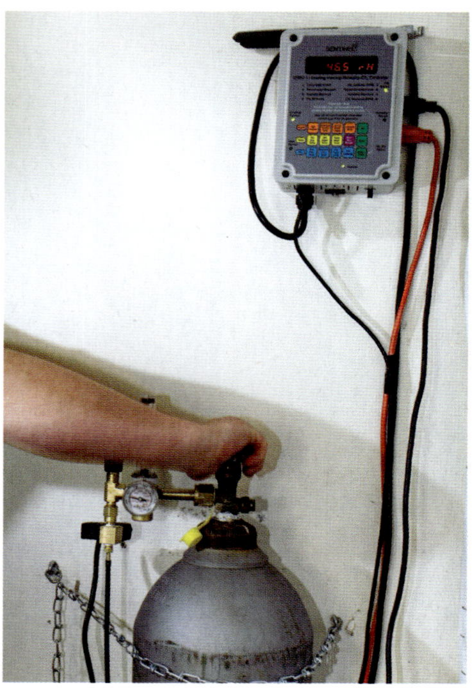

Carbon dioxide controllers regulate the amount and timing of CO_2 emissions.

PHOTO: JEFF GOLDBERG

Plants and trees can absorb more CO_2 when it is readily available. However, genetic and environmental conditions may limit their uptake. Scientific evidence suggests that by absorbing higher levels of CO_2, plants and trees can experience increased vigor and faster growth rates. Cannabis, in particular, has demonstrated its capacity to absorb and use excess CO_2 to achieve optimal growth. As a result, CO_2 supplementation is widely used in horticulture, from plant nurseries to medical cannabis cultivation facilities.

Your air circulation system can help replenish the CO_2 that plants consume. Adequate air circulation alone can outperform CO_2 supplementation in environments with poor air quality, so it is crucial to address air circulation before considering CO_2 supplementation.

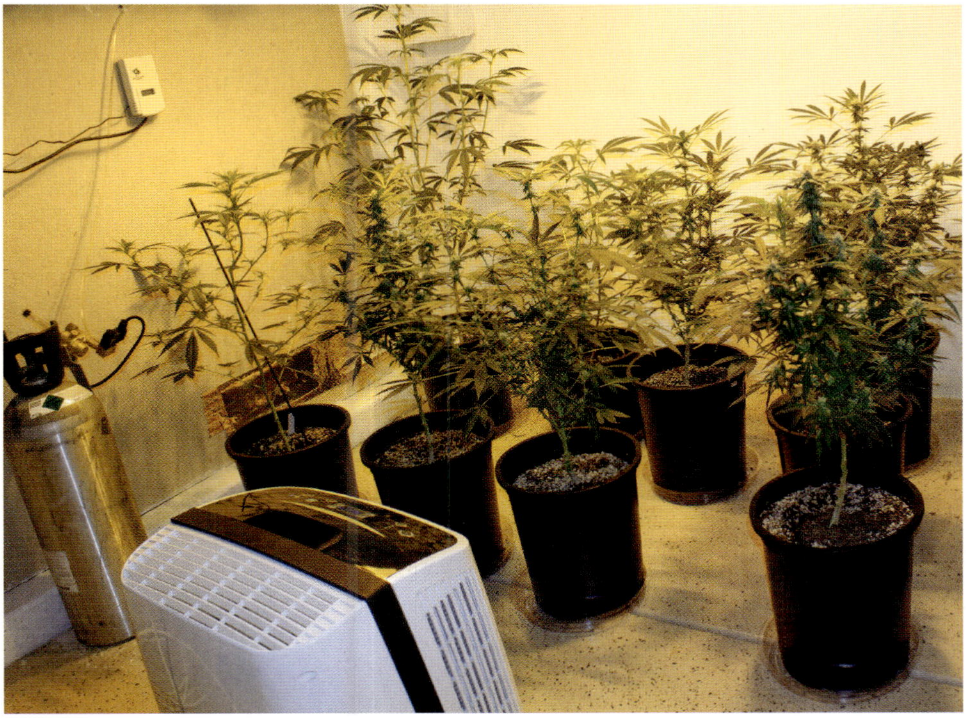

Combining carbon dioxide and humidifiers can help push plant genetics to their limits.

Many growers have reported significant increases in yields after improving air circulation and introducing CO_2 supplementation. This approach doesn't transform an already optimal plant into a super producer; rather, it maximizes the potential of a system that previously used up this available resource. The outcome may vary based on the genetics of the plant; every cannabis strain has a genetic limit for bud production. This limit can be exceeded through breeding or the use of growth boosters, although the latter is a subject of controversy. Organic growth boosters, on the other hand, can offer safer alternatives to optimize growth.

The introduction of additional CO_2 can help ensure that your plants achieve their optimal growth rates. While you can grow high-yielding plants without supplementary CO_2, the noticeable impact on growth speed and bud quantity places CO_2 in the same category of importance for high yields as plant genetics and light source. If you are already optimizing these aspects, CO_2 supplementation is the next logical step.

PHOTO: PURE BRED GROWERS

CO_2 is generated on an industrial scale by burning fuel, resulting in greenhouse gas emissions, and contributing to climate change. CO_2 production for horticulture differs significantly. Plants absorb CO_2 during growth, and the gas becomes sequestered as a solid within plants and does not contribute to greenhouse gas emissions in the Earth's atmosphere. Nonetheless, the overall carbon footprint depends on the source

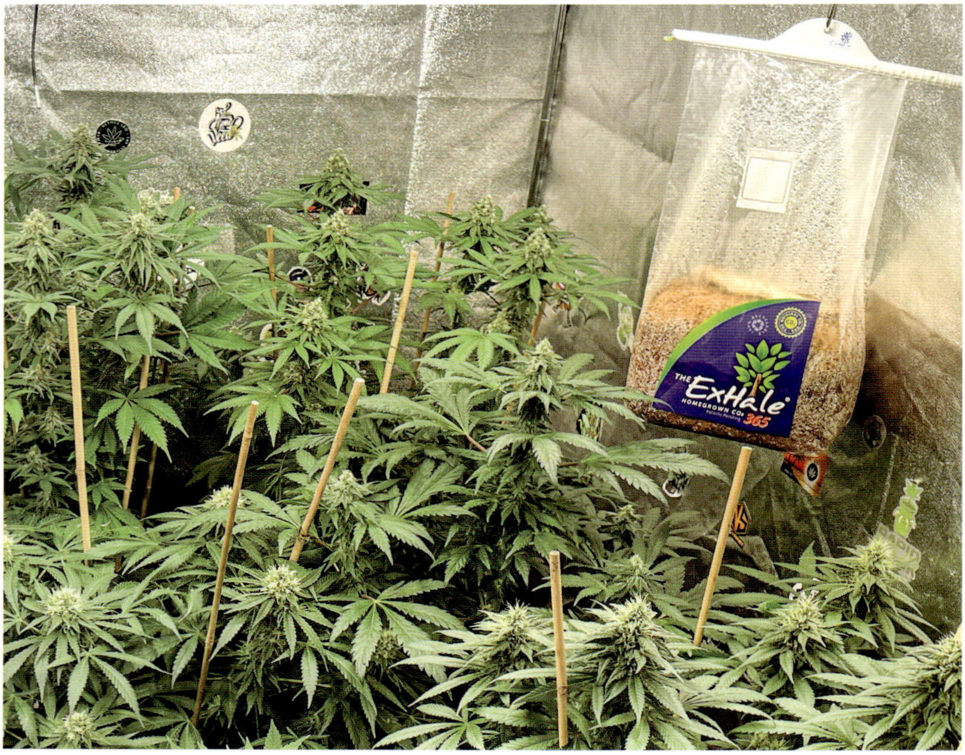

The Exhale 365 is a self-activated CO_2 bag for those who don't have the space for a carbon dioxide system.

PHOTO: TANYA PETERSEN

of energy used. Cultivation can contribute to greenhouse gas emissions when it relies on non-green energy sources, a significant concern.

In the grow room, CO_2 is emitted on a timed-release basis. This is achieved through a device attached to the tank nozzle, which controls the release of compressed CO_2 at predetermined intervals. To ensure precision, you may need a tank regulator, which can be either an infrared sensor or a flow meter. The regulator manages the quantity of CO_2 released, while the timer dictates when it is released. Some units incorporate both functions; combined or separate is a matter of choice.

CO_2 tanks are readily available and can be refilled at welding supply stores, although many horticulture stores now stock them. Welding supply stores, convenient locations to refill your CO_2 canisters, possibly offer more security than gardening suppliers. Tanks are available in various sizes and shapes, but for larger grow spaces, opt for multiple 20 lb (9 kg) tanks or the 50 lb (22.7 kg) variant to ensure a sufficient supply of CO_2. Choosing 20 lb tanks is recommended, as they are easier to handle and fit well in your grow room. Have at least two tanks to enable you to refill one while the other continues to release CO_2 into your grow room.

Calculating Carbon Dioxide

How much CO_2 should you introduce into your growing environment?

The calculation of required CO_2 involves two steps.

1. Calculate the volume of your grow area in cubic feet by multiplying the room's length, width, and height.

There is already some CO_2 present in the room, typically around 300 ppm. Since the optimal level for cannabis is 1,500 ppm, you'll need to increase the CO_2 levels by 1,200 ppm.

2. Multiply the cubic foot size of the grow room by 0.0012 to determine the amount of CO_2 needed to supplement the room to reach 1,500 ppm.

For example, in a 10 × 10 × 10 foot–room (1,000 cubic feet):
1,000 × 0.0012 = 1.2 cubic feet. Therefore, introducing 1.2 cubic feet of CO_2 will raise the room's CO2 concentration to 1,500 ppm.

That covers the basic calculation. However, the challenge lies in controlling the rate of air circulation.

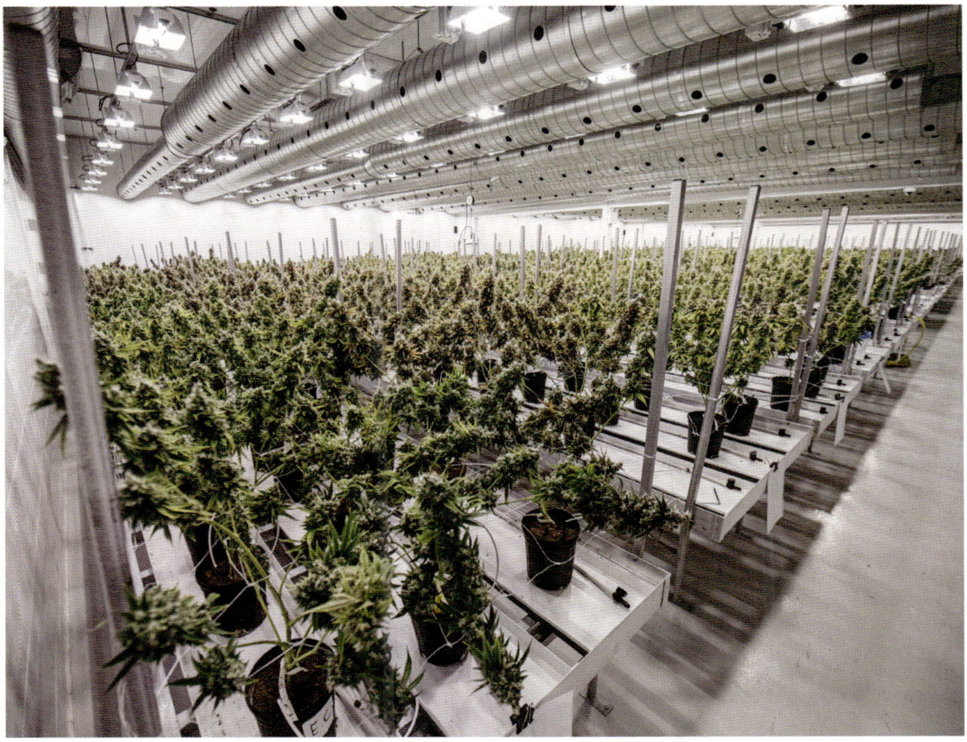

PHOTO: TWEED

Calculating carbon dioxide uses the same formula for any sized space.

You can reduce the speed of your active vent fan to prevent excessive expulsion of CO_2. You're paying for it, so you don't want to waste too much. When you reach 1,500 ppm of CO_2 in your grow room, you can raise the temperature to 95°F (35°C) without causing stress to the cannabis plants.

If this higher temperature does stress your plants, try increasing the CO_2 concentration to 2,000 ppm, which should be more suitable for your plants at that temperature. However, if slowing down the vent fan's speed still leads to heat stress in your plants, you'll need to regulate the frequency of CO_2 release during each air change. The more frequent the venting, the more CO_2 you must release to replace vented CO_2. To achieve this, use a hose with your regulator to ensure that the CO_2 is distributed at a distance from the vent, to allow the CO_2 to effectively flow through your plants, similar to fresh air.

Heat stress can stunt growth and negate the benefits of CO_2 supplementation. So before introducing high levels of CO_2 into the grow environment, optimize your air circulation system. A well-designed air circulation system offers the flexibility to facilitate a slow CO_2 release system, allowing you to control the timing, amount of CO_2, and ventilation required to maintain the desired temperature range. CO_2 supplementation should not continue during the 12/12 light cycle, as photosynthesis does not occur without light. Furthermore, additional monitoring may be required during this period since temperatures may drop during the dark period.

Climate Controllers

Climate controllers, also known as environment controllers, climate monitors, or climate sensors, are immensely helpful in the cannabis grow room. These are available

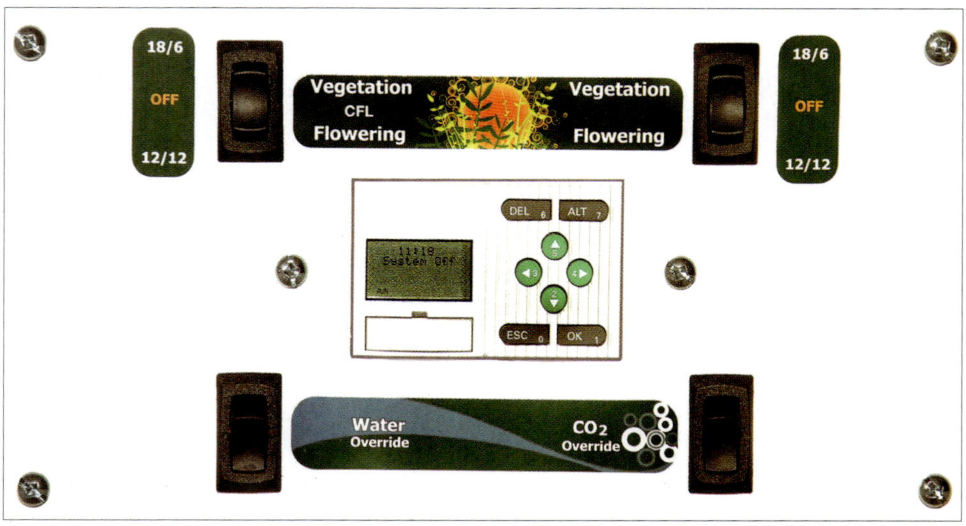

PHOTO: BC NORTHERN LIGHTS

Advanced climate controllers are small computers that can handle several streams of data and perform calculations to regulate the grow area's equipment.

in both analog and digital formats, with more expensive models offering greater functionality and control over various devices. Like timers, climate controllers regulate the operation of electrical devices, though they also handle a wide range of tasks. In your grow room, a climate controller can manage: Lighting; timers; ventilation and extraction; CO_2 distribution; humidity; and pumps for hydroponics, the last often separate. The controller for fluid-related tasks should be kept separate from the one handling other functions.

A climate controller is typically mounted on the grow room wall, with the devices it controls plugged into dedicated slots. The controller itself is then connected to the electrical mains. High-end climate controllers are self-regulating and come equipped with built-in sensors that detect when specific tasks or sets of tasks need to be activated. These controllers are robust, featuring numerous dials, displays, sensors, and socket connections. Some systems offer USB interfaces for configuration via a PC, while others are cutting-edge smart devices. Consequently, climate controllers can be some of the most expensive components in your grow room.

An advanced climate controller can be programmed to perform like this:

During the flowering phase with a 12/12 photoperiod, the climate controller manages the lights, ensuring they are on for 12 hours and off for 12 hours. It constantly monitors the room's temperature, which fluctuates when the lights cycle on and off. Heat sensors in the controller adjust the speed of the extraction fans to maintain the desired temperature settings. If the temperature falls below the predetermined level, the controller activates an attached heating device to achieve the desired temperature or temperature range. Simultaneously, the controller can regulate CO_2 systems and humidifiers in the grow room, and alert you to humidity-related issues. Additionally, it can control a hydroponic system, ensuring that the correct amount of liquid medium is replenished on a timer basis using pumps.

When opting for a climate controller, you are investing in a sophisticated, customized unit. Read the specific instructions for each controller to understand its capabilities and operation fully.

Emergency Flushing

Emergency flushing is a last-resort option for when all else has failed. It is not a routine practice but rather an emergency procedure when a simple transplant won't suffice due to excessive nutrients in the medium surrounding the roots. An example: You're using soil with high water retention. In a moment of impatience while feeding your plant, you pour the feeding solution directly onto the soil, spilling a substantial amount of the undiluted feeding liquid. Panic sets in as you realize that your plant's life is at risk due to this chemical overload.

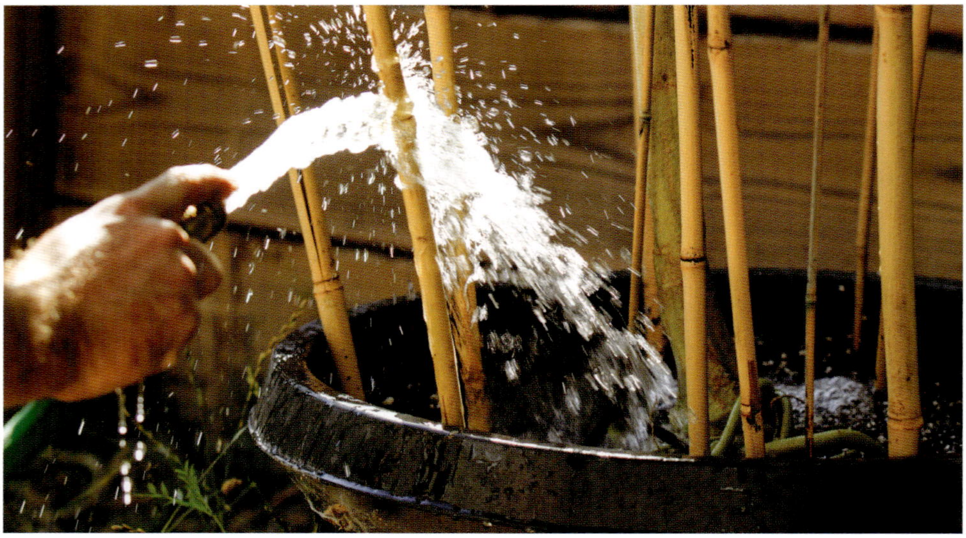

Water can also be used to drain a plant of unwanted nutrients.

PHOTO: JUSTINCANNABIS.COM

In this situation, you can either flush the soil or transplant the plant. Flush first, then consider a transplant, but remember to prepare the new medium beforehand.

If your plant is a large sativa, you may require assistance to flush the soil. Smaller plants are easier to handle. These steps will serve as a guide for urgent situations:

Step A

Sometimes, it is possible first to tip out some of what went in.

1. Carefully transport the potted plant to a suitable area for emptying, preferably a white sink that allows you to monitor the fluid's color.
2. Gently lay the plant on its side, taking care not to bend or break the stem.
3. If the stem seems fragile, use a stake or bamboo to support the plant.
4. Tilt the potted plant so that the top of the pot and the soil faces the sink at an angle.
5. Continue tilting until the liquid stops draining out.

Step B

If your pot has perforations, proceed with these steps. Otherwise, skip to Step C for transplanting.

1. Raise the plant upright and place it in the sink.
2. Pour a generous amount of water onto the soil, using a tap, hose, or watering can.
3. Allow the water to flow out from the bottom of the pot, paying attention to the color of the runoff as in Step A.
4. Repeat this process until the water runs clear. The soil will become muddy during this process, with some mud being carried away with the water.

5. Once the water runs clear, tilt the plant on its side again and wait for complete drainage.
6. Flush water through the plant multiple times to ensure all nutrients are eliminated. A three-gallon pot usually requires about seven flushes. Monitor the color of the water to know when to stop flushing.
7. Promptly move your plant to a warm, dry location and wait for the soil to dry out. You can use a fan on the soil but avoid directing it at the plant.
8. Proceed to Step D.

Step C

Familiarize yourself with the transplant section in Chapter 4. Ensure that you have the new medium prepared in advance, as you don't want to handle a flushed plant while simultaneously setting up the new medium.

1. Remove the plant from its pot as described in the transplant section.
2. Hold the soil together with your hands over the sink and position it near the drain. You may require assistance if dealing with a large root mass.
3. Allow the water to trickle slowly over the soil without squeezing or crushing it. The soil will become muddy and break apart, which is expected.
4. Repot the plant into a new medium.

Step D

1. Monitor the soil's pH daily. If the flush was successful, the pH should gradually return to the near-neutral 7 mark, assuming your water source is pH-neutral at 7 or that you've adjusted it if needed.

A soil flush is a make-or-break procedure, which some plants do not survive. The flush involves overwatering your plant to the extent that most minerals and nutrients are removed from the soil. If your plant does not manage to recover, view it as a learning experience for future endeavors. Since a soil flush can be shocking to the plant, use it only as a last resort when no other solution is viable. Even if it survives, your plant may have suffered some damage.

Recovery time depends on the extent of the damage, though it usually takes around two weeks for the plant to begin to recover. After the first week of recovery, you can trim away any burnt or damaged leaves. You can resume feeding after the first week of recovery if the disorder was not severe, but should wait two weeks if it was.

Clean and Store

Cleaning is a vital aspect of cultivation to prevent future issues such as contamination. Maintaining cleanliness also leads to better results. Consider purchasing cleaning products and assembling a cleaning box to reduce time spent searching for a cleaning rag and water. You can easily obtain packing boxes, so there's no reason to leave

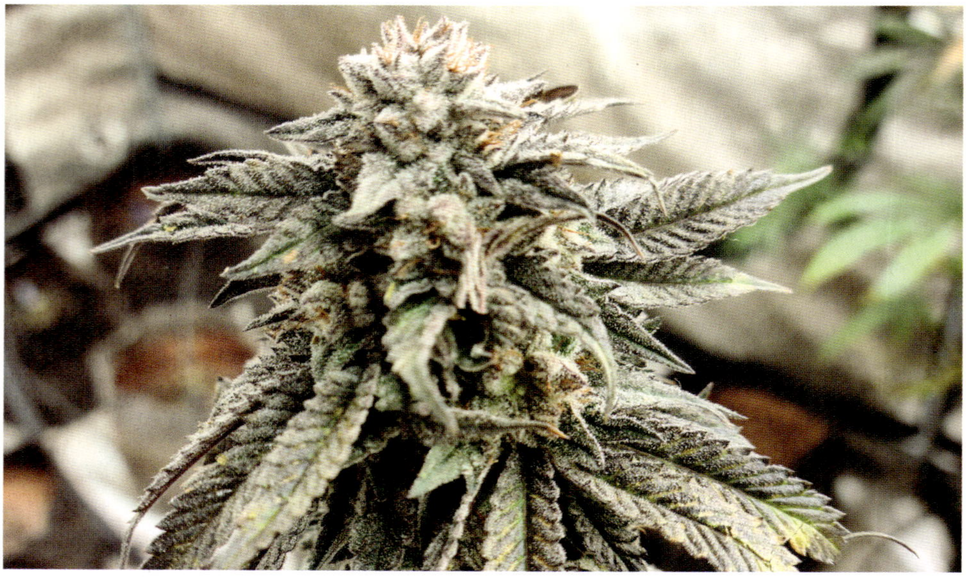

This plant has been well flushed before harvest to make the bud easier to cure due to the lack of chlorophyll.

PHOTO: CZECHBAYAREA

open nutrient containers on your garage floor, a possible safety hazard and unsightly as visible chemical reactions occur. Clean your tools and containers and put them in a designated storage place to keep them safe and in a pristine condition.

Making the Most of Experimental Trials

Designing smaller trial experiments in your grow is an excellent way to improve your results. Once plants are well-rooted, you can experiment with nutrient control, pH, watering, aeration techniques, temperatures, humidity, CO_2, pruning, flushing, topping, and anything else you plan to do in your main grow area. There's no need for your entire grow space to be subject to any experiments that can be conducted on a much smaller scale. Clones are ideal for these experiments. Creating them can take some time, but, once you have clones, you can establish a small mother plant, as explained in Chapter 13, from which you can take all future cuttings.

Your experiments will likely be strain-specific, so you may need to repeat the same tests if you introduce a new strain, especially if you're transitioning from one extreme, such as a pure indica, to another, like a pure sativa.

Conducting trials can help prevent any harm to your crop. Moreover, it can save you time, effort, and expenses in the long run. You can begin by maintaining a small trial grow area, such as a dedicated tent for clones with an LED. If you start your growing journey in a smaller tent and plan to expand, you can then keep that smaller tent for working with mother plants, taking cuttings, and conducting experiments.

Inside a Grow Tent

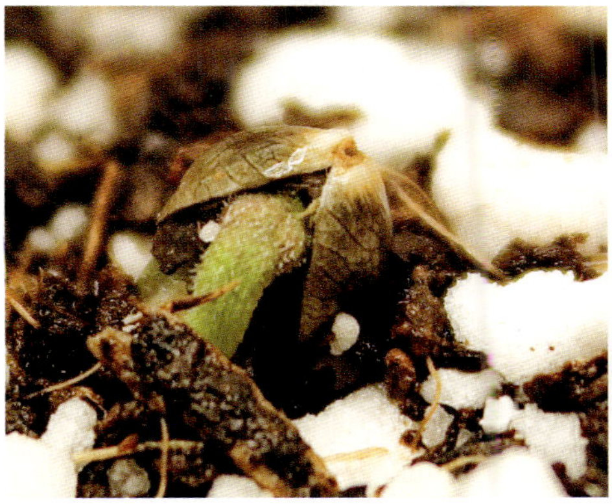

Seedling pushing the shell away from it.

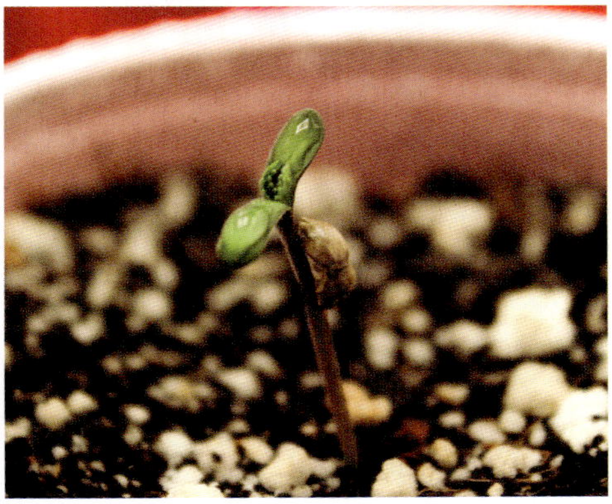

Breaking the surface to receive the light.

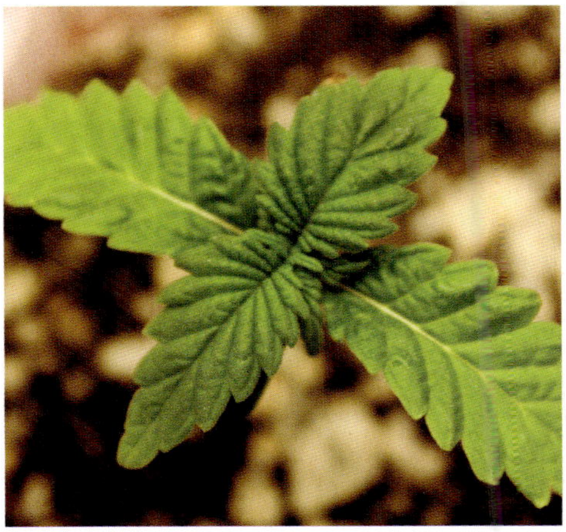

The first true leaves emerge, and the seedling is ready for more.

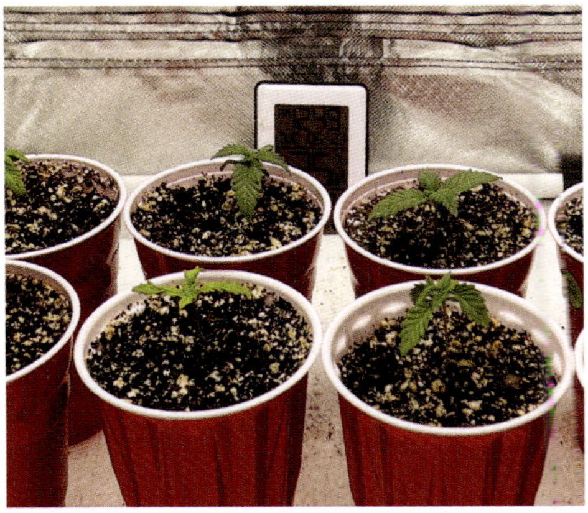

Seedlings are already in the grow room and benefiting from the environment.

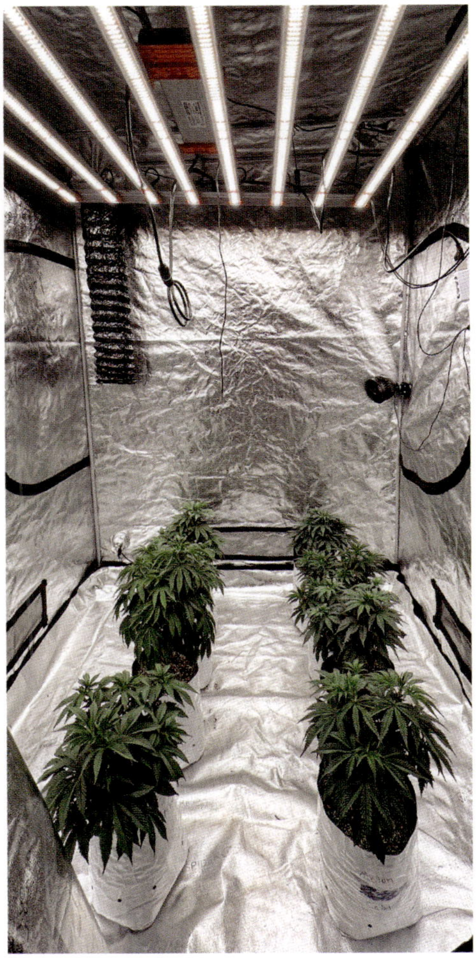

Vegetative growth is at a healthy early stage as these plants will grow more. *continues...*

PHOTOS: TEE ROBERTS

Inside a Grow Tent *continued*

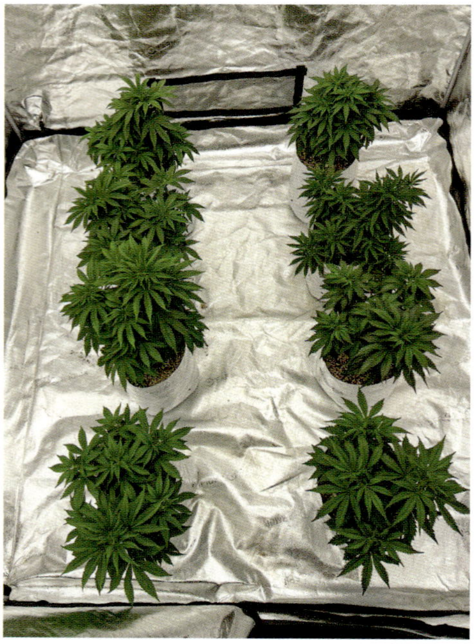

The gaps between plants will fill in over time.

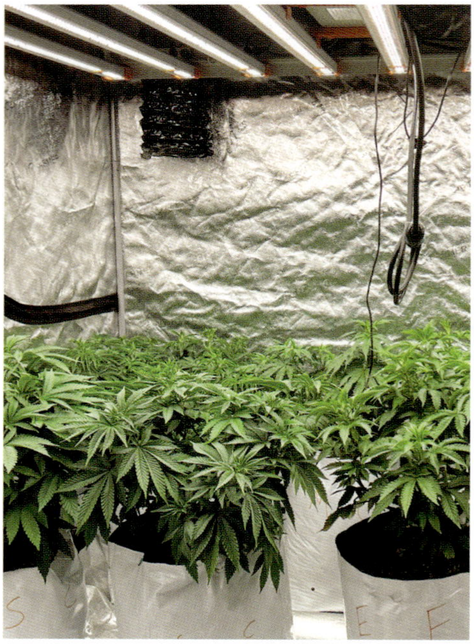

Grow bags allow the plants to be shifted around if needed.

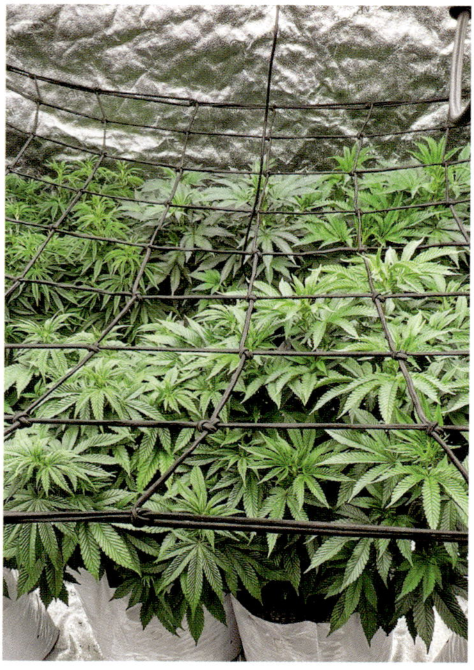

A netting is used to help support the plants and keep them upright.

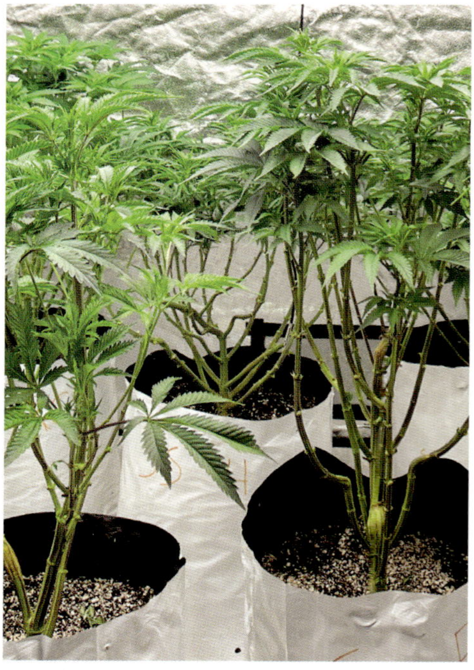

These plants have been pruned, especially the lower branches.

PHOTOS: TEE ROBERTS

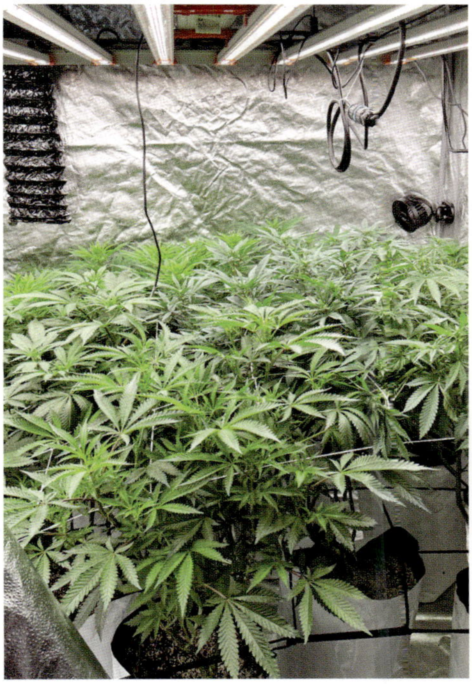

Plants have reached a satisfactory size for pre-flowering.

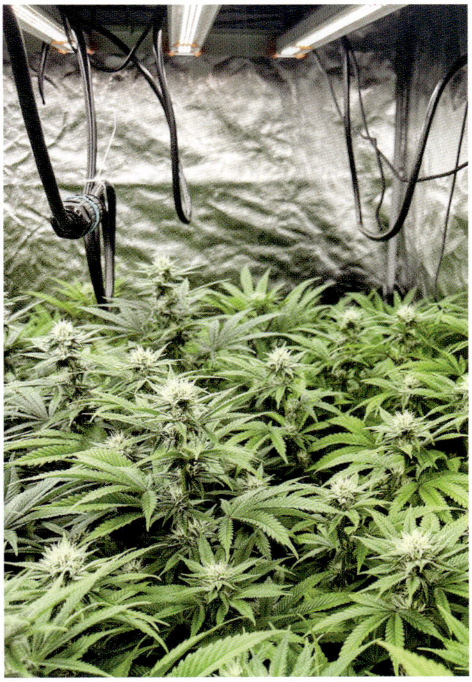

Already a few weeks into flowering, and the top colas are showing.

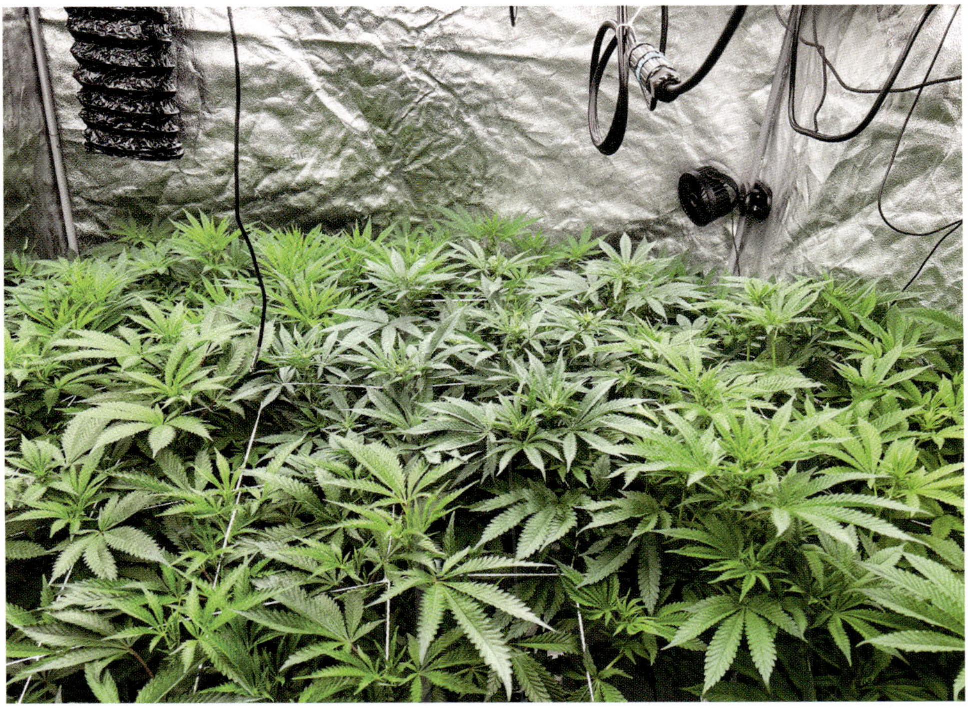

This canopy is even and is just above the netting which holds everything in place.

continues...

Inside a Grow Tent *continued*

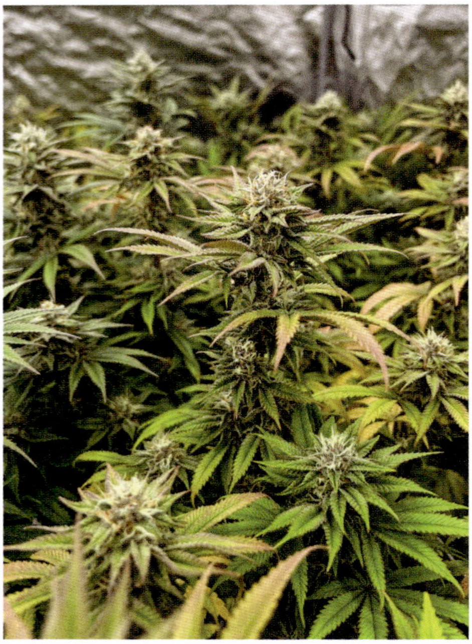

The internode spaces fill in with flowers to make the colas more evident.

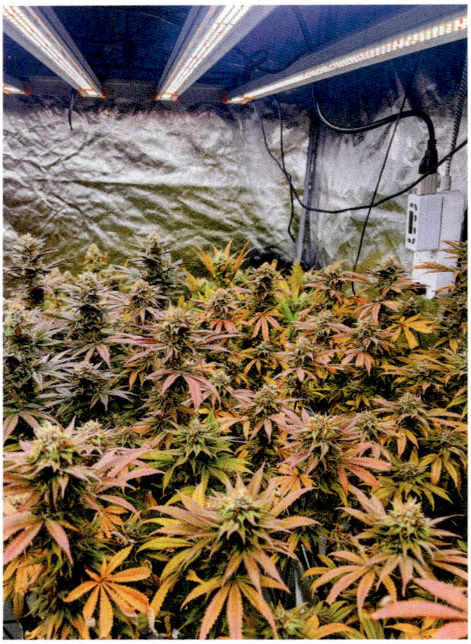

A room full of flowering female plants kept upright with the netting.

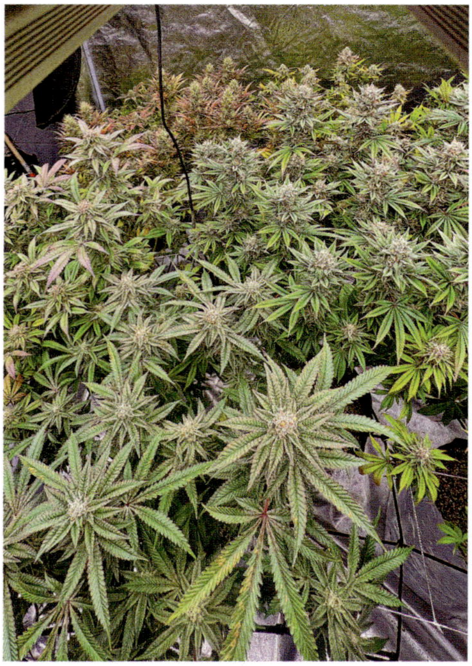

It isn't hard to see that these plants would collapse without the netting.

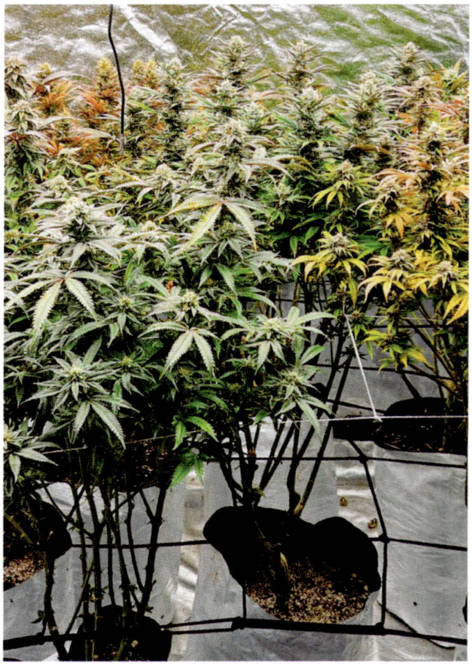

How much you want to bunch your plants with nets depends on you.

PHOTOS: TEE ROBERTS

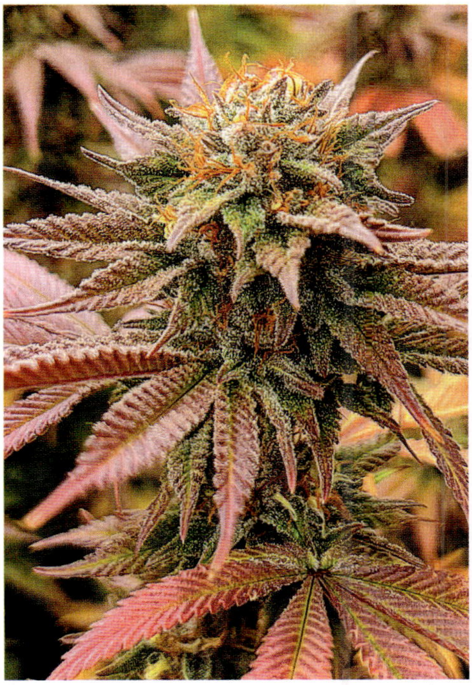

At the end of flowering, there can be some radical color changes.

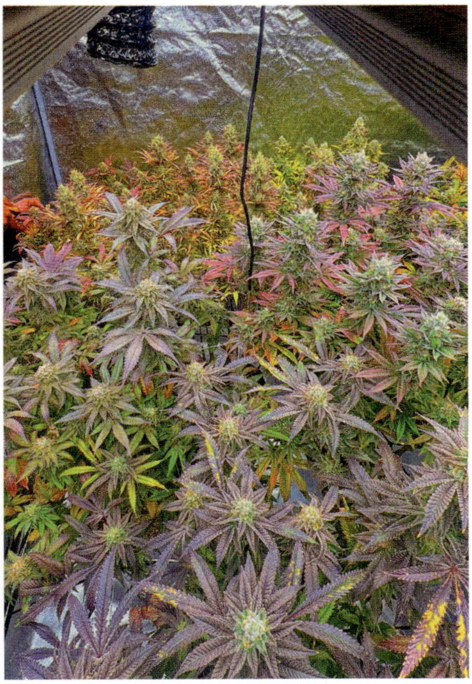

Flushing plants will also cause them to change color in most cases.

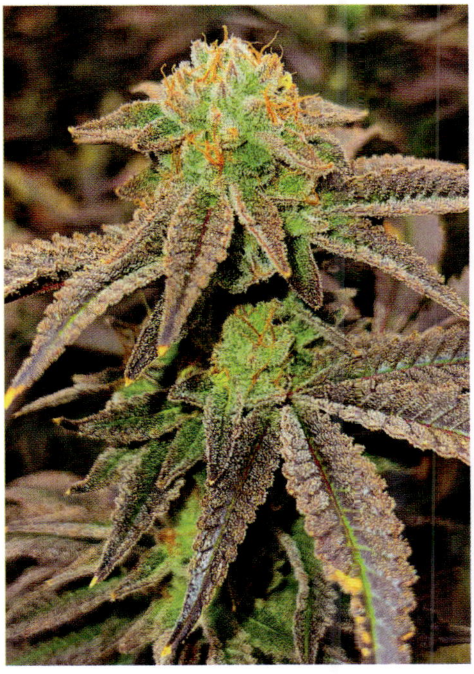

The expected frosty look of trichome-covered flowers and leaves.

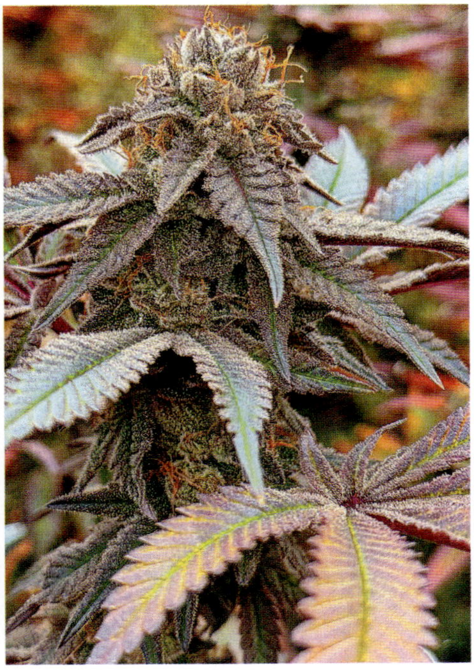

This plant is ready for harvest as most pistils have changed color.

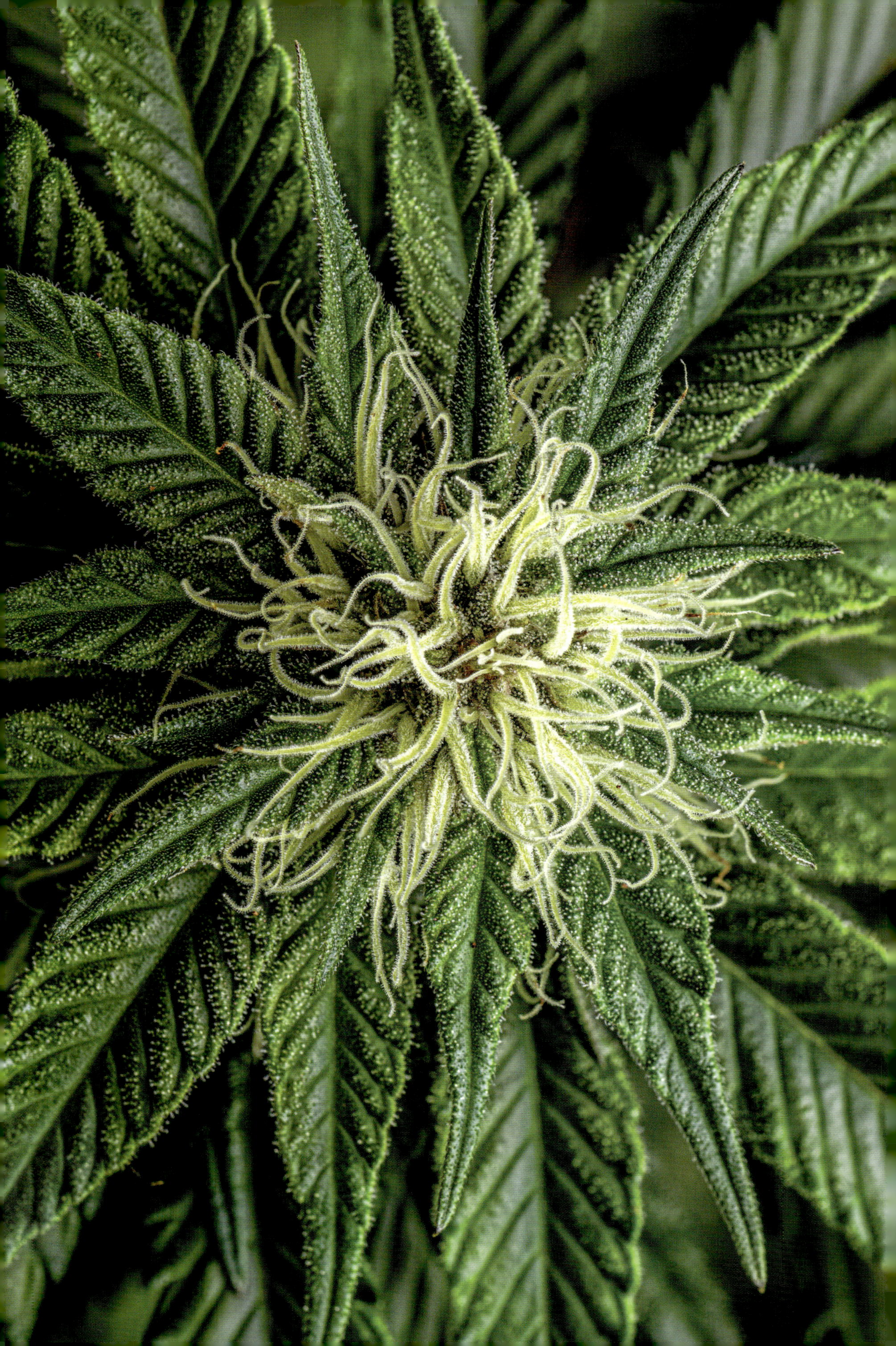

9

Pre-Flowering and Flowering

Once you have set up your central growing environment and modified controls for optimal plant growth, your vegetative plants will develop multiple nodes and a small leaf mass at the top. These leaves should be flat and spread out to capture maximum light across their surface area, indicating that your plants are thriving. If you notice any issues, such as leaves not spreading out as they should, consult Chapter 15 to identify and address any problems before the flowering phase. Resolving these issues quickly is crucial to achieve the best possible results.

Failure Rates

Nearly every grower encounters challenges along the way. Few beginners reach the pre-flowering and flowering stages without experiencing at least one significant problem. Don't be discouraged if you do face difficulties in your initial attempts. The key to successfully growing healthy and potent plants is to persist in your cultivation efforts and continue learning from your mistakes—and from resources like this book.

Experienced growers also encounter general failure rates due to genetic factors, such as seeds that fail to germinate and clones that fail to root. Despite the right conditions, some plants may not progress to the flowering stage, and there is nothing that can be done to save them. These outliers are sometimes referred to as the "runts of the litter," as they possess the opposite of hybrid vigor. Such occurrences are more likely in large populations. If everything else in your grow is in order and only one or two plants exhibit these issues, it's probably due to genetic variability.

Failures will always happen when you're experimenting with different growing methods, environments, and strains. Even experienced growers lose one or two plants out of every ten when experimenting, so there is no "acceptable" failure rate. As you gain experience and optimize your techniques, failures will become less frequent.

PHOTO: ROB BRAMHILL

It's important to distinguish between occasional losses due to genetics and those due

Healthy Vegetative Growth

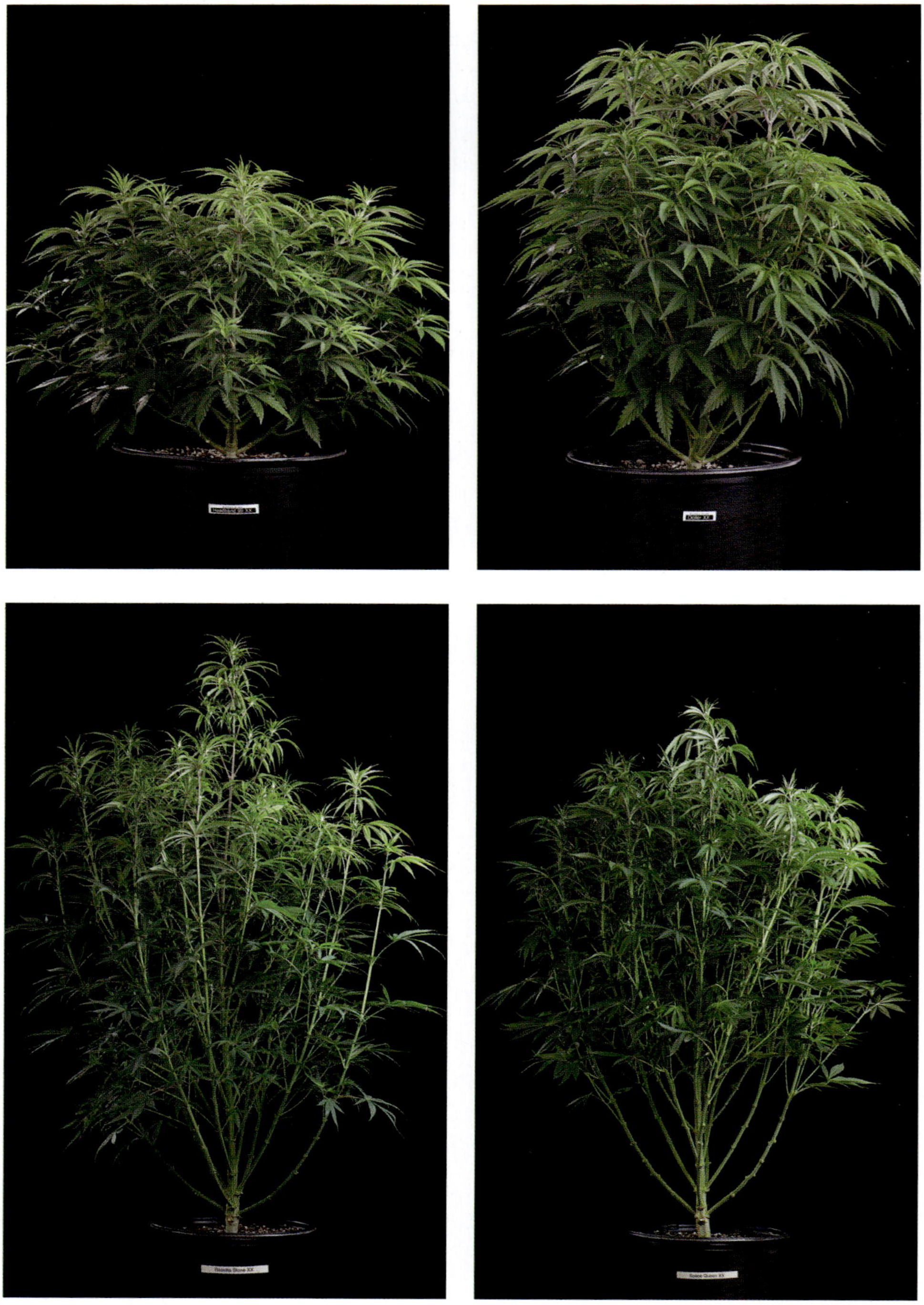

PHOTOS: RUSSELL-HOWLAND PHOTOGRAPHY

An example of how expansive the cannabis plant can get during vegetative growth before pre-flowering. Understanding that the plant will get even bigger while flowering is essential for space considerations.

to a problematic batch of seed stock. Seed banks may recognize a bad batch if many growers report problems. If you suspect you have problematic stock, contact your seed bank and inform them of this. Document the problem with photographic evidence. They may replace the seeds if there are enough concerns. Outdoor growers must acknowledge that external environmental factors, such as climate change, challenging pests, or aggressive fungi outbreaks, can lead to high failure rates. However, following the guidance provided in this book will ensure you a substantial number of successful plants.

In conclusion, issues with seeds usually stem from cultivation methods and environmental factors. Through experience, you'll gain a deeper understanding of the causes of failure and be better equipped to assess whether genetics are a contributing factor.

Lateral Branching

During the vegetative growth stage, plants increase in size, producing more leaves and new branches. Their stems grow thicker and leaves expand, so they resemble typical cannabis plants. Once the plants exhibit new leaf growth at most node regions between the stem and branches, they have reached a stage where they can efficiently

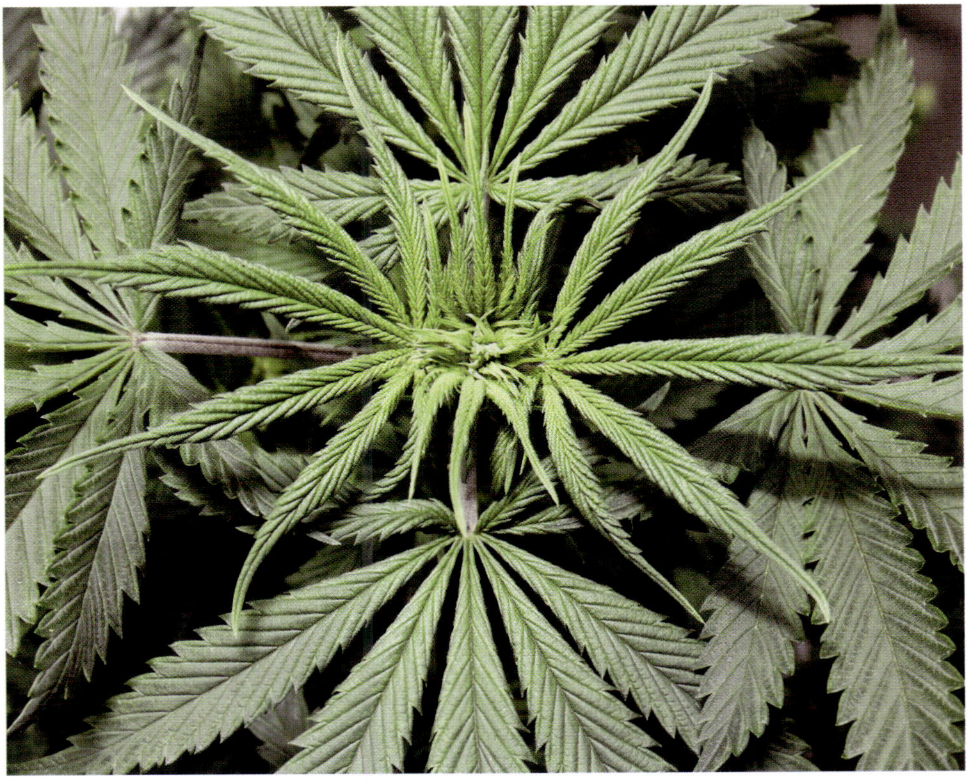

PHOTO: DAVID STRANGE

The top node displays new formations that become branches with leaves. This plant is looking healthy and strong.

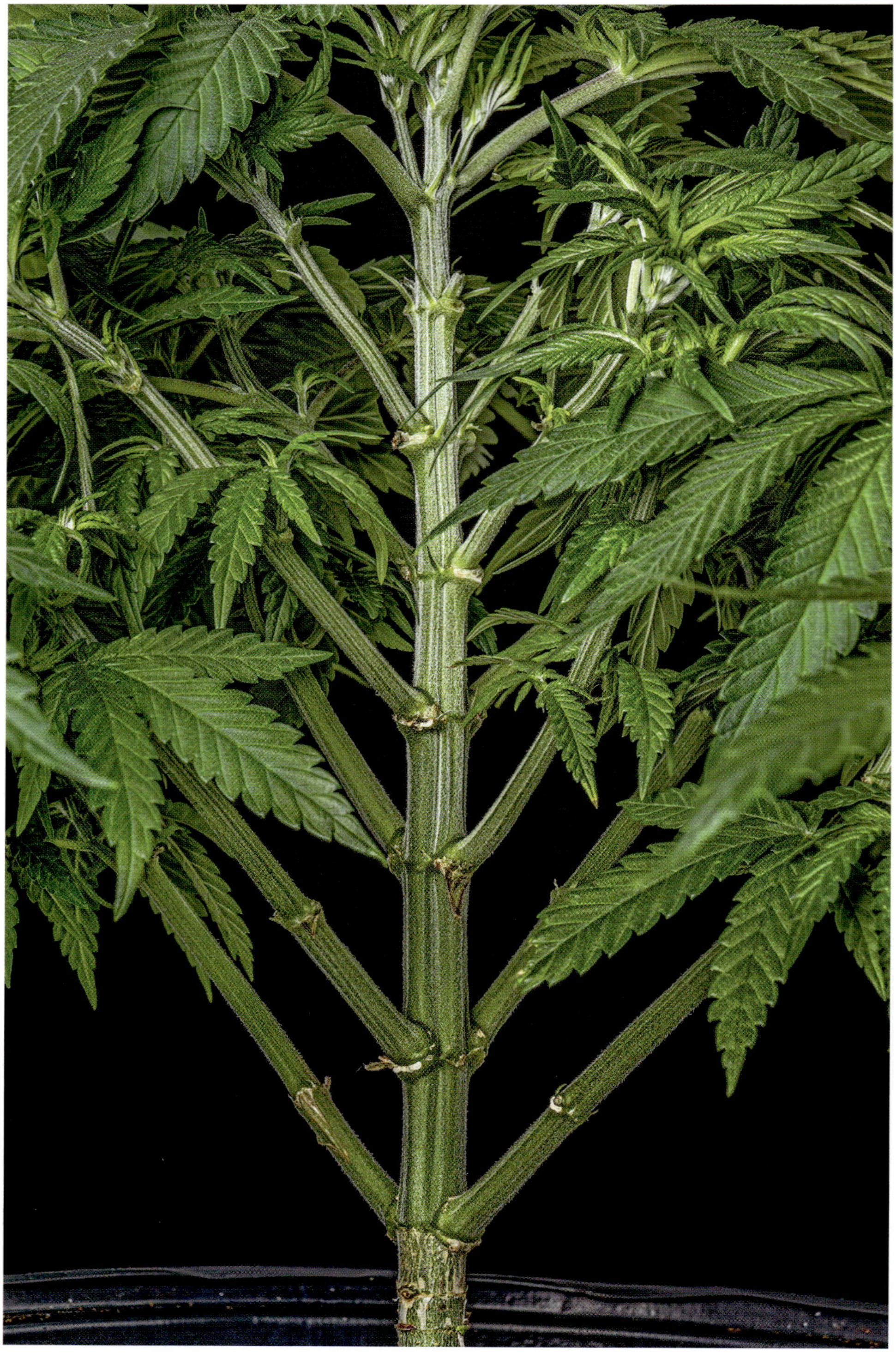

PHOTO: ROB BRAMHILL

You can keep internode lengths short by employing shorter distances to the light. This way, your plant reaches its genetic minimum height.

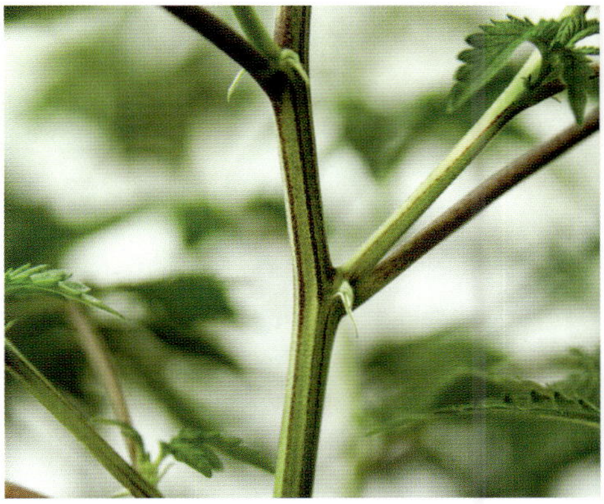

Pruning can produce more branches at node regions.

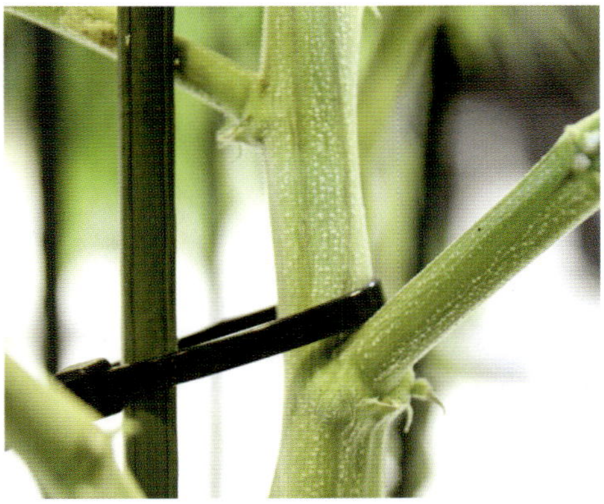

Pruning can cause alternative, not opposite, branching (next to rather than across from).

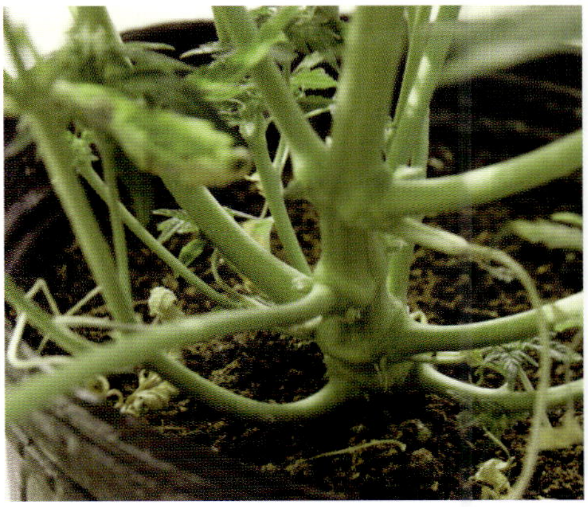

A heavily pruned supercropped plant.

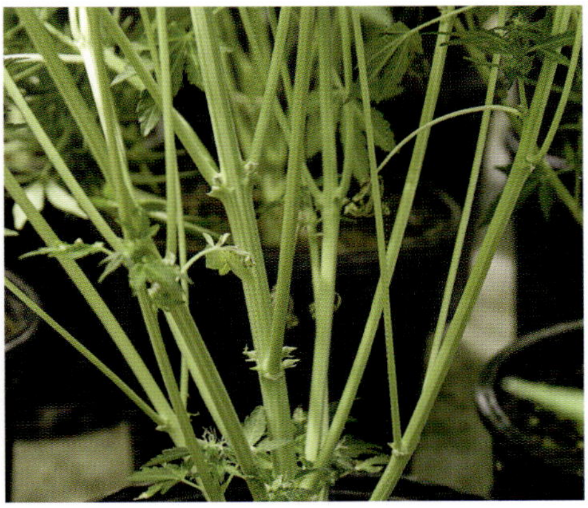

Extensive supercropping and pruning to produce multiple branches.

convert light energy through photosynthesis into additional side branch growth. These lateral, or secondary, branches are essential for achieving a bushy plant structure. While indica plants are naturally bushier than sativa varieties, manual pruning can also help create a bushier appearance.

As your plant continues to develop, more node regions will appear, accompanied by increased branching. Eventually, pre-flowers will appear in these node regions, marking the progression toward the flowering stage. You can generally expect four to eight weeks of vegetative growth after completing the seedling stage, though the specific timing depends on the strain you are cultivating. For sativa strains, this period can be longer. Recognizing this transition in your plant's development is crucial, as it signals the onset of the pre-flowering phase. This new stage requires adjustments to your grow space and gardening approach. The following section will guide you on how to identify the pre-flowering stage.

PHOTOS: DAVID STRANGE

Pre-Flowers: Females

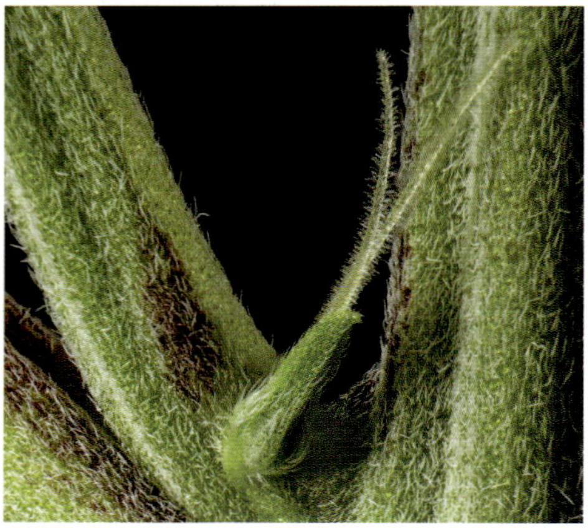

Two pistils grow from a calyx.

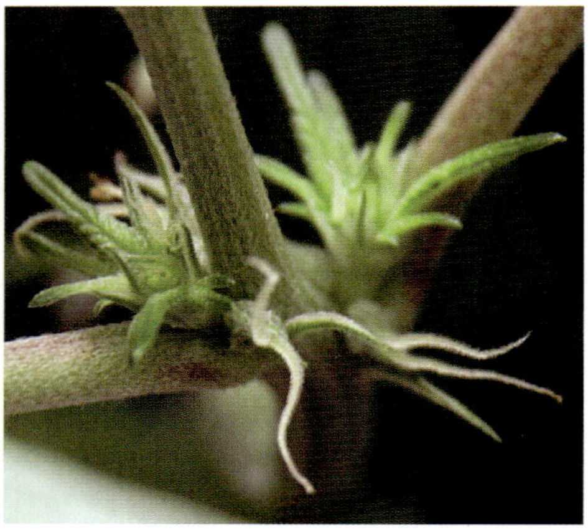

A few pistils appear at a node region.

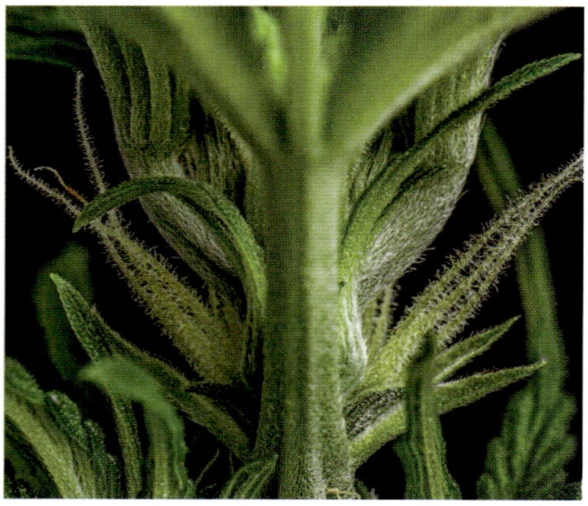

If you placed a mirror halfway vertically, it would reproduce the same image.

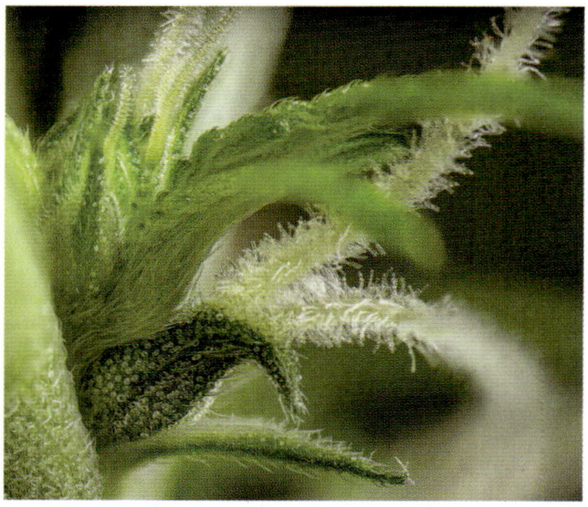

Trichomes develop on the calyx and pistils.

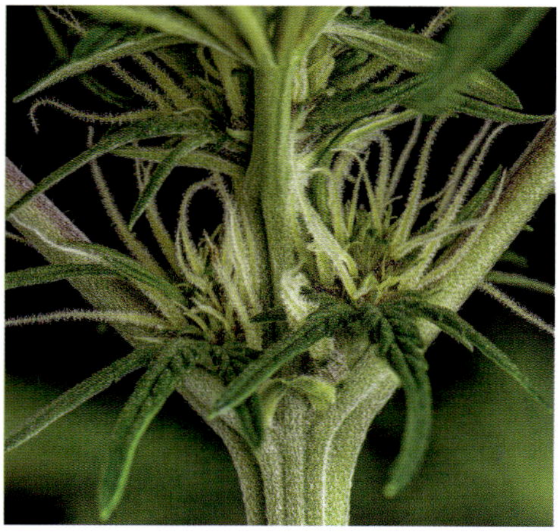

Flowers at nodes will extend outwards.

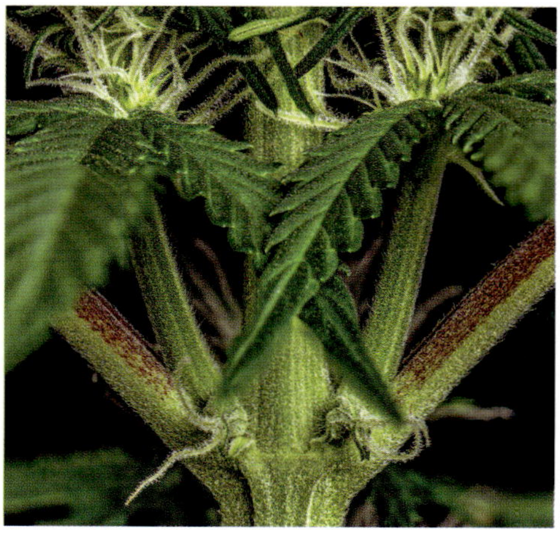

Flowers extend outwards on branching.

PHOTOS: ROB BRAMHILL, HANNA BLISS (MIDDLE LEFT)

Pre-Flowering and Early Sexing

As a grower starting with standard seeds, you should aim to grow as many female plants as possible. Because clones inherit the genetic makeup of the plant they originate from, you can predict the sex of your clone if you have information about its history. You can identify a plant's sex during the pre-flowering stage by examining the node regions for calyx development. Note that male plants generally pre-flower before females.

Checking for Calyx Development

1. Select a plant and carefully examine the node regions where the lateral branches meet the stem. Look for tiny, pod-shaped structures in these areas. A magnifying aid can make them easier to spot.
2. If you don't find any calyx development in the initial node regions, proceed to check other node regions along each branch until you reach the tip.
3. If you still don't find any calyx development, check other plants in the same population. If none of them show calyx development, it indicates that the population hasn't reached its pre-flowering stage. Calyxes can appear suddenly and within a day, so be patient. However, if you find calyx development in some plants within the same group, it's likely that all of the plants are entering the pre-flowering stage.

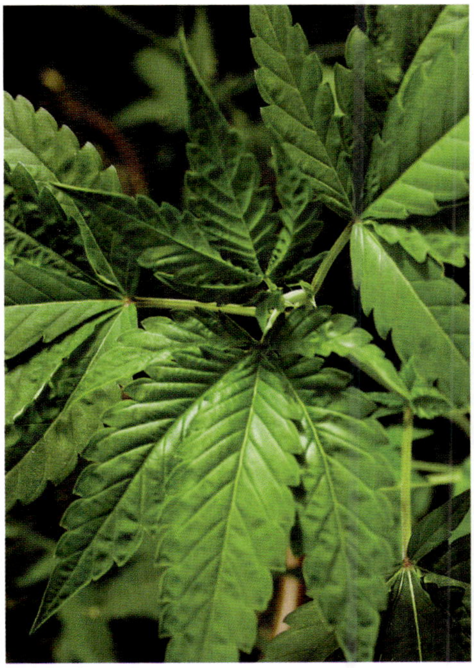

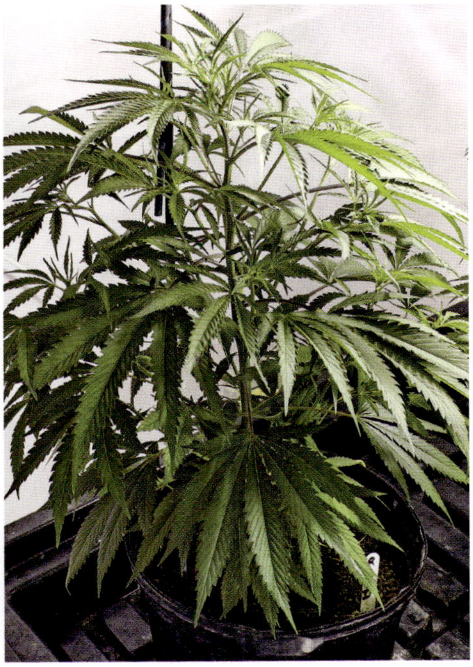

PHOTOS: DAVID STRANGE

A single young plant can produce 100 node areas for checking during pre-flowering. Start high and work down. Physically get in there and move leaves around searching for calyx development if you must.

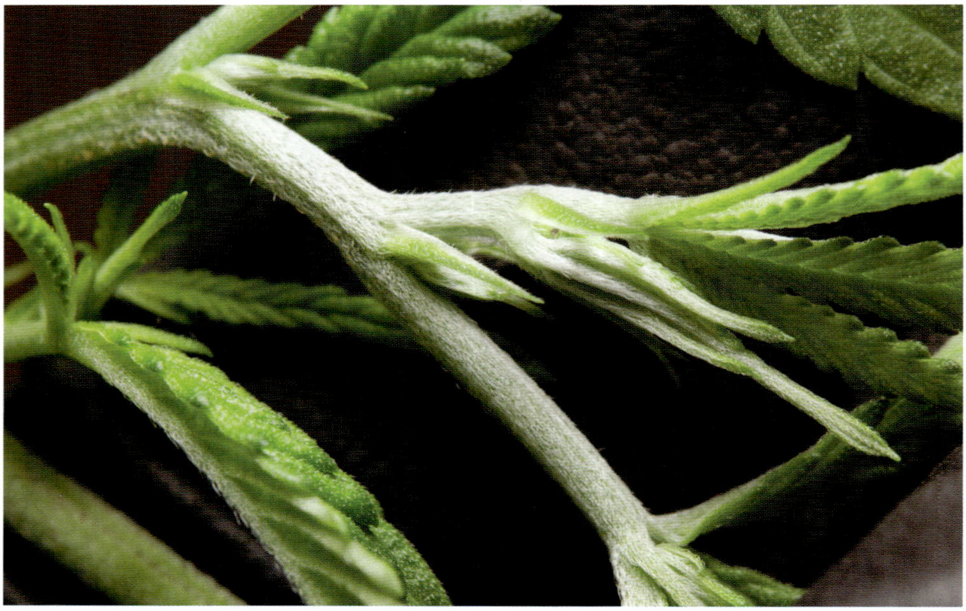

A closer inspection of the node area reveals both new leaf growth and possible calyx development.

PHOTO: DANKSHIRE PHOTOGRAPHY

Early Sexing Methods

There are three early indicators of plant sex. Though they are not 100% accurate, these methods are often reliable predictors of your plant's sex:

1. Calyx Sexing:
   An effective method to identify plant sex early is to closely examine the calyx using a magnifying glass. If the calyx is raised on a short stem, it's probably a male. Otherwise, it's likely a female.
2. Height Sexing:
   Some plants may be taller than others, even though you started growing them at the same time. Smaller plants tend to be female, taller ones male. You can segregate these plants into two groups and check the accuracy of your assessment when sex becomes definitively identifiable. As you gain experience with a particular strain, you can more reliably sex by height.
3. Force Flowering Sexing Test:
   Forced flowering is a precise early-sexing technique used by experienced growers who seek to induce the flowering stage as early as possible. However, this technique may lead to sexual issues, such as hermaphroditism. Forced flowering is initiated by using a 12/12 light cycle at the end of the vegetative growth phase to induce a photoperiod change without waiting for calyx development. Some plants may react more quickly to this change, causing them to flower a few days earlier than they naturally would. Forced flowering is not advised for your main grow room. Instead, it should be used with a plant cutting for testing purposes.

Forced flowering in testing involves taking a single cutting from the plant whose sex you want to identify instead of forcing an entire grow room to flower.

1. Take a cutting at the end of the vegetative stage, as you would when making clones, and place it in a cup of water or a cloning medium like Rockwool. The plant should be bushy enough for you to take cuttings without stunting growth.
2. Expose the cutting to 12 hours of light followed by 12 hours of total darkness, following the forced-flowering method.
3. Observe whether the cutting begins to flower and displays its sex. However, for this method to work, you must ensure that the plant the cutting came from is mature enough. If this is your first time working with the strain, the timing can be difficult to guess. That is why this test is for experienced growers. You can check for the breeder's recommendations if they are specified. If not, you can ask the seed bank for an estimate. You can also research the strain online. An immature plant will not show its sex because photoperiod changes do not influence initial calyx development.

In most cases, you will be able to observe a flowering response from the test before the plants in your main grow room begin to flower. The corresponding plant from which the cutting was taken will have the same sex. This method may not always result in flowering before the main grow room plants do. In some cases, the cutting may prioritize root growth over flowering. But keep in mind that you're not trying to grow a full-sized bud from this cutting; you're simply determining its sex. All you need is one sex organ to be visible, and the clone can then be discarded or planted for a small yield.

Calyx observation can be combined with height estimates, which eliminates the need to cut your plants. If you do choose to prune your plants, label the cuttings and try to root them as clones to use for a sex test later on.

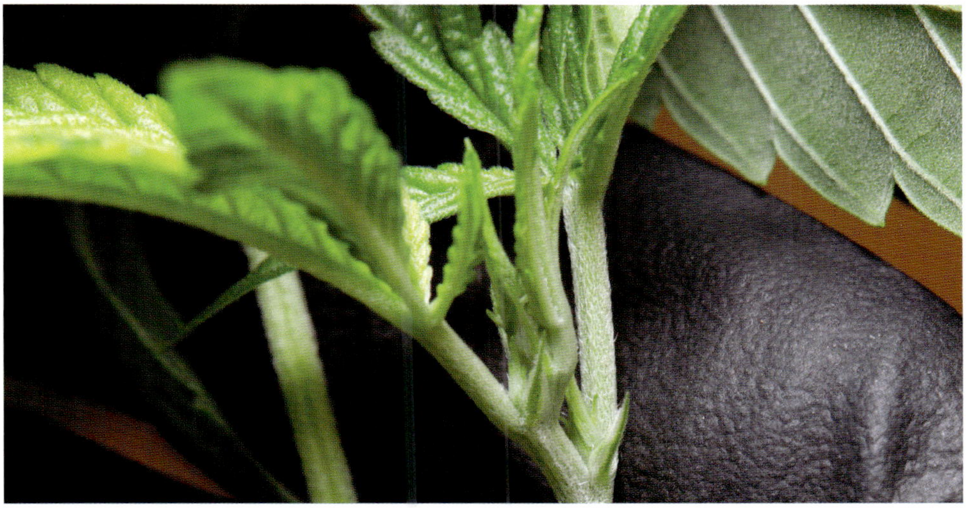

PHOTO: DANKSHIRE PHOTOGRAPHY

Holding a node region for inspection. A background color helps.

Pre-Flowers: Males

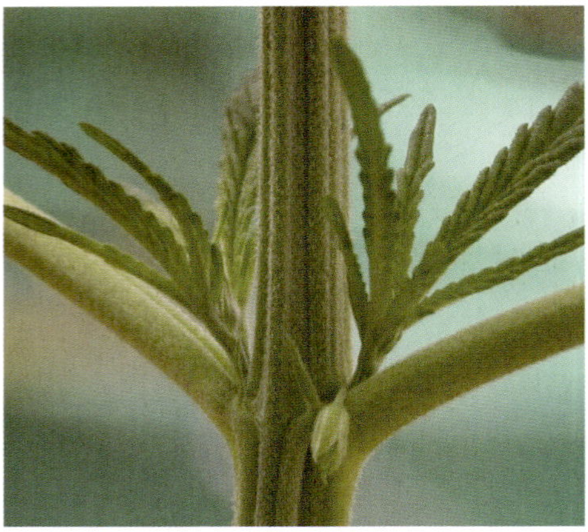

A raised calyx indicates possible males.

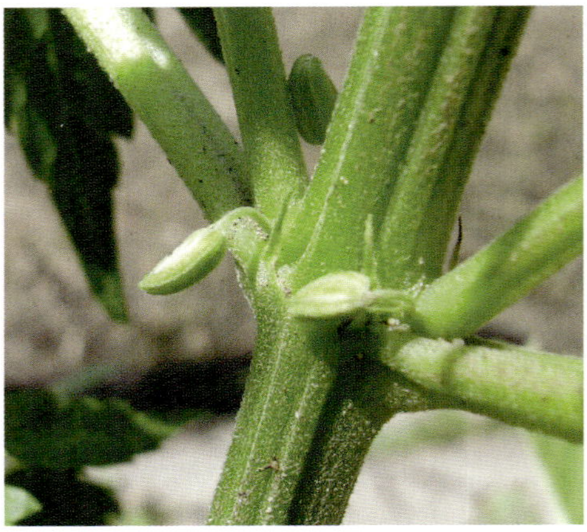

Calyx raised on the stem are males.

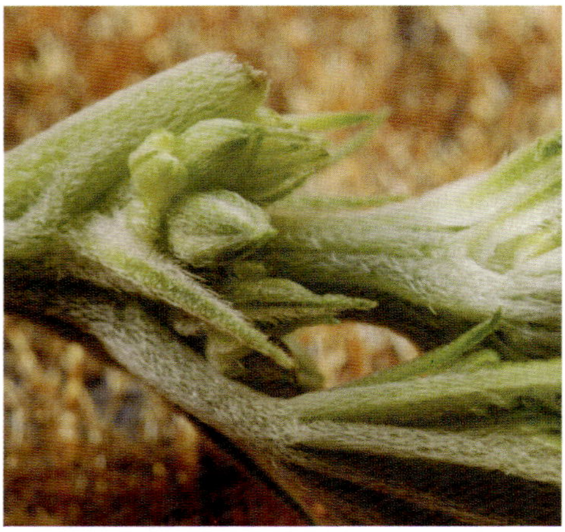

Male flowers show very quickly after calyx development.

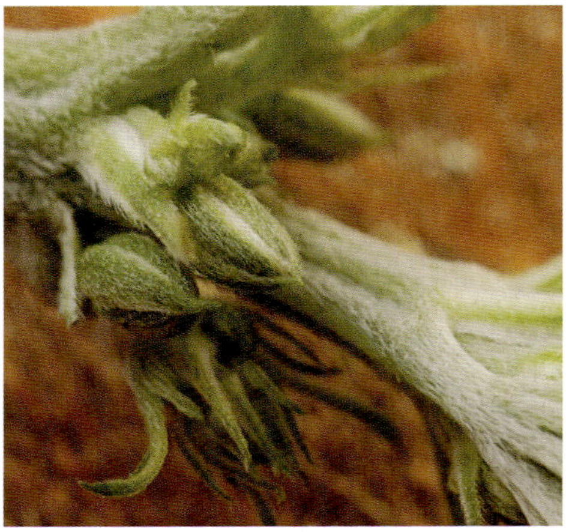

Even these males can start shedding pollen soon.

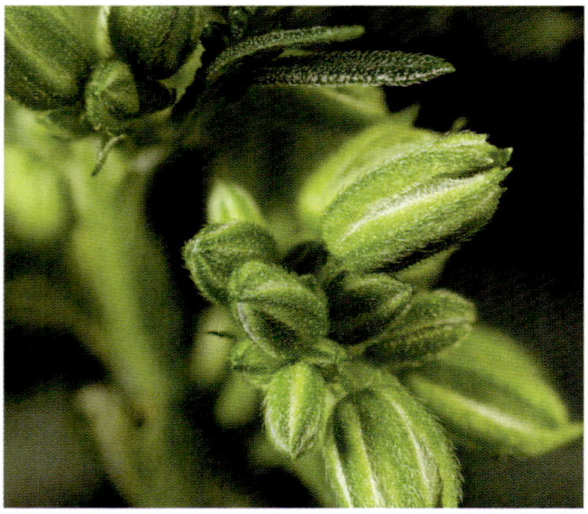

Male cluster ready to burst.

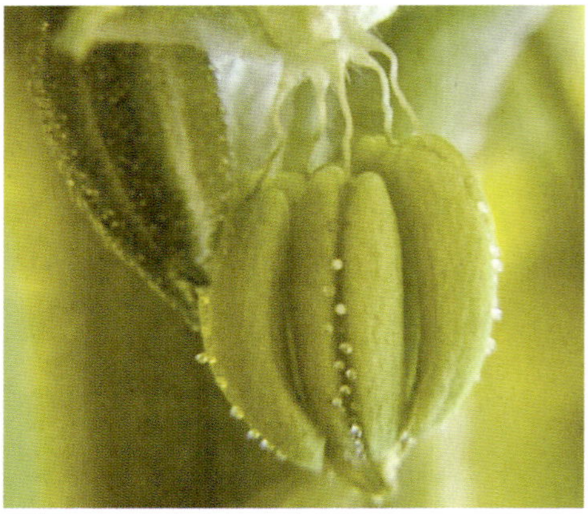

This male is almost finished releasing pollen.

PHOTOS: HANNA BLISS (TOP LEFT, BOTTOM RIGHT), MEL THOMAS (TOP RIGHT), ED BORG (MIDDLE ROW), ROB BRAMHILL (BOTTOM LEFT)

When to Flower

Determining the optimal time to transition to the flowering stage is crucial in cannabis cultivation. Your cannabis plant will remain in the pre-flowering stage until you initiate flowering by implementing a 12/12 photoperiod. Most growers initiate this transition two weeks after the pre-flowering stage begins. During these two weeks, the plant continues to grow vegetatively, expanding in size. The timing of when to switch to flowering primarily depends on how large you want your plants to become.

Calyx development is an indication of the plant's readiness to flower. Flowering immediately after calyx development might lead to faster results but may result in shorter, less bushy plants, and lower yields, possibly a good option for your grow environment as there will be less crowding.

However, you could continue vegetative growth for a few weeks after you identify calyx development to enable the plant to generate more node regions, resulting in taller and bushier plants and potentially larger yields. The outcome varies based on the strain's genetics. Repeated experience with a particular strain will help you determine which approach works best.

Bud production doesn't increase at the same rate as plant growth. It depends on such factors as the growing environment, strain genetics, and the number of nodes on the plant. While all nodes have the potential to become bud sites, every strain has a genetic limit to its capacity for bud production. Pruning and topping plants can create more node regions, potentially increasing yield, but it takes some time for the plant to respond to pruning. Ultimately, bud production will be distributed across all regions, so the total yield may not significantly exceed that of an unpruned plant.

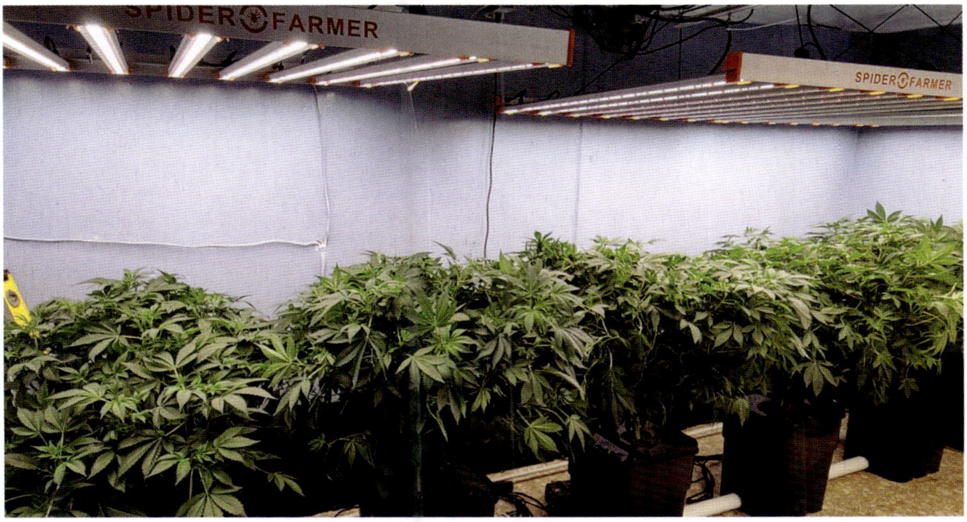

At the end of vegetative growth, multiple node regions are present on these pruned plants.

PHOTO: SPIDER-FARMER.COM

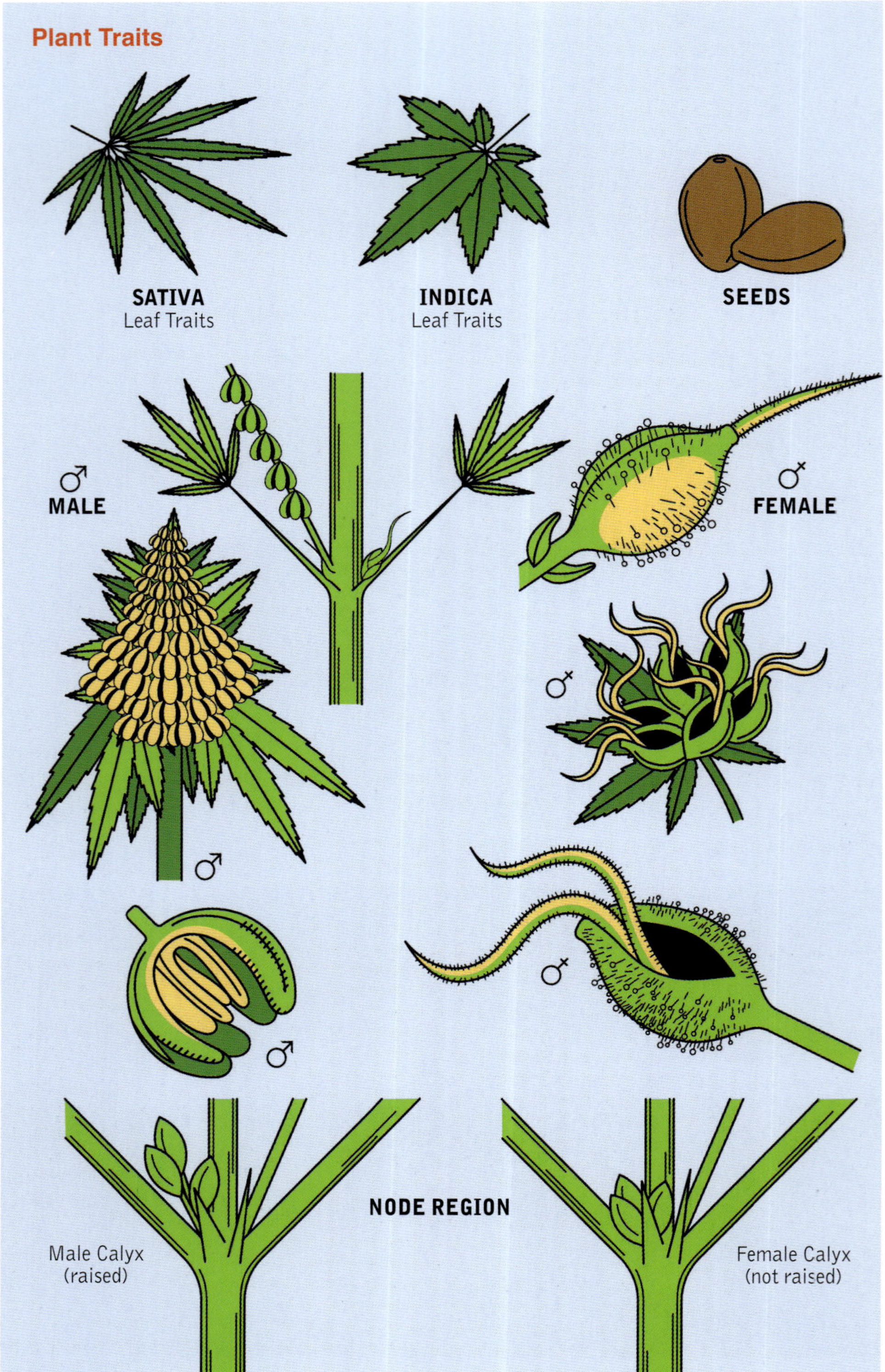
Plant Traits
SATIVA
Leaf Traits
INDICA
Leaf Traits
SEEDS
♂
MALE
♀
FEMALE
♀
♂
♀
♂
NODE REGION
Male Calyx
(raised)
Female Calyx
(not raised)

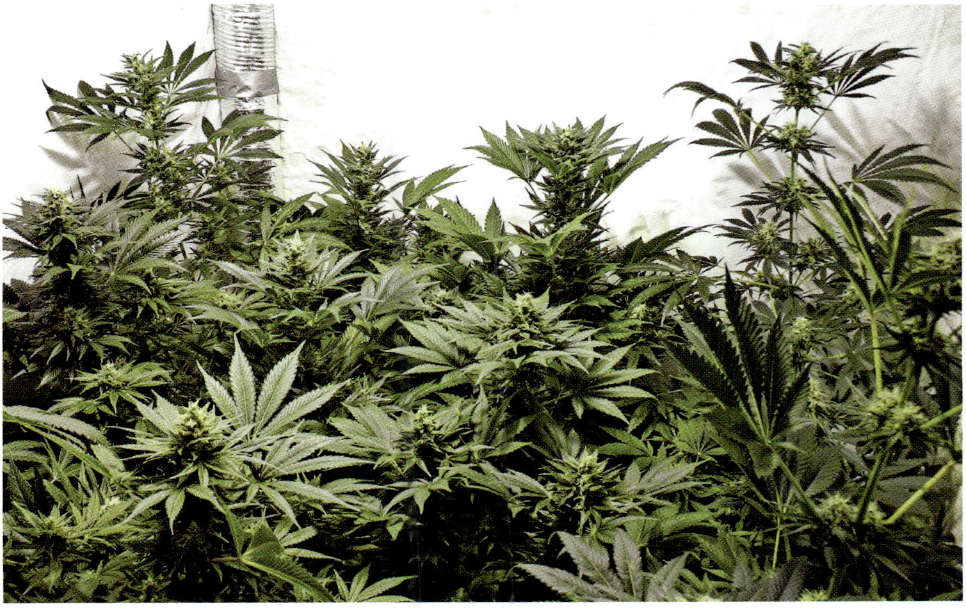

Even a small indoor flowering grow room can still pack a lot of colas inside.

PHOTO: DAVID STRANGE

Whether you prefer less bud sooner or more bud later, you can achieve more bud by flowering a larger number of plants as soon as they mature rather than flowering fewer plants that have undergone extended vegetative growth to reach their maximum height and size. If you choose to prune your plants, factor in an additional week or two for recovery and development. Pruning won't affect sexual development because plants mature based on age. Pruned plants will be shorter and bushier than unpruned plants by the end of flowering. Extending the vegetative phase will result in larger bushes.

Larger plants don't always equate to bigger buds, especially in the case of strains bred for attributes other than high yield, like taste. While some strains respond well to pruning, most large cannabis plants with substantial top colas and bud masses have undergone the entire vegetative growth phase without pruning.

If you choose the longer route with extended vegetative growth, ensure you have ample space, as some cannabis strains can grow more than double in height and width during the flowering stage. To initiate flowering, all you need to do is introduce a 12/12 light schedule.

The Importance of the 12/12 Photoperiod

The 12/12 photoperiod is a critical factor in achieving high yields from cannabis plants, a fact that became widely accepted knowledge in the mid-1980s. In their natural outdoor environment, cannabis plants typically grow between April and October or November in the Northern Hemisphere and August to April in the Southern

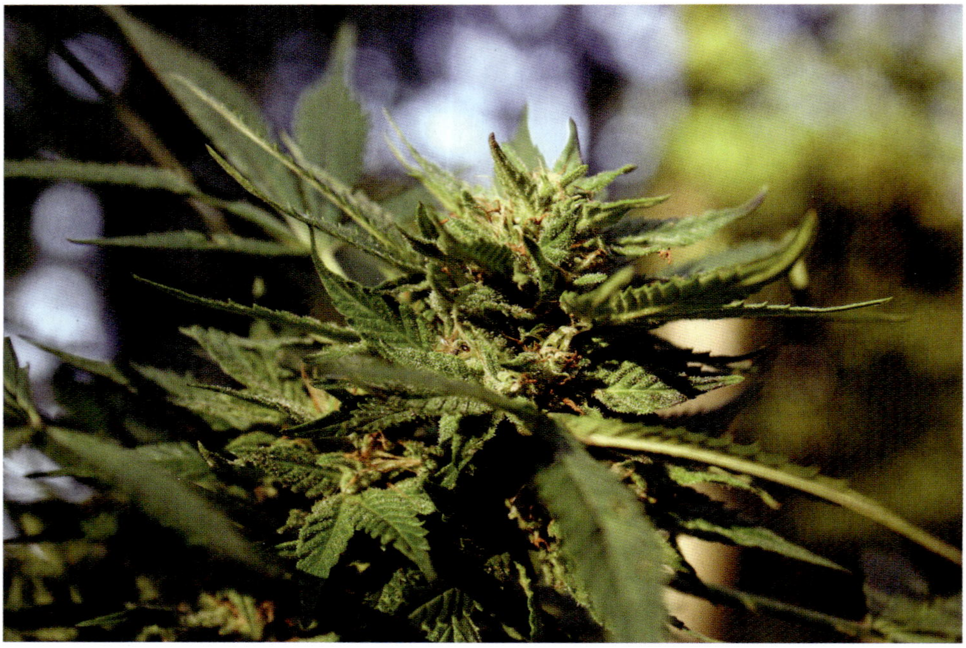

Traditional Skunk#1 is a popular hybrid chosen by growers for both indoor and outdoor growing.

PHOTO: DAVID STRANGE

Hemisphere. In the Northern Hemisphere, plants enter the flowering stage between September and November, as the days become shorter and the nights longer. When the 12/12 photoperiod occurs naturally in the changing seasons, mature cannabis plants are stimulated to flower. As long as this 12/12 light cycle continues, the flowers will continue to grow larger and more abundant. Extending the light hours beyond 12/12 does not increase yield; in fact, it can decrease your results.

To promote the flowering stage indoors, you can manually switch your lights on for 12 hours and then off for 12 hours each day, or you can use a timer to automate this process. During the 12 hours of darkness, maintaining total darkness in your grow area is essential. Even seemingly innocuous sources of light can disrupt the flowering process, including a low-intensity reading lamp or the "on" indicator light of an electrical appliance on the other side of your room. In such cases, you may experience continued vegetative growth, but it will occur for only 12 hours a day. To avoid this, your grow room must be completely sealed to ensure it is entirely lightproof. Even a tiny pinhole can allow photons to pass through.

Preventing Light Leaks in Your Grow Space

To prevent light leaks, you can use grow tents, many of which are labeled as guaranteed lightproof. Many growers opt to use tents, even if they have an entire room, to divide it into compartmentalized grow areas. Grow tents allow you to have a 24/0 light cycle in some tents and a 12/12 cycle in others. They are inexpensive and quick to set up.

In the past, growers copied photographers who often used readily available items from hardware stores to make their film-processing rooms completely lightproof, such as thick black screening around door frames and any open light points, hanging black strips at entrances and exits, and so on. Darkroom photographers now use grow tents that have been rebranded as darkroom tents.

If you've covered your grow room with Mylar, you should already be well on your way to preventing light leaks. To check for potential light leaks, enter your grow room and turn off the lights. Wait for at least three minutes for your eyes to adjust to the darkness. Once they do, you should be able to identify potential sources of light leaks. Some pinpoint-sized light leaks can only be detected using light sensors, also called quantum light sensors.

Any light leak can compromise your results dramatically. Seal it up.

Unlike simple light meters, light sensors offer the most reliable assessment of light leaks. They are typically USB-powered, allowing you to run a cable from the sensor to the outside of the tent, where you can take readings. Place the sensor in the tent just before you close the zipper and seal it off for the test. While the sensor can detect the presence of a light leak, you'll still need to locate the actual leak by moving the sensor around until you find the highest reading, indicating the proximity of the light leak. Mylar can then be used to seal the leak effectively.

In getting this step right, you achieve two objectives that lead to significantly better yields: You ensure that all the photons emitted from your light source remain within the grow area for absorption and you prevent any external photons from entering the room during the crucial 12/12 flowering photoperiod.

Pre-Flowering Considerations for 24/0 and 18/6 Photoperiods

With the use of LEDs, running a 24/0 light cycle has become very cost-effective, making it accessible even for budget-conscious growers. In the past, some growers opted for an 18/6 vegetative photoperiod instead of a 24/0 cycle, the 18/6 cycle considered more natural. It also reduces the carbon footprint of cannabis production, especially if the upstream energy source used is not environmentally-friendly. However, studies

PHOTO: STONED ROSIE

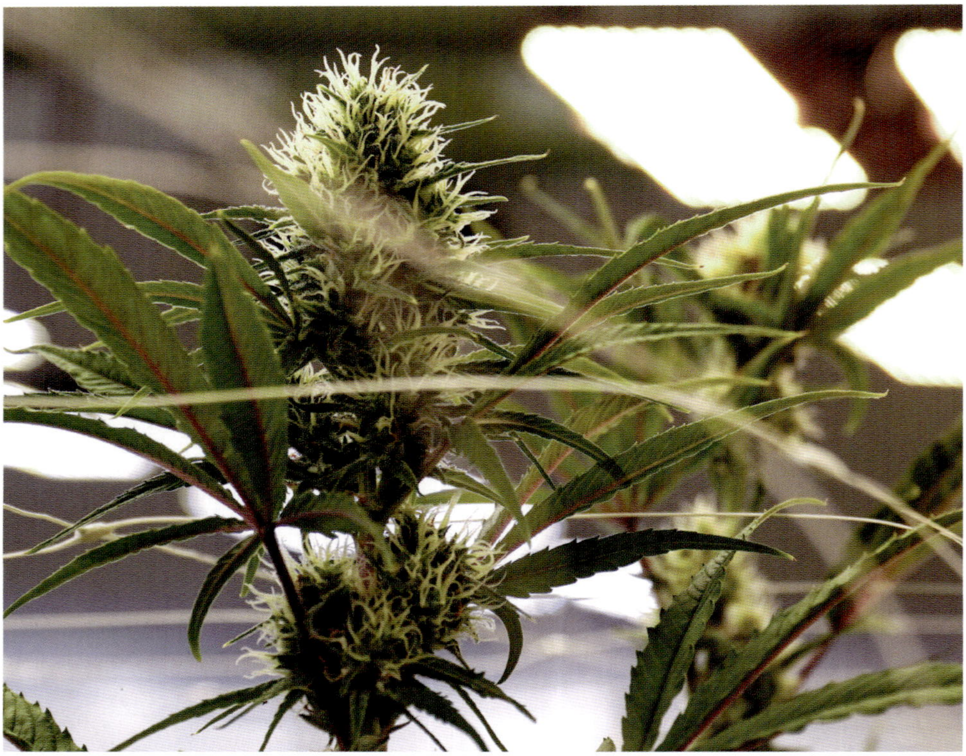

A few weeks into flowering, these plants look healthy under LEDs. A 12/12 photoperiod allows these plants to flower as they naturally would outdoors in late summer/autumn.

comparing growth outcomes have consistently shown that 24/0 leads to higher yields. Note that a photoperiod below 18/6, such as 17/7, is not recommended,[1] as it tends to result in reduced yields and is associated with an increased risk of hermaphrodites.

Flowering Female-to-Male Ratios

After nurturing your plants, you might find yourself in a situation where all your seeds have produced male plants. If this happens, write a letter to the seed bank, explaining that all of your seeds turned out to be male and include photographs as evidence. Seed banks and breeders are not in control of male-to-female ratios, so it's not their responsibility—but if you're genuine in your communication and a bit lucky, the seed bank may send you some free seeds or offer a discount on your next purchase.

Some growers may get 100% females, and others may end up with 100% males, though such extreme cases are rare. Typically it's about half. Five or more females from a pack of 15 seeds is considered acceptable. Ending up with fewer than five females is disappointing, but you require only one female plant if you intend to clone and preserve that particular genetic line. This is when you buy standard seeds; if you are buying feminized seeds, ending up with hermaphrodites is a risk that comes with the territory.

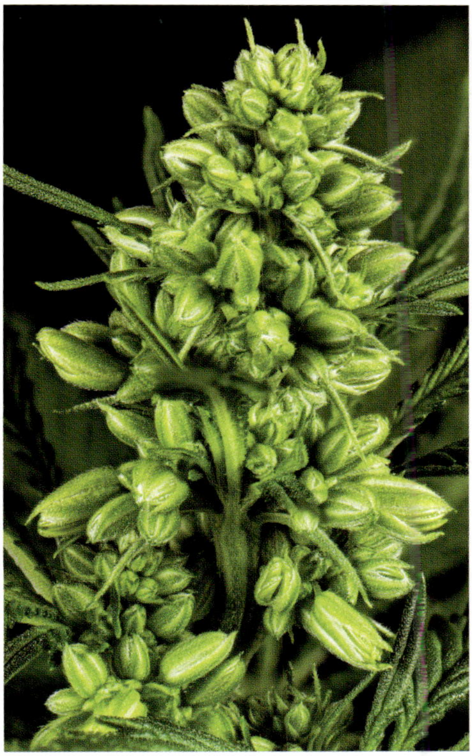

These male flowers are ready to open and release pollen.

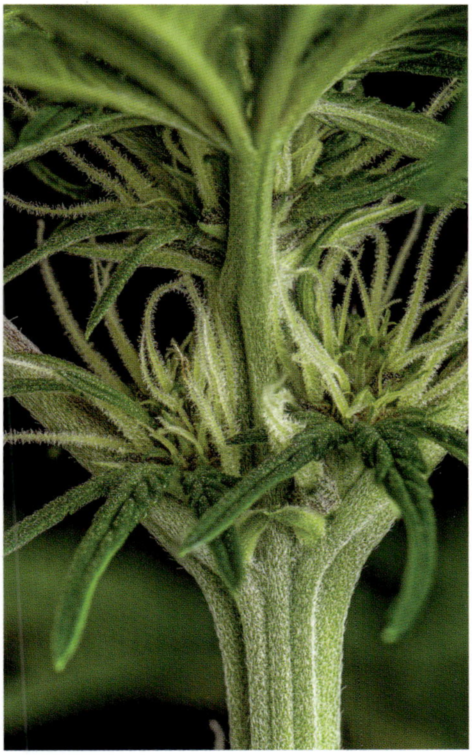

Day 34 of flowering. It is a slow process, but it is worth it for the ending.

Growing a larger number of female plants is beneficial for a broader selection when choosing a clone cutting. Getting an unfavorable percentage is a common occurrence in cannabis cultivation and is random. There will be times when the odds work in your favor.

Bracts Are Not Calyx Development

The circle in the illustration highlights the location where growers should initially look for calyx development. It does not depict calyx development, but shows two new sharp-looking points emerging from the nodes. Novice growers often mistake these early-stage shoots for calyx development. While the illustration highlights the right region, actual calyx development occurs right next to these spine-like structures, which are called "bracts." Bracts protect the cannabis flowers. In other plant species, bracts may attract insects for pollination with their colorful appearance.

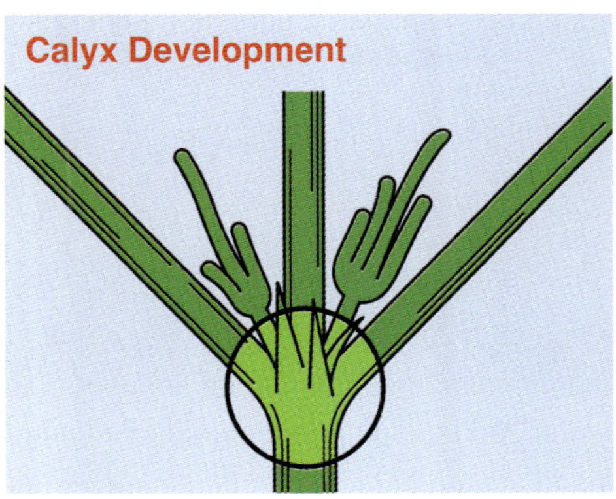

PHOTOS: ROB BRAMHILL

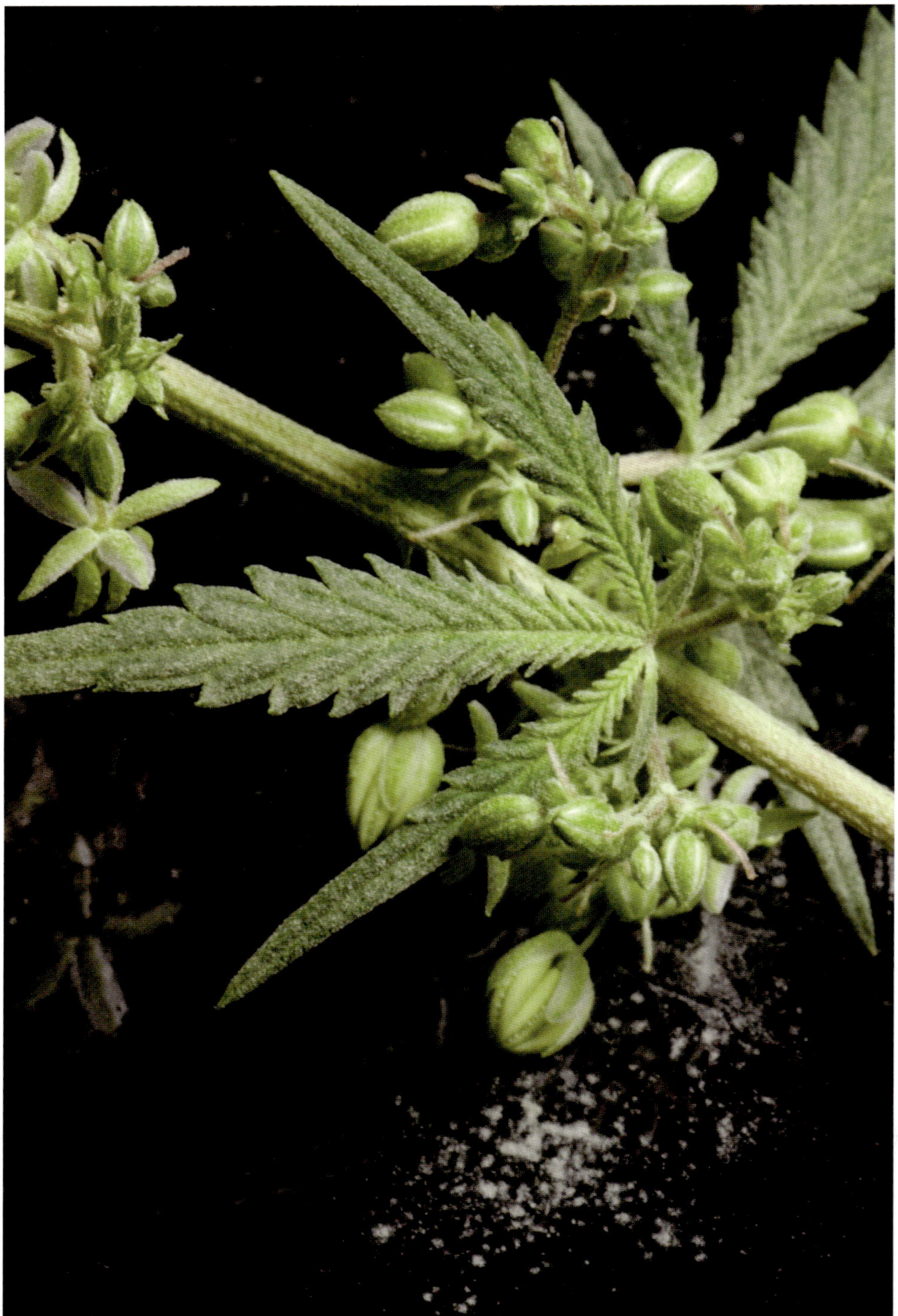

PHOTO: ED BORG

Any movement of a male plant with open male flowers will drop pollen. This can be helpful when recovering pollen that you want to use on female plants later.

Male Flowering

Male plants do not require a specific photoperiod to release pollen. Male flowers can emerge within a few hours or days of calyx development, regardless of whether you're using a 24/0, 18/6, or 12/12 photoperiod. However, male flowers tend to grow more vigorously and abundantly under the 12/12 photoperiod. The rapid onset of male flowering is a critical concern for growers aiming for a sinsemilla harvest, and demands their active attention.

Once a male plant begins to flower, it continues to do so through its flowering period, producing new calyx formations and more male flowers. It can take anywhere from 12 hours to one week from the initial calyx development for male flowers to appear and release their pollen. Therefore, it's essential to separate male plants from female ones as early as possible if you intend to grow a sinsemilla crop. Males tend to appear before females, but thorough inspection is necessary as there are always exceptions.

Pollen

Collecting pollen can be done in several ways, depending on how much control you want over the dispersed pollen. When collecting pollen, turn off all fans, as they will spread the pollen throughout your grow room. Clear grip seal plastic bags of different smaller sizes offer the best way to capture pollen in a controlled manner. Use these reclosable bags to cover the male flowers. They are also transparent, allowing photosynthesis, but pollen release doesn't need light now. The main advantage of the transparency is seeing the pollen gathering in the bag. If you don't want to use plastic, you can use a cheesecloth tied into a sack around the male flowers, but you will likely need to cut away the branch and open the sack on a table to gather the collected pollen. You can also cut away the branch with the plastic bag method. In many cases, preparing every male flower to capture pollen is too much work, but you can still acquire falling pollen by placing down sheets of white paper to surround the plant's stem when the first pollen falls so that you gather the rest. Pollen not captured in bags can be shaken from the leaves onto the white sheets where other pollen will have fallen. You can fold sheets with pollen in them. More techniques for pollen collection are covered in Chapter 17 on breeding.

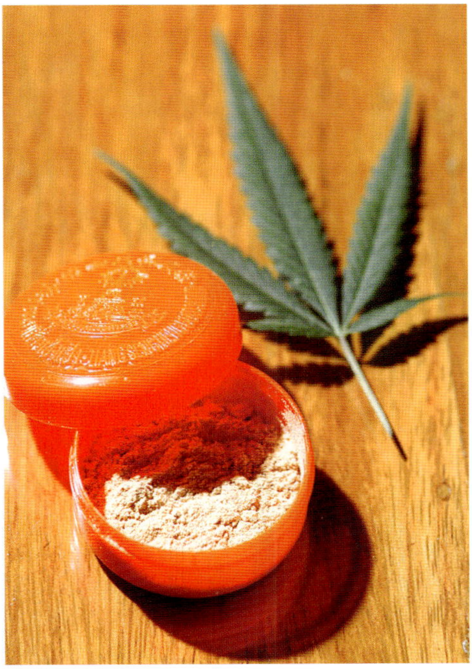

PHOTO: ED BORG

Save your pollen in containers for future use.

Moisture is detrimental to pollen and can cause it to deteriorate. Proper storage methods, discussed in Chapter 16, are essential to preserve pollen quality. If you wish to produce seeds, you can pollinate female flowers by brushing pollen onto them. Female plants can be pollinated at various stages, but the best time is 15 to 30 days into their flowering period. Pollinating plants less than three weeks before harvest may result in immature seeds, although this can vary with the strain.

Flowering

Assuming everything has gone smoothly and you've removed the male plants, the female plants will now enter the flowering stage of their life cycle.

During flowering, male cannabis plants produce pollen sacks that, when ripe, burst open, releasing pollen and fertilizing the female plants. The female plants develop white hairs, or pistils, at the internodes and the main bud, or top cola. The top cola typically carries the most pistils. These pistils start to curl slightly and grow longer and thicker as flowering progresses. They are sticky to the touch and become covered in resin during the flowering period. Their resin serves the dual purpose of catching pollen and providing UV protection. Avoid disturbing the pistils, as they contain valuable THC and other medicinal cannabinoids. If the female plant isn't pollinated, she will attempt to produce more resin to capture pollen, resulting in the desired sinsemilla crop, with bigger and better buds.

During the strict 12/12 light cycle, female plants will experience more growth, producing more leaves, branches, and flowers until they reach the peak of their flowering period. The lower leaves will stretch out to maximize light absorption, and the plant will take on a cone shape with a wide base and a narrow top.

Peak of Flowering

The breeder's recommended flowering times and a strain's specific characteristics can guide you in determining the optimal time for harvest. During the peak flowering period, the pistils at the tips of the female flowers will swell. As this swelling occurs, they will change color, typically transitioning from white to shades of orange, red, or brown, a sign that they are ready for harvesting. Chapter 16 provides detailed instructions on proper harvesting techniques.

Do not interfere with your plants during this stage. Minimize the time you spend with them and avoid unnecessary contact, as excessive handling can drain energy that should be directed toward bud production. Give your plants room to grow.

Dehumidification During Flowering

While not essential for beginner growers, experienced growers often use a dehumidifier to reduce humidity to prevent or slow down mold issues during flowering. By

Peak Flowering

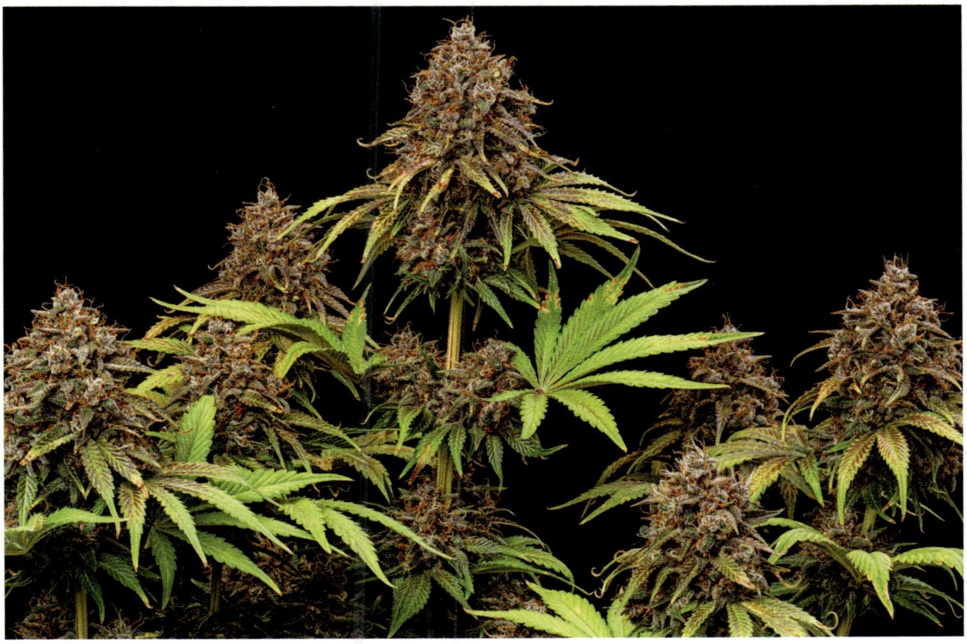

This is what it is all about: Many colorful colas at their peak of flowering and ready to be harvested. Leaf discoloration is common around this time.

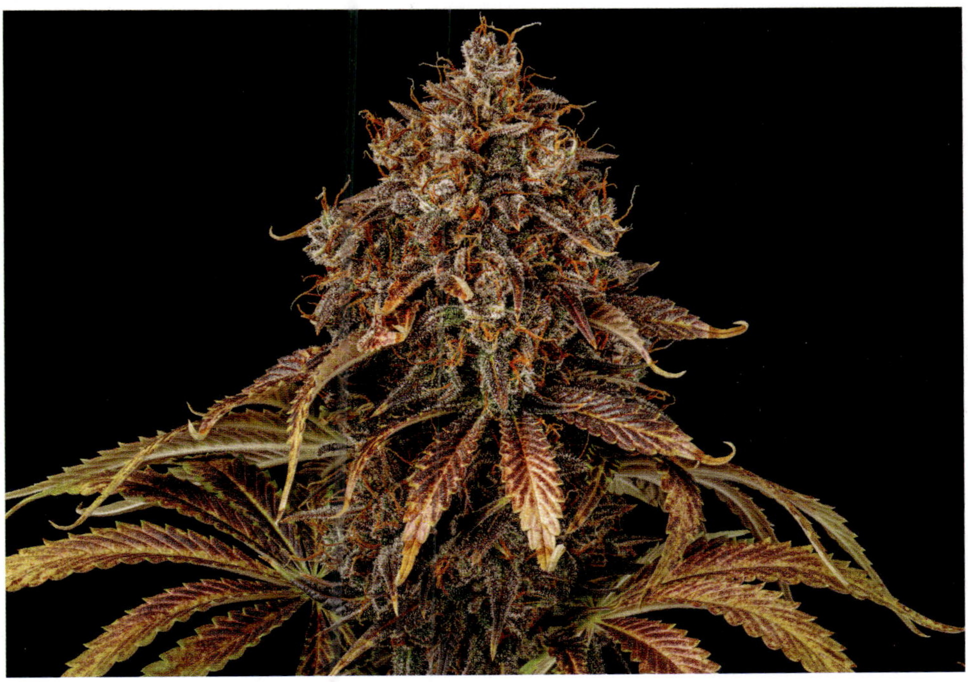

The flowering plant has used up its stored nutrients by peak flowering, which causes the leaves to change color. Most of the pistils have become amber, signaling time to harvest.

PHOTOS: ROB BRAMHILL

reducing the moisture in the air, they also encourage more resin production, as the plant generates additional trichomes to protect against dry conditions. This form of mild stress can yield better results. If successful, it can significantly enhance the frosty appearance of your buds. The increase in trichome numbers is a good thing, but this is at the risk of possible stress-related issues. Flowering cannabis plants tend to thrive with a relative humidity (RH) range of 40–55%, though lower RH levels are even more favorable. If you lower humidity levels during the final weeks of flowering, aim for as low as possible, even below 25%. Other mild stress techniques include gentle airflow or plant movement, which should already be occurring with proper ventilation.

Stress-Related Sex Issues (Hermaphrodites)

If you switch to a 12/12 light cycle before pre-flowers have appeared, you may encounter stress-related sex issues (hermaphrodites) and/or abnormal bud growth.

Cannabis plants are typically not self-pollinating. Instead, they are dioecious, which means they produce male and female sex organs on separate plants and require cross-pollination between plants to reproduce. A single plant that possesses both male and female sex organs is referred to as monoecious and produces seeds rather than the coveted sinsemilla. Dioecious plants evolved from monoecious ones by segregating the sex organs between separate male and female plants. Some cannabis strains may still exhibit monoecious traits due to specific genetic or environmental factors.

Cannabis exhibits a high degree of genetic plasticity, including variability in sex determination. Cannabis chromosomes typically follow XY sex-determination, where a plant with XX chromosomes is female and a plant with XY chromosomes is male. Using a microscope to observe the cannabis plant during meiosis can help you determine the plant's chromosomes.

There are two possible causes for the monoecious, or hermaphrodite, trait in cannabis:

1. Chemical Induction: Some chemicals, such as silver thiosulfate and silver nitrate, can induce the monoecious condition by influencing plant hormone regulators. These chemicals are typically used in controlled scientific experiments.
2. Environmental Stressors: Stressors like photoperiod irregularities and low temperatures may trigger monoecious sexual expression in cannabis plants because phytohormones, like auxins, and their jasmonic acid ratio are stimulated by these environmental factors.

Research has identified over 10,500 differentially expressed genes, with about 200 potentially responsible for male flower development on female cannabis plants. Various hormones influence sex expression; however, additional research is required.

Hermaphrodites

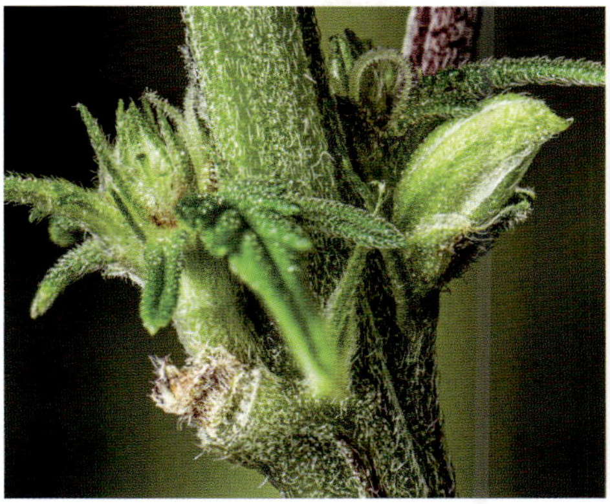

Hermaphrodites can be difficult to determine in the early stages of pre-flowering.

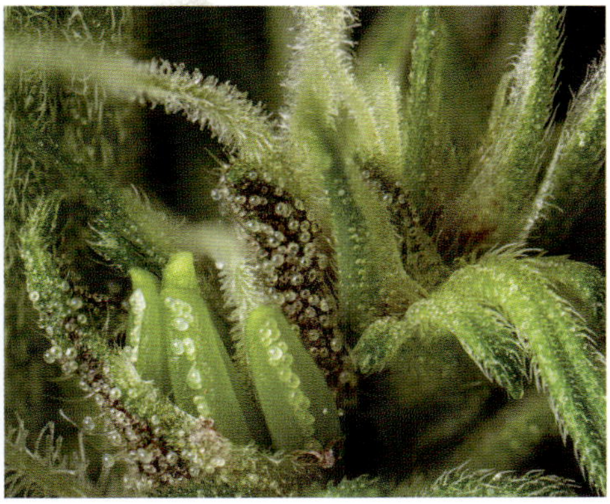

Pistils and male banana shapes indicate hermaphrodites.

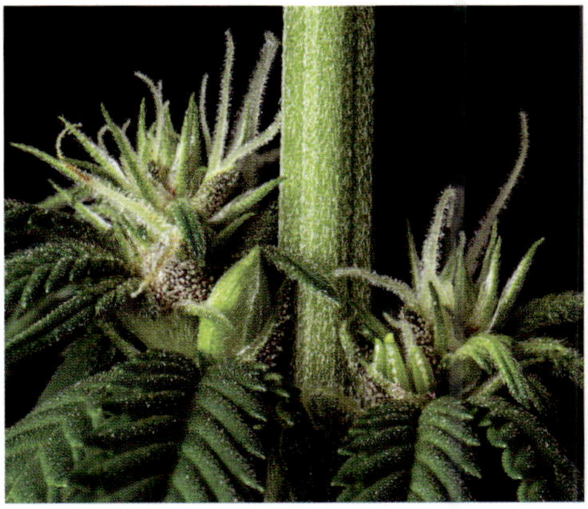

Male flowers are hidden among the females.

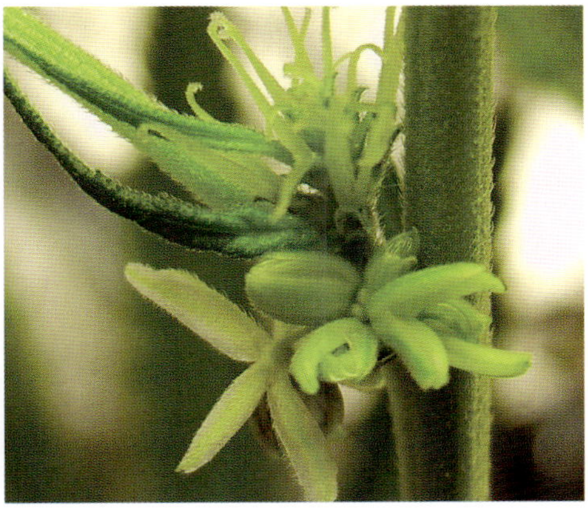

Male flowers are very apparent among the female pistils.

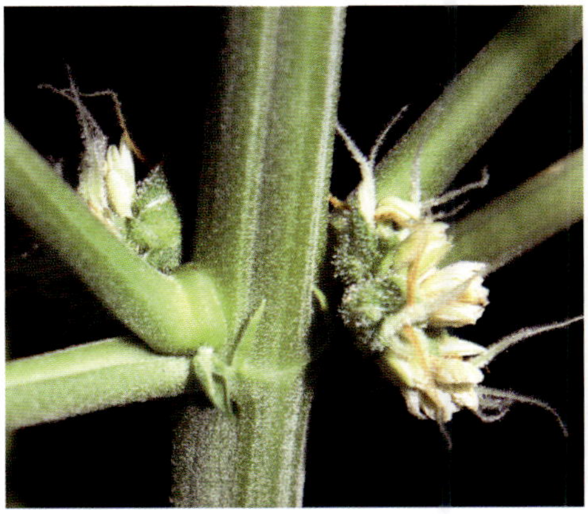

Male-to-female ratios on hermaphrodites can vary.

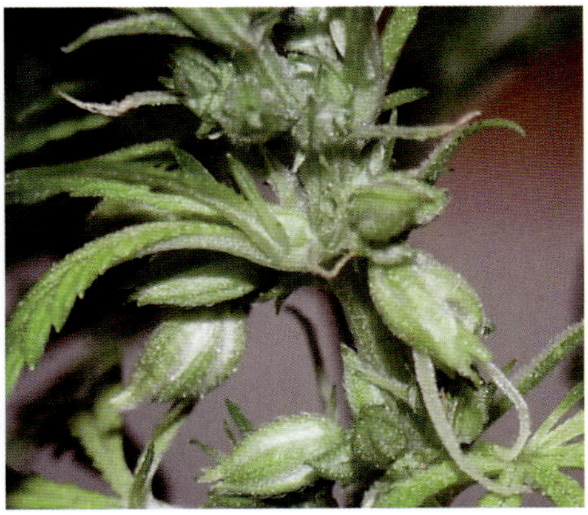

Mostly male flowers with some female pistils.

PHOTOS: ROB BRAMHILL (TOP ROW AND MIDDLE LEFT), NMS (MIDDLE RIGHT), DAVID STRANGE (BOTTOM LEFT), HANNA BLISS (BOTTOM RIGHT)

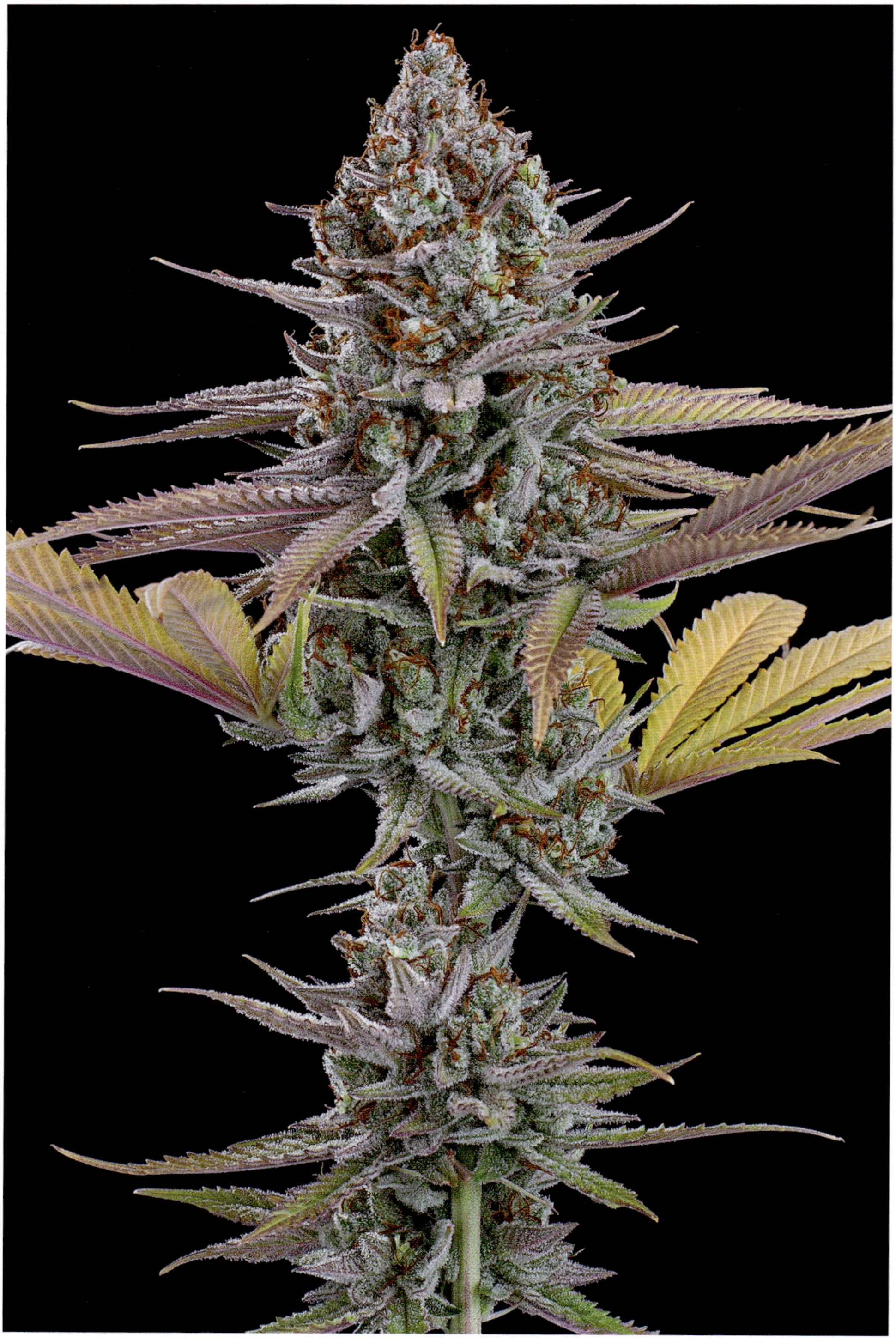

PHOTO: RUSSELL-HOWLAND PHOTOGRAPHY

Enormous top cola with no gaps between internodes indicates this plant was grown with the love and care it needed.

Hermaphrodites can produce seeds even if all male plants have been removed from the grow room. These seeds can be collected and grown. They usually result in more females than males, often exceeding the expected 1:1 male-to-female ratio. This bias may be attributed to mutations or variations like single-nucleotide polymorphisms (SNPs) and genetic sequence deletions. Copia-like retrotransposons, which are a class of recurring DNA sequences that change their position on the plant's Y chromosome, may play a role in altering sexual expression.

The hermaphrodite condition typically manifests between the fourth and seventh week of the flowering period and continues until harvest, allowing for self-pollination and seed development. To mitigate these tendencies, environmental stressors such as photoperiod disruptions and low temperatures must be addressed.

For further information, refer to the 2020 study by Zamir K. Punja and Janesse E. Holmes, "Hermaphroditism in Marijuana (*Cannabis sativa L.*) Inflorescences – Impact on Floral Morphology, Seed Formation, Progeny Sex Ratios, and Genetic Variation"[2] in *Frontiers in Plant Science*, Volume 11.

Abnormal Bud Growth

The hermaphrodite condition is by far the most common form of abnormal bud growth you will come across. Genetic diseases caused by mutations are rarer, so look for hermaphrodites if something doesn't appear right with the flowers. Additionally, self-pollination creates seeded buds, so the crop is no longer sinsemilla because pollen spreads. One hermaphrodite plant can seed the rest of the crop. The plant needs to be removed.

Photoperiod disruption, cold temperatures, pests, or a nutrient disorder will not directly cause hermaphrodites, but indirectly, the stress induced by these conditions may lead to the development of hermaphrodites. Some strains may be more genetically susceptible to conditions that stimulate the disorder. The bottom line is that good practices can avoid issues promoting hermaphrodites.

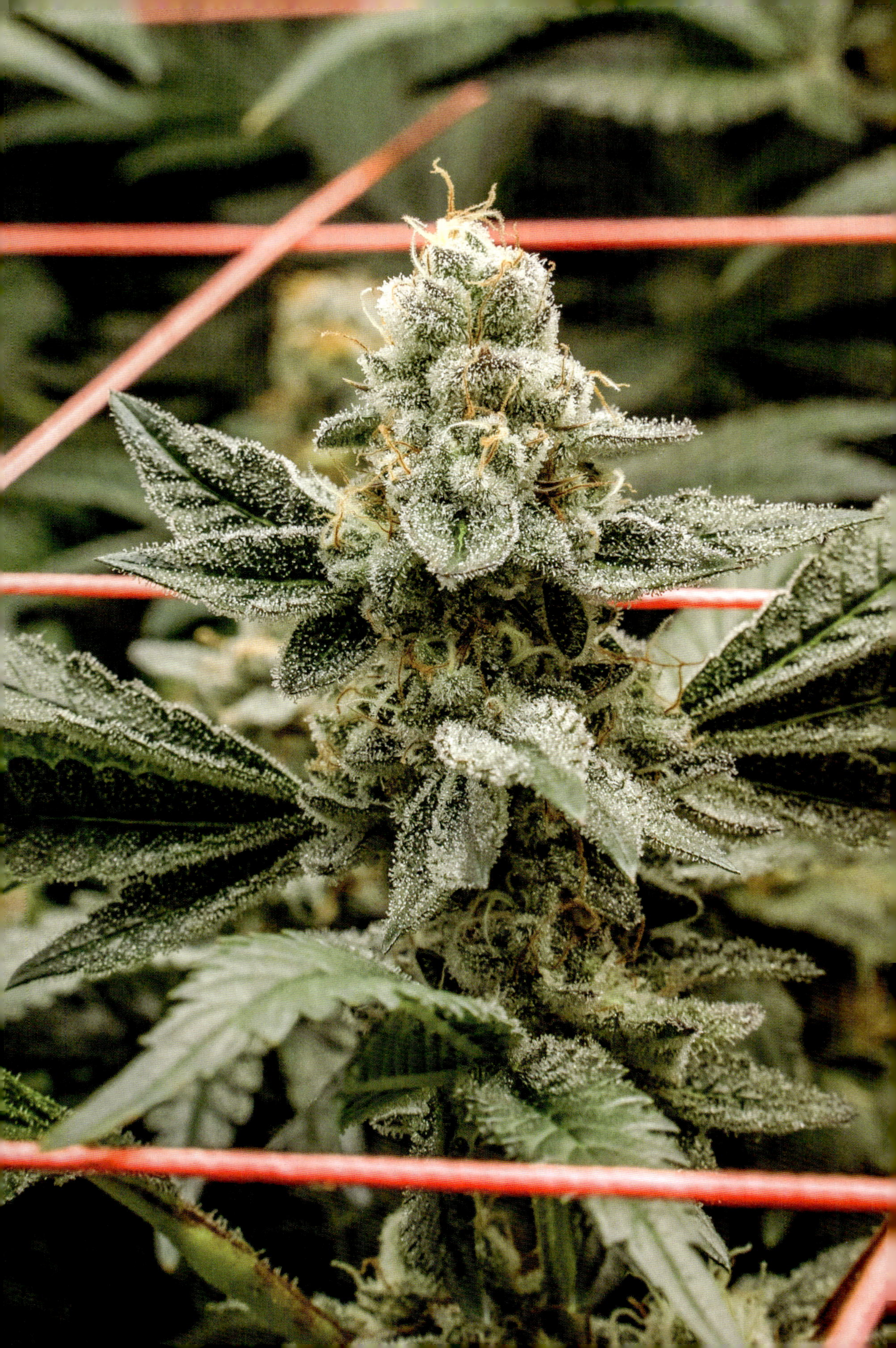

10

Indoor Grow Methods

Indoor growing may seem complicated to the beginner, but learning the advanced information on indoor growing in this chapter will guarantee your success in an effective, cost-efficient indoor grow space.

One-Light-Per-Plant System

In experiments to gauge a strain's potential, the golden lighting ratio is one light per plant, which allows each plant to maximize the available light and grow in optimal conditions. Placing multiple plants under one light results in them sharing the same available energy. The combined yield from a multi-plant setup is generally expected to be comparable to that of a single plant grown under the same light. This concept is rooted in the conservation of energy and aligns with the calculations discussed in Chapters 7 on daily light integral (DLI) and photosynthetic photon flux (PPF).

Most growers aim for a balance of yield, potency, and flavor. Many award-winning or photo-worthy plants have been grown under the one-light-per-plant system. However, your yield per plant will often appear lower than the advertising picture, which was likely done under a one-light-per-plant system intended for a specific type of photo shoot. All plants aren't under a one-light-per-plant system because while using this method to maximize yield from a single plant, you must also consider efficiency and cost. Getting a higher yield from more plants under the same amount of light is something we can do.

Instead of cultivating one visually impressive plant, many growers opt to grow multiple plants using techniques to optimize space, light, and time. Their objective is to maximize yield with a smaller financial investment, which can be done by growing multiple plants under one light to fully use the available energy. Dedicating a 1000-watt HID light to a single plant is not cost-effective. A single plant in a one-light-per-plant setup may produce around 1 pound of bud, whereas three plants, when managed effectively, can yield 1.5 or even 2 pounds. Achieving this level of productivity involves advanced

PHOTO: JOE'S CANNA GROWS

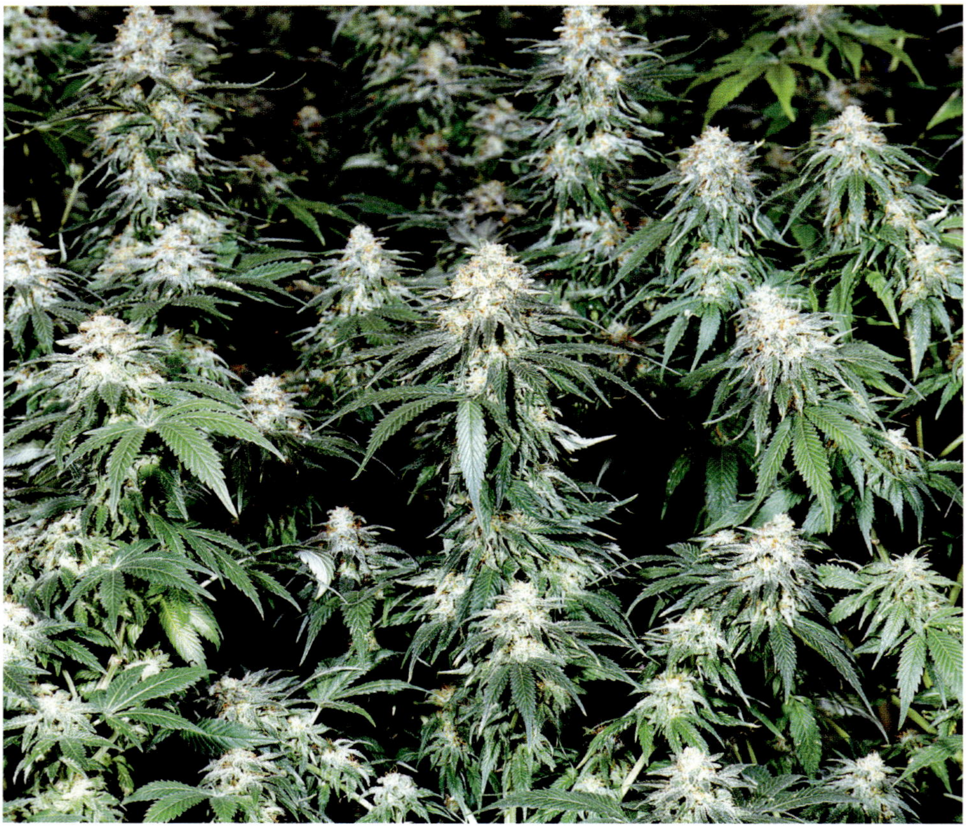

A 6 X 6-foot room in full bloom demonstrates that patience and time can produce top-quality bud.

PHOTO: ED BORG

techniques to boost yields. These methods have evolved over the last 25 years and are more manageable and cost-effective today due to the advent of LED lights.

The four primary systems commonly used by indoor growers are:

1. Sea of Green (SOG): Focuses on maximizing the number of plants in the given space, emphasizing efficiency.
2. Screen of Green (ScrOG): Involves training plants using a horizontal mesh screen, or trellis, to maintain an even canopy. ScrOG also focuses on producing substantial top colas while potentially using upper and lower branches to fill the canopy.
3. Tent Growing: Grows several plants in an enclosed, confined space.
4. Cabinet Growing: Like tent growing, but uses a solid structure, which can be assembled, built from scratch, or modified.

Tent and cabinet growing can be combined with SOG and ScrOG techniques. While cabinets offer the advantage of concealment, they require renovation work for air intake and outtake, Mylar lining, odor control, and light-leak management, making them less popular than tents, which are easier to set up, dismantle, and relocate.

Sativa Hybrid Growing

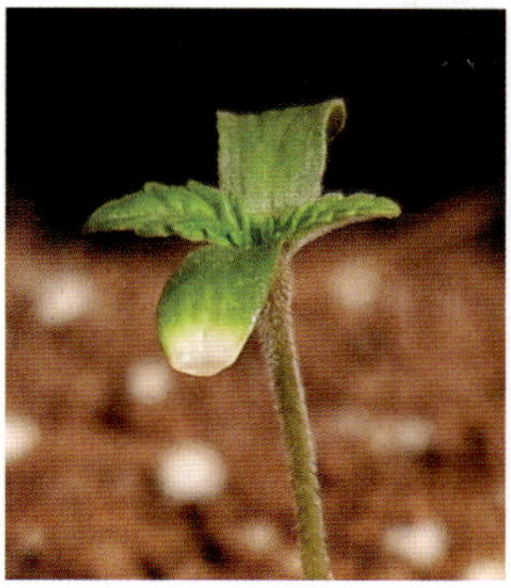

Seedling shows promise.

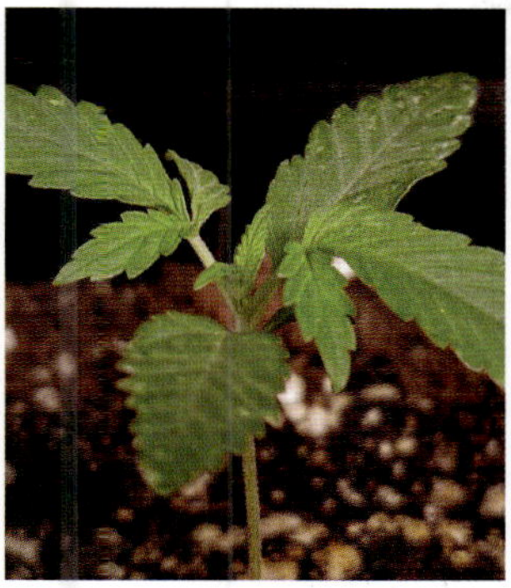

Healthy new formations.

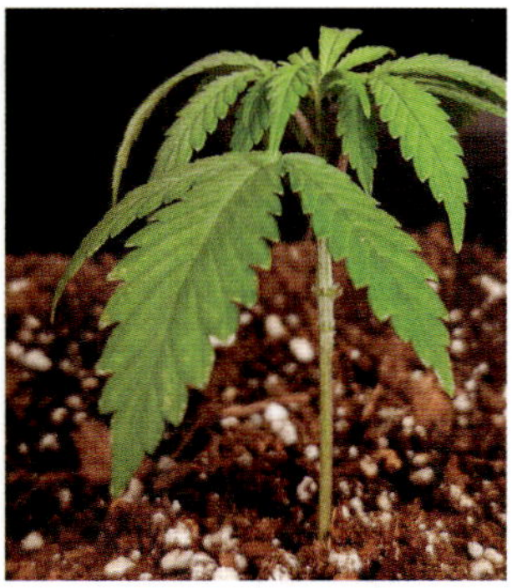

Seedling shows more new leaves.

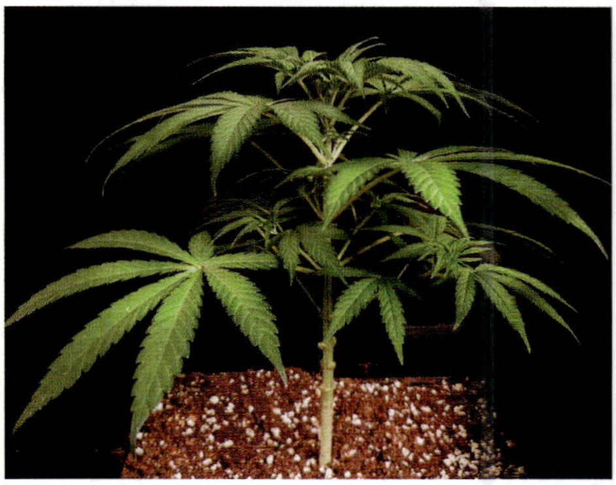

Vegetative growth is bushy. This trend of growing leaves continues.

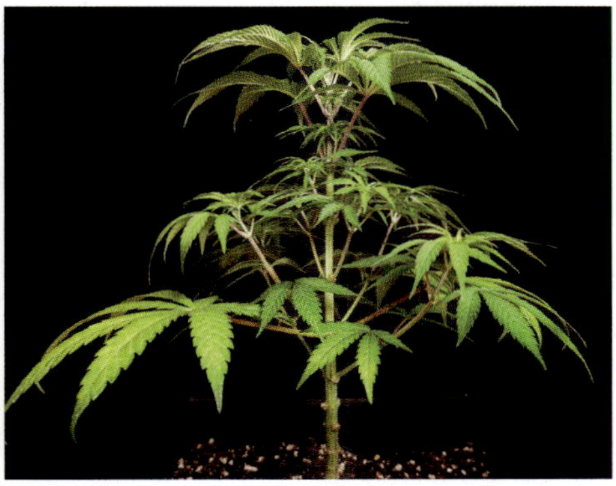

The plant grows more side branches and makes a push upwards.

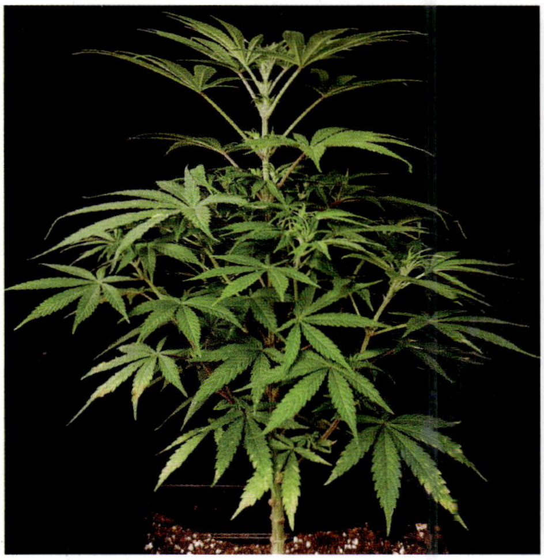

Vertical growth is going to dominate later vegetation.

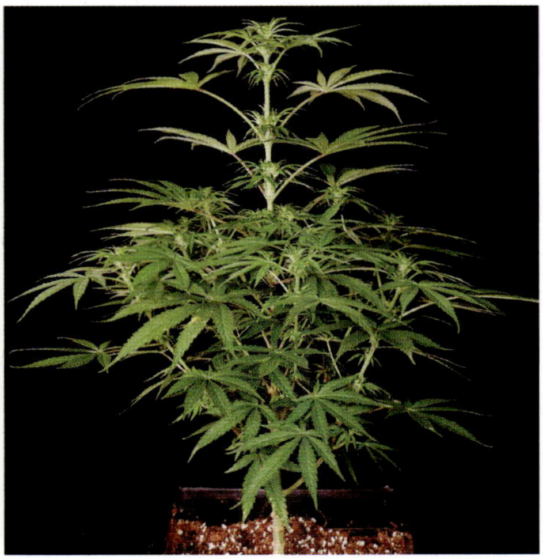

The plant has reached the height for pre-flowering.

continues...

PHOTOS: DOCTORSCHOICE.FARM / PHOTOGRAPHED BY FRANZ JANYR

Sativa Hybrid Growing *continued*

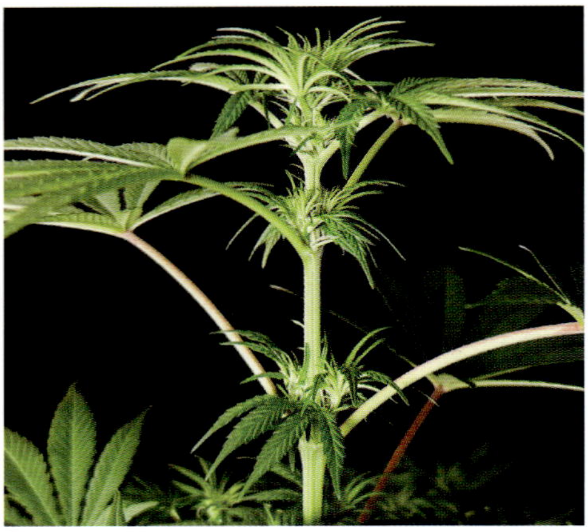

Pre-flowering initiates. Node regions fill in.

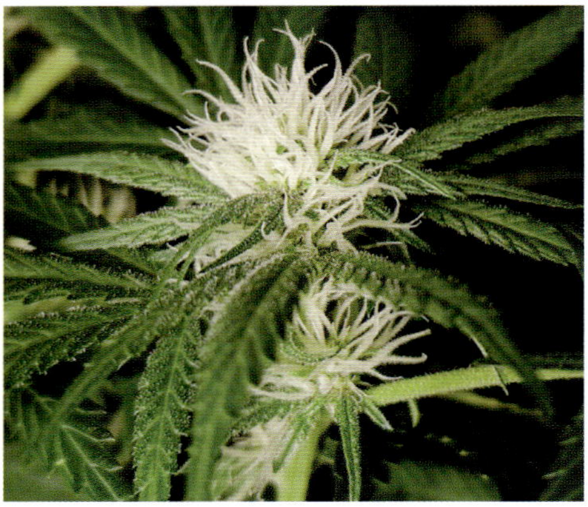

More pistils grow at the flowering nodes.

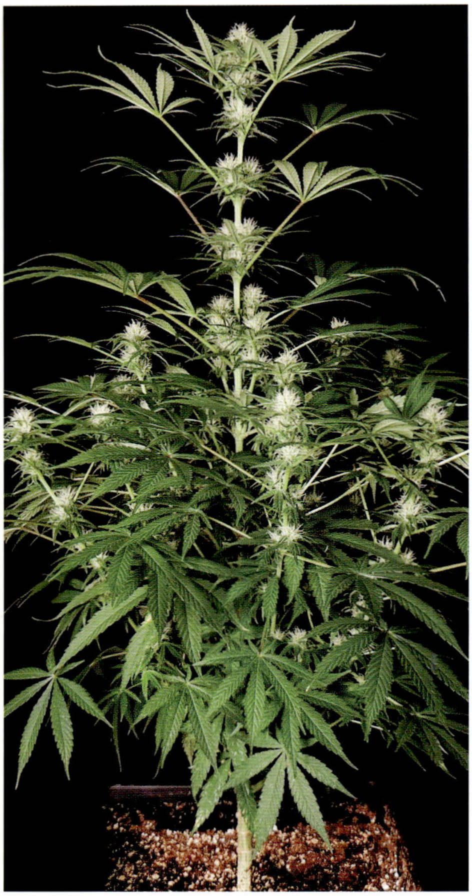

The pre-flowering plant continues to grow upwards.

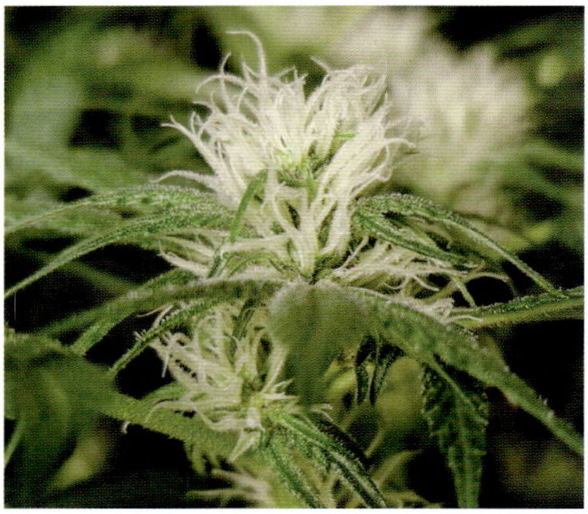

Trichomes begin to show on the flowering leaves.

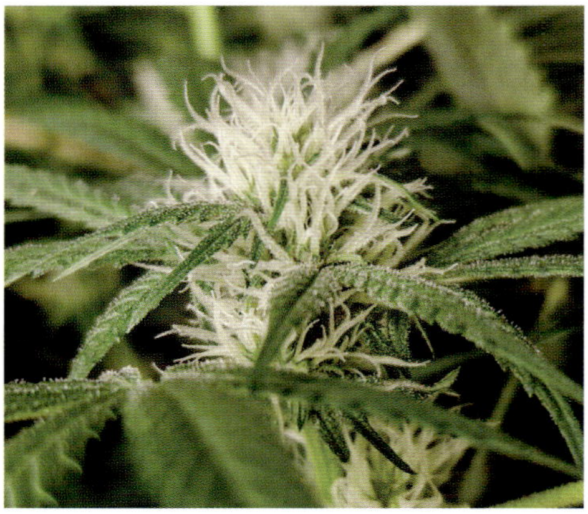

All flowering cannabis plants start with cream-colored pistils.

PHOTOS: DOCTORSCHOICE.FARM / PHOTOGRAPHED BY FRANZ JANYR

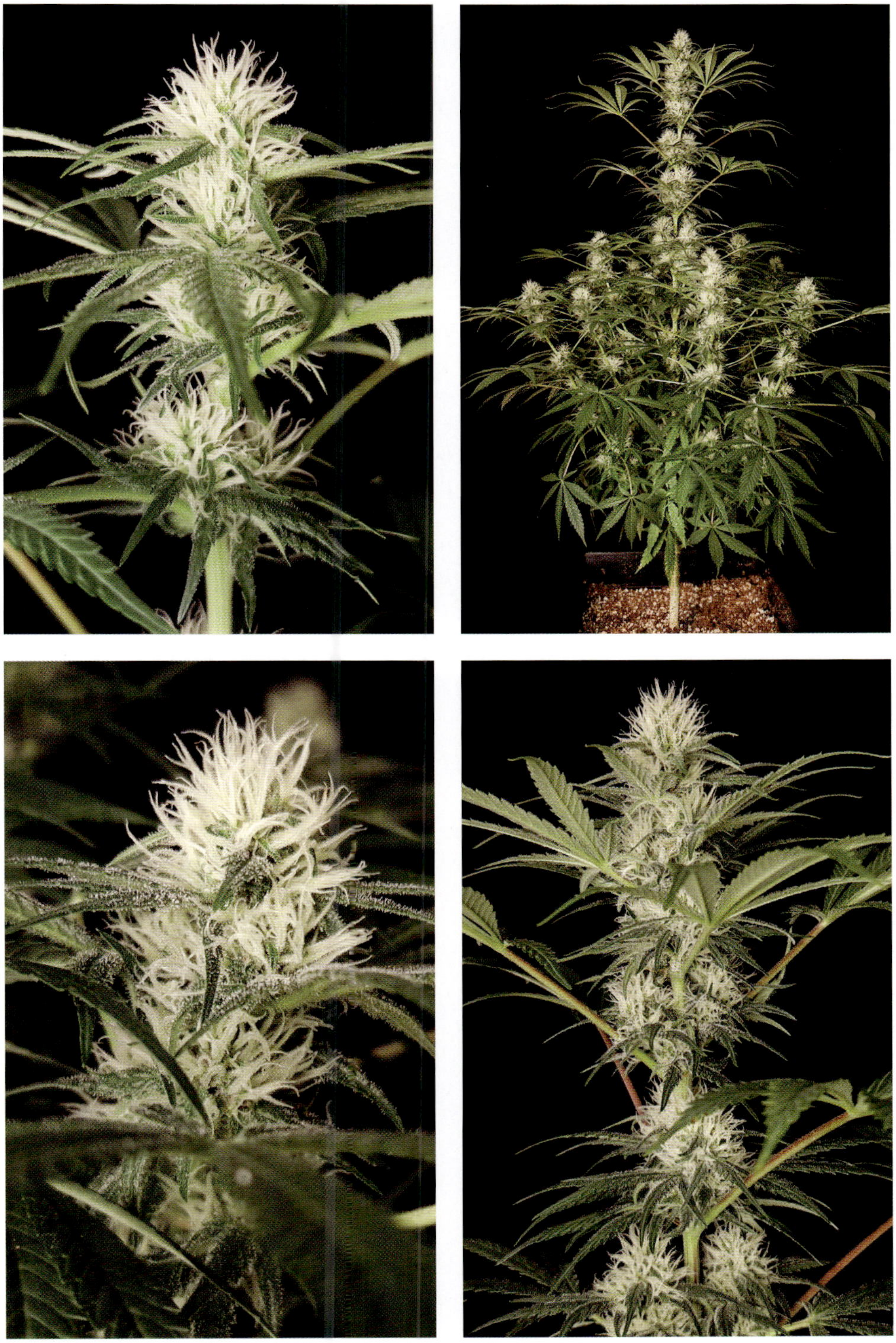

There are many benefits to growing your own cannabis, but the pleasure you get from seeing your hard work paying off with beautiful flowers like these should not be underestimated. *continues...*

Sativa Hybrid Growing *continued*

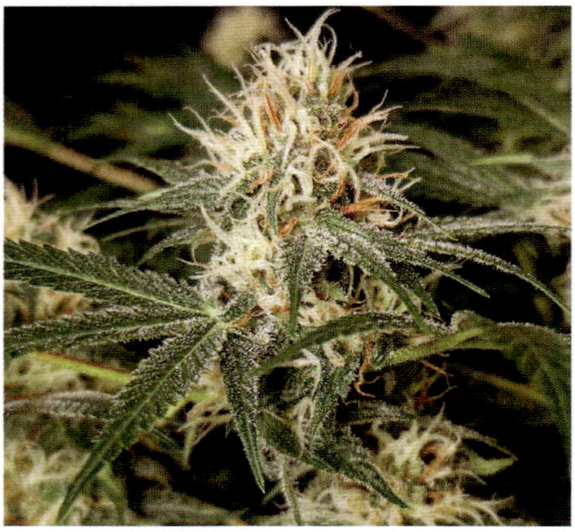

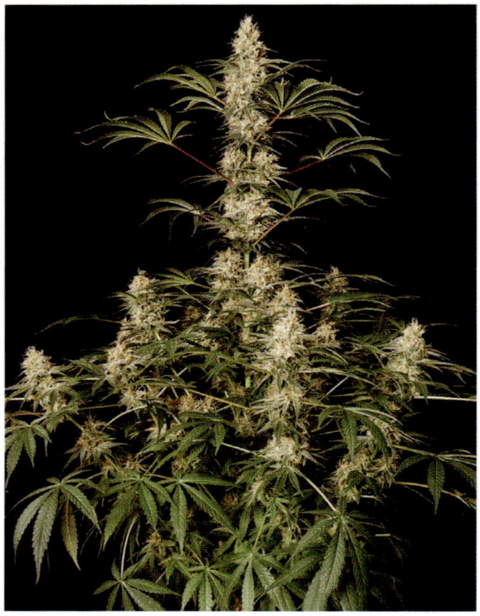

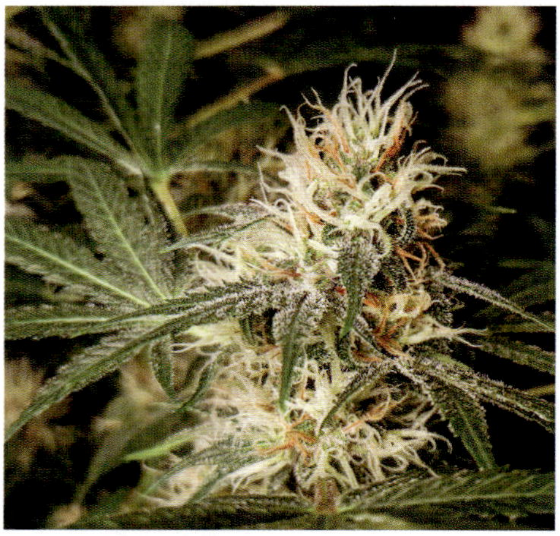

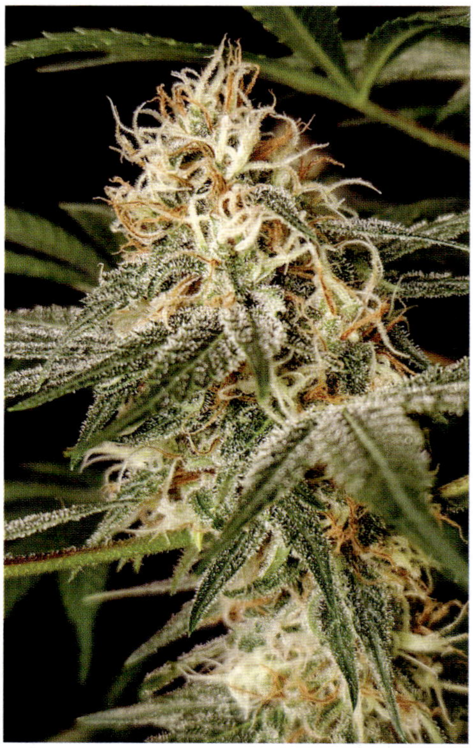

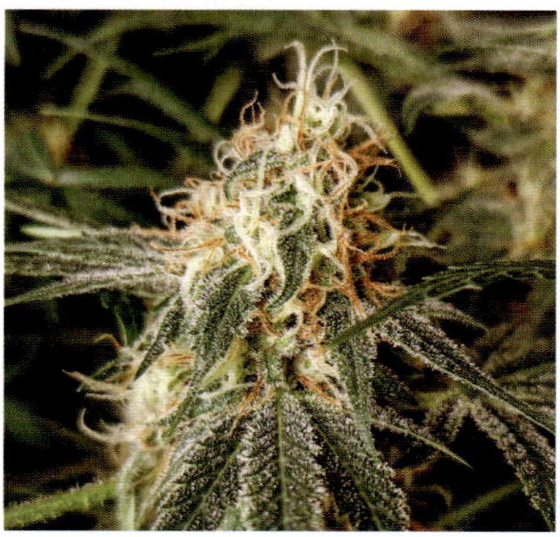

The flower combines complexity and simplicity, showcasing beauty at every node. When the trichomes become this frosty, it's like they're coming straight out of a freezer. The pistils curl more each day and begin to change color.

PHOTOS: DOCTORSCHOICE.FARM / PHOTOGRAPHED BY FRANZ JANYR

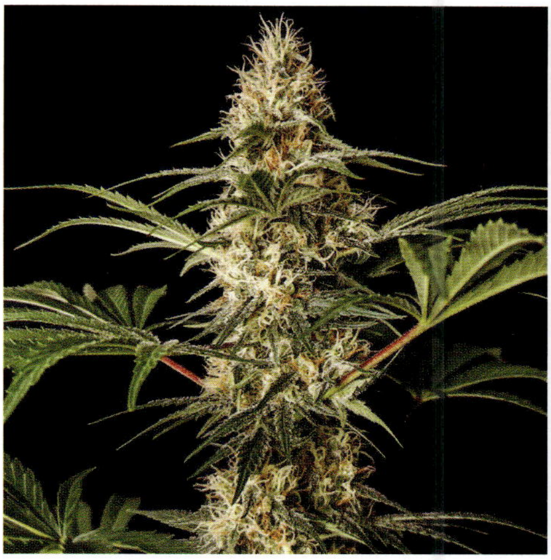
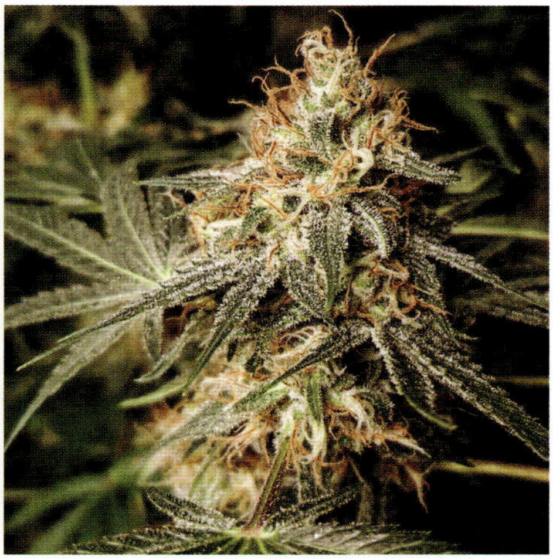
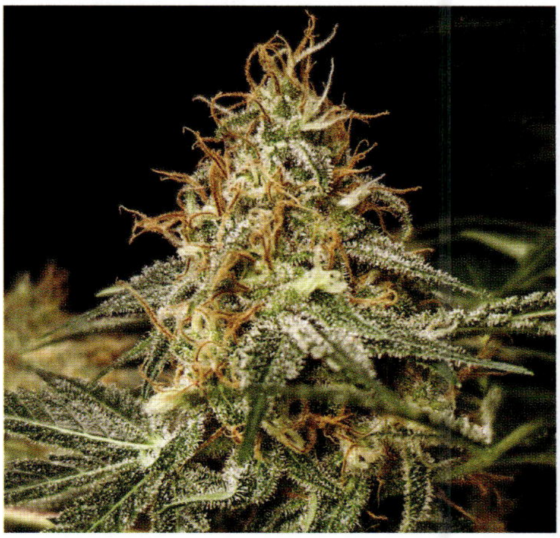
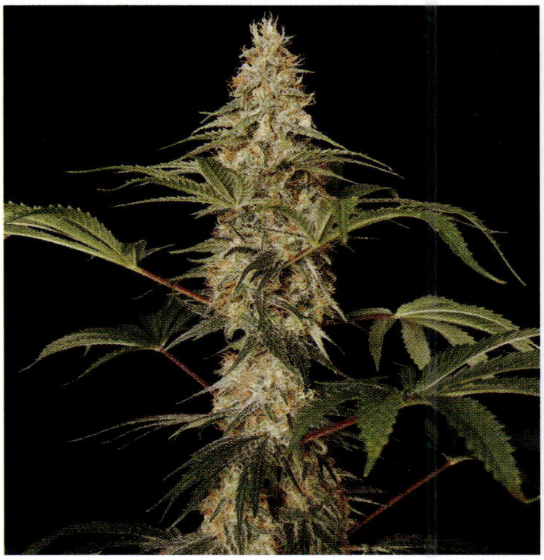
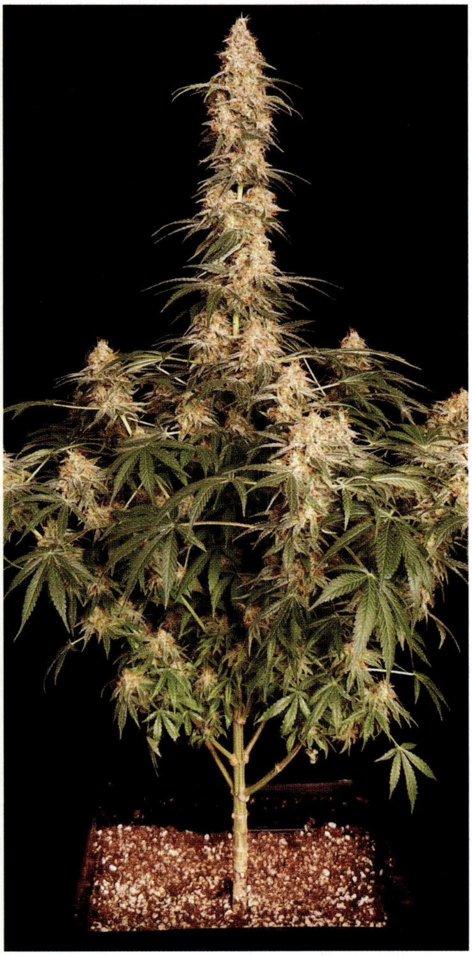

Every bud bursts with pistils, revealing nature's secrets. The pistils turn amber, forming a major top cola with buds at each node. Towering skyward, the sativa genetics shine through. *continues...*

Sativa Hybrid Growing *continued*

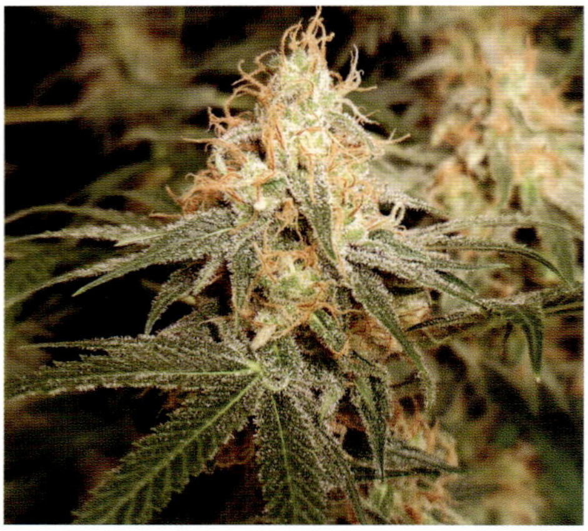

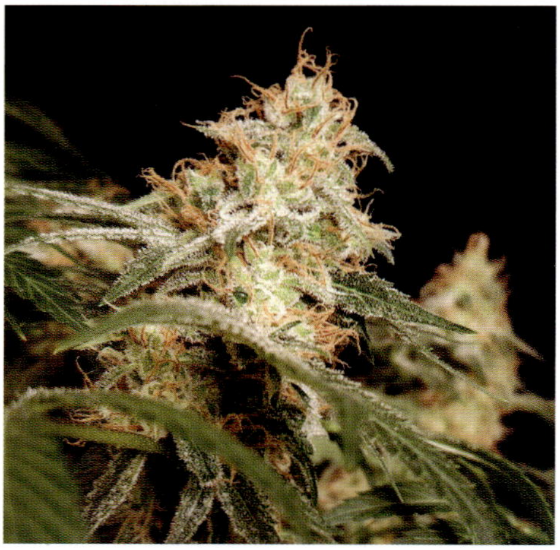

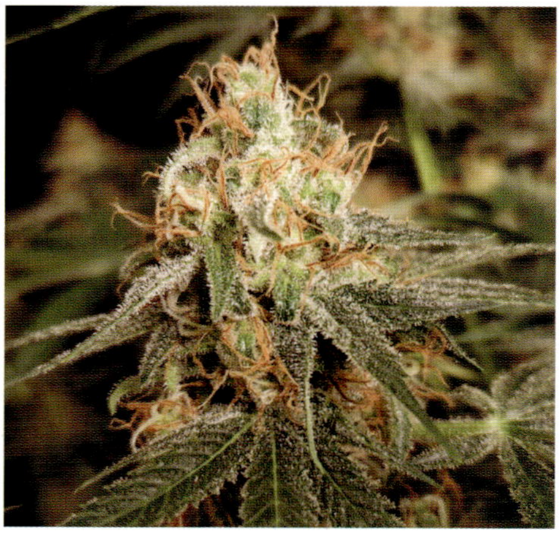

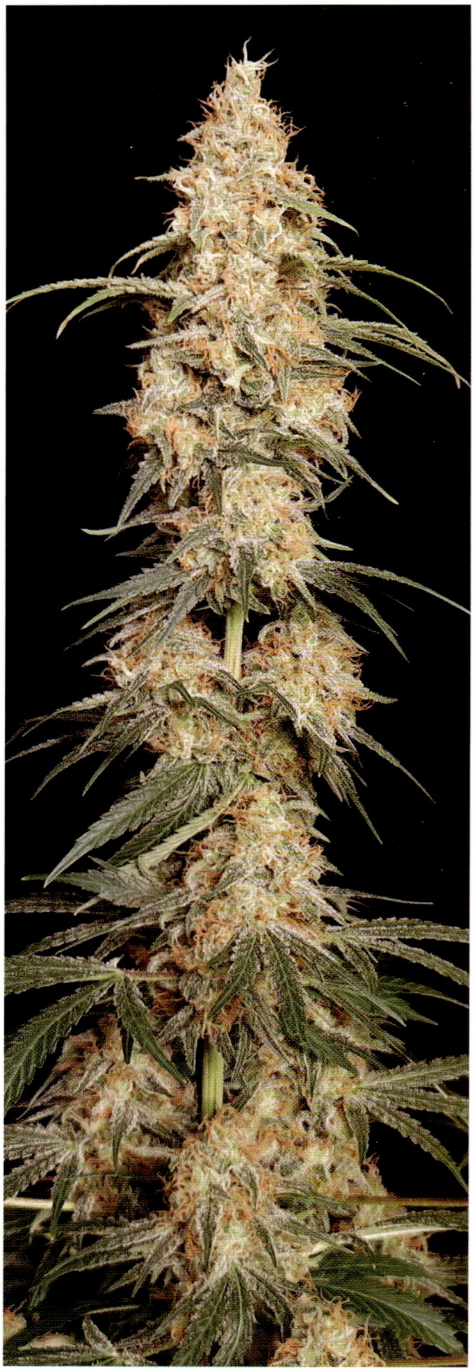

Nature's brushstrokes of vibrant colors and textures speak the universal language of flowers, making us feel good. Each day of flowering brings peace and calm to the grower, with happiness blooming at every node.

PHOTOS: DOCTORSCHOICE.FARM / PHOTOGRAPHED BY FRANZ JANYR

Soil or Other Growing Medium

Starting with soil is recommended for less experienced growers venturing into SOG or ScrOG cultivation. These methods can be adapted for use with hydroponics, but soil remains the most commonly used medium and will be the primary focus of this chapter. If you already have experience with soil, you may want to explore alternatives such as coco coir, vermiculite, perlite and Rockwool, many of which also feature in hydroponics.

Soil is compact, making it well-suited for SOG and ScrOG techniques by providing stability to the plants. Soil-based cultivation allows you to adjust plant spacing by simply relocating pots. In contrast, most hydroponic systems require predetermined plant spacing at fixed positions.

It's typical to have one pot per plant in soil-based SOG setups, while ScrOG can use multiple plants per pot. With both SOG and ScrOG methods, reaching every plant becomes

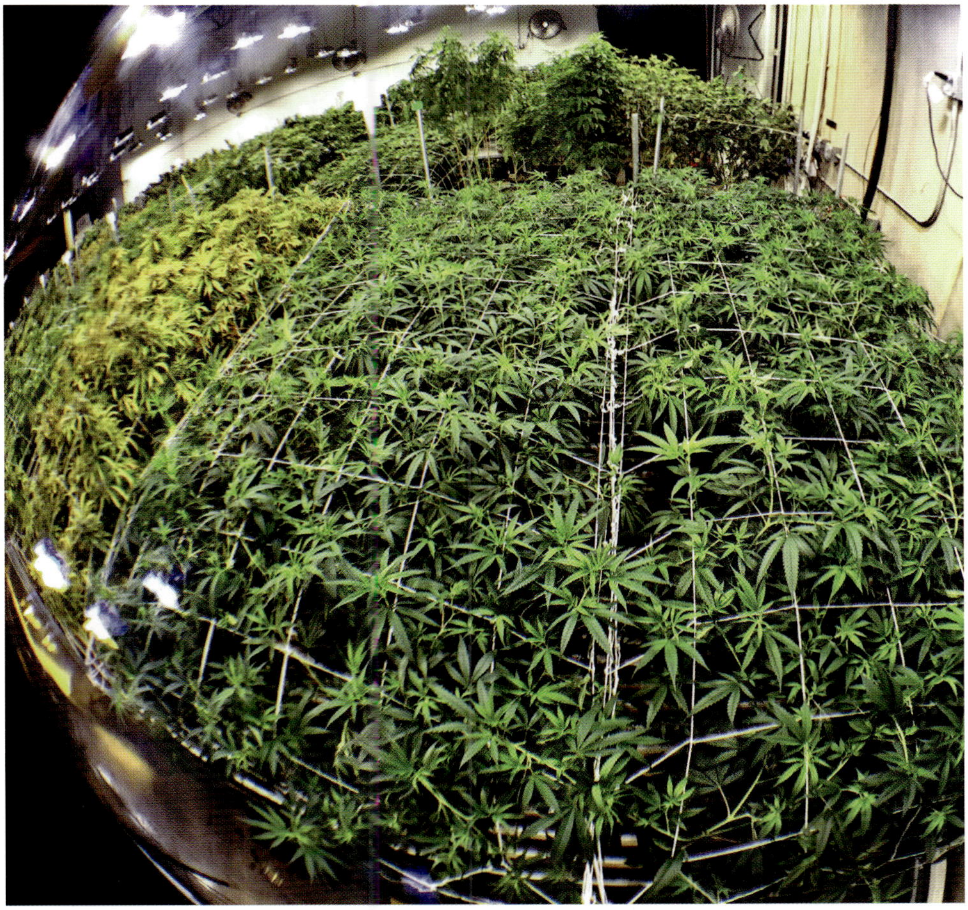

PHOTO: HIP2THECROP

A wide-angle view of a ScrOG showing how the net curves somewhat as the plants push against it while growing. You should attempt to keep the net down by training plants within it.

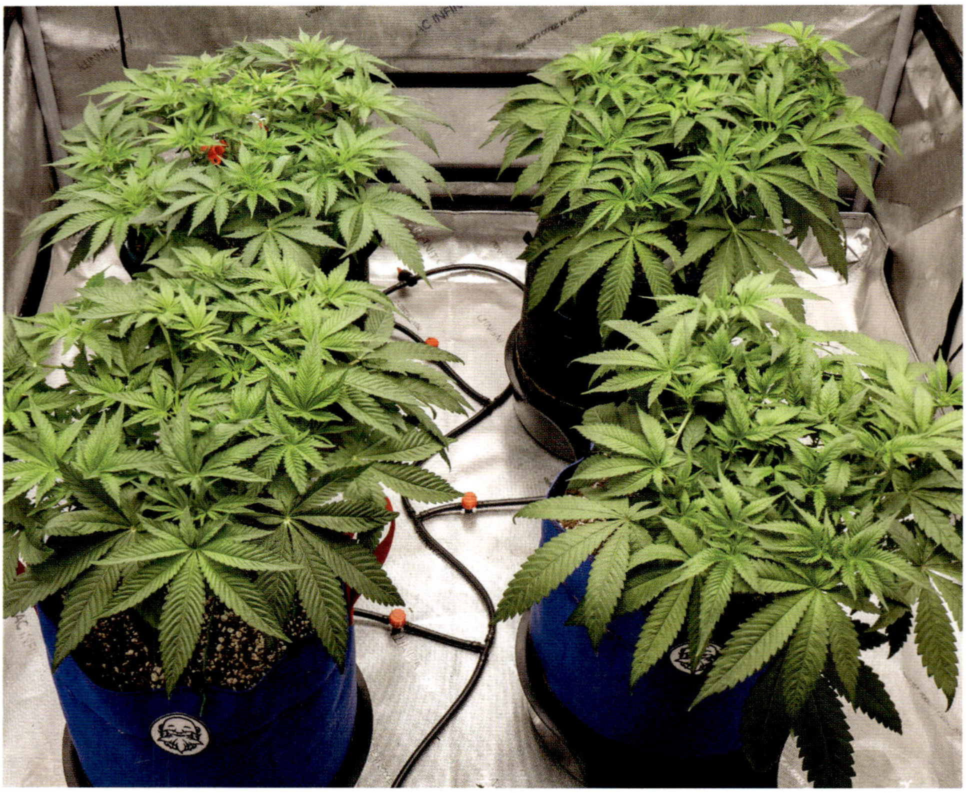

These four plants will expand during flowering to fill the gaps between them. Leaving room for that expansion is essential.

PHOTO: JOE'S CANNA GROWS

increasingly difficult as the canopy becomes denser and plants grow taller. This is particularly problematic when electrical equipment is involved. Even if you can reach all sides initially, central pots often become less accessible. To address this, you can use a watering can with an extended spout to reach under the canopy and access each pot.

Accessing each plant is far more manageable with a tent-based or smaller area cultivation setup. Experienced growers eventually explore irrigation systems, using pipes positioned over each pot with nozzles to dispense fluids. Because this irrigation setup begins to resemble hydroponic systems, growers may transition to hydroponics as they gain experience.

Experiment before you introduce the irrigation system. Use empty pots to test and determine the appropriate watering schedule. Your goal is to achieve even fluid distribution within the soil, ensuring uniformity across all plants. If you're using a watering can with an extended spout, you can further extend the spout's reach by modifying a clear hose, allowing you to observe the fluid's flow and its reach within your grow. We will delve into irrigation techniques in more detail later.

Why Not One Pot for Multiple Plants?

While it's possible to group plants into one large pot, one plant per pot is preferable. If one pot experiences a nutrient issue, such as lockout, overfeeding, or a pH imbalance, it will affect only one plant and can be addressed without an impact on other plants. Transplanting also becomes more straightforward without interfering with other plant roots. In multi-plant pot systems, precise measurements and adjustments are crucial to maintain uniformity. These concerns apply to most hydroponic systems as well. While hydroponic systems offer easy access to the entire compact crop, feeding and watering typically originate from a central reservoir.

The Significance of the Cannabis Canopy

Our advanced indoor cultivation methods center on the cannabis cola, the main bud site typically located at the top of the stem. In most cases, this cola produces the largest quantity of buds, so that indoor growers create an environment that emphasizes its growth. In outdoor settings, the sun's movement causes the lower branches of a plant to receive less light, while the top part consistently receives more.[1] As the plant grows, this top section increases in height. Our goal is to achieve an even canopy of uniformly growing top colas, diverting light away from the less essential side branches. This does not mean side branches and leaves are unimportant; they just hold less significance in these advanced systems. A dense canopy will shade these lower branches, more light being retained above the canopy.

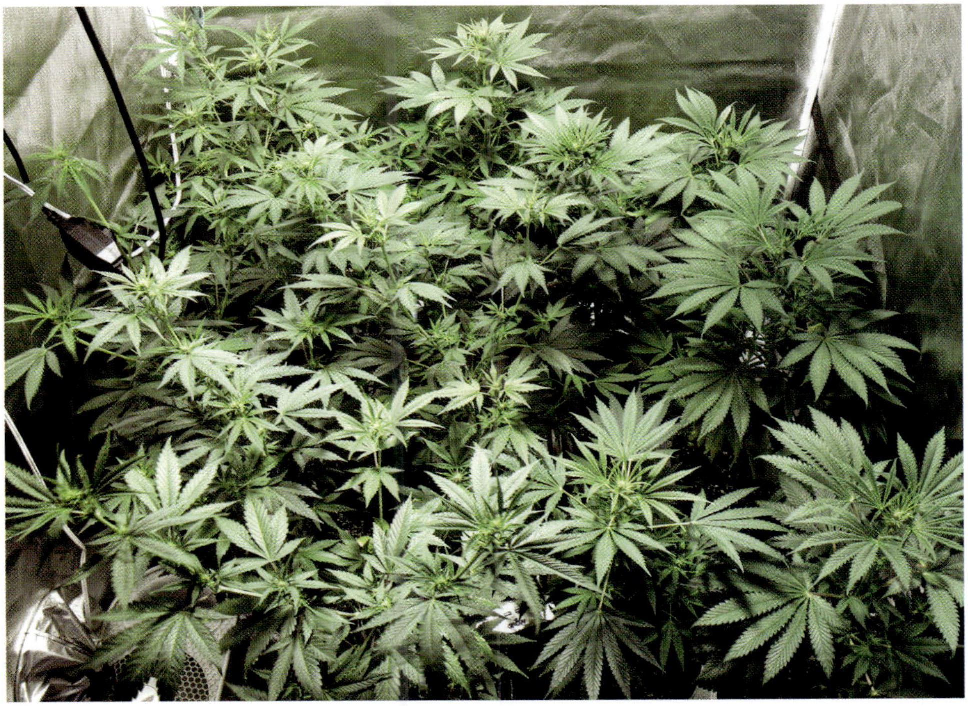

PHOTO: DAVID STRANGE

The gaps are filled with more growth, especially side branching.

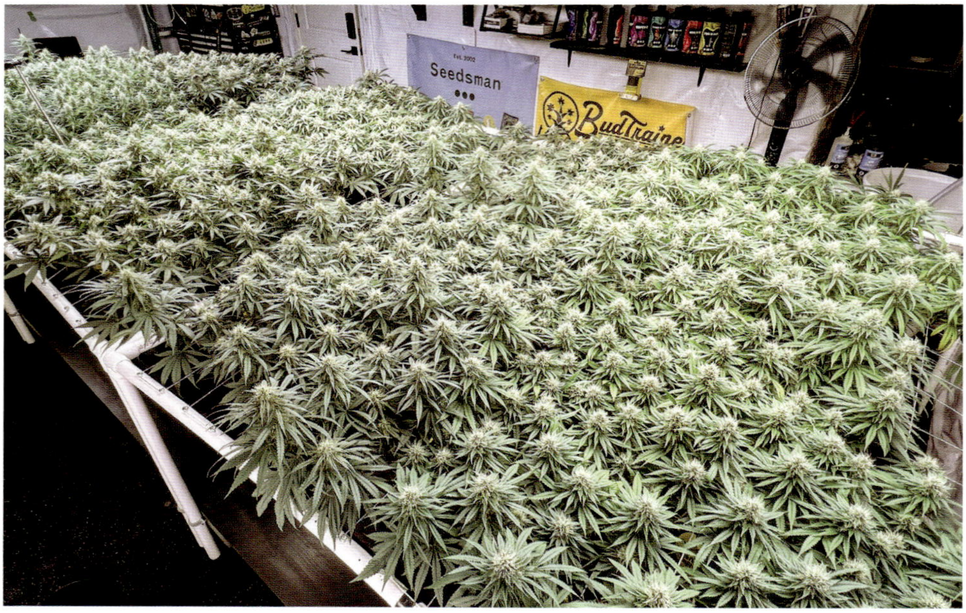

By applying the practices laid out in this book, you can achieve an even canopy all the way to harvest time.

PHOTO: NORTHERNSCROGGER.COM

This is where the SOG and ScrOG techniques are useful. SOG maximizes the growth of top colas under a single light source, while ScrOG achieves the same while also optimizing lateral branch growth. Both methods aim to grow an even canopy. To achieve this, even light distribution across the top of the plants is crucial.

Attempting the SOG method with new hybrids is not recommended. Variability within such a population can result in an uneven top canopy. Even one hybrid outperforming the others in light competition results in reduced yields for the other plants and, eventually, a drop in overall yield. Stable genetics are essential to address potential variability issues. Most experienced growers eventually turn to clones, as they offer the greatest stability.

If you have limited cannabis cultivation experience, start with seeds, and avoid cloning. Understanding the cannabis growth cycle will better prepare you for future endeavors involving mother plant selection and cloning.

Preparing the Special Clone Mother

Cloning plays a crucial role in advanced cannabis cultivation. Before selecting a plant for replication through cloning, grow a test crop from seeds or obtain clones from another source. Take cuttings from all the test plants during the third and fourth weeks of vegetative growth and label each one. Details on taking and growing cuttings are discussed in Chapter 13. Do not initiate flowering in any of these cuttings.

If a cutting grows too large to manage, reproduce it by taking additional cuttings and labeling them accordingly. Continue growing the test plants until they mature, at which point you can induce flowering by manipulating the photoperiod if they are not from autoflowering strains. Remove the males and corresponding male clones. By the end of the flowering phase, you should be able to identify a mother plant that outperformed the others. Allow the corresponding cutting from this plant to grow to full size in a vegetative state under a 24/0 light cycle to serve as the source for additional clones. To maintain a clone, it's best to provide 24 hours of light a day, as any period of darkness may induce flowering. Be mindful of how many cuttings you require. The other cuttings are no longer relevant to this project and can be disposed of.

Follow this simple step-by-step guide for selecting a mother plant:

1. Grow a large test crop.
2. Take cuttings from each plant and label them meticulously.
3. Do not flower these cuttings.
4. Continue to grow the test crop.
5. Identify males and females during pre-flowering/early flowering in the test crop. Eliminate the males. Refer to the labels created in step 2 to remove clones from the clone room that correspond to the males.
6. At the end of flowering, select the best female plant and locate the corresponding clone.
7. Cultivate the corresponding clone, now the clone mother plant, but do not flower her. A clone mother can also consist of a collection of clones, not just a single plant.

Once the clone mother develops numerous branches, take multiple cuttings from her. You can prune to increase branches. Use these clones as the genetic source for your next crop. Reserve at least one clone without flowering it, so that can serve as the next clone mother, in case you lose the original. Strains have been lost before, so having a backup is essential.

Reputable breeders often assess thousands of plants to find an outstanding specimen. Aim to grow more than 20 plants to ensure you can identify a suitable clone mother. While outdoor cultivation allows for a broader selection, indoor strains must ultimately be adapted for indoor conditions.

Take your cuttings before flowering to prevent having a batch of flowering cuttings that need to revert to a vegetative state, a process not applicable to autoflowering strains. Reverting to a 24/0 light cycle can be time-consuming and stressful. If a clone exhibits pre-flowers, it can immediately be induced into flowering by adjusting the photoperiod to 12/12. The outcome will resemble a small bud on a shorter stem. Age is conserved in clones, meaning clones are the same age as the parent plant they were taken from. Therefore, they are sexually mature enough to flower if taken from a

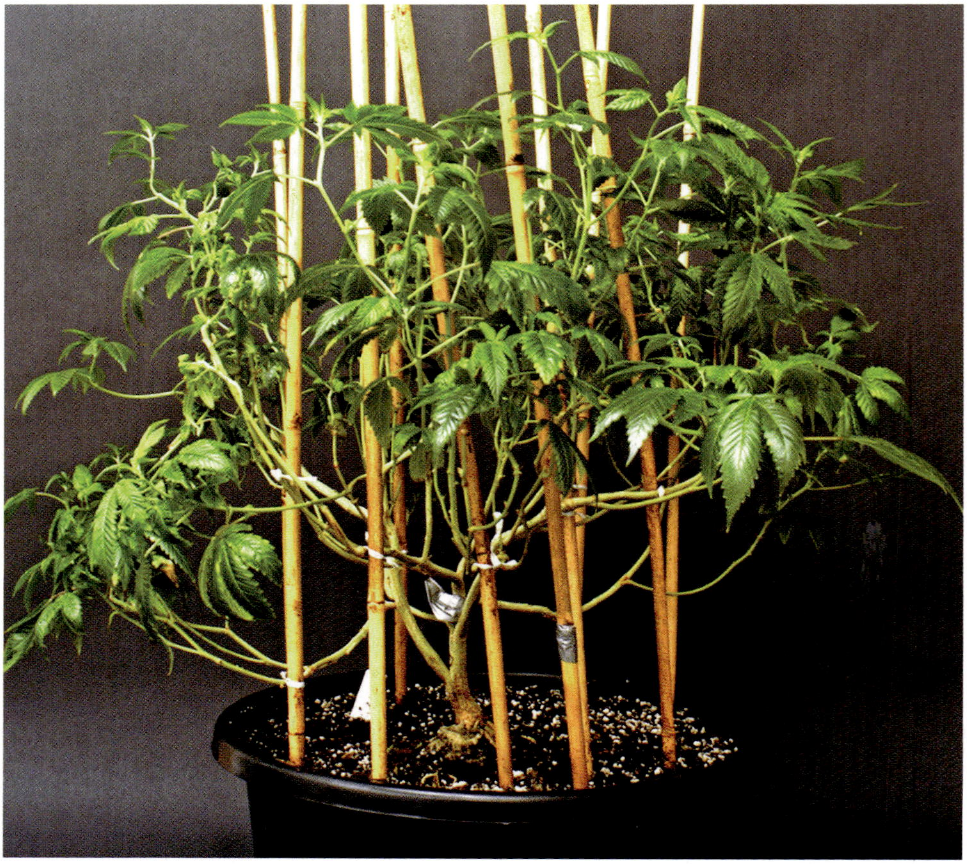

Pruning creates more branches and keeps the plant squat. This clone mother donor has been staked and pruned multiple times by taking cuttings for clones.

pre-flowering or flowering plant. If you take a cutting from a plant just a week before it flowers, you may need to wait another week before you can initiate flowering. Even two-inch clones can be flowered if taken from a plant during its flowering cycle. However, the bud quantity will be lower as the clone didn't have the opportunity to grow larger during the vegetative phase and develop more node regions, creating additional areas for bud formation.

To create more clones, allow the clone of the selected female plant to undergo vegetative growth to develop more branches suitable for cloning. You can prune to stimulate additional branching. Taking a cutting in the vegetative state gives you greater control over the clones. Always take multiple cuttings from the mother plant and grow these clones to create a room full of high-quality female plants. Though this requires time and may temporarily reduce yields, the exponential replication of genetic material turns a single plant into populations of that same plant. Because these are clones, they are not just plants in the same strain, but identical copies of the mother clone.

PHOTO: ED BORG

A clone mother is the source for all future clones of this specific plant. When cloning is integrated with advanced indoor techniques, the desired traits become more prevalent than in a population with trait variations, leading to superior outcomes. However, we strongly recommend using this method only after gaining experience with the complete life cycle of a cannabis plant, from seed (or clone) to harvest. Beginning with this knowledge provides a stronger basis for subsequent improvements using these techniques. While it is possible to purchase clones, creating them yourself provides valuable learning experience.

Clone Cuttings

To obtain a substantial number of mother plant cuttings, grow the designated mother plant in vegetative conditions under a 24/0 photoperiod for three weeks before taking multiple cuttings from her. Take as many cuttings as you intend to grow to full maturity. You might need to repeat this process or establish a second mother plant to produce a sufficient number of clones. Once your cloning operation is in full swing, it becomes a circular process, making up for the time you invested initiating a mother plant. A grow filled with clones is essentially the same mother plant duplicated multiple times. Every clone you take from a mother plant with the intention of further cloning effectively becomes a mother plant itself. In this process, no genetic information is lost, as clones are genetically identical.

Consider pruning to stimulate the growth of additional branches to create more potential regions for cloning. We will delve into pruning techniques for enhancing branching shortly. Once you've invested the time to establish a system that continually generates clones, you'll significantly increase productivity in a shorter timeframe. The advantage of using clones lies in their uniform growth. By selecting and cultivating a clone that exhibits higher yields than other plants, you can potentially double your yield in a specific grow space. Remember that clones inherit the same issues as the clone mother, such as susceptibility to pests, nutrient requirements, or genetic disorders. If a problem affects one clone, it can affect the entire batch equally.

Clones provide a head start for growers. Furthermore, they are a crucial asset for future breeders, as discussed in the breeding Chapter 17. Some growers choose to swap or purchase clones to bypass the time-consuming process of identifying and preparing a special female plant, although this may require communication with other growers, potentially posing security risks. Medical cannabis clubs often offer clones for sale to medical users.

Entire grow rooms can be designated for the cultivation of clones, leading to exponential growth. To sustain these clones effectively, you'll need to divide the plants into different areas in your grow room based on their stage of growth.

Cutting a Clone

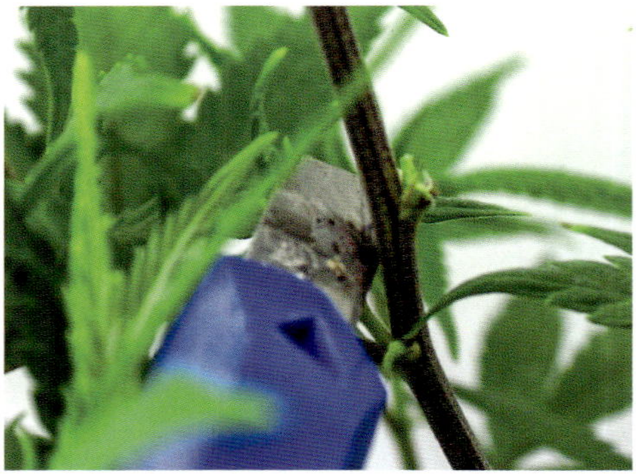

A slice is made above the node.

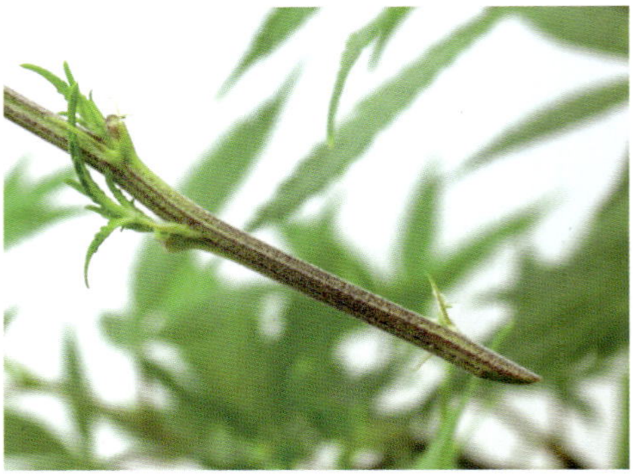

Above the node leaves a longer stem.

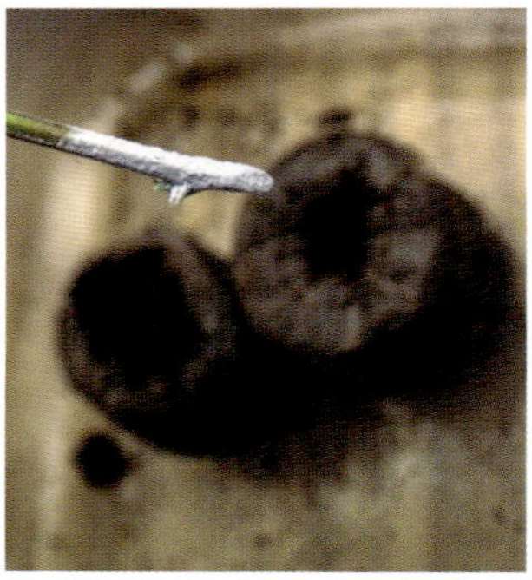

Rooting hormone is applied to the sliced tip.

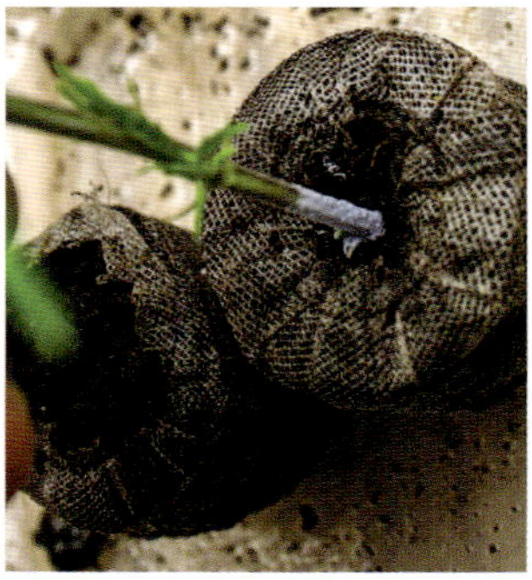

The treated end is then inserted into a peat cube.

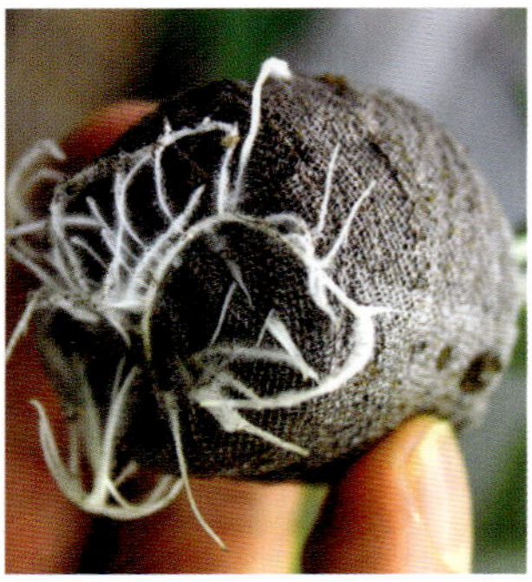

After a few weeks, roots will show through the cube.

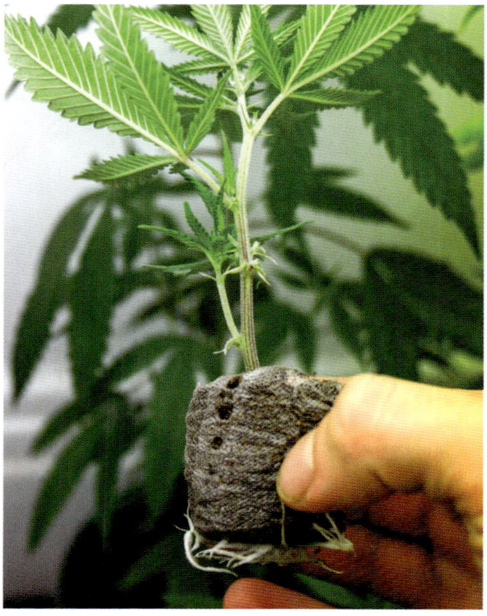

The clone should be ready for transplanting.

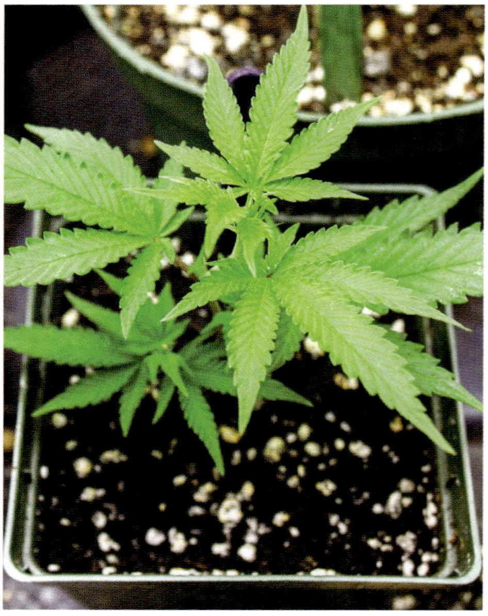

The clone is transferred to its new grow medium.

PHOTOS: DAVID STRANGE

Two- and Three-Stage Systems

Implementing a two- or three-stage system, separating the plants by their stage of growth into separate grow areas, can be advantageous to a cannabis grower. However, setting up the system can be time-consuming and requires additional grow spaces. Tents are a practical solution, even for SOG and ScrOG growing, as they can be equipped with low-wattage LEDs suitable for maintaining clones in their vegetative state. A 2 × 2-foot tent provides about 4 square feet of cloning space, which can comfortably accommodate several small plants without heat-related issues using LED heat sync cooling technology. You can maintain a continuous batch of clones in this space and transfer them to the primary grow area when they are ready.

Both two-stage and three-stage systems involve a clone stage in the first tent, so the distinction is that a three-stage system has separate tents for vegetative growth and flowering. A two-stage system is, therefore, 1 clone tent + 1 shared veg/flowering tent. The veg/flowering second stage tent switches to 12/12 when the plants are finished with vegetative growth. After harvesting, the clones from the first stage are relocated to the now-empty second-stage area for vegetative growth and eventual flowering. This is a type of perpetual system, but the three-stage system next has an even faster perpetual turnover.

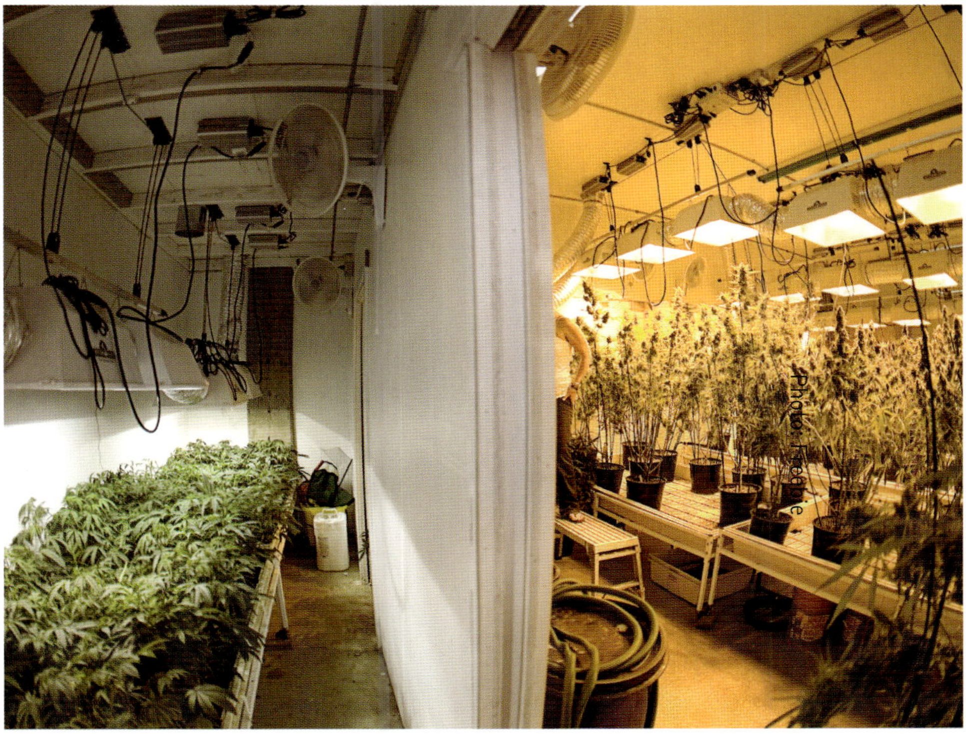

Here is a two-stage system. The room on the left is for vegetative growth, and the room on the right is for flowering.

PHOTO: TRICHOME TECH / PHOTOGRAPHED BY FREEBIE

A three-stage system introduces an additional tent into the process: 1 clone tent + 1 veg tent + 1 flowering tent. You would think plants complete vegetative growth and are transferred to the vacant flowering area, followed by clones taken from the clone area and placed in the vegetative area, but this is not what happens in a three-stage system. There is no physical movement of the plants required between the veg tent and flowering tent. Those designations are only temporary. Instead, you change the photoperiod in the tent. For example, you switch from a 24/0 photoperiod for vegetative growth to 12/12 for flowering. After harvesting, the 12/12 stage changes back to 24/0, and new clones are moved in to repeat the process. Unlike the past when switching metal halide (MH) bulbs to high-pressure sodium (HPS) bulbs was necessary, LEDs remain in place, and in some cases, they may even include a selector to switch between vegetative and flowering modes.

This is also how plants are moved between stages in a ScrOG or hydroponic system; they are not physically moved at all. The photoperiod of the grow areas is changed instead.

Perpetual Growth Cycles

The goal of a perpetual growth cycle is to maintain a continuous flowering process. There are several compelling reasons to adopt a perpetual growth cycle. They are cost-effective in the long run and provide an opportunity for gradual improvement in your cultivation methods, particularly when you focus on a single strain. Since perpetual cycles continuously replicate the natural cannabis plant life cycle, you gain substantial experience with the entire growth process relatively quickly. You also safeguard against the failures that you may encounter, such as mold, pest infestations, or nutrient imbalances. With a perpetual grow cycle, these issues are compartmentalized, minimizing potential losses. And you have a consistent and uninterrupted supply of cannabis, eliminating the risk of running low or running out. Perpetual growing also allows you to fine-tune your timing, enabling precise decisions on when to start new clones, move them, and initiate the flowering stage. Notably, there's no need to determine the sex of your plants when using clones. The additional investment is well worth the benefits; perpetual growth cycles offer optimal efficiency in terms of space, energy consumption, and time.

SOG or ScrOG?

SOG refers to a growing setup of densely packed, untrained clones that naturally form a sea of green canopy, while ScrOG uses a screen to train plants to fill the growing space—two fundamentally distinct cultivation methods, and the distinction goes beyond just the use of a mesh screen. We can distinguish these methods by understanding that SOG involves adapting the light to match the growing canopy, while ScrOG adapts the clone's tops and branches to match the light. Therefore, SOG typically requires more frequent light adjustments compared to ScrOG.

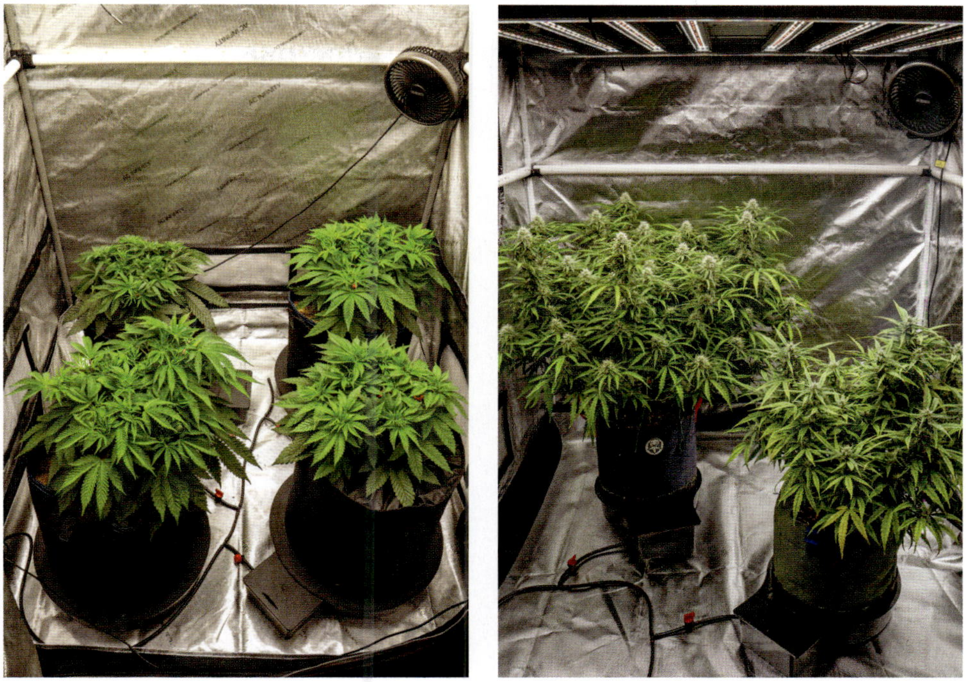

SOG growing is used to utilize a small space without the need for a mesh screen. You don't have to use all the space for a neat grow.

SOG, when used with stable strains and proper preparation, can efficiently fulfill your cultivation goals. However, if you begin with seeds, particularly with variable hybrid strains, ScrOG offers better control over the average canopy height. Many growers initiate their cultivation journey with ScrOG using seeds and then transition to SOG for subsequent rounds after selecting clones from the ScrOG grow.

The uniform canopy in a SOG grow is achieved by starting with identical clones at the same growth stage. If each clone is cultivated uniformly in a controlled environment, the only expected variation is due to the plant's access to light, which depends on its proximity to the light source, whereas growing a variety of strains in a SOG grow often leads to an uneven canopy due to genetic variations in plant height. Some plants may be shaded by others and forced to stretch and compete for light, wasting energy that could be channeled into bud production, particularly during the flowering phase. SOG can tolerate some variation, but is generally more efficient when all plants grow uniformly. Strains with a tendency to grow bushy are better suited for ScrOG systems, since it relies on training branches around the mesh to fill the screen, maintaining an even canopy height. ScrOG is an effective method for controlling plant height and is particularly useful when growing naturally tall outdoor sativa strains indoors. When executed correctly, both SOG and ScrOG can be equally productive cultivation methods.

PHOTOS: JOE'S CANNA GROWS

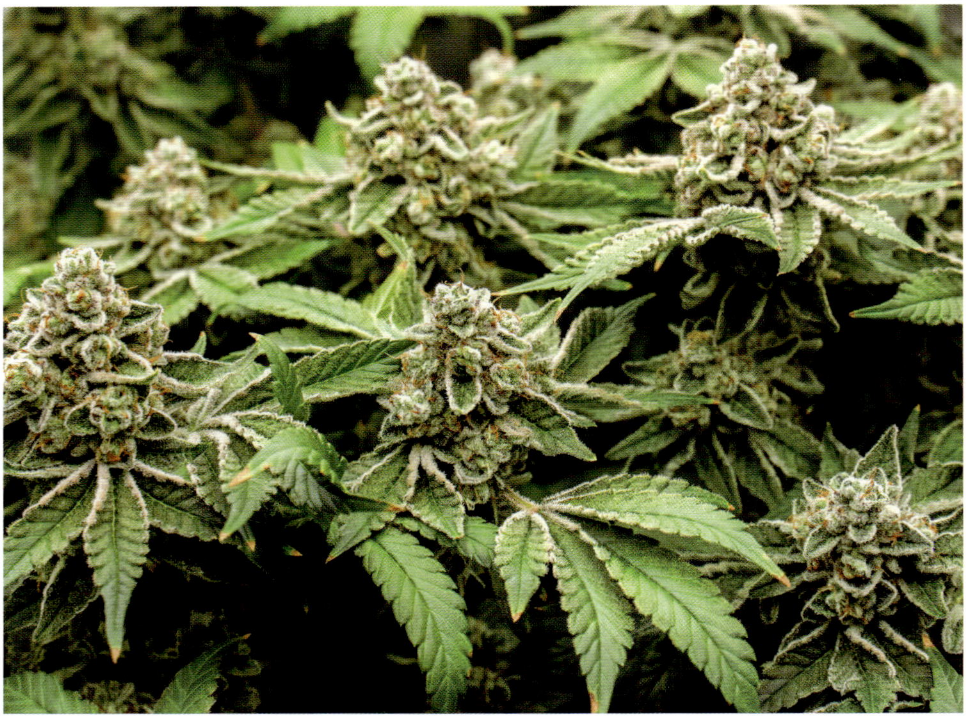

Some strains are dense, meaning you can have many colas in a smaller area. Density and resin often go hand in hand.

Sea of Green Setup

In SOG cultivation, your goal is to have one plant per square foot. Indica strains are favored for their compact size and shape, although most indica strains can be comfortably grown in less than 1 square foot, in an average of 0.5 square feet per plant. For exceptionally compact setups, short indica plants, especially clones, can thrive in as little as 0.1 square feet of space. Pure sativa strains generally do not require more than 1.5 square feet. SOG setups fall somewhere between these two values. This information should help you determine the number of clones needed for your growing area. The key to a SOG setup is to densely pack the plants.

SOG Pots

Pots for a SOG setup differ from pots used in other cultivation methods, being tube-shaped and deeper than they are wide. They come in various materials, from economical plastics to more expensive ceramic versions. Some growers have devised cylinder-shaped pots using everyday items. If such pots are not readily available, you can use pots with equal width and depth, as long as they are not wider than they are deep; you want to encourage root growth downwards rather than sideways. This approach minimizes lateral root development, which restricts bushy growth, as the two are interconnected. Plant density is the primary objective of the SOG setup.

PHOTO: JOE'S CANNA GROWS

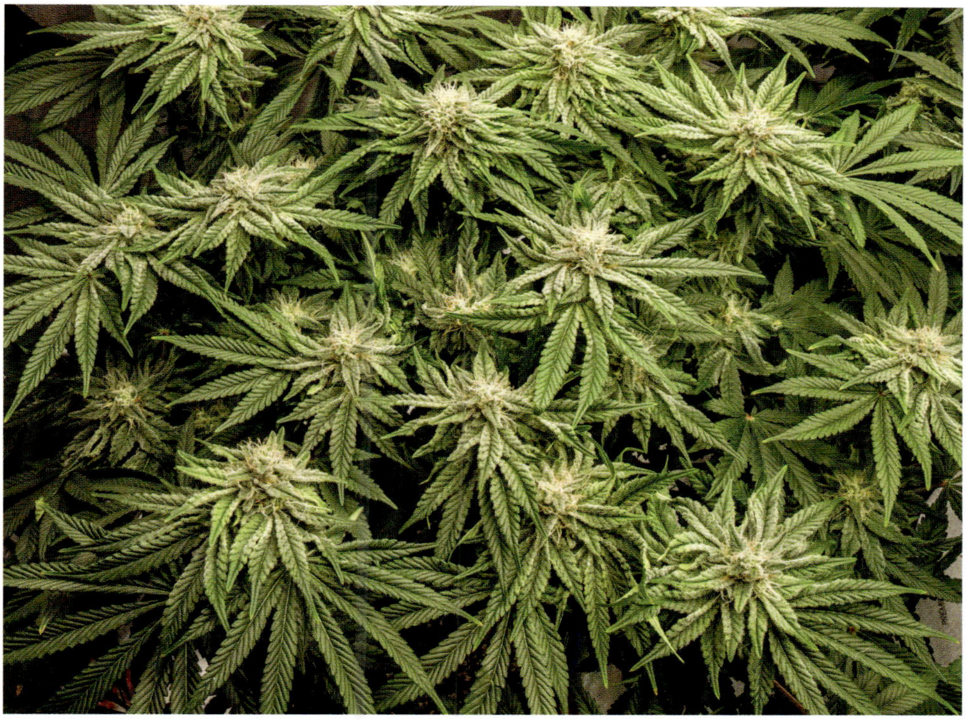

SOG fills the canopy with flowers without the use of a mesh screen. Good genetics and even light distribution help achieve uniformity.

You can also use grow bags, which come in many sizes to fit nearly any setup. Deeper bags with small diameters work well with SOG. Many grow bags are biodegradable.

SOG Timing

Prepare your clone selection before transplanting them all into the vegetative growth room to eliminate the need for pruning to maintain a flat canopy. Rooting usually takes around two to three weeks from cutting to well-rooted clone. In your SOG, keep plants tightly together, as we shall not be extending vegetative growth. When the plants reach the desired height after an additional two to three weeks of vegetative growth, initiate flowering. Your goal is to grow from clone to harvest as quickly as possible without sacrificing overall yield, so keep your rooting and vegetative growth time as short as possible. Achieving this efficiency demands experience and repeated attempts with clones; guesswork won't suffice. Innate abilities won't guarantee optimal results on your first attempt. However, if you are patient and keeping learning, your second grow will almost certainly be more successful.

Indica strains tend to fill gaps in the canopy more rapidly than sativa. A reliable indicator for time to flower indica strains is when the canopy of leaves appears ready to achieve full coverage within a week. When growing from clones, consider initiating

PHOTO: JOE'S CANNA GROWS

flowering when an additional week of vegetative growth would complete the canopy. Clones offer more flexibility than seed-based cultivation, which requires waiting for the pre-flowering stage. Clones carry the age of the mother plant from which they were derived. If they originate from nearly flowering plants, clones will initiate flowering as soon as you introduce the 12/12 light cycle. This eliminates the need for a vegetative growth stage.

Sativa strains typically require earlier flowering than indica due to internode stretching during the flowering phase. Keep detailed records of your timing and adjust it as needed for subsequent grows. These records will eventually enable you to pinpoint the precise day to switch to the flowering phase based on your past data, rather than relying on visual cues.

The result is a lush, dense canopy of buds, or sea of green. If you use perpetual harvesting, you can anticipate a significant yield of buds every few months, especially with promising strains.

SOG Productivity

SOG uses clone plantlets in combination with a PPF-to-surface area ratio to maximize the rate of bud production in a given grow space. The photosynthetic photon flux (PPF) is a measurement of photons in the photosynthetically active radiation (PAR) range that are emitted by a light. A surface area ratio can be calculated by dividing the PPF by the surface area; see Chapter 7. SOG increases the production rate using minimal space because the primary focus is always on the top colas rather than the flowers on side branches.

Larger SOG setups can benefit significantly from a drip irrigation system, which ensures that plants in the middle of the crop, which become difficult to access due to the density of the plants, receive proper water and nutrients.

If your canopy becomes uneven when growing from clones, it's likely due to excessive light in one area. You can achieve better light distribution by raising the light by a foot or more if the canopy is very uneven, or a couple of inches if it is not. Adding supplementary lighting can also help. Avoid pruning, as it redirects the plant's energy toward branching instead of bud production. Instead, use fans aimed at the canopy, not just below it. Remove any necrotic leaves that fall during the late flowering stage.

SOG plants ideally require no tying or training. The canopy's density should naturally keep the plants in formation without bending. If excessive bending occurs, initiate flowering earlier in the next cycle. For harvesting, refer to the methods outlined in Chapter 16, and explore Chapter 13 for techniques to stimulate root growth using cloning gels.

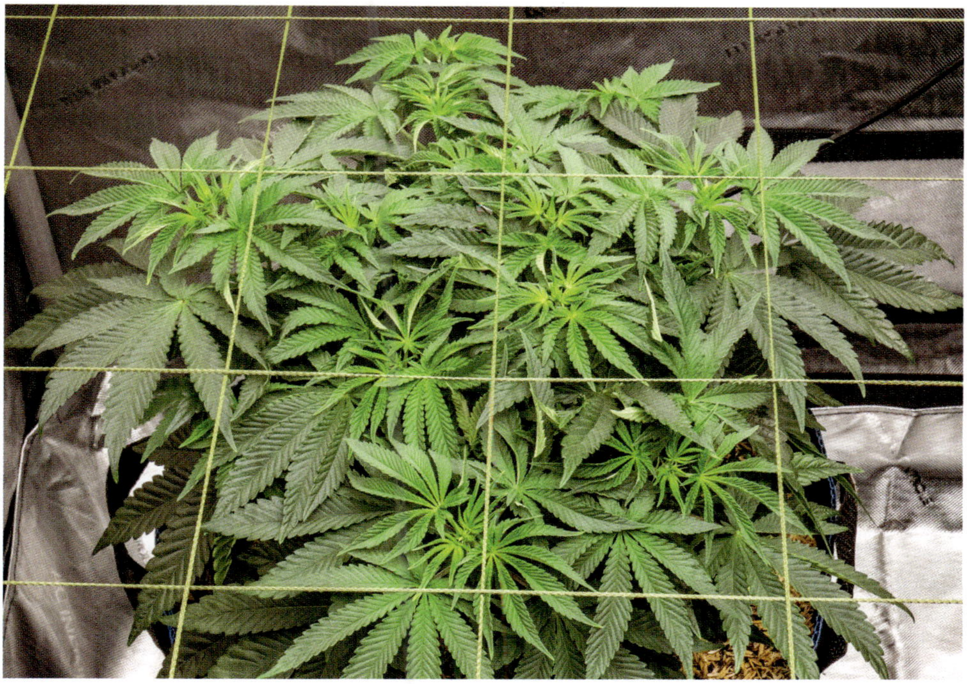

ScrOG uses a mesh screen to keep the plants' flowers upright and pointing to the light instead of growing outwards to the sides under their weight.

Screen of Green

The ScrOG is like the SOG technique, with the key distinction being that fewer plants are required. In ScrOG, you place a mesh screen between your plants and their light source to create a canopy of dense colas, or a screen of green. The mesh is typically about the size of regular chicken wire, each square roughly one square inch.

This method works exceptionally well for growing from seed and dealing with variations in a population. For clones, SOG may be a more suitable choice. In ScrOG, provide at least one square foot per flowering plant. ScrOG uses large pot sizes as lateral root growth and branching is desired to create bushier plants, which are trained through the screen to produce more colas.

As the plants grow upward through the mesh, ScrOG growers gently guide them around the netting to create an even canopy. The plant's branches penetrate the mesh openings and grow above the wire lattice, allowing you to bend them down safely through another opening. Do not overbend, as this can cause a stem or branch to split. Experiment with gentle bending; if you encounter resistance, wait for further growth of the stem or branch before attempting to bend again. Gravitropism, the biological process that compels the plant to continue growing upward, will eventually guide the plant upwards again, and the process can be repeated.

PHOTO: JOE'S CANNA GROWS

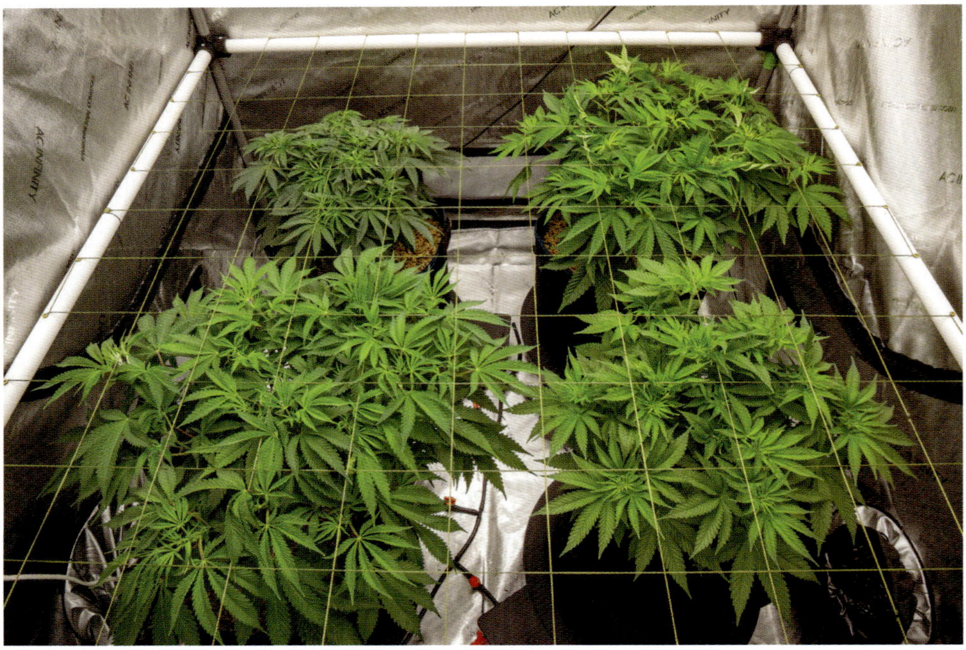

Most tent growers use a screen because the tent shape and frame allow for the easy assembly of one. Why not have the screen? It makes sense.

PHOTO: JOE'S CANNA GROWS

Plants should not be flowered until the entire mesh is covered with green growth. Timing depends on the strain and screen height. Once you become more familiar with the strain you're working with, you can determine the best mesh height. Even if you haven't trained the plants around the ScrOG before the flowering stage, flowering will promote further growth, and the mesh will help support the colas and branches. The canopy is manually created in ScrOG, unlike its natural formation in SOG. Since ScrOG entails more bushiness, you'll likely need to prune and top during the vegetative growth stage before flowering. Pruning and topping are covered in more detail in Chapter 13.

The height of your screen depends on the strain and growing conditions. Your experience with that specific strain will help you determine the ideal height, but you can use these ballpark estimates for the first round. Indica require lower screens than sativa strains. Measurement begins at the top of the pot. The heights are roughly: 6–8 inches (15–20 cm) for indica, 16–20 inches (40–50 cm) for hybrids, and 25 inches (60 cm) for sativa. A reasonable estimate if you are uncertain is 10 inches (30 cm). Do not be concerned if your plants don't appear to grow near the mesh during the vegetative stage; they'll catch up during flowering. Shorter plants might not require as much training, but taller plants or those competing noticeably may benefit from it. Without the mesh, branches and colas may bend due to their weight, and branches may even touch the ground. ScrOG addresses these issues, the screen preventing the colas and branches from bending over.

Try to direct your training inward toward the center of the light source, rather than away from it. Place plants closer together if you have extra space, but avoid overcrowding. Your judgment will improve with experience. There's no need to train fan leaves or the lowest branches through the mesh if there isn't sufficient space for them. Concentrate on the top colas first and then work your way down each branch.

If any leaves beneath the canopy develop necrotic areas, remove only the affected portions, not the entire leaf. Even if a leaf is partially damaged, it is still receiving some light which contributes to flower production. Adjust the mesh to accommodate plants on the outer rim, redirecting them toward the light. Some ScrOG mesh configurations may resemble a cage shape, sloping down at the sides to support lower branches that cannot reach the canopy; however, if you use this shape, you'll still need space to access your plants underneath the screen.

You can also use elastics, strings, or nylon filaments tied into a netting instead of a wire mesh, but it must be tight and thick enough to support the flowering plants. Using nets provides the advantage of easily reshaping the screen; wire mesh can be more challenging to manipulate. Some netting can be tied to allow the knotting to slide and adjust the trellis mesh sizes, which can help customize the screen. If you use elastic trellis netting and want to reuse it, you will need to cut the plants away from it without cutting the netting itself. In the past, HID lights generated heat, warping nylon filaments, which popularized metal screens. LEDs do not heat netting; however, we are now using more nylon plastics that are not environmentally-friendly.

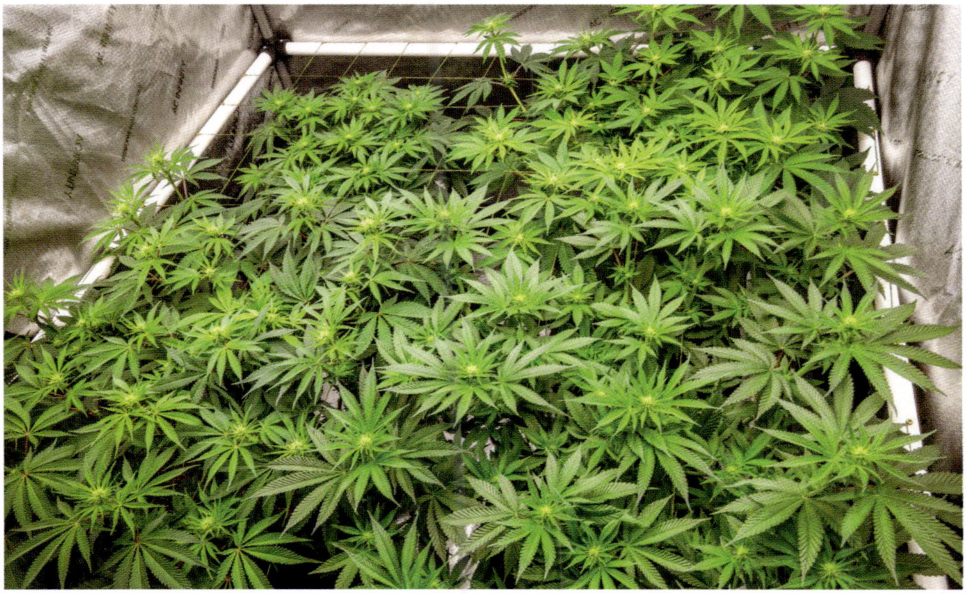

PHOTO: JOE'S CANNA GROWS

Sativa-leaning genetics can become unwieldy in a tent grow, so a mesh helps train those branches and top colas into as even a canopy as possible.

ScrOG Tips from the Northern Scrogger

youtube.com/northernscrogger

Screen of Green is a tried and tested technique that many growers of all experience levels have used with great success. But! There are a few tips that can make your life easier when you're just getting started, or when you want to improve. These are nothing new; in fact, the top tips below are all built off the traditional way to use this growing method, which is being lost as people move away from the fundamentals. As my grandma used to say: If it aint broke, don't fix it!

Early Training

Don't wait too long to start training your plants. Early training means shorter ScrOGs and a shorter veg time, which means you can start growing that bud without delay. I start training once my plants have been moved into their final pots, and once they're big enough for me to bend without stressing them out. It's a lot easier to get a handle on training when you focus on just one thing, so focus on getting the top branch to the same level as the bottom branch. This will open up the node sites to the light, and encourage more branching, so a better ScrOG eventually. This will be the only topping I do on the main branch, otherwise it can become too thick to work with.

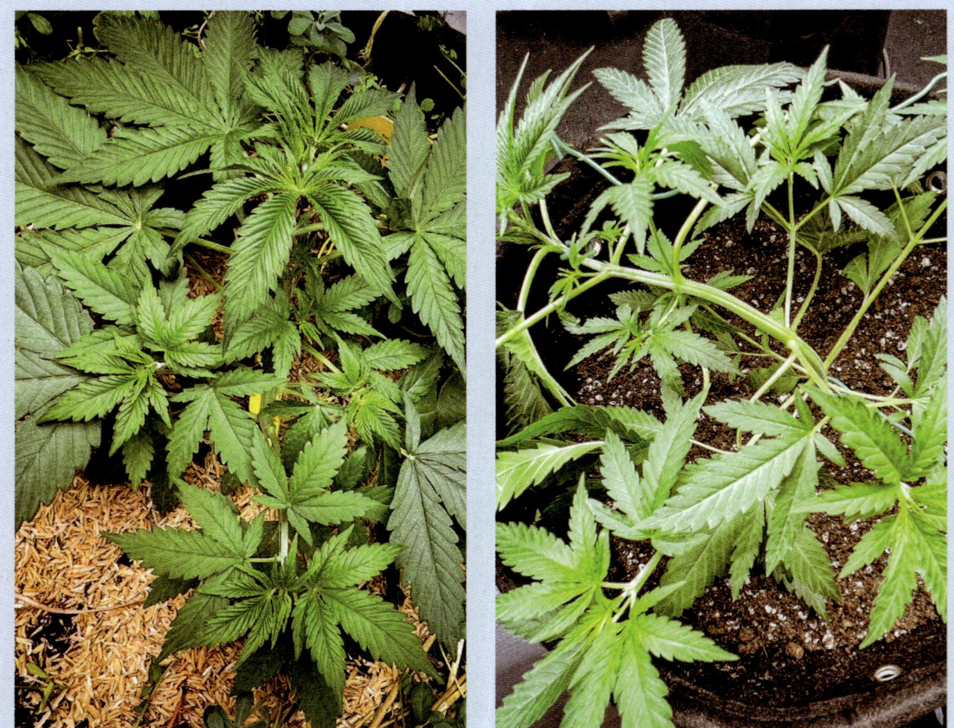

You can start training when the plants are big enough to withstanding bending.

PHOTOS: NORTHERNSCROGGER.COM

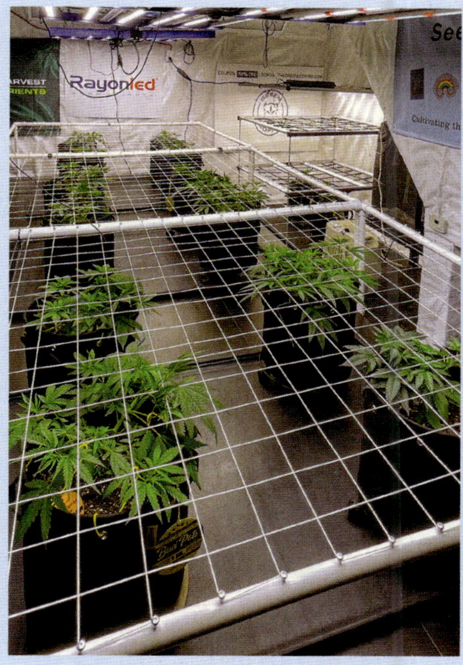

Screens should be installed 4-8 inches from the top of your plant's final pot.

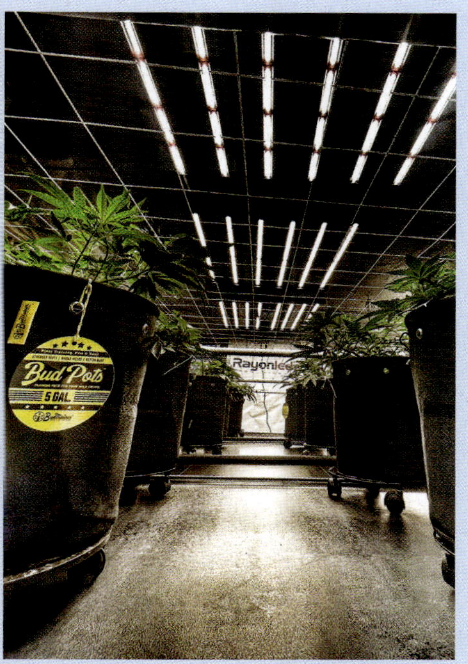

Don't force the screen onto your plants!

The best material to use, when training, is the plant itself: The big fan leaves on indicas and indica hybrids. The rubbery soft tie down material works great on the stems—they're gentle on the plant and avoid hurting it.

This early training takes place for about a full month before installing your ScrOG screens. When you do install them, make sure they're between 4 and 8 inches from the top of the pot. This will let you train your plants into the screen, not your screen into your plants. You may not get everything right first time—but that's okay. The most important thing when using ScrOG is to learn from your mistakes. Trust me: There's no other way!

Understanding Tucking

When I use the term 'tucking', what I mean is the process of bending the branch back under the ScrOG screen. Let me clarify: You are just tucking the branch underneath the screen to the adjacent hole, in order to keep it growing under the screen, horizontally. This is a canopy management technique, and should result in the most even, lush carpet of bud at the end of the whole process. Take the opportunity to tuck large leaves as you go, to keep it even more neat. Keeping a neat, even canopy will help to maximize your space, lights and yield.

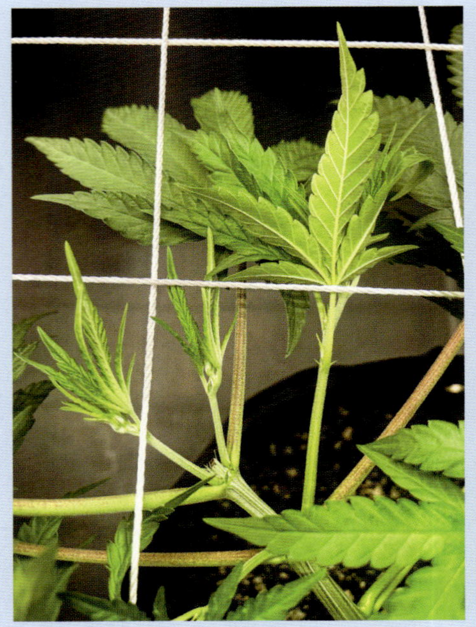

You can tuck your plants once they are reaching into the next square of the screen.

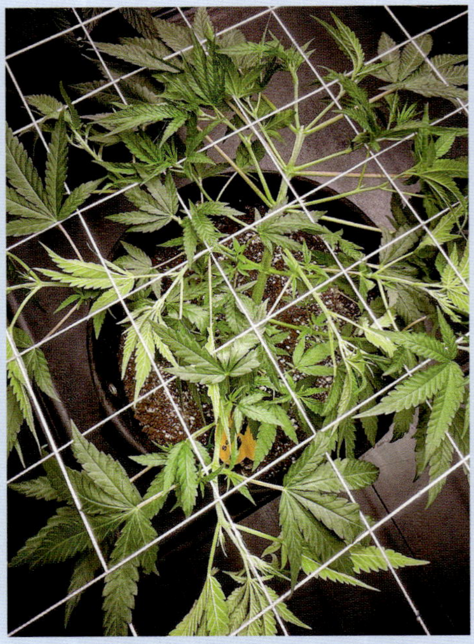

You are not weaving the plant in and out of the screen; you are keeping it tucked below it.

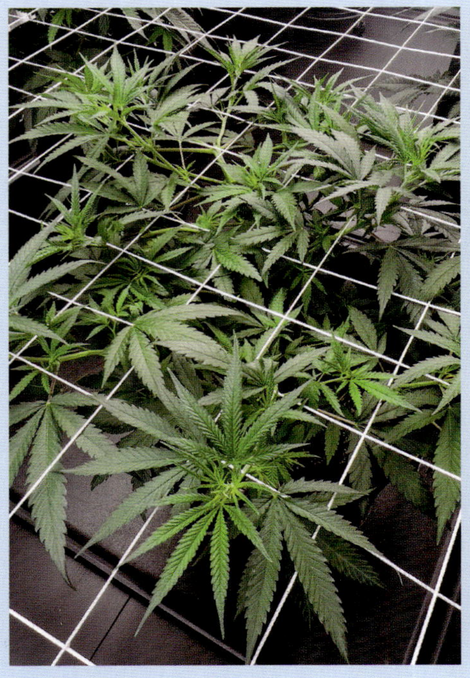

This leaf is prime for tucking.

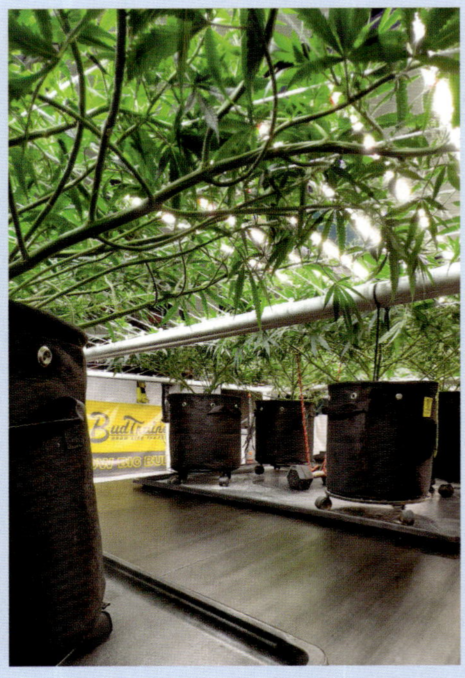

This has been well tucked and will grow a very neat canopy.

PHOTOS: NORTHERNSCROGGER.COM

As above, you should start tucking your plants as early as you can—as soon as they reach adjacent holes. Tuck your branches until your screen is over half full, and looking strong, to ensure a full canopy. Once your screen is looking 60%-75% full, flip your grow room into a 12/12 light cycle and watch those babies stretch! For the first few weeks or more (strain dependent) they will stretch like crazy, and during this period you must keep tucking. Don't lose the benefits of all your hard work by getting lazy now.

At about three weeks or a little later, the plant will begin the work of growing its colas, and you will have the pleasure of watching them grow up from the screen in an even, beautiful single layer. Because all these buds will be receiving an equal amount of light, your yield potential will be maximized and your cola development should be incredible. Your efforts at keeping your plants tucked will have been more than worth it.

Defoliation

Now we get onto more controversial territory: Defoliation.

Defoliation is the removal of plant growth and it's a topic that divides growers. Some call it pruning, but it amounts to the same thing: Cutting off healthy growth for the

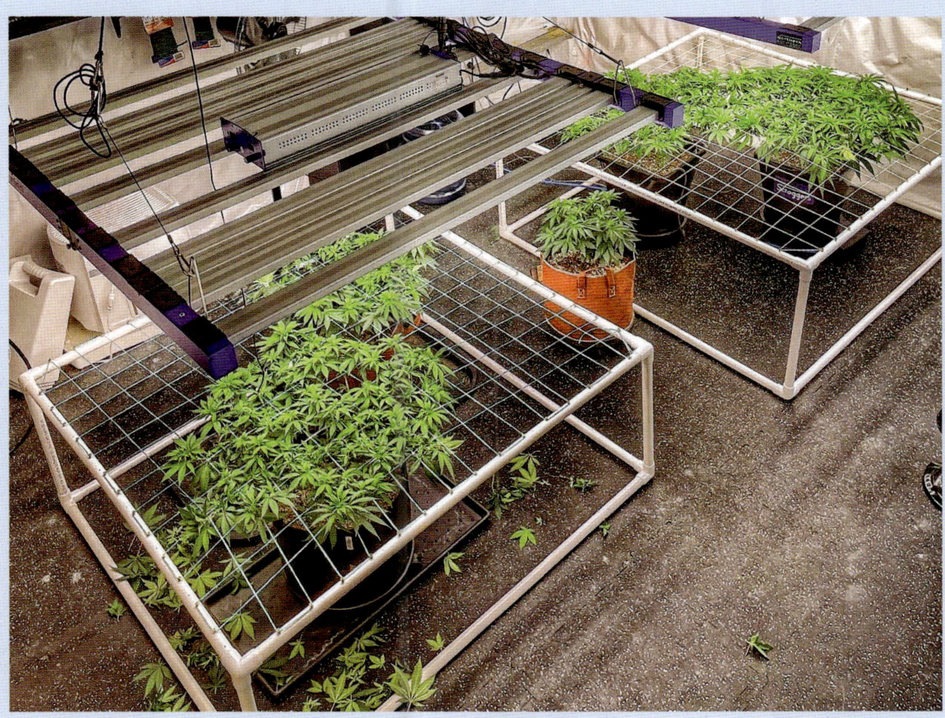

These plants have been defoliated—and they're thriving.

purposes of training. It's easy to understand why some hate the idea—why would you cut off any healthy plant matter if you didn't need to?—but my personal experience has shown me that defoliation is actually pretty essential in order to get the most out of your ScrOG grow.

It should be remembered that if you can tuck a leaf instead of cutting it, you should. This isn't a technique that's supposed to be used instead of tucking; it is supposed to compliment all the tucking you learned about above. Both have the goal of allowing the maximum light to reach the nodes and eventual bud sites.

Timing is key when it comes to defoliation. Tucking should happen all the way through the vegetative period. Two Major Defoliations should happen. First: One week before you flip the room to 12/12 light cycle, strip all foliage beneath the screen; yes, I mean all of it, down to bare sticks. It will take a few days at most for a healthy plant to recover, but they come back stronger than ever. The first time you do this, it will freak you out. Don't worry; have faith in the process.

Second: Flip the grow into 12/12, and then after 20 days, strip everything below the screen again. Be incredibly thorough this time; get small stunted buds, leaves,

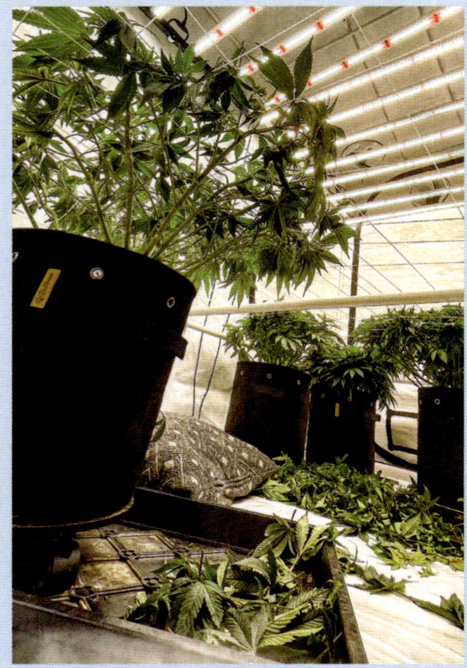

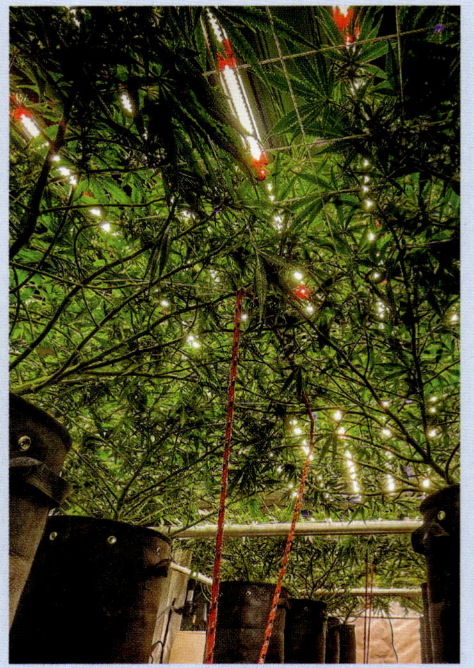

These plants have had all foliation below the screen removed, and are sending all their energy towards bud growth.

PHOTOS: NORTHERNSCROGGER.COM

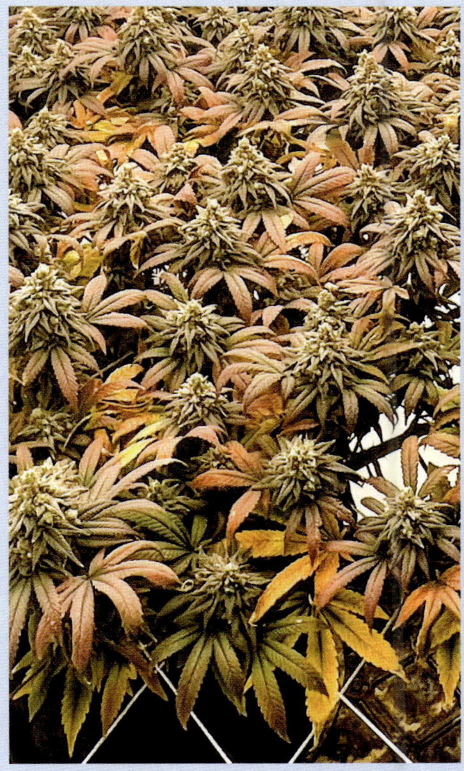

The results of these three methods are very clear to see!

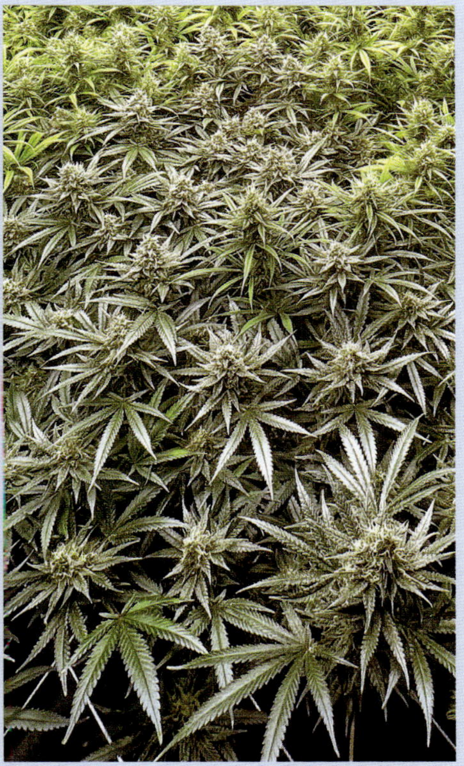

You can achieve this kind of canopy with just a little bit of work.

anything that's taking energy away from those main colas. Not only will you direct the plant's energy to the right places, you'll also help avoid mold and mildew by ensuring good airflow around the bud and main grow sites. The downside of tucking is that it blocks up the screen; this defoliation helps clear all that out.

For many growers, stripping their plants back like this can be a difficult thing to do. If you're not convinced, try it with only one of your plants and compare its final yield, and overall health, to the plants that you didn't defoliate. I'm certain you'll see more growth, with stronger, bigger colas, a neater canopy and no mold at the end of it. The important thing is to give your plant time to recover after that first defoliation.

By utilising these three methods, you'll be tapping into the traditional ScrOG methods that made the technique so popular to begin with. You'll also be giving your plants the best possible conditions in which to grow strong, even canopies with beautiful bud.

Keep on Tuckin'

Sweet Seeds® Guide to Plant Bending

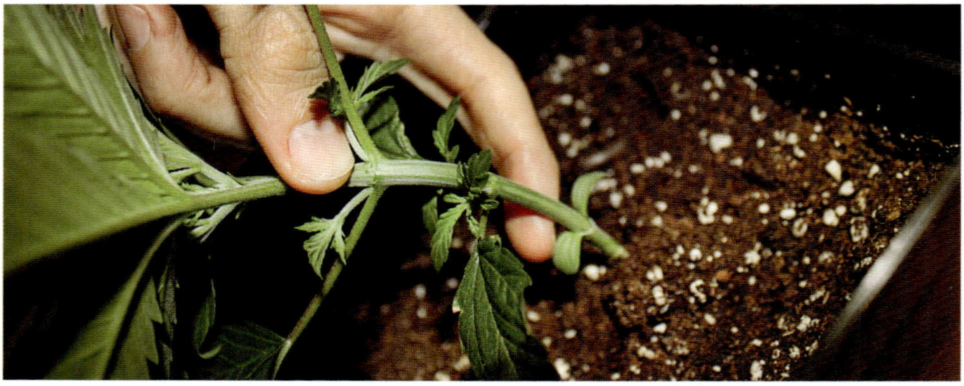

You can bend a young plant easily without breaking the stem.

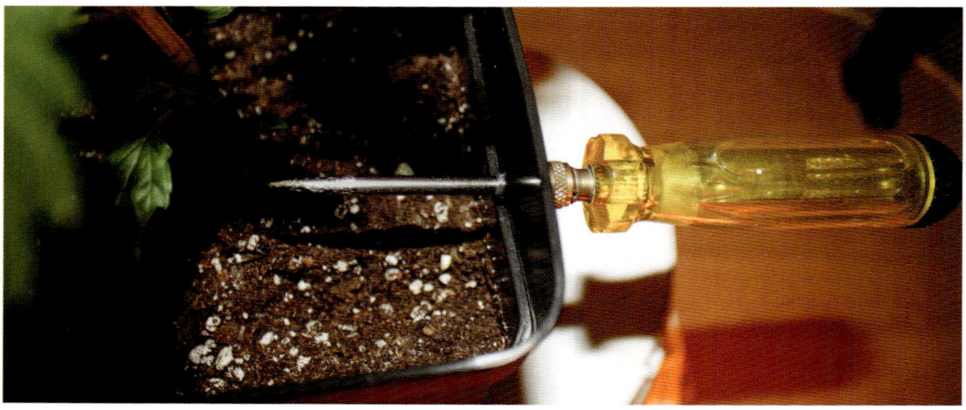

Make a hole for a tie point for the top part of the stem. Keep this hole as far away from the plant as possible.

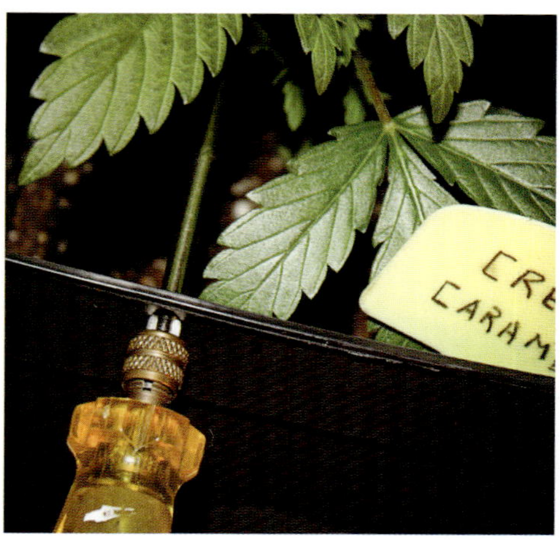

This lower stem hole should be as close to the stem as possible.

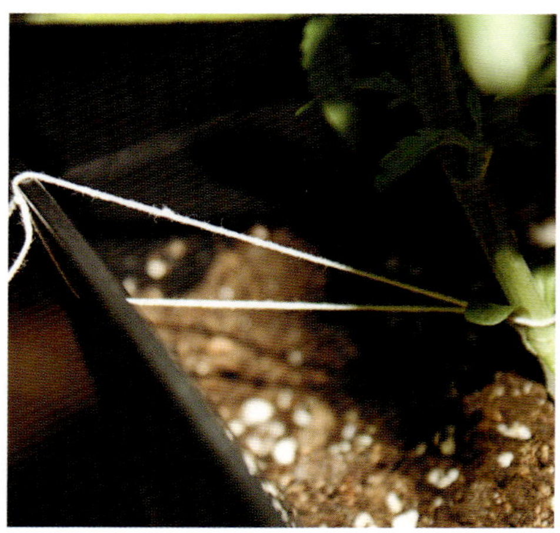

First bend occurs by looping "around" the lower stem and low stem hole.

PHOTOS: WILD ROSE® AND CREAM CARAMEL® / PHOTOGRAPHED BY TOMMY L. GOMEZ

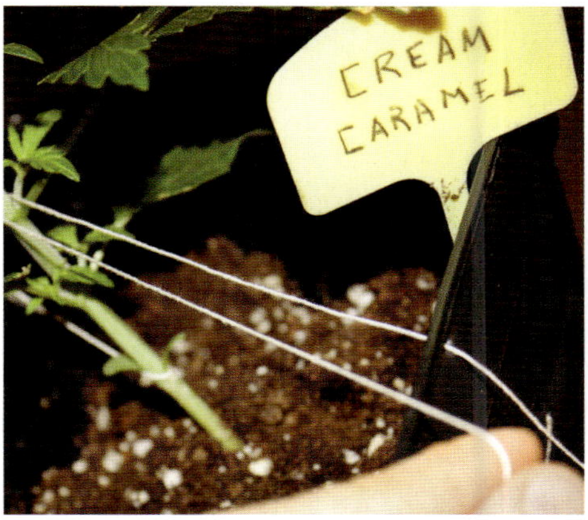

Do not tie a knot on the stem. Stems grow in width. Loop it.

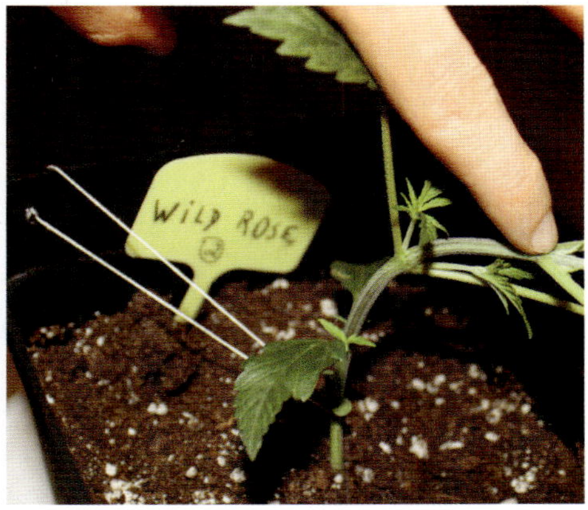

The second bend occurs on top.

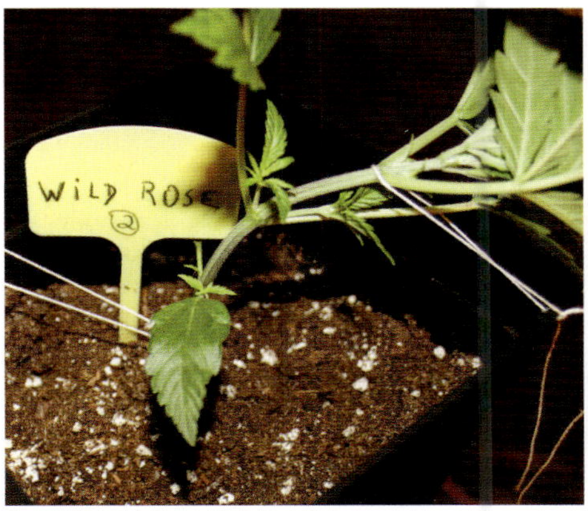

Fix the top to the furthest hole.

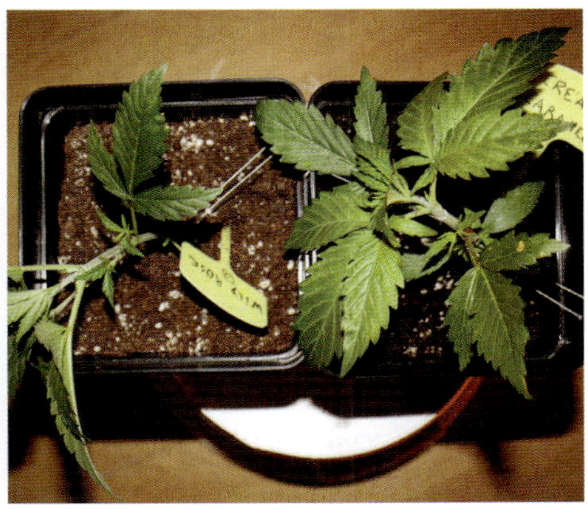
Overhead view of the shape of both bends.

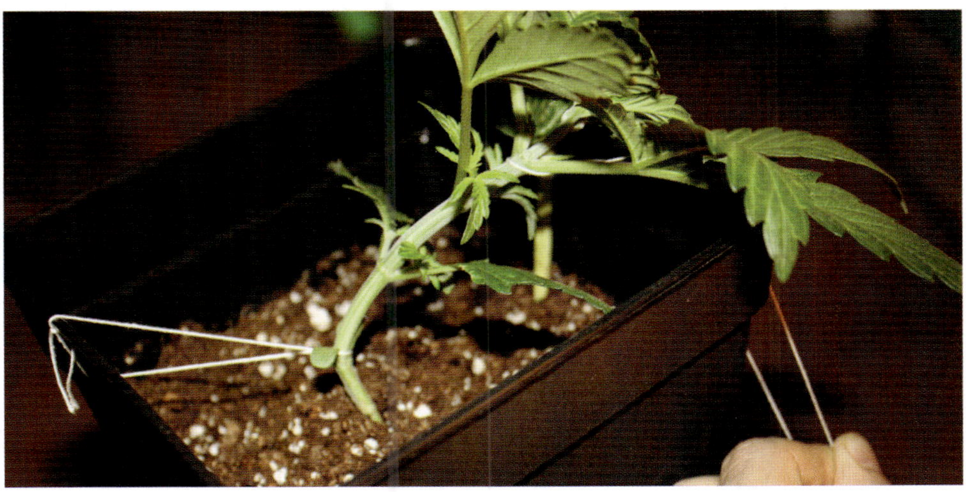
You can pull and shorten this top loop to shape your plant.

Central Point Screen Fixing

Some ScrOG growers prefer to tie and stake down the center of the screen to prevent it from being pushed up by the central canopy of buds, as the buds directly under the light tend to be more vigorous. While these plants may not grow tall, they are likely to yield the most bud per unit area. If they were to push the screen upward, it would cause uneven light distribution, as well as lead to stems and branches breaking if not handled with care. To avoid these issues, do not let your plants remain in vegetative growth for too long, as the development of more leaves than buds makes the ScrOG method less effective. To secure the center of the screen, use a line to fasten it to a point on the floor and a weight with a suitable attachment point to hold it down.

Leaning and Bending Techniques

If you find that your plants are naturally bending too much, raise the screen for the next cycle or invest in a stronger mesh. If you've crafted your own screen, you can enhance its thickness with thicker wire or a sturdier line. Adjusting the screen's height and thickness in this way allows you to fine-tune your setup.

If you have many branches to contend with, you can guide them over and under the screen, directing them inward or in a clockwise or counter-clockwise direction. Your objective is to prevent one cola from casting a shadow on another. This deliberate positioning of plants is more efficient than allowing them to grow in various directions. For support, secure plants diagonally against each other, using the tension created by the weight of adjacent plants. Although diagonal tying is better suited for standard grow room setups than SOG or ScrOG grows, it is an option. When the screen effectively does its job, additional tying becomes unnecessary.

Experiment with different screen shapes and observe their impact on your overall yield. Some ScrOG growers use a stadium-shaped screen to match the curvature of light dispersion, although it's unclear how much this affects the final yield. A slight yield improvement may not always justify the extra effort required. Nevertheless, shaping and training the plants in different ways can be exciting, and can help put some fun into growing.

Training, Not Pinching or Breaking (yet)

Be careful not to crush or pinch the stems, as this can lead to the development of branches around those areas. While this "supercropping" isn't necessarily a bad thing and can even enhance yields, the growth of additional branches directs the plant's energy toward leaf and branch development rather than bud production. When a branch undergoes supercropping and manages to recover, the healing process stimulates further branching. These new branches tend to emerge in irregular locations around the injury site, and these nodes may become filled with bud. Supercropping is an advanced technique for ScrOG setups, but it's not as effective for SOG, which prioritizes vertical growth rather than lateral. More information about supercropping can be found in Chapter 13.

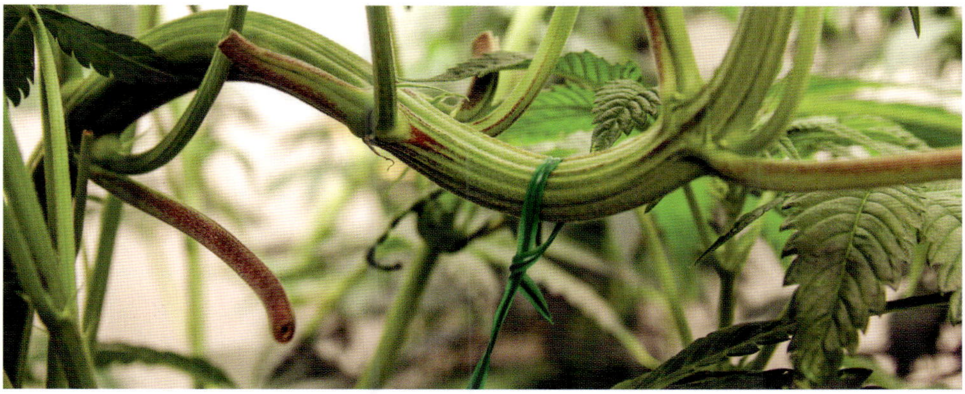

Notice how the loop allows the stem to grow without strangling it. This is important; otherwise, the twist tie will cut through as the stem expands.

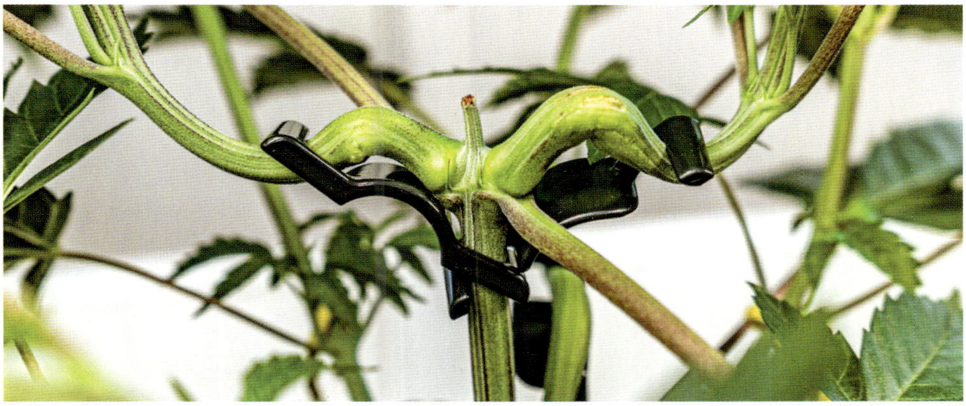

BudTrainer's BudClips are becoming increasingly popular not only for bending branches with their curved bracing technique but also as a useful tool for topping your plants.

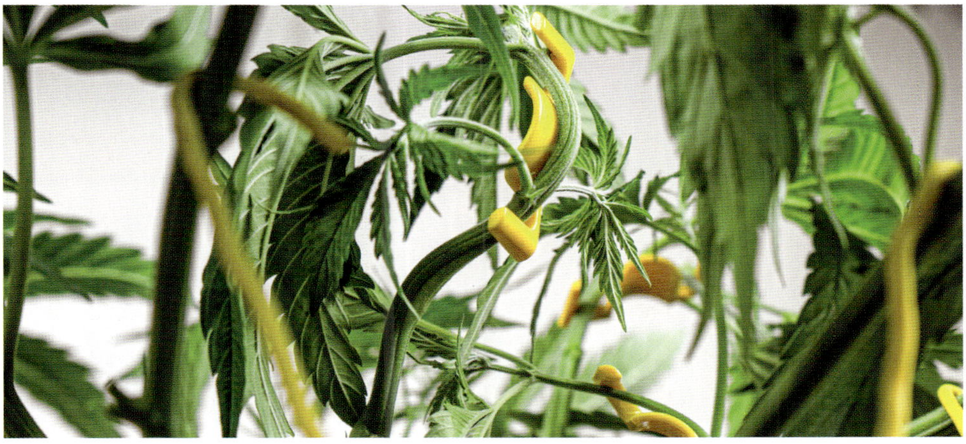

A combination of BudClips and BudHuggers can shape a plant any way you want. As long as you bend down, the plant will try to grow back up again.

PHOTOS: DAVID STRANGE (TOP), BUDTRAINER.COM (MIDDLE AND BOTTOM)

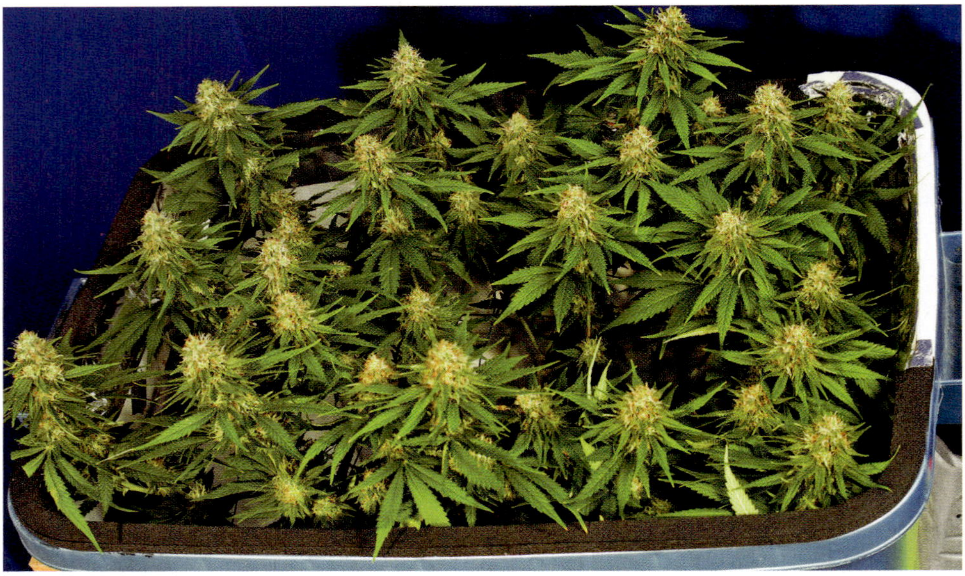

In this photo, we have a single Jack Herer plant grown using ScrOG.

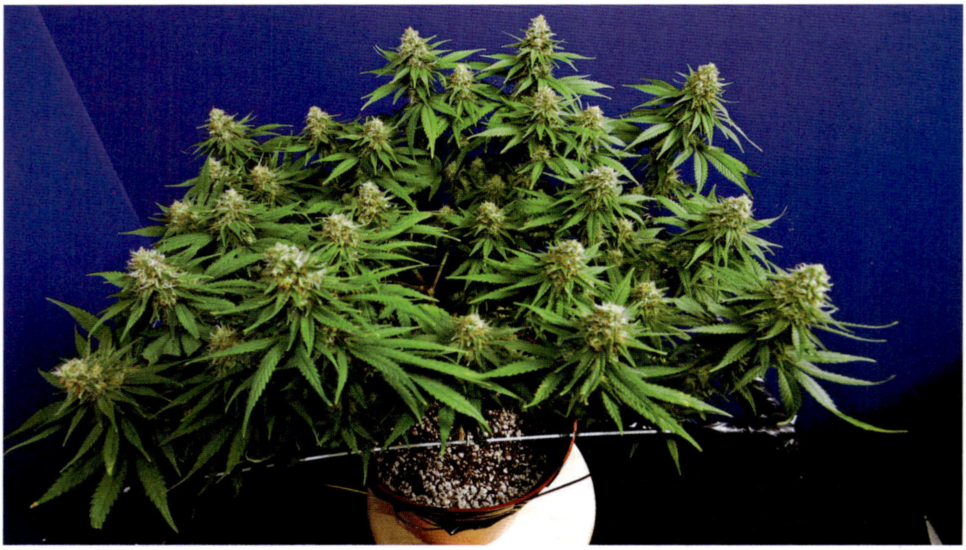

This ScrOG set up demonstrates how much bud one plant can produce.

Single-Plant ScrOG

It's possible to create a lush green canopy using the ScrOG technique with just a single plant. In our ScrOG photos, you can see examples of a single-plant ScrOG setup, showcasing the potential to achieve over 20 colas from a single plant through careful branch pruning. You may find it necessary to prune a branch multiple times to encourage further branching, though be aware that each round of pruning extends the growing time.

PHOTOS: WEADO

The ScrOG pruning technique can induce lateral growth even in strains that do not naturally exhibit bushy growth. This makes single-plant ScrOG particularly well-suited for promoting extensive canopy coverage. However, the more you repeat prunings, the longer you have to wait for recovery and growth in the vegetative phase. During the flowering stage, these newly formed smaller branches will expand, producing additional leaves and flowers.

With careful pruning, each branch should occupy a section of the mesh. You can train branches in various directions without weaving them over and under the mesh. First, guide each branch through an open square in the mesh. Once you anticipate sufficient coverage, you can initiate the flowering phase. The mesh will provide the necessary support as the flowers develop, allowing them to lean in various directions while maintaining the planned positions. This flexibility allows each branch to bend more freely, enhancing overall plant structure and bud development.

SOG and ScrOG Lighting Considerations

Lighting plays a crucial role in these advanced growing techniques. Incorrect light placement can lead to uneven canopy heights. Placing the light too close causes stretching at the periphery of the canopy. Placing the light too far away causes excessive stretching throughout the entire canopy, which will negatively impact yield.

HID lights, especially those with higher wattages, can be excessive unless you're working with a sizable SOG or ScrOG area. Given the compact nature of these setups, often in grow tents, a high-quality LED light is optimal. LEDs offer reduced electrical costs, generate less heat, and provide the flexibility to train branches closer to the light source, effectively directing the maximum available light onto your canopy.

While it's still possible to use HID lights in these systems, anything above 600 watts is overkill for tent setups and can lead to higher expenses. As mentioned in the lighting section in Chapter 7, some growers opt for HPS bulbs throughout the entire growth cycle rather than switching from MH to HPS, necessitating investing in multiple types of lights.

Although MH lights are better suited for vegetative growth, they are not used to extend the vegetative phase in budget SOG and ScrOG setups. Therefore, if you choose to use HID lights, use smaller HPS lights like the 250-watt and 400-watt series to reduce electricity costs and heat generation while still achieving satisfactory yields.

While LEDs are generally recommended for these growing methods, the choice of lighting and the balance between expenditure and heat management is ultimately up to you.

Sweet Seeds® Micro ScrOG

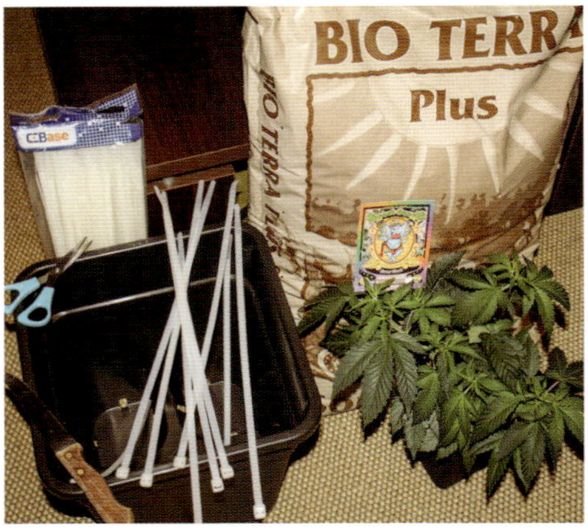

Items needed: Thick locking strips create the mesh.

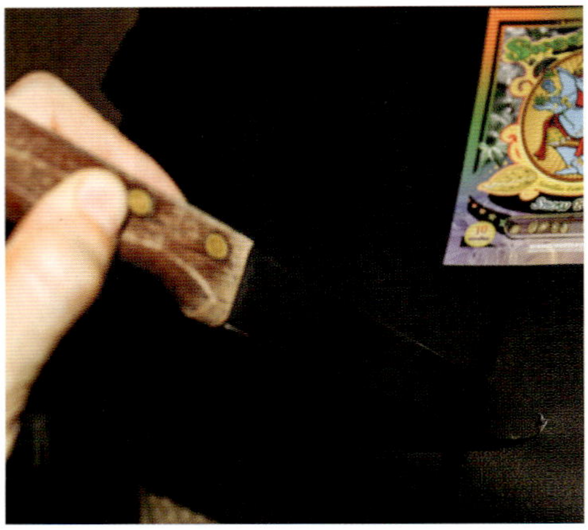

On opposite sides, puncture the upper rim to slot the strips.

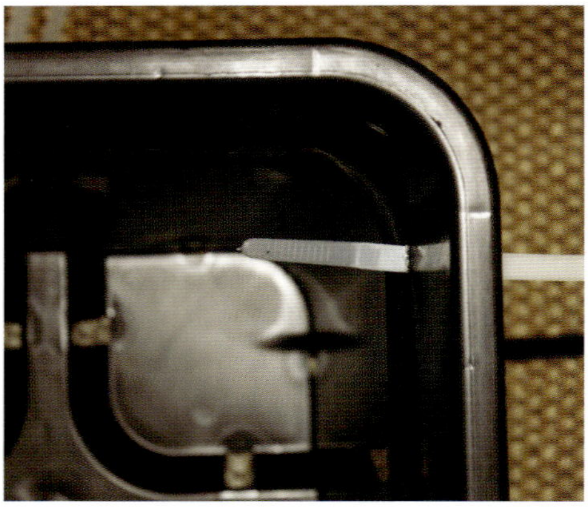

Check to make sure the strips can go through.

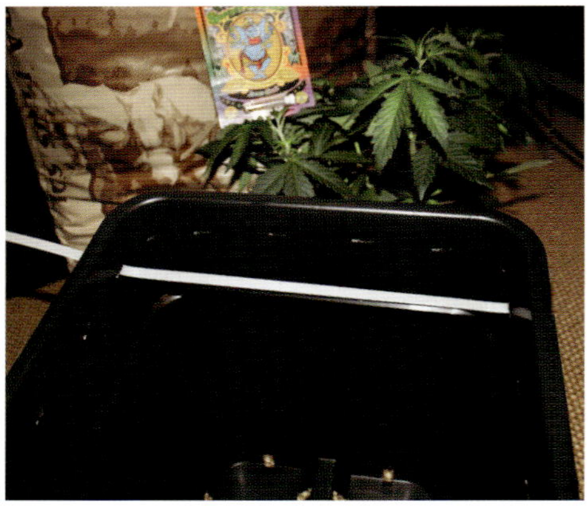

Punctures should be opposite each other for a through slotting.

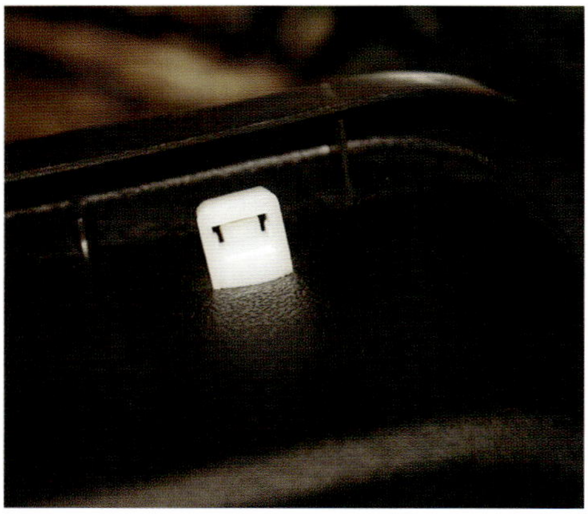

Pull it right through to the clasp point.

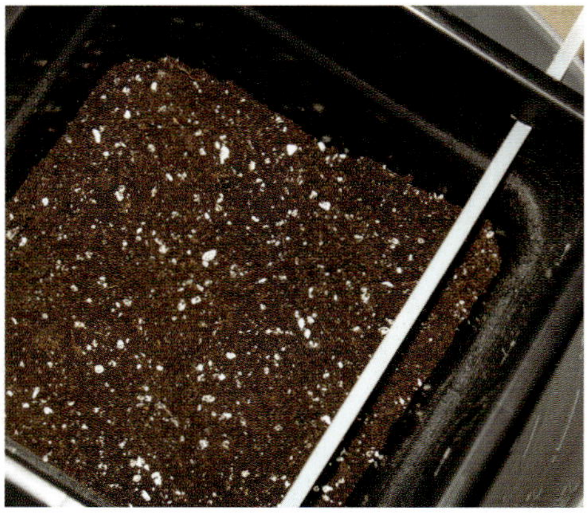

You now have one strip of the mesh in place.

PHOTOS: SWEET SEEDS / PHOTOGRAPHED BY TOMMY L. GOMEZ

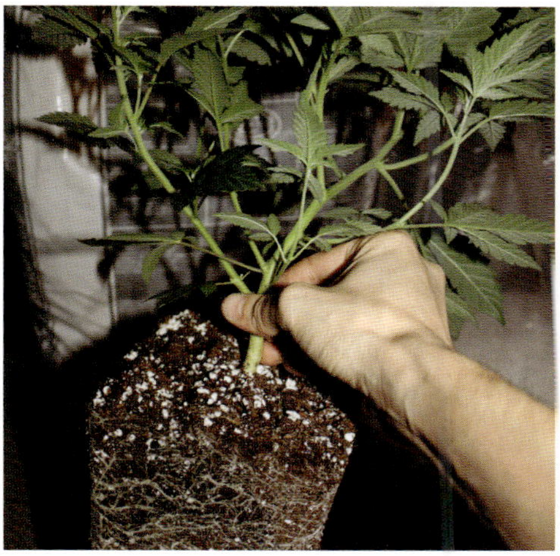

Get your clone ready for transplanting.

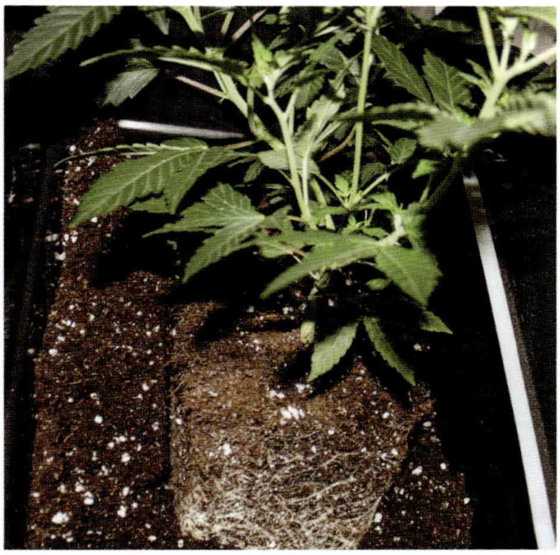

Clone medium needs to be well below the strip.

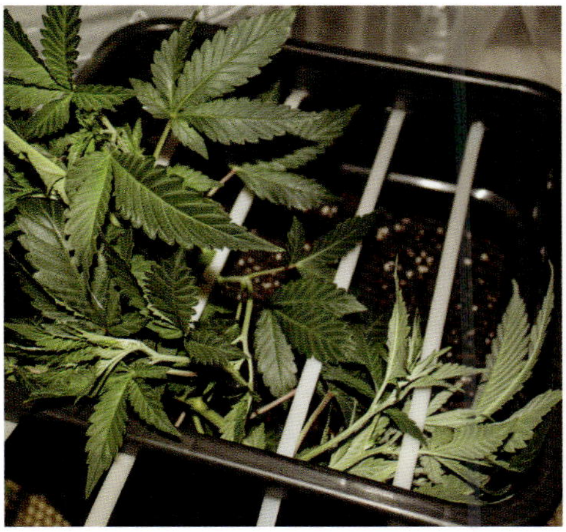

Complete more strips.

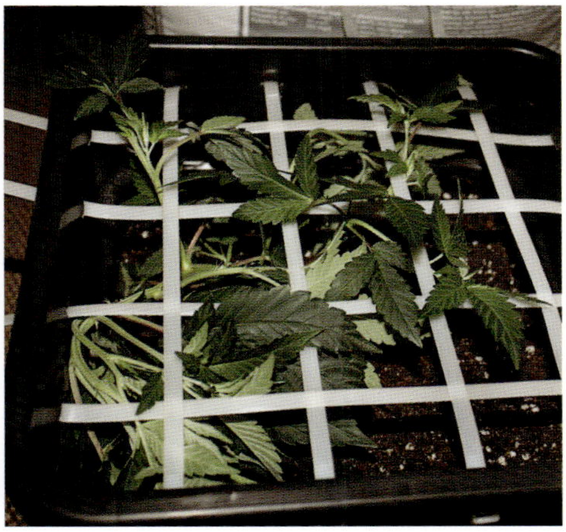

After adding more soil, complete the strips.

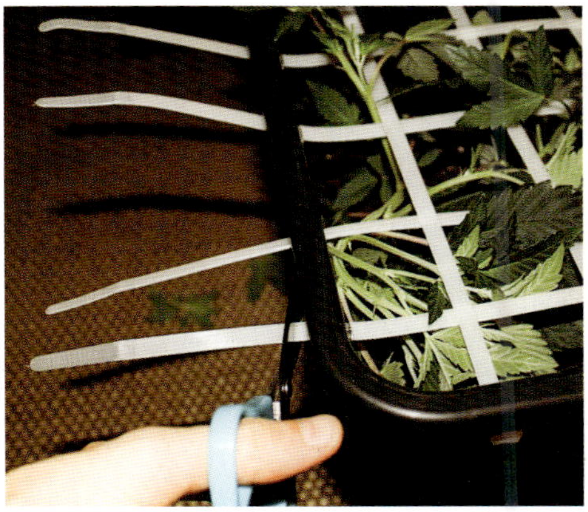

Cut away the ends and tape them down.

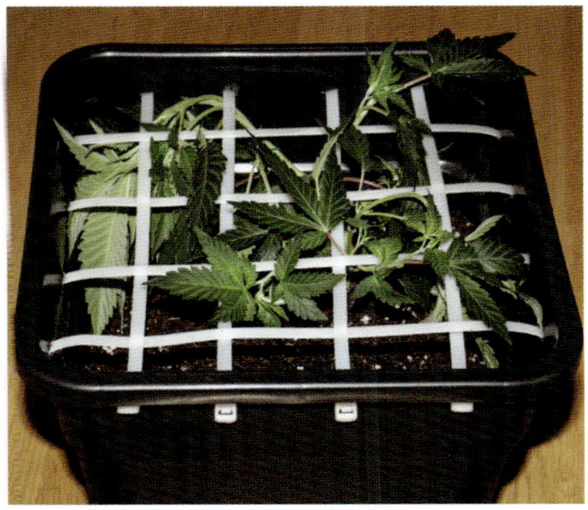

You now have a single plant ScrOG setup.

continues...

Sweet Seeds® Micro ScrOG *continued*

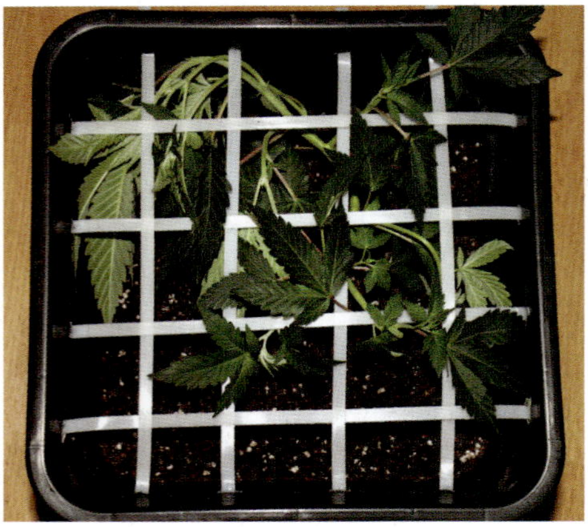

Bend branches under the strips.

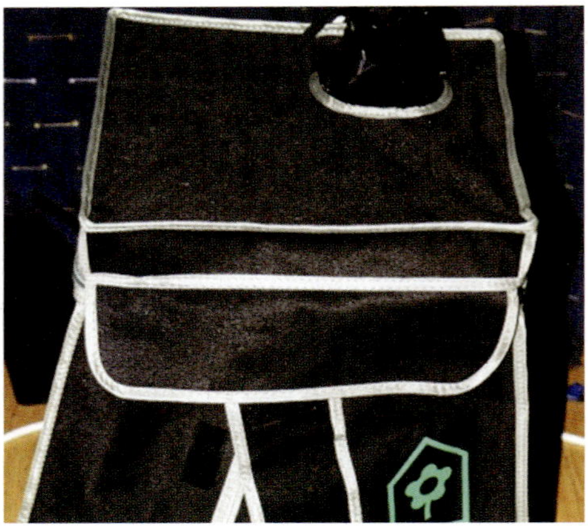

It easily fits into a small grow tent.

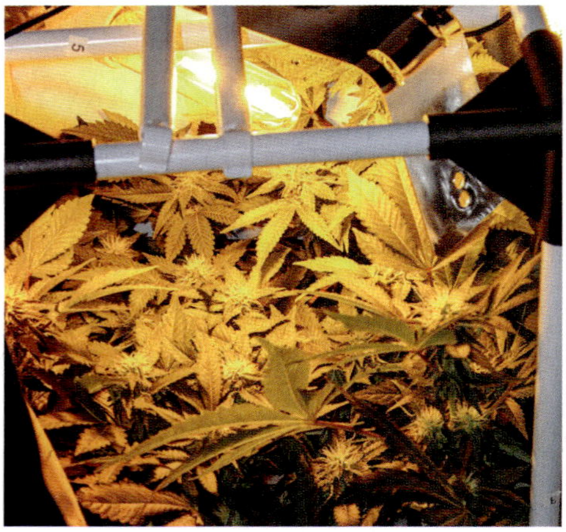

Mini ScrOG in a grow tent.

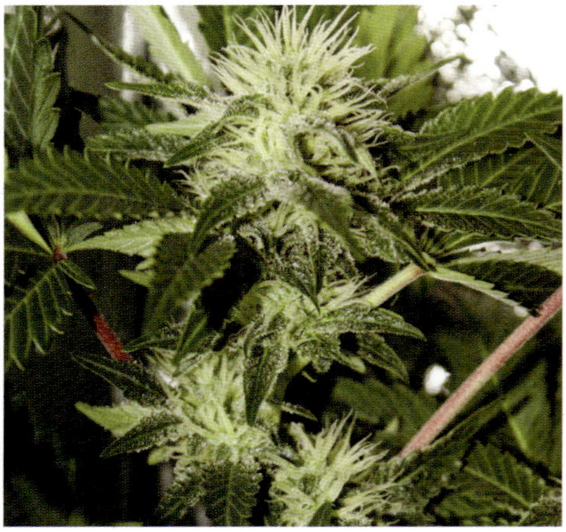

Flowering in a grow tent.

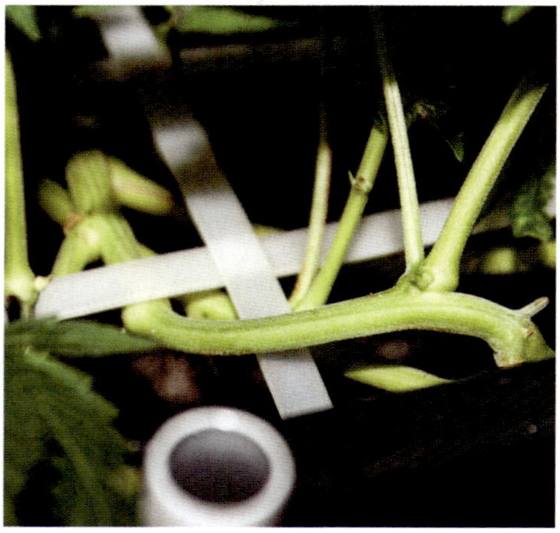

Branch bending using the strips.

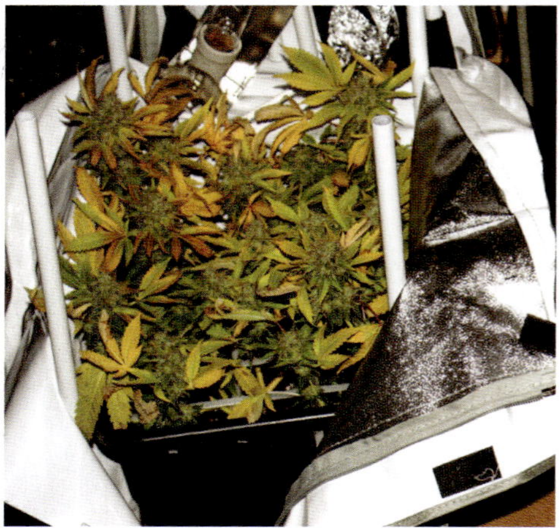

End of flowering.

PHOTOS: SWEET SEEDS / PHOTOGRAPHED BY TOMMY L. GOMEZ

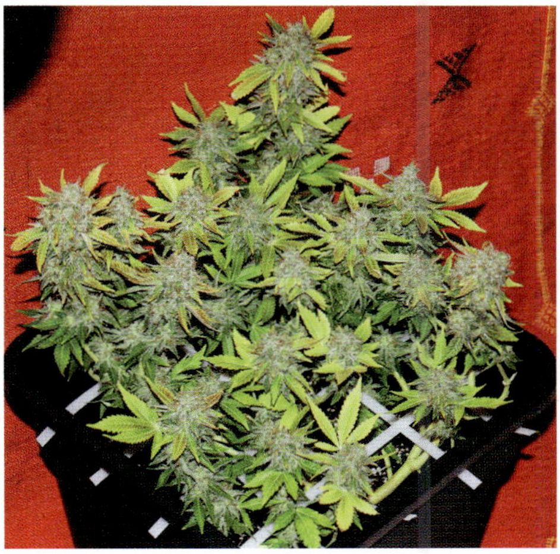
Single plant ScrOG results.

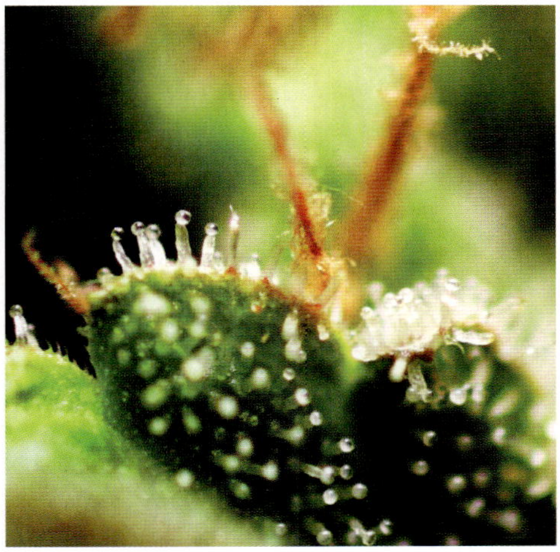
Trichomes aplenty.

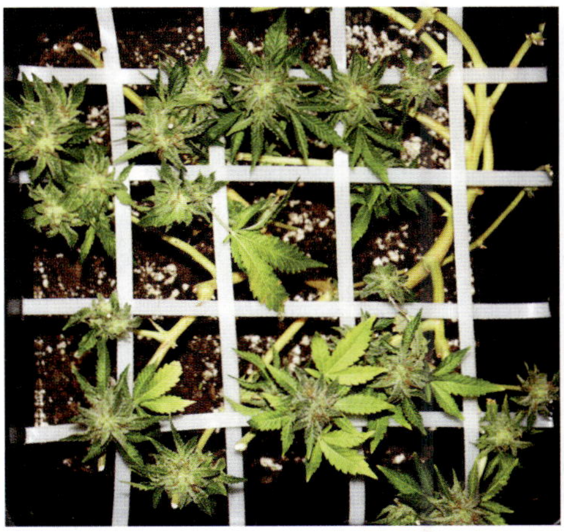
Removal of leaves to demonstrate plant shape.

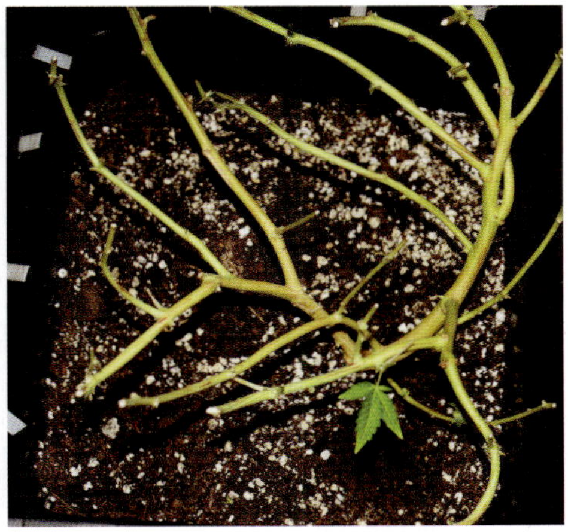
Only branches left show bending results.

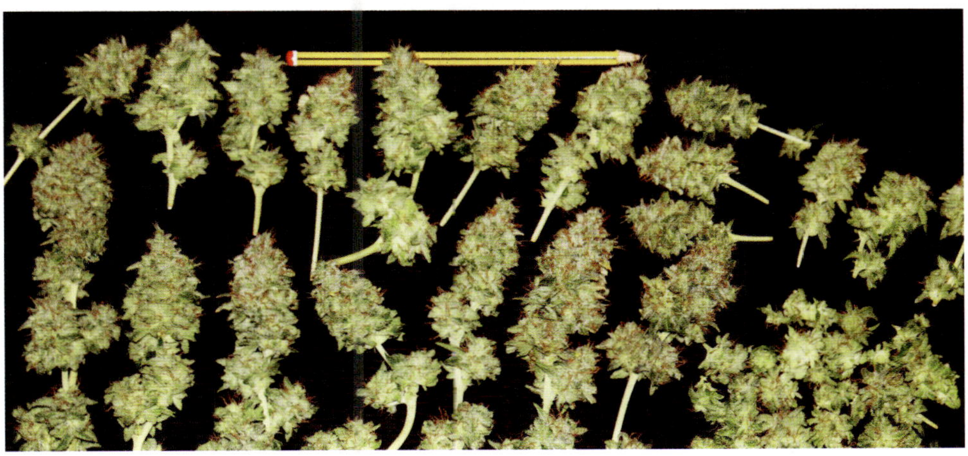
The rewards of a single small ScrOG system.

PHOTOS: TOMMY L. GOMEZ

Closet Growing

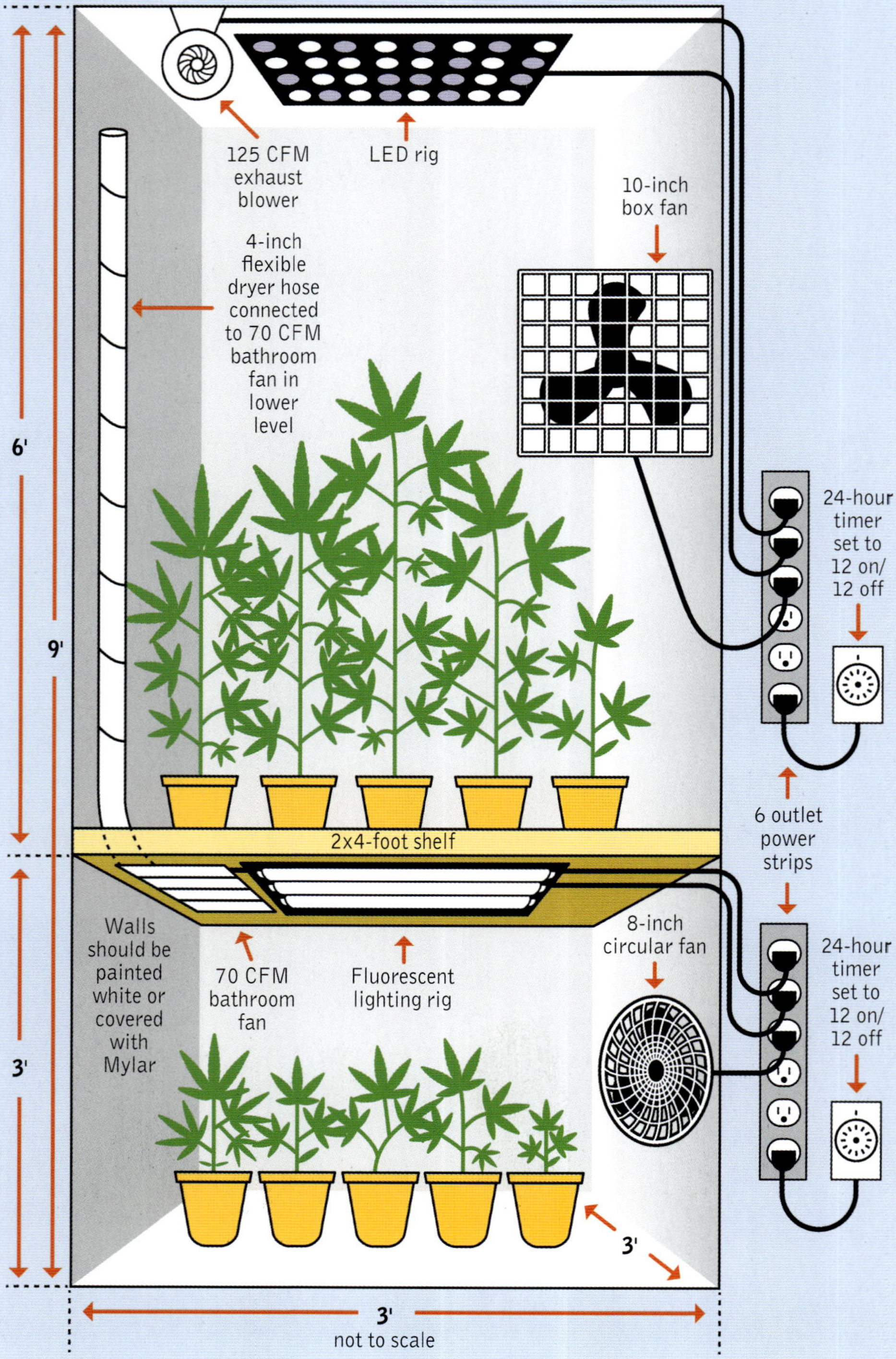

Tents and Cabinets

Tents and cabinets can be combined with SOG and ScrOG techniques for more advanced cultivation. Tents rely on rigid plastic or metal supports with canvas walls, while cabinets are typically constructed from wood or metal. Neither tent nor cabinet growing falls under the category of highly advanced cannabis cultivation, but they offer remarkable effectiveness. They are easy to use, result in high yields, and allow for stealthy growing. They are also compact and do not require an entire room, making them pet safe and more effective at pest control.

A cabinet may be a small closet, old refrigerator, a customized box, or even a simple cupboard. Tents are commonly made of multiple layers of polyester canvas and polyethylene (PE), making them both highly waterproof and tear-resistant. These growing environments provide exceptional stability, enabling growers to have complete control over nearly every aspect of the cultivation process. Some models even feature observation ports, eliminating the need to unzip the entire front of the structure to observe the plants. You can make your own grow tent or buy one that is relatively affordable and accessible online. Tents are typically equipped with internal reflective materials, such as Mylar, and are designed to be light-leak proof.

Both tents and cabinets typically accommodate anywhere from one to 12 plants, although larger tents can be as big as a small greenhouse. These setups can be divided into sections to facilitate the separate cultivation of clones and flowering plants. You can also buy or create smaller cabinets or tents and partition them to achieve this division. The primary advantage of tent and cabinet grows is your ability to maintain a continuous cycle of plant growth.

To get started with a tent or cabinet setup, you'll need three components: Tent or cabinet, lighting, and an air ventilation system.

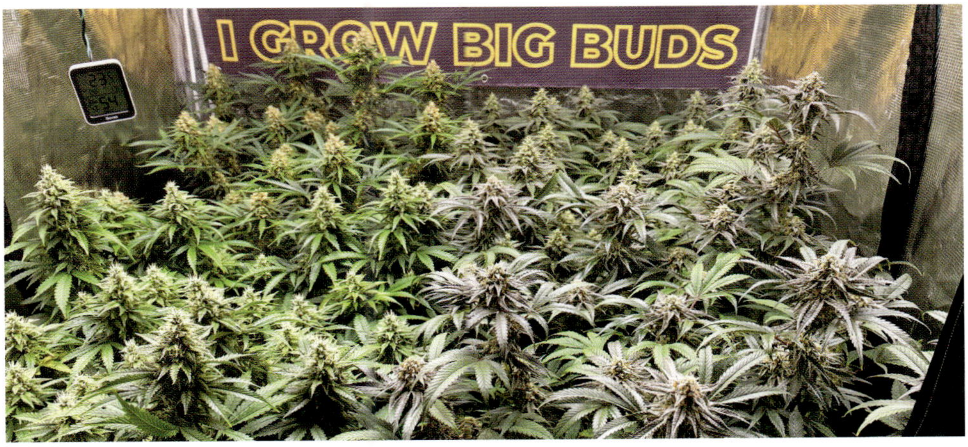

PHOTO: BUDTRAINER.COM

Grow tents are genuinely just as innovative as LEDs for modern indoor cannabis cultivation.

Hydroponic and Soil Grow Cabinets

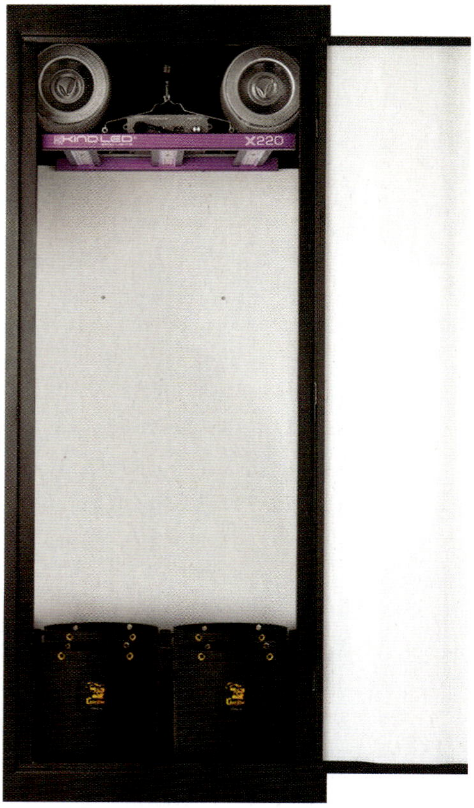

Modern grow cabinets pack a lot into a small space, including carbon filters.

Hydroponics can also be used with a grow cabinet just as much as soil.

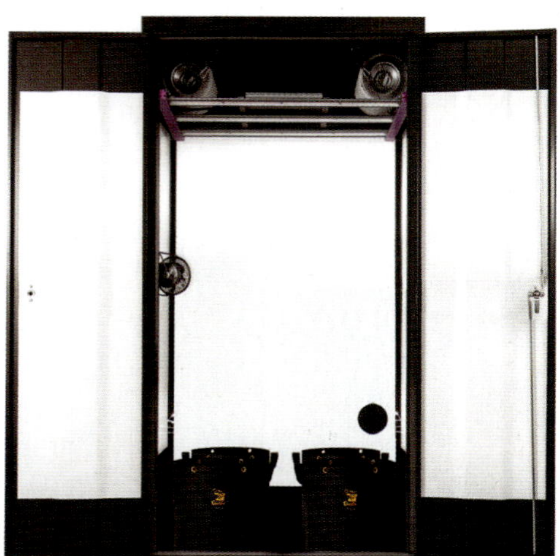

Many cabinets come in different sizes to give you various space options.

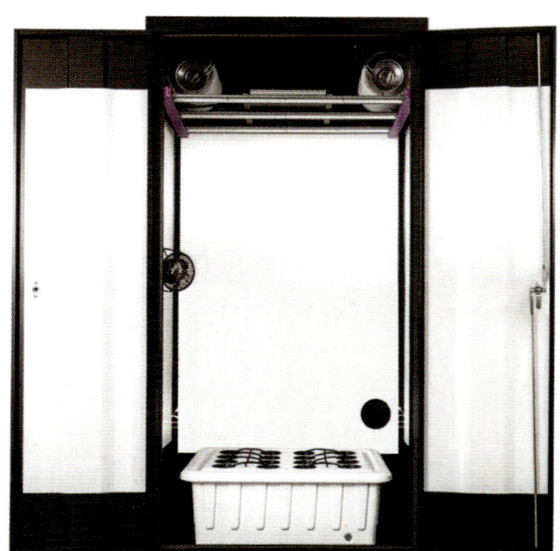

Unlike tents, the structure of the cabinet doesn't bend with air movement inside.

PHOTOS: GORILLAGROWTENT.COM

Most growers use adjustable straps, chains, or spring-type cords to set up their lights. For ventilation, growers typically make a large hole low in the cabinet or tent to allow air intake and another higher up for air extraction, though tents often come pre-designed with these openings. An extractor fan placed near the top hole removes the heat generated by the light. LEDs require less ventilation due to their lower heat output.

The intake hole should be located on the opposite side, with the intake fan operating at a faster speed than the extraction fan. This ensures that a fresh supply of air circulates before exiting the grow space. Passive intake, while quieter and less disruptive, can create a vacuum effect, potentially allowing unfiltered air to seep in through any cabinet leaks. Keep the fans active and the intake operating faster than the extractor to maintain effective air filtration and control.

When using carbon dioxide supplementation as discussed in Chapter 8, make careful calculations to avoid excessive venting. If you are using HIDs, you can mount a four-inch dryer flange on the light hood and connect it to the exhaust fan flange with a four-inch dryer hose. This setup pulls air through the light, cooling it before it exits the grow space. Because LEDs generate less heat, temperature management is simpler.

A cabinet can be painted white inside or lined with Mylar to reflect light. Most tents come pre-fitted with Mylar-type reflective surfaces.

Similar to tents, cabinets can be equipped with compartments for clones. Horizontal shelving is better than vertical shelving for non-professional setups. Because vertical systems may stack rows of clones one above the other, this presents two significant concerns: Potential spills and rising heat. Liquids from an upper shelf can leak or spill, posing a danger to the electrical components of lights or ventilation systems underneath. Even if plants are enclosed in humidity domes, there is still a risk of electrical hazards from liquid drips. Trays can mitigate this risk and capture potential spills, ensuring safety. The use of hydroponics further compounds the risks associated with vertical setups.

Vertical divisions are also prone to temperature disparities, with the upper compartments being warmer than the lower ones. While LEDs help manage heat more effectively, HIDs generate heat and contribute to this heat imbalance. In cabinets where the flowering compartment is located below the clone compartment, it's vital to extract warm air and introduce cool air. Horizontal compartments are better for most tents because they are typically safer. For additional safety, segregate clone cultivation using a separate smaller cabinet or smaller tents.

After harvest, well-rooted clones can be transferred to the grow tent or cabinet, continuing the perpetual growth cycle. Keep in mind that cabinet shelving must be sturdy enough to support the weight of potted plants after watering as well as flowering plants.

Tent Screen of Green

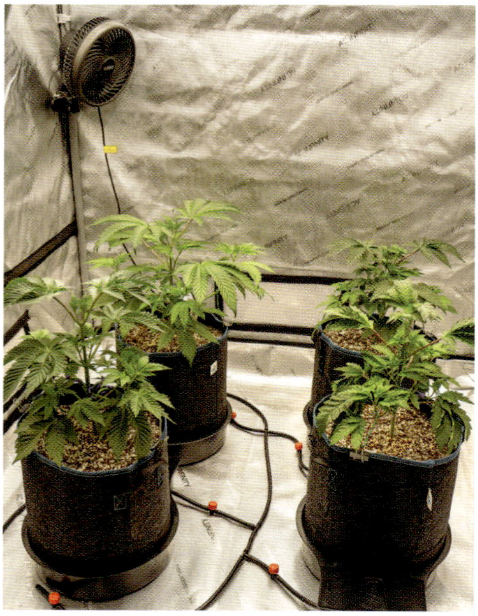

Your focus with ScrOG is to get lots of branching, so topping and pruning are helpful here.

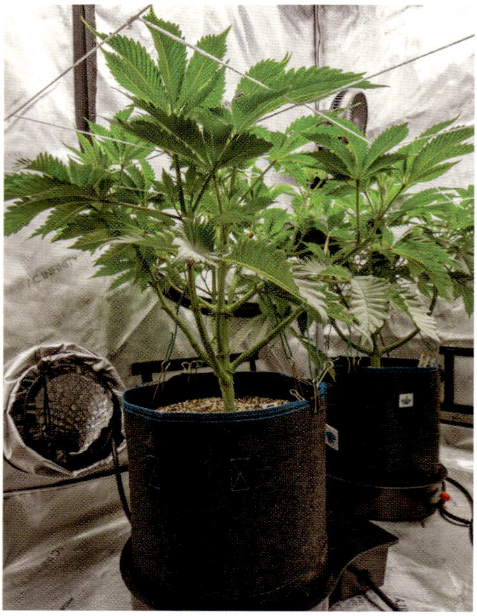

A squat plant in vegetative growth is ready for the screen. Place it so that several gaps are over the one plant.

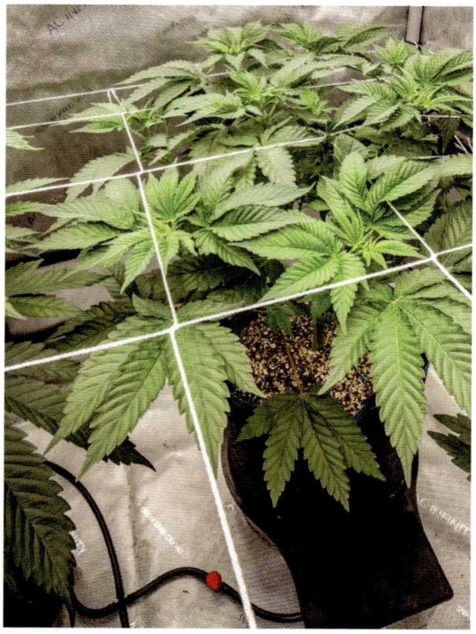

You can see how the sides of each screen square will support future branch growth.

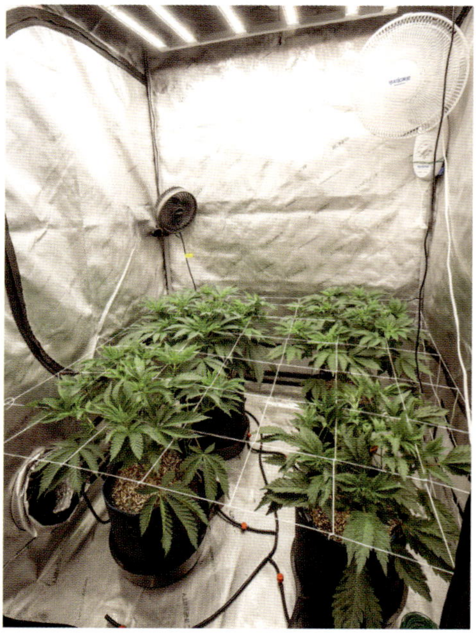

As vegetative growth continues, the plant will fill in the squares of the screen above branch growth.

PHOTOS: JOE'S CANNA GROWS

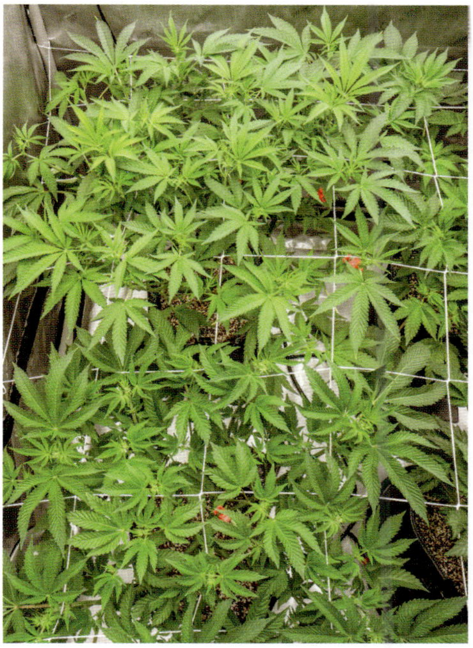

This overhead view of a ScrOG gives you an idea of how the plants will move through it. The gaps will fill in during flowering.

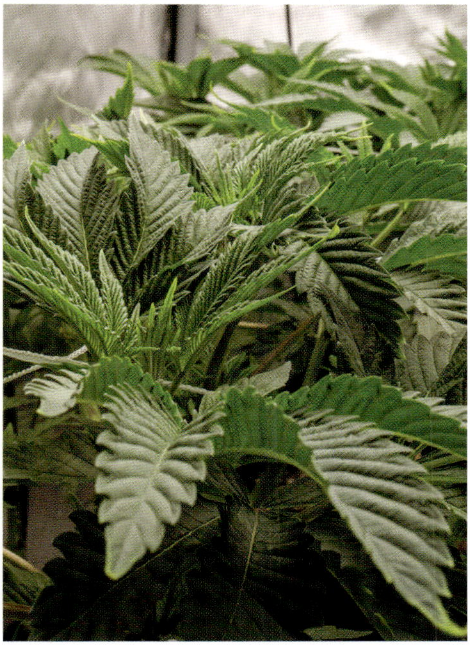

An even canopy is already emerging because of the screen. Check to make sure the screen doesn't bend too much.

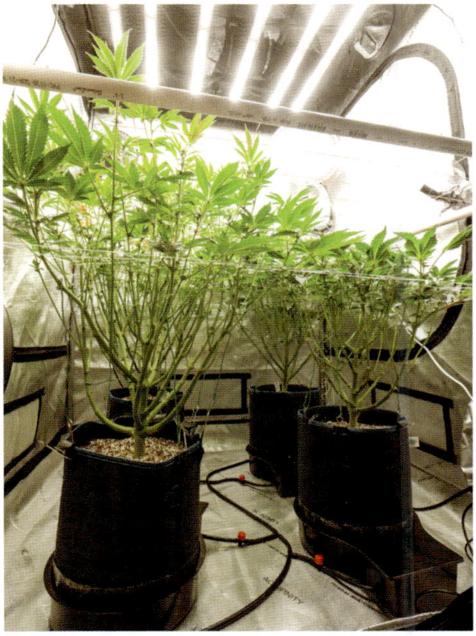

This ScrOG has undergone some defoliation of leaves under the mesh. You can see how these have been pruned for shape.

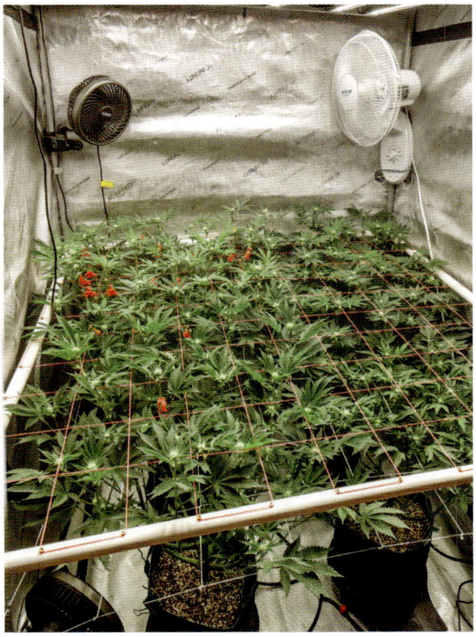

The flowers in the early weeks of growing will be thankful for the screen as it keeps them pointing upwards.

continues...

Tent Screen of Green *continued*

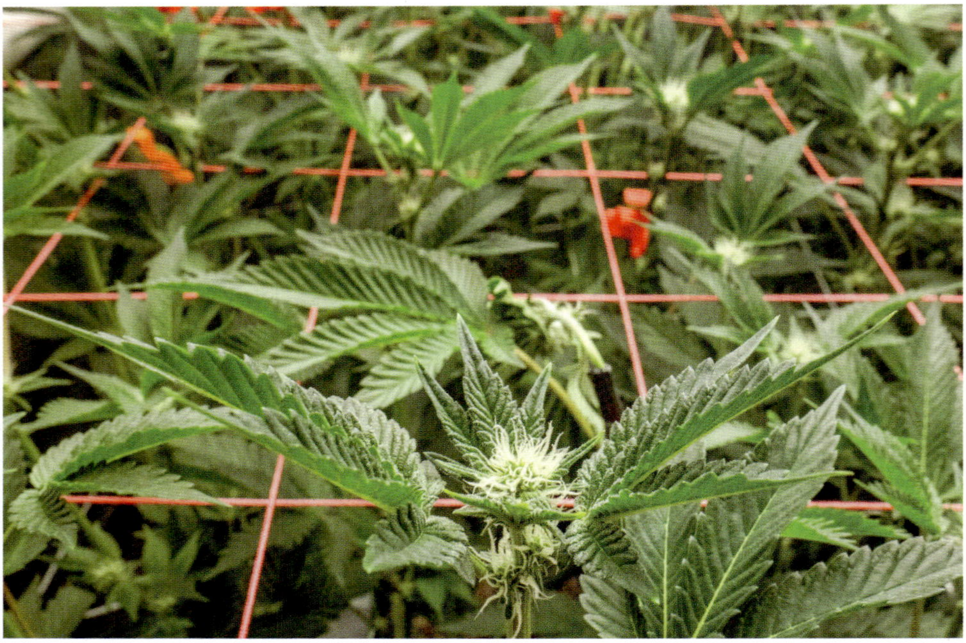

The screen encourages an even canopy and will help maintain that flatness as much as possible throughout vegetative growth and flowering.

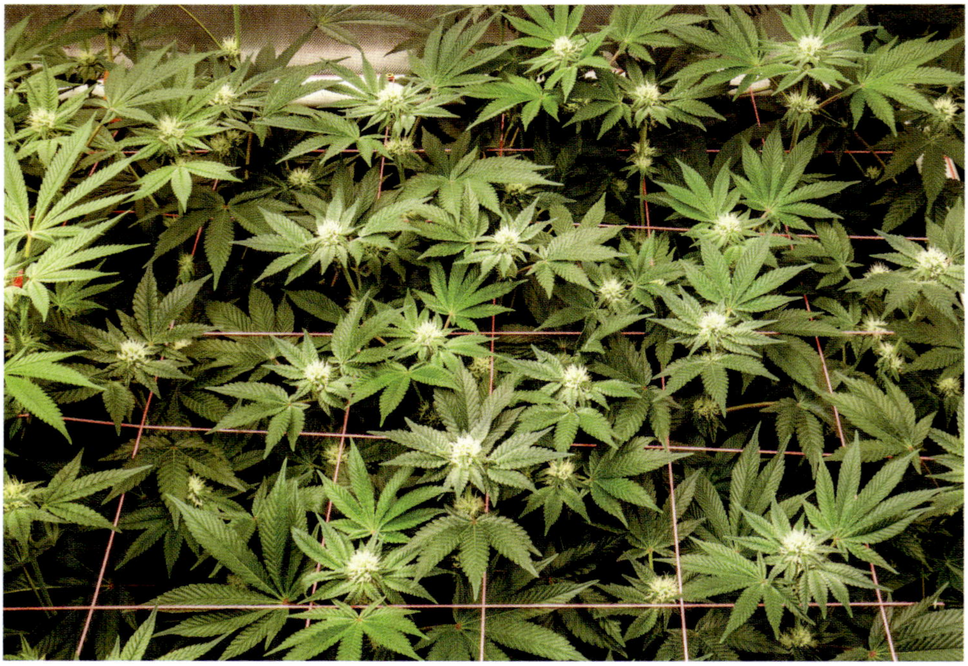

An overhead view of the ScrOG at the start of flowering. This height at flowering is perfect for where your screen should be.

PHOTOS: JOE'S CANNA GROWS

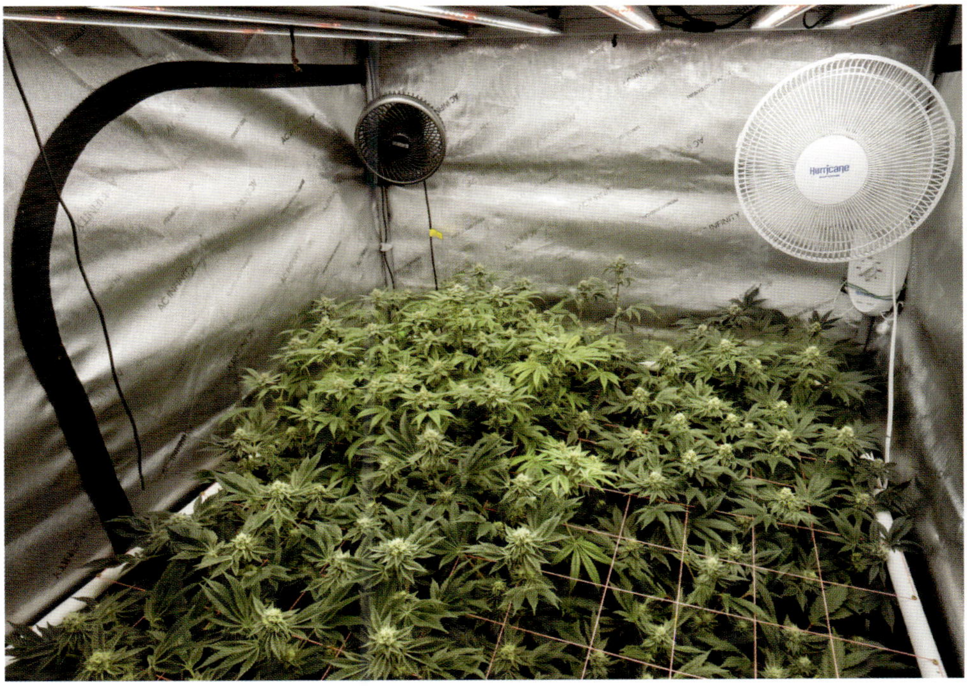

A ScrOG is perfect for new hybrids or strains with a lot of variation because the screen prevents taller plants from collapsing onto the shorter ones.

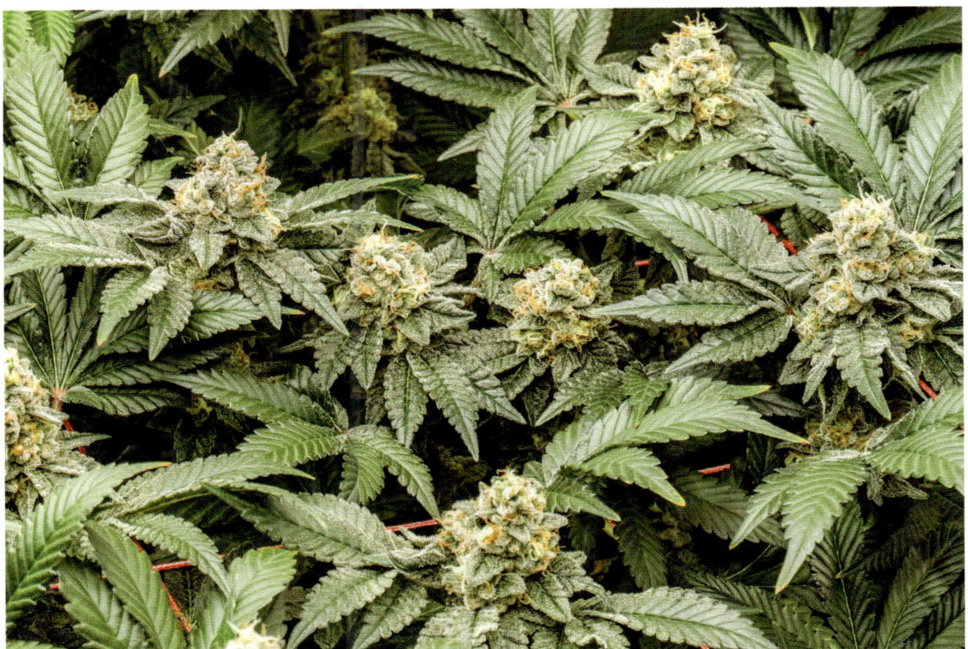

In a well-designed ScrOG, many colas per square foot emerge. Amazingly, something as simple as netting can increase yield.

Autoflowering Strains and Perpetual Harvests

The emergence of autoflowering hybrids has made perpetual harvests more complex. If you're cultivating autoflowering strains, you'll likely rely on seed-based propagation rather than cloning because their flowering process is tied to their age. When you take a cutting or clone from an autoflowering plant, the genetic predisposition to flower remains intact, regardless of your attempts to keep it in a vegetative state; the duration of the vegetative growth phase is beyond your control. Autoflowering hybrids have not demonstrated an ability to revert to the vegetative state effectively. Therefore, it's essential to carefully consider whether autoflowering strains are suitable for your SOG or ScrOG setup.

When dealing with autoflowering strains that have been crossed with regular strains, predicting and controlling the flowering process becomes more challenging. Experimentation may be necessary to determine the best approach.

Customizing Your Growing Setups

The advanced growing methods discussed in this chapter are highly customizable. Many cannabis growers have transformed entire rooms into ScrOG or SOG setups, but those content with a monthly yield of about four ounces of dried bud may prefer a small SOG in a tent. The choice between these methods ultimately rests with you. ScrOG works best when dealing with diverse strains, while SOG thrives when using uniform clones. Under optimal conditions, growers can harvest as much as 30 to 50 ounces of

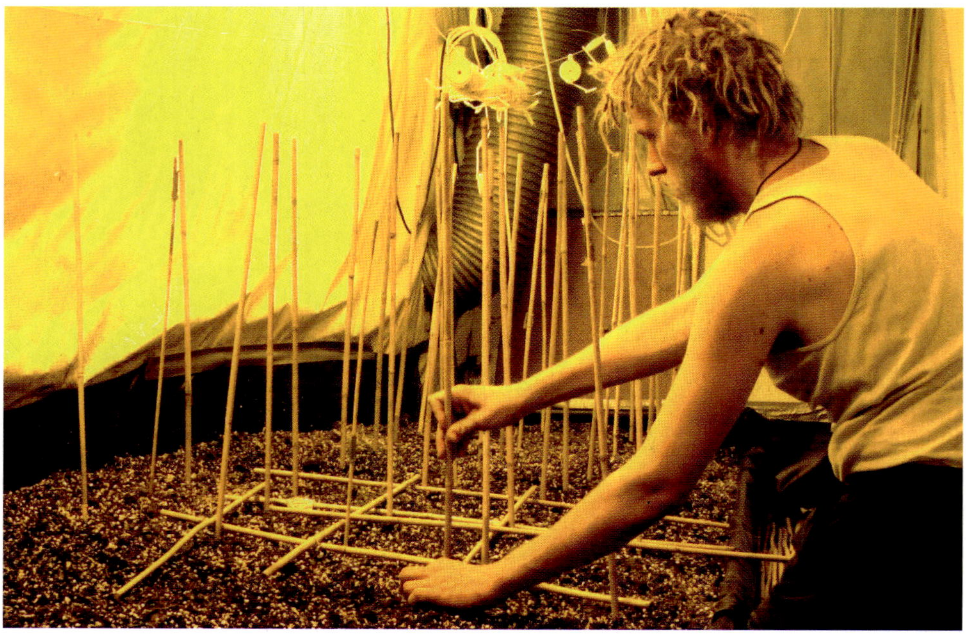

PHOTO: ED BORG

Bamboo stakes can be used to create a grid with support stakes. These can reinforce side branches so that they remain upright and do not bend under their weight.

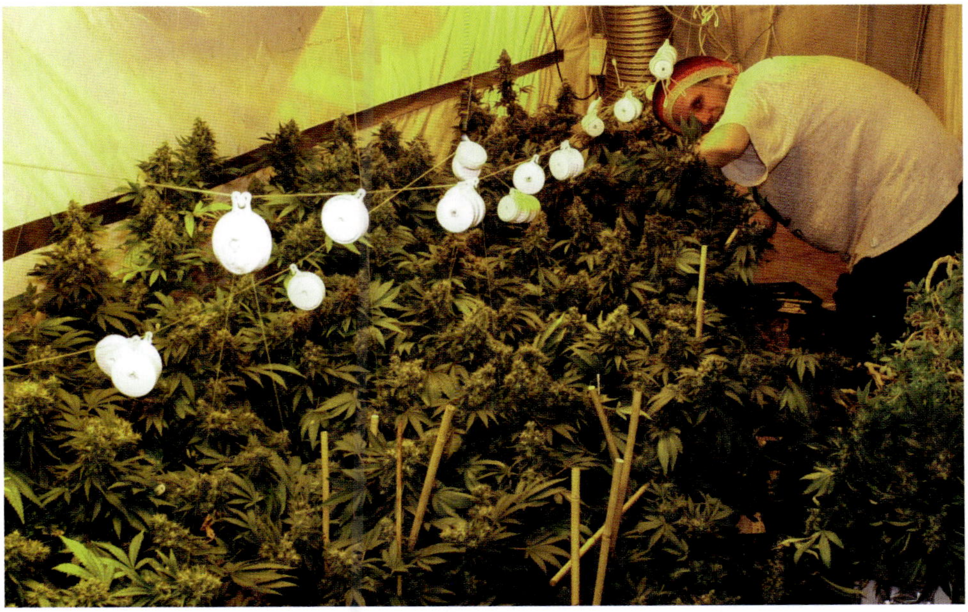

The branches rest against the bamboo stakes, sufficient to keep them from falling sideways. Bamboo also allows for points to tie up the plants.

cannabis every two months in a medium-sized room from either setup. However, each ounce of cannabis translates to one square foot of space. For example, to achieve a 30-ounce yield, you would need around 30 square feet of space, or a 5 x 6-foot room with one plant per square foot.

Like the growers who have contributed to this book, you can continually experiment to maximize the use of your growing space. For you, cannabis growing could evolve into an intense hobby, and a highly rewarding one at that. Over time, you may delve deeper into plant genetics, potentially developing your own strains from breeding and stock. You might even consider entering competitions, or end up producing some of the finest seeds available on the market. For a comprehensive exploration of breeding and genetics, refer to Chapter 17.

Another avenue worth exploring is hydroponics. While soil growers can achieve comparable results, hydroponic growers often find it easier to manage densely packed spaces due to the way nutrient reservoirs feed plants through a network of pipes. Hydroponic systems also often lead to slightly faster grow cycles than soil-based cultivation. Many portable hydroponic systems, like Nutrient Film Technique (NFT), seamlessly fit into grow tents and can be assembled effortlessly. All you need to do is fill the system with nutrients and cultivate your rooted clones with no need for pots, soil mess, or concerns about overwatering. Zip up the tent, and you're good to go. If hydroponics piques your interest, Chapter 11 is dedicated to hydroponic systems.

PHOTO: ED BORG

Autoflower Devotchka: Seed to Flowering

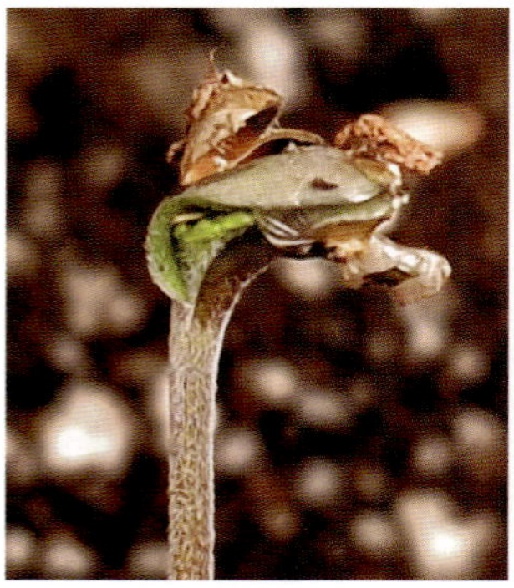

Autoflowering germination is the same as standard seedlings.

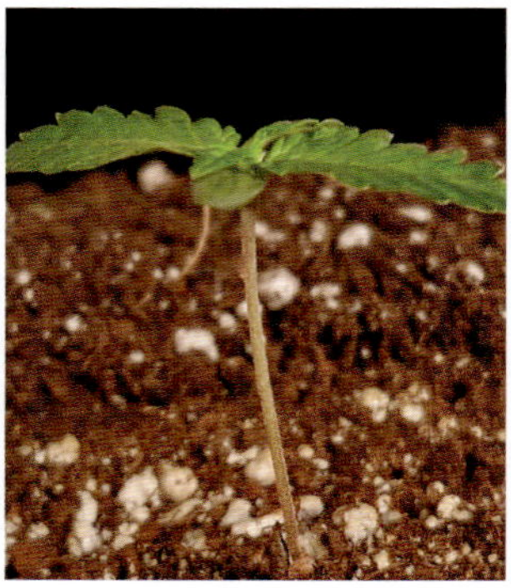

Autoflowering seedling breaks the surface.

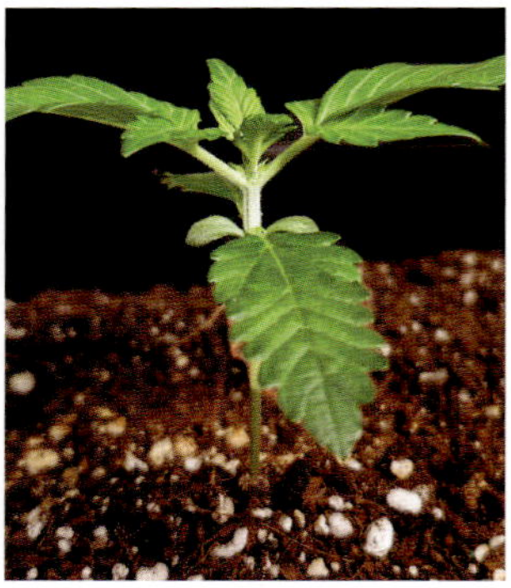

Autoflowering seedlings reaching for the light.

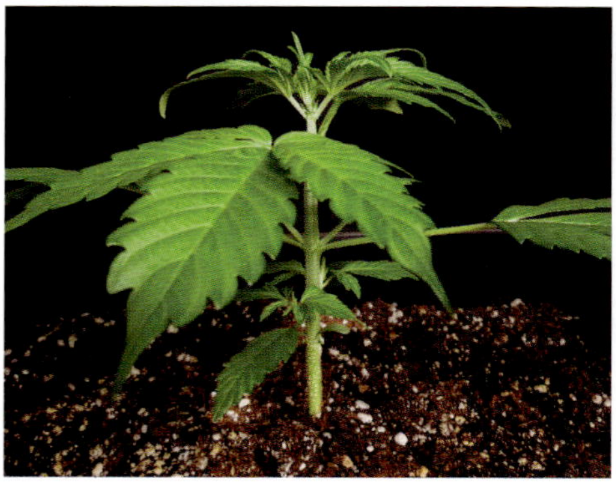

Autoflowering genetics have been hybridized with standard plants.

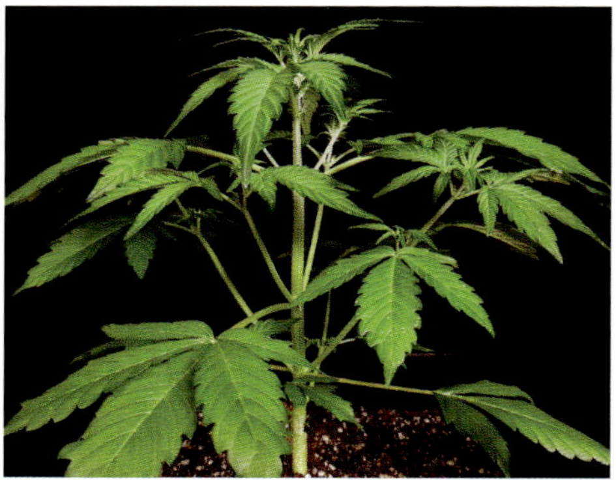

You can expect autoflowering plants to be shorter than usual.

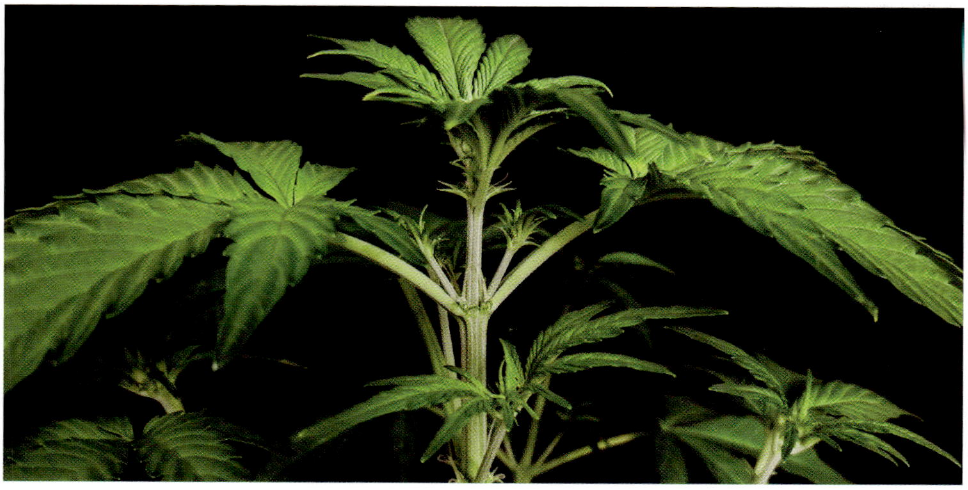

Autoflowering plants will mature based on age, not the photoperiod—but still need 24/0 and 12/12 like standard genetics.

PHOTOS: DOCTORSCHOICE.FARM / PHOTOGRAPHED BY FRANZ JANYR

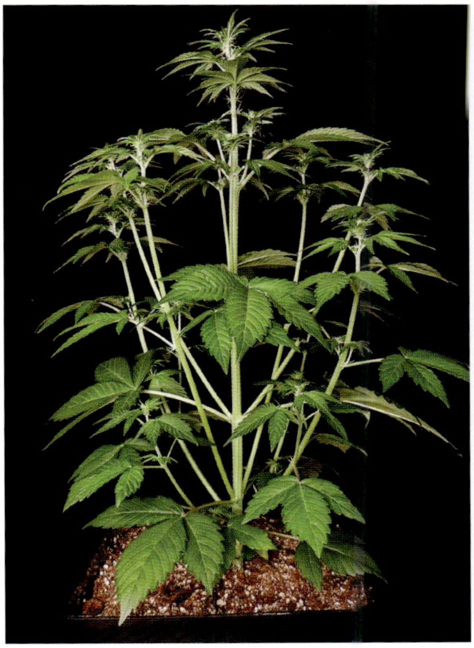

Autoflowering in pre-flowering and ready for 12/12 and to put on some height.

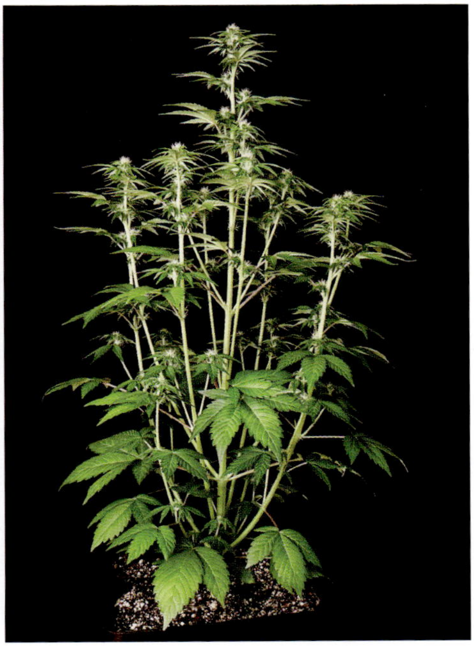

The size of your autoflowering plant largely depends on the genetics of the hybridization.

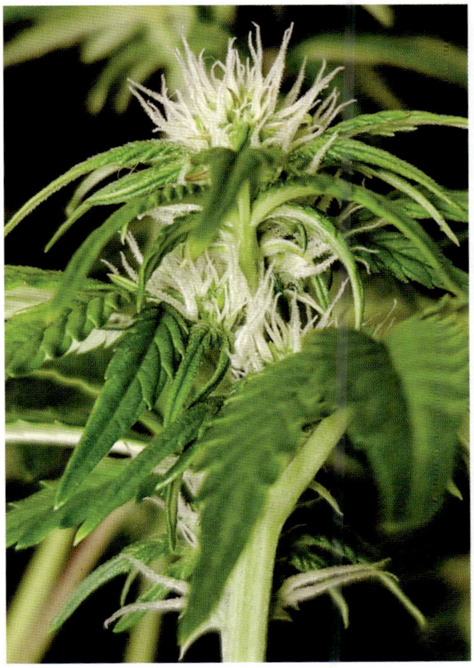

It doesn't matter if you use 24/0 lighting or 12/12; autoflowering plants will flower according to age.

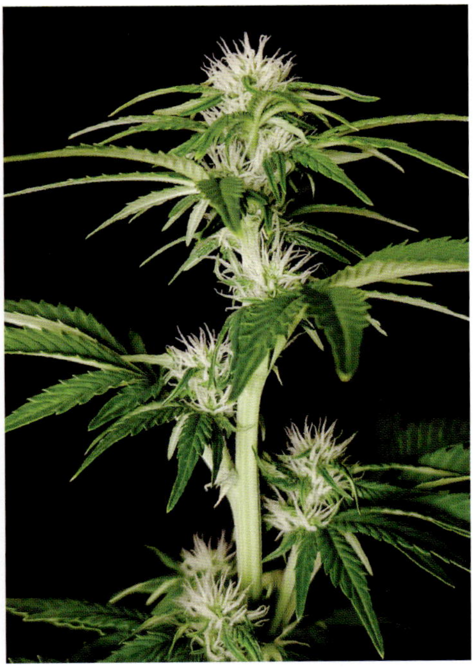

Switch to 12/12 when signs of flowering show.

continues...

Autoflower Devotchka: Seed to Flowering *continued*

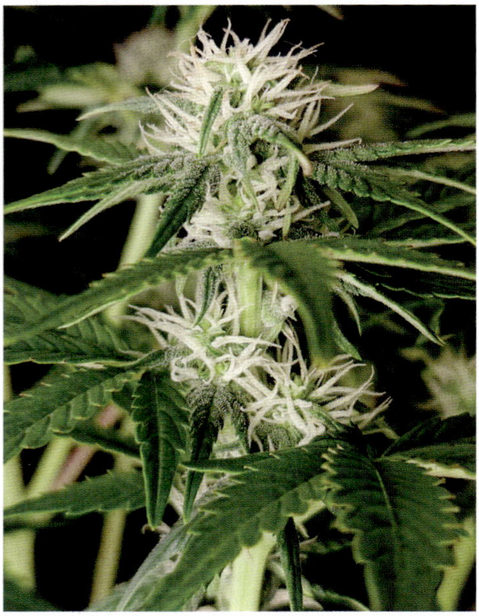

Autoflowering plants only need 12/12 of light, just like standard seeds.

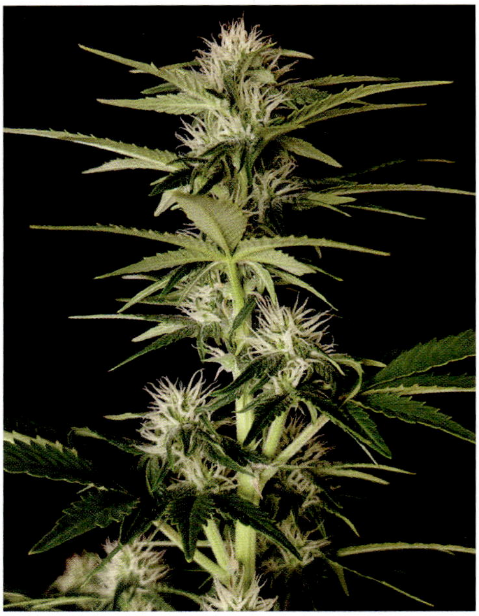

Autoflowering plants should start to fill in at the internodes midway through flowering.

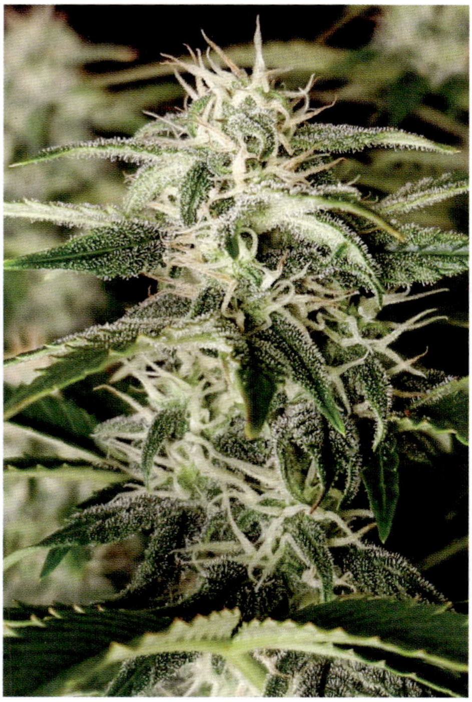

Like standard genetics, you can expect frosty trichomes to show on the flowering leaves.

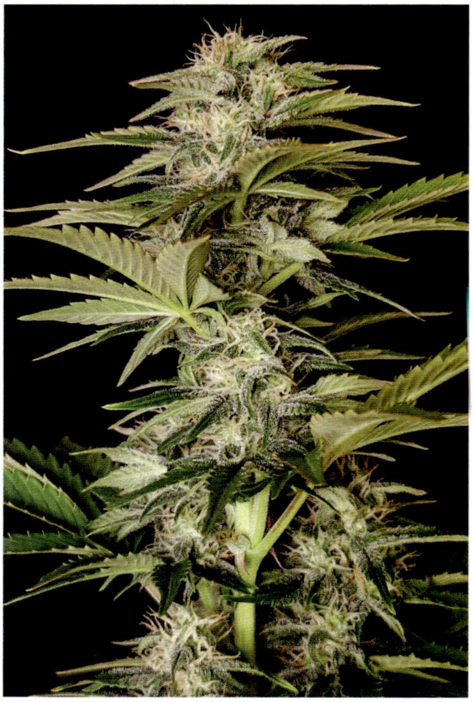

Results might involve lower yields than from standard, but maybe not by much.

PHOTOS: DOCTORSCHOICE.FARM / PHOTOGRAPHED BY FRANZ JANYR

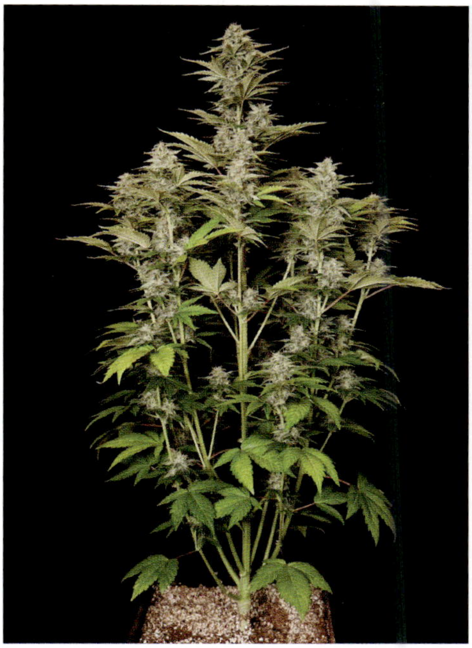

Anyone would be happy with the results of autoflowering genetics.

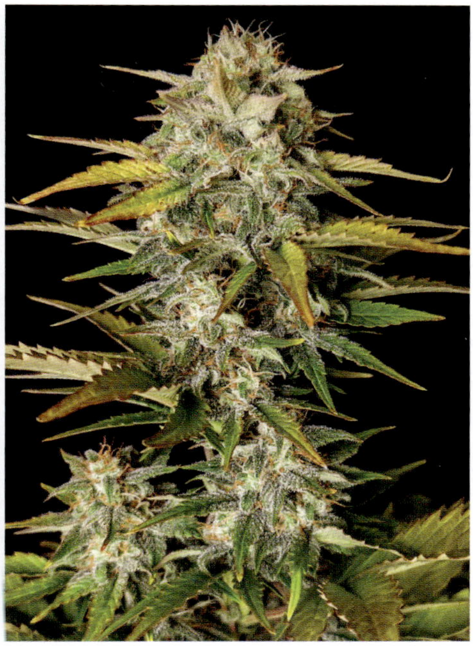

Can you tell if this bud is from standard or autoflowering? Probably not.

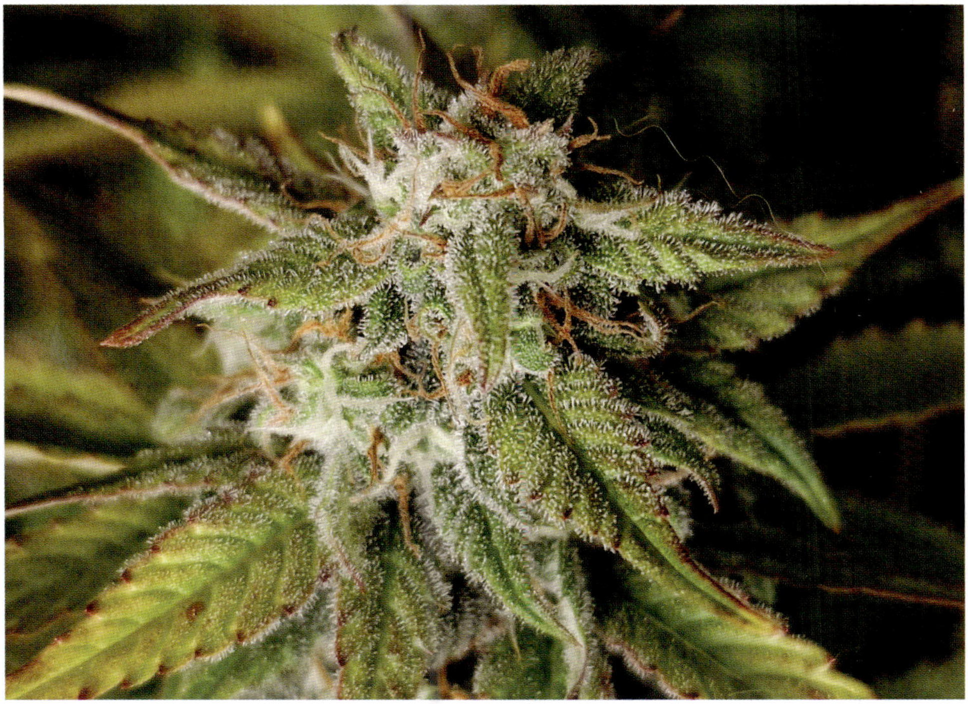

Ultimately, the user cannot determine if the bud is from standard or autoflowering. Only the grower knows.

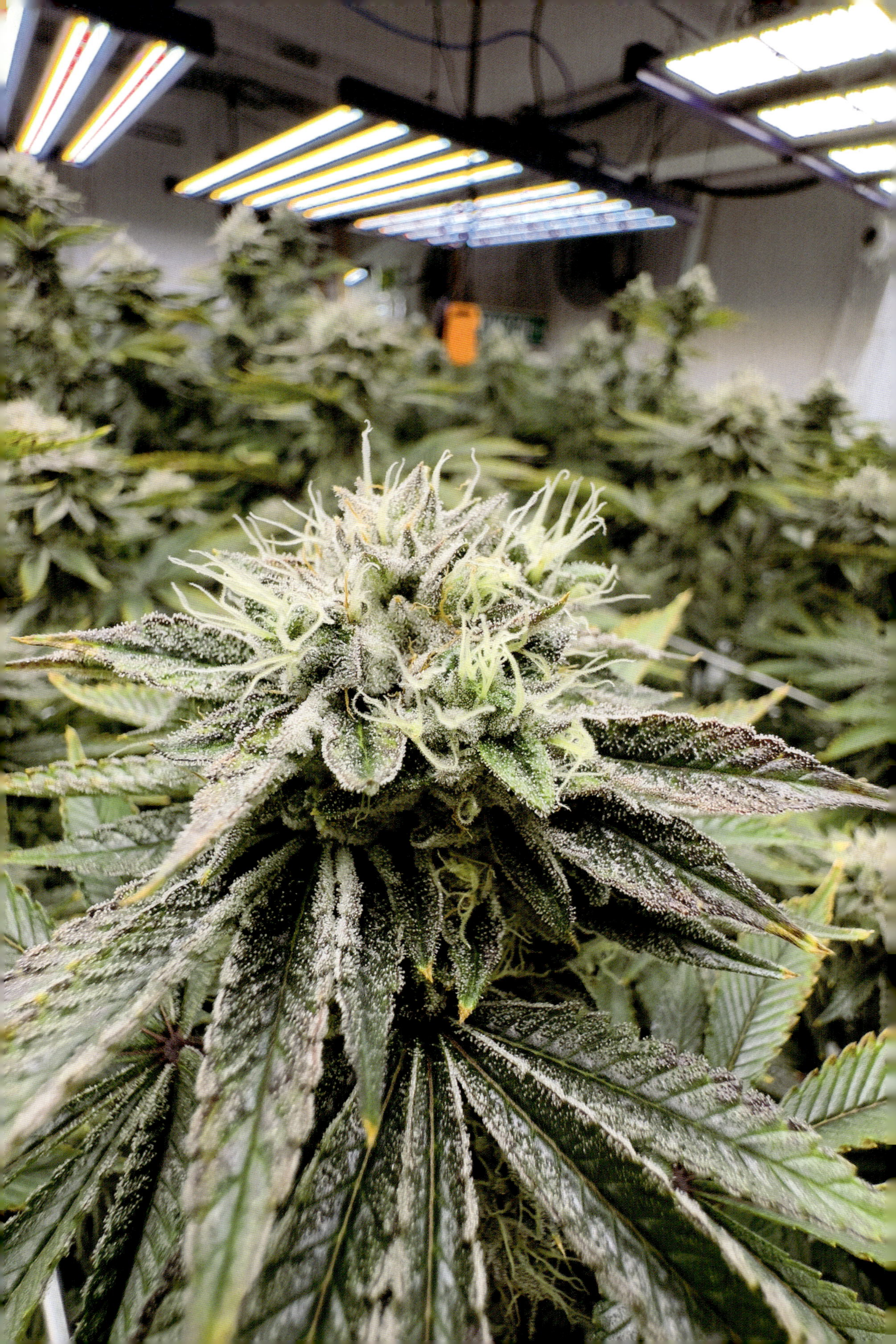

11

Hydroponics

Hydroponics is a very successful way of growing cannabis if you're looking for large bud quantities at faster growth rates. Because the liquid medium surrounding the plant's roots provides nutrients at a molecular level, roots do not have to seek them out, and plant energy is spent on other areas of growth. Hydroponic systems do not necessarily make plants grow faster, but rather allow for a high degree of energy optimization. Another advantage of a hydroponic system is a reduced threat of pests; most pests need soil and can't thrive in hydroponic substrates.

The main disadvantages of a hydroponic system are that it does require a certain degree of expertise, maintenance, and a large work area. Your work area should be larger than the hydroponics unit, to ensure the unit is accessible on all sides. A poorly maintained hydroponic system will kill your plants quickly. Hydroponics is rarely a 'one plant per pot' setup. All your plants depend on a single reservoir, meaning overfeeding will affect the entire grow. On the other hand, the results of a hydroponic grow can be remarkable. The skills obtained by using hydroponic systems can also be transferred to indoor soil-based grows, as good soil-based growers often optimize the soil's nutrient composition to achieve optimal results.

Attempts at water-based cultivation have been documented since the Middle Ages. In the mid-1800s, scientists began to identify the main elements that plants need to grow, and it became apparent that soil contains many of the nutrients a plant needs. But a lot of what makes up soil is not used by the plant, as soil is also important for supporting the plant to stay upright. Some plants, such as the water lily, have adapted to living in water; they are lightweight so they can float on water, and allow oxygen and other gases to reach submerged parts of the plant through air channels. Plants growing near rivers, streams, and in the deltas near the sea have root masses that are either fully or partially submerged as the waters lower and rise with rainfalls and the tide. This demonstrates roots' ability to obtain nutrients without the presence of soil. Understanding this led to the development of hydroponics.

PHOTO: PRESTON BJORNSON

For our purposes, it is also important to understand that nutrients from the soil can leak into the river. Fertilizer leakage or spills can have disastrous consequences for rivers and deltas. This includes nitrogen and phosphorus pollution. The ecosystem becomes destabilized by a rapid growth of algae as a result of excessive nutrient content. Algae then absorbs oxygen from the water, which causes fish to suffocate in this oxygen-deficient environment. The same problem can occur in aquariums and hydroponic systems: Algae can starve our plants of oxygen. Thus, algae growth needs to be stopped and eliminated immediately when we are growing in hydroponic systems.

Soil is composed of many things. Once we understand what a plant requires to grow in soil, we can modify the natural growing conditions by maximizing our control over each plant's needs individually; we can develop a culture. The development of 'cultures' entails creating an environment that delivers the plant exactly what it needs while eliminating what it does not. These environments tend to be aqueous and can be carried out in something as small as a petri dish. As the use of aquatic horticulture cultures grew in popularity, the practice became known as hydroculture. The development of hydroculture has rapidly increased in recent decades, and we are now able to cultivate plants to full maturity on entirely hydroponic setups.

Hydroponic Cultures

The most popular type of aquatic horticulture is hydroponics. There are two popular forms of that in cannabis cultivation: Solution culture and medium culture hydroponics. Solution culture hydroponics means the roots shall not be within any solid type of medium, like perlite, vermiculite, or Rockwool. So if we use those, we are doing medium culture hydroponics, with the substrates being the medium.

Solution cultures are more challenging to manage than medium cultures but can produce better results. Medium cultures are more like soil grows, but the medium is entirely replaced by another medium other than soil, such as large slabs of Rockwool or vermiculite/perlite mixes. These tend to soak up the solution, and the roots stay within the slab or mix. They are easier to do because once the amount of air-to-solution ratio can be balanced for the roots, it behaves as a soil grow would. Medium culture hydroponics is often used with decorative plants for indoor fountain displays. It requires less care when set up, but cannabis growers usually find it lacking the control offered by solution cultures. The basic concept of solution culture is that a reservoir tank holds the solution, and we control when and for how long this solution meets the roots. Solution cultures are more suitable for cannabis cultivation because their precision and accuracy facilitate optimization.

Hydroponic Substrates

There are many hydroponic mediums to choose from. Rockwool is the most popular because it is easy to work with. Rockwool comes in either slabs or cubes; the cubes vary in size from 1 to 6 cubic inches, while the slabs can be cut to suit the shape of your pot or container.

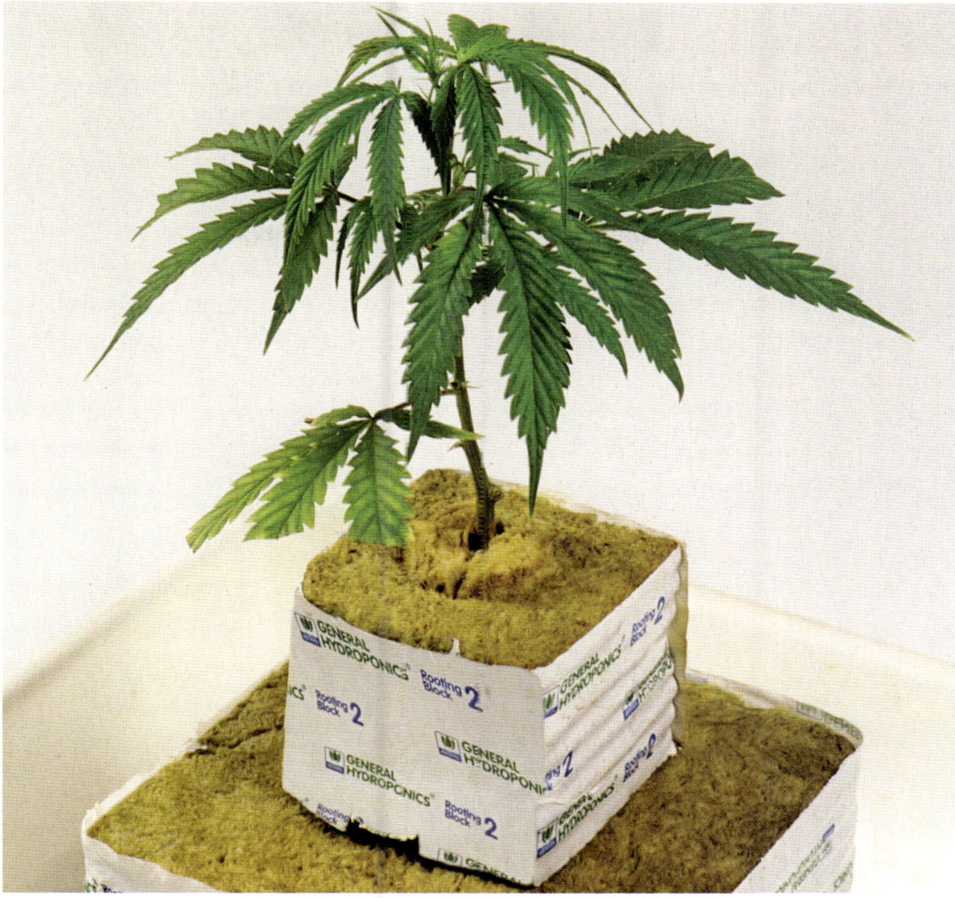

Rockwool cubes can be stacked or inserted into one another. Roots will grow through both.

Rockwool

Many growers already like to use Rockwool cubes for seed germination and rooting cuttings. Some growers pre-soak Rockwool for 24 hours in water with a pH level of 5.6 (7.0 for soil grows) to stabilize the Rockwool's pH level, which can be slightly alkaline. If you decide to do this, let the water reach room temperature. Your substrate pH should be within the 6–7 range.

Expanded Clay Pellets

Expanded clay pellets, also known as "grow rocks," come in various sizes. They are an ecologically sustainable medium, usually manufactured into round shapes by baking clay in a rotary kiln at very high temperatures so that the clay pops like popcorn and becomes porous. Because clay pellets are full of tiny air pockets, they are very light and will float. They are inert, pH-neutral, and contain no nutrients, meaning they can be used in hydroponic systems to support to the cannabis plants' stems. Clay pellets can also be reused; just mix 10 ml of hydrogen peroxide with 1 gallon of water

PHOTO: ANDRE GROSSMAN

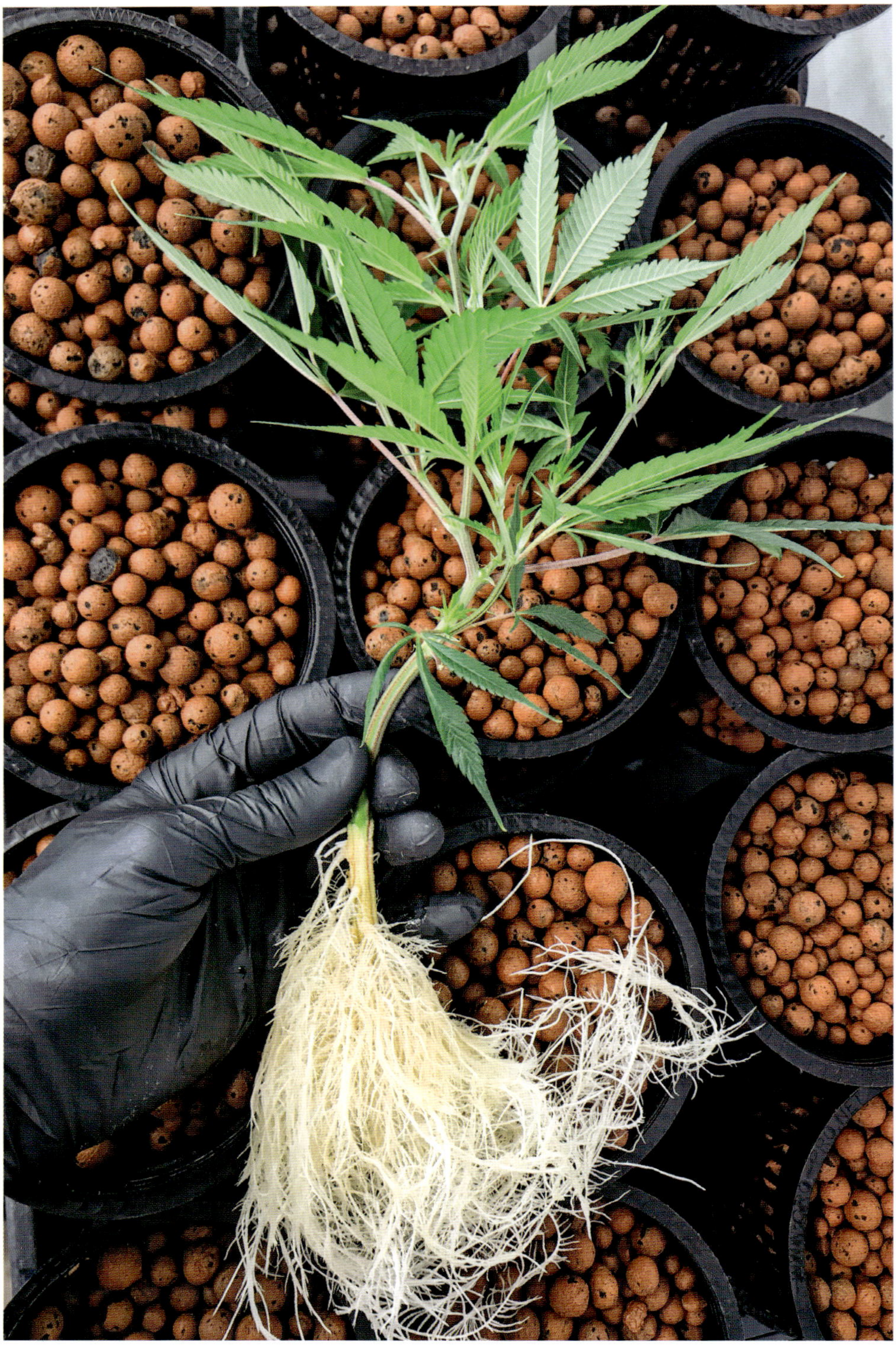

PHOTO: HIP2THECROP

The gaps in clay pellets allow nutrients and water to splash against the roots without drawing dirt in, creating a clean medium for hydroponic growing.

and let the pellets steep in the mix for a few minutes before drying them out. After a few hours, they should be ready for reuse. Expanded clay pellets tend to be a bit more expensive than most other soilless substrates but the extra expense is worthwhile since they can be reused. They can be used on their own as a growing medium in a hydroponic system but should be mixed with another substrate when used with other growing techniques because they drain quickly.

Oasis Cubes

Oasis cubes come in several formats, including Horticubes and Rootcubes. They are similar to Rockwool cubes, but are made from different materials, namely phenolic and floral foam. Before use, Oasis cubes should be completely saturated with water. If you use a tray to soak them, you can drain away the excess water by tilting the tray over on its side, leaving about an eighth of an inch of water in the tray. Feel the weight of the tray—it should feel heavy. Oasis holds a lot of water! The cubes should never be allowed to dry out completely. Like Rockwool, growers can expect a high success rate using Oasis cubes. Because they retain warmer temperatures better than Rockwool, they are favored by growers who need to keep their grow warm.

Coconut Fiber

Coconut fiber provides added protection from root diseases and fungus infestation, promotes rooting due to its natural hormones, and retains moisture well, preventing the roots from drying out between watering cycles. Coconut fiber is dry and usually comes in a compressed, block format that needs to be rehydrated. When rehydrated, compressed blocks can expand to roughly nine times their original size, and have a texture similar to wet ground coffee. A typical coconut fiber mat is around ½ an inch thick and 24 to 36 inches wide, but different sizes are available. These mats are very suitable for hydroponic systems as they can be placed directly into the tray without requiring much shaping.

Soilless Mixes

Soilless mixes are pre-packaged bags of combinations of soilless substrates. The substrate types and their ratios are usually printed on the bag. They can include the following: Vermiculite, screened peat, peat, perlite, composted bark, fine silica sand, quartz, construction-grade sand, and coconut fibers. Most growers prefer to prepare their own soilless mixes because it is cheaper and offers them more control.

Perlite

Perlite is a naturally occurring, silicon-based rock. Perlite is distinguished from other rocks by its ability to expand to 20 times its original size when heated, due to water present in the raw rock. When heated, the rock "pops" like popcorn into large pieces of nutrient- and water-retaining, puffy perlite. Perlite is a form of natural glass, is chemically inert and usually has a neutral pH of 7.

Hydroponic Grow Chamber

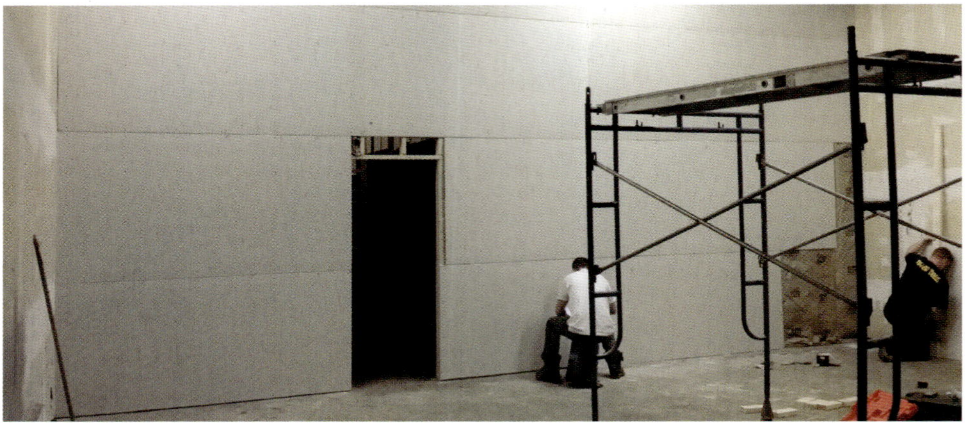

Preparing panels for reflective white walls.

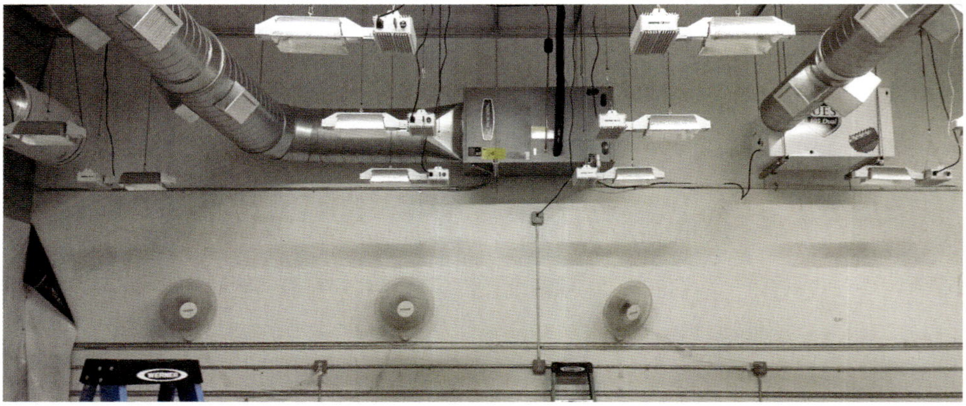

Similar lighting rig as a soil-based grow.

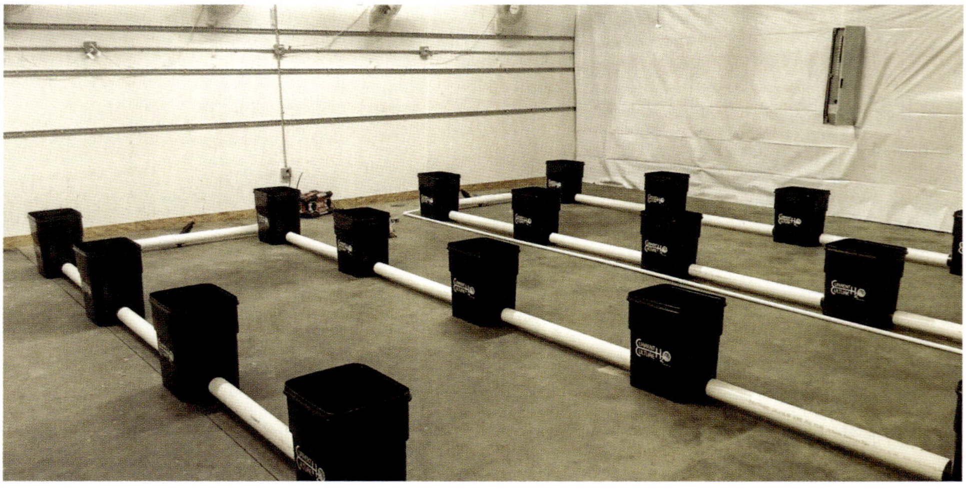

The big change. Hydroponic tubing and containers for the growing medium.

PHOTOS: @BEAM401 / CH9 FEMALE SEEDS

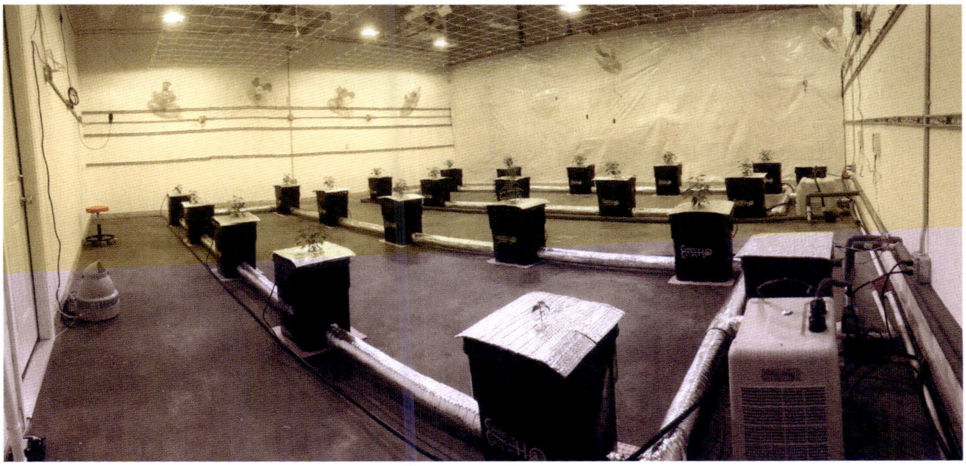

One clone per hydroponics container. These will get big.

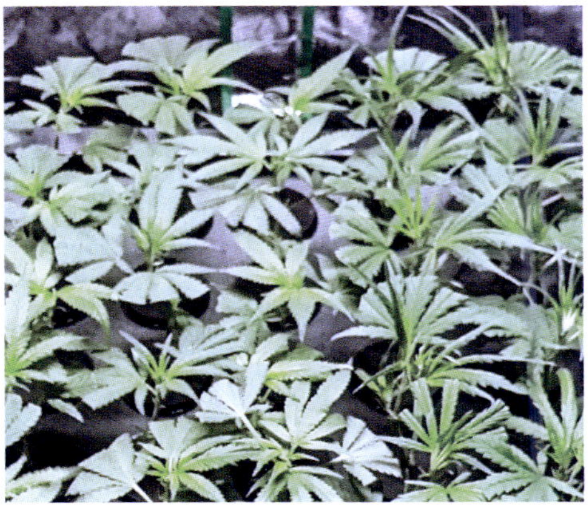

Clones prepared for transplanting.

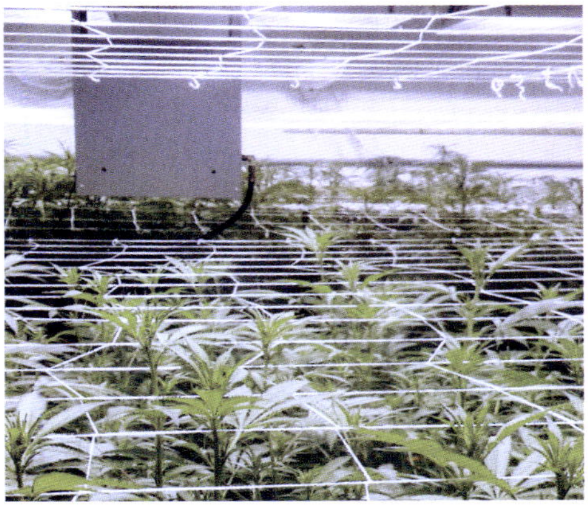

Clones in vegetative growth under a mesh.

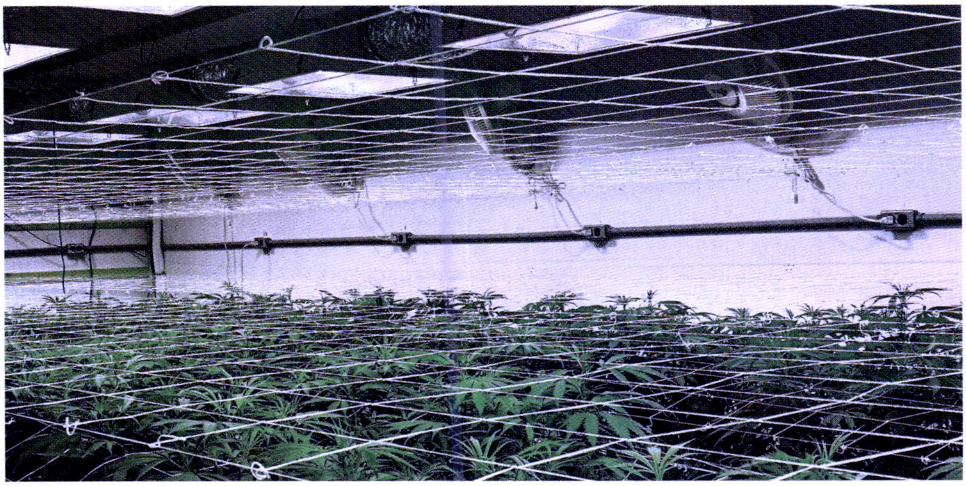

The even canopy of clones in vegetative growth in hydroponics.

Basic Hydroponic Systems

You know that plants need a base material, the medium that holds nutrients and minerals that drains well and allows air to get to the roots. In the early days of experimenting with artificial grow mediums, growers discovered that plant roots didn't always respond well to soilless mediums like Rockwool and clay pebbles, and that soil still outperformed them. Why? Is it because soil is inherently better? It can't be this, because we already know that soil is mostly structure. Yet we also know there are poor and excellent soil types for growing in. Sandy soils drain too fast, and silty soils become too soggy. It seems that using soilless substrates may also suffer from these disadvantages. This is one problem we have with medium cultures. We need more control than this.

The basic model for solution culture is the ability to segregate nutrients and water from roots. A container holds water and nutrients separate from the plant and medium, only combining them when necessary. One way of doing this is to have a soilless medium hold a plant in place but allow roots to grow out from the medium and into a container, with the solution flowing or pumped into this unit at timed intervals, which leaves the roots exposed to air in between. This is similar to how plants on a riverbank will operate, with their roots exposed to air in low waters and submerged during high waters. Nature regulates the conditions and the plant adapts. This is what we want to achieve.

There are many ways to do this. For example, a plant can absorb a measured amount of solution and expose its roots to the air when it is used up. Alternatively, we can pump the nutrients both in and out of the container. Roots are then left dangling in an empty system for dry periods. Hydroponic systems do produce significant root clusters. One can easily pick up a three-gallon bucketful of root growth from a single plant.

There is another type of hydroponics in which roots are kept entirely out of a solution and, instead, are misted with a nozzle and spray bottle to feed the plant roots; unsurprisingly, this is called aeroponics. We will explore this method later.

Sizing for Hydroponics

You will need to be prepared for the size requirements of hydroponics; you will probably need floor space larger than the dimensions of the hydroponic system. Buying a 4 x 4-foot hydroponic unit for a 4 x 4-foot grow tent means you can only access the unit through the tent opening. While some systems can work with only one access point, most require access to all sides. Another factor in size considerations is lighting coverage.

You will likely be able to find a kit, light, hydroponic system, and tent all in one purchase bundle. In this case, the necessary sizing of each part will have been worked out by the person who assembled the kit. Look at these bundles, note the sizes and download some assembly manuals; you can probably obtain the system parts individually, or if you have DIY skills, you can make it yourself. You may want to consider environmentally-friendly alternatives to PVC piping, though many "environmentally-friendly" alternatives to petroleum-based plastics are not actually good for the environment. If you must use PVC, make sure it is made from recycled materials, especially ocean plastics. 3D printing typically uses polylactide resin (PLA) made from renewable resources. Most metals like copper, cast iron, and galvanized steel are okay, as long as the joints have not been soldered with lead. While we aren't drinking the water in our hydroponic systems, our plants are absorbing elements from them, and certain toxins can stunt growth. Pipes can also be made from pulp composites, although make sure you choose a material that doesn't degrade quickly. When degradation occurs, try to recycle the parts you need to replace. Glass and ceramics are environmentally-friendly, but fracture and break easily. Growers have been quite creative here, even using bamboo. Once you gain experience and learn how the systems work, you may be inspired to make your own from recyclables.

White Kits

Most hydroponics kits are white on their external or surface parts, to reflect the light back at the plants. A good kit will have no light leaks, so light does not interact with fluids, encouraging algae to grow. If you decide to build your own kit, ensure you are buying white materials or painting them matte flat white after you buy. Use white tape too, or spray paint it white after you have applied it. This will make any system more energy efficient while optimizing harvest results and preventing algae.

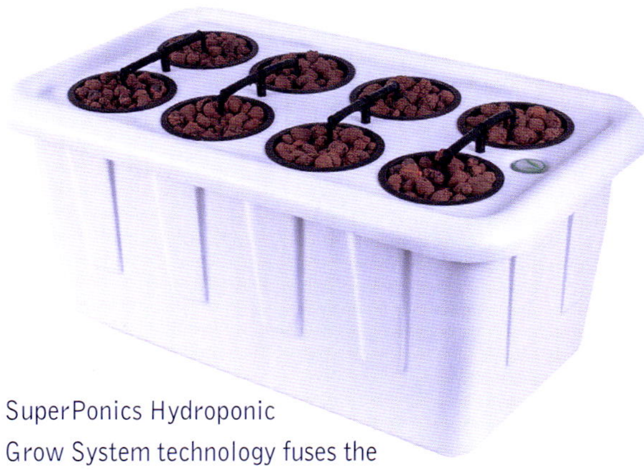

SuperPonics Hydroponic Grow System technology fuses the best of hydroponics by combining automated top feeding, Deep Water Culture, and bubble and aeroponics.

PHOTO: GORILLAGROWTENT.COM

Static and Flowing Systems

We now understand that immersed roots can't access the gases in the air, but they can access nutrients and water. When dry, they can access gases in the air but don't have access to nutrients and water. So we understand that there has to be a balance here, and hydroponics can do this.

In a static solution, roots are exposed to the air after the plant absorbs some of the solution, exposing parts of the roots to air as the solution level drops. The solution is topped up when half or more is used up. The solution is static because it does not move out of this chamber. Instead, it enters manually by watering, and its only exit is absorption by the plant and evaporation.

In a flowing solution system, the liquid moves in and out of the feeding chamber. An external reservoir holds the solution during the dry period, releases it to the hydroponic pots when the plants need nutrients, then the same solution is returned to that same reservoir after the wet period. It is therefore possible to determine how much solution the plants absorbed, which is why NASA uses hydroponics in space test labs. A flowing system gives the grower more control over the hydroponic system than a static system, but a static system requires less maintenance and movement. Pots for hydroponics are called net pots because they have a lot of openings for roots to grow through and fluids to penetrate. We will discuss these later in this chapter.

Air Stones

Air stones are used by many hydroponic growers to ensure their reservoirs are properly aerated. While pumps are usually sufficient to have the water bubble at some point, thus capturing air, the further use of these stones ensures better aeration. Air stones rest at the

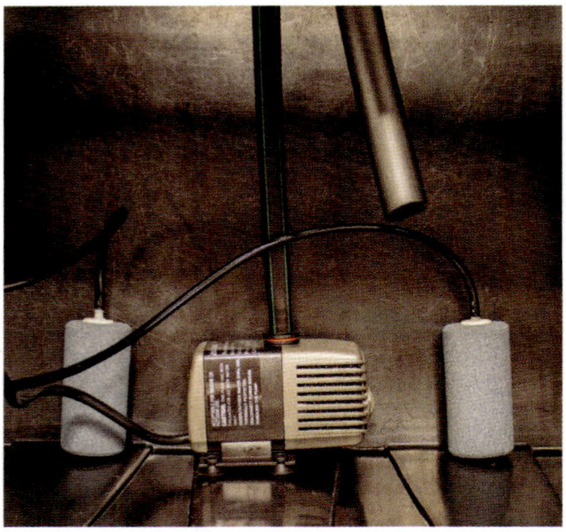

Two air stones on either side of a pump inside a hydroponics unit.

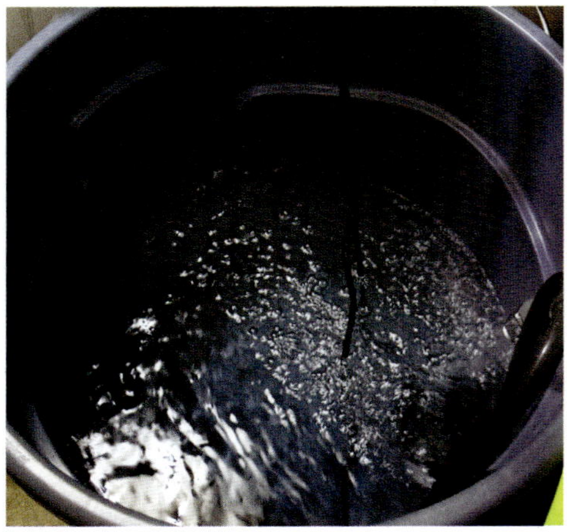

Air stones bubbling in a bucket. The surface splashes are important.

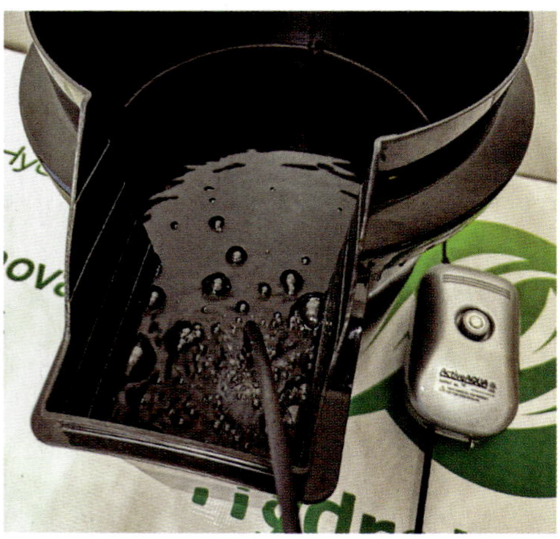

Air bubbles pop at the surface, and particles of nutrients strike the exposed roots.

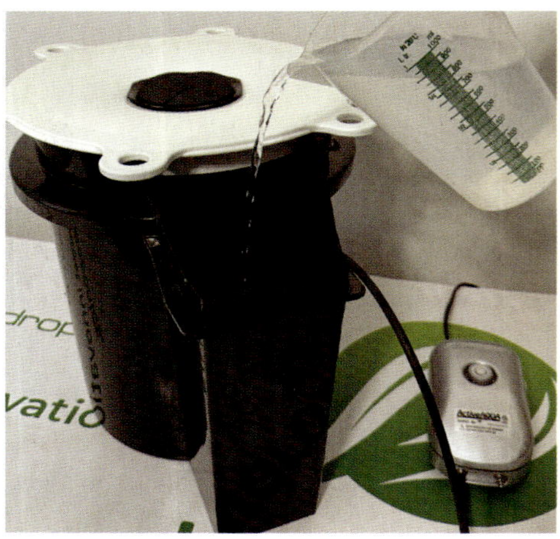

A premade side compartment means you don't have to lift out the plant to refill.

PHOTOS: @TREETRUNK422 (TOP), THEHYDROBUCKET.COM (BOTTOM)

bottom of feeding chambers and reservoirs, with an air line connecting them to a pump. As a result, air gases defuse through the air stone as many air bubbles. They can quickly solve problems caused by a lack of air gases in water: Bubble the water, and you introduce more air-related gases into the water in the tank. Air stones are essential for static systems, because a steady stream of constant bubbles in the solution-feeding chamber is necessary. One pump per plant for an air stone can become expensive, so growers can split the line. Hydroponic air pump splitters are inexpensive and very effective.

For flowing systems, we want the solution reservoir to be bubbling. This way, you can have an aerated solution in both systems and shorter dry periods in flow systems. Air stones are important, so factor them into your system or ensure the kit comes with some.

Root Mats

In solution medium hydroponics, the root mat is the thick mass of roots that grows throughout the plant's life.By the end of harvest, root mats usually fill whatever system they are inside. If we expand the solution container, root mats will often grow larger into the new space. It is not uncommon to find the root mats adapting to the same shape as the container they are inside. The situation is precisely the same as using pots with cannabis plants to restrict the plant size. Smaller pots lead to less lateral growth and less bushy plants. Wider pots encourage lateral growth that result in bushier plants. In solution medium hydroponics, the chamber for the root mat will restrict how bushy a plant can get. Don't worry about root mats clogging a system; root mats are permeable with a low density but high volume. Most hydroponic systems operate perfectly with full root mats already developed.

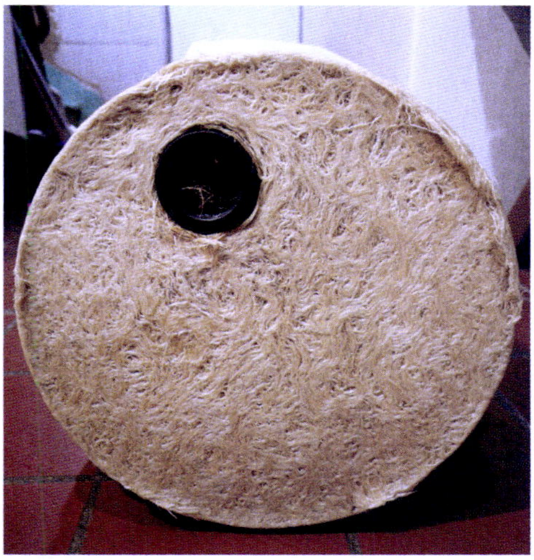

A root mass can easily fill a portion of a hydroponics bucket.

Clone Tanks

A clone tank is a mini hydroponic bucket that houses new clones prepared for hydroponic systems. Clones can be transported over short distances by rooting in Rockwool and wrapping in paper but should be transplanted into a clone tank as quickly as possible. In such a tank, several net pots share the same container and an air stone will be present in the low-strength solution. When the tank is under LED lights, the pumping system activates surface-bubbling of the solution, causing it to splash up and nourish the clone's roots. Using a clone tank may seem unnecessary if you can obtain clones

PHOTO: @TREETRUNK422

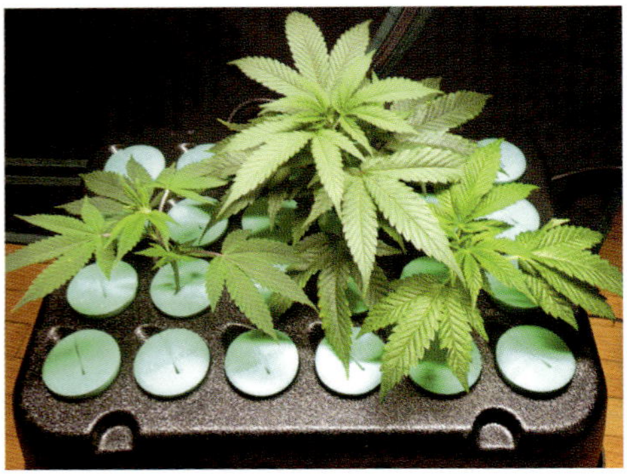

A hydroponic clone starter kit for later transplanting.

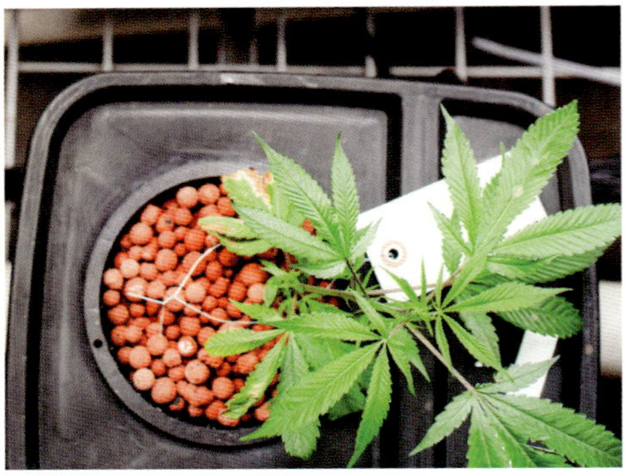

Clone hydroponic starter kits allow the root pot with plant to be moved to a bigger tank.

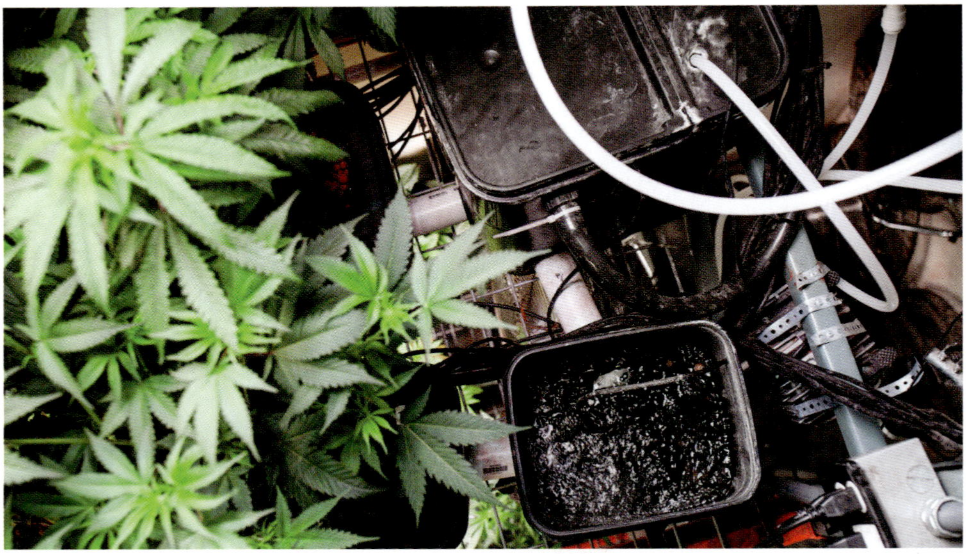

Clone hydroponic starter kit with the top off. Notice the bubbling of the nutrient solution? Don't open it too long. Algae tends to grow where light is exposed to the water.

PHOTOS: @TREETRUNK422 (TOP LEFT), KRISTEN ANGELO, GREENRUSH LLC (TOP RIGHT AND BOTTOM)

immediately upon assembly of your hydroponic units. However, this unit makes sure you can obtain clones whenever you want throughout the process. You should keep them on a 24/0 photoperiod and prune them.

Flowing Systems

Once you understand a flowing system, a static one is easy to follow. Static systems use the same principles as flowing systems, though on a larger scale.

A moving or flowing solution system is an improved hydroponics method due to the extra control it provides. When the solution flows through the plants, it is perfectly aerated. You may hear the terms "active" and "passive" used in hydroponics. In an active flowing system, fluid movement is achieved through gravitational forces and the use of a powered pump. On the other hand, static systems are considered passive, even when using powered pumps with air stones, because the solution isn't moved, it stays static.

Flow Adjustment

It is harder to adjust the solution with solid mediums once the medium has absorbed it. That is why we perform emergency soil transplants in case of overfeeding. With flowing solutions, the fluid is almost always reclaimed by the pump back into the reservoir where adjustments can be made, such as adding pH-up/down products or adjusting the nutrient ratio. These changes are much easier and doable in flowing systems, as a problem can be addressed and treated quickly by stopping the flow and reclaiming the solution back into the reservoir.

Testing Hydroponics

There is no point in adding plants to a system that you haven't tried to run without plants first. You need to test the system to make sure it works properly. First, try to adjust the pH. Then, go ahead and add nutrients. Let the system run without plants for a week. During this time, you can detect and solve problems, such as potential algae buildup due to light leaks, wide pH fluctuations leading to transplant shock, or potential rot areas where water pools instead of moving. Run everything as you would if plants were in it. If you need to run it for a few additional weeks, then do so. Keep notes. This is a crucial part of any successful hydroponic system, and will help eliminate potential problems from wide pH fluctuations, leading to transplant shock. pH imbalances will cause chemical reactions with your nutrients, making them no longer accessible to your plant's roots. You can also try out the pH adjustments recommended in the next section during this test phase.

pH Adjustment

Generally, hydroponic systems thrive at a pH level of 6. Some strains might respond well to a pH of 5.5 and some to a pH of 6.5. If your plant isn't responding well to a pH of 6, first try to bring the pH down, as many systems may need a pH slightly lower than this. Use a pH-down product to reduce the pH to 5.8. If things get worse, you have gone the wrong way and need to go back to 6 and slowly increase the pH level instead. If things don't change at 5.8, then reduce by another 0.2 to a pH of 5.6. If things get better, try 5.5 and compare between that to 5.6. Do the same when increasing the pH, going by increments of 0.2 and closely observing the results.

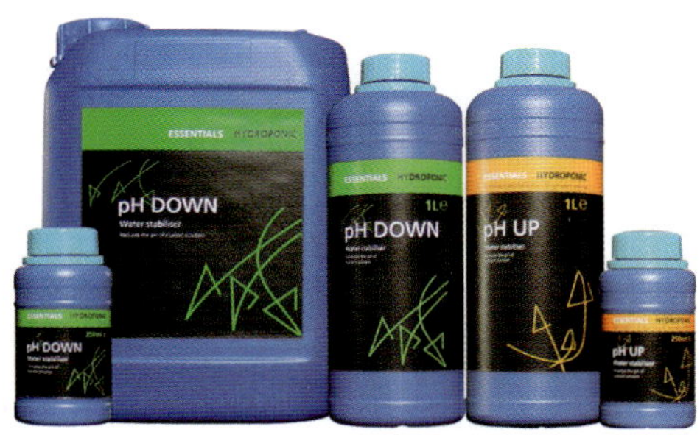

pH-up and pH-down solutions bring pH back to neutral.

PHOTO: HYDROGARDEN.COM

Hydroponics is at its most tricky here. You can go a little below or over the ideal, but not by much. Changes must be made

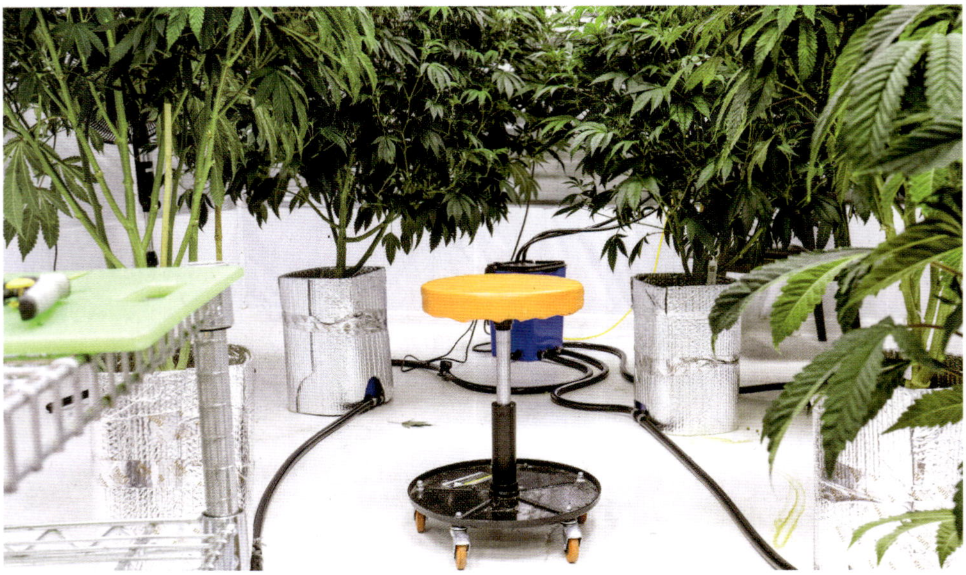

Hydroponics can optimize growth quickly. Look at the vigor of these plants.

gradually, with a maximum change of 0.2 at any time. A change of 0.5 pH can create problems and a change of 1 pH can be disastrous if the strain is sensitive. These problems can be mitigated by using a good pH reader and pH-up and pH-down products.

Water Hardness

Limescale is a white, chalky substance that appears when the water's pH is too high and mineral-rich. Limescale is a common problem in domestic water supplies. Water is classified as "hard" if it contains minerals in amounts above 1 grain per gallon (GPG) and "soft" if it contains amounts below that. Very hard water reaches levels above 7 GPG. Your local water company can provide information about your tap water's pH and mineral content. If you find that your water source has an unsuitable pH level, try using a reverse osmosis water-filtering system to clean it and produce distilled water with a neutral pH level of 7.0. Beginning with a pH of 7 makes it easier to adjust to the levels using pH-up and -down products. You need to treat hardness problems before the water enters the hydroponic system. Avoid using agents like water softeners in your system, and try to solve the problem before it requires the addition of something. If you try to treat the problem with softening agents, you won't know how the chemicals will react with nutrients in the solution. Filtration systems that remove calcium, magnesium, and other chemicals are the best treatment method for hard water in horticulture. You can add them back later as secondary nutrients as needed. This gives the grower far more control.

PHOTO: KRISTEN ANGELO

Tweaking Hydroponics

The key to a successful hydroponics grow is testing your setup before placing plants in the system. You should test all the feeds you are planning to use. Measure and compensate for any pH changes. The better you tweak your system, the fewer adjustments you will need to make during the actual grow. The system's temperature will adjust under lights and fluids in the hydroponic trays will warm up due to surface heating on the covers. The situation is much easier to test for if you are only using clones. For example, a flowering feed test can be done on clones, but a flowering test will have to be skipped when you are growing the strain from seed for the first time. You won't have a chance to experiment here, but go with trial and error for flowering. You can experiment with the flowering feed on the clones though for future grows. You can also test the vegetative feed or vegetative and flowering on clones transplanted from the clone tank to the hydroponic system. Clones allow for any test you can conceive. You won't be able to foresee every event, but early tweaks will provide you with experience and strategies to tackle any new hydroponic system.

Experimenting with a test grow can be the difference between a grower who is forewarned and a grower who is not. This is not always ideal, and requires some patience, but it will give you invaluable knowledge for your real grow. While you can try to grow right after assembling your hydroponic unit, you will not be able to fix the imbalances quickly. In that situation, you would be experimenting simultaneously with fixing problems and growing a plant in an advanced cultivation system.

Hydroponic Meters and Readers

Meters and readers are essential in hydroponic systems to ensure proper nutrient levels. Close observation and documentation are just as important. Failure with hydroponic systems is nearly always because of a fault with the mixture and rate of flow, so we need to measure our mixtures closely. An Electrical Conductive (EC) meter will measure the amount of nutrients in your solution. EC meters can also read Total Dissolved Solids (TDS), but you can invest in a separate TDS meter for added safety. These are science classroom-grade devices; some have digitally displayed readings and smart devices. Advanced readers may come with analytical reagents for testing samples in tubes. Some test kit systems use a color grading system with a matching card. An aquarium thermometer is useful for observing water temperature; place an aquarium thermometer into every reservoir of your system. This is an ever-expanding field of new technologies, so research is required before investing.

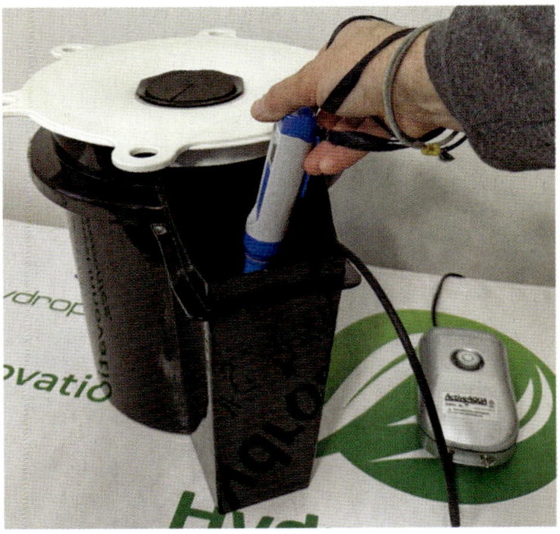

A meter is used to take a reading from a hydroponic medium.

PHOTO: THEHYDROBUCKET.COM

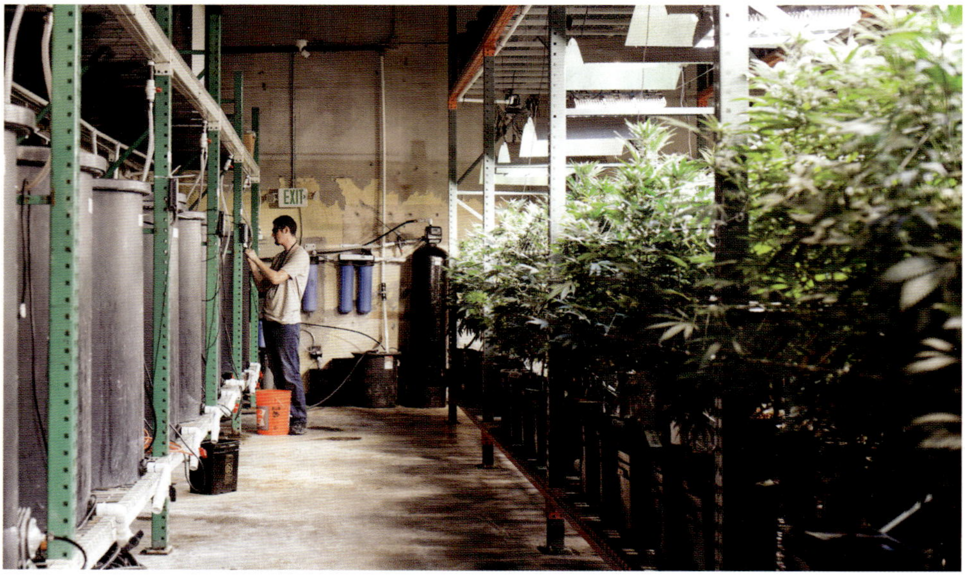

Water stored in large tanks for pumping to large grow areas.

Hydroponic Nutrients

Nutrients are a crucial part of your hydroponic setup. Nutrient solutions come in several different forms. It is vital to check that the solution you use is the best for your type of plant and setup. Some supplements and fertilizers should only be used with soil as they contain the wrong elements for hydroponic use; while you can use hydroponic feeds for soil grows, you cannot use soil feeds for hydroponics. However, organic foods can and do blur these boundaries. So why not just use hydroponic feeding solutions exclusively, then? Most hydroponic nutrient solutions are complete nutrient solutions, meaning that they provide every element and compound needed for proper plant growth. Because of this, hydroponic nutrients can be pricey. You can, of course, decide to use hydroponic feeds exclusively, and you will know you are spending your money well. The most important point here is not to use substandard feeds because shortcuts can be expensive in more ways than one: They could lead to the total devastation of your crop.

Hydroponic Nutrient Strengths

When nutrients are mixed at full strength, cannabis tends to suffer from a chemical burn. It's suggested that when using any hydroponic formulations with cannabis, you do so in moderation—at least for your first grow. Many cannabis growers have bought these products anticipating the production of great big buds only to end up with great big plant burns. Even medium-strength formulas have the power to burn your plants.

PHOTO: KRISTEN ANGELO

Always consult the information on the packs, but generally 3.5 ml of the primary, secondary, and micronutrients per liter is referred to as 100% strength. The same amount mixed with 2 L of water is 50% strength. Cannabis grows very well with 25%

to 35% nutrient strength solutions. Start with around 30% strength and adjust as needed. You'll be surprised at how rich a bud cortent you can produce with a nutrient strength of only 30%.

The most common problem associated with hydroponics is plant burns. Underfeeding plants is a rare issue. Over time, you'll get to know your strain and what it likes. The better you know your strain, the better you'll be able to control the feeding amounts.

Single versus Multipacks

In hypdroponics, different nutrients are segregated into separate bottles to avoid the elements combining into new compounds. In such a s tuation, the unintended chemical reaction is precipitation and it often produces powders around the bottle caps and residues within the mixture. If the elements combine, the solution will likely become unbalanced, making it useless to you and your plants. This is why many growers opt for nutrient multipacks. If you want to try a single bottle, Formulex has managed to hold all the elements in a single pack using specific chemicals to prevent precipitation. It is very good for starting clones or seeds in a Rockwool SBS tray and it can also be used in soil grows. However, you are more likely to encounter multipack nutrients for your hydroponics.

Twin/Triple Multipacks

In multipacks, the chemicals are separated to prevent precipitation. The most comment multipack nutrient solutions are Optimum, Power Gro, Ionic, Earth Juice, and General Hydroponics (G.H.) Flora Series. The G.H. Flora Series, a three-part system with Gro, Micro, and Bloom components, is the most popular one for cannabis cultivation. Some double nutrient packs come ir two sets: Grow, which is used during the plant's vegetative growth stage, and bloom, which is used during flowering. The bloom formulas contain more phosphorus and potassium and less nitrogen.

An experienced grower can adjust these nutrients to get optimum performance from their plants. These packs have instructions on the bottles on how to mix the nutrients in water to create different strengths.

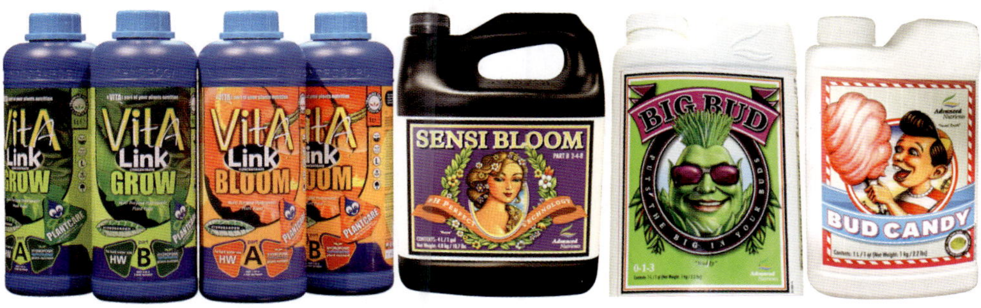

Various nutrients in different ratios allow the grower to choose what to use for each stage of the growth process.

PHOTOS: HYDROGARDEN.COM (LEFT FOUR), STONED ROSIE (THREE RIGHT)

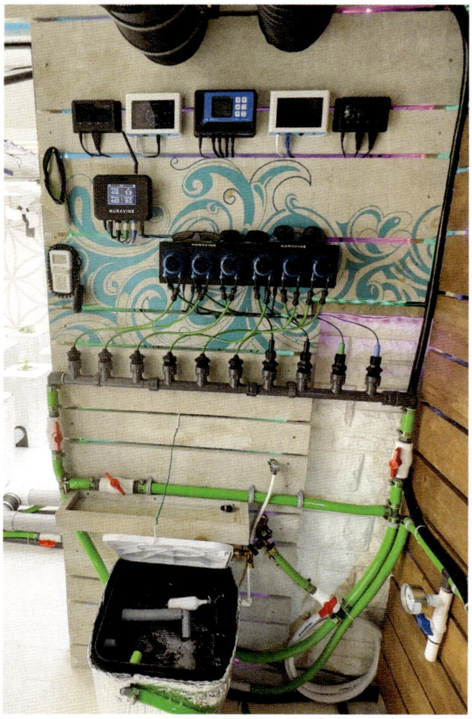

An automated grow room monitoring system that also controls nutrient mixtures.

Mixing Hydroponic Nutrients

Always follow the instructions on the products, but dilute to the strength that best suits your strain by using the calculations we provide. You will need a container and a stirring rod to mix the nutrient solution.

Each of the packs should have the letters A, B, and C written on them. A usually represents the primary nutrients, B, the secondary nutrients, and C, the micronutrients. However, in some cases, A represents the vegetative food, B, the flowering food, and C, the secondary nutrients or a secondary and micronutrient mixture.

As per the note above, in most cases, the mixture takes about 3.5 ml of each (A, B, and C) per liter of water to make a 100% strength mixture. As we said earlier, 100% strength is too strong for cannabis, and should be reduced to around 30%.

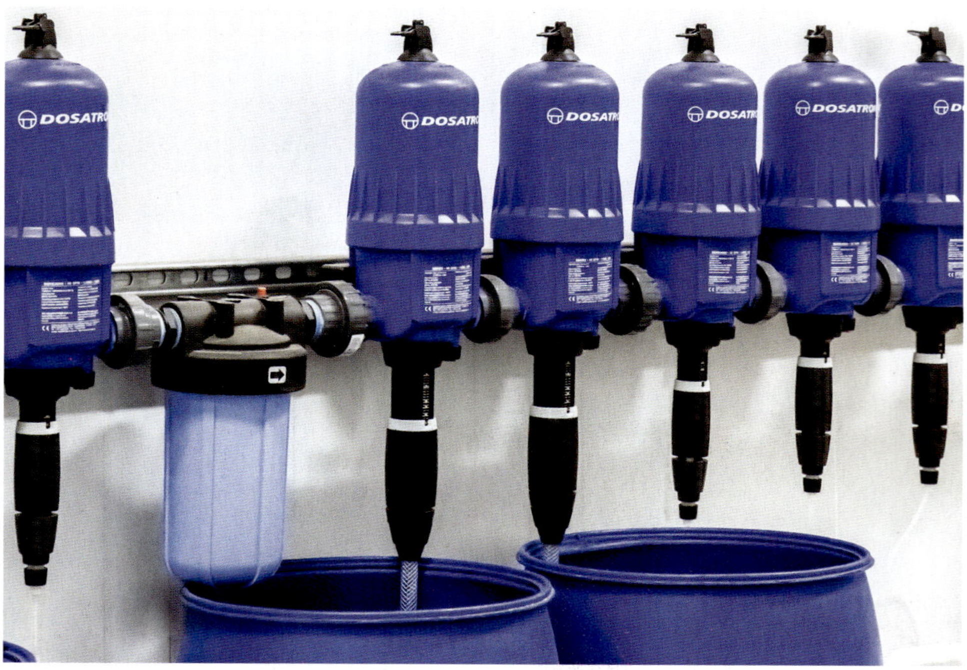

Non-electric water-powered dosing pumps.

PHOTOS: PRESTON BJORNSON (TOP), DOSATRON.COM (BOTTOM)

Adding More Nutrients?

When it comes time to feed your plants, I suggest you refresh yourself by reading the soil feeding chapter, as well as the chapter on organic foods, as the methods and information are similar. These three categories of soil, hydroponics, and organics provide an extensive overview of how to feed cannabis.

No one can tell you exactly what a plant will use in your system. The plant may not absorb all the nutrients. Some nutrients are siphoned by the plant and used immediately, while others are stored. A ppm reader can be used to measure exact amounts of nutrients in the reservoir, but they aren't strictly necessary. As long as you are keeping records of your nutrient dilutions and feeding routine, you will be fine; growers have managed for decades without meters. The plant will reveal if it has too much, too little, or just enough of a nutrient. It takes a few grows to learn to read the plant, which is part of the growing experience and is especially true regarding hydroponics.

Make sure to record your nutrient mix ratio from the start and carefully measure subsequent additions. For example, if you used 1 L mixed with 3.5 ml of nutrients and the plant absorbed half of it, you would need to mix 1.75 ml with ½ L to top the reservoir up. You can make a mixing chart to learn how to mix exact amounts as needed. Now and again, you will need to mix a fresh batch of nutrients as topping up becomes increasingly inaccurate.

Refreshing Fluids Completely

Maintaining good practice involves completely refreshing fluids from time to time. That is because, in many cases, the problem solver is to start afresh with a new mixture and get a workable pH. The ability to throw out your solution and start again is a significant advantage of hydroponics; in soil grows, you have to transplant the plants when something goes wrong. A hydroponics grower can easily adjust nutrient values with a new solution. Furthermore, you can throw the solution out in your garden as it is organic and helpful for anything growing there.

Hydroponic systems need to be kept clean as bacteria develop quickly in water. They should also be sealed against light leaks to avoid algae buildup. However, keeping the water devoid of problem pathogens is challenging, especially over extended periods. Regular maintenance is essential: Turn off the pump, empty the reservoir, clean it as per the methods below, depending on what is required, and then add a fresh, room-temperature solution. We need to be economically aware of the dump methods of hydroponics, and we shall cover more about this as we go through the process.

Cleaning

You may need to physically clean your system if you get a lot of algae growth. Hydroponic solutions that are well-maintained will self-clean somewhat automatically.

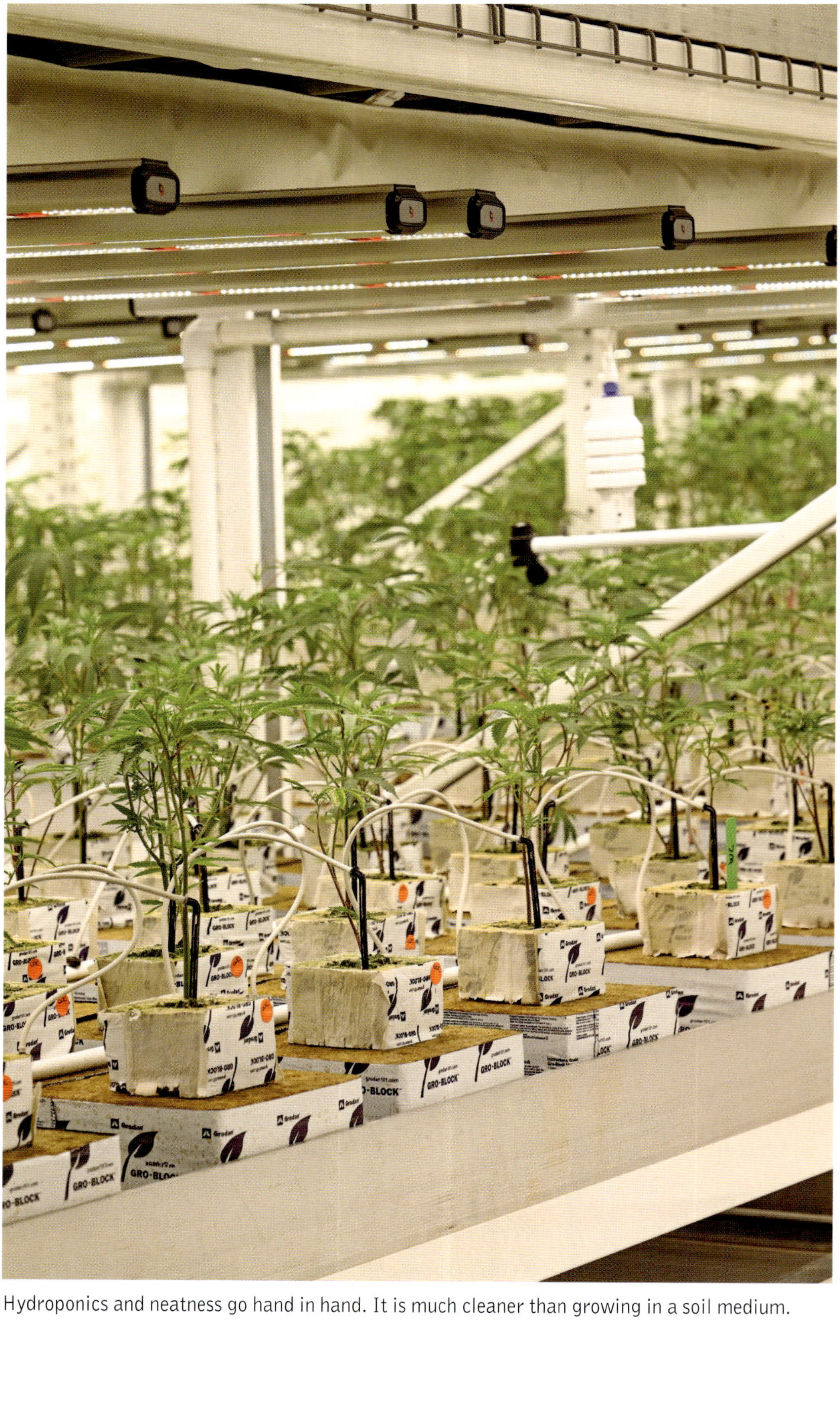

PHOTO: MIAMIMANGOCA.COM

Hydroponics and neatness go hand in hand. It is much cleaner than growing in a soil medium.

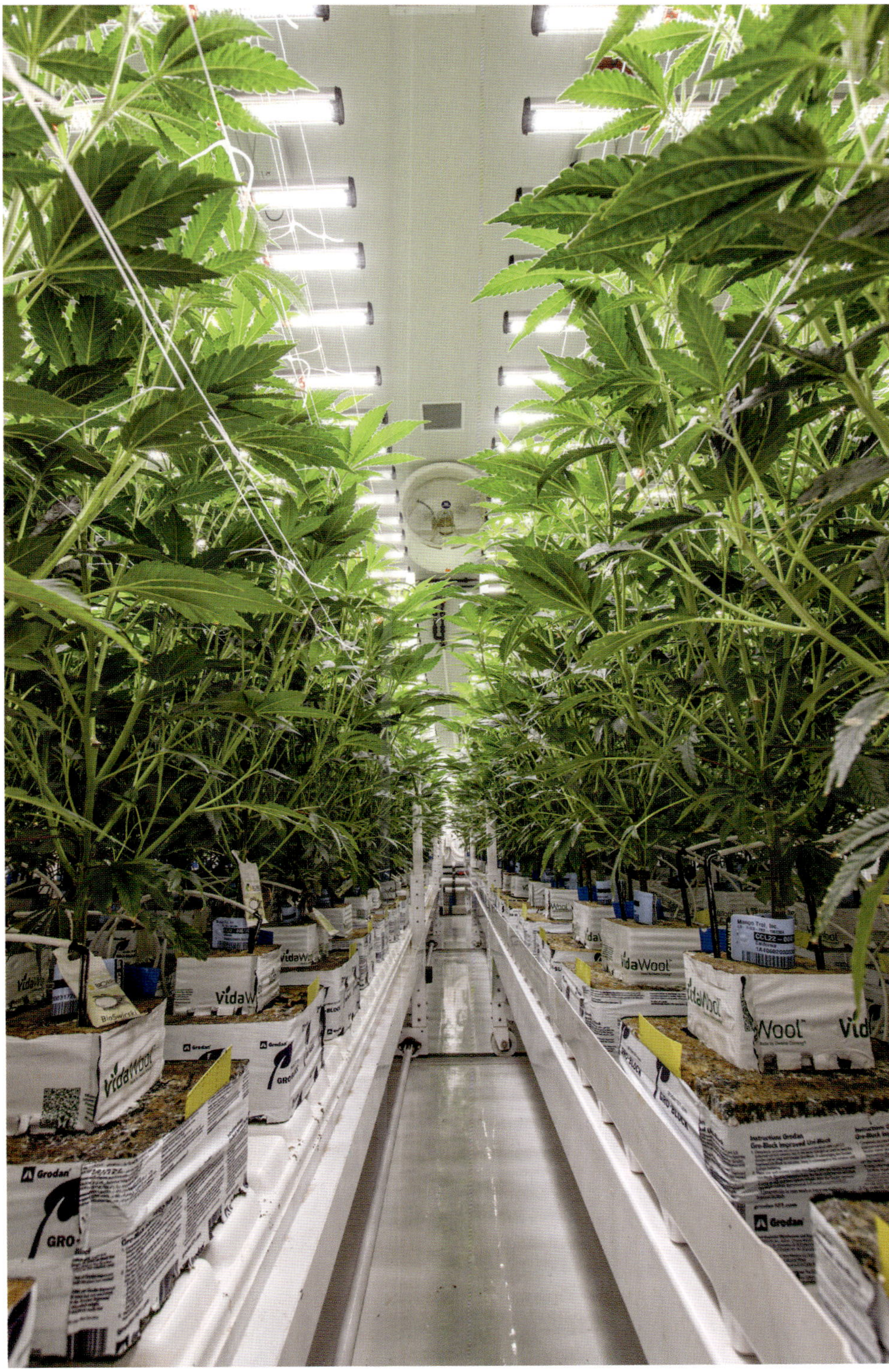

The scientific precision of hydroponics makes it easy to duplicate the process over and over again.

PHOTO: MIAMIMANGOCA.COM

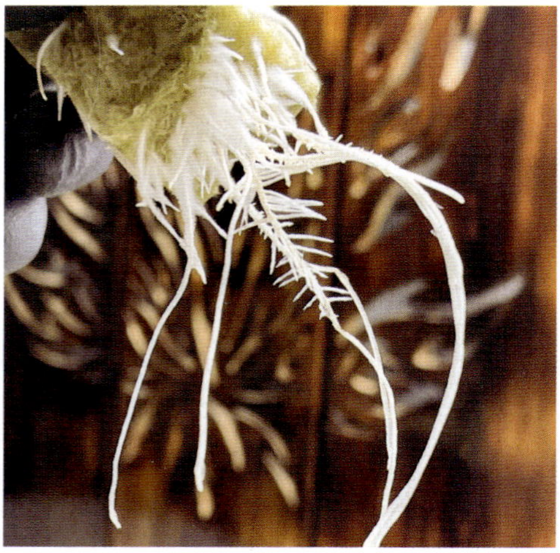

Roots are occasionally left exposed to air within the hydroponic medium.

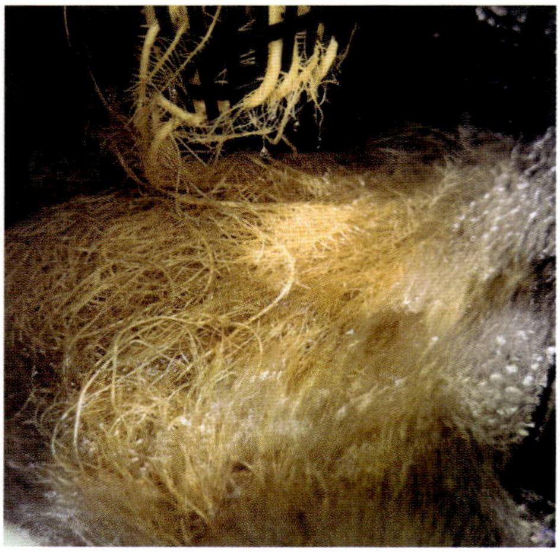

Usually, the lower part of the roots is submerged, while the upper part receives only splashes of water and nutrients.

If you are carefully maintaining the system, then the only extensive cleaning you will need is sterilization between harvests. Bleach cleaning is not mandatory but is recommended in the case of severe fungal or pest problems. To do this, dissemble your system and clean it with bleach. Wash off the bleach, let it air dry, and wait for it to dry fully before starting the system again. Bleach is the most commonly used cleaner but hydrogen peroxide also works. You will want to run the system for a day with plain water to clean it and ensure it is working properly before replanting. Follow your notes from the previous grow to make any adjustments to your solution as needed.

Debris Unclogging

If you have a clean, enclosed system, there will not be any foreign matter; problematic matter can only come from within the system. Clay pebbles are a common cause of a clogged hydroponic system as they can spill out of the net pot and float to a point in the flow that causes a blockage. If these clay pellets are constantly jamming up your system, you might want to try Rockwool cubes or another soilless plant support medium instead. There are many organic alternatives that are just as efficient at holding the plant in place. Fallen plant leaves can also cause clogging.

PHOTOS: PRESTON BJORNSON

Algae

Algae is one of a large group of non-vascular, mainly aquatic eukaryotes capable of photosynthesis. Avoid exposing your fluid containers to direct light over extended periods to prevent algae growth.[1] Most hydroponic kits are manufactured to be light-proof to eliminate this problem. If you build your system like the Deep Water Culture (DWC, also known as The Bubbler) described later in this chapter, seal your reservoir with white duct tape. Avoid using black tape or garbage bags as black absorbs light.

If you plug light leaks, algae will stop growing, and you can maintain a balanced system. After harvest, you can clean out the system to ensure no residual algae remains. In some cases, like with DWC, it is possible to wash part of a system and replace the nutrient solution with a fresh mix without disturbing the plants. Always throw out all old, algae-infested nutrient mixtures and water.

Selecting a Hydroponic Kit

The main consideration when choosing a hydroponic kit is your grow space. Bucket systems are best for smaller areas, whereas tray systems are better for spacious areas. You should also get a system you feel you can use confidently. Read the instructional manual and follow it carefully when assembling, and consider watching any videos about it that you can find online. Many of you may be using a tent as well, so your system won't be extensive. Buckets and tents are great.

The complexity of your system will depend on the choices you've made. Most small- to medium-sized systems will not require excessive assembly time. Running the system can be complex, but all systems can be automated with pumps and timers. However, automating a system requires calculations, pump timers, and programming. Most growers will still interact with the grow even in an automated system, checking for pH changes, mixing new feed batches, and looking out for diseases and pests.

Timed pumping is at the core of hydro-irrigation systems; you will need a powered pump set to specific on and off times. Timed pumping can be done with an all-in-one timer and pump unit, or you can add a timer between the power cord cable and the pump's power line. Then you do the math, fine-tune through time and get into running your system efficiently.

You may come across terms like "wick system" or "gravity system." These are easy to assemble but are more complex than many other setups because they need a reasonable degree of testing to get right and vigorous maintenance to keep running.

If money is no object and you want the expert's advice, get a Nutrient Film Technique (NFT) system. On the other hand, if you want to save money, build your own and go for DWC (Deep Water Culture; The Bubbler) first or look at building an NFT. These systems tend to be manageable for everybody who has had success with hydroponics and cannabis. Even experienced growers stick with these. If it works, then it works.

There are many different hydroponic systems: NFT, DWC, wick, automatic hydroponic pots, gravity-fed, Flood and Drain (also known as "Ebb and Flow"), drip irrigation, and nozzle spray systems such as aeroponics. The more automated systems require more technical gear. Understanding how NFTs work will provide the basic knowledge for all the other systems.

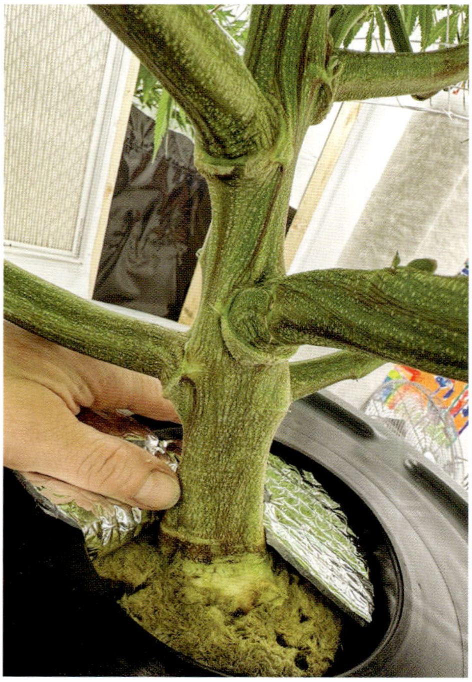

Cannabis can thrive in hydroponics, as demonstrated by this tree of a plant.

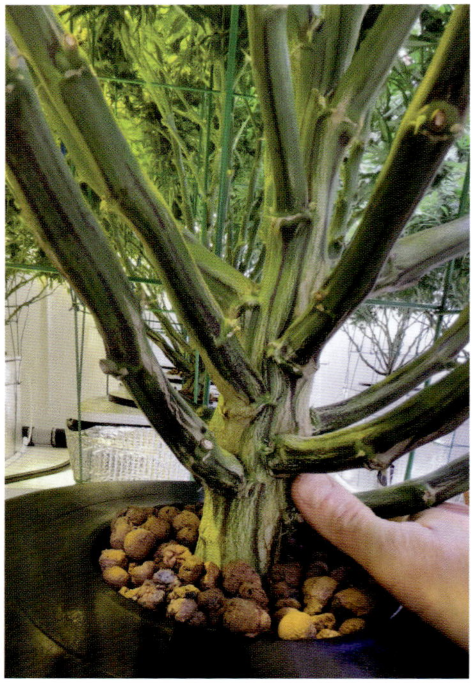

This plant's branches are thicker than most plants' stems.

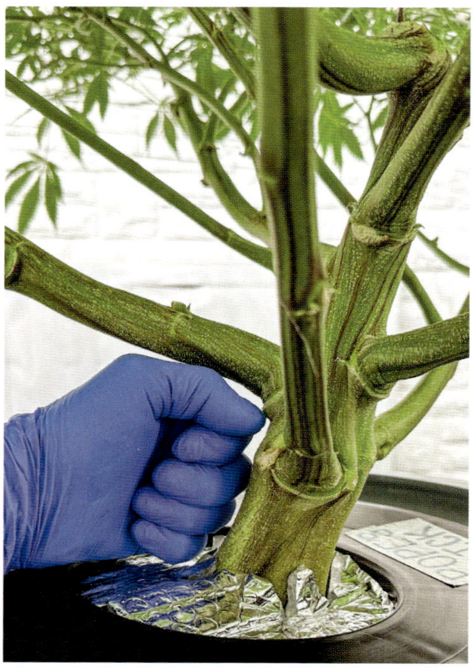

The thickness is due to the demands of this sativa that bushes big.

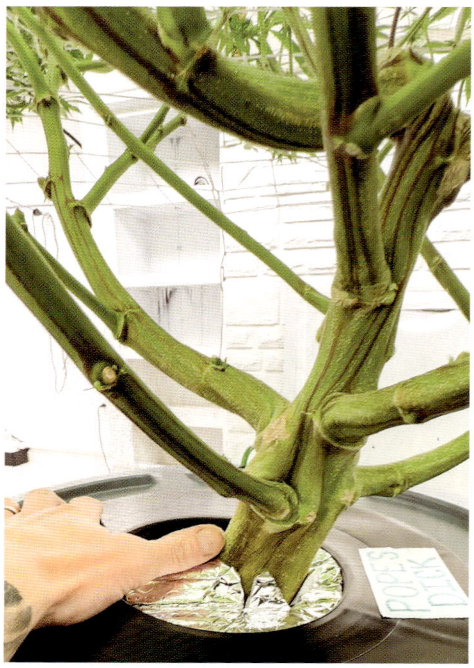

The right genetics and hydroponics can create the hulk.

PHOTOS: PRESTON BJORNSON

Nutrient Film Technique (NFT)

Nutrient Film Technique (NFT) systems divide the roots into different roles: The upper portion of the roots are for air and the lower are for the solution. A shallow film of the solution runs down a slight gradient slope past the roots, which become moist with uptake. The pump returns the gathering solution to the start of the slope. As long as the pump is powered, a film of solution will repeatedly flow past the plant's roots. If the pump is on a timer, then NFT systems car keep the roots out of the film solution for the scheduled period.

Nutrient Film Technique System

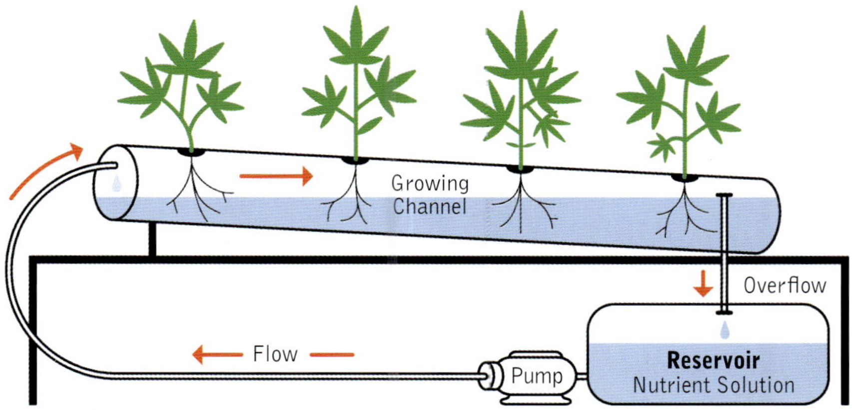

Notice the flow direction, which is active (pumped) and inactive (gravity at the overflow), to complete a circuit.

Optimal growth is achieved by calculating the best flow rate. A fast flow rate will not allow the roots to take in the nutrients it reeds while a slow flow rate will cause buildup. You should consider the slope angle and the tray size in your calculations, which is something we will cover in detail later in this chapter. Sometimes, the NFT kit's instructions will account for this, so calculations are not needed.

NFT systems are usually bought as all-in-one hydroponic tray systems. In other words, the reservoir that holds the pumps and nutrient solution is contained in the same system, although sometimes the grower can separate them. The unused nutrients are recycled to create a constant flow to the roots and back into the reservoir. In addition, they may feature a water-resistant submersible pump.

Fixed vs Adjustable Slopes

An NFT kit, when assembled, will have a slope most likely fixed by the angle of the trays when locked in place. Because NFT is a gravitational system, it is ideal for long, continuous setups. The slope should be minimal to allow the nutrients to slowly run towards the base, through the plant's roots and medium. Some kits will allow you to shift that angle a few increments. If you make your own, you can make it adjustable to give you more options. You can use pins to move a tray up or down, giving you several possible angles per tray. You can adjust a tray's slope by propping blocks under one end—or, indeed, previous editions of this book.

Slabs and Net Pots

In an NFT Rockwool slab system, the plants sit on a Rockwool slab cut to meet the NFT tray's planting holes. Most of these NFT systems come with a lid that divides the space between the medium and solution to allow root growth. The depth of the block often depends on the maximum height of your fluids. You integrate two Rockwool slabs by inserting one into another. Slabs can be shared or individual.

Growers often start clones in Rockwool cubes and insert the cubes into a Rockwool slab with spaces made for them. This makes it a continuous medium, as fluids are absorbed across that row of inserted plantlets. While Rockwool is not the only slab medium that can be used, it is the most popular.

Net pot systems minimize the amount of substrate used as they place the plant directly over a fluid channel. It can take large pellet substrates such as clay pebbles or dense organic fiber to occupy enough space around the plant's base to hold it steady. This simultaneously allows roots to grow through the spaces between pellets, through to the channel underneath them.

Net pot systems are recognizable at a distance because the trays have visible spaces between plants when seen from above. These spaces are occupied by nutrient films flowing between the net pots. The nutrient film is enclosed in the trays to keep light away from the solution. Net pots are not designed for absorption. Instead, the plant depends on the nutrient film.

The trays, when white, will reflect light on the plants. If you have algae growth, wasted light is absorbed by these cyanobacteria. Pack pellets tightly in the net pots to block light from entering the fluid channels. Yes, it does look awe-inspiring to lift a plant from

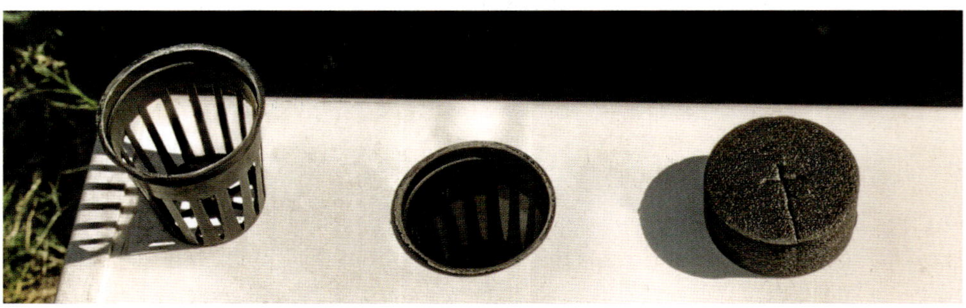

PHOTO: PETER ALVA

This aeroponic unit uses foam to block light from entering in the net pot.

a hydroponic unit exposing the root mat to see, but we should do that as little as possible. Transplanting is simply a case of moving the net pot and clone from the clone tank to the NFT tray in one move. Though cloning tanks will not have the same nutrients or strength as the NFT system, you should maintain the same pH. Another reason for lifting plants is to check for root rot problems. However, for the most part, you will not disturb them too often, if at all.

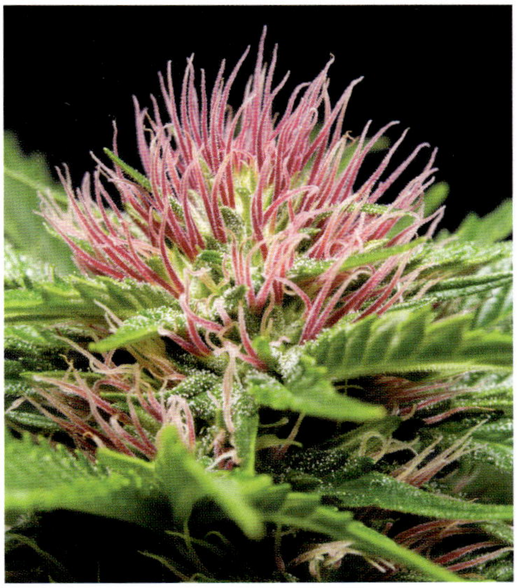

Very few strains show such colorful displays during early flowering; usually the pistils are cream-colored.

PHOTO: DANKSHIRE PHOTOGRAPHY

NFT Maintenance

Ensure the water pump is always working. If you have an outage, the water will gather instead of being pumped, which can cause root rot. However, it is possible to have the NFT self-contained if you aren't running fresh water piped in all the time. It won't flood anything, even with a pump off. All you can have going wrong is all your fluid gathered at a tray's base, going nowhere fast. If you prevent leaks, use a controlled amount of fluid on a timed schedule, and regularly check the pH, you will only need regular top-ups. The system is safe if you get your calculations right.

If, for some reason, you do want to use fresh running water in a hydroponic system, you will need to factor in overflow to manage any potential flooding. Water needs a pathway to drain out of the system if there is a potential for flooding. Some trays have "overflow" systems built in. You need to work out potential risks and safety features with electrical components like pumps and LED lights.

Rot and Inactivity

Plants in hydroponics are susceptible to root rot when a system allows stagnant, inactive water to gather around the roots. Water can become stale and develop pathogens in case of an inactive pump or blockage. Any fluid that doesn't eventually move through the system will have pH fluctuations and generally change its constitution at the molecular level, causing problems like rot to appear around the roots.

Root rot can be prevented by adjusting the tray to a sufficient slope and preventing blockages. You can use a capture area at the bottom of the trays to gather the solution, but you want it moving again during the day. Next to light leaks, stagnant water is the main cause of bacteria. Lift the plant out with the net pot and observe the roots to ensure there is no gunk buildup.

NFT Trays

"Trays," "troughs," and "channels" are used interchangeably to refer to the receptacle under the plants where the solution flows. NFT systems can be upscaled by adding modular trays and link systems with T-junction pipes. More pumps can be added to control higher volumes of flowing solution. It is possible to run multiple trays from a single reservoir. NFT systems often have flat trays instead of curved ones because they allow for a narrower flowing film. Many homemade systems use recycled, curved pipes. Curved trays have more depth at the center and less at the side of the channel.

Solution Temperature

The ideal solution temperature for hydroponics is room temperature. The solution should settle to room temperature (68-72°F / 20-22°C) after a few days of running. If the hydroponic system is self-contained, the reservoir is shallow, and the grow room's temperature is adjusted to cannabis cultivation environment conditions, the temperature of the fluid should be perfect. The solution will also absorb any heat present in the tray due to the heat emitted from the lights, especially if you are using HIDs. The test phase covered earlier will help ensure everything in the grow chamber is operating correctly and being cooled by the active airflow.

Any fresh solution batch should be allowed to reach room temperature before being added to the system. We expect some cooling when the two are mixed due to the solution at lower depths being cooler than the surface, but they should achieve room temperature soon after. Use an aquarium thermometer in the reservoir and measure the grow area's temperature to record any changes. If the reservoir water temperature is significantly warmer than 78°F (26°C), air circulation should be adjusted to cool the grow area down. Warm seasons will require proper airflow, as rooms get hotter, air intake is warmer, and the system's temperature increases. Heating mats for water tanks can help increase fluid temperatures if cold is a problem. These are available from aquarium shops. However, heating the grow area is a safer idea first, as well as considering options for better insulation.

NFT Flow Rates

There are no deep waters in NFT. The goal isn't to have the roots submerged in the fluid. Instead, a thin layer should flow through the roots. The fluid volume is estimated using the hydroponic system's instructions and some ingenuity. A basic guideline for NFT systems is a flow rate of 1 L/minute. It is not uncommon to start with a 0.5 L/minute flow rate for new plants and increase the flow rate as the plants grow. Flow rates can go from 1 L/minute to 1.5 L/minute. Beyond 2 L/minute is challenging to manage. The faster the flow, the more difficult it is for the plants to absorb nutrients. The slower the flow, the greater the chance of water pooling and root rot, but this is more a design flaw than a growing technique problem.

Alternatives to NFT

As we stated initially, NFT systems provide a foundation for almost every other system in hydroponics. Some alternatives may function as part of an NFT system or they may be combined. You should first consider DWC (The Bubbler), which is popular because it is straightforward to make from a few DIY store items. In addition, DWC is compatible with tent growing due to its method of growing plants close together.

Wick systems use capillary action and molecular forces to provide constant, slow-release nutrients directly to roots through the wick. They are the most minimal static system but offer the least control.

"Automatic" hydroponic pots are units advertised as all-in-one, self-watering pots. There is a wide range available to meet a grower's needs. They are primarily for ornamental plants but can be used for fruits, vegetables, and herbs. Some automatic hydroponic pots can also be used with soil. The technology varies, but the idea behind them is minimal maintenance. Unlike the other systems, they are not modular, and you follow the instructions that are provided. Automatic pot systems are more efficient when they follow the basic principles of NFT or DWC systems.

Gravity-fed systems mean that the solution reservoir is held above the feeding trays, connected by a pipe and controlled by a floating switch valve, much like a toilet cistern ballcock or ball float valve. When the cistern is flushed empty, the ball drops down, and the valve opens. Gravity releases the solution from a pipe and feeds into the cistern. It is also an automated system, as the water level drops when the roots absorb the fluids. Intermittently the valve opens, replenishing the feeding tray.

Flood and Drain systems (also known as "Ebb and Flow") have similar mechanics to NFT, but instead of a thin film of fluid, a larger volume of solution is used. More noticeably, the solution is completely drained from feeding trays to the reservoir and pumped back again, usually through the same pipe with the aid of a timer. Due to the larger volume of liquid, there tend to be more overflow outlets with the trays and drainage points for spills.

We will need to go through some drip irrigation theory before considering how nozzles are used with advanced spray systems such as with aeroponics. These systems tend to consume the least amount of liquids, but calculating the spray rate can be tricky.

You may not find any alternative more suitable for your situation than NFT, but we shall go through them all the same because you may come across parts of them in some NFT systems. For example, floating valves are only found in some systems. More likely than not, you will try a DWC system, which is highly recommended for ease of use and portability.

Inside a Hydro Tent

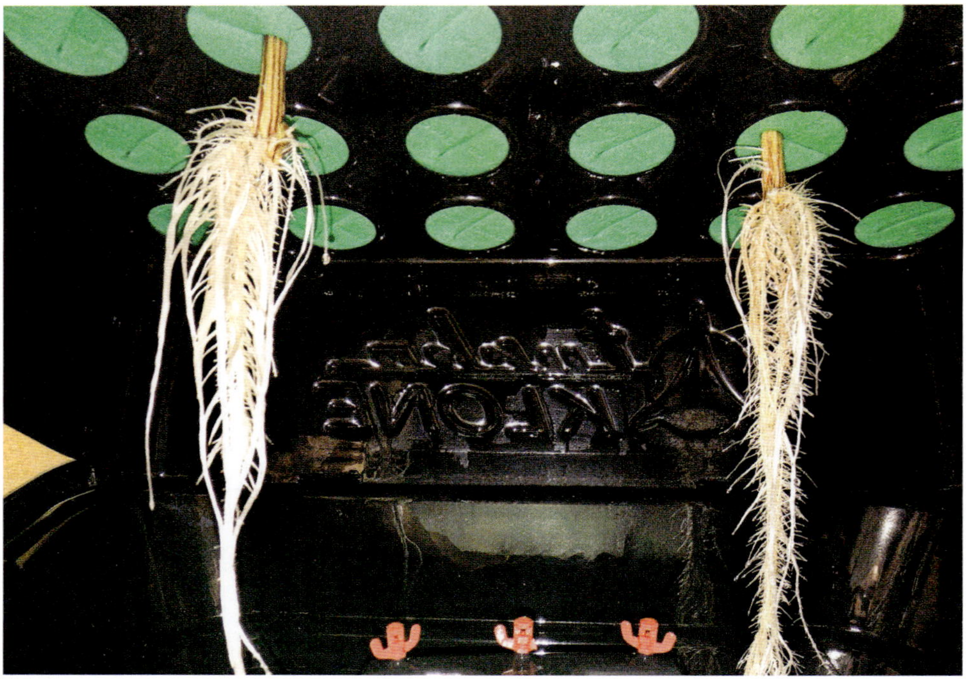

Foam without net pots can be used with different systems depending on what you want to do. The system must be light-leak-proof.

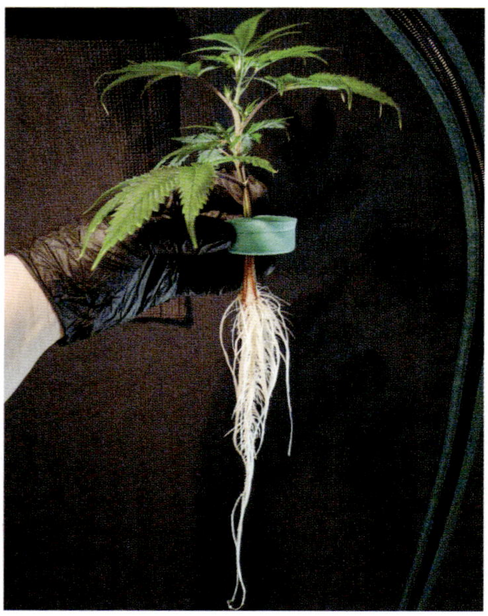

The foam cap supports the plant stem and the root mass underneath because the disc is jammed into the rim of the hydroponics lid.

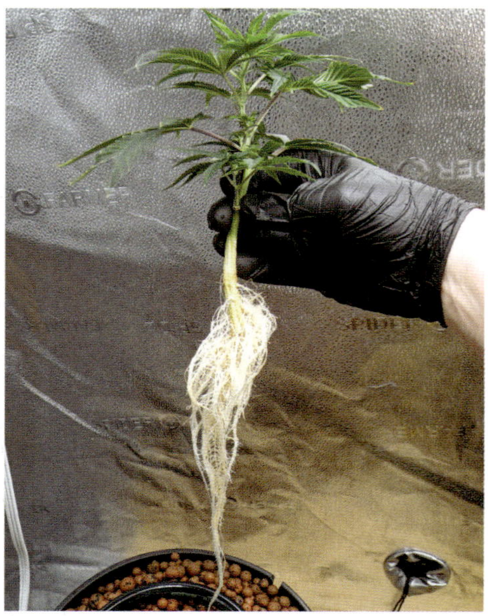

Hydroponics can stimulate quite a quantity of root mass to grow even in the early stages of growth.

PHOTOS: @TREETRUNK422

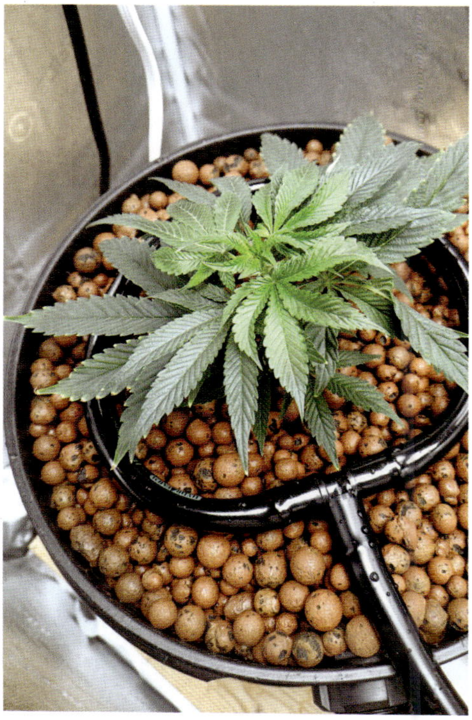

Closed loop drip irrigation system. It makes watering easier.

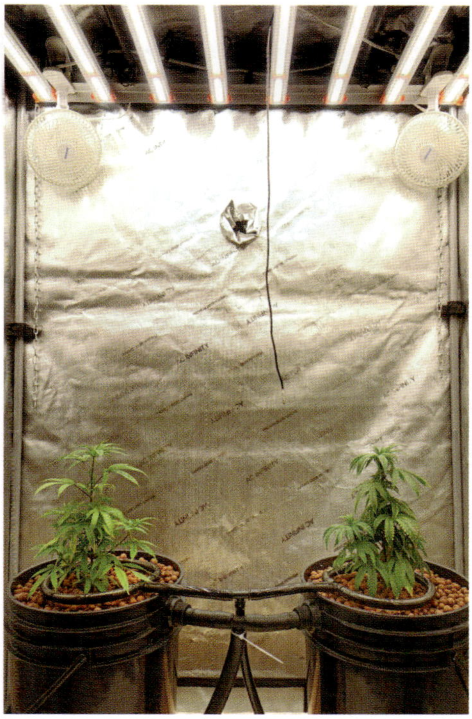

Don't underestimate how big plants can get in hydroponic systems.

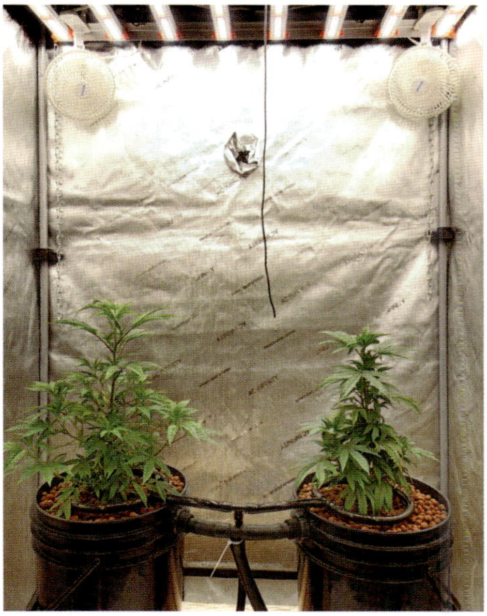

Plants can put on more height than expected within a few days.

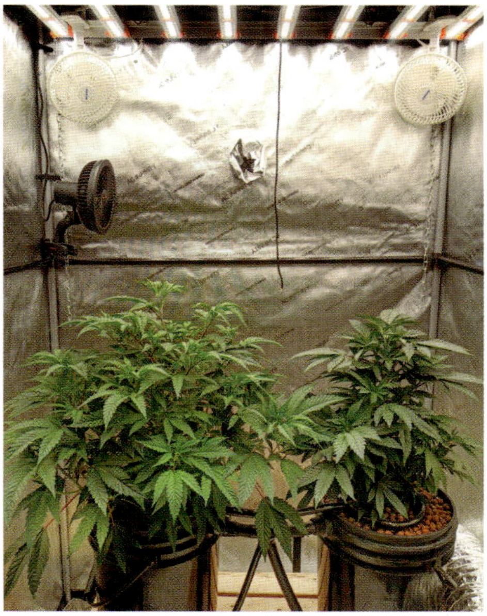

At the end of vegetative growth, the bushy capabilities of cannabis are on display.

continues...

Inside a Hydro Tent *continued*

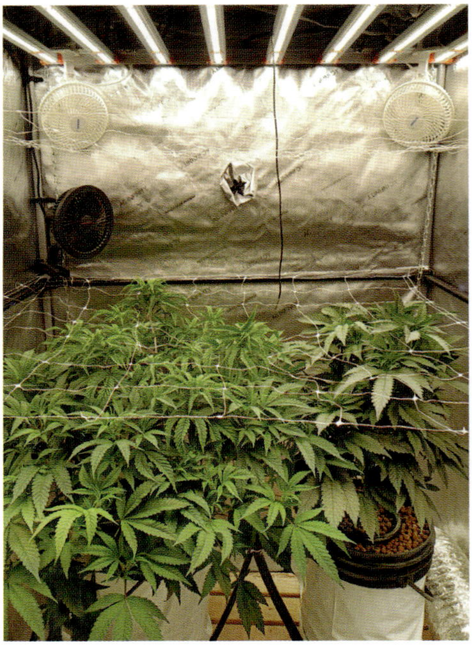

At this time, a net screen has been introduced to keep the canopy even.

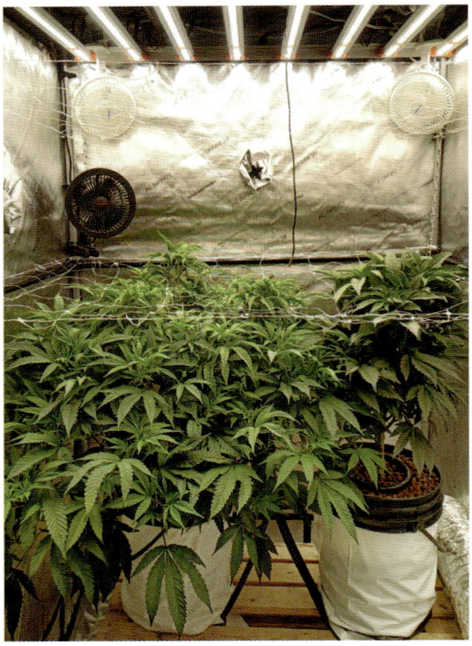

This hydroponics grow is a vigorous one and will need more maintenance.

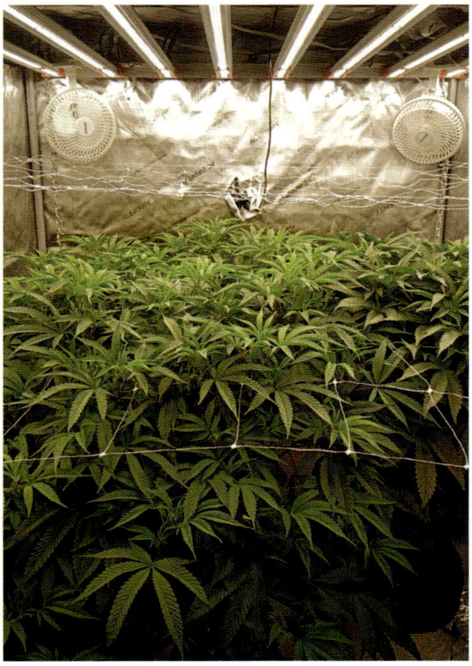

A second screen is introduced to control the canopy.

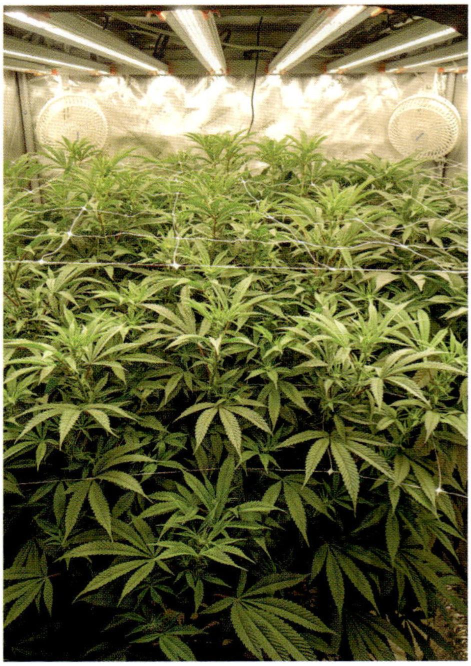

The first will hold the plants midway, and the second will support the upper foliage.

PHOTOS: @TREETRUNK422

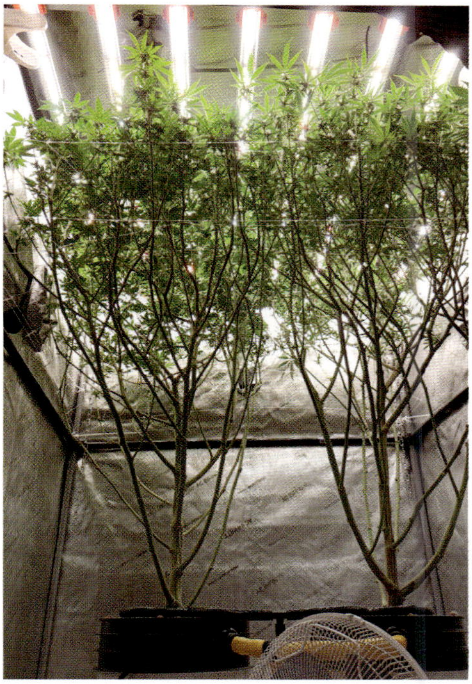

These plants have been defoliated in the lower foliage regions.

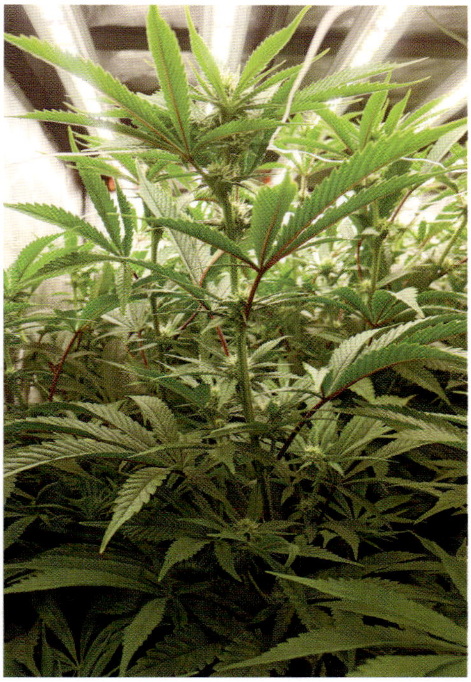

The second screen will be used to keep the flowering canopy even.

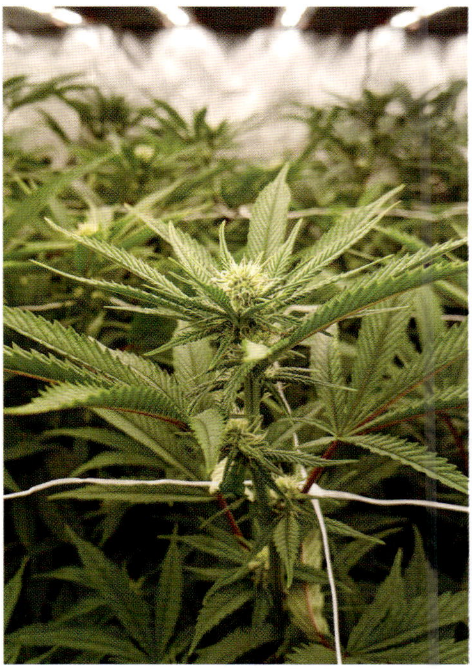

Early flowering looks like it is going to be quite intensive.

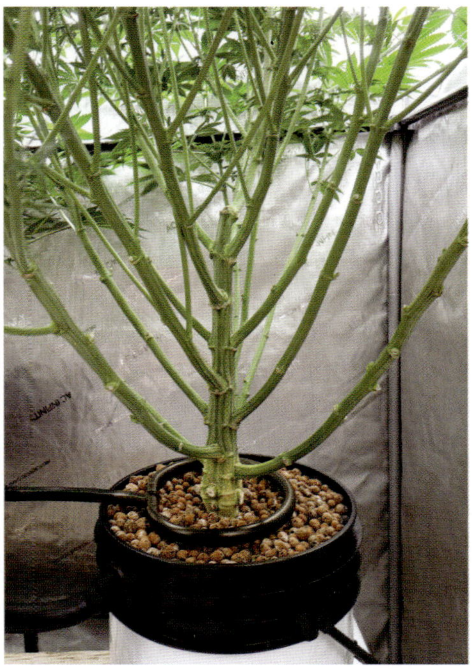

Heavy defoliation leads to a clear area beneath the first screen. *continues...*

Inside a Hydro Tent *continued*

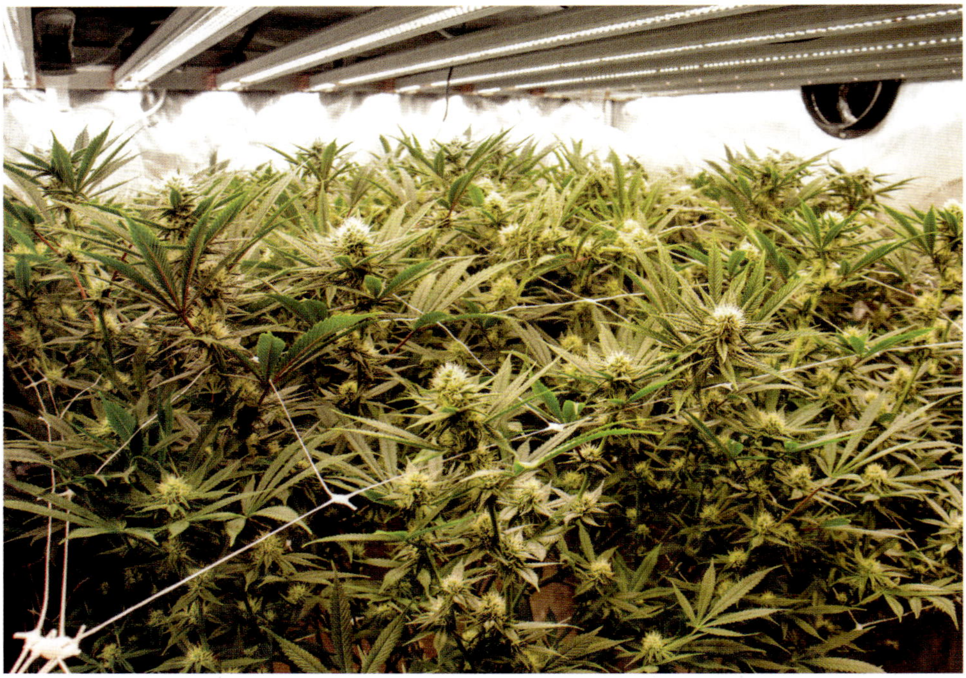

The second screen was the right choice for the intensity of this plant's growth and flowering.

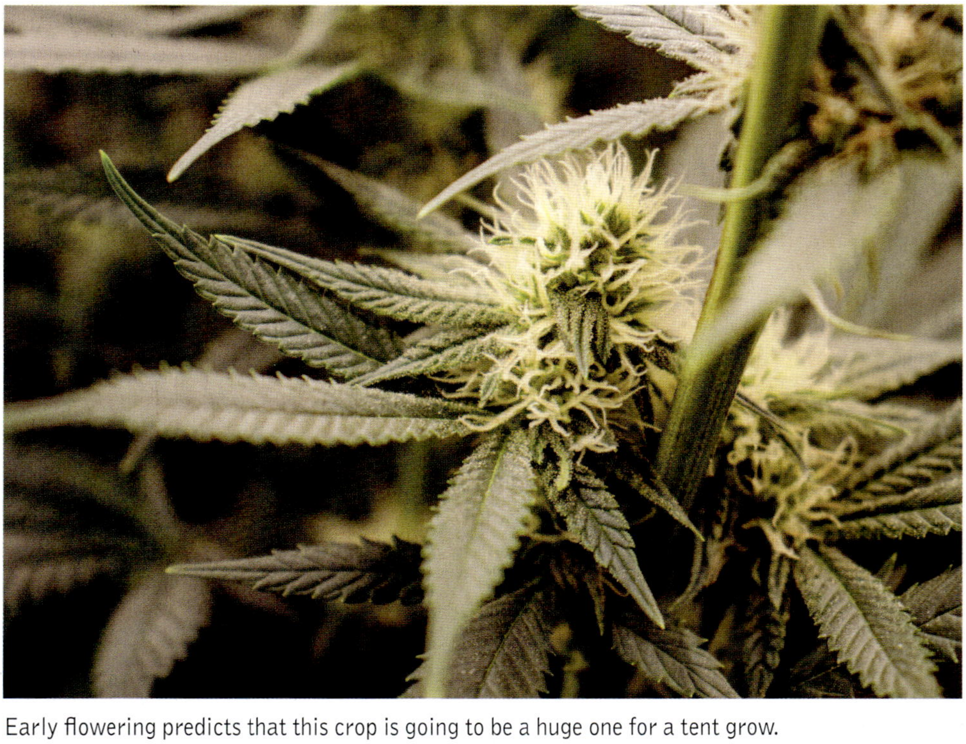

Early flowering predicts that this crop is going to be a huge one for a tent grow.

PHOTOS: @TREETRUNK422

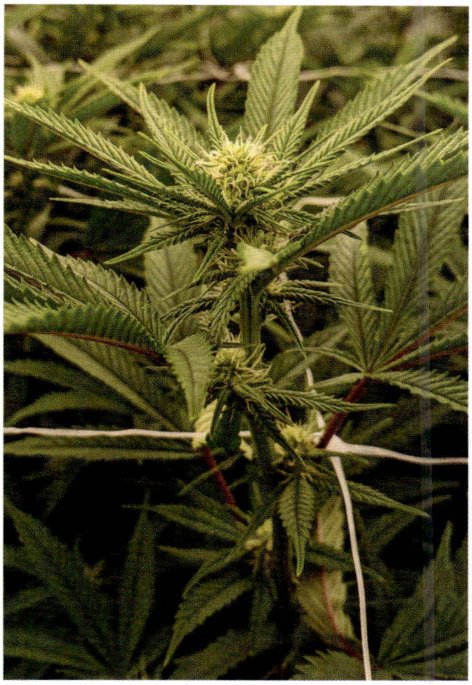

The cannabis flower promises nature's relief and tranquility.

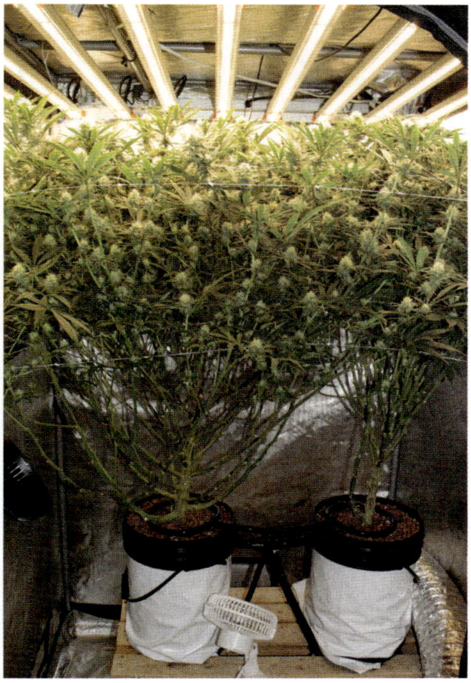

LEDs allow plants to be closer to the lights as there is no heat.

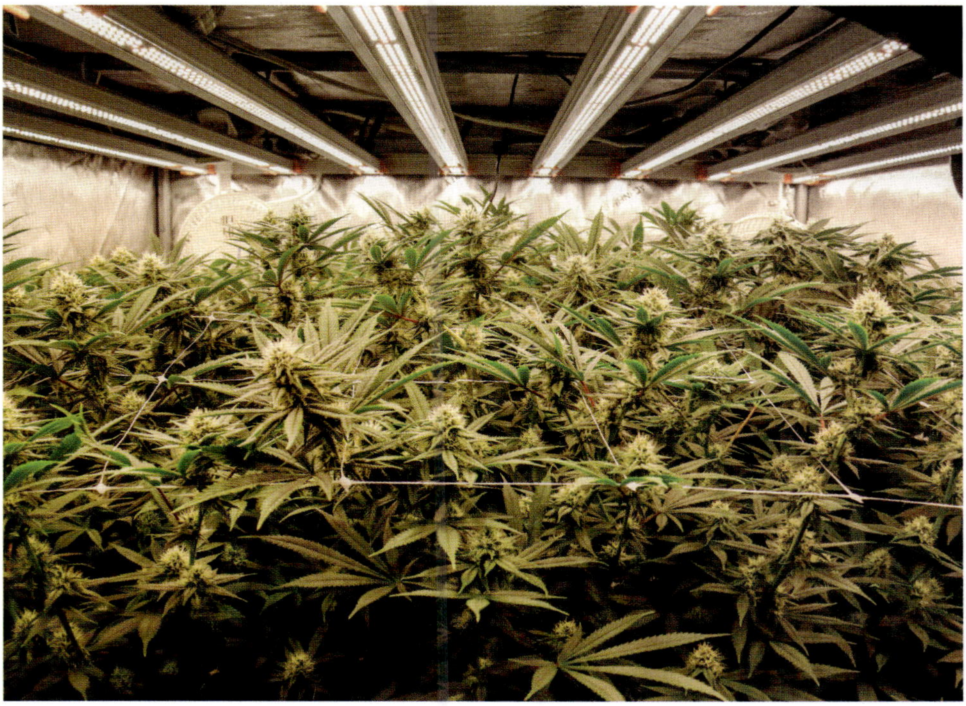

The second screen is keeping the canopy under control. LEDs are cool.

continues...

PHOTOS: GREG GREEN (TOP LEFT), @TREETRUNK422 (TOP RIGHT AND BOTTOM)

Inside a Hydro Tent *continued*

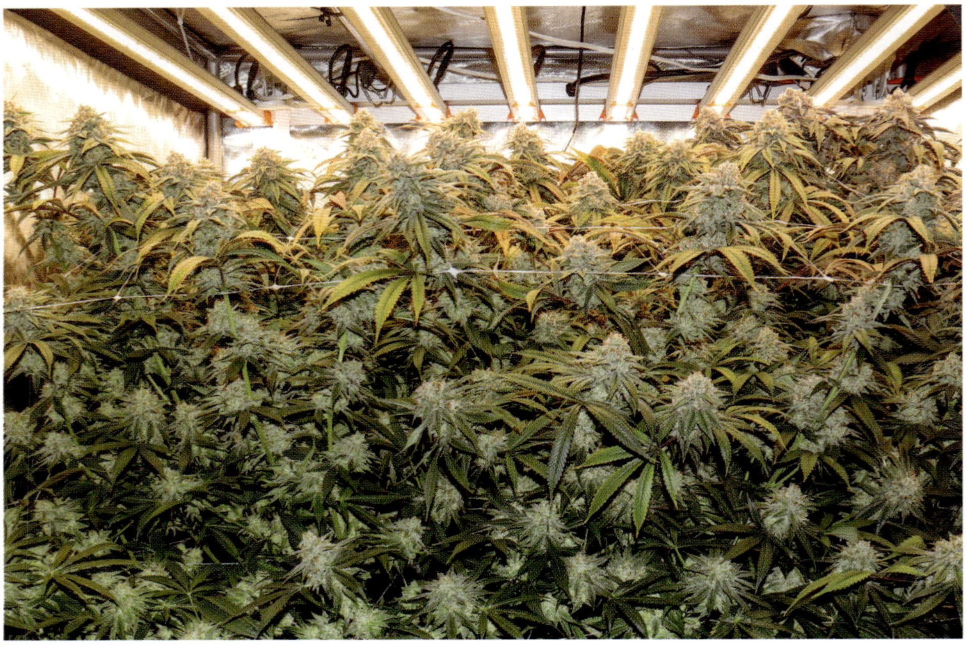

The limited space available makes screening important for this bountiful harvest. LEDs paid off for this tent's hydro growth.

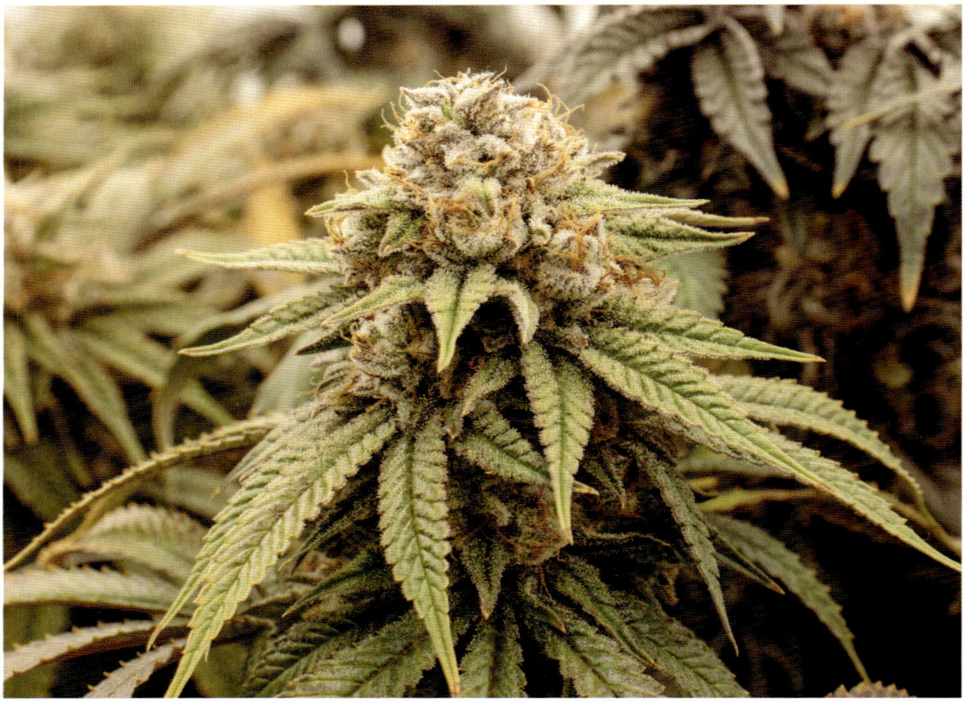

PHOTOS: @TREETRUNK422

Hydroponically grown, thick, juicy buds and lots of frosty side leaves make this grow appealing.

DWC A.K.A. The Bubbler

The Bubbler is simply an all-in-one nutrient and plant-holding bucket with a lid and a pump, but it produces extraordinary results! The pump will send air through the tube to the air stone, releasing air into the solution. The pumped air "bubbles" the solution causing it to splash at the surface, wetting the bottom of the net pot and roots. As the bubbles pop, they spray the underside of the net pot and roots. The net pot isn't sunk into the fluid here; it operates on the principle that the bubbles provide a spray of liquids. Eventually, root mat development and size means that roots will be sunk into a static feeding solution. Using the bubbler method, you can produce optimal growing conditions for top-yielding strains, as long as it is maintained and managed well by you, the grower.

The key to the system is to have the air movement near the surface of the fluids at the start of DWC, which can be done in two ways. The first is to move the air stone nearer to the solution's surface, and the second is to have a powerful pump that disturbs the water enough to cause surface splashing.

DWC is very similar to a cloning tray, where the clones live off the nutrients and water splashed onto the clay pebbles. As the roots grow down, water bubbles will come into contact with them. They will gradually grow through the net pots and down into the nutrient solution, where they will drink until the unit is dry or the roots no longer touch the nutrient solution. Check the Bubbler every day to see how much your plant has absorbed.

Let your roots get air periodically by letting a root zone form. Let the solution level drop a few inches below the net pot to do this. Do not constantly top up your reservoir; it is sometimes better to let the water level drop. When you need to refresh your

Bubble Bucket System

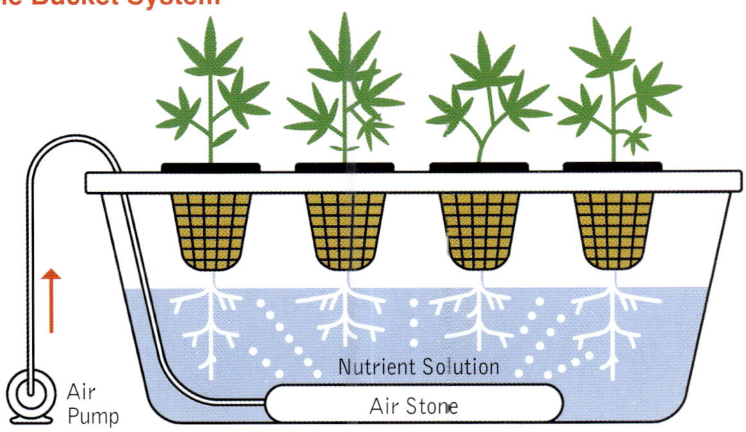

The ingenuity of the bubbling bucket is that surface bubbles splash against the exposed roots, allowing them to receive air.

Build Your Own Hydro Bubble Bucket System

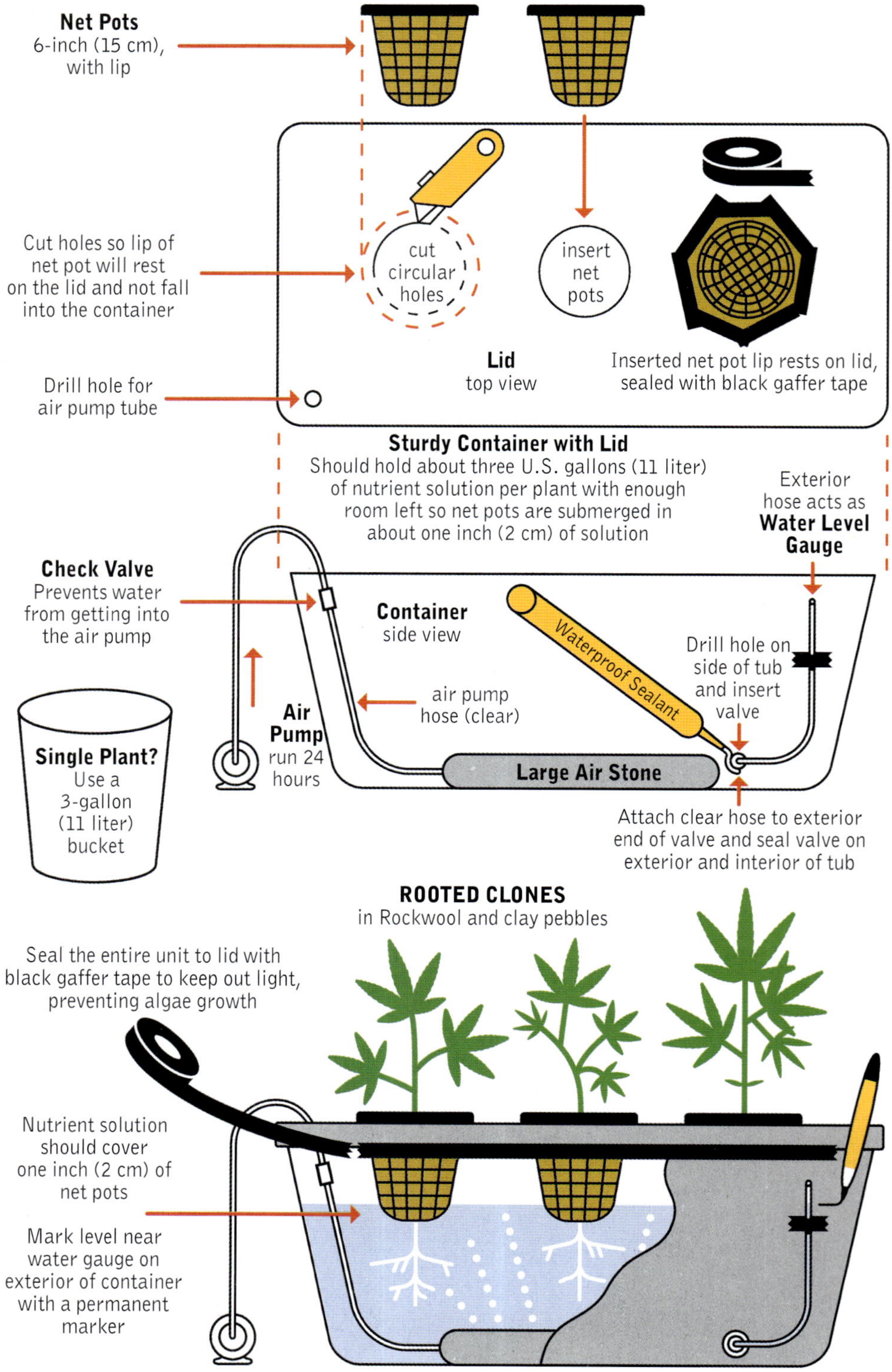

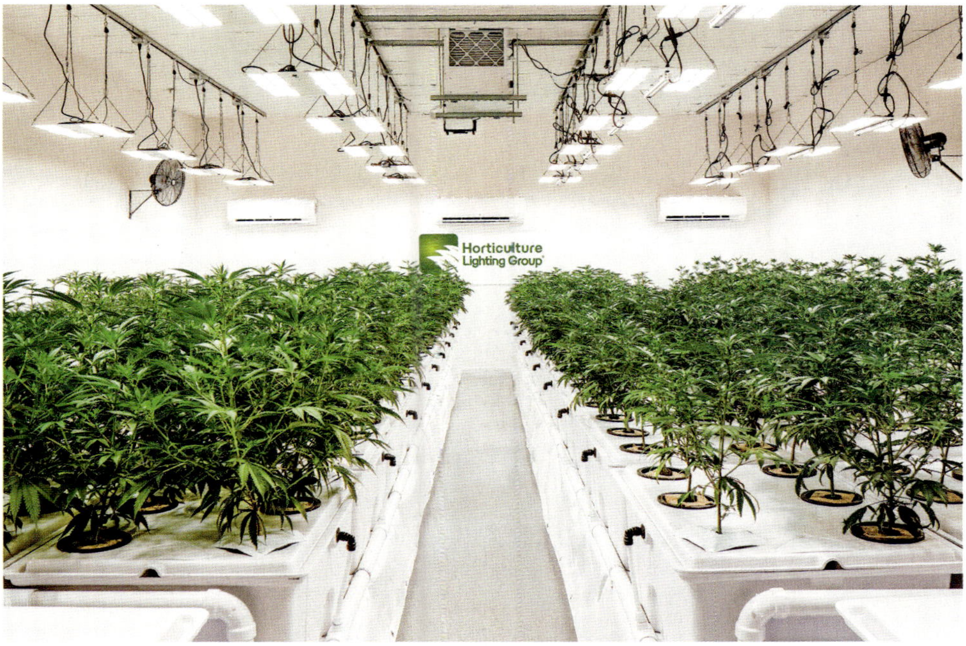

Deep Water Culture and bubbling buckets share a lot in common. Both show tremendous results when applied correctly.

PHOTO: HORTICULTURE LIGHTING GROUP, HLG.COM

nutrient mixture completely, simply lift the lid that holds your plant and carefully scoop the root mass into another container filled with the new mixture. Once a good root mass has developed, your plants will exhibit unprecedented growth!

You can wrap any bucket in white masking tape to make it reflective and avoid light leaking into the solution. This budget-friendly hydroponic system is highly recommended if you don't have enough funds for something expensive. It is very popular with tent growers as you can pack the buckets closely together. Constant maintenance and management are required to produce optimal growing conditions for top-yielding strains using this method.

Wick

Wick systems require minimal maintenance but they are tricky to set up, as controlling nutrient uptake requires trial and error. In a wick system, the nutrient solution is held in a reservoir (a nutrient solution container) above which another container—the grow container—is placed. The grow container holds Rockwool, another type of soilless substrate, and the plants. Try experimenting with a wick on clones to approximate how a wick hydroponic system works. This system doesn't require electricity as no active pumps and timers are involved. Instead, it relies on capillary action to move solution up one or more wicks to feed the plant, making it one of the most straightforward hydroponic systems to make.

Wick System

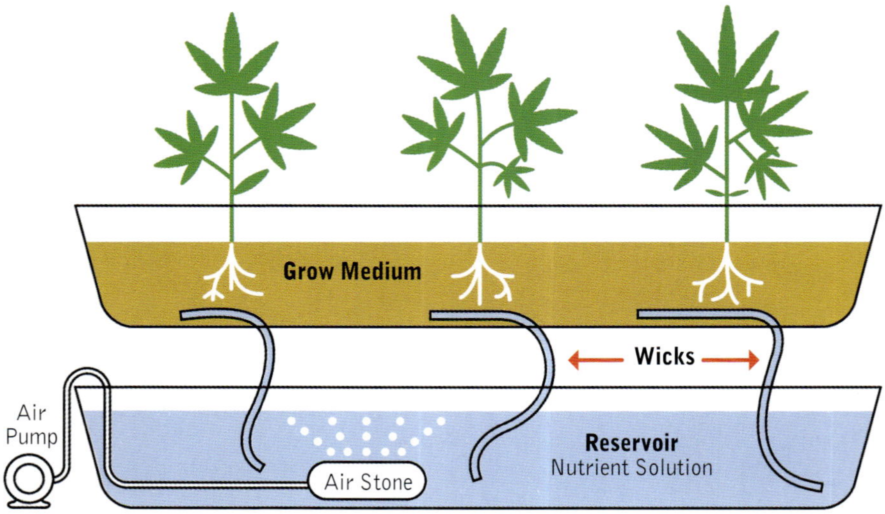

The wick system is simple and direct once you figure out the setup. The wick pulls water into the grow medium using capillary action.

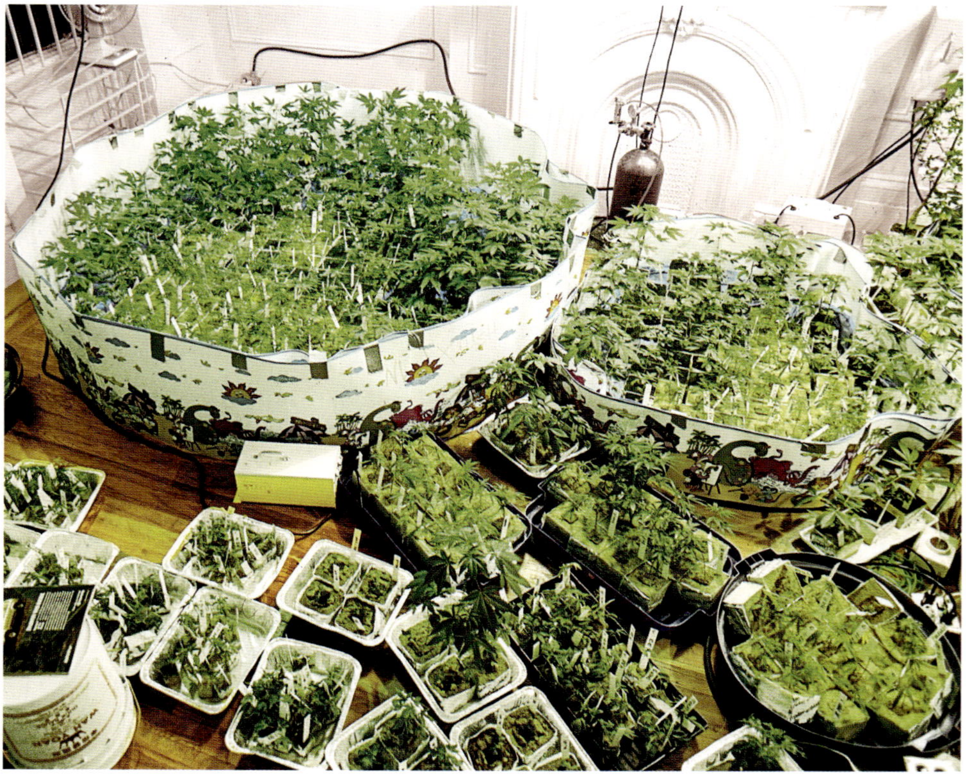

PHOTO: ANDRE GROSSMAN

This clone nursery setup uses a wick system. At the back of the grow room you can see a large cluster of plants in a kiddie pool.

How to Build a DIY Wick System

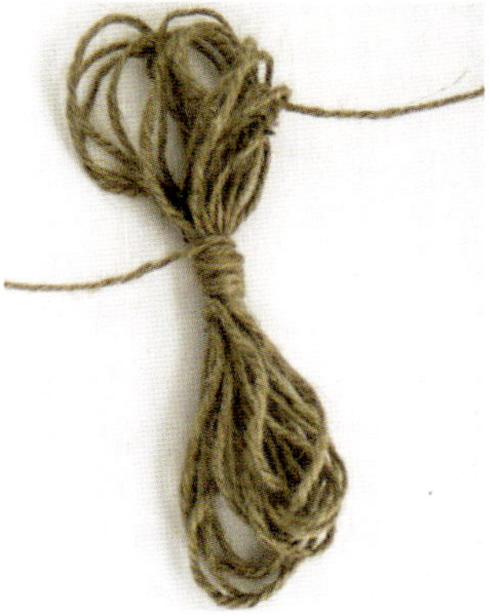

As long as the cord is absorbent it will work.

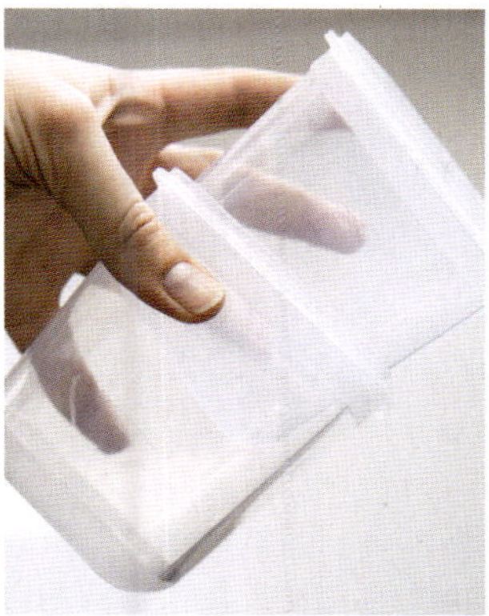

Two containers that nearly fit into each other.

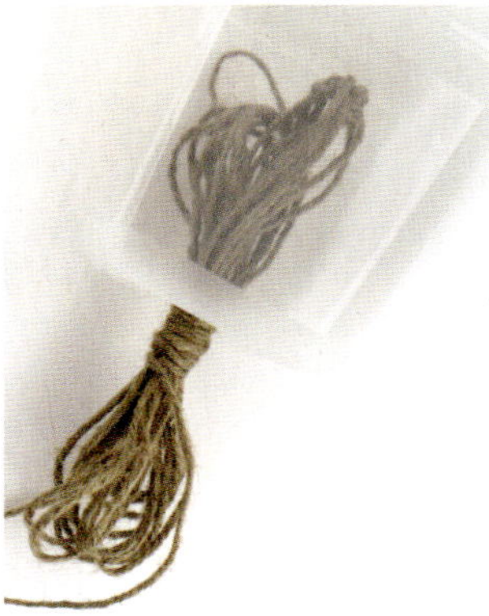

Feed the cord into a bottom hole made in one.

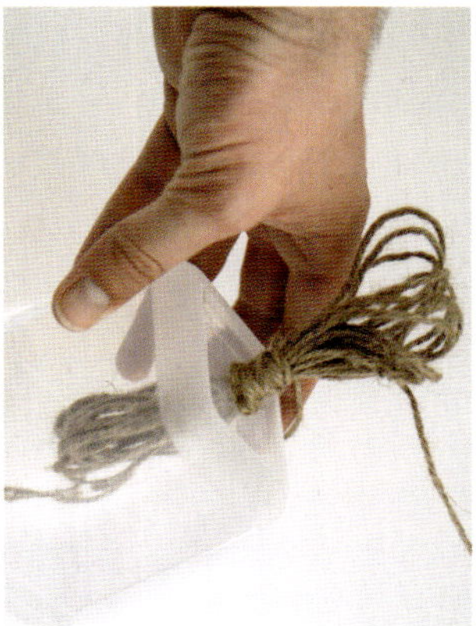

A knot can prevent it from slipping through.

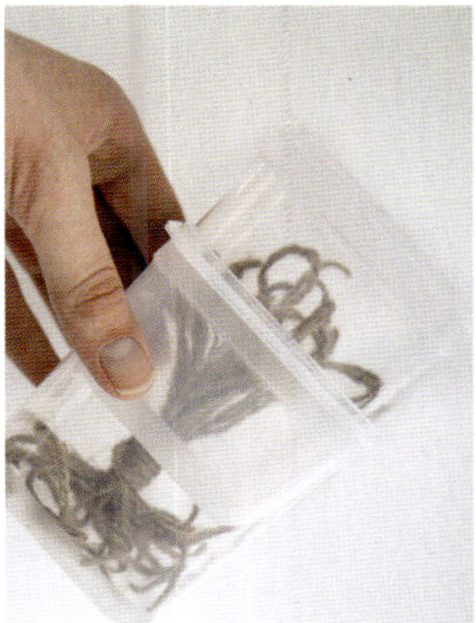

Connect the containers so the cord is contained.

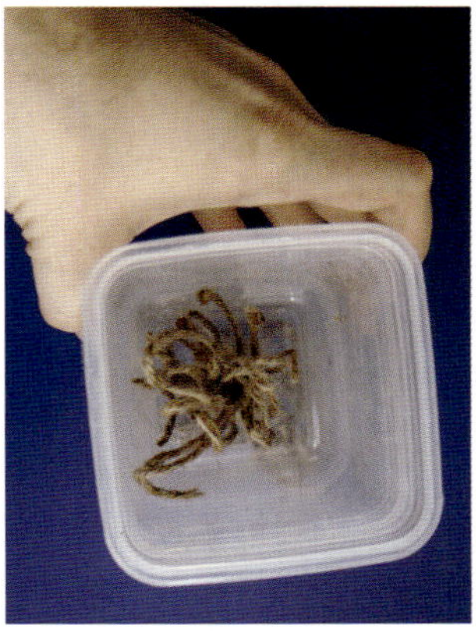

Absorbed nutrients run upwards into the top part.

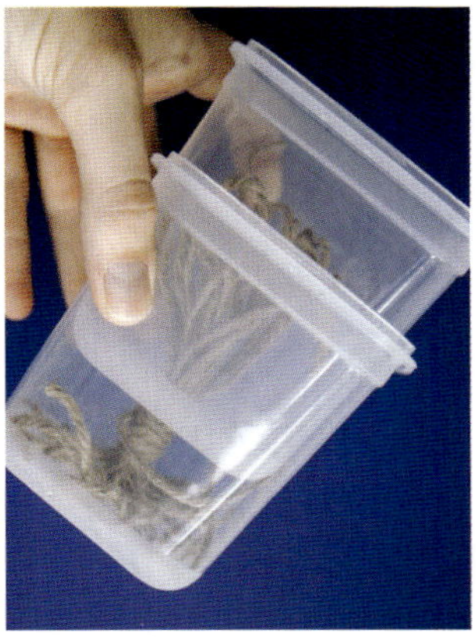

Next step is to pack medium into the top part for a seedling.

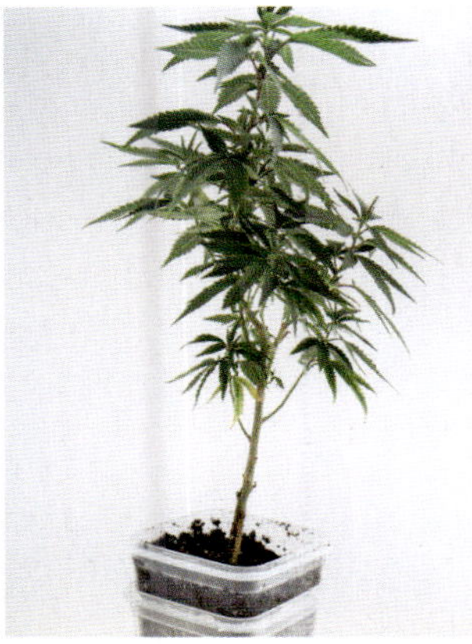

You can also transp ant a clone into it.

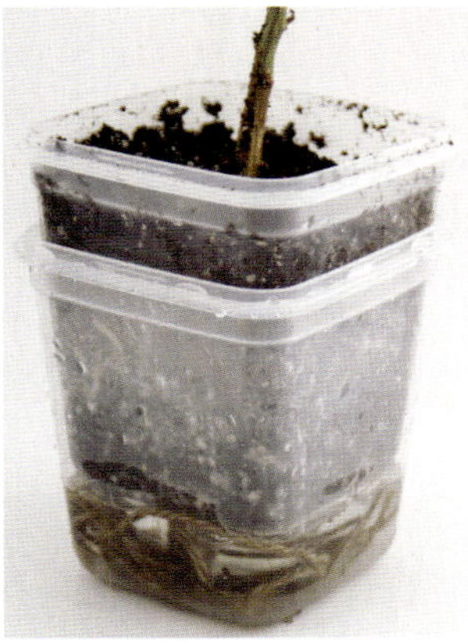

Nutrient top-ups done by refilling the bottom part.

PHOTOS: WEADO

Building the system is simple. Before adding substrate or plants, make several holes in the bottom of the grow container. Then push the wicks down through the holes into the nutrient solution below. Something as simple as cotton strips from an old T-shirt can be used as wicks. The tops of the wicks are secured in place in the grow container to guarantee that the nutrients absorbed are evenly distributed to all areas of the substrate. This ensures that your plants have access to adequate nutrients and water.

The wick system does not offer growers much control over the feeding rate. The problem with capillary action is that the amount of time it takes for the nutrients to travel up the wick and into your medium may be much less than the time it takes for your plants to use those nutrients. You will need to add or remove wicks to control nutrient delivery to your plants. Too many wicks may result in overwatering or overfeeding. Wick system growers often have to hand-water the plant from above to compensate for the slow capillary action of the wicks. The more water your plants need, the harder this is to get right. However, plenty of growers have grabbed some clones and sat them in a net pot in a container with a nutrient solution under and a wick going into it—a simple outdoor solution to growing a clone. The sun and topping up the system do the rest. Once you have experience using wicks, you can adapt them to almost any growing situation.

Automatic Hydroponic Pots

These pots grow one plant at a time and are usually bought as an all-in-one hydroponic setup. In each pot, a pump delivers the nutrients to the bottom until they reach the roots (or they are manually fed by hand, so they are not "self-watering"). The roots then drink as much as they can until they're dry—and once the roots are exposed, the pot is fed with more nutrient solution. The performance of the pots depends on the system you buy. Automatic hydroponic pots best suit growers who want to unbox a system quickly, put it under a light, and stick their ready-bought clones into the unit. The idea behind them is minimal setup and minimal maintenance. You may see these more used with showcasing displays rather than for optimized production. The DWC (Deep Water Culture; The Bubbler) shares much in common with these automatic pots. However, the Bubbler is a DIY system, whereas buying a DWC system usually results in something more like an automatic hydroponic pot.

Auto Pot System

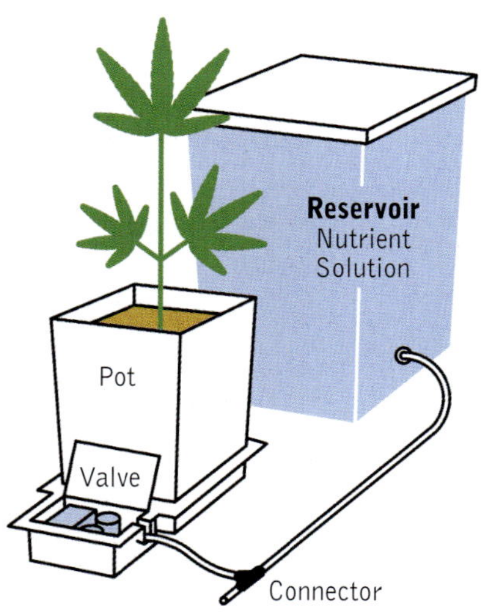

Notice this system is for a single plant. This is often sufficient for growing one big one.

DWC with Hydrobucket

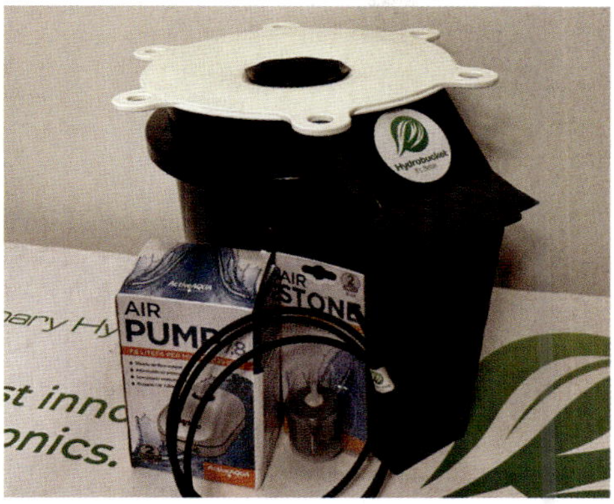

DWC is simple yet has remarkable results. Buy or make your own.

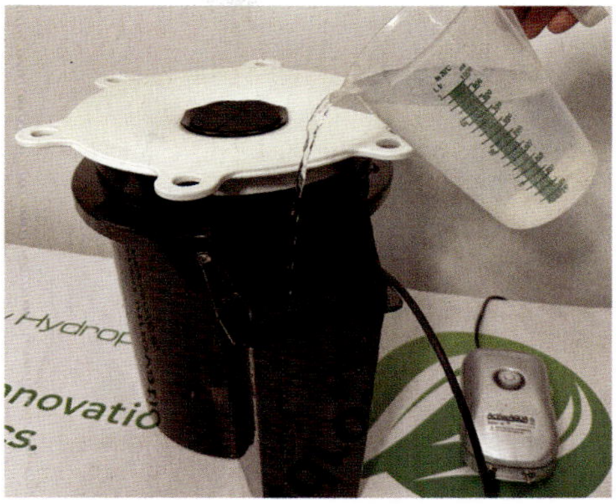
Everything is in one unit and requires active powering (pump).

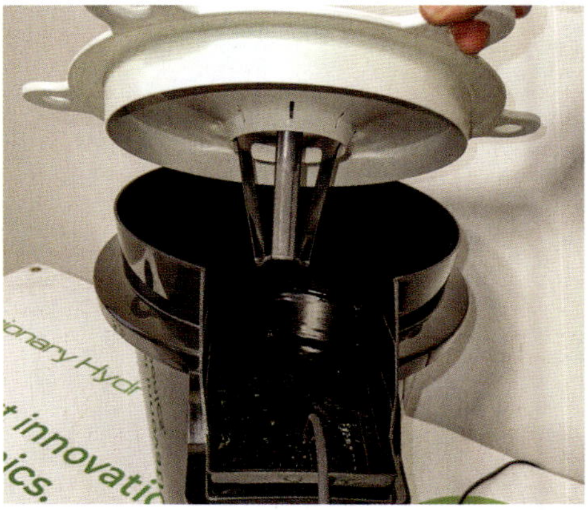
A lightproof lid is important to prevent algae growth.

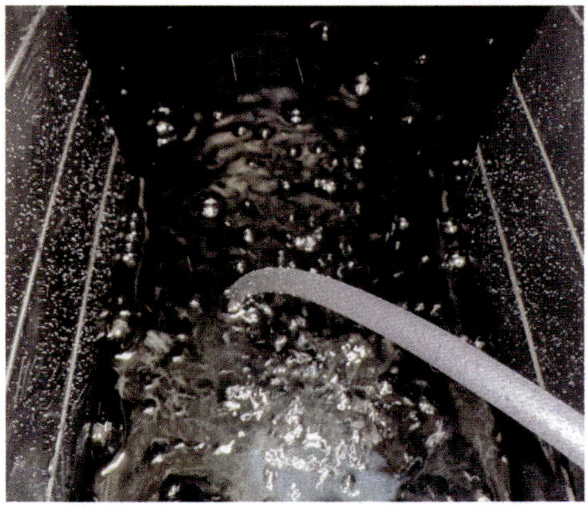
The solution is to constantly keep it aerated.

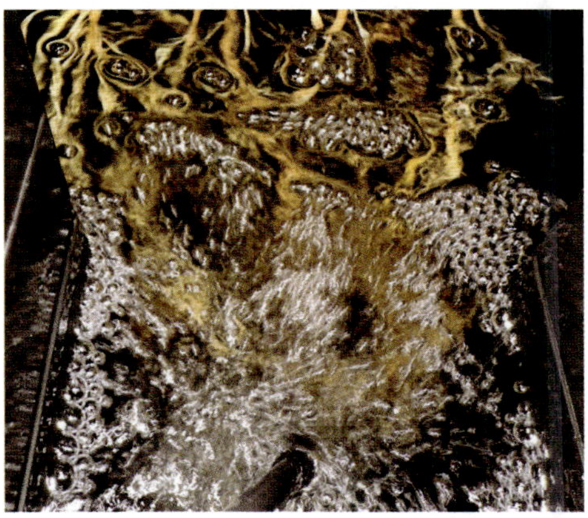
Bubbles of nutrients splash against the roots exposed to the air.

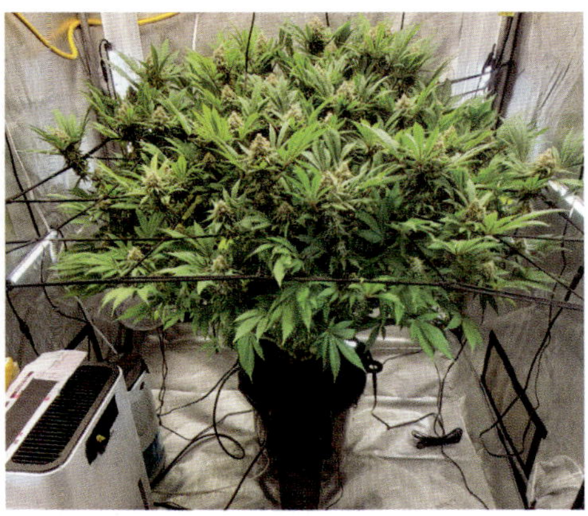
A double screen is needed to control this massive bush.

PHOTOS: THEHYDROBUCKET.COM

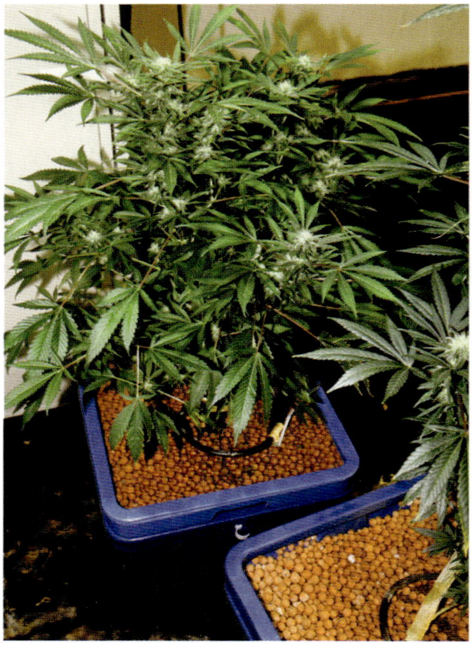

YouTube features hundreds of different homemade and commercial stand-alone hydroponic systems. Viewing them is a good idea.

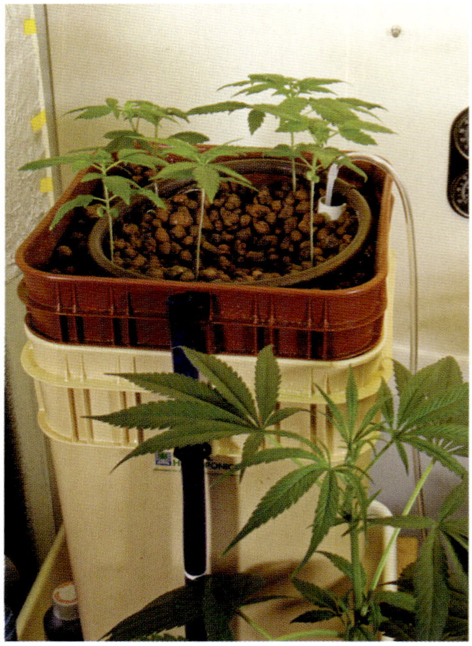

A single stand-alone hydroponic system might just be what a novice or low-key grower is looking for.

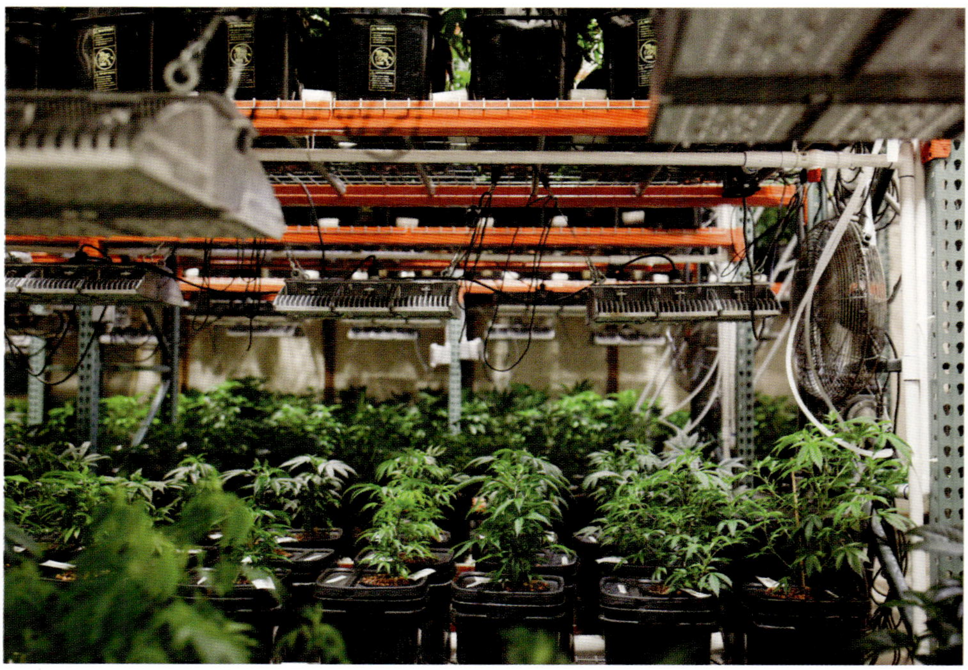

One hydroponic bucket per plant set up.

PHOTOS: ANDRE GROSSMAN (TOP), KRISTEN ANGELO (BOTTOM)

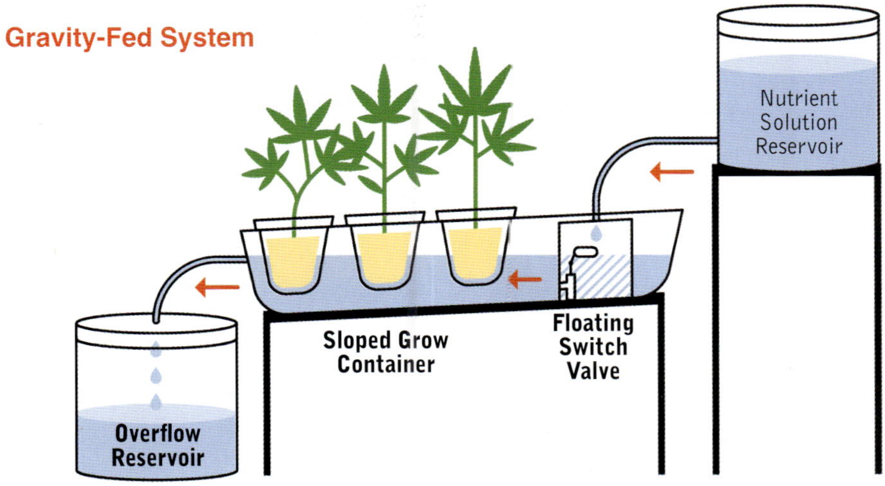

A gravity-fed system is a one-way system manually changed when the overflow is full and the nutrient solution is depleted.

Gravity-Fed

While many of these setups require gravitational forces to create a flow, a gravity-fed system is different from your typical NFT. Gravity-fed systems use a floating switch valve, like the one in a toilet cistern. This system is automated; when the level of the feeding solution decreases, the floating ball drops, causing the valve to release more liquid. In addition to the floating switch valve, there is also the positioning of the units that clues us into it being a gravity system, namely either the grow tray or the reservoir above the other. These will be connected to a pipe that, with a pump, will return gravity-dispensed fluids to the reservoir again.

Instead of pumping, manual systems must physically move the reservoir above the grow tray to dispense fluids. If you find that you are using a system where you empty and refresh your reservoir entirely, you can manually swap reservoirs by disconnecting the empty one and replacing it with a new full one. If you do this, then you can place that new reservoir above the feeding trays to make use of a gravity-fed system. A popular version of a gravity-fed system is a flood and drain system, also known as ebb and flow. These system are some of the most complex to run, but you can learn a lot from it.

Flood and Drain (Ebb and Flow)

Many gravity-fed principles are used in Flood and Drain (or Ebb and Flow) kits. These systems work the same way as NFT systems but have a deeper tray that holds a larger volume of solution and requires less pumping. In some cases, Flood and Drain systems only need to pump nutrients to the plants two or three times a day. Unlike NFT, which has a shallow film of solution running down the tray, Flood and Drain systems require a greater depth to ensure the roots are flooded in the plant tray. This tray is called the flood tray in these setups. Like gravity-fed systems, the flood tray and the reservoir can be connected to a hose that, with a pump, will return gravity-dispensed fluids to the reservoir again.

These systems should have overflow holes due to the potential for spills. The tray bases are generally flat and not curved to ensure nutrients reach all the plant roots. A curved tray system is not ideal because it may result in some roots needing more nutrients, as there is less solution available in the curve towards the base. The area at this base receives the lowest volume of fluids. You can imagine it as just a trickle running down a thin line. In addition, gravity forces roots downwards, even in a horizontal position, compressing them, which can produce a denser root mass than what is on top. The result is that the densest area of roots receives the least solution at the base of the curve. A flat tray without curves helps to find the solution to root mass distribution in the face of these gravitational forces, which you can't compete against. You are going with the flow, literally.

The timing of Flood and Drain systems must be adjusted according to the growth stage. For example, during photosynthesis, the plant will be more actively taking up solution than during dark periods. That means that in a 24/0 photoperiod you will need more solution than in a 12/12 photoperiod; the flowering stage usually gets one flood less than the vegetative stage. If possible, avoid flooding during the dark period; try to time your flood during the light part of the 12/12 cycle. Flood and Drain timing is based on exposing the roots to air but not letting them dry out.

Ebb and Flow System

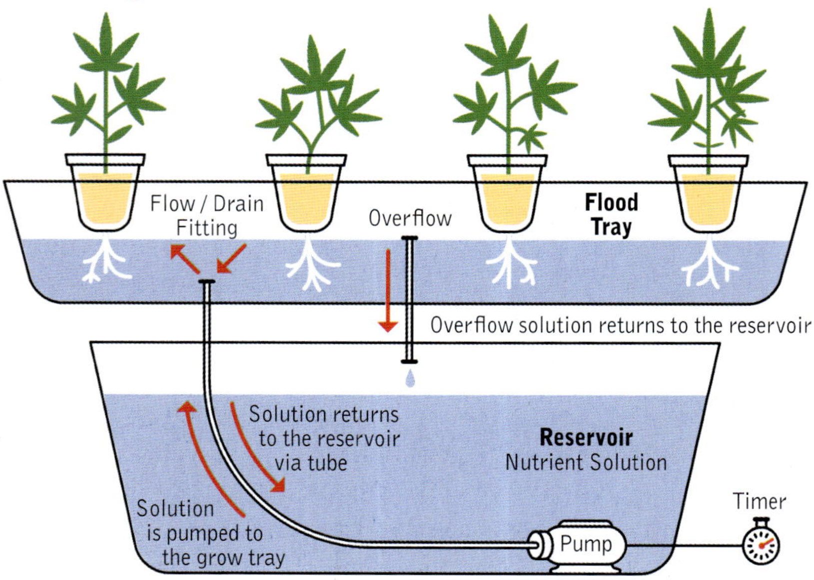

Notice that there is a two-way system with the flow/drain tube. It almost works like a tide.

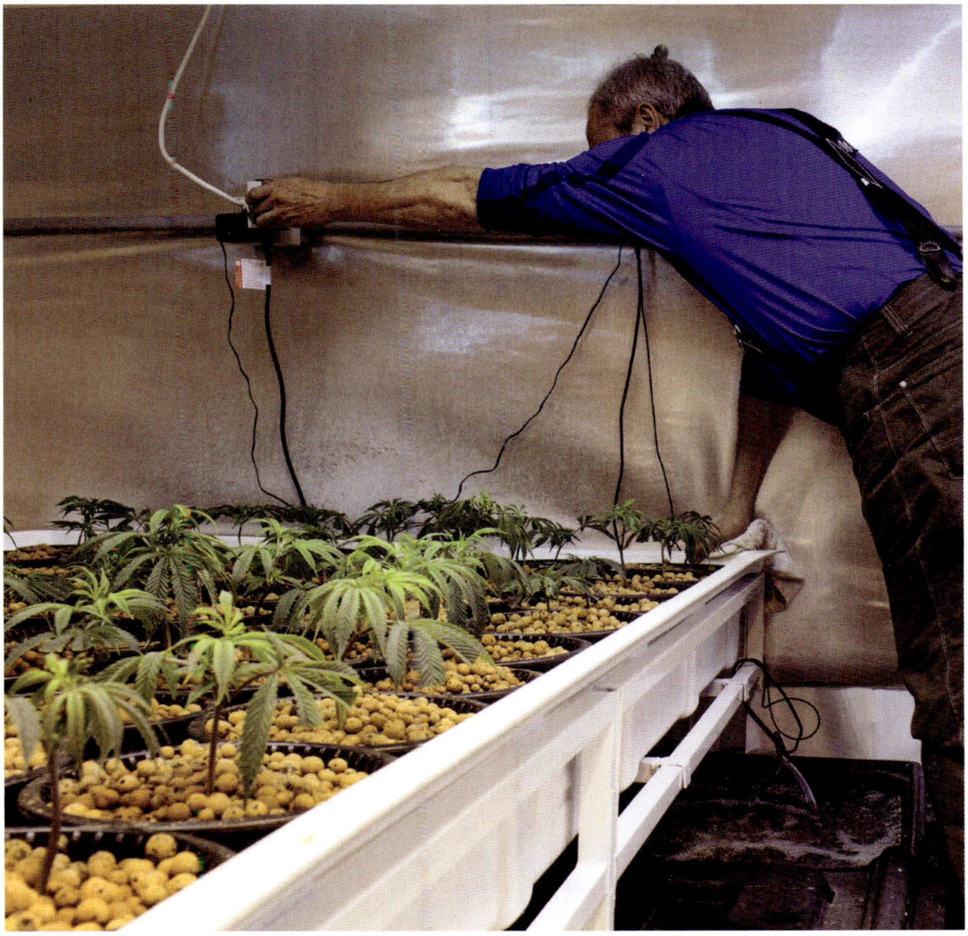

Releasing used nutrients back into the reservoir on the ground.

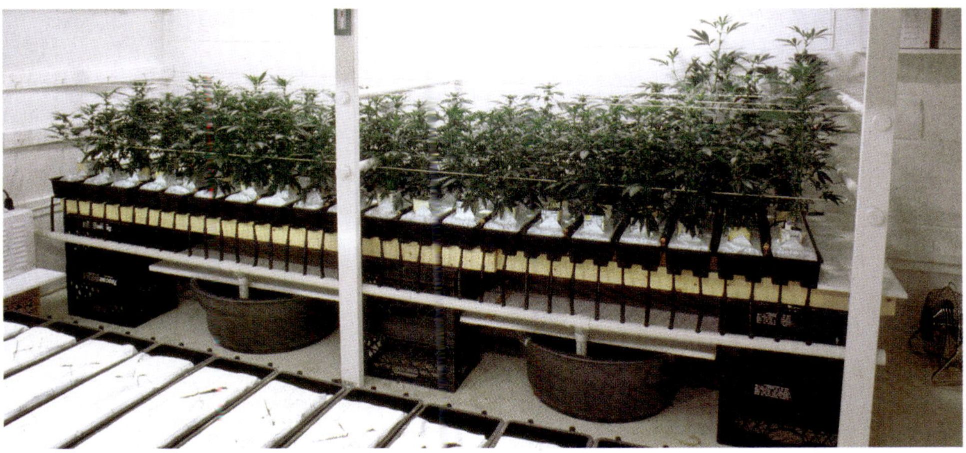

This is an advanced Ebb and Flow system. There is plenty of space to manage water recirculation, and like the best systems, it is well organized and free of clutter.

PHOTOS: KRISTEN ANGELO (TOP), ANDRE GROSSMAN (BOTTOM)

Ebb and Flow System

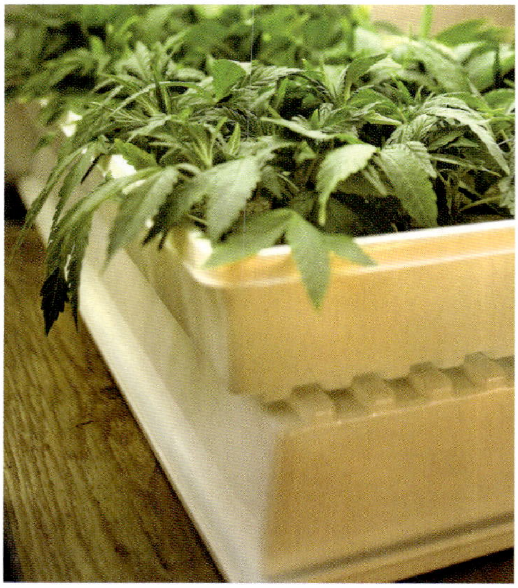

Cleanliness is important at these early stages to prevent any disease-producing agents (pathogens) from infecting cuttings. Keeping them healthy is half the battle.

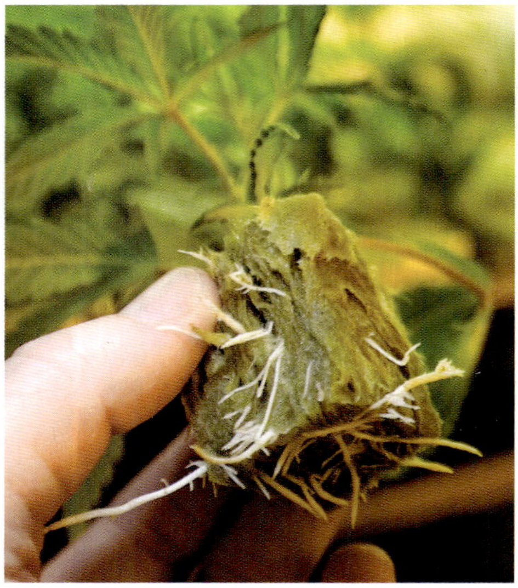

Healthy cuttings in Rockwool show their vigor, as the roots are abundant and tightly packed with very few going out for a longer reach than others.

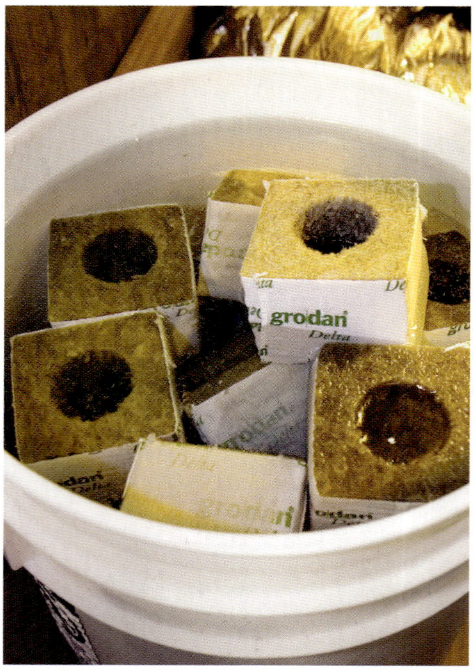

Propagation products like these Rockwool blocks with hollow cores are reliable aids to successful cloning techniques.

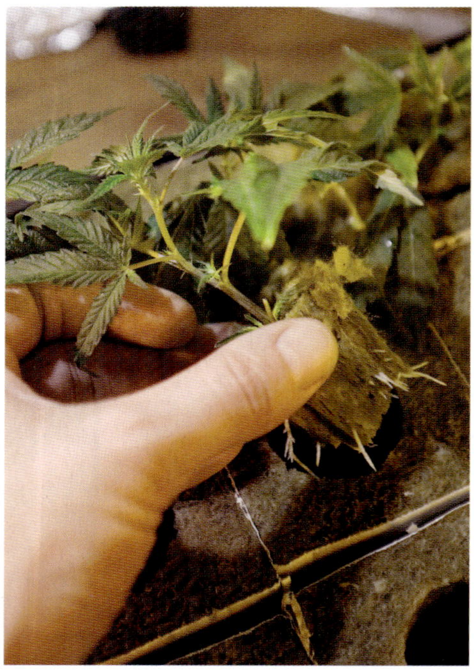

The mini version of the Rockwool block can be inserted into the hollow blocks sometimes called delta blocks.

PHOTOS: JEFF GOLDBERG

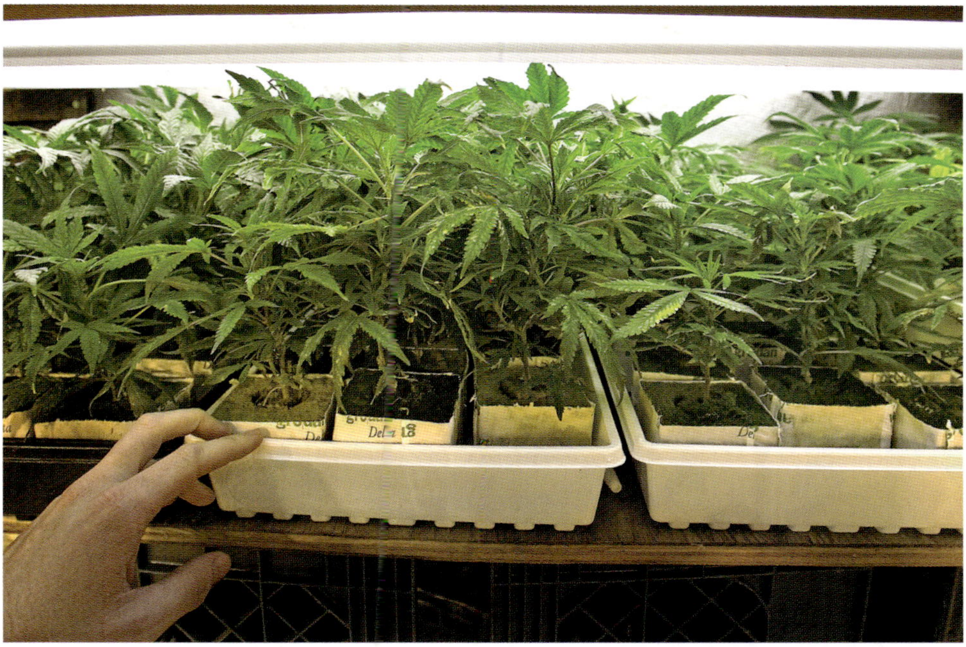

A very important part of cutting propagation is to keep them from stretching and creating long internode length. Less crowding and low-hanging lights help deter this.

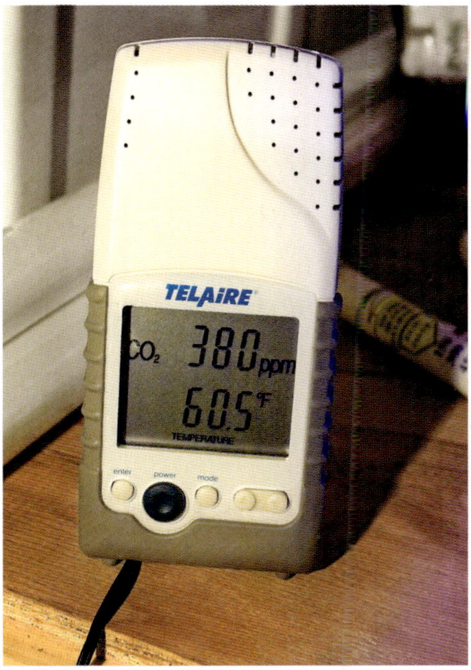

Digital measuring devices offer a higher degree of accuracy when maintaining control of nutrients, CO_2, humidity, and temperature.

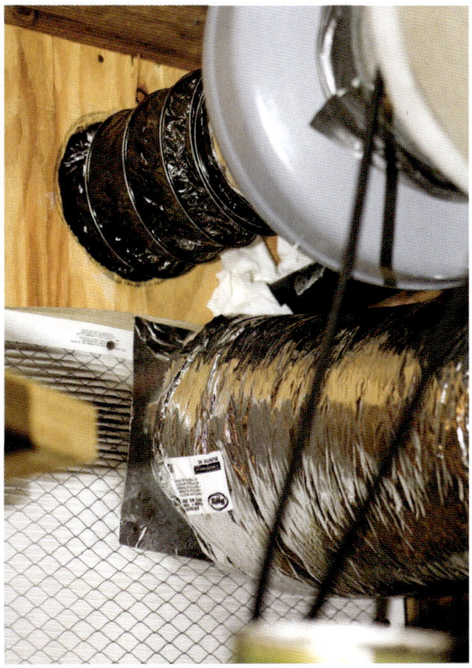

Here the vent outtakes are well sealed to prevent light and smell leakage. The tight fit helps to keep airflow under your control. *continues...*

Ebb and Flow System *continued*

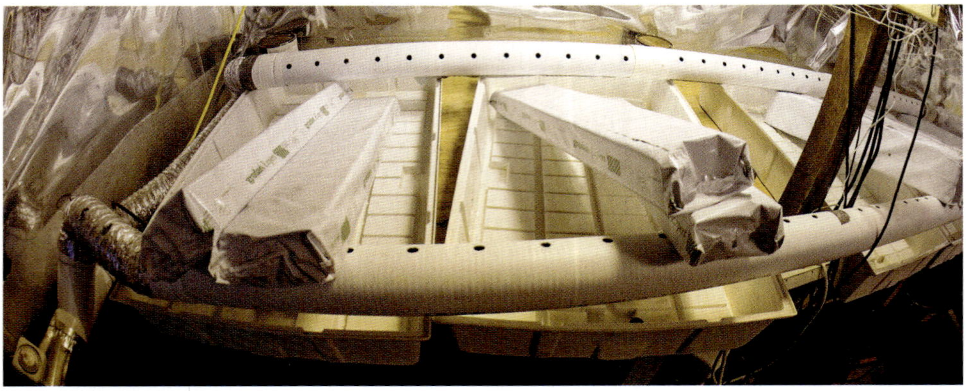

If you have trouble visualizing any hydroponic design then visit YouTube. All hydroponics are somewhat similar but vary in design.

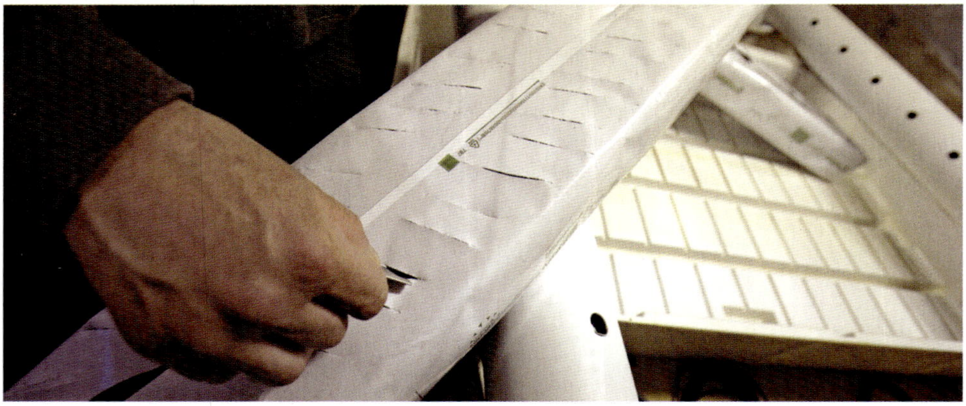

Here the substrate is being prepared. In the background the trays are waiting for a nutrient solution to be added.

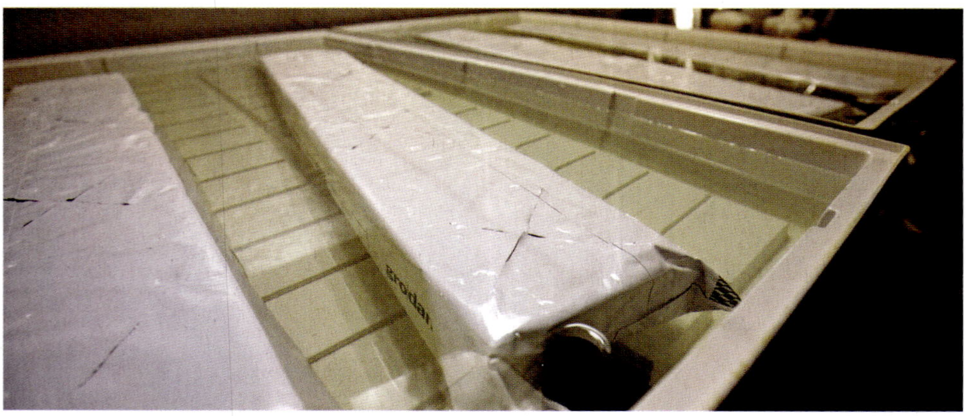

The substrate is placed in the nutrient solution in the tray. Notice how they might float? Adding plants will weigh them down.

PHOTOS: JEFF GOLDBERG

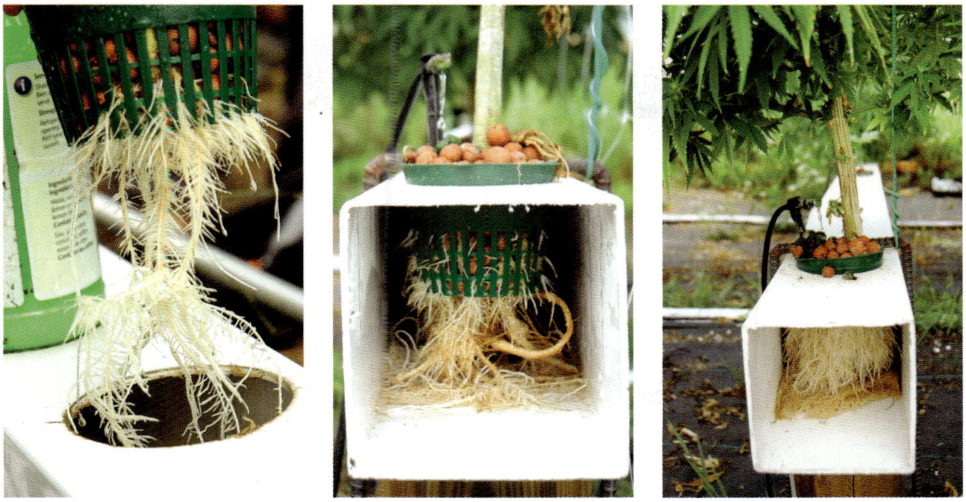

Aeroponics works based on intermittent misting of a nutrient solution against the plant's roots inside a chamber.

Drip Irrigation System

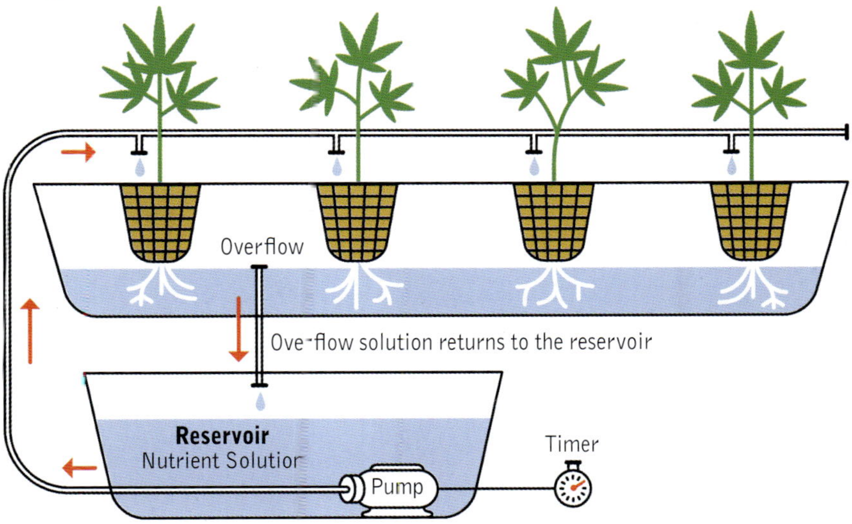

The trickle-down effect from the top makes the drip irrigation system work.

pumps the solution through a central line that splits into lateral lines. Sand filters are standard for drip irrigation. Some pressure valves and backwash controllers may be needed for the system to work correctly.

The key to a drip irrigation system is to keep the solution local, around the plant. Plant spacing is crucial. The feed points along the lines need to be kept close to each plant. In most soil and hydroponic systems, the solution can move around the plants

PHOTOS: STONED ROSIE

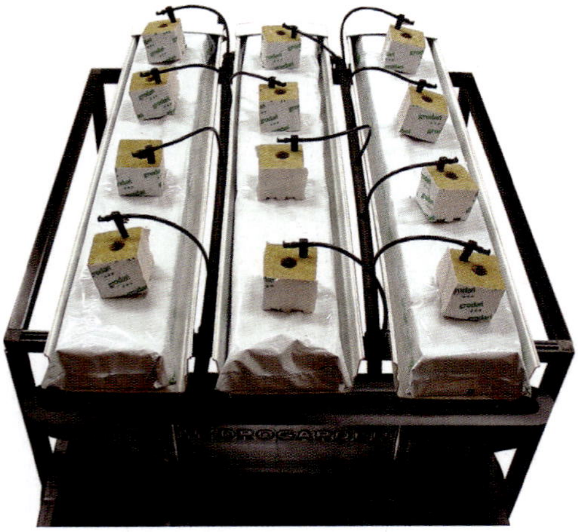

While setting up may take a while, maintenance is minimal afterward.

and in places where no roots have grown. Drip irrigation puts the solution where the roots will access it right away, which conserves nutrients and water.

Drip irrigation resembles a sprinkler watering system, but without a sprinkler and with less pressure. The fluid emitters are either holes in a hose, nozzles, or top droppers next to each plant. Top feeding is the most obvious identifier of a drip irrigation system. The more complex a drip system, the more it is like an emitter rather than just a pipe dripping at regular intervals.

Hydroponic growers have adapted drip irrigation to hydroponic systems with great success. You can use it with any hydroponic medium, from clay pellets to Rockwool. It may seem like drip irrigation is overly complex for our needs, but the system is invaluable because it can help with water conservation, which can be legally enforced in many places due to draughts likely brought on by climate change. Hydroponics users transition to various drip irrigation systems for these environmental reasons.

Due to the wide variation of drip irrigation models, it offers a quick fix to potential problems. Adding a dripper to a system can help it in myriad ways, including dripping secondary nutrients that the plant has been missing.

Aeroponics

Aeroponics is a branch of hydroponics that has steadily developed into a field of its own. It is a form of spray irrigation with an internal misting system. These systems are generally expensive and thus are used mostly by professional growers. Aeroponic systems use spray nozzles within deeper containers, such as buckets, pots, basins, or deep trays. The plants are grown in net pots. A grid with adjustable nozzles is placed into the container and the nozzles are pointed toward the root mass of each plant to mist with the solution at regular intervals. The nutrients are pumped from the reservoir to the nozzles. The spray from the nozzle is generally fast and powerful, hitting the roots with enough pressure to make them move slightly. The spray sends enough particulates for roots to become enveloped in a film. The remaining solution that drips from the plant roots is retained for reuse.

The depth of aeroponic systems allows for more root dangling and, by keeping a static solution away from the roots, encourages liquids to drip down into the nutrient-gathering chamber. The container inside will be damp and misty, with droplets dripping

PHOTO: HYDROFARM.COM

Aeroponic System

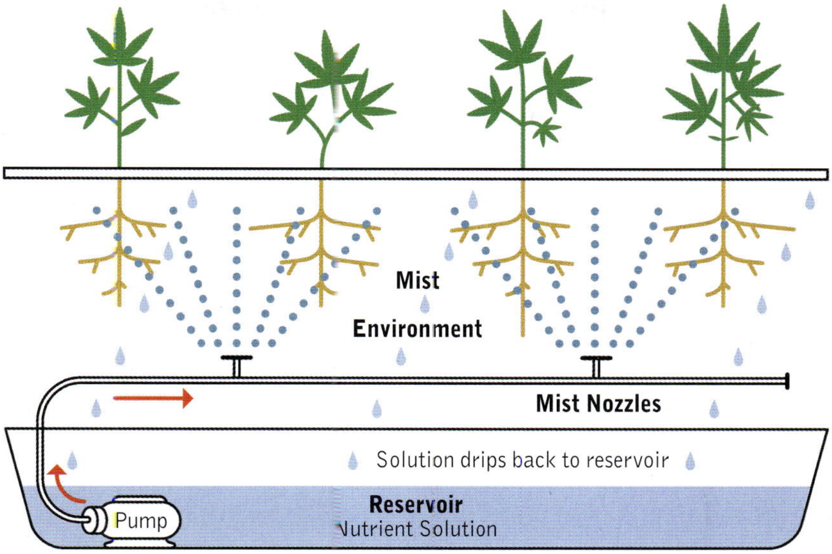

The solution in aeroponics is to only ever touch the roots with a mist, never with a running liquid.

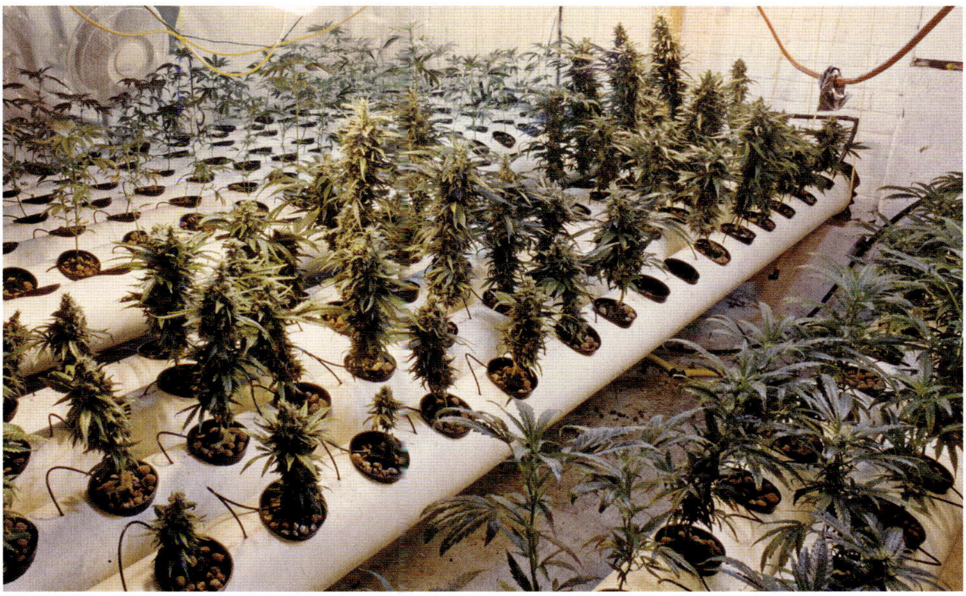

NASA brings us one of the most important revolutions in hydroponics-type cultivation. This is called aeroponics and many hydro growers are turning to it for better results.

PHOTO: ANDRE GROSSMAN

down the sides and from the roots after each automated spray. Because of this, a small amount of solution will gather at the bottom of the container. An air stone may be required to keep this water aerated. The roots will absorb this leftover solution when they reach the bottom of the tank. This absorption helps the plant get extra nutrients.

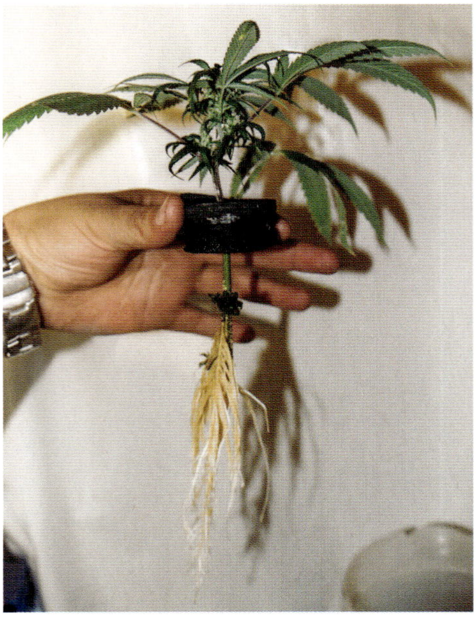

A typical-sized root mass for an aeroponics clone. Roots grow fast in aeroponics.

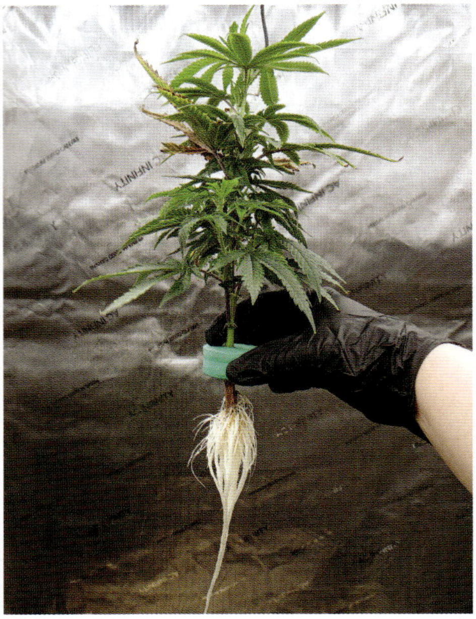

This clone will explode with root growth in aeroponics in the coming weeks.

Overcoming problems in aeroponics is easy, as you can supplement with another delivery system, such as watering and feeding the roots manually or running the trays as NFT. Create a plan to deal with supplement issues should they arise. As roots grow and the mats thicken, the nozzle arrangement may have to be adjusted. While this adjustable spray system offers easy fine-tuning, it is also why aeroponics is more complex to set up.

Hydroponics and aeroponics can be combined to offer better chances of success for first-time aeroponic growers. A suboptimal hydroponic system will usually still produce a bounty of buds but a suboptimal aeroponic system can fail quickly, producing nothing. Exclusively using aeroponics is a very efficient way to use water and nutrients. It also provides optimal air intake (the "aero" in aeroponics) and optimal amounts of nutrients due to the small, absorbent size of the mist droplets.

It's Your Hydroponics

In the end, most of these systems use hoses and pipes for fluid and air control across a plant root network, powered by pumps and synchronized with a timer. Reservoir containers sometimes hold the solution, and the growing unit is either a tray, basin, or bucket that gets flooded with fluids bubbled with air stones for aeration. Precision root misting systems are known as aeroponics. These systems vary within each model group. Many are DIY customized and hybridized. Hydroponics is advanced but can also be fun. Once you learn the principles of NFT and DWC, everything else opens up to you quickly, and the possibilities of hydroponics become endless.

PHOTOS: PETER ALVA (LEFT), @TREETRUNK422 (RIGHT)

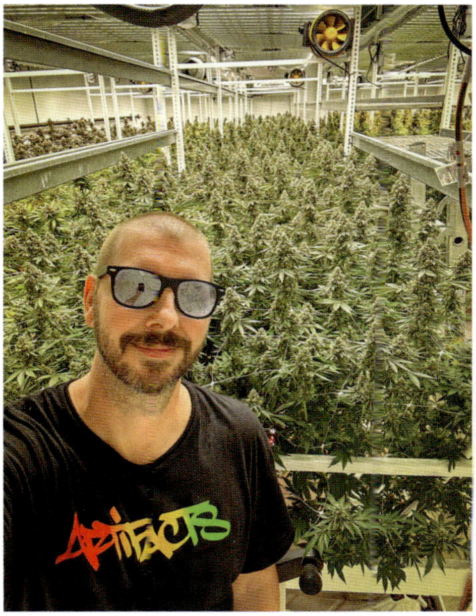

A symphony of green bloom stretches almost as far as the eye can see with this harvest.

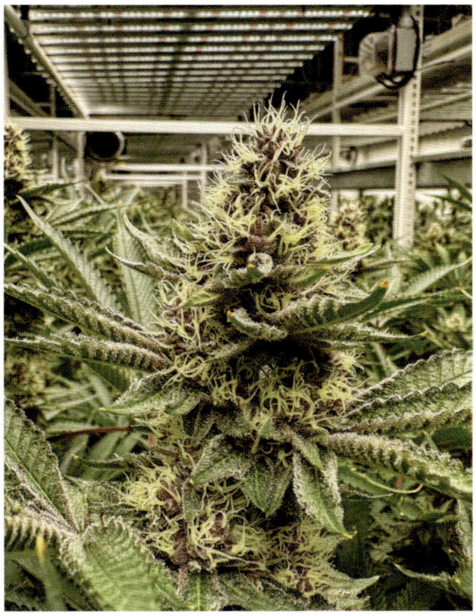

You can almost smell the overpowering sweetness of cannabis in this beautiful photo.

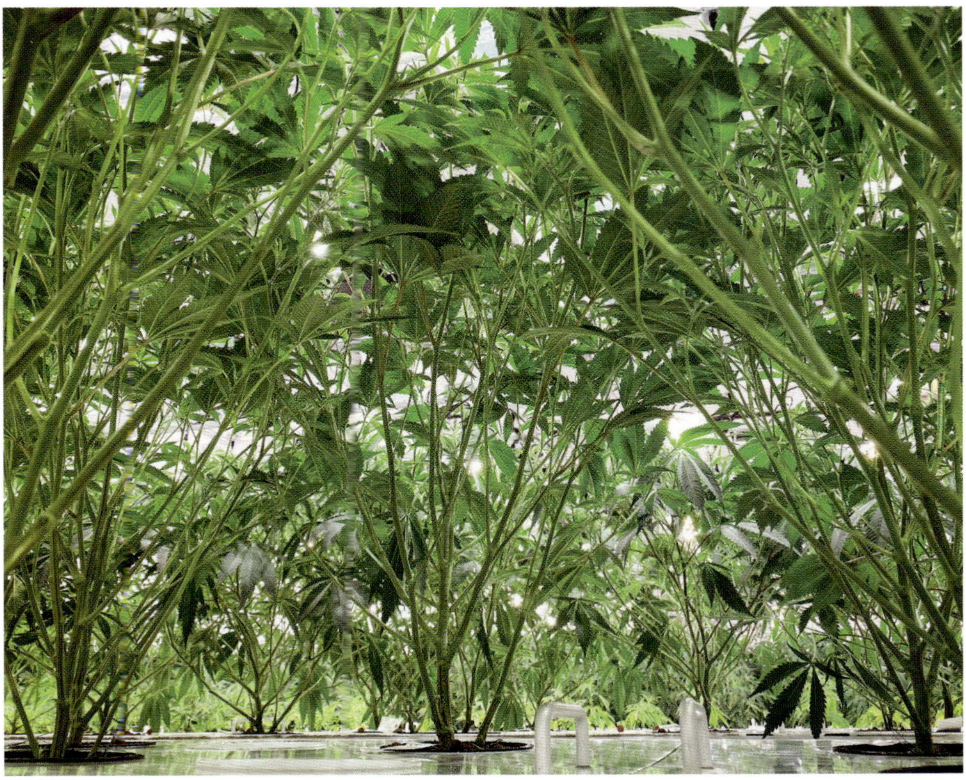

Growing hydroponics is so neat that you don't need to defoliate the lower branches and leaves.

PHOTOS: HIP2THECROP

Building a Hydroponics Grow Room
by Preston Bjornson

My growing career started in a test facility that I built for an 23,000-square-foot licensed producer (LP) our family had dreams of operating. Things went south, and our LP facility never got to operational phase—but I learned a lot during the build and running the little test facility. Let me share some of those learnings with you.

After purchasing a house, I was able to start up my own little grow operation. The grow room I have right now is a mini version of what our LP facility was going to look like. I was originally running one large tent and two small tents in this room. Growing in a tent comes with a set of difficulties when it comes to environmental control and height restrictions. I decided to put my plumbing, HVAC and carpentry skills to work and build my own sealed room to combat environmental fluctuations, so that I could fully express the plants that I was growing with total control of my environment. I had a lot of fun designing the layout of my hydroponic system, including lighting, dehumidification, and CO_2 supplementation, adding an artistic touch to the room to make it very eye-catching and pleasing to work in. The first step for me was the layout plan, equipment placement and power ratings. Once I had my rough blueprint I hired an electrician to come in and check out my panel. I had enough space to run everything I wanted and I gave him the go ahead to run dedicated lines to power the grow, with plugins in specific spots for a clean look. This whole build took me approximately three weeks, working full time to complete it.

I decided to run a hydroponic system due to my professional background as a plumber. As soon as I saw the Under Current RDWC Hydroponic System from Current Culture H2O, I was immediately hooked. The design is simple, efficient, and very pleasing to the eye; I just had to have it! We ordered a large system for our test facility and I ran it very successfully. When I went off on my own, I decided to DIY the system using

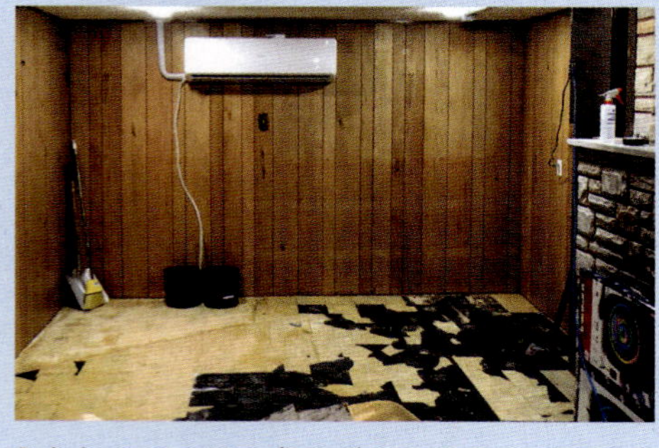

It is important to clean the grow room, or you will run the risk of having mold issues and pests.

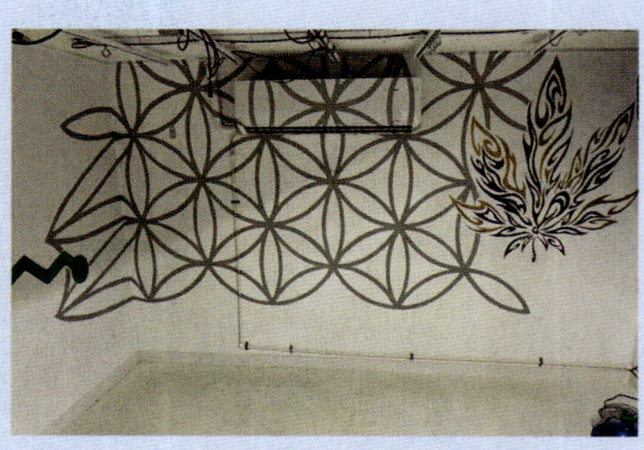

The same room, renovated and cleaned, will produce far better results.

PHOTOS: PRESTON BJORNSON

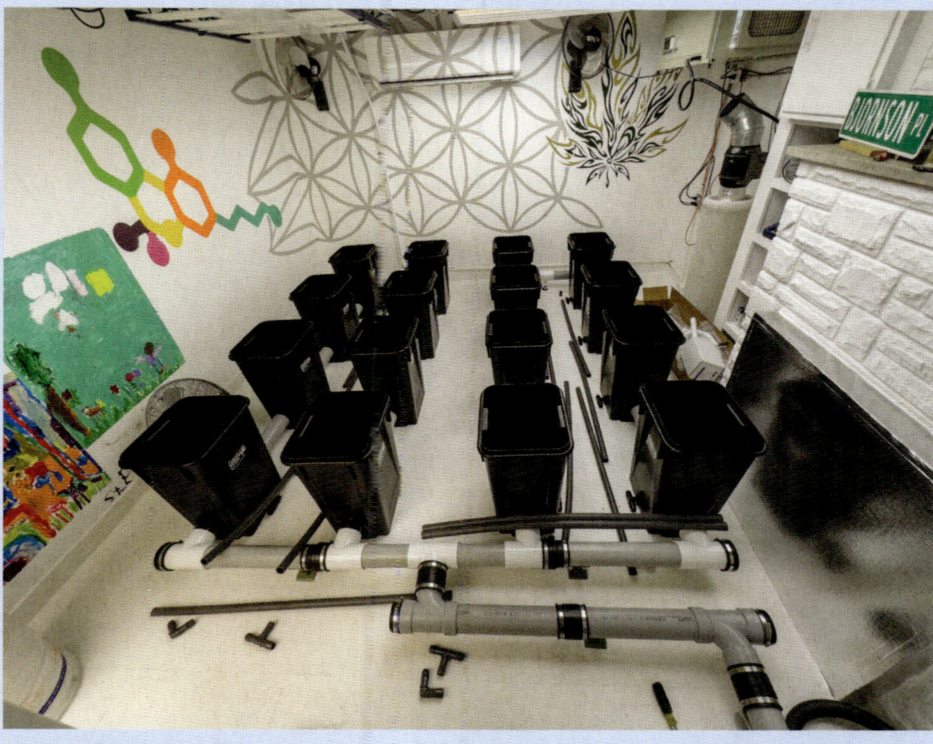

Halfway through installing a 4x4 bay DWC system. Wrapping and hosing are connected next.

13-gallon EZ Store buckets to save money. It was approximately half the cost but took lots of time to source all the parts and build it. It was very rewarding but time consuming. I ran the DIY system for several years before it started showing its age. Several buckets had cracks in the bottom and I just could not salvage the system. It was a losing battle. Every time I fixed a bucket or replaced it, I found another leak. Ultimately, I had to take the plunge and after getting a commercial account with Current Culture I made the investment to get a brand new professional system so I could get running.

Another great advantage of an Under Current system is the ability to run very low nutrient strength solution with automation and consistency. I feel that Under Current is the best type of hydroponic growing system on the market. The explosive growth and yields are absolutely phenomenal.

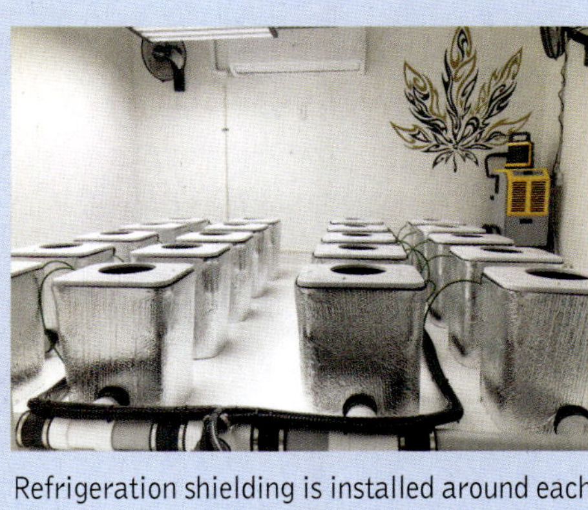

Refrigeration shielding is installed around each DWC bay. Hosing is then connected.

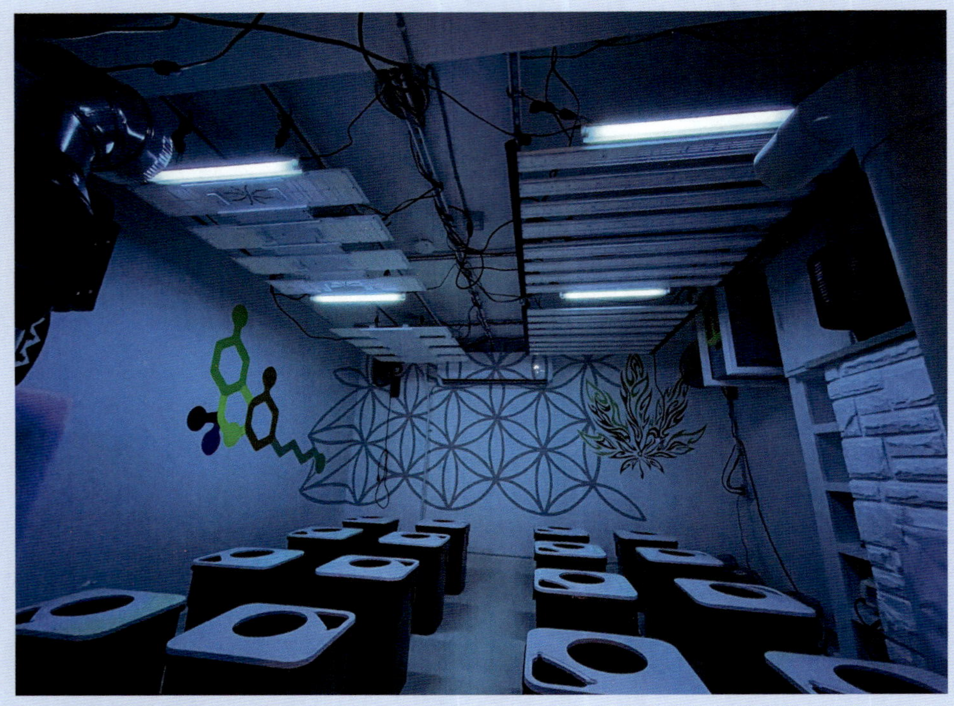

LEDs will more than suffice to grow an abundance of cannabis using hydroponics.

Lighting is probably one of the most important considerations in your garden. I grew with HPS lights for some time before making the switch to LEDs. I built my own LEDs using COB LEDs and was very impressed with the yields I was getting compared to HPS. There was a learning curve involved in the switch, but it was fairly easy to get dialled in using a PAR meter. After having success with DIY lighting, I decided there was a risk factor involved, as these lights were not electrical stamped and approved. For my personal grow I bought high-end LEDs for safety and reliability. I was getting awesome yields from those lights and was fairly happy with the results I was getting. I was contacted by Grand Master Level LEDs to see if I'd be interested in making a switch to their lights. I was reluctant at first as it was a new company. I got on a Zoom call with the owner Thomas Gibson and we completely hit it off. We have a lot in common and his company's origin story really impressed me. I'm all about feelings and I knew right away I wanted to be a part of his team. It was one of the best decisions I made in the garden: I got a pound and a half increase per light compared to the lights I was running previously. His new spectrum tuning lights are changing the game in the growing industry, using top bin diodes. The lights being sleek, easy to clean and waterproof were major selling points for me. Being able to run the Emerson effect was key to bringing out the full expression and efficiency of my plants.

PHOTOS: PRESTON BJORNSON

Over the past four years, I have been able to do several lighting tests. My first test was HPS versus LED. The test came back from the lab and LED won hands down: Higher yields, THC and terpene levels. The second test was implementing UVB in my room. Lab tests came back and UVB did boost THC and terpenes, but only by one percent. For me, that is not enough of an increase to take the risks involved with UVB, especially in a home grow. If you're looking for that edge and getting ahead of your competition in the legal market, UVB might help you get an advantage over your competitors.

When it came to deciding how many plants my room could comfortably hold, I kept changing system layouts to find the perfect amount of plant sites to fit the room without too much crowding. I went from 20 sites to 12, 16, three and finally back to the magic number of 16. This setup seems to absolutely fill the room. There's no wasted space whatsoever and the yields are massive at an average of 3.5 dry lbs per light.

The Control Room is where all the magic happens. Of course, the flower rooms are magical but this control room sets it all into motion. There's a lot going on in here. It's my office, nutrient mixing room, and storage area. It's built with efficiency in mind; cleanliness is something I've always taken very seriously. Due to all the controllers I had lots of wires that needed to be tidied up. I built my own custom gear

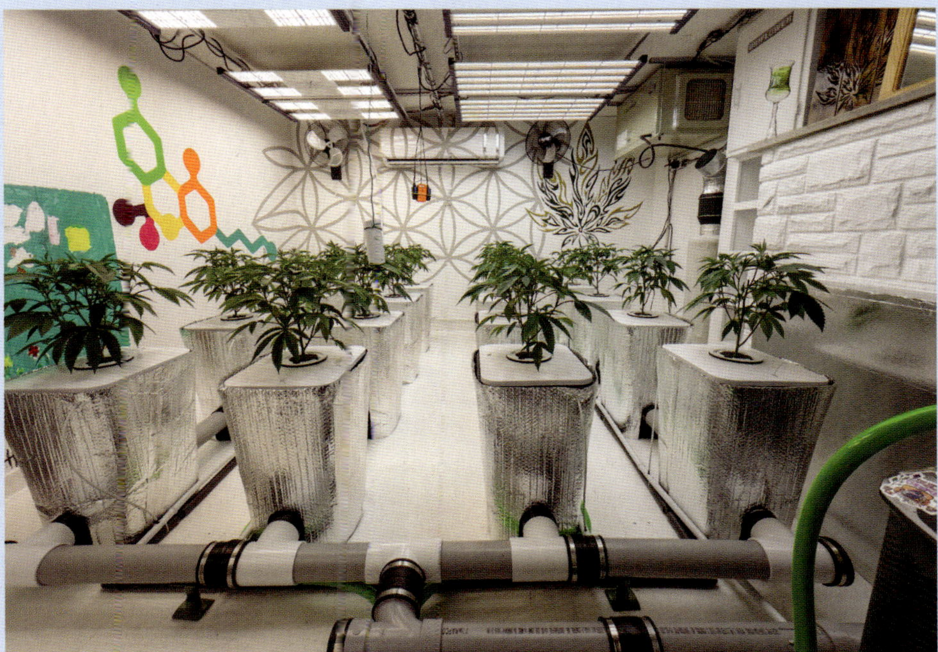

These plants are nature's canvas; indoors, they live and breathe if conditions are optimal. We are expecting a magnificent bloom.

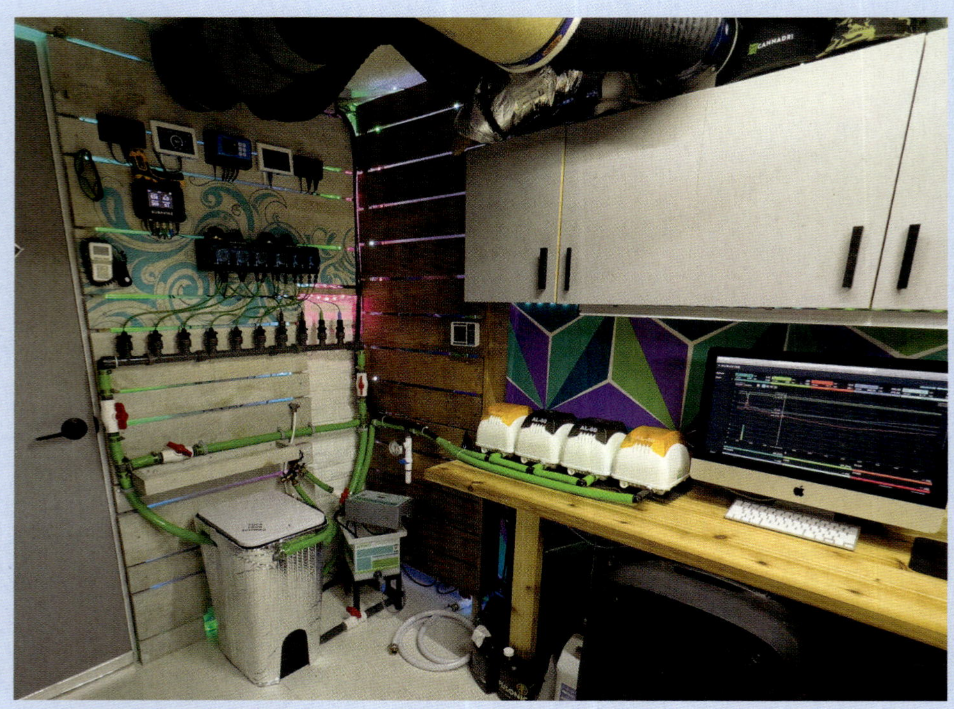

A sophisticated monitoring station for controlling a hydroponic system.

board walls with backlit led strips that allow for hidden wires and a very sharp look. LEDs can change the mood since they are fully customizable; painting some waves to match the hydro theme was also a lot of fun. All the paintings you see in the grow have been done by hand. I've even given one of my daughters, Stella, a blank canvas to paint whatever she desired.

Automation is a huge part of my success and on this front, Nuravine has hit the ball out of the park. Their dosing system is mind blowing and can adapt to any type or style of growing with complete customization. Having a family and a demanding plumbing career takes up a lot of my focus, and the garden gets attention when it's appropriate. It's all about balance; a busy mind is a peaceful mind. Automation is how I've saved my relationships outside of the grow. The labor savings are very noticeable. I could step away for two weeks and the plants would be fine. The only downside is it would be an absolute jungle in there without plant canopy management which is my number one source of labor. The growth is crazy and pruning and de-leafing is absolutely essential. You have to be a bit brutal at times and this is not for the faint hearted. Shaping plants and pruning will come second nature as a necessity with an Under Current system and as bad as it might feel removing some large branches, the plant will reward you for it!

PHOTOS: PRESTON BJORNSON

Mixing dry nutrients into liquid from Cropsalt is also done in this room, with a magnetic stirrer with heat plate. I make concentrated solutions to feed my nutrient doser. I've tried many brands of nutrients and my favorites are Cultured Solutions liquid and Cropsalt powder. They are the purest form, non organic and run super clean!

I have had the great pleasure of working with some great breeders and pheno hunters over the years. I'm all about supporting local! Growers Guild has been supplying me with absolutely amazing genetics for the most part. I've become a grower that showcases breeder cuts. The best of the best. I'm not set up for popping seeds and hunting. There's too much on the line with a system like this. It's gotta be a winner every time. My most recent run of the true Death Bubba from GML, Covert Valley Craft and Lifecycle Botanics has been a challenge with stunning rewards. The next breeder on my radar is Scallywag Seed Co: Paul Martin. He's a great Canadian breeder with an old school library of genetics. He has the ethics to work plants thoroughly, rather than chucking pollen. I admire his approach with breeding and stabilizing genetics.

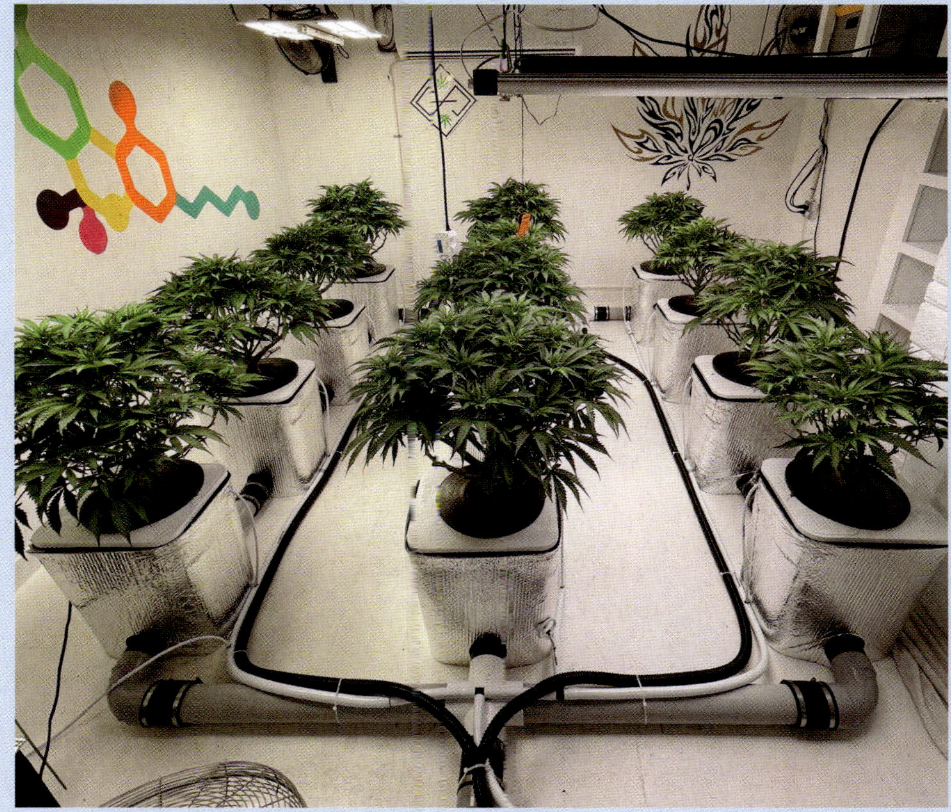

A well-set up hydroponic system will run itself with little maintenance.

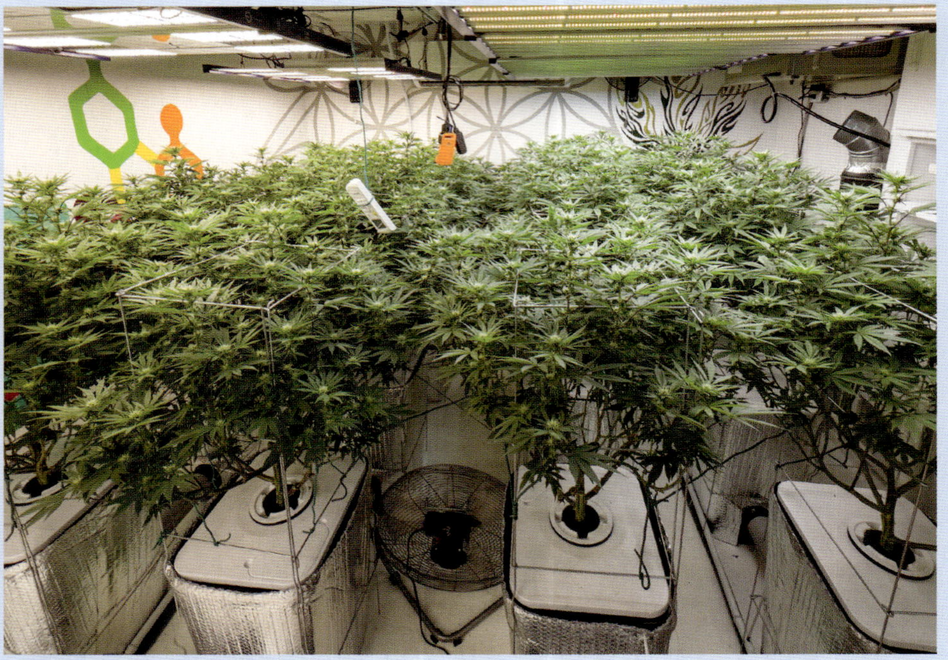

Judging by how pre-flowering has taken off, some serious buds will grow in the later stages of flowering.

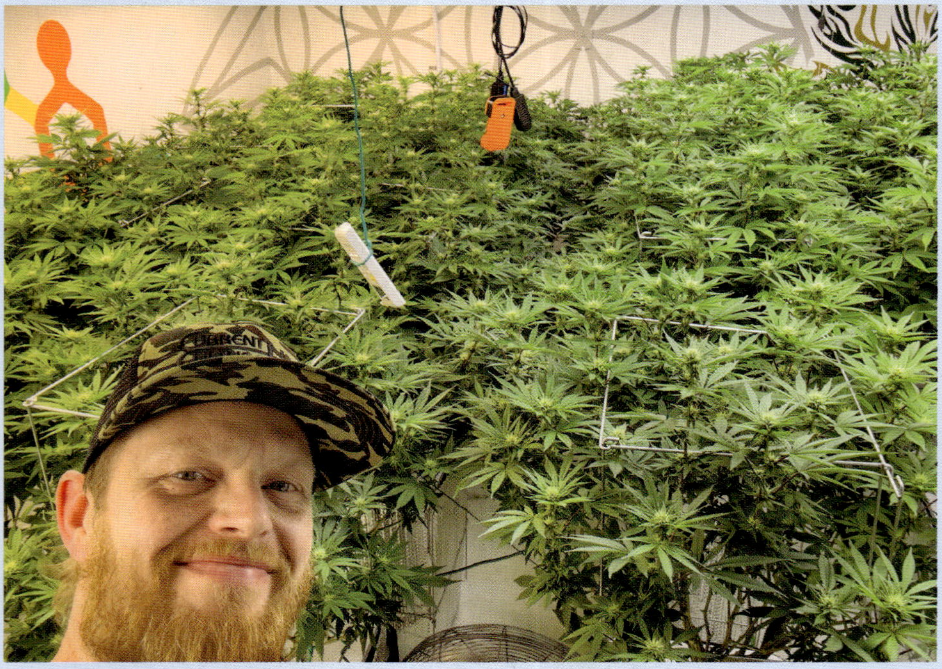

An automated system allows inaccessible areas of the grow to receive everything they need.

HOTOS: PRESTON BJORNSON

Harvest is when most new growers find out the hard way that they are not done, not even close! With my setup, the day I chop the plants is extremely hectic with lots of moving parts. Cages need to be carefully removed first, then I chop the whole plant and temporarily hang them all in the 5x5 room while I dismantle the Under Current system, sweep and sanitize and mop the floor. I set up my DriFlower drying racks and start to remove fan leaves and buck the plant down. I prefer a dry trim over wet: Cutting leaves releases chlorophyll and can greatly affect the taste and smoothness of the end product. Dry trim preserves and allows for a slow, natural release of chlorophyll.

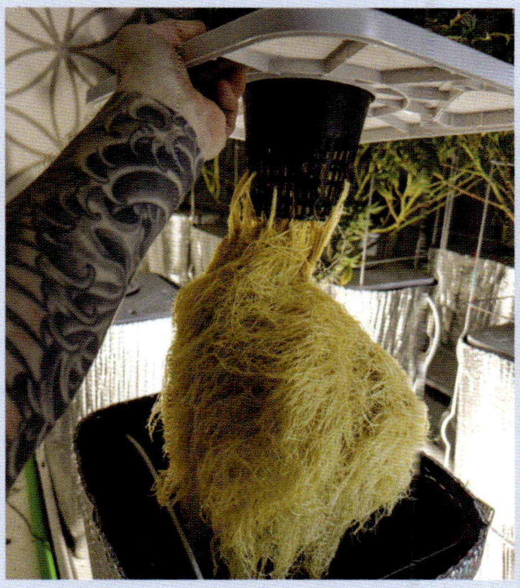

DWC produces an enormous root mass by the end of harvest. Most of it will be submerged.

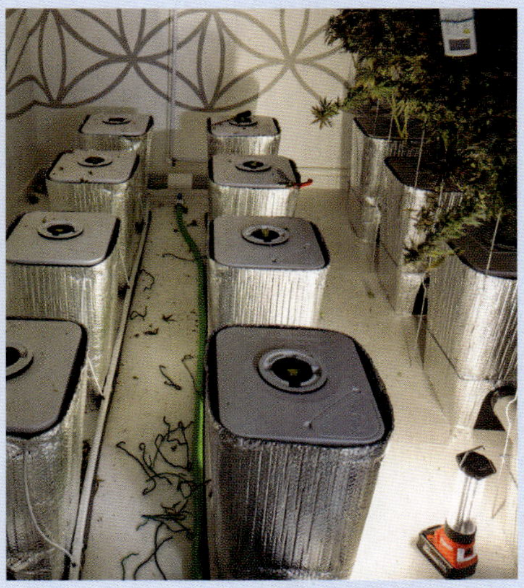

Harvest time means chopping the plants at their base to remove the bounty.

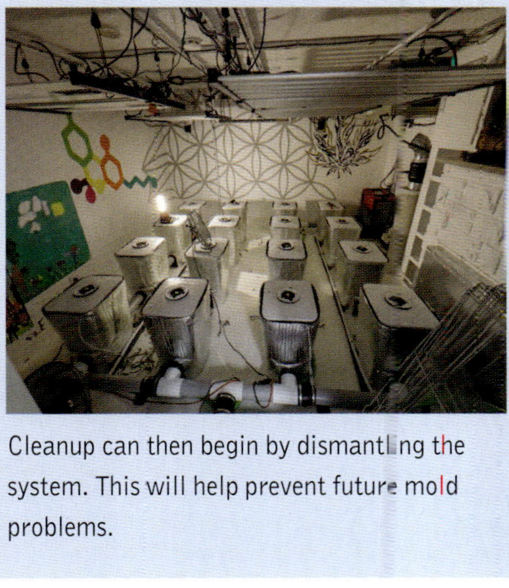

Cleanup can then begin by dismantling the system. This will help prevent future mold problems.

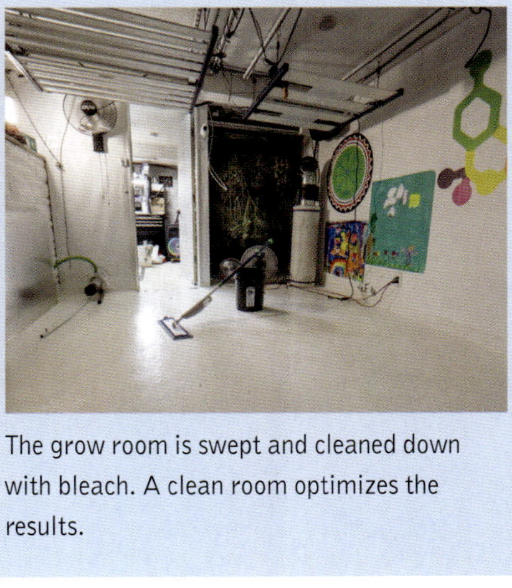

The grow room is swept and cleaned down with bleach. A clean room optimizes the results.

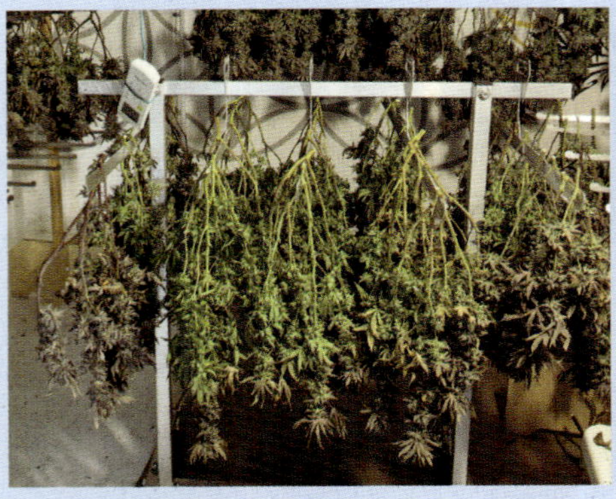

Freshly harvested plants are hung upside down to dry out.

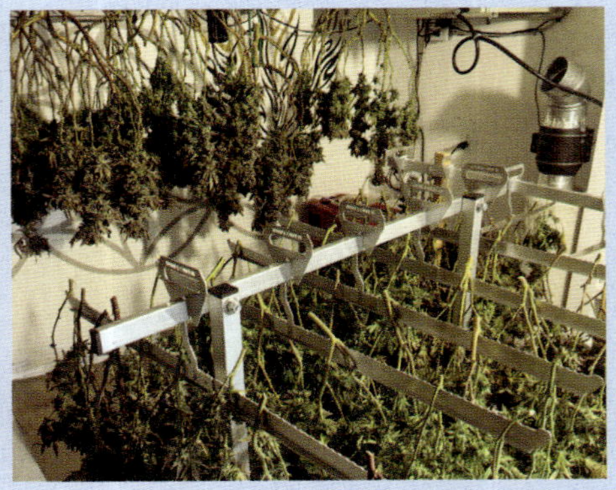

All of these flowering branches contain lots of pieces of bud.

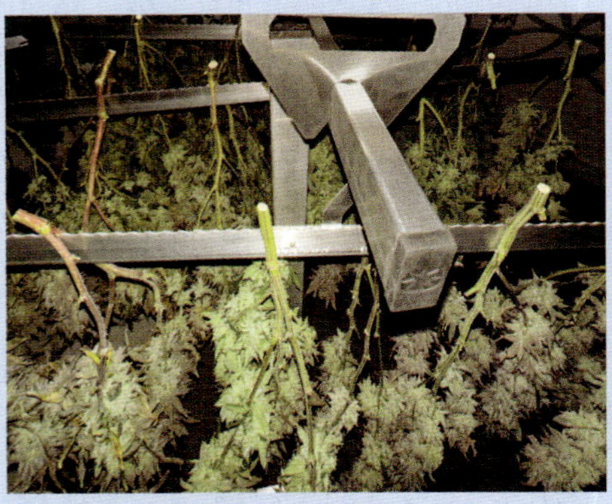

DriFlower is a "get it and go" horticultural drying solution using racks.

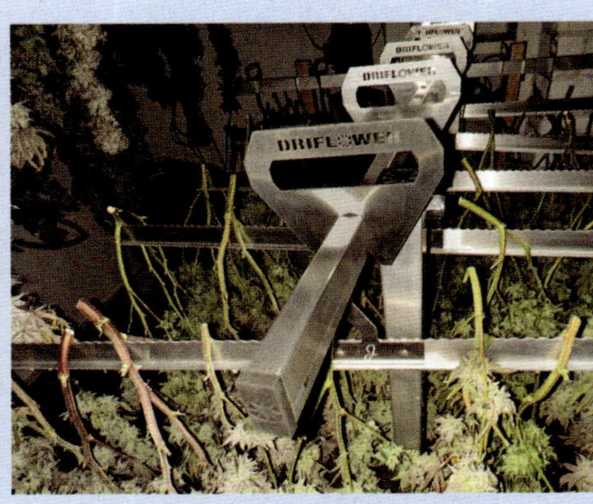

These can support whole plants or cut branches, as is the case here.

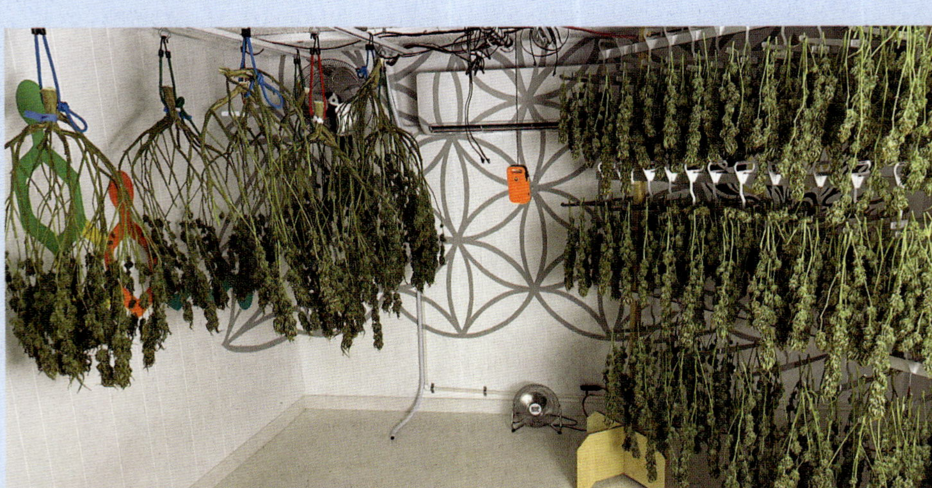

Hangers and brackets make this drying system work.

PHOTOS: PRESTON BJORNSON

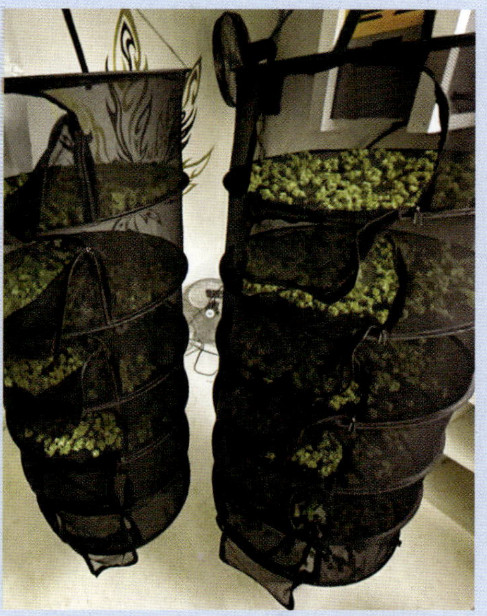

Hanging baskets are used to manage the buds for curing.

Drying and curing is the last and most important step to preserving the taste and smell of the buds you just worked so hard producing over the past few months. Environmental control is key and should not be overlooked. When drying your plants, you need a consistent environment to prevent mold and preserve cannabinoids. My method is low and slow: My dry consists of a 2-3 week period at at 55-57°F (13-14°C) and a swinging relative humidity (RH) of 55-60%. At week two, the small lower buds will be dry and ready. They either get hand trimmed or thrown in the hash bucket. This gives me a week to trim. By week three of the dry I'm on all the big beautiful colas that are a breeze to trim for the most part. After that, all the product it gets cured either in 5-gallon food-grade pails or, as full colas, in turkey bags or large Mason jars. If you haven't tried trimming and curing whole colas on the stick, you gotta try it out! The terpenes are preserved further this way. The cool temperatures are also a key factor of preserving the terpenes. If you dry too quick your buds will have that hay taste and odor and that's no fun at all. Do the best with your budget and add equipment each grow, when you can afford it, to help with environmental control.

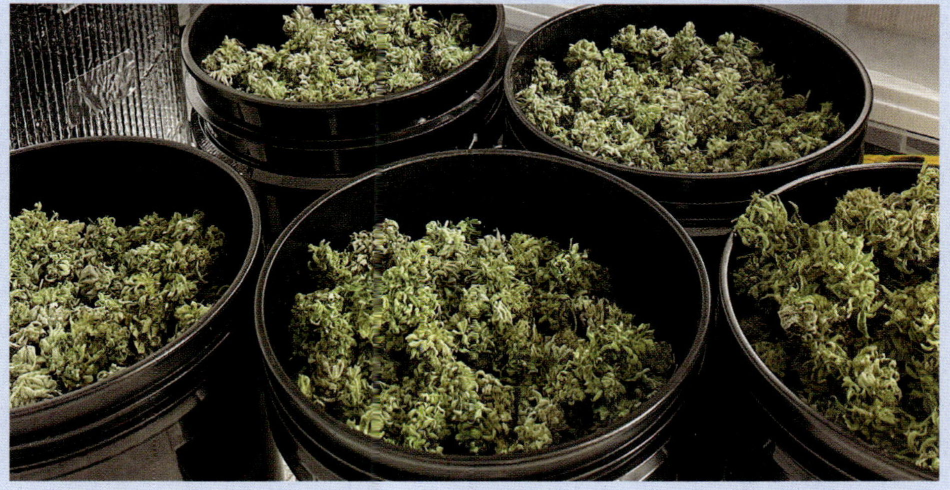

Literally buckets of bud from growing using hydroponics.

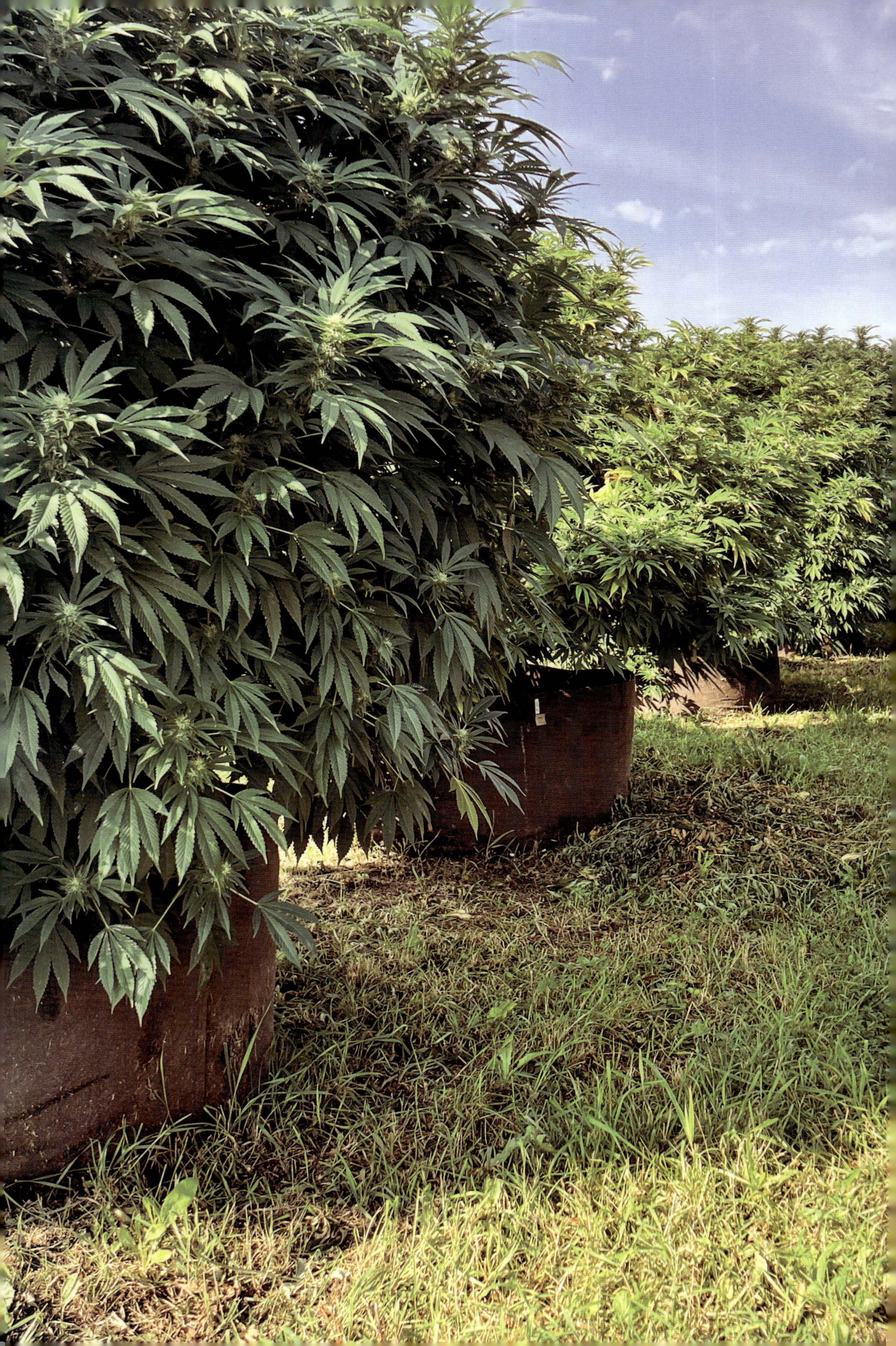

12

Outdoor Growing

Outdoor cannabis cultivation can be highly rewarding, provided you have the right climate and conditions. Outdoor growing is a planned agricultural activity, on selected and prepared land, aimed at producing specific cannabis crops, with the expectation of a yield superior to that of wild cannabis plants growing naturally in the same area. Outdoor growing encompasses grows from small-scale personal gardens to large farming operations. It requires careful management and is similar to indoor growing in terms of tasks and requirements.

Many essential elements for a successful outdoor grow site are covered in the indoor growing chapters of this book, so revisit those chapters, paying close attention to topics such as genetics, germination, soil types, and feeding, as they provide valuable information about your cannabis plants' fundamental needs. The principles of successful cannabis cultivation remain consistent regardless of method. The scope of outdoor cultivation varies significantly, depending on such factors as whether you are transferring indoor plants outdoors. Greenhouse cultivation is also a form of outdoor growing. When outdoor growing occurs on a property without proper authorization, such as on public land, it's often referred to as guerrilla growing.

Some cannabis enthusiasts state that the best cannabis they've ever encountered was grown outdoors. If you reside in a climate where tomatoes thrive, you likely have the ideal environment for outdoor cannabis cultivation. In regions with hot weather and extended summers, it may be possible to cultivate high-yielding sativa varieties like Haze, African, and Skunk hybrids, which, despite their longer flowering periods, can yield over 2 lbs of bud per plant when allowed to reach full maturity outdoors.

Why do some people find that cannabis grown outdoors offers a superior finished product? One possibility is that the natural light spectrum influences cannabinoid content differently than artificial indoor lighting, which can affect the chemical composition of the plant. Outdoor harvests may also exhibit higher levels of terpenes and terpenoids, which can contribute to differences in taste and aroma. Clones grown outdoors often have a darker appearance and a distinct taste. Expressed traits are not solely determined by genetics, but are also influenced by the environment.

PHOTO: ROOTPOUCH.COM

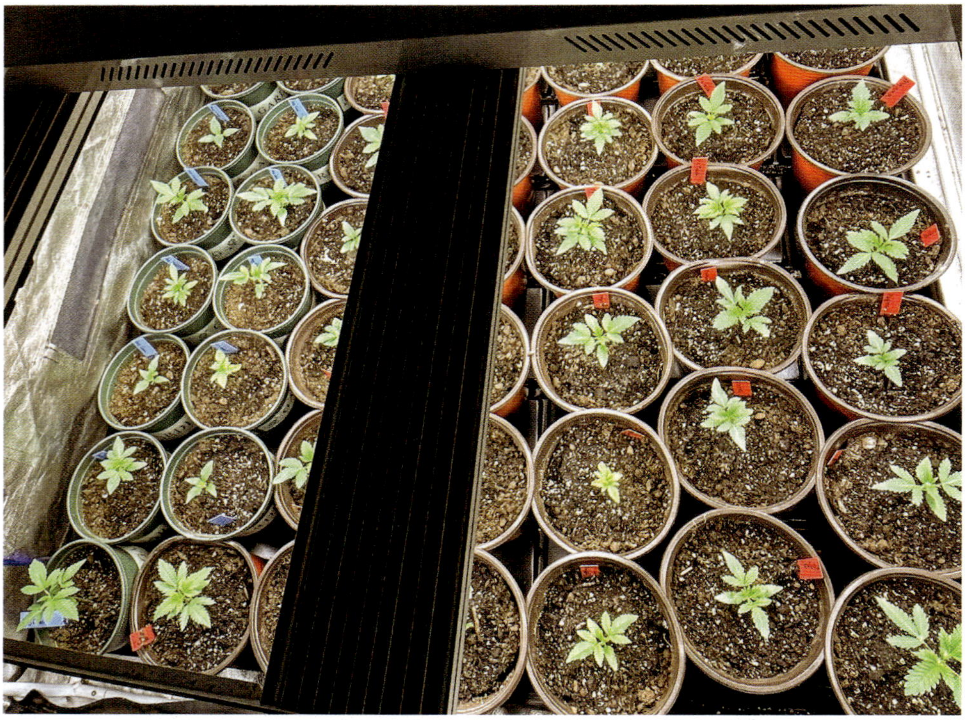

Seedling preparation for outdoor planting. If the environment isn't too harsh, these seedlings should be ready to be at one with Mother Nature.

Transplanting for Successful Outdoor Cultivation

Before you embark on outdoor cannabis growing, you must make the necessary preparations. Planting seeds directly in untreated soil can result in a low germination rate. However, if planting directly in untreated soil is your only option, transplant seedlings instead. Many outdoor cannabis growers initiate their plants indoors first, by germinating and nurturing seedlings in a batch before transitioning them to the outdoor environment. The process of moving a seedling or cutting from indoor to outdoor settings is similar to transferring plants from a clone room to a grow room. For more detailed guidance on transplanting from indoor to outdoor settings, revisit Chapter 4, particularly the section on hardening off cannabis seedlings.

Prepping for outdoor transplanting is not a small undertaking, but it pays off when you find a suitable system. The key to success is perforations in the pot. Some growers cut away the base of plastic pots and use a piece of cardboard held in place with masking tape to secure the bottom. They then transport plants to the outdoor grow patch, remove the cardboard, and plant the entire setup directly into the ground. As the roots grow, they extend downward through the opening at the pot's base. Drilling perforations in plastic containers isn't overly complex, provided you have a drill and a hole saw drill bit. Alternatively, you can use grow bags.

PHOTO: TANYA PETERSEN

Direct air exposure can inhibit root growth. If a root extends out from the side of a soil bank and detects air without moisture, it will slow down and eventually cease growth in that direction in a process known as air pruning. Roots near perforations in containers tend to avoid growing through them when only air is present.[1] When you transplant a container with a perforated base into the ground, the compacted soil prevents direct air exposure, allowing roots to grow through the perforations and into the surrounding soil. It is best to leave the pot in the ground in this situation, as attempting to remove it may tear the roots that have grown into the surrounding soil. Beginner growers may prefer the bottomless pot method, while experienced growers can tip the plant out, much like a transplant, and place it directly in the ground.

Fabric seedling grow bags provide a convenient and biodegradable solution because roots can penetrate the pores in them. Again, direct air exposure prevents excessive growth. When you transplant the grow bag into the ground, the roots will extend into the surrounding soil. With grow bags, instead of planting directly into the ground, you can insert seedling grow bags into larger grow bags or containers. Some bags even have handles, allowing for limited movement of the plant. You may have seen them marketed as non-woven grow bags. Growers can then choose to either regularly manage the grow for optimal results or intervene periodically, allowing nature to take its course. However, consistent management typically produces the best results. This method offers the added advantage of easier cloning of all-female plants for transplantation to the outdoor patch, resulting in an ideal all-female, sinsemilla outdoor crop.

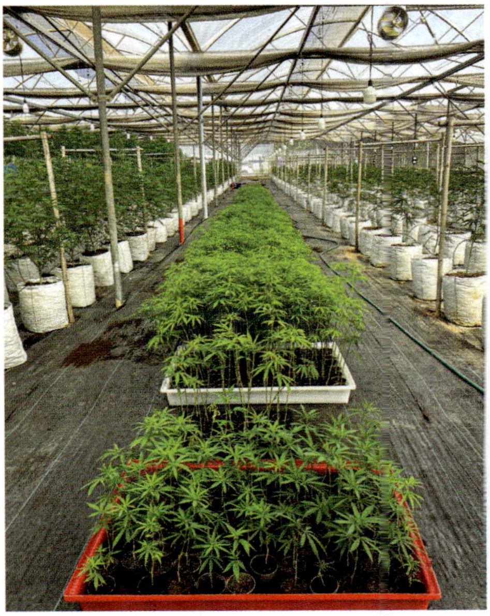

A greenhouse is the middle ground for outdoor strains but with indoor protection.

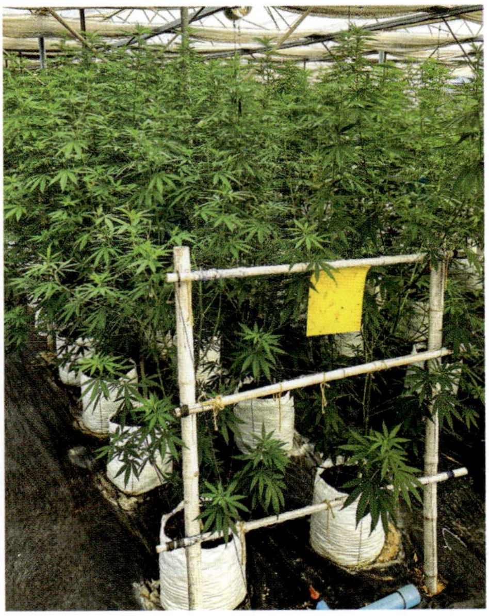

These outdoor sativa plants are too big for indoor cultivation without lots of training and pruning.

PHOTOS: HIP2THECROP

Outdoor Transplanting

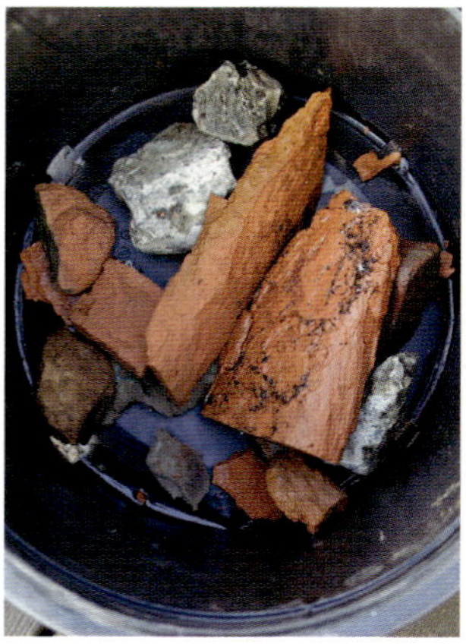

Place rocks on bottom.

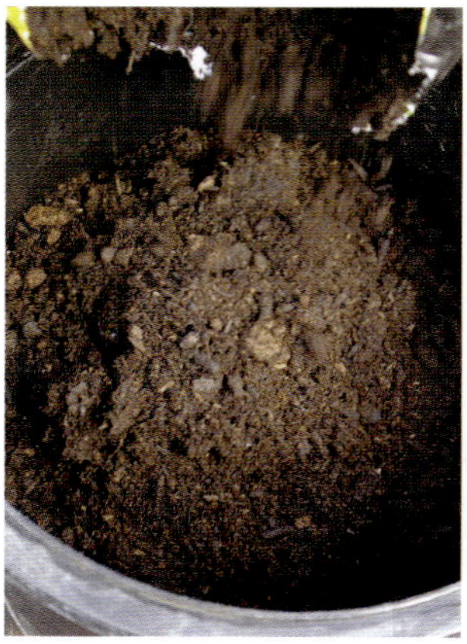

Fill ¾ of pot with soil.

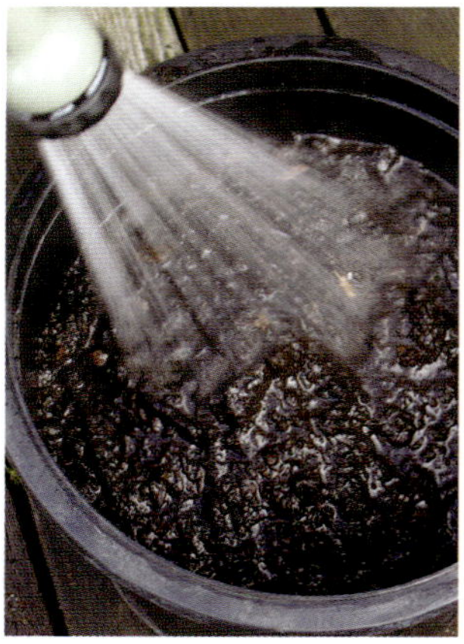

Thoroughly water soil.

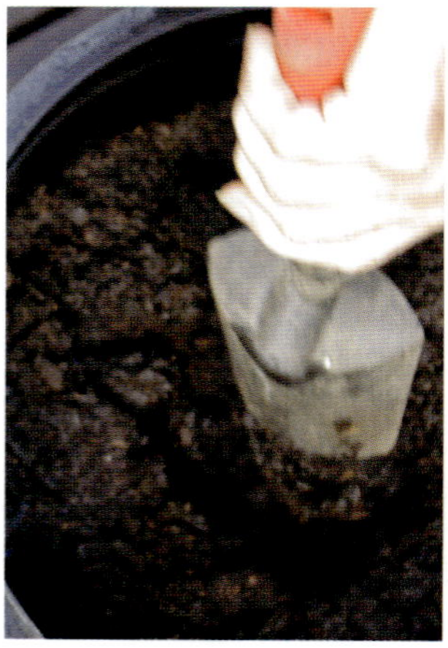

Create a hole for plant.

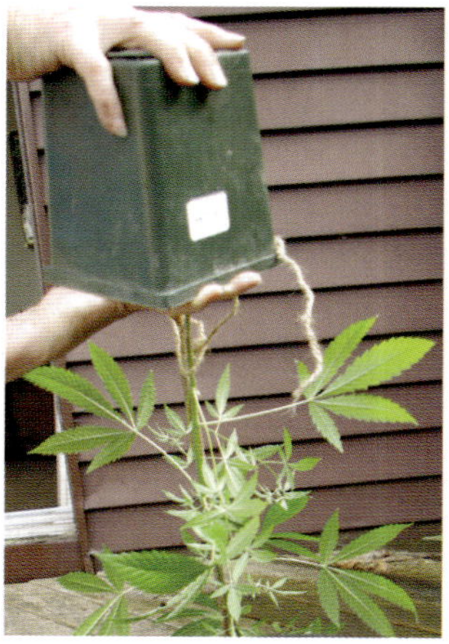

Gently remove plant.

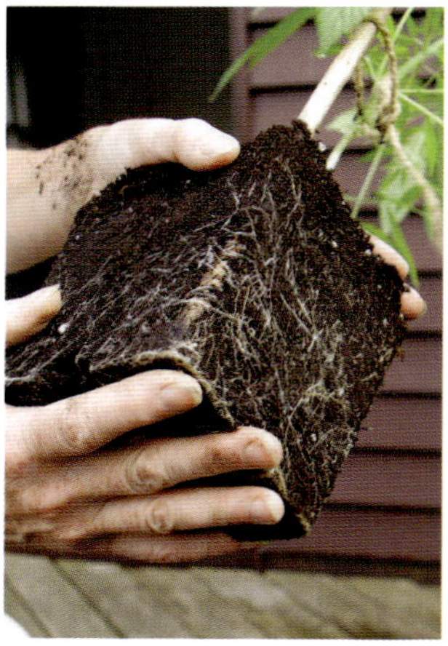

Prod soil to loosen roots.

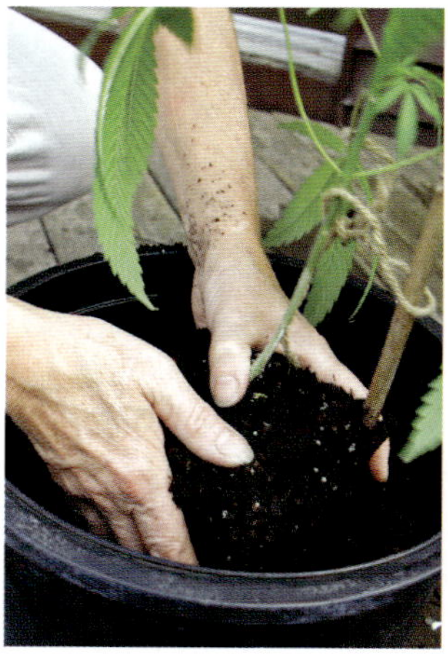

Place plant in new pot.

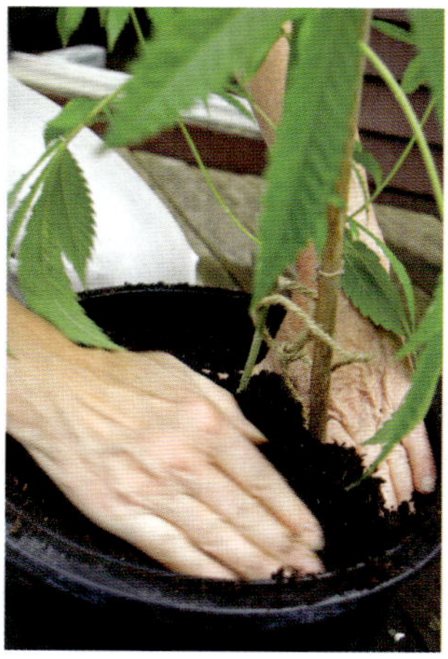

Tamp down to secure plant.

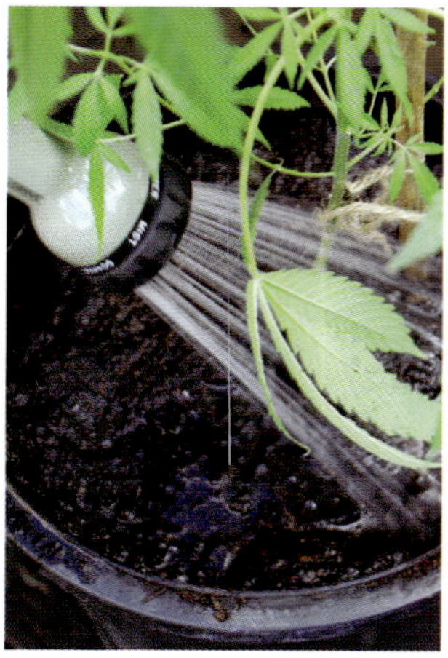

Water regularly.

PHOTOS: GCP

Cannabis Growing Season

In the Northern Hemisphere, the Earth tilts toward the sun around the end of March before tilting away again around the end of September. This period, from March to September, forms the prime window for outdoor cultivation in the Northern Hemisphere. The Southern Hemisphere experiences its growing season from September to March, following the same tilting pattern. For many plants, the growing season is defined by the absence of frosts, spanning from the end of the last frost to the onset of the first frost. In theory, cultivation can occur year-round in frost-free tropical climates. However, because cannabis is photoperiod-responsive, there is an additional layer of complexity. Cannabis cultivators plan their flowering periods around a 12-hour day and night cycle, with vegetative growth ideally completed before daylight decreases to 12 hours.

The Earth's orbit around the sun results in varying lengths of daylight depending on the season. As the Earth orbits, the sun's path across the sky, or its diurnal motion, changes. Regions tilted toward the sun are warmer because they receive more than 12 hours of daylight a day. Growers aim to ensure their plants complete vegetative growth and initiate flowering as daylight hours decrease. Cultivation typically begins during the summer period when more daylight is available.

The ideal time to initiate growing outdoor plants from seeds for the Northern Hemisphere is generally March and April which allows them to mature and commence flowering by August or September, when daylight hours are decreasing. Planning your grow spot and starting your garden by April is generally crucial for optimal results. If you're growing pure indica or an indica hybrid strain, planting in May or June is ideal due to indica's shorter vegetative and flowering periods compared to sativa strains. Growers in the Southern Hemisphere should push these timelines by six months.

Localized strains typically perform predictably due to their history as specific cultivars. Hybridization plays a pivotal role in expanding outdoor growing options and breeding activities. This process often involves crossbreeding pure sativa with indica strains to reduce plant size and flowering time. As a result, while many pure outdoor strains remain localized, breeding efforts have enabled new outdoor strains to adapt to various geographical regions.

Clones should be transplanted just before the flowering season begins, as they require only a week or two of growth before initiating flowering. Autoflowering strains are a valuable option for growers in regions with insufficient darkness to trigger flowering, enabling cannabis cultivation to occur in regions where it was previously impractical. Autoflowering plants should be should be planted at the start of the summer for flowering when your location has the most sunlight. You can plant as late as you want, but you must avoid frost before the end of flowering. Optimization is discovered by experimenting with your location and autoflowering strains.

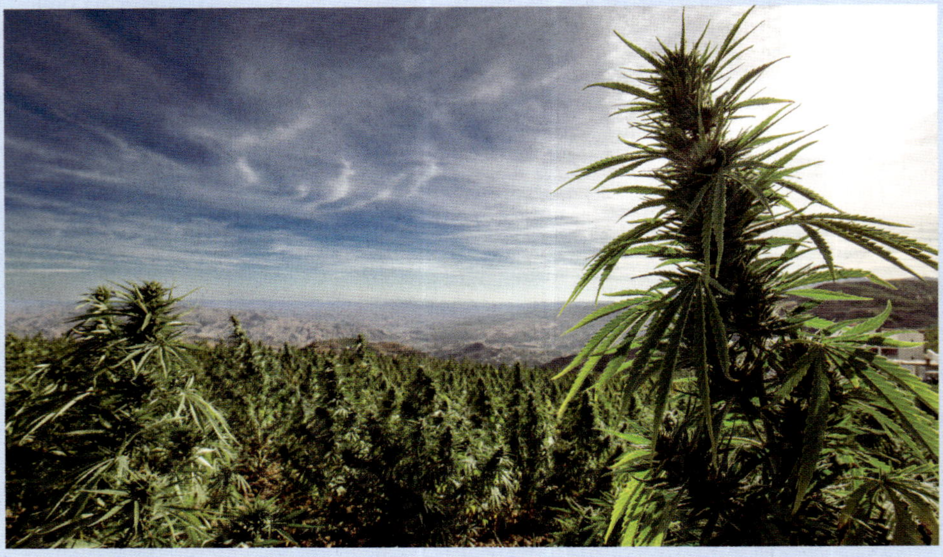

Outdoor Moroccan top-heavy colas are like an ocean of green across the landscape.

Growing in Extreme Conditions with Dinafem Seeds

Growing cannabis in extreme environments can be challenging, requiring both knowledge and tenacity. However, it can be an opportunity to delve into the fascinating art of cannabis cultivation. Dinafem Seeds invites you to explore the different ways to adapt your cannabis grow to these challenging environments.

Cannabis is a highly adaptable plant. From its original beginnings in Asia it has spread throughout the world, acclimating and changing its morphology to survive in new environments. If you live in an area with environmental conditions that can be extreme for cannabis plants, there's no need to worry. You can overcome obstacles to reach harvest time successfully.

Growing Cannabis in High Mountain Regions

High altitude can present several challenges, including extremely cold temperatures, exposure to high winds, and rapid temperature changes. Although not ideal for growing cannabis, these conditions can be mitigated through careful management.

The first step to growing cannabis in mountainous areas is to choose strains that are native to areas with the same conditions or strains whose genetics contains a clear dominance of these landrace varieties (e.g. Afghan strains). These cannabis genetics are sturdier, with shorter internodes and stronger branches. They showcase a morphological structure designed to withstand high winds and adverse conditions.

PHOTOS: DINAFEM SEEDS

Exposing your cannabis plants to temperatures that are too low can negatively impact their development and affect their yield. To counteract the drop in night temperatures, you can use temporary greenhouses and, if necessary, propane heaters.

If you decide to grow at high altitude, you may find it difficult to transport water to your grow. However, you can take advantage of the water that flows downhill from melting glaciers. As a bonus, glacier water collects nutrients and minerals along its way down the mountain, so is a great nutritional source for your plants.

To collect water for high-altitude grows in the mountains, whether from glaciers, snow, or rain, you must use water collection and storage systems. These can be as simple as catchment surfaces, such as roofs or tarps, which direct water to storage tanks, helping you save money and ensure sustainable irrigation.

Advantages of High Mountain Areas

Studies have proven that growing cannabis in high mountain regions increases production of terpenes, cannabinoids, and flavonoids. This means that the buds from plants grown at high altitude could be of higher quality and showcase more potent aromas and effects. Also, the pollution-free air in high altitudes results in higher-quality buds—and getting away from the pollution of the city and being surrounded by nature has benefits for your physical and mental health. *continues...*

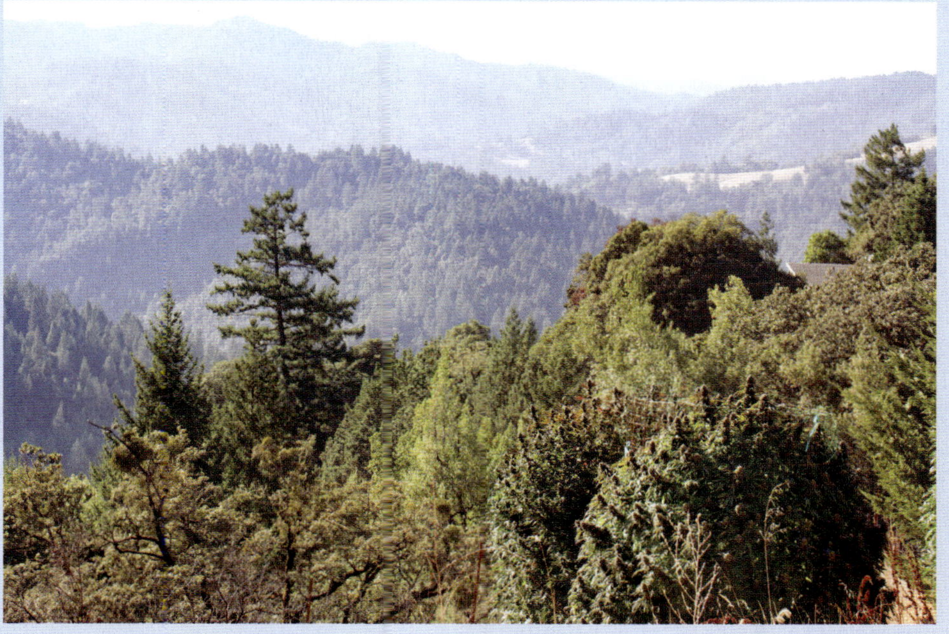

Higher altitude outdoor cultivation in the mountains of the USA.

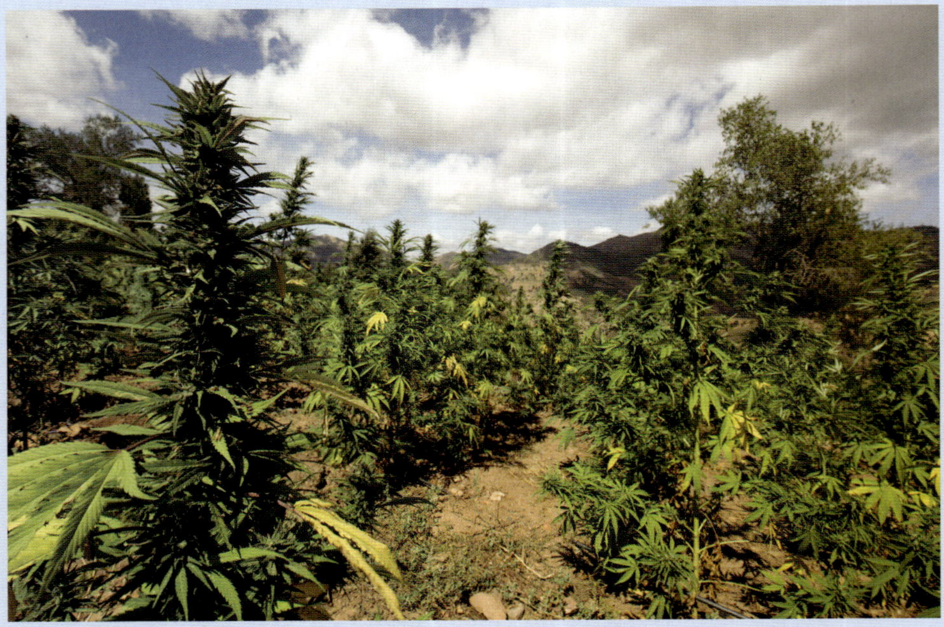

Climate and conditions will cause some nutrient disorders in these Moroccan outdoor plants due to their sheer size but they'll still produce lots of buds.

Growing Cannabis in Arid Regions

Arid climates are characterized by low humidity levels, which lead to considerable temperature fluctuations between the day and night. The key to growing cannabis successfully in these environments lies in effective heat management and water intake.

In the hours when the sun is most powerful and temperatures exceed 85°F (30°C), provide your grow with partial shade and ensure that the plants are hydrated.

Reducing water evaporation from the substrate is crucial. To do this, you can use mulching, covering the soil with a layer of materials such as straw or bark to retain moisture and isolate the roots from excessive heat.

Another good way to keep your plants hydrated is to add super-absorbent polymers or hydrogels to your soil. These materials retain large amounts of moisture and nutrients, releasing them slowly into the substrate.

The lack of vegetation in arid regions results in warm and dry winds. The onslaught of hot, powerful wind can burn your cannabis plants and even break branches. Building a windbreak around your grow or at least near the most vulnerable parts is a good solution. Selecting drought-resistant strains that easily adapt to arid climates is vital.

PHOTOS: DINAFEM SEEDS

Growing Cannabis in Polar Climates

Although it may seem far-fetched to some, growing outdoors in countries like northern Norway and Sweden is possible, but only in the summer months. The biggest challenges in these regions are their low temperatures and short summers.

Choosing plants with short flowering times is key to ensuring a successful grow without the cold getting in the way. Autoflowering strains are an excellent option. They were created using ruderalis plants, a cannabis subspecies that adapted to the Siberian climate and developed the ability to flower without a photoperiod.

If you prefer growing photo-dependent plants, you can use the light deprivation technique, placing a canvas cover on a structure made of greenhouse poles to reduce the hours of light your crop receives. This way, you can initiate flowering earlier by subjecting the plants to a 12/12 photoperiod. This method is used by some growers who are looking to have product ready by late August to get ahead of dispensaries' end-of-season market flood.

Successful cannabis cultivation in extreme conditions requires greater effort on the grower's part. However, with the right strains and appropriate knowledge, it can be a gratifying activity. There's no better feeling than the reward of reaching the finish line after having overcome obstacles along the way.

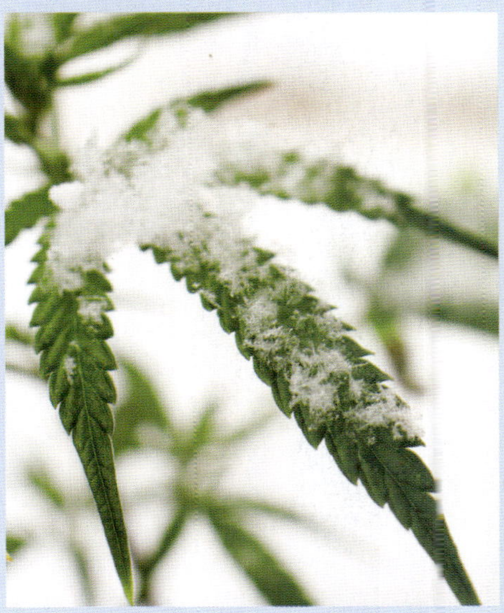

Frost is usually the death knell for many plants, including cannabis, but they may survive a short duration of extreme weather.

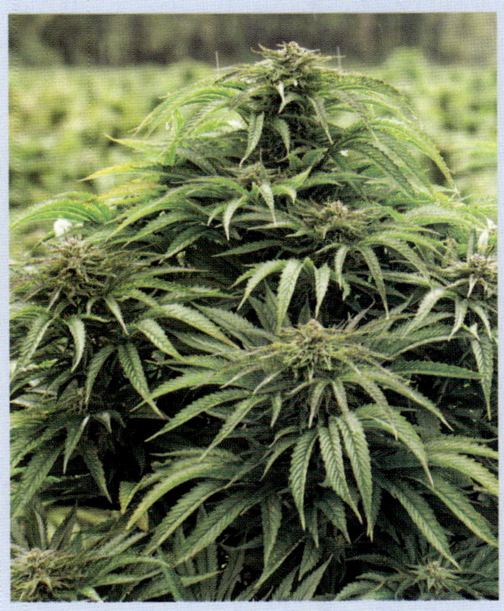

Rain does not impact cannabis flowers because water does not mix with cannabis oils.

Outdoor Cultivation in Australia

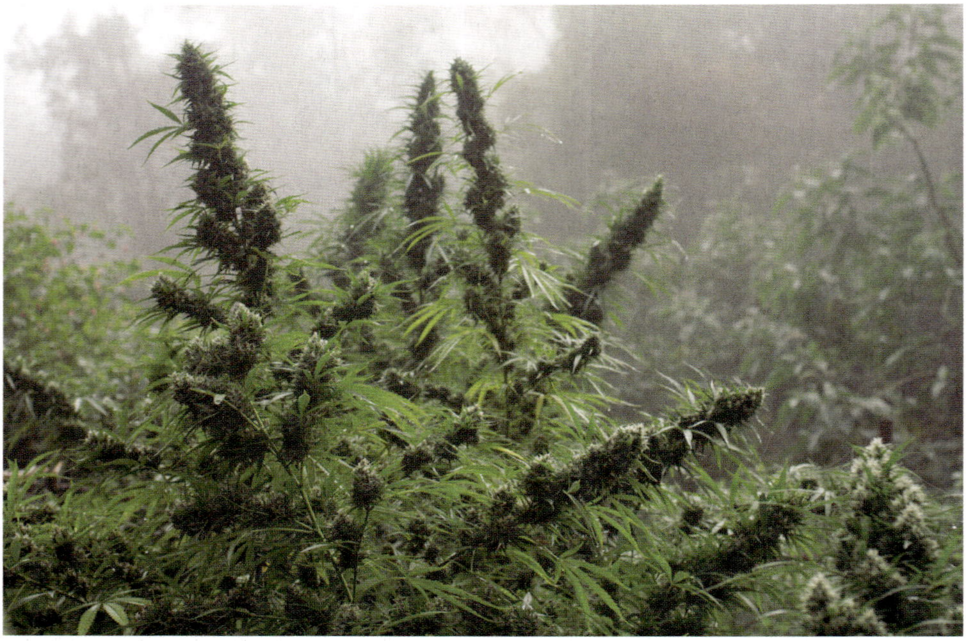

High humidity causes mold. Check buds regularly and clip any sites you suspect of mold.

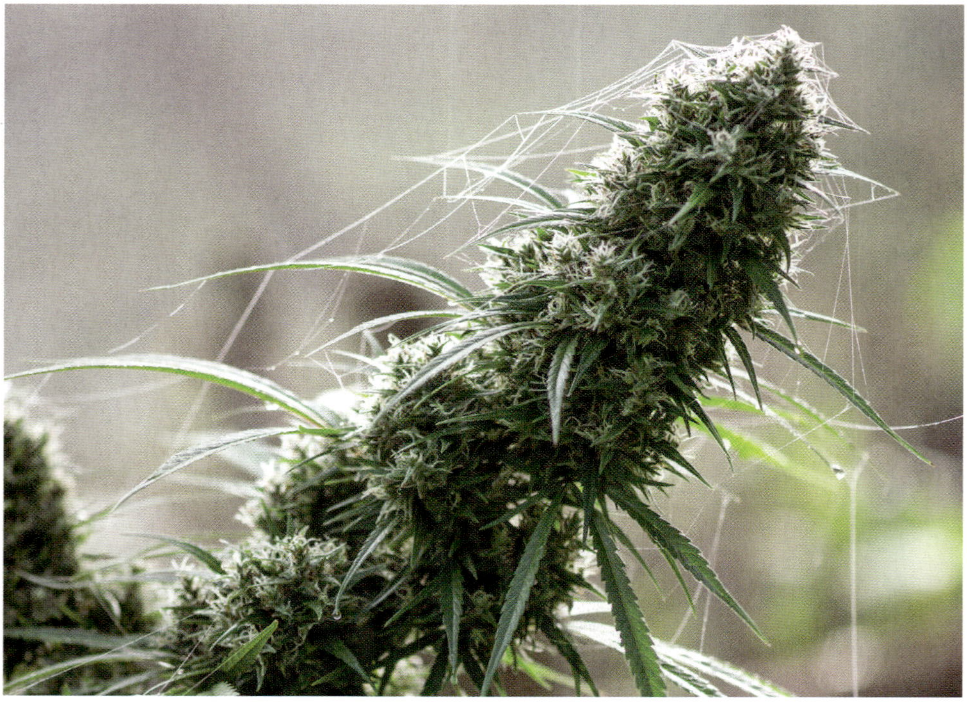

PHOTOS: MARK HEINRICH

Luckily these are regular spiderwebs, not from mites. Regular spiderwebs have wide spaces. Mites' webs don't.

Outdoor Cultivation in Africa

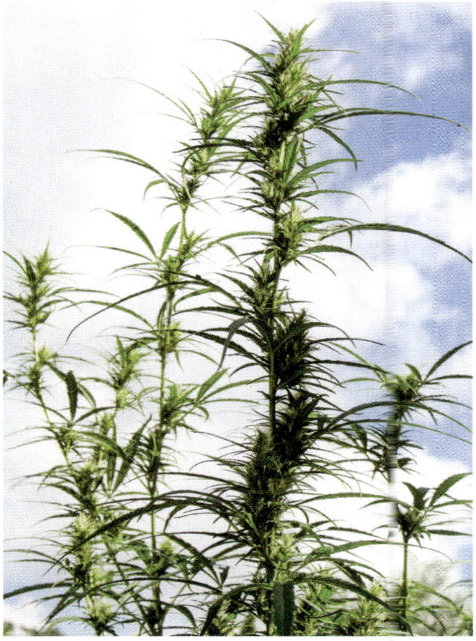

These sativa landraces are lower yielding but the quality is the best.

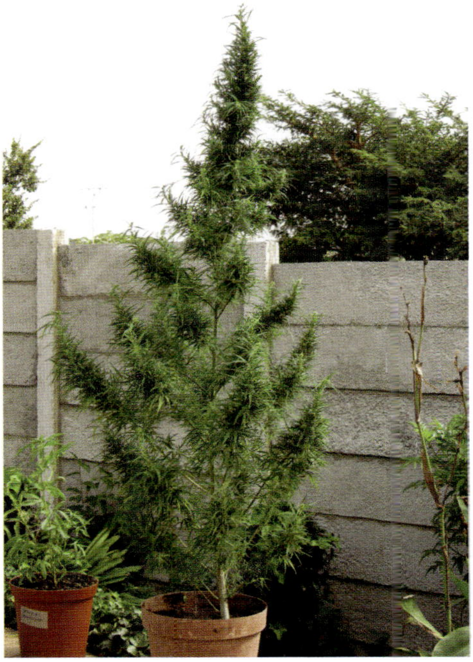

Durban Poison is an outdoor sativa that performs well in a good sized pot.

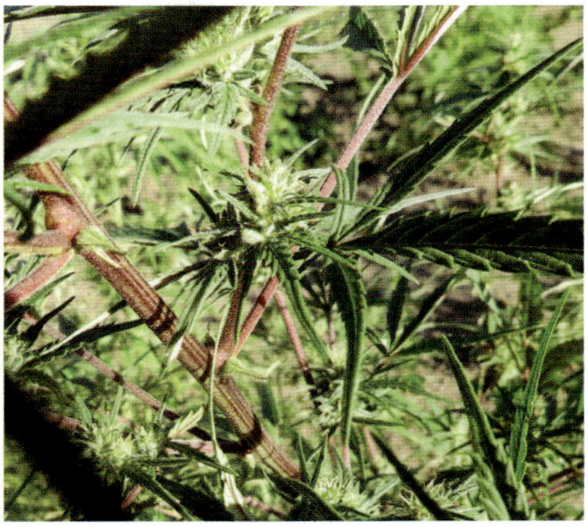

What is interesting about this is the color of the plant stem; it's more common now but used to be specific to foreign landraces.

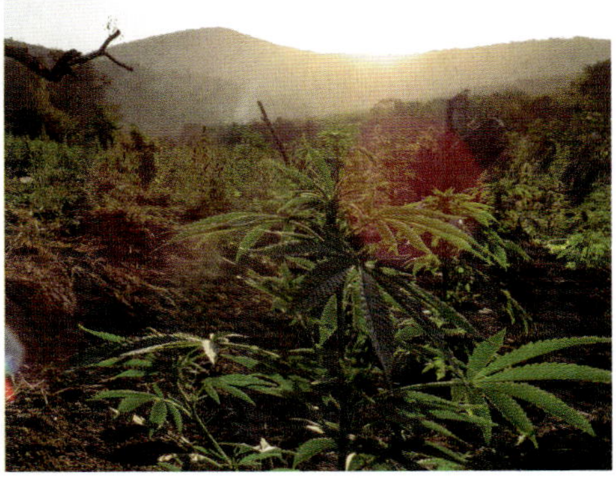

Having outdoor plants is a vision to behold at sunset/sunrise.

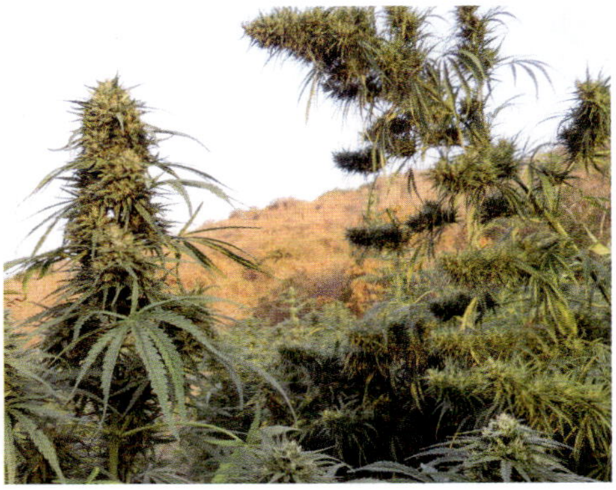

The sun moves so all parts of the plant receive light.

PHOTOS: WEED.CO.ZA (LEFT COLUMN), SEEDS OF AFRICA (RIGHT COLUMN)

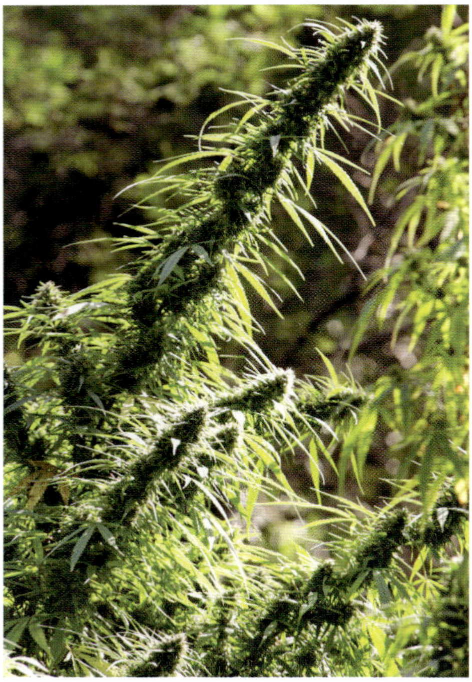

Outdoor harvest sizes are often vast and bountiful, with staggering yields.

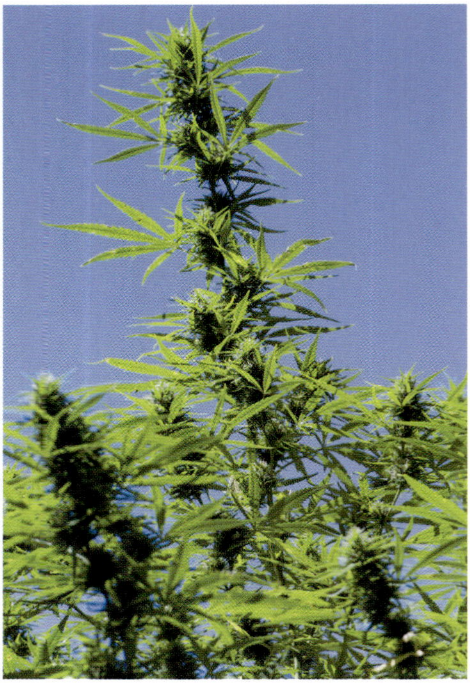

Soaring into the sky. This cola is towering. Outdoors, an uneven canopy is common.

Outdoor Flowering and the Photoperiod

A natural transformation occurs in the outdoor environment towards the end of summer that greatly influences cannabis plants: The change in photoperiod. The cannabis plant orchestrates its flowering process through intricate biochemical reactions, which continuously monitor the changing duration of daylight and the uninterrupted darkness at night. The key player in this floral symphony is the plant hormone known as phytochrome.

In the summer months, daytime is longer, resulting in more hours of daylight; as the year progresses, nights grow longer and days shorten. Phytochrome closely observes this gradual transition and signals to the plant that it's time to begin flowering. However, for flowering to commence, the plant must be sufficiently mature. If it isn't, the photoperiodic changes won't yet influence the plant's ability to express its flowering genes phenotypically.

PHOTOS: MARK HEINRICH

The specific photoperiod required for initiating flowering may vary slightly among outdoor strains due to the different amounts of light and darkness available at different latitudes across the globe. Some plants need as little as eight hours of darkness to trigger flowering, while others require more. Nevertheless, the majority of mature cannabis plants will naturally commence flowering when the photoperiod shifts to a

12-hour day and 12-hour night cycle. Autoflowering plants operate differently, basing their flowering initiation solely on their age, independent of environmental cues.

Outdoor growers must anticipate when this natural photoperiod change will occur, ensuring they don't miss the onset of the flowering phase due to late outdoor cultivation. Early spring is the optimal time for growers to plant their outdoor cannabis crops.

The plant's photoperiodic response is deeply ingrained in its genetics and is a fundamental part of its lineage. Reputable seed banks often provide information about whether their strains necessitate special adjustments to the photoperiod, especially for outdoor varieties. Mature cannabis plants will transition to the flowering stage when confronted with the natural changes in photoperiod.

Researching Outdoor Strains

Successful outdoor cannabis cultivation begins with meticulous planning. A crucial aspect of this preparation is selecting the right outdoor genetics for your growing environment. To make an informed choice, you must conduct thorough research. Follow this step-by-step guide to navigate this process effectively.

1. Seek Local Knowledge: Start by seeking information from local growers or online communities about which strains thrive in your region. Their experiences can provide valuable insights into what works best in your specific climate.

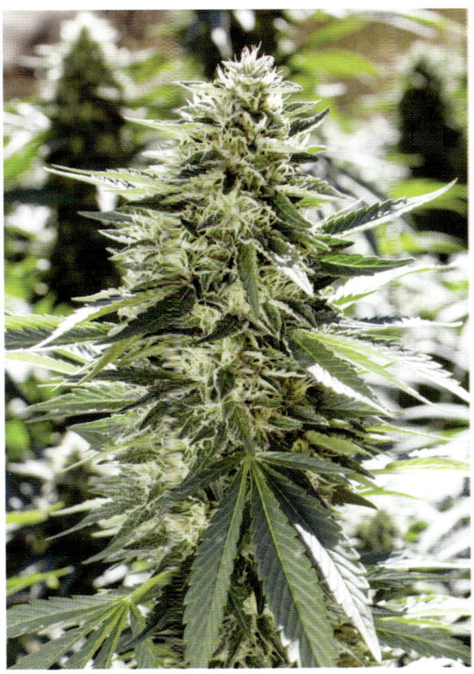

Lemon Diesel grows milky white flowers before they change color in the final stages.

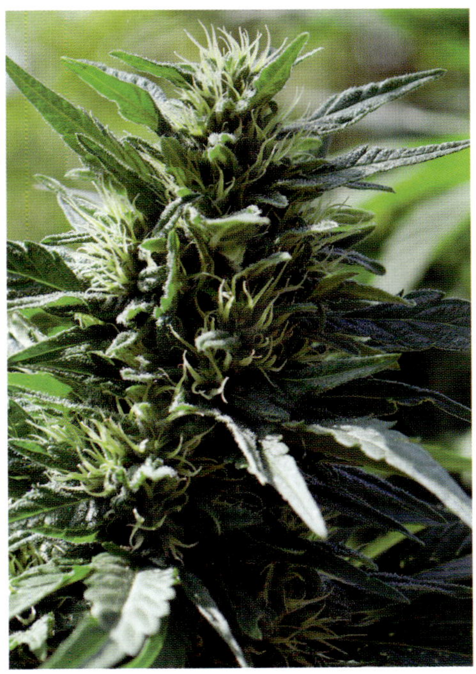

Haze strains like this Lime Haze are best grown in locations that have longer summers.

PHOTOS: EMERALD TRIANGLE SEEDS (LEFT), GREEN HAVEN GENETICS (RIGHT)

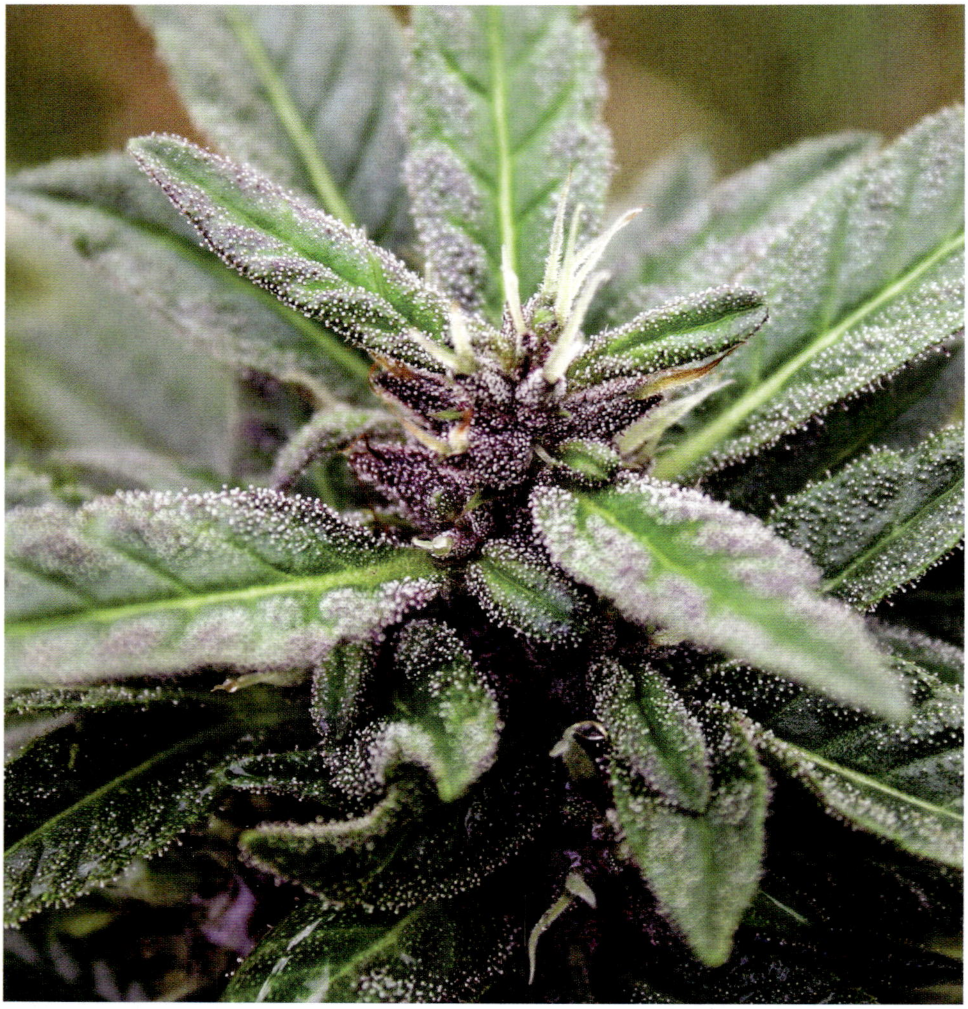

Autoflowers like this Purple Ryder are a great choice for outdoor growers with a short growing window. Connoisseur quality flowers.

PHOTO: DAVID STRANGE

2. Check Climate Compatibility: If local information is limited, look for regions with a similar climate and gather information on which strains are successful there. This can help you identify strains that will likely adapt well to your conditions.
3. Research Modernization Trends: Outdoor strains that have historically performed well in your region are often modernized through hybridization with popular strains. These modern hybrids may offer variations in taste, cannabinoid content, plant size, and flowering times. Be prepared for some genetic variability with these strains.
4. Decide Breeding Goals: Understand the breeding goals of outdoor strains. Breeders often aim to reduce flowering times, plant height, and odor.

5. Consider Local Favorites: Established regional strains, while not always the most stable, can be a good starting point for new outdoor growers. These strains are sometimes freely shared within the local growing community.
6. Avoid Bag Seed: Differentiate between established local strains and bag seed. Bag seed is often the unwanted hermaphrodites from a partial sinsemilla grow: Cured bud with seeds. Be careful about using bag seed, as it may result from hermaphrodite self-pollination and is not always reliable for outdoor cultivation. If you know the source and it doesn't have seeds, then it's better than bag seed.
7. Consult Seed Banks: Contact seed banks that cater to your region and inquire about their outdoor genetics. Seed banks usually provide information on the strains they offer, including details about their suitability for different climates.
8. Check Seed Bank Feedback: Many seed banks have feedback from customers regarding how their strains have performed in various regions, which can help you in making your selection.
9. Read Online Reviews: Explore online forums, grower communities, and strain reviews to gather additional insights on specific strains. Pay attention to the experiences of growers in environments similar to yours.
10. Trust Performance History: Prioritize strains with a proven performance history in your region. While it's exciting to experiment with new genetics, starting with reliable strains increases your chances of success.

Comprehensive research is a crucial step in selecting the right outdoor cannabis strain for your cultivation project. By leveraging local knowledge, climate compatibility, and feedback from seed banks and growers, you can make an informed decision that aligns with your specific growing conditions and goals. Success often begins with choosing genetics that thrive in your region.

Open Patch Preparation

The ideal patch is not just about the soil, but rather encompasses the entire environment where your plants will thrive. The first consideration for your patch is whether it receives adequate sunlight. Observe how the sun moves throughout the day and take note of where shadows are cast. An ideal outdoor patch should remain mostly shadow-free during daylight hours.

An open patch that receives an abundance of natural light is the most productive. Whether it's a small garden plot or a large commercial field, it will have the potential to grow substantial cannabis plants. These plants can achieve impressive dimensions, surpassing those grown indoors with the same floor area. Outdoor cultivation is eco-friendly, benefiting from the cost-effective use of natural light, so is appealing to those seeking responsible cannabis cultivation. To ensure success in your outdoor cannabis project, assess your patch thoroughly and choose a location with minimal shade. Proper patch preparation is the key to promoting healthy plant growth and maximizing your yield.

Preparing a Plot

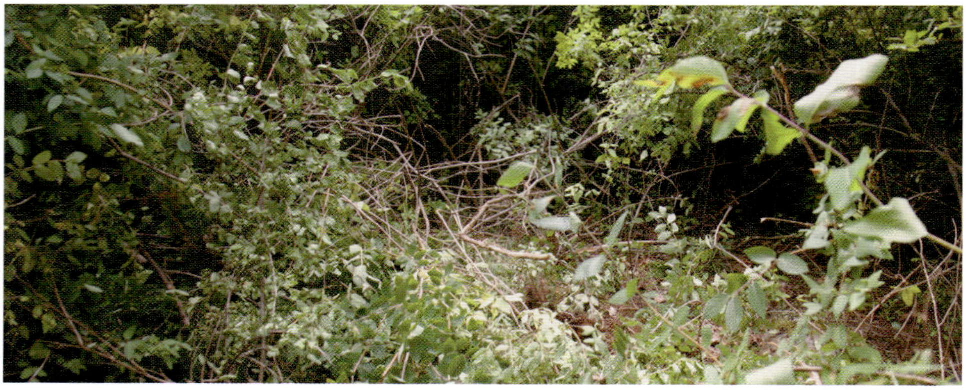

This could be a guerrilla grow or an outdoor area you want to grow in. The area is covered in thickets and weeds.

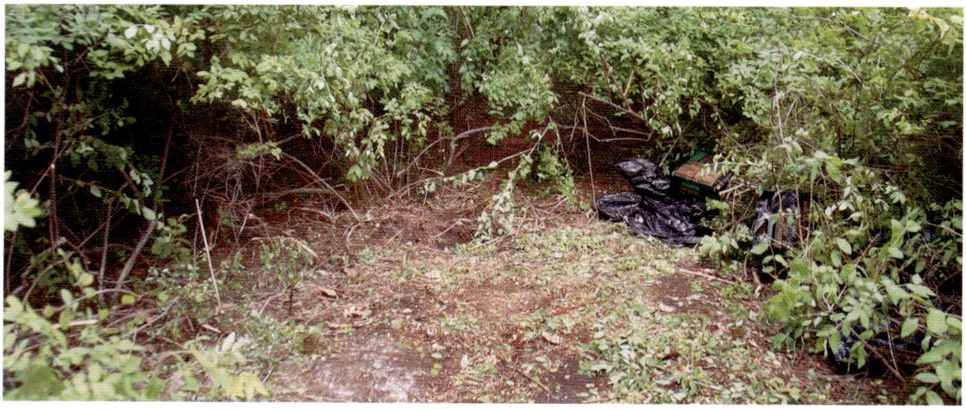

Here the thickets and weeds have been cleared back. The soil has not been touched or replaced though. Grow bags can be placed here nicely.

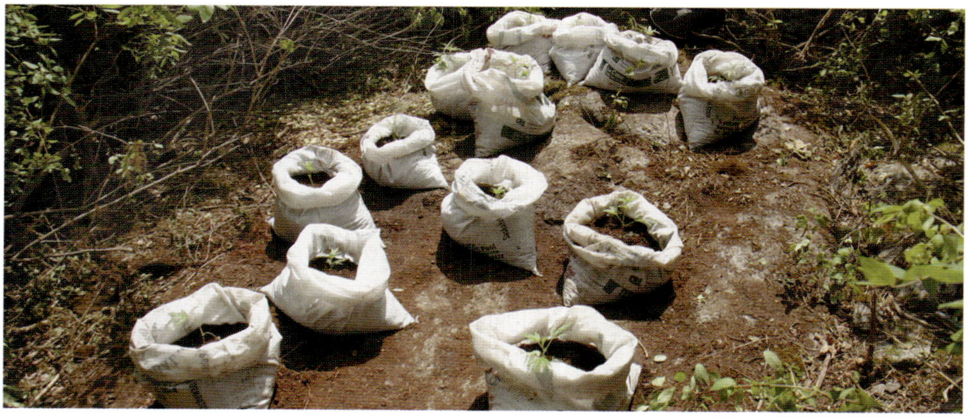

Here the transplants have been brought to the grow site. They are spaced out to judge how they will eventually go in.

PHOTOS: DAVID STRANGE

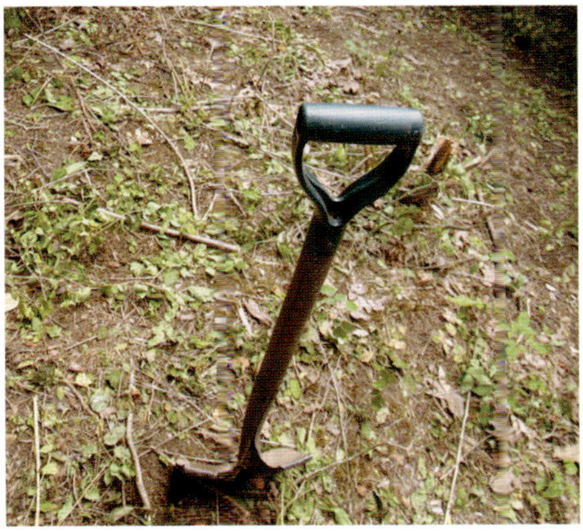

Replacing the soil is a good idea. You can either just turn the soil or bring in your own.

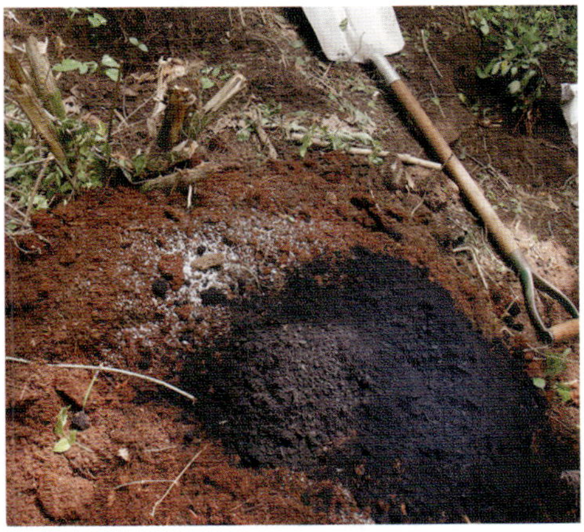

Combining soils gives growers more control over the medium in which their plants will grow.

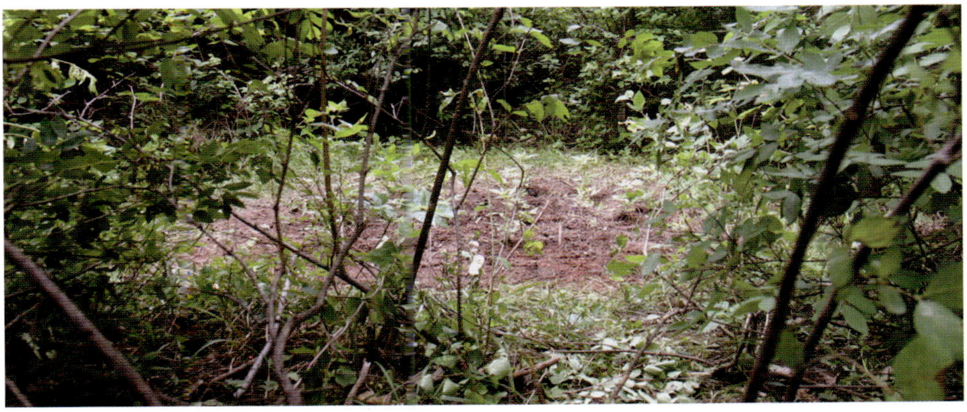

This plot is semi-camouflaged. It is deep in the woods where people are less likely to trek through but at the same time can be spotted if close enough.

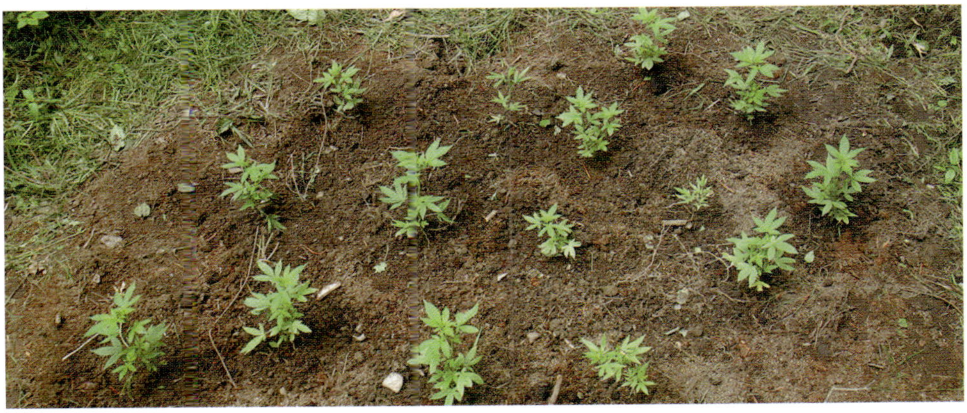

Note the wide spacing between plants. Outdoor plants tend to get big and bushy, so they need the space. Use harvest time to judge if you got the spacing right. Make note of this for future grows.

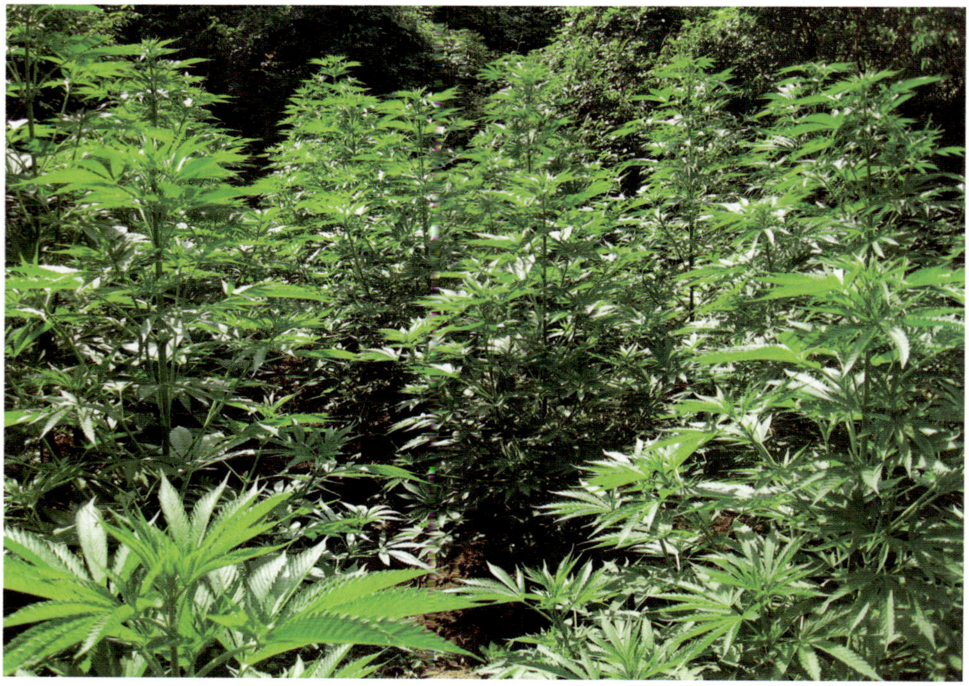
PHOTO: CH9 FEMALE SEEDS

The space between plants allows the grower to move through the plot to water, feed, and check where needed.

Perimeter Losses

One significant concern with open patches is their vulnerability to the elements, particularly grazing animals and strong winds. Plants on the outer edge of the patch are often the first to encounter these hazards. In cases of severe storms, your crops can be at risk of damage. If possible, aim to grow crops in areas where adverse conditions are less frequent or severe. Some growers plant a larger number of plants so that the plants on the outside can be sacrificial, safeguarding the plants in the center. In such cases, the anticipated yield is based on the plants inside the perimeter, and any survival of the perimeter plants is a bonus.

Calculating the number of plants on the perimeter involves adding the sides together. For instance, if your plot measures 5 feet x 5 feet, the total area is 25 square feet and the perimeter is 20 feet. However, if you plan for one plant per square foot, the number of plants on the perimeter would be 16. You can use squared paper with 25 squares to represent a 5 x 5 area and number each square. To count the perimeter, start by going around the edges. The fifth square on each corner serves as the first square of the adjacent side, so do not count it again. Consequently, the number of plants along the perimeter will be 5 + 4 + 4 + 3. This totals 16 plants. You can apply this method to various plot shapes. Your plot doesn't need to be symmetrical for you to determine its perimeter.

By subtracting the plants along the perimeter from the total plants in your plot, you can estimate the potential perimeter losses. For example, in a 5 × 5 open plot with 25 plants, 16 plants on the perimeter may topple during a severe storm, representing a worst-case scenario just short of complete crop failure. More commonly, one side of the perimeter would be affected by the storm, the others unaffected. A 10 × 10 plot of 100 plants has 36 plants on the perimeter, resulting in an effective count of 64 plants within the plot. As the plot size grows, this ratio increasingly favors the plants in the interior.

Strong winds are not the sole environmental challenge, and even greenhouses may not suffice as protection. Another consideration is the need to address unwanted and competing plants, commonly referred to as weeds.

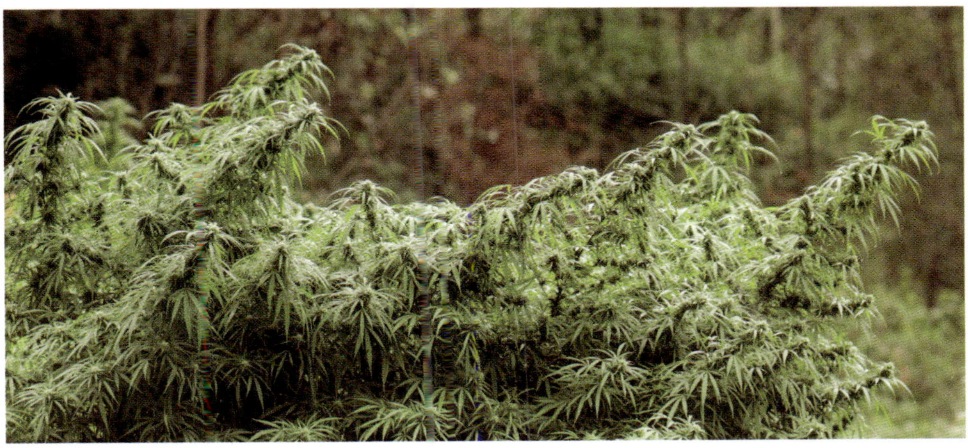

Outdoor strains demonstrate how much top colas and branches can bend with the weight of flowers on them.

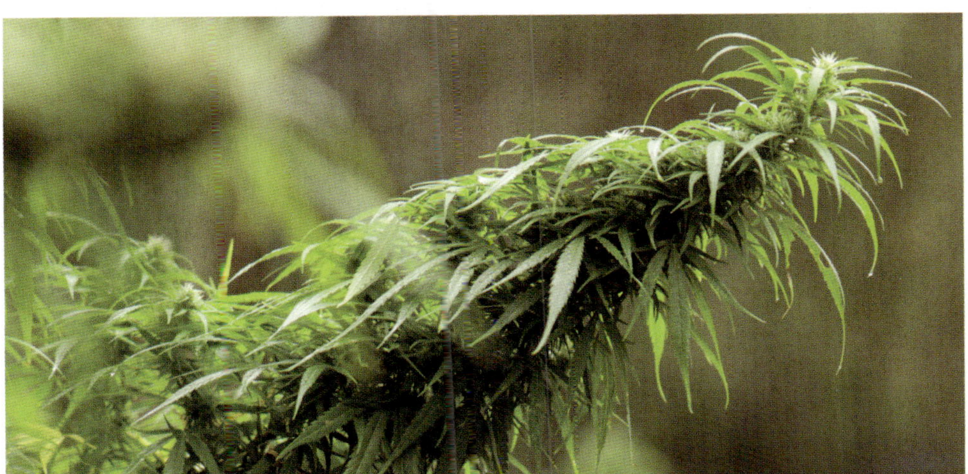

Outdoor strains can often have quite a lot of leaf. A higher leaf-to-calyx ratio is quite normal for some outdoor strains.

PHOTOS: KANGATIVA / PHOTOGRAPHED BY MARK HEINRICH

Backyard Organic Grow

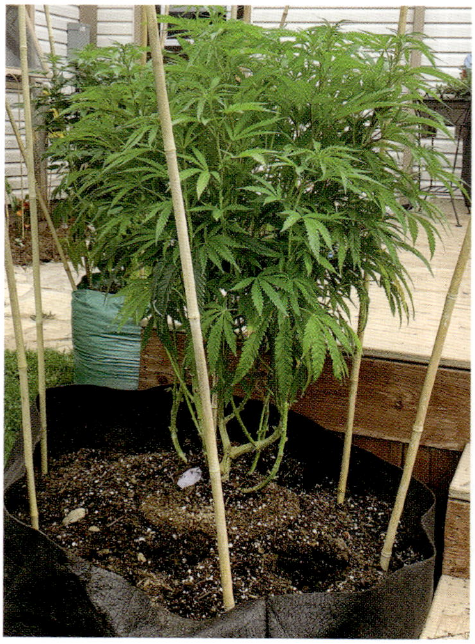

Several bamboo sticks can be used for upright support by placing them around the plant.

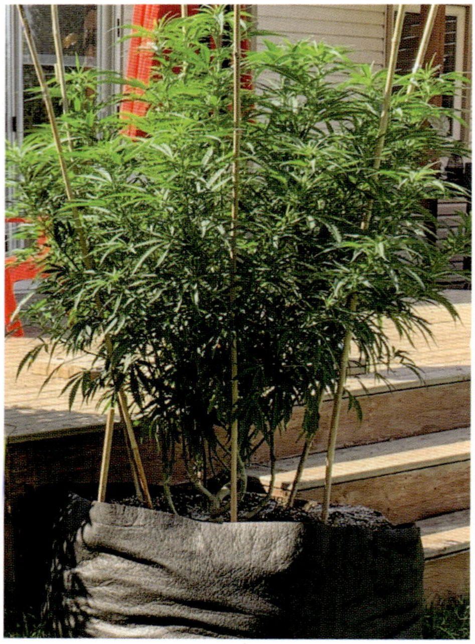

As the plant grows, the bamboo catches on the branches and holds them upright.

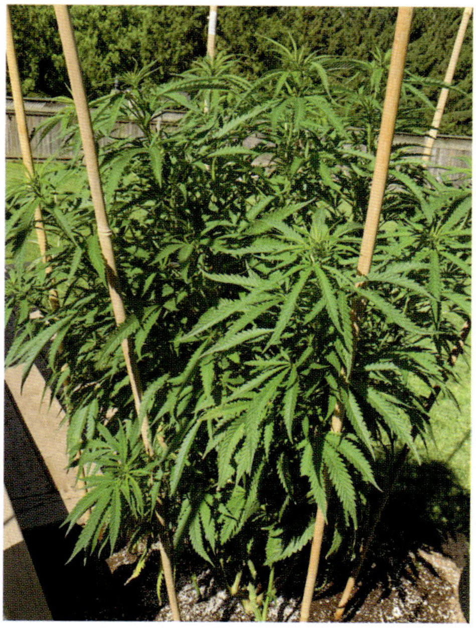

If they miss it, you may need to guide a branch onto a bamboo stick. Don't force anything.

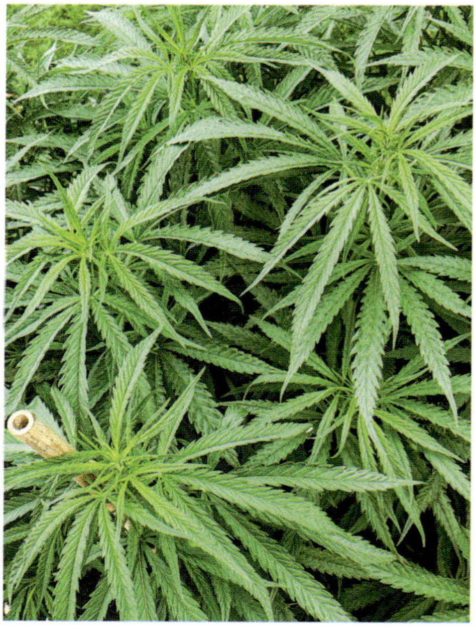

You can also insert a bamboo stick to hold a branch upward. Try to keep them on the outside to avoid disturbing roots.

PHOTOS: TANYA PETERSEN

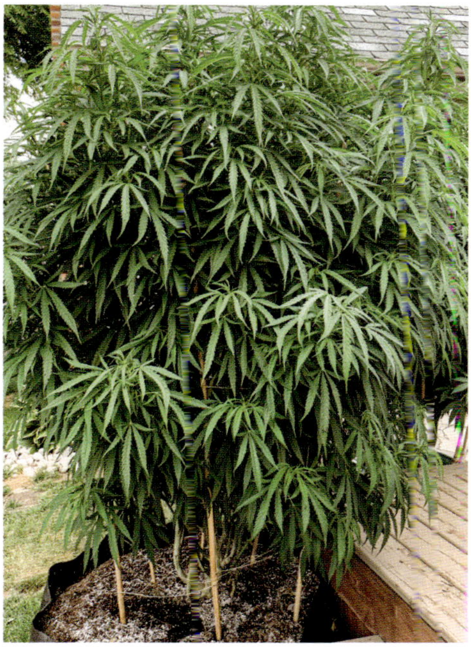

As the plant grows, the bamboo becomes an inner circle. More may need to be placed on the outside.

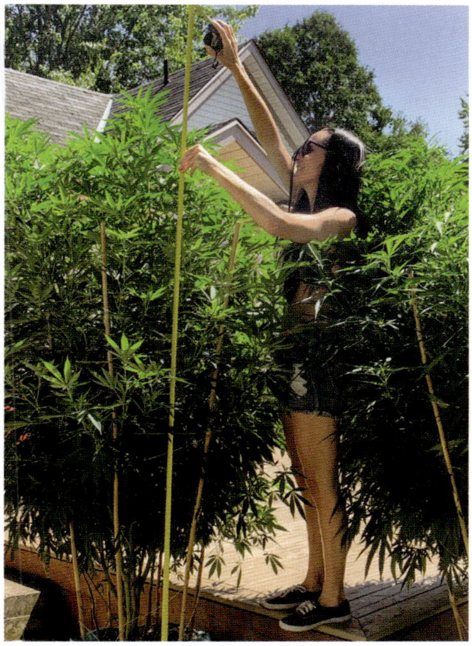

These outer bamboo sticks are usually longer than the inner ones because the branches are higher.

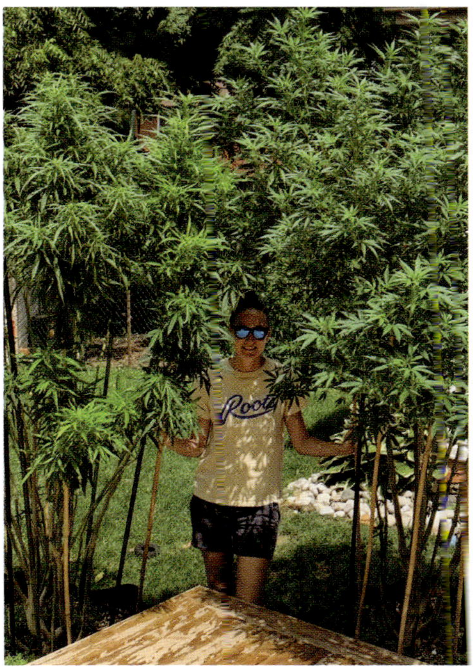

Without the bamboo sticks the branches would be bending downwards due to weight.

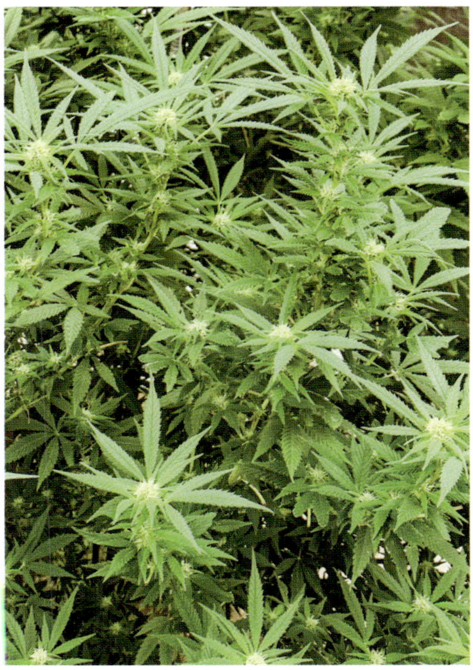

The bamboo keeps the colas facing the sky and not the ground.

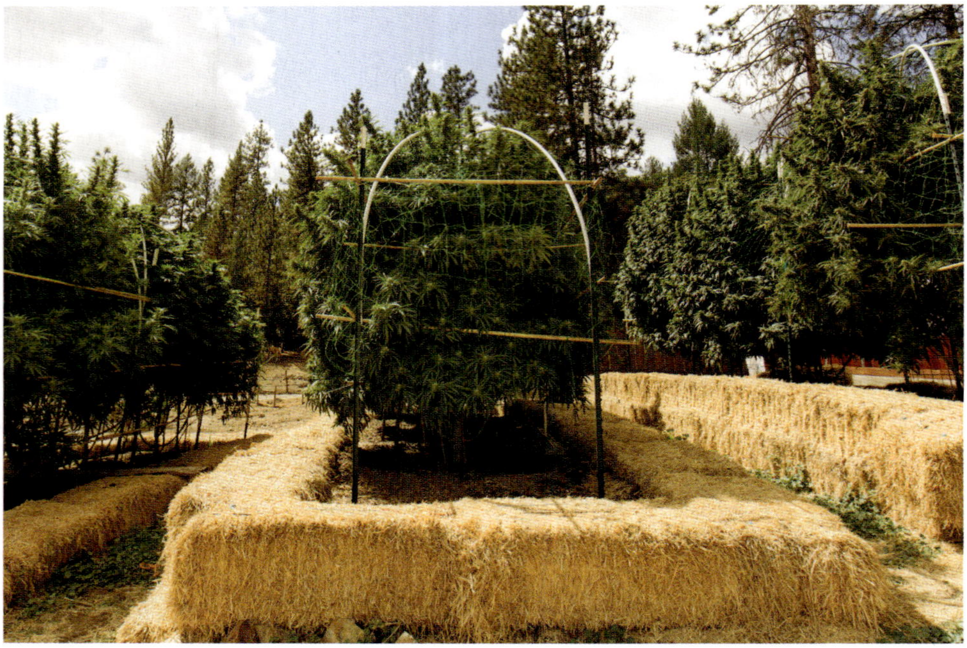

Surrounded by bales of straw, the inner section holds fertile soil for big cannabis plants.

Weeds

Effective preparation of your plot includes land clearing, which can be undertaken a year in advance. Clearing the land of unwanted plants, debris, and other obstacles can significantly enhance the success of your cannabis cultivation project.

Weed management is a crucial aspect of successful cannabis cultivation. Effective weeding involves addressing the issue before these unwanted plants become a significant problem. While cannabis often outcompetes most weeds due to its vigorous growth, taller weeds force competition that can divert the plant's energy into extending internode lengths rather than efficient leaf production or energy storage for flowering. Consequently, weeding is not about cannabis's inability to coexist with weeds but rather about eliminating factors that cause unnecessary competition and conserving the plant's energy.

When preparing your grow patch, physically remove as many weeds as possible. Be discreet and avoid leaving piles of soil and weeds that may attract attention. You can transport the excavated soil in bags to another location since retaining this soil isn't necessary. The patch becomes more manageable after laying down your soil mix. Manual weeding is more practical for smaller patches, though using organic weedkillers is also an option. Replacing the soil helps reduce weed content. Maintaining a weed-free patch is essential to ensure optimal conditions for your cannabis plants. This means regular weed removal.

PHOTO: DINAFEM SEEDS

There are two approaches to weeding: Planned weeding and visit weeding. Planned weeding involves scheduled sessions, typically on weekends or as part of general garden maintenance, while visit weeding is conducted during regular visits to the patch, removing a few weeds each time to prevent them from proliferating. Your objective always is to remove potential sources of competition and, as certain pests may be attracted to certain types of weeds, potential pest vectors.

If your patch is densely infested with weeds, consider using ground cover, particularly mulch. Mulch prevents weeds from receiving adequate light for growth. Moreover, you can water mulch, allowing the water to seep through to the soil below. Mulch can also be used in greenhouse grows.

Another method of outdoor growing involves using a bag of soil laid sideways with openings to transplant a few clones. Growing in such a bag ensures that the soil is pre-treated and free of viable weed genetics. The bag's cover prevents sunlight from reaching the soil, reducing the risk of weed germination. You can add your preferred soil mix to a grow bag. Plastic soil bags are generally not recommended due to poor air exchange and soil structure issues.

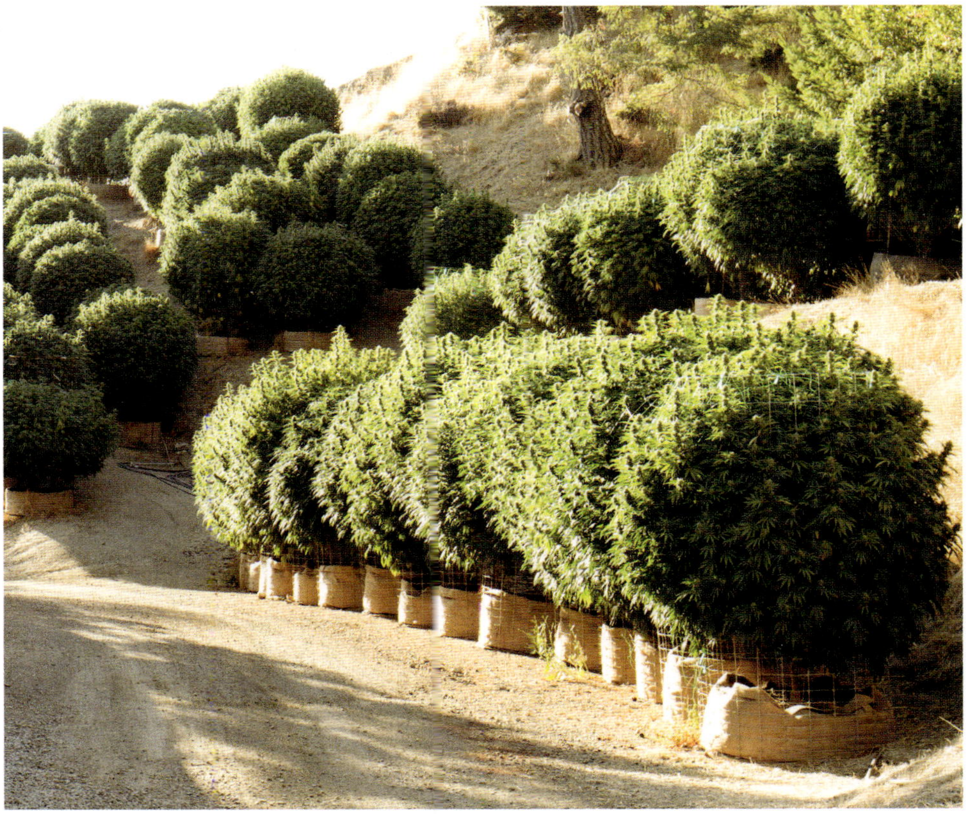

PHOTO: DINAFEM SEEDS

Spheres of cannabis. Just look and appreciate the beautiful shape on display here.

Building a Commercial Greenhouse

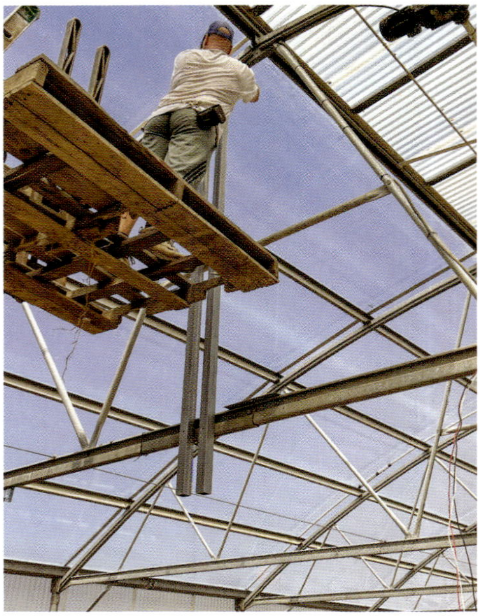

Mounting support for the blackout drive shaft. 12 hours of darkness is strictly maintained this way.

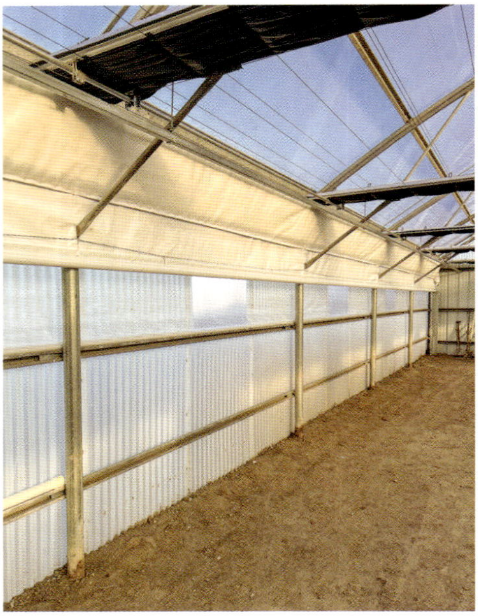

Additional structural support means 12 hours of 100% darkness.

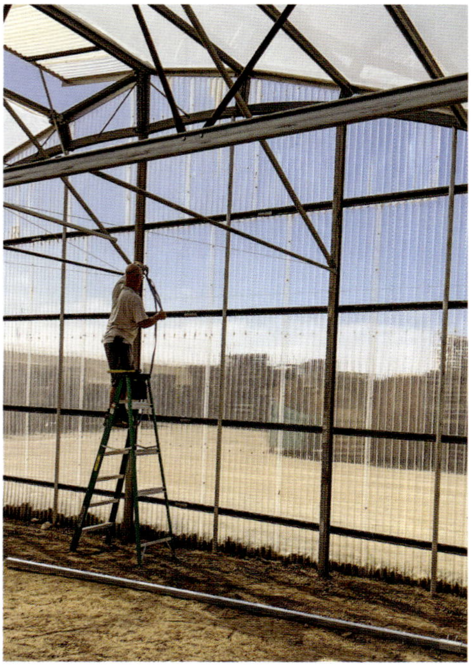

Blackout reinforcement to make sure that everything stays above our heads.

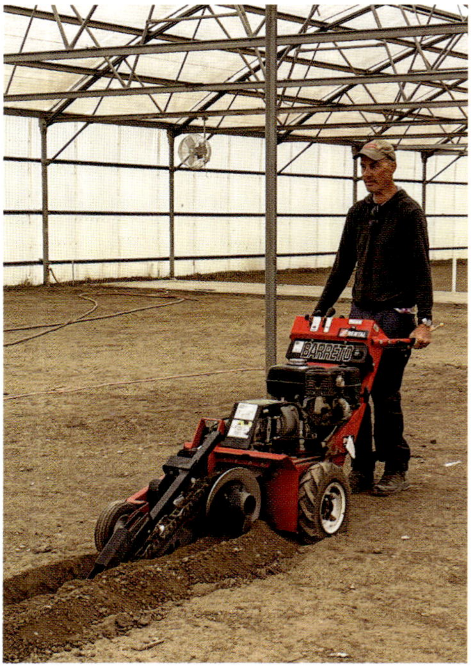

Irrigation lines can be dug manually but a trenching machine is better and faster.

PHOTOS: GREENHOUSE BY ISAAC PABST AND HENRI VAN DEN BOS

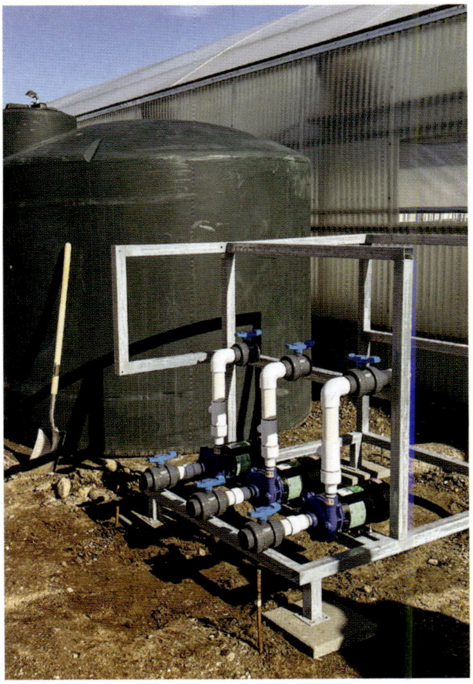

Pumpset for irrigation. Calculate daily usage, pump flow rates, and tank sizes if needed.

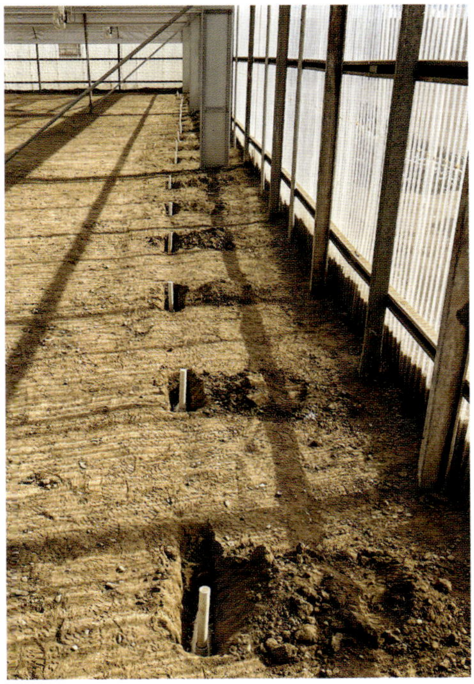

Stub in your drain lines, flush lines, and collection lines.

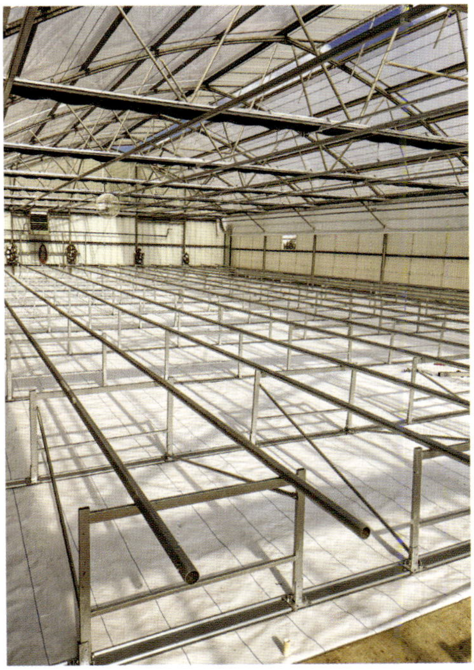

Lay ground cover and install rolling benches. Here we see the legs and rollers.

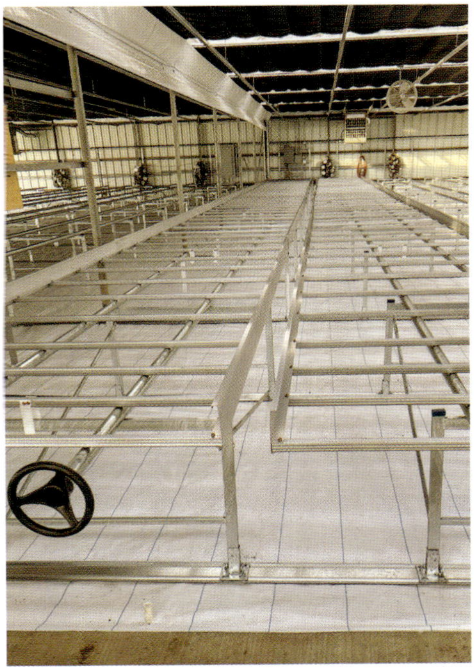

Assemble tops for tables and attach them to the legs or bases.

continues...

Building a Commercial Greenhouse *continued*

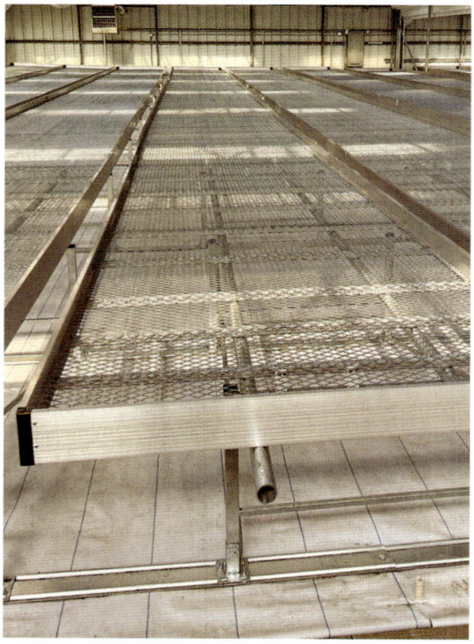

Install table tops, mesh or expanded metal for drainage and airflow.

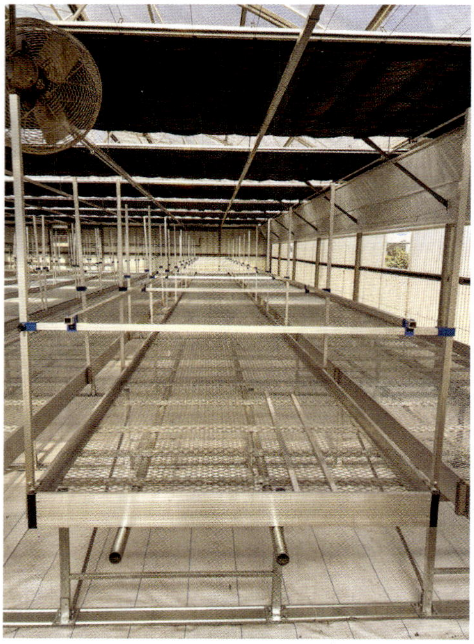

Install trellis system to accommodate the plastic trellising.

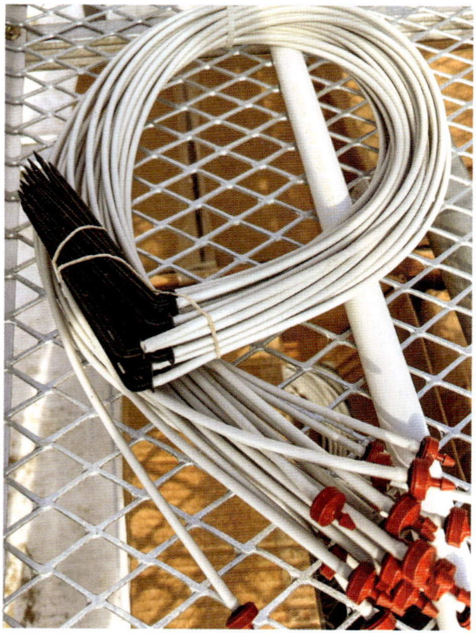

Drip lines with emitters. 2 gallons per hour with four lines per emitter, for ½ gallon per hour per plant.

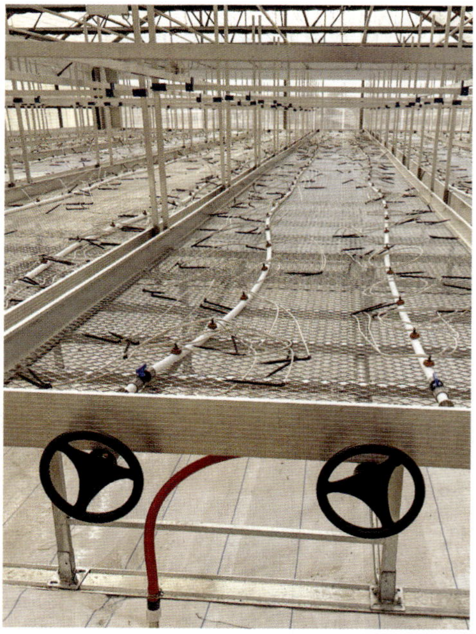

Install irrigation lines, custom punch emitters, and attach spaghetti drip lines.

PHOTOS: GREENHOUSE BY ISAAC PABST AND HENRI VAN DEN BOS

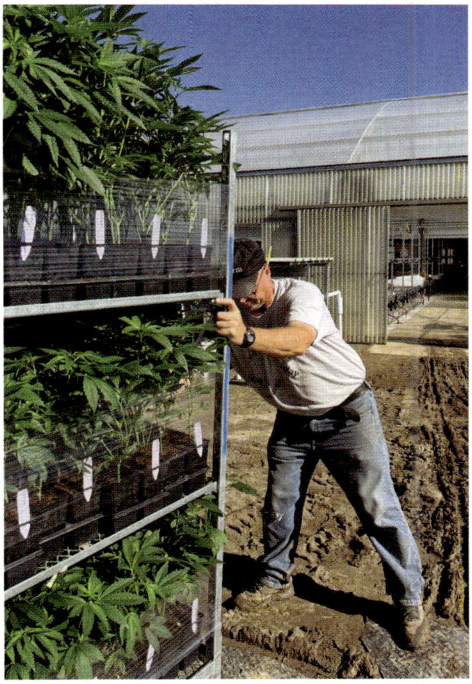

The plants' arrival after starting indoors at the nursery for outdoor/greenhouse use.

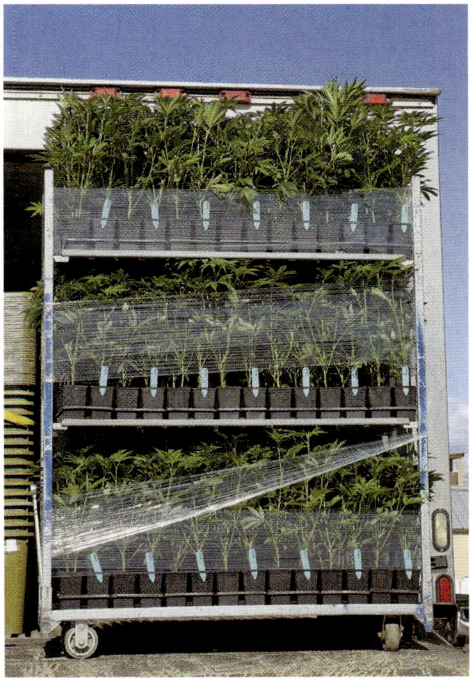

2436 plants per bay, 14 tables with 174 plants per table.

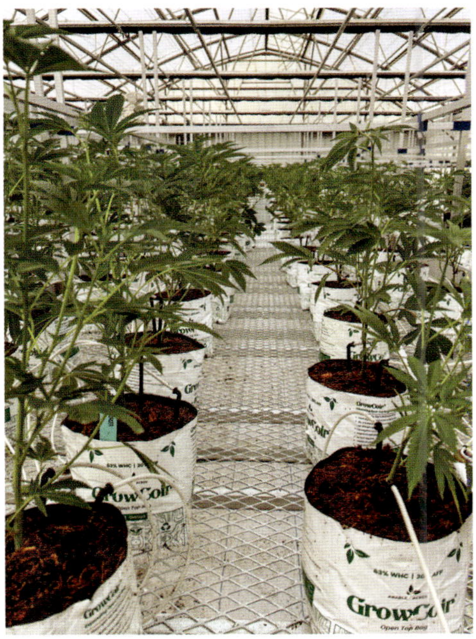

Transplanted into 1 gallon coco bags. In summer, these bags should be 2 gallons to make use of additional production.

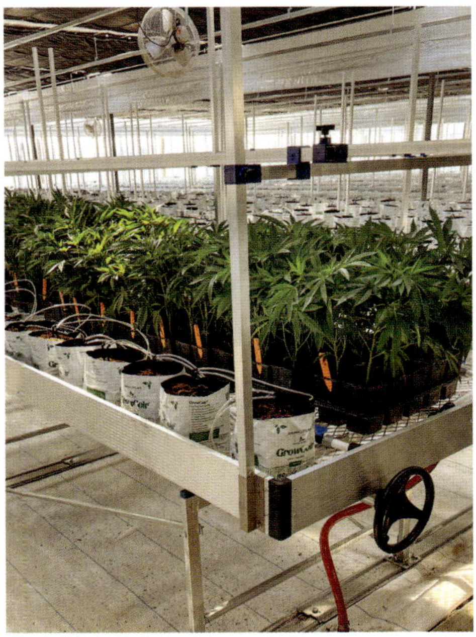

4-inch trays on each table where the coco bags are pre-set and wet, ready to accept the new plants.

continues...

Building a Commercial Greenhouse *continued*

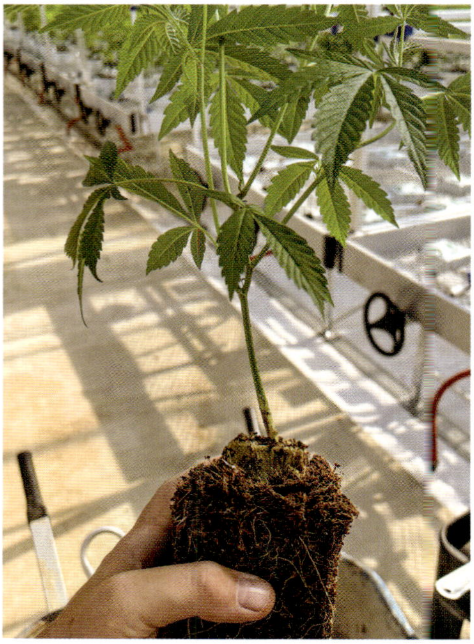

Transplanting using 4-inch square with peat starter for support.

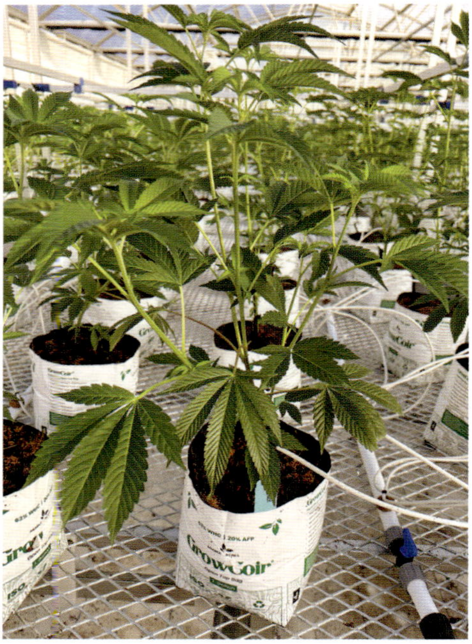

Use two irrigation spikes at opposite sides of the plant to ensure even dispersal of fluids.

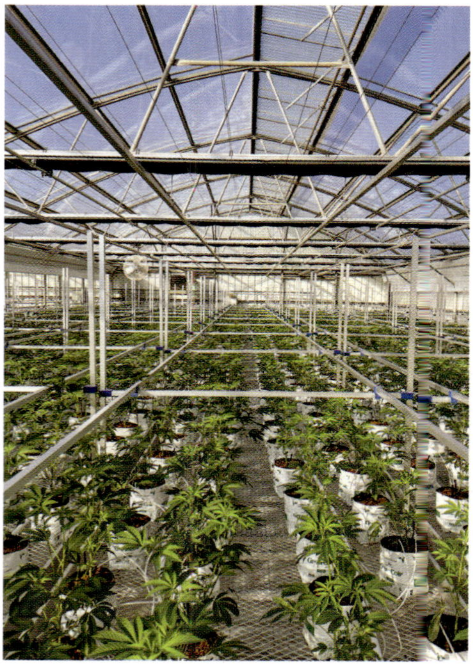

The transplants in this half bay will go through eight weeks of flowering.

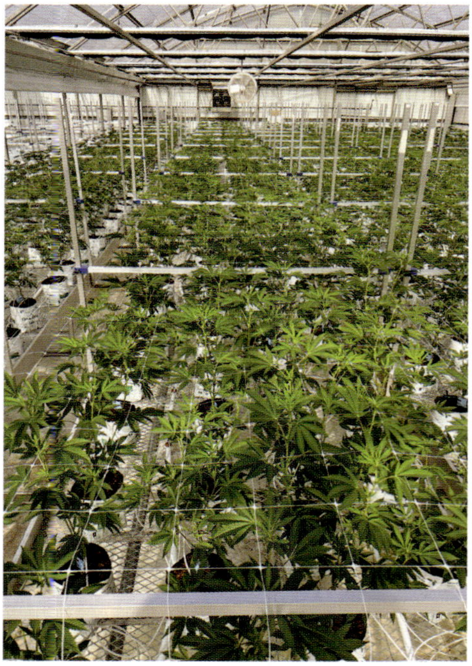

"Trelliscoping" uses a trellis to hold the branches and colas upwards. It is similar to a ScrOG.

PHOTOS: GREENHOUSE BY ISAAC PABST AND HENRI VAN DEN BOS

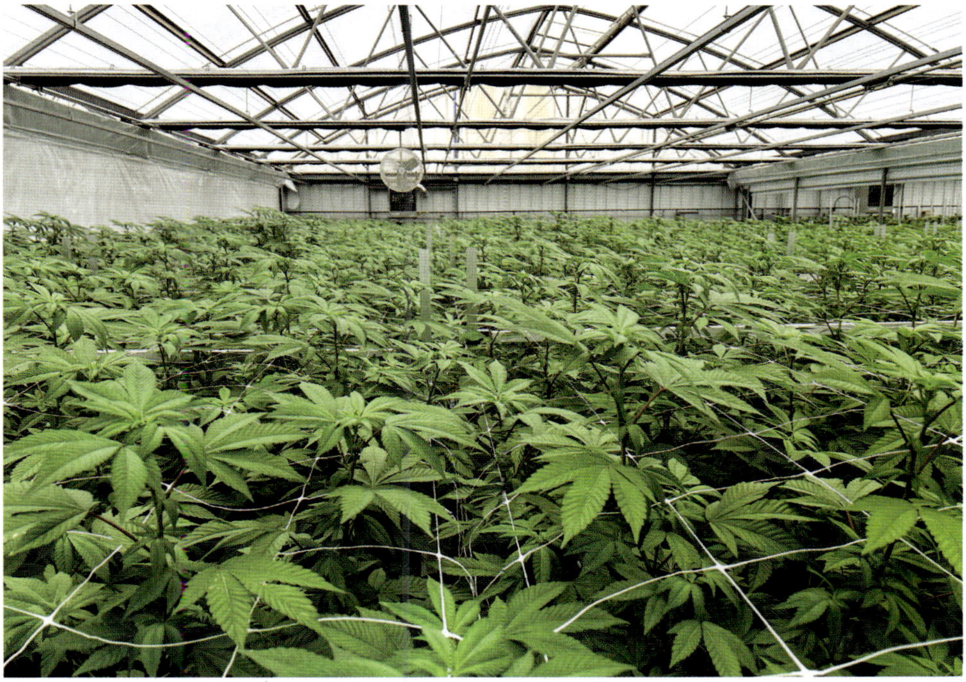

Two weeks into flowering, these plants have doubled in size and are already forming an even canopy through the trellis.

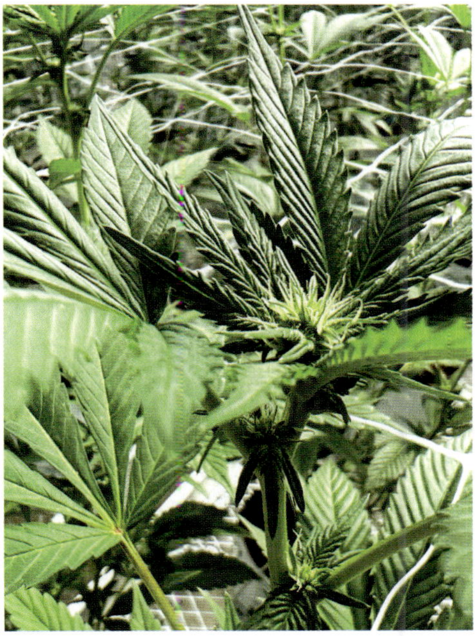

About three weeks for pistil formation. No spraying anything after these three weeks to avoid contamination.

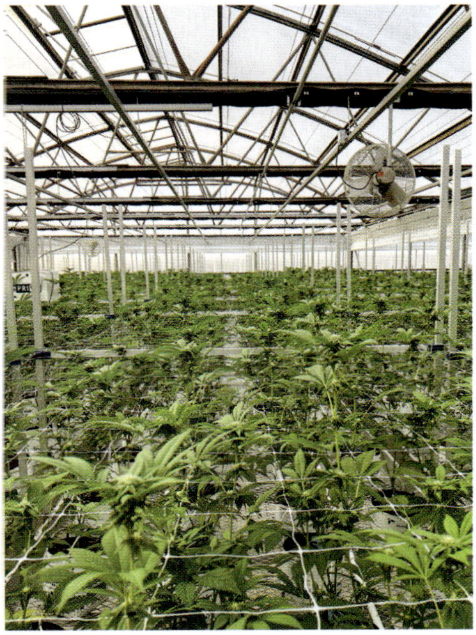

Four weeks into flowering in this bay, resembling the flowering of plants the way they should be done.

continues...

Building a Commercial Greenhouse *continued*

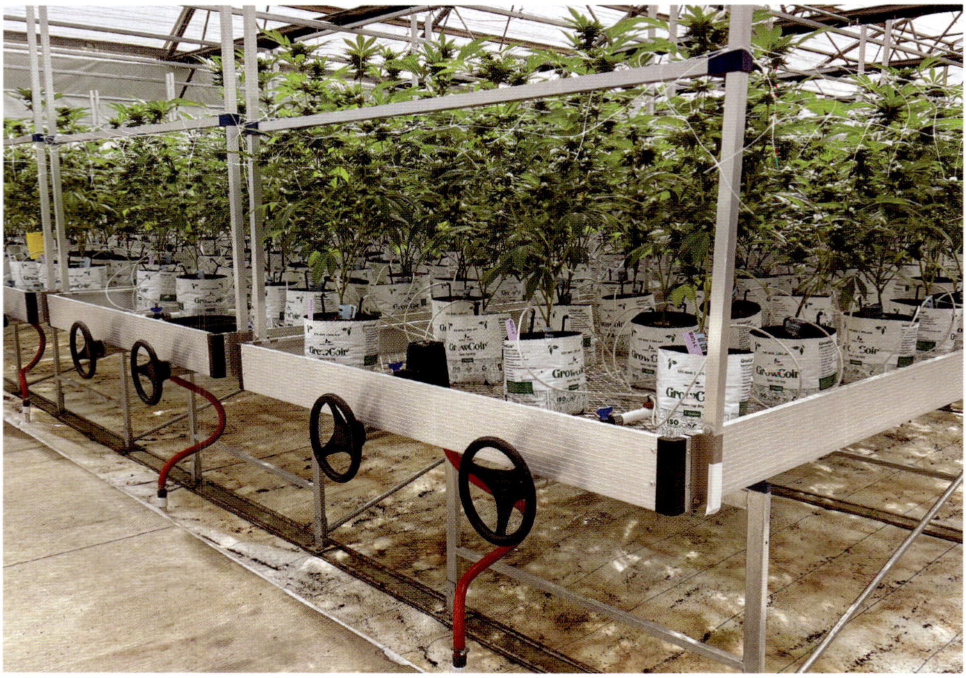

Five weeks into flowering, we are now seeing the bud formation.

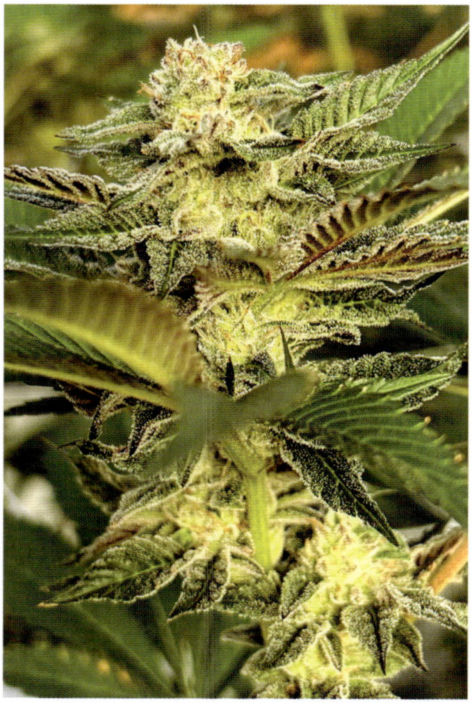

Almost seven weeks into flowering Hashburger.

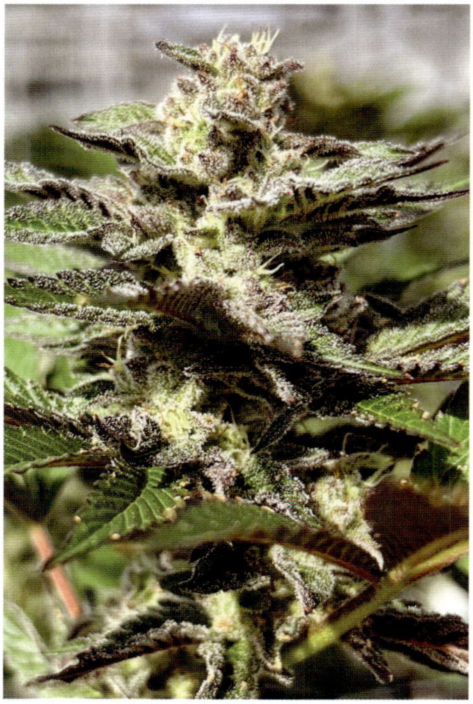

Hashburger is done at eight weeks flowering.

PHOTOS: GREENHOUSE BY ISAAC PABST AND HENRI VAN DEN BOS

Advanced Weeding

Good outdoor practices will involve manual weeding. In the initial stages of preparing your grow area, weeding by hand is safer and more controlled. Typically, you'll need to weed the patch every week for the first two to three weeks, followed by monthly maintenance throughout the plant's growth cycle. Weeds can proliferate rapidly. We've all experienced the frustration of returning from a two-week vacation to discover fully grown weeds in our gardens, seemingly out of nowhere. Avoid the use of organic weed killers unless absolutely necessary. If you're considering using them, understand the specific product you plan to use and how it interacts with cannabis. Some weed killers claim to protect your cannabis plants while targeting only surrounding weeds, but they may not be compatible with your grow. To make informed decisions, research the products commonly used by experienced cannabis growers.

If you wish to experiment with weed killers, do so with clones rather than your main cannabis crop. The cannabis you're cultivating will ultimately be consumed or inhaled, so, if you must use a weed killer, exercise caution and opt for one that is certified as food-plant-friendly and organic.

Autumn/Winter Cleaning

To enhance the quality of your patch, clear it at the end of the growing season, ideally before the first frost, which usually occurs well after your last harvest. Removing dry

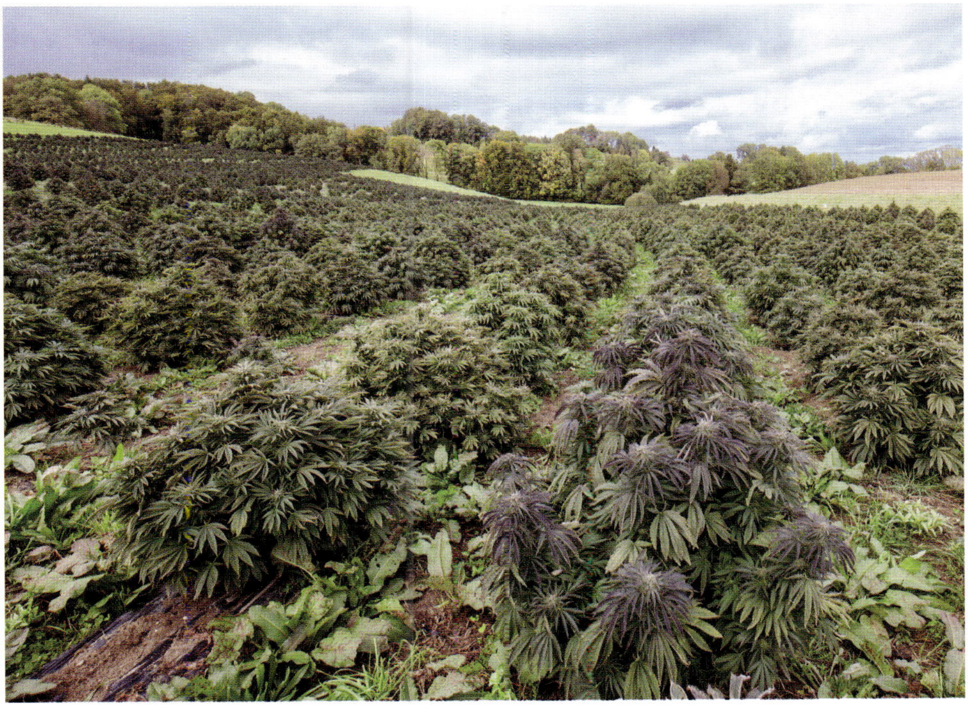

PHOTO: DINAFEM SEEDS

There are other weeds around, but they are not causing much competition for our plants.

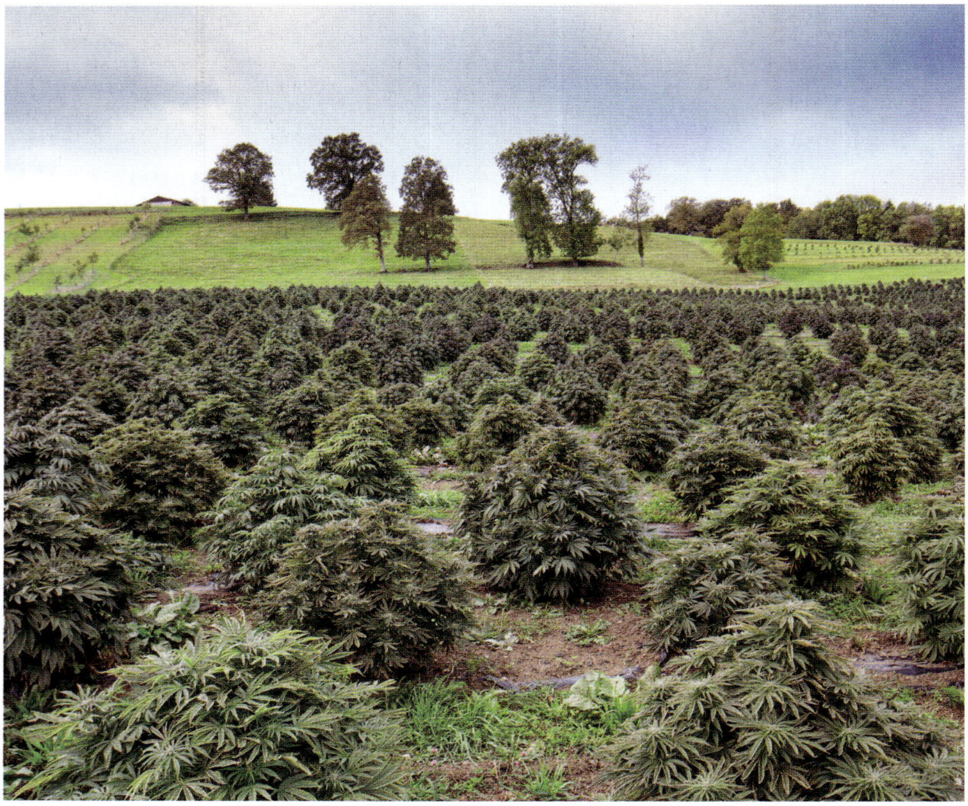

Weeding clears pathways around our plants.

PHOTO: DINAFEM SEEDS

organic debris, such as leaves, branches, and dead plant material, before the onset of winter is more efficient than contending with the thawing and decaying layer of compost in the springtime. In spring, a new ecosystem of pests eagerly invades and feeds on this decaying matter, and weeds germinate prolifically. By clearing the harvest beforehand and allowing the winter to maintain your cleared area in a state of stasis, you can effectively slow down these processes. This method is one of the simplest yet most effective approaches to transforming any potentially overgrown outdoor site into a well-prepared plot.

This practice offers a distinct advantage to outdoor growers, as patches that receive abundant sunlight and boast fertile soil often become densely populated with weeds and vegetation, even in the heart of thick forested areas. Such growth can also obscure potentially favorable growing areas. Therefore, the period following the end of the harvest season presents an opportune moment to locate and prepare your patch.

Outdoor Soil

Natural outdoor soils vary in composition, necessitating analysis to ascertain factors such as nutrient content and pH levels which are pertinent to cannabis cultivation.

Farmers typically enlist agricultural firms to assess their land, making adjustments and using soil turning techniques as necessary to maintain fertility. Left untreated, soil often harbors weeds, fungi, and unwanted pests. While the winter cold acts as a killing frost for cannabis and other plants, it doesn't eradicate all living organisms. Some species have evolved defense mechanisms and reproductive strategies to endure the winter months. The frozen land effectively holds seeds from weeds, fungal spores, and dormant pests, awaiting the arrival of spring thaws.

You can reduce initial weeds, potential fungi, and unwanted pests by starting with prepared soil. This approach ensures that the soil type is suitable and the macro and micronutrient levels as well as the pH balance are correct. Your primary task during cultivation will be adjusting the phosphorus levels during flowering, managing pH fluctuations, and replenishing nutrients. Although you may still encounter weeds, fungi, and pests later on, you have effectively eliminated the immediate source of these issues: The soil that held them in stasis during winter.

For many outdoor growers, their plot is a manageable patch or a greenhouse, allowing for complete soil replacement by excavating and using soil obtained from a local plant nursery. The soil types discussed in Chapter 6 for indoor cultivation apply equally to outdoor scenarios, so the advice for mixing up a loam-based substrate suitable for cannabis is also the same. Following the guidelines on soil composition permits creative approaches to outdoor patches. Revisit the indoor Chapter 8 for more detailed instructions.

Indoor growers typically use fresh soil for each growth cycle. They sift the soil after harvesting to separate it from the roots and either reuse it or place it in a garden for composting, to use for future cultivation projects. Outdoor greenhouse and manageable patch grows often use the same soil for several seasons before replacement. However, outdoor soil can be reused in a similar manner if it proves suitable for plant growth without encountering issues like weeds, fungi, and pests.

To identify topsoil, dig down at least 1.5 to 3 feet to expose the root-supporting layer. If the soil doesn't appear to be an ideal loam, particularly if it contains excessive clay, the topsoil should be broken and turned over. It's generally more effective to replace the soil initially and perform this topsoil turnover in subsequent seasons. You will still need to replenish nutrient levels, particularly nitrogen. However, the fundamental structure and composition of the soil will remain the same as the loam you initially introduced. Completely changing the soil is not necessary on an annual basis for a plot and should be done only when establishing the plot initially. After harvesting, you can aerate the soil by turning it with a pitchfork. This process brings roots to the surface, allowing you to manually remove larger sections by shaking the soil off them and placing the remains into your plant compost.

Amending Soil

Organic Additives

Blood meal has a very high concentration of nitrogen and is therefore a popular choice for the vegetative growth period.

Bone meal is high in phosphorus, and is most suitable for the flowering period. It is a slow-release fertilizer so most growers add it during the later stages of the vegetative growth stage.

Fish emulsion is a liquid solution made mainly from decomposed fish and other ingredients. Most growers use this when their plants are still young as it is gentle and provides a nice balance of nutrients.

Worm castings may be the best all-purpose fertilizer. While not being high in any one nutrient they contain micronutrients, which aid the soil generally, and a very balanced mixture of the three basic nutrients (N-P-K).

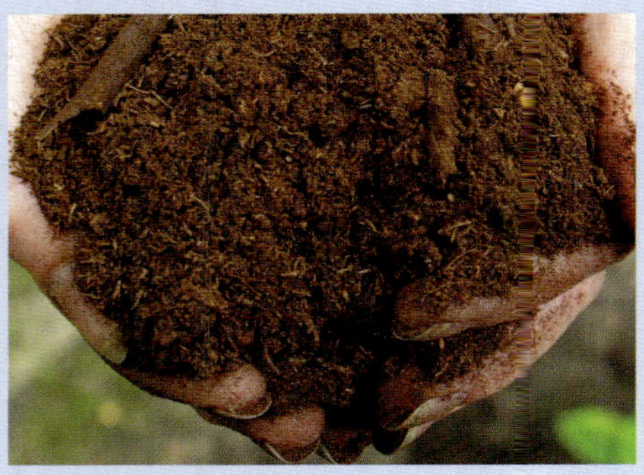

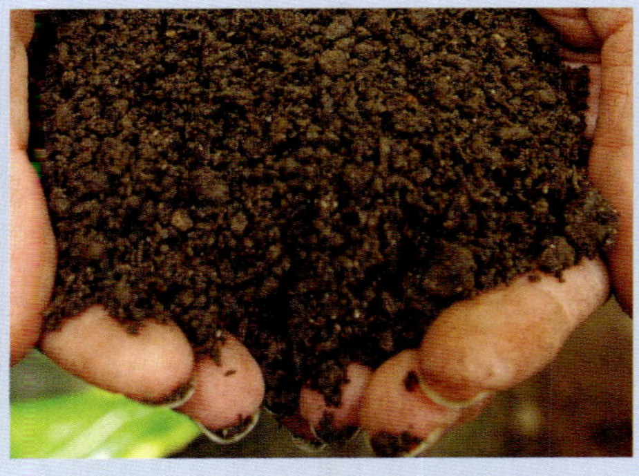

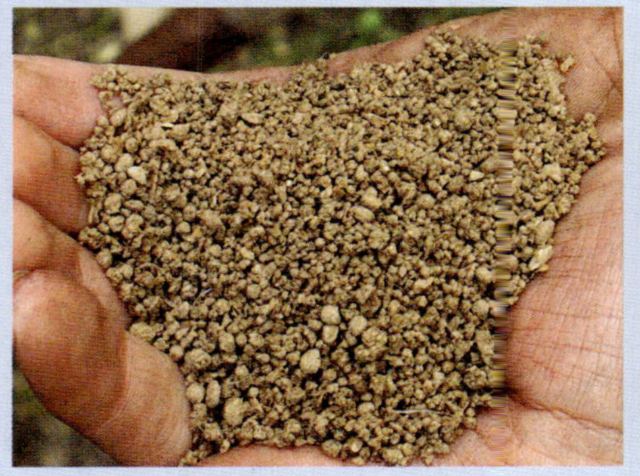

Correcting soil deficiencies before planting will greatly increase the likely success of your plants. For the example photographed here, we have chosen a sandy site.

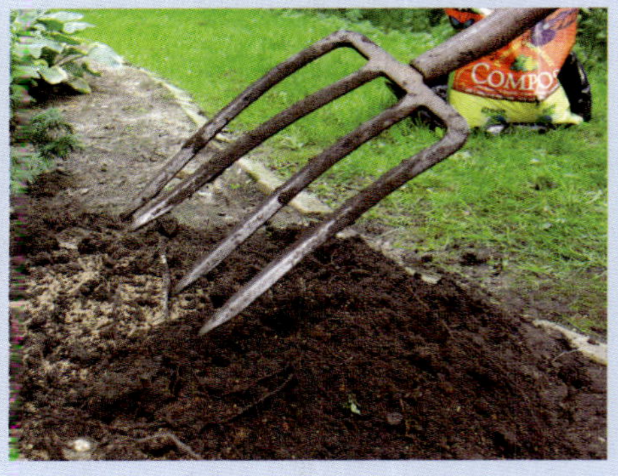

To correct the composition of the soil, we have added organic compost, bone meal, and peat moss. Use a pitchfork to combine and break up the soil.

PHOTOS: STONED ROSIE

Kelp meal is best when used as part of the general soil or composting mix as it is rich in many elements and ensures an abundance of micronutrients.

Manures, these are a mixed lot, with the excrement of different animals having slightly different effects. In general though, rabbit, cow, chicken, horse, and bat manure provide excellent bases for any composting mix but should not be added directly to soil.

Coffee grounds are highly acidic and are generally used to rapidly change the pH of soil or compost.

Eggshells when ground down are another often-used household substance that is great in the compost pile. They usually have an alkaline affect.

Lime is sworn upon by many organic growers as a quick way to raise the pH and render formerly acidic soil alkaline. Other growers, though, dismiss it since it takes a while to break down and cause the reaction. This is probably best added to compost or early in the season if you have good reason to believe your soil might need an alkaline boost.

Wood ashes work very quickly to raise the pH, are high in micronutrients and are, in general, just good for the soil.

No matter which soil base you choose, remember that once your plants have begun to flower, you should flush the soil with water. This rids the soil of excess nutrients and greatly enhances the taste and size of your harvest. If you are using store-bought fertilizers it is, generally speaking, a good idea to flush your plants every three to four weeks. Check the pH levels at least once a week for the first month after planting your seedlings, and twice per week after that or any time something seems amiss. Cannabis does a good job of letting you know when something is wrong since it will discolor, droop, or lose excessive amounts of leaves. If your soil mix is good, that is just one less thing to worry about during the growing season.

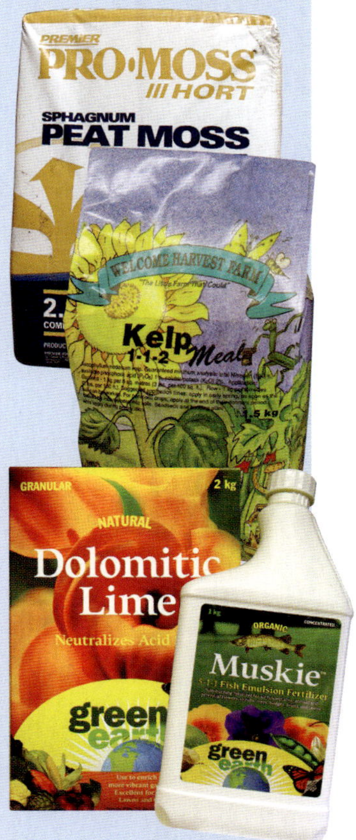

Soil amendments can improve your soil but unnecessary use/overuse can backfire and create more problems. Even organic materials can cause problems if used incorrectly. Increasing the soil pH can create a nutrient imbalance while lowering the pH can create toxic conditions.

PHOTOS: GCP

You want a topsoil that is close to the composition of a loam and not full of stones and roots from grass and weeds. Sometimes, the topsoil is nearly suitable but requires enhancement to become an excellent loam. Mixing store-bought soil with the turned topsoil can help achieve this. As you dig down and turn the soil, note changes in its composition and sift through it to determine necessary adjustments. You can create a custom mixture using sand, silt, and clay if you don't want to use store-bought loam. Test a portion of topsoil in a bucket to calculate the adjustments required for the entire plot. When soil is added, it results in raised mounds, potentially altering the plot's level. Removing some soil from previous growth cycles, such as root masses with some attached soil, can help maintain a level plot.

One challenge when excavating a patch is maintaining its natural appearance, especially when security is a concern. If you use vermiculite, perlite, or other colorful soilless substrates, ensure they are positioned well below the surface. A sprinkling of coconut-based grow medium across the surface can blend the patch seamlessly into its surroundings. When mixed into the soil , coconut fibers also enrich it with nutrients and give roots additional space to grow and breathe. Outdoor growers often favor coconut substrates, readily available at grow shops in the form of coir blocks. These blocks, when immersed in hot water, expand into a substrate that retains moisture, making them preferable to mulch.

Outdoor Challenges

Outdoor growers face a range of challenges when nurturing their plants. Every lesson learned can refine your strategy for future seasons, as even seemingly minor adjustments, such as altering your planting time by a week or adjusting watering frequency, can have a significant impact. Unlike indoor cultivation, where you have control over

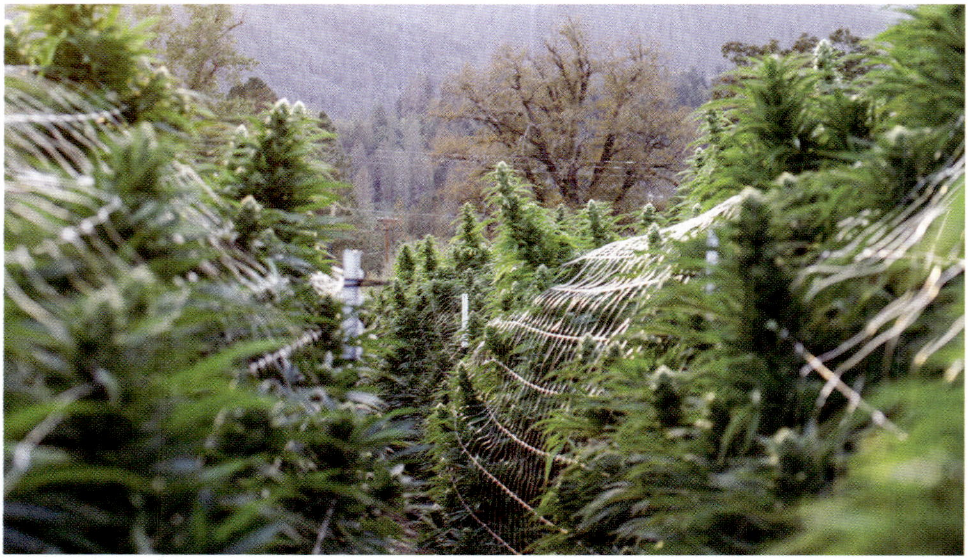

PHOTO: DINAFEM SEEDS

Outdoors in Oregon, this is a CBD crop with netting to keep the branches upright.

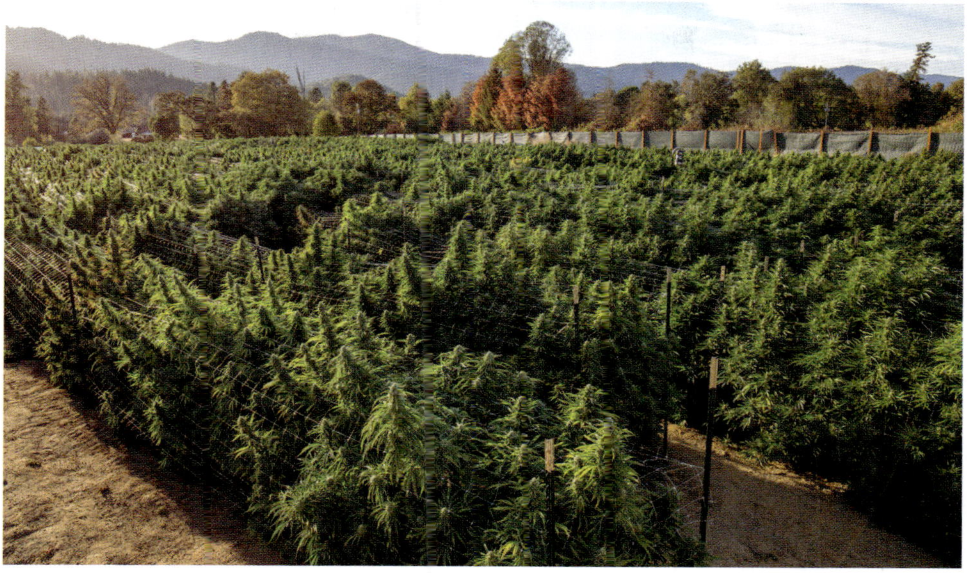

CBD is just as important as other cannabinoids for medical use.

the environment, outdoor growers must maintain records and plan diligently, as each growing season is subject to environmental fluctuations.

Growing outdoors typically begins with preparing your chosen patch and then sowing seeds or transplanting seedlings or cuttings. Do not bury seeds too deep; a depth of ½ to 1 inch below the soil's surface is ideal. Seeds buried too deep may fail to germinate as the seedling has to break through more soil to reach the sunlight. However, when seeds are buried just an inch below the surface, they become easily accessible to birds that probe the soil in search of worms or other potential food sources. Birds may also consume seeds directly from the plant. While commercial systems use such methods as automatic crow bangers, sound discharge systems, or kites resembling predatory birds to control birds, these solutions are not always effective, and they generate noise that may not be neighbor-friendly. In situations where bird interference significantly hampers crop success, consider germinating indoors and or using a greenhouse.

Watering and Irrigation

After you sow seeds or transplant, a gentle sprinkling of water in the initial stages is all that's required to start your plants. There's typically no need to adjust soil pH or introduce soil additives, especially if you've refreshed the patch.

To assess underground moisture levels, dig a small hole about a foot deep in your grow patch, taking care to avoid significant roots. Insert your hand into the hole and judge if the soil feels dry, or cool and moist. If it's the latter, the soil has retained moisture below the surface, providing a water source for your plants.

If rainfall doesn't adequately supply your plants, you'll need to provide water as needed to ensure optimal growth. Natural irrigation techniques can be effective but may reveal the location of your plants to others. If you wish to direct root growth away from a dry side of the plot, you can dig a trench there to air-prune the roots, guiding them toward moist areas while discouraging growth in the arid direction. Using runoff to channel water toward your patch can also be an effective approach. Many outdoor growers eventually turn to hoses and pipes after experimenting with different garden plots or greenhouses.

The water requirements of your plants will depend on their size, with larger plants potentially needing at least a gallon of water per day. Natural loam soil can retain moisture for two to six weeks before becoming extremely dry under the sun. Some regions even have underground water reservoirs. Visual inspections are an effective way to gauge whether your plants require watering; if they appear significantly wilted, they need water.

Polymer Crystals

In arid conditions, you can incorporate polymer crystals with water-retaining properties into your soil mix, providing plants with access to water during dry spells. To prepare, fill a plastic bottle with water and polymer crystals and allow them to expand overnight as they absorb water. These swollen polymer crystals assume a gel-like consistency and gradually release stored water throughout the season. These crystals also improve soil

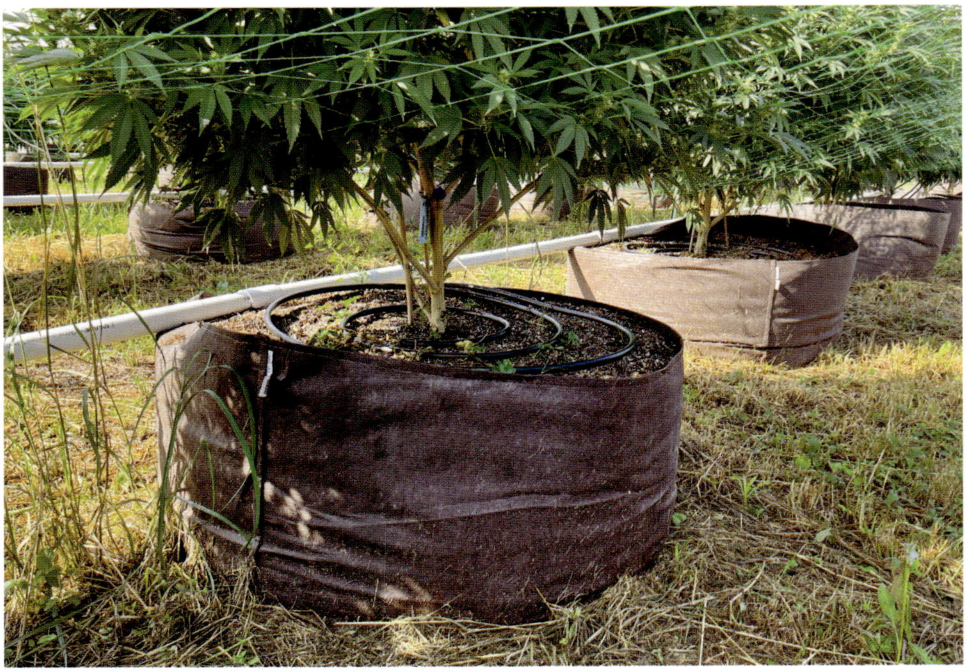

PHOTO: ROOTPOUCH.COM

Drip lines encircle the plant to ensure an even spread of feed and water.

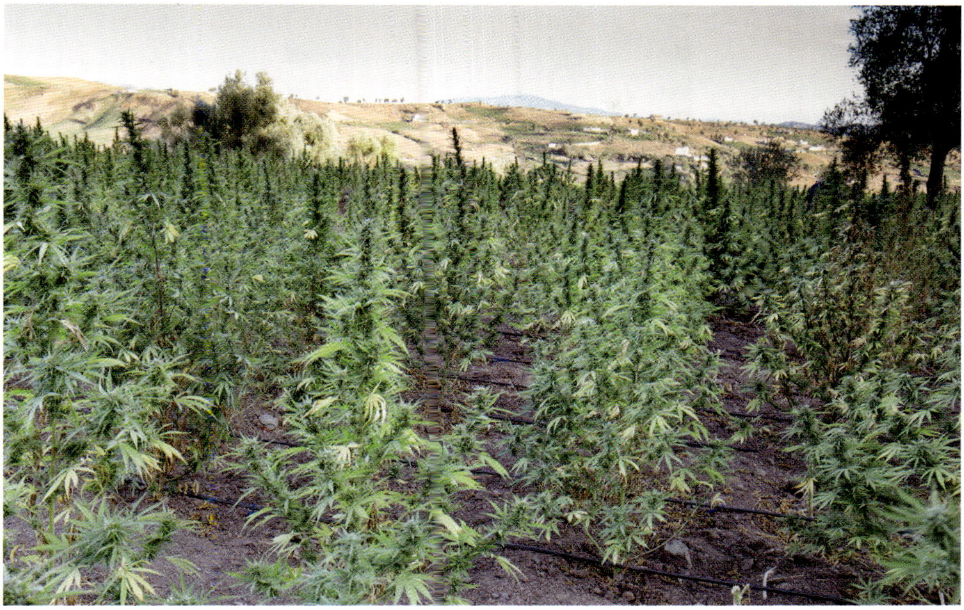

Towering colas into the distance. You can still make out the irrigation lines.

PHOTO: DINAFEM SEEDS

aeration by occupying space, which reduces soil density. Some outdoor growers have reported up to 20–40% reductions in water requirements for their plants. The crystals will continue to absorb water from rain, providing a consistent water source.

Rain, Water, and Resins

When it comes to rain, water, and resin management, it's essential to consider your watering methods. While sprinkler-type systems can function automatically with a timer, it's generally better to water the base or lower sections of your plants while keeping the upper parts as dry as possible. Water can't wash away cannabis resin, but direct contact with water on the flowers and leaves can introduce unnecessary stressors. Avoid direct contact between water and the flowers because watering can dislodge resin glands if the water pressure is too strong.

The flowers will naturally dry out following rainfall and should recover well. However, prolonged rains toward the end of the flowering phase may impact the final yield's quality. Unfortunately, there's little growers can do to prevent rain from hitting outdoor flowers, except for transitioning to a greenhouse setup.

Most cannabinoids are not water-soluble but may exhibit solubility in water to some extent. Any loss of resin due to rain is primarily a result of direct physical interaction. Though cannabis plants have naturally developed defenses to cope with such conditions, most growers prefer to minimize exposure of their outdoor flowers to rain by growing in a greenhouse instead.

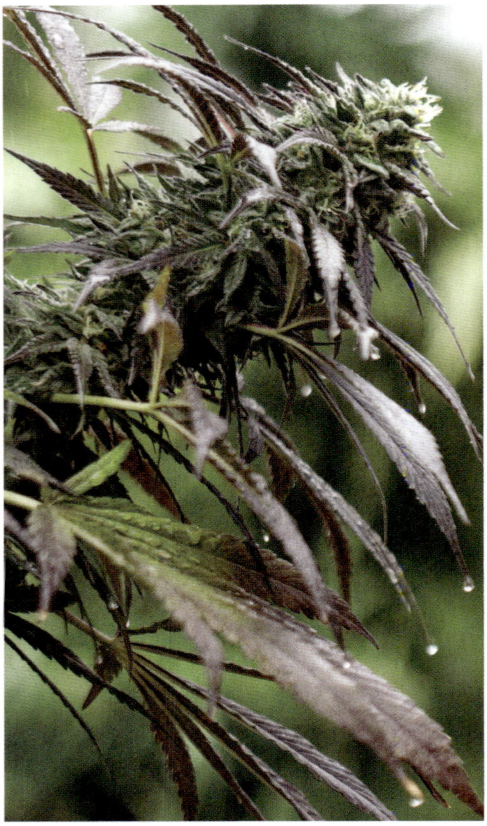

Rainwater flows to the leaf tips and drips down. They dry up when the sun comes out.

Pests and Fungi

Ensuring your outdoor plants remain healthy and free from unwanted predators is crucial. During the second week of vegetative growth, consider spraying the area with an organic pesticide. Detailed information on dealing with pests and predators is covered in Chapter 15.

Observation, Measurement, and Response

Outdoor plant care involves careful observation and measurement to ensure appropriate responses. Consider not only your plants but also the entire environment, including soil conditions, weather, and surrounding vegetation. Take note of any animal presence, mold, or encroaching ivy. Asking questions and taking precautions can prevent issues down the line.

Observation provides valuable insights, but measurement is necessary to obtain precise data. Measure moisture levels, nutrient feeds, and pH levels, and track the number of weeks or days your plants have been in the vegetative and flowering phases. Use appropriate tools and calculations to make accurate measurements to help you stay on track with your growing plan.

Customize responses to address specific problems based on measured data, never relying on random guesswork or untested experimentation. Later chapters discuss various response strategies in more detail.

Adding Nutrients

You can add nutrients at any point during the plant's life cycle. For example, shifting to a higher phosphorus feed during the flowering phase can promote bud growth. Outdoor soil treatment closely resembles indoor practices, except for the weeding process. For more information on feeding throughout the plant's life cycle, refer to Chapter 8 on indoor plant feeding. You can also explore organic growing techniques such as the use of slow-release feeds that can be mixed into your soil. Trial, error and good note-keeping will be your friends in this endeavor.

PHOTO: DINAFEM SEEDS

Guerrilla Outdoor Gardening

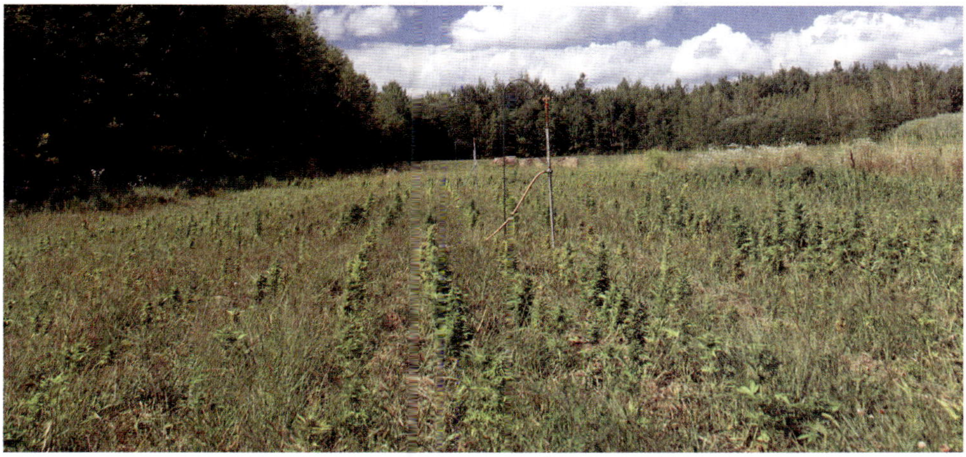

Autoflowering plants plotted alongside weeds and grasses. The grass and weeds help hide the short autoflowering plants.

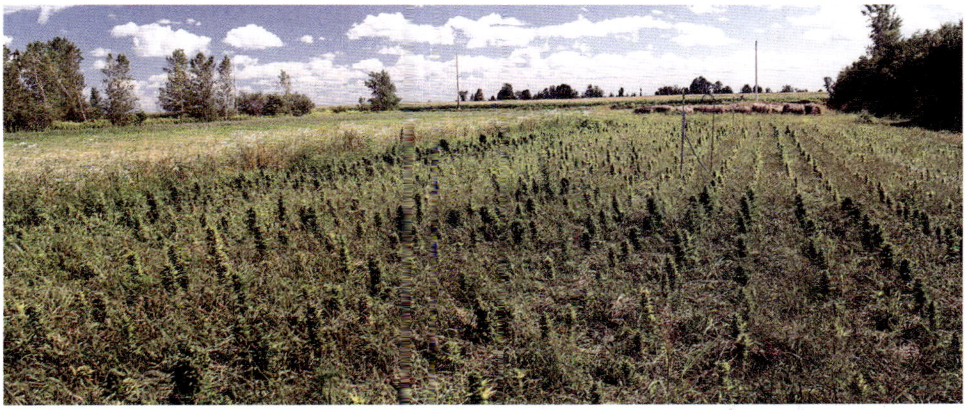

Autoflowering plants will stay short and flower quickly.

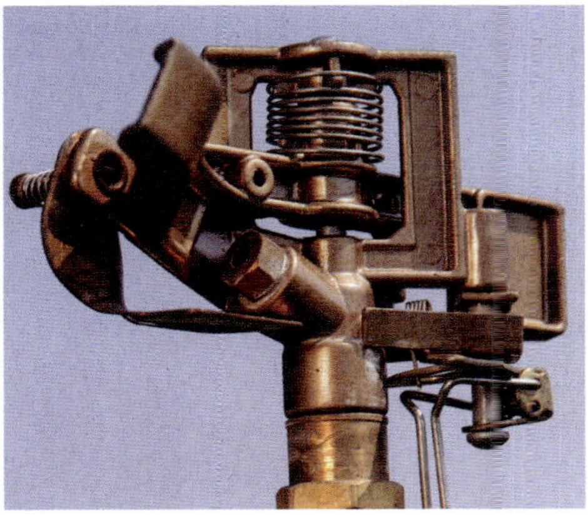

Outdoor sprinkler system.

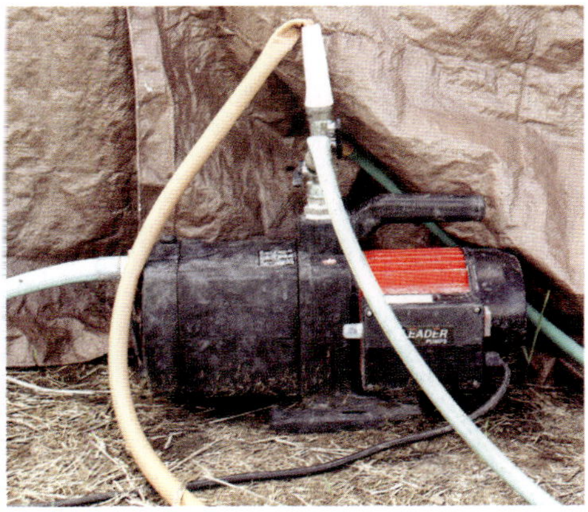

A pump for irrigation.

PHOTOS: DAVID STRANGE

California Snow: Seed to Harvest

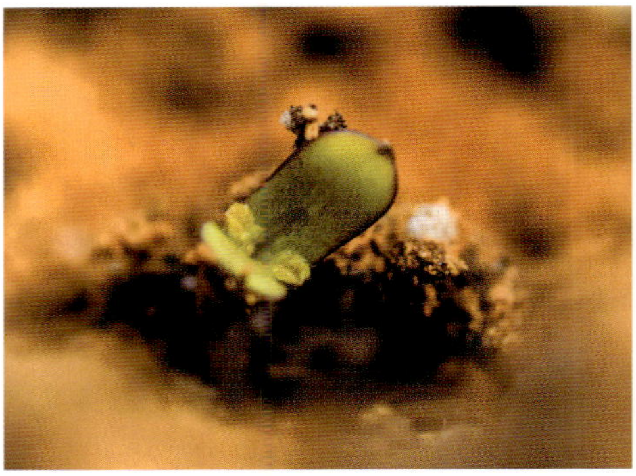

Tender roots push down into the soil as the seed breaks open.

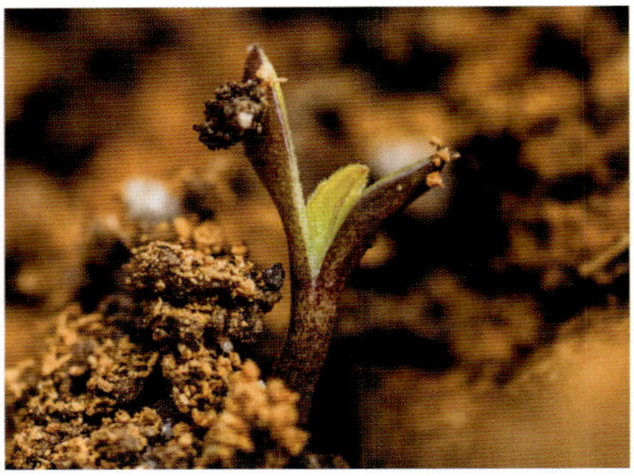

The seedling sprout is delicate but willing to grow into a bigger plant.

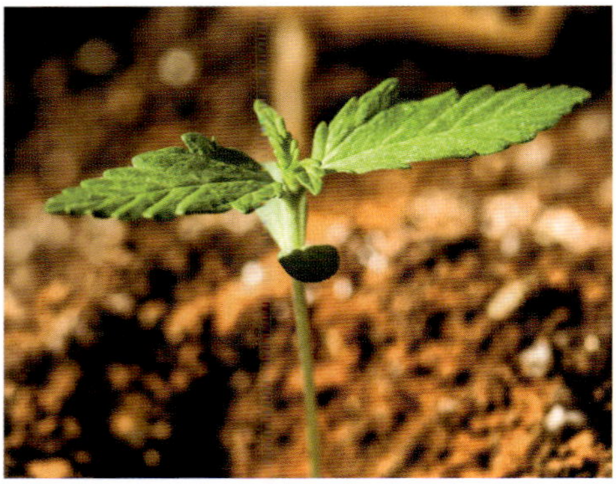

The leaves unfurl, reaching up to soak in the light.

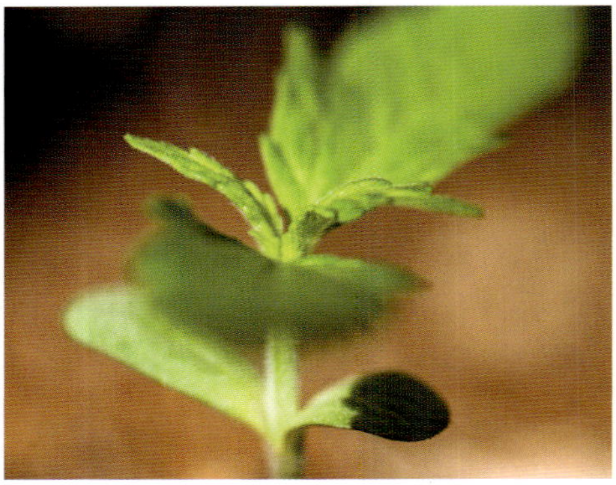

The plant grows more vibrant green leaves.

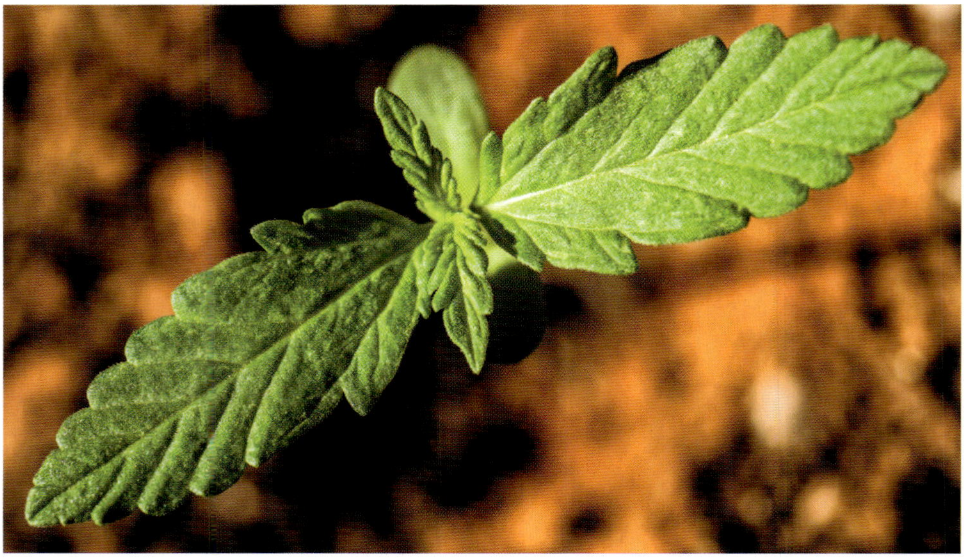

The promise of becoming a mature cannabis plant. This seedling looks healthy and strong.

PHOTOS: ERIC PALMER

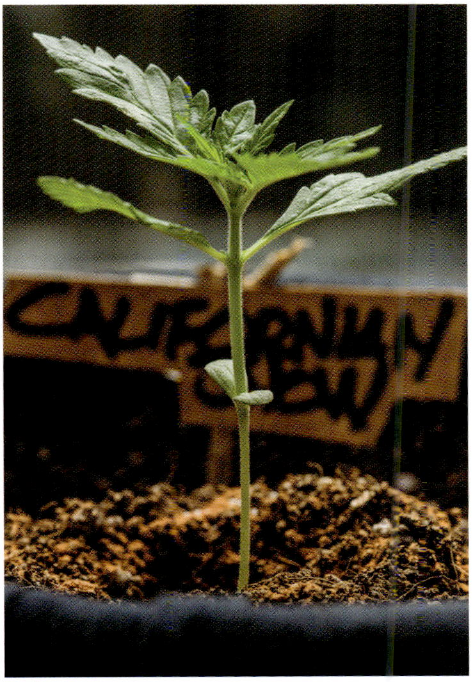

Light, nutrients, and water all fuel the seedling's rise.

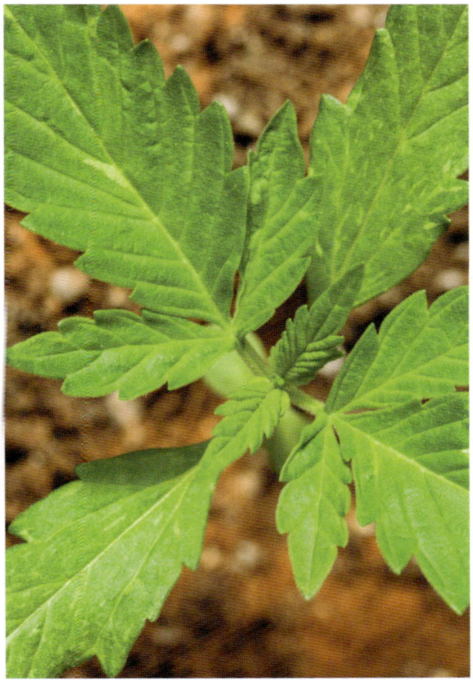

The seedling's perseverance means it stands resilient on its upward journey.

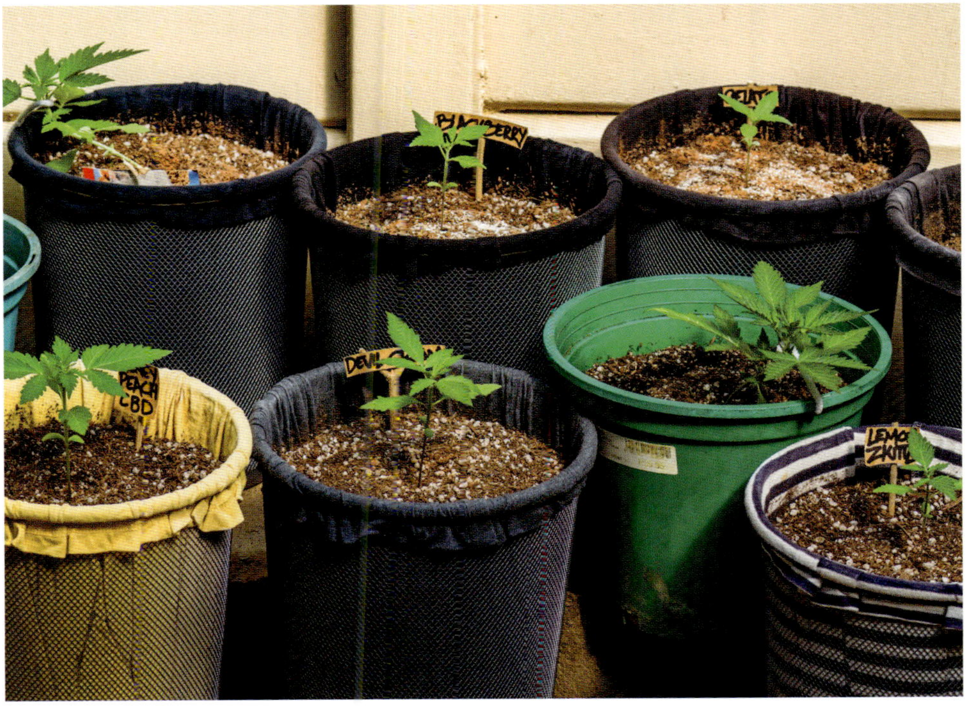

No matter the strain, they all start the same way: From a seed to a seedling.

continues...

California Snow: Seed to Harvest *continued*

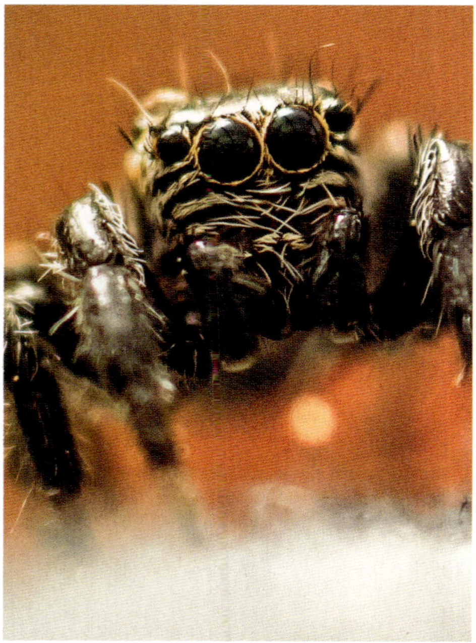

A friendly spider comes along to catch any pests that might harm the seedling.

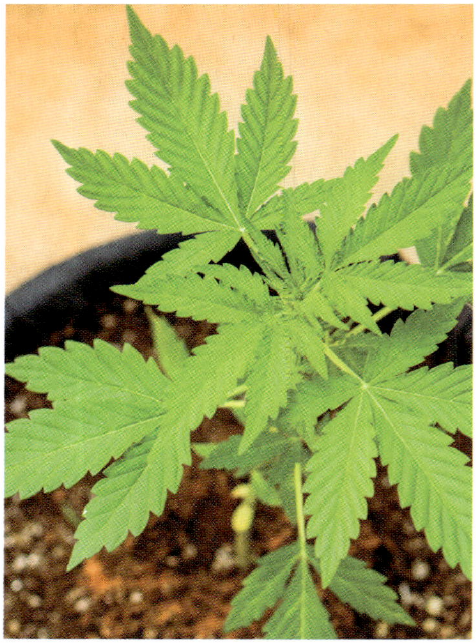

Branching out with purpose, these new shoots add strength to help the plant thrive.

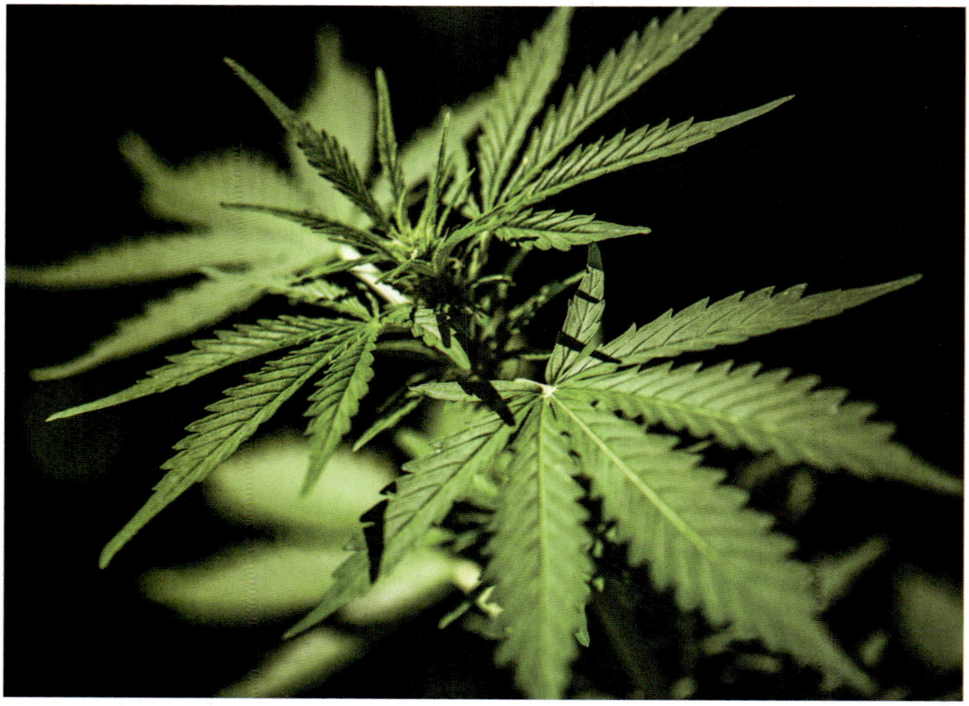

The leaves grow broader to take in more light. The plant starts looking less fragile and more vigorous.

PHOTOS: ERIC PALMER

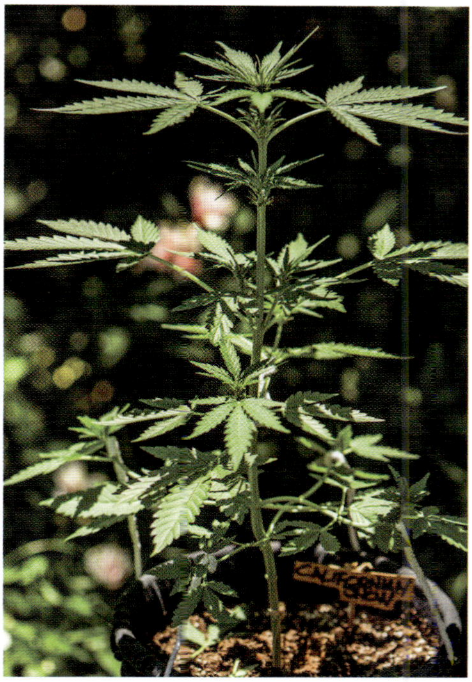

Promising flowers to come, buds will start to appear at the end of vegetative growth.

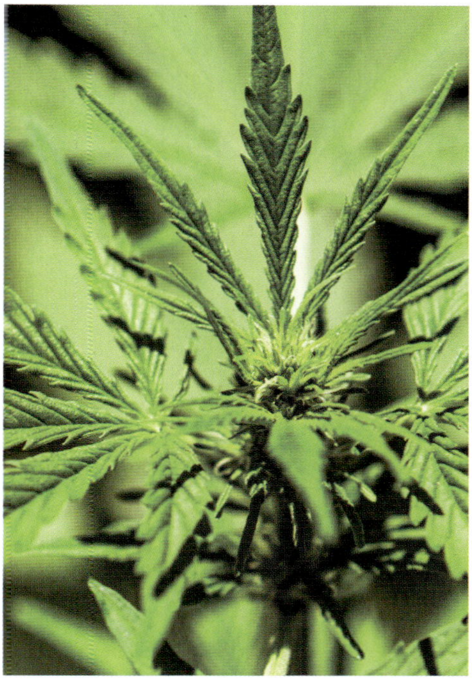

Blooms appear at the nodes, signalling vitality.

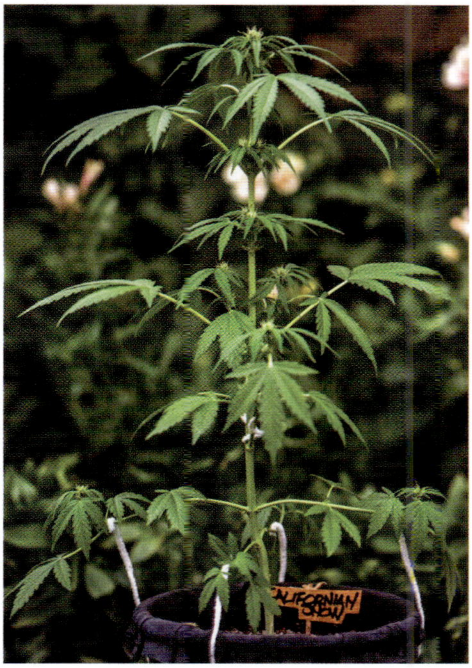

The lower branches are being trained with pipe cleaners.

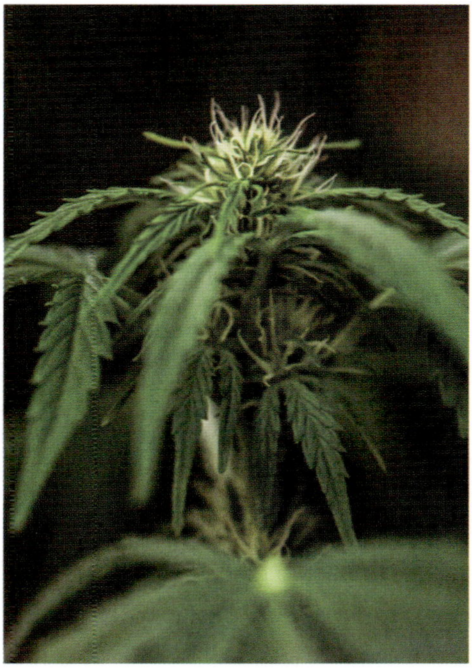

The early flowering stage shows pistil growth protruding at the nodes.

continues...

California Snow: Seed to Harvest *continued*

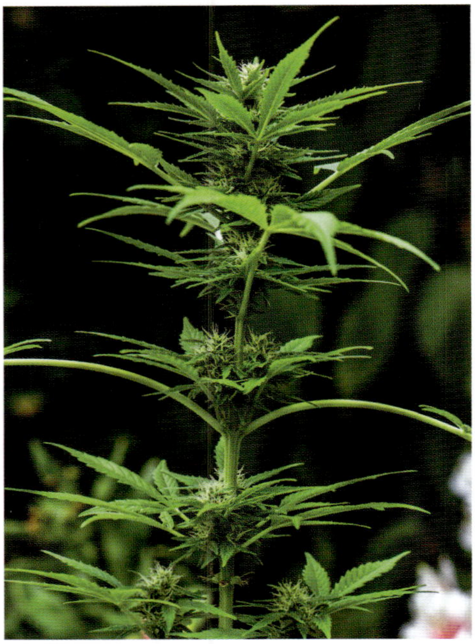

Cannabis fragrance fills the air as days pass with pistils curling and swelling.

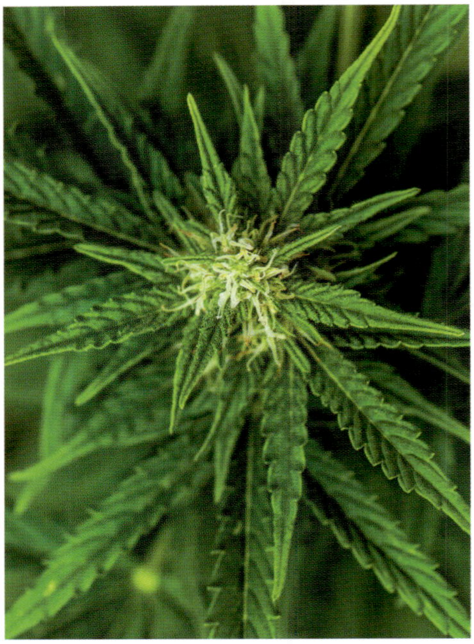

The beginnings of a top cola are small at first but will grow much more prominent in time.

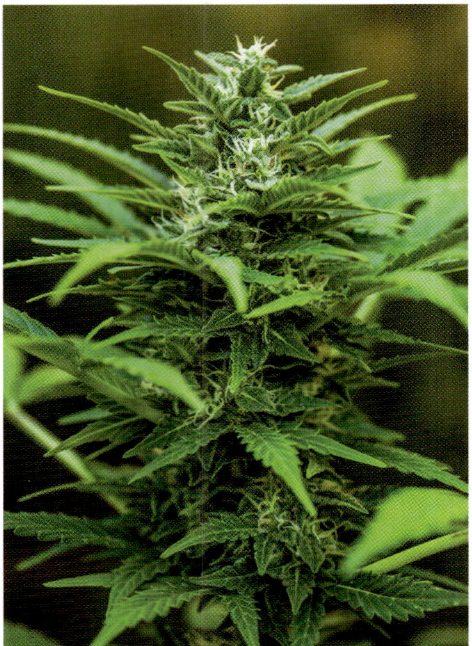

Flowers turn a creamy color in contrast to the lush green of the cannabis plant.

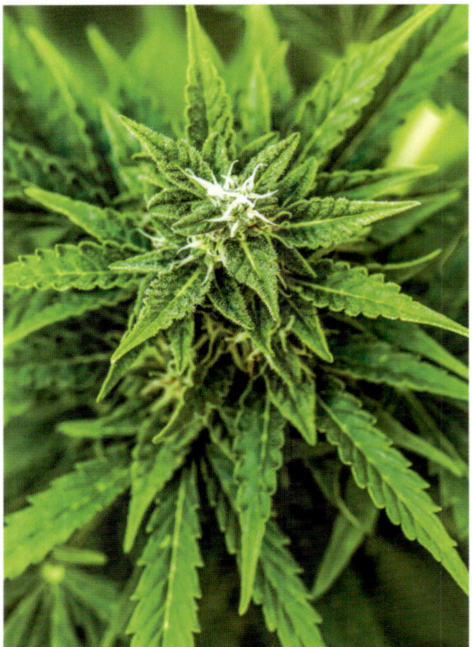

The natural beauty of the cannabis plant is a living work of art and symbolic of life.

PHOTOS: ERIC PALMER

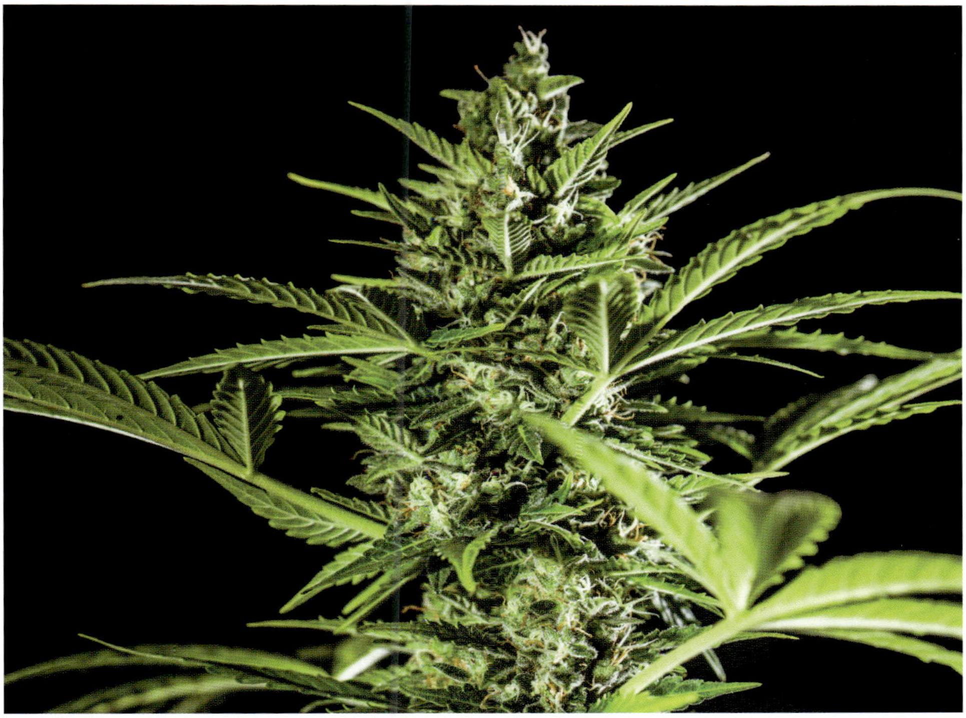

The top cola fills in as its flowers explode in a mass of sticky, trichome-covered pistils.

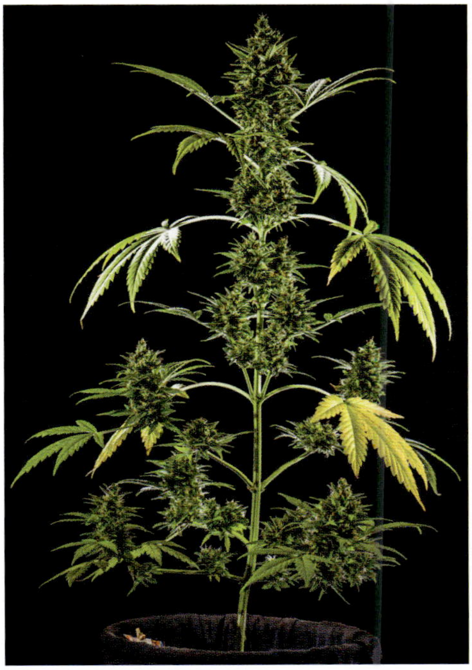

The node gaps between branching fill up with more flowering clusters of dank buds.

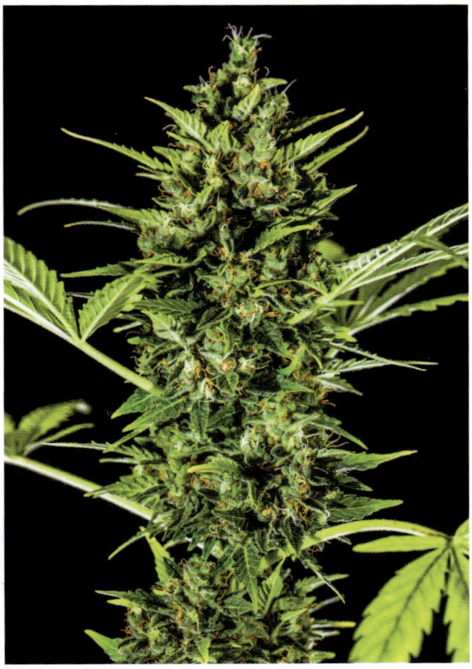

The top cola stands as a testament to the attractiveness of cannabis flowers. *continues...*

California Snow: Seed to Harvest *continued*

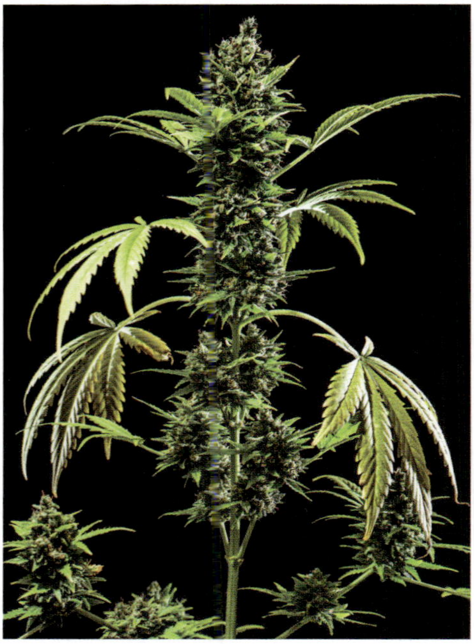

The flowering symmetry spreads evenly to more parts of the plant.

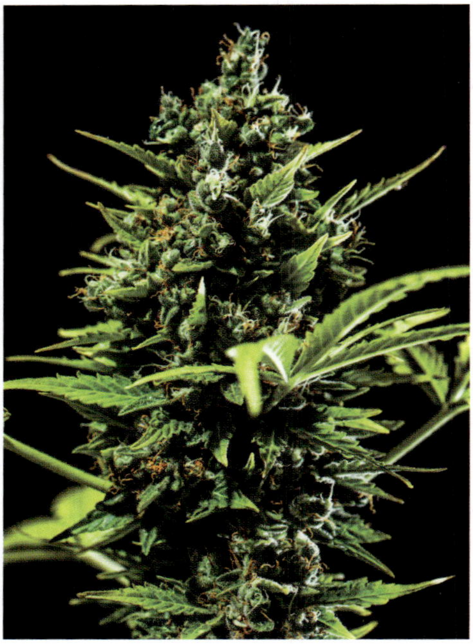

Getting wider as significant flowering growth pushes genetics to their limits.

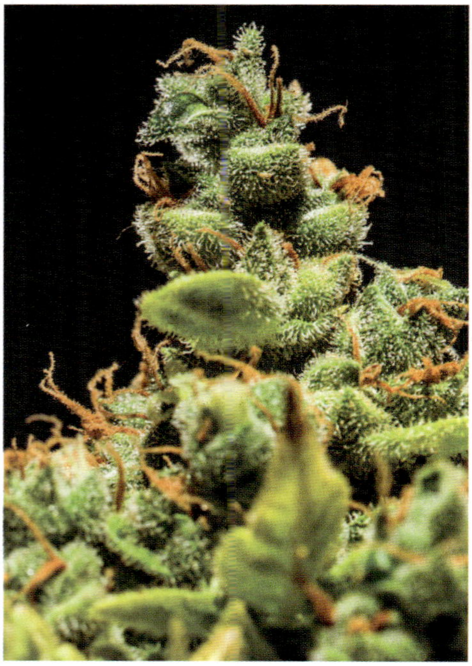

Pistils turn amber as the flowering plant nears harvest time.

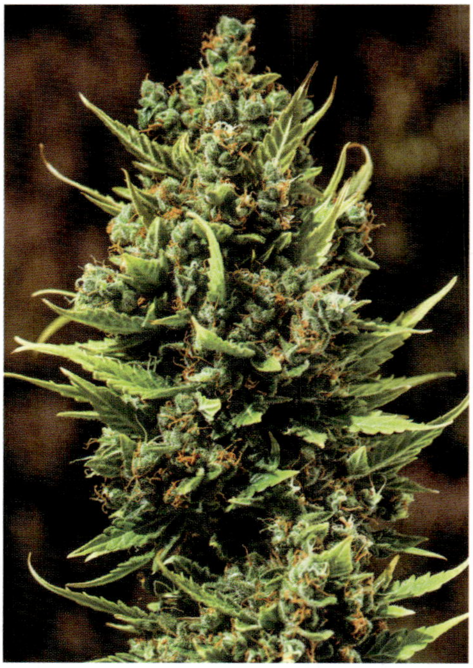

The top cola is in full bloom and is as thick as an arm.

PHOTOS: ERIC PALMER

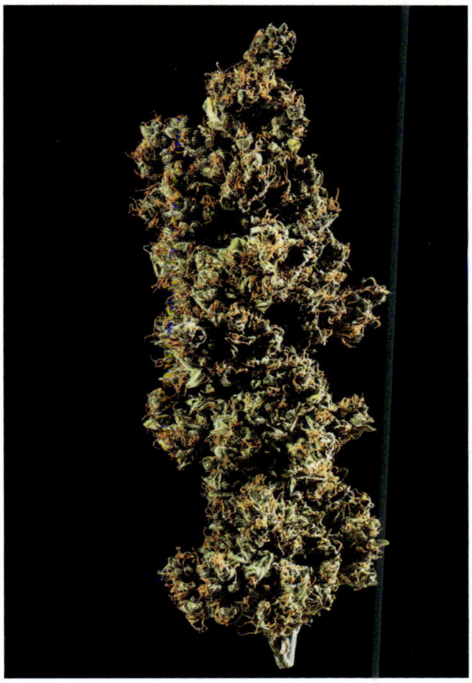

After harvesting and manicuring, the amber colors overtake the green.

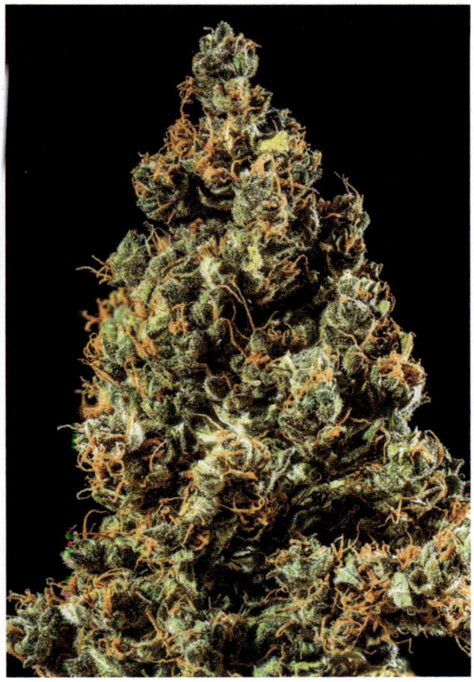

A closer look reveals the extensive mass of flowers blooming.

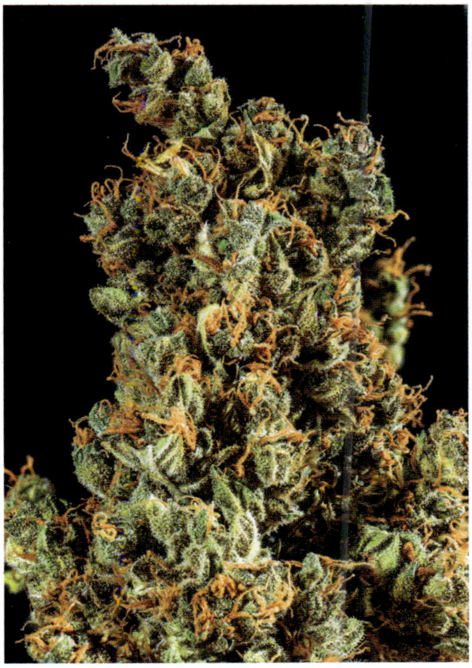

These pistils are full of resinous trichomes bursting with cannabinoid oils.

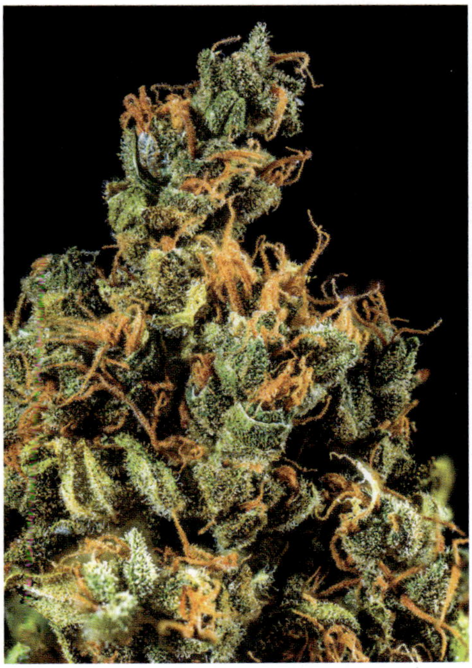

Trichome and pistils cover this spectacular bud.

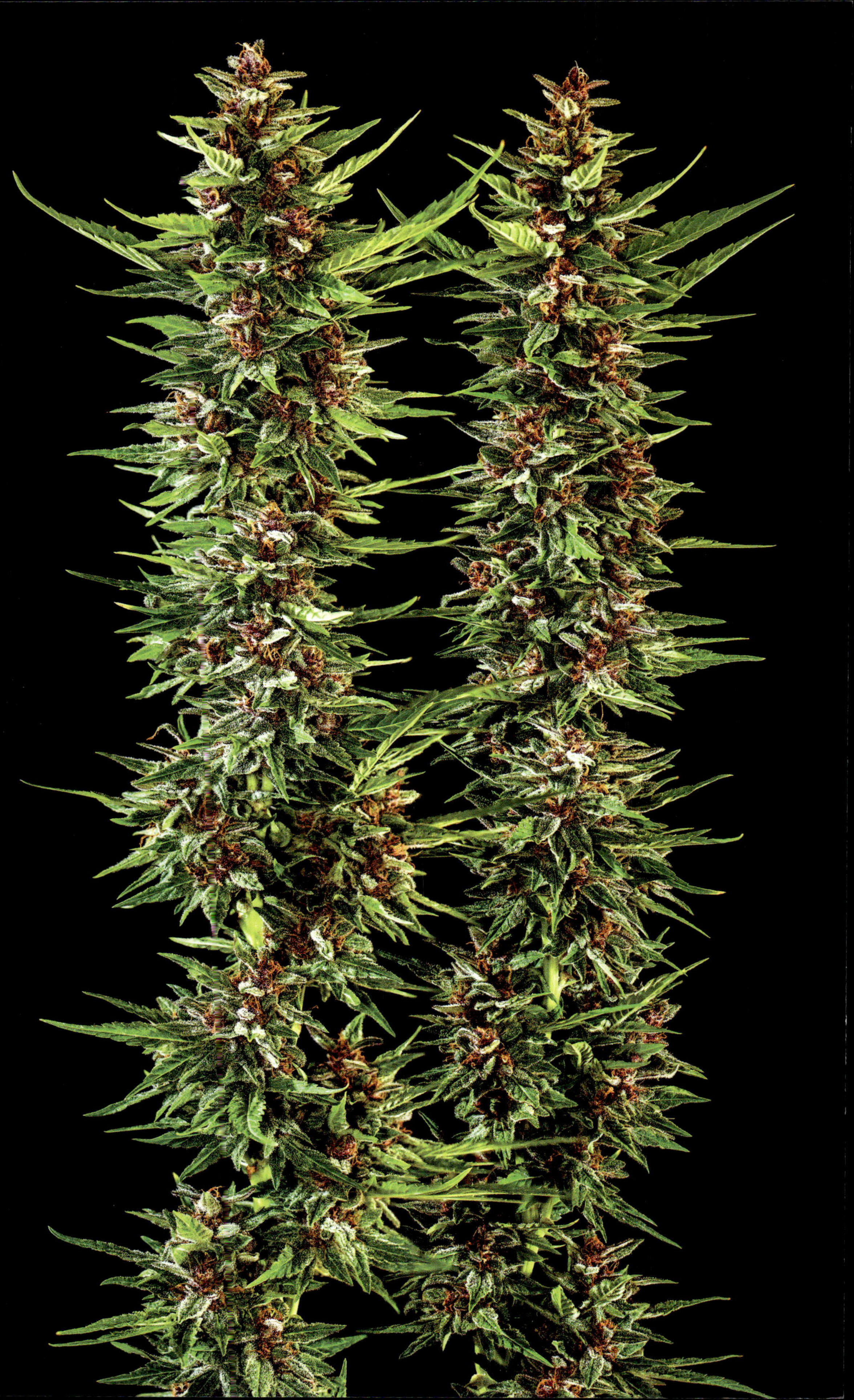

13

Caring for Mature Cannabis Plants

This chapter generally concerns plant shaping techniques to increase your chances for success and optimization. Plant management is part of cultivation. There will sometimes be direct intervention between the grower and the plant to achieve a desired outcome. Plant manipulation is important for growers who choose methods such as SOG and ScrOG, or want the plants to do something particular that they wouldn't normally do under natural outdoor conditions.

Toward the end of the flowering stage, your cannabis plants will fill out into the traditional Christmas tree shape. From vegetative growth to the end of flowering, the cannabis plant develops in three main sections: the top cola, mid-section, and base. The top cola will develop a large amount of bud. In most cases, it will be the highest yielding part of the plant, if allowed to grow without pruning. However, plant manipulation allows the grower to achieve a more even dispersal of bud.

The mid-section of a plant contains stems with old and new leaves, and as the plant progresses this should fill in, with buds growing between the nodes. Although these buds will generally be smaller than those found at the main cola, they should be just as potent. Growers who find that bud taken from the mid-section is less potent have likely not allowed their flowers to develop enough before harvest. Finally, towards the base of your plant, you will find large fan leaves and a small amount of bud. Growers, especially SOG and ScrOG growers, should treat each section differently to get the most out of their plants.

Defoliation

If your plant is growing under an artificial light source and the fan leaves are not receiving much light during flowering, you may be tempted to prune them away. This is called defoliation. Should you defoliate? This is a topic of heated discussion in the cannabis growing community. In this book, you will see some plants that are defoliated and others that are not. Here, we explain the advantages and disadvantages of defoliation.

PHOTO: ERIC PALMER

Defoliating Your Plants

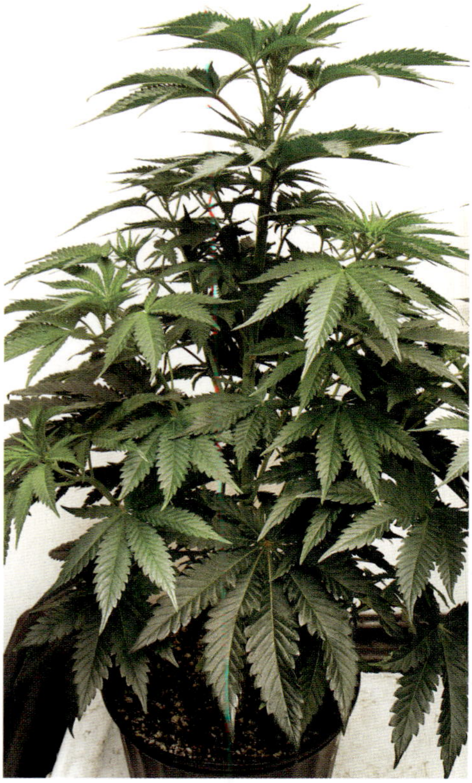

Some growers prefer to remove the lower leaves. This is called defoliation.

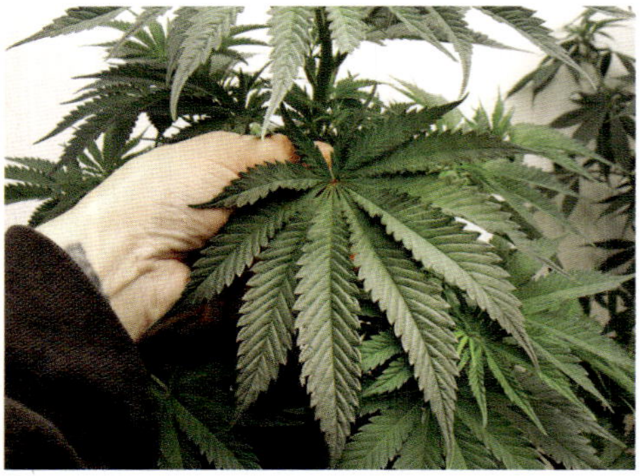

Defoliation is done by extensive pruning, including hand-picking leaves off.

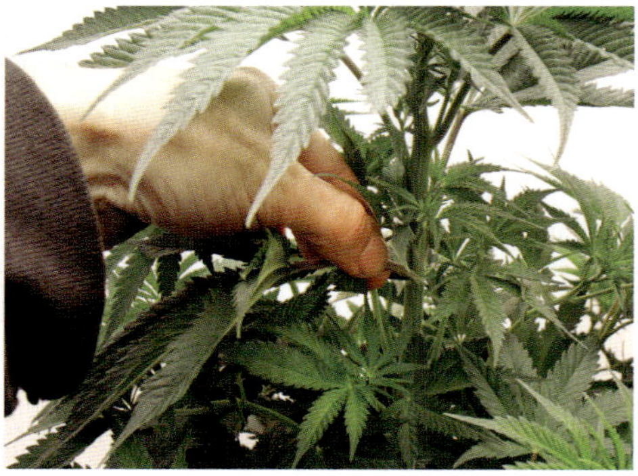

Some lower leaves will snap off if you bend them at their base.

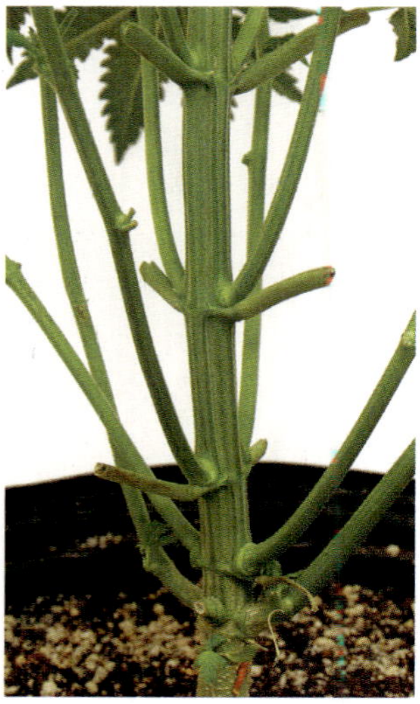

The lower part of a defoliated plant.

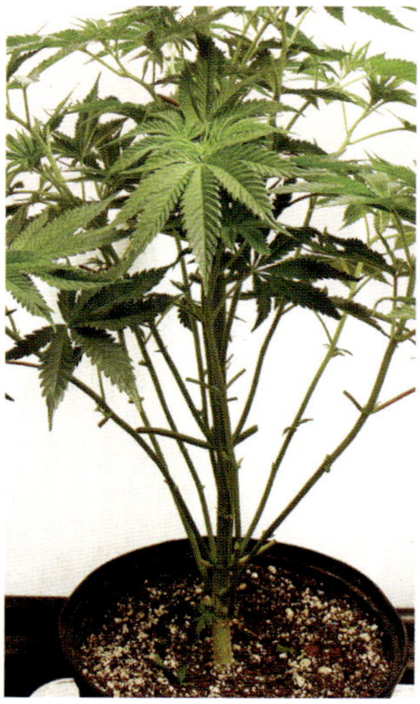

A defoliated plant will show signs of having prior leaf.

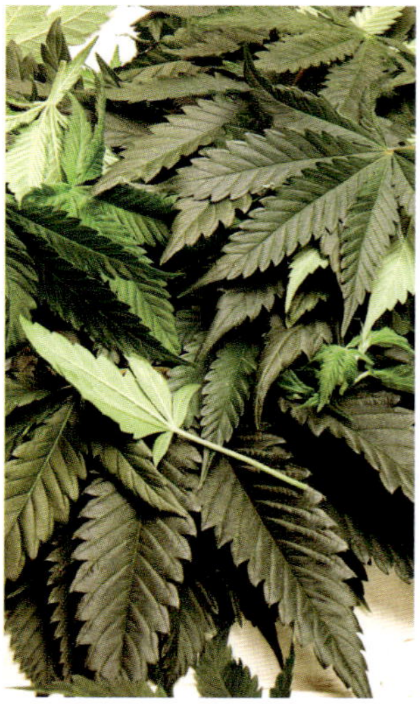

Defoliated leaves can be used as compost.

PHOTOS: DAVID STRANGE

Fan leaves produce sugar, stored as starch, used in bud production. Cutting away the fan leaves may cause stunted bud growth, resulting in a smaller yield. This implies that the only time you should remove fan leaves is when the leaf is moldy, badly burnt, or covering a large bud mass. Clipping a leaf in half along the blade is better than removing it. Partial clipping is a strategy growers use to keep as much leaf as possible. That also goes for other leaves, but fan leaves are generally the ones growers like to remove, especially during the late stages of flowering. You still can and should remove dead leaves from your plant and throw them away. Never leave the dead matter on your soil as a fertilizer, as it attracts unwanted pests while decomposing.

The other side of the argument is that plants naturally shed these leaves in nature, so we should remove them to allow light to penetrate the shaded flowering sites. Lower leaves may wilt in the late stages of cultivation and reveal shaded flowers. Maybe the plant will have a sufficient amount of stored starch to finish flowering, even after this loss. Light is a crucial factor in bud development, and if the lower leaves prevent light from reaching a bud due to an uneven canopy, you will want to tie them back or remove them. Refer to the ScrOG section for information on clipping fan leaves and defoliation.

You can experiment with both methods to find which produces better results for you. Maybe the results will be the same, indicating that the pros and cons cancel each other out. If you see improvements with a method, maybe that is the way to go for that strain in that environment. We keep an open mind on both methods.

Types of Plant Manipulation

This chapter covers essential aspects of caring for mature plants, including thinning, pruning, light bending, training, topping, bushing, increasing yield, and cloning. Using these methods, you can directly manipulate your plants to achieve optimal growth. However, before we discuss this, we should address the sun's natural manipulation of the outdoor cannabis plant.

Light Bending (Phototropism)

Light bending occurs when a plant grows at an angle towards the light; you might have seen this happen with the plants on the perimeter of your grow area. If you filmed your plants with a time-lapse camera, you would see a slight sway in the population from East to West as they reach for the sun. However, plants outside are able to "reset," bending in both directions throughout the day. For plants indoors, the bending is only in the direction of the light source. If your plants bend too much, they may eventually grow into another plant and block the light, a form of competition you don't want in your grow area. It is also a sign that your lighting system is not delivering enough light to your whole grow area. There may be some bending in all systems as the outer area of the grow receives lesser light due to the spherical spread of intensity. Even systems using reflectors will have areas where less light is being spread than in others. Chapter 7 will give you more information on lighting.

During flowering, the buds will become heavy. This may cause the stems to bend to the point of hitting the ground, resulting in uprooting and possible breakage where the stems and branches haven't been strengthened enough through wind or fan-related resistance. Of course, genetics also plays a role in susceptibility to breakage, but overextending can happen for many reasons, and uses too much energy that could be devoted elsewhere.

If you don't have a fixed system, like a fixed hydroponics setup, you can avoid light bending in an indoor grow environment by turning your plants around. If a plant leans too much in one direction, move it toward the middle of the grow space or turn the pot around. It only takes a day or two for the plant to straighten. If your plants can't be easily moved, as with fixed hydroponic setups, ScrOG, and outdoor gardens, you may have to tie plant to plant or branch to branch to prevent bending. If the plants aren't bending into each other, the competitive impact is minimal and it isn't really a problem. However, it can signal that your grow space has too many plants, insufficient light, or both.

If you are growing outdoors and have a significant problem with light bending, you may have to cut away surrounding foliage to allow more light to reach your plants. The outdoor section in this book will help you find a better outdoor patch to prevent this problem from occurring. If surrounding foliage can't be reduced or objects are in the way, try using string, plant stakes, or bamboo to keep your plants upright. You can use a natural biodegradable hemp cord to minimize waste. Tying is also how we get additional benefits from pruning techniques.

Pruning for Yield

Pruning is the process of manipulating the number of node regions, or potential bud sites, on your plants. It has nothing to do with thinning, which involves removing whole plants to eliminate potential competition. Pruning is accomplished using clippers held at a 45-degree angle to the shoot being cut; this cut area will go on to develop two more branches. You can see this process occurring naturally by looking at a tree, and noticing how the stem divides into branches which sub-divides into more branches which divide into new shoots and leaves. Some pruning methods involve cutting branches or stems to cause more flowers to grow. Cutting a plant at the stem will automatically result in "topping," which results in growth of more than one top cola; we'll discuss this below.

Branches can break naturally due to environmental conditions, causing more branches to grow near the damaged area. Why do plants do this? A branch that breaks may have too much weight for its environmental conditions. So if it breaks, would it not make

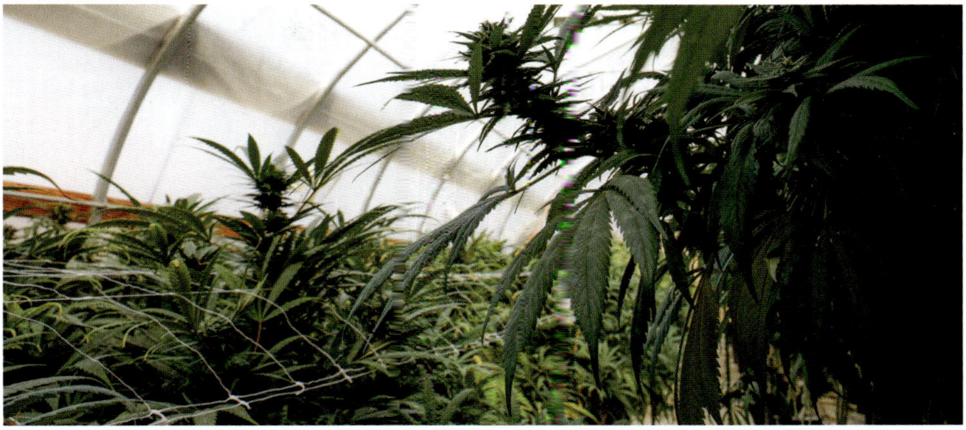

Plants will always compete for light by growing where they can find enough of it.

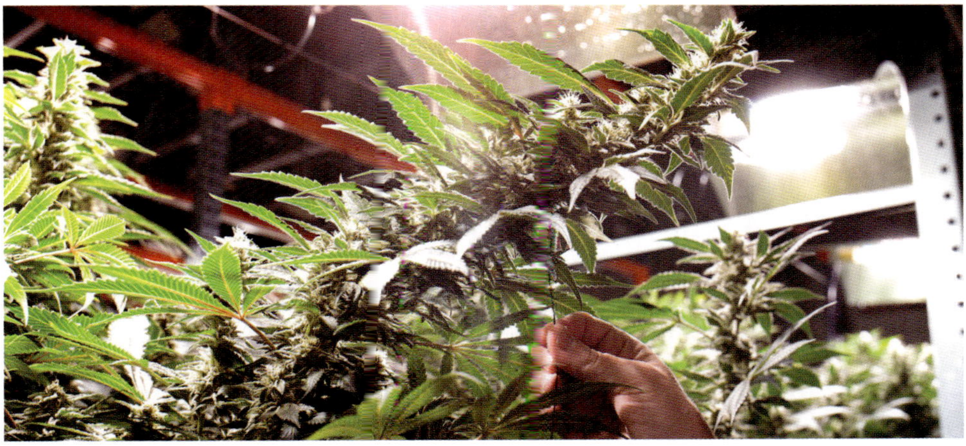

You can check your flowers by bending branches and stems carefully.

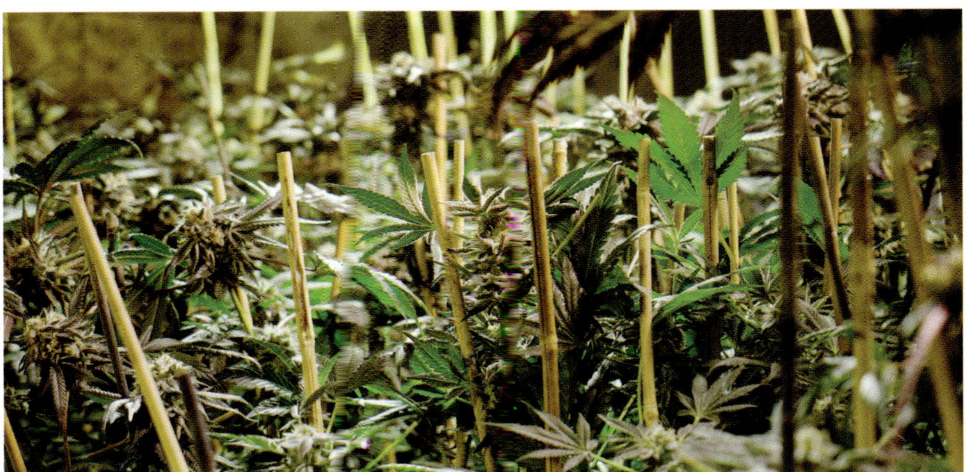

Planning is half the work for dealing with densely packed flowering plants.

PHOTOS: KRISTEN ANGELO (TOP AND MIDDLE), TRICHOME ART (BOTTOM)

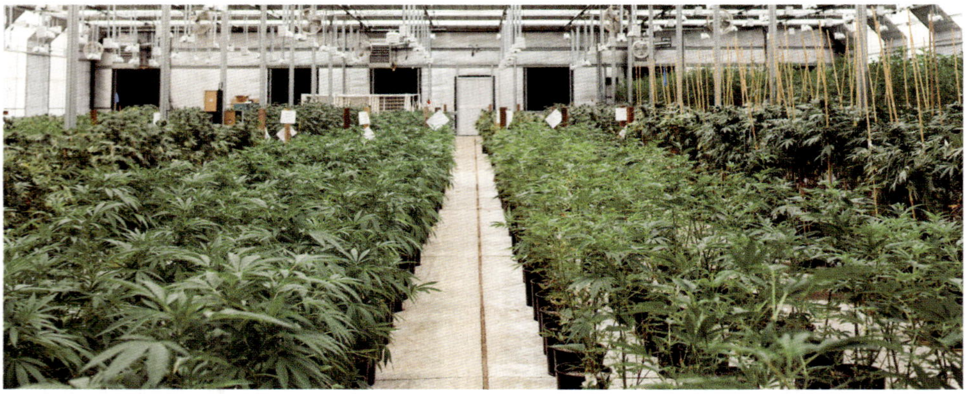

Pruning is done during vegetative growth when the plant has developed enough branches and so removing some doesn't stunt growth dramatically.

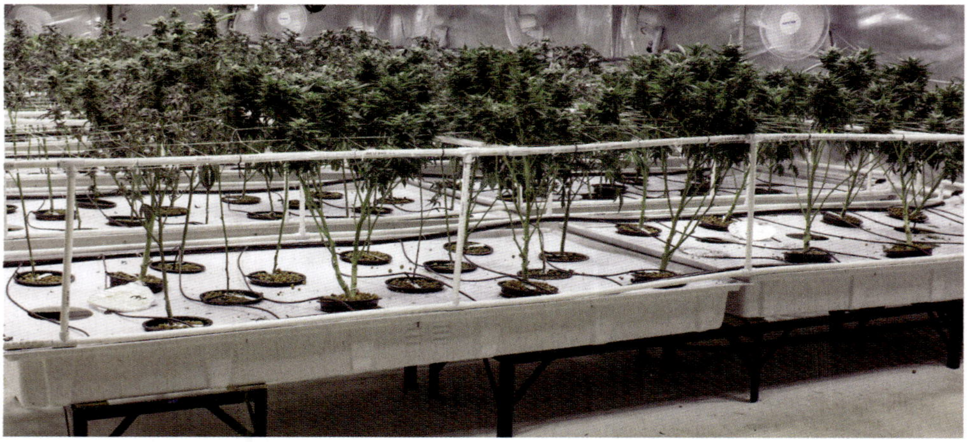

Pruned plants have a lower center of gravity which promotes stability for hydroponic systems.

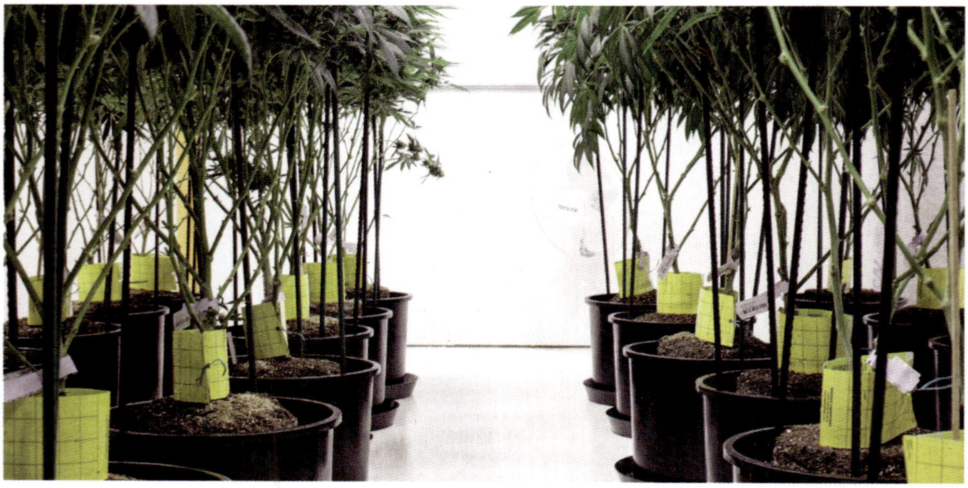

Branching can get complex with pruning.

PHOTOS: KRISTEN ANGELO

sense for the plant to spread that weight more uniformly over two branches instead of one? That is precisely what natural selection has selected: The ability of plants to respond to stresses in ways that can spread their branch, leaf, flower, and fruit weight around more after branch splitting or breaking. Pruning is a method of deliberately forcing a plant to do this. If you prune above a node region with the leaf side being above and the stem side below, branches will develop there to replace the missing branch. This division spreads the bud weight, which is determined genetically; rather than being entirely on a single branch it is instead shared between two or more branches. It's important to note that pruning should not increase the production of flowers, as double yield in that area could potentially cause more branch failure. However, you can sometimes get more out of pruned plants depending on the strain. These plants are considered favorable to pruning. You will find them suitable for ScrOG grows as well.

Cannabis plants grow branches out from the stem. The bushy look is due to development of new leaves and branches at the node regions. Some of these new branches may develop new shoots, but those are somewhat smaller and thinner, and don't support as much bud growth. Node regions produce the most branching from pruning techniques.

Indica plants tend to be smaller than sativas. As you learn about pruning your plant, you can produce small, bushy sativa or sativa hybrid plants that grow in smaller spaces. Without pruning, a sativa plant can stretch to five feet or more.

There is a limit to how much you can prune a cannabis plant. If you prune a stem or branch, it will split in two. You can prune these new branches, and end up with four. You can try to prune each of these four to try to create eight, or prune some lateral branches, but the results will depend on the strain and its genetically predetermined branching limit. If the plant has reached its threshold, it will not produce more branches. All strains are different in this respect. We can understand more about these constraints by looking closely at "thinning" and "topping," particularly the latter which is probably the most popular form of pruning among cannabis growers.

Your plants can be categorized into regular plants or bushy plants. Regular cannabis plants will bush somewhat naturally, but bushy plants that have been pruned are much broader. We will first discuss some processes that retain a regular shape.

Thinning

Thinning involves reducing the density of plants in a group by cutting the plant at the stem to manipulate plant height or removing plants from the grow altogether. Plants naturally compete for light, and plants that grow taller than the rest can easily prevent light from reaching other plants in the group. This competition is especially noticeable with unstable strains and new hybrids in which some of the population may grow more vigorously than others.[1] Thinning also occurs when you remove males for sinsemilla.

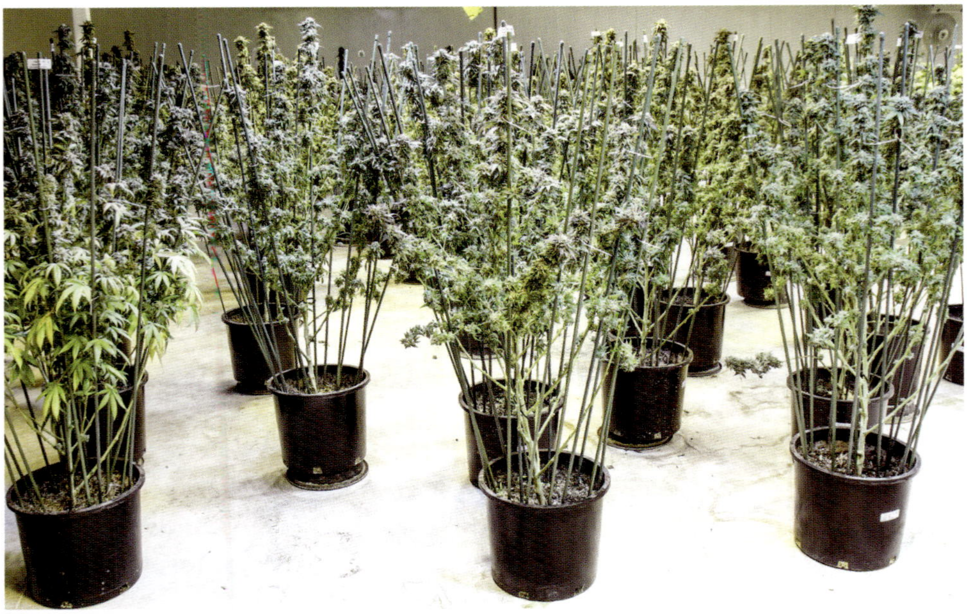

The spread in this shot is due to the removal of males. These plants have been thinned out by pruning and defoliation.

PHOTO: DAVID STRANGE

When growing from seed, thinning your crop either by cutting or removing plants creates a more even canopy and allows light to penetrate every top cola without some plants getting in the way of the other plants' light requirements. SOG growers know about this because it is an important part of that method.

A crop of clones taken from the same mother should not need to be thinned because they will all possess the same genetic makeup. However, clones will not grow uniformly if light dispersal is uneven or each plant doesn't receive the same environmental conditions (including water, nutrients, and air). The clones that receive more light have a better rate of photosynthesis and will grow more vigorously. Growing from clones is an excellent way to achieve optimal uniform results.

It is not unusual for outdoor growers to thin their plants, since the sun is not under their control. Thinning can be avoided somewhat in the next grow season by predicting space issues and planting better, which is why growing the same strain again and learning from prior experience achieves better results.

What is the best course of action if a big, vigorous plant is doing better than all the others, but you don't want to chop it down to even the canopy? You might decide that the increased yield from the huge plant is worth its negative effect on those around it; you won't know for sure until it completes flowering. If it is easy to move the plant, you might consider that. If it's a potential mother, you might take cuttings.

In most cases, however, the large plant will prevent uniform growth and optimal results from your crop. You may be tempted to thin the "other way" round, leaving the taller plants and removing the smaller ones. However, statistically, height is a general indicator of potential plant sex; if you have started from seed, the taller plants are generally male, and the smaller ones are female. This dimorphism probably evolved due to gravitational forces, allowing taller male plants to drop pollen onto the smaller female plant's flowers underneath. Taller male and shorter female plant genes have more reproductive success in this model. Do not give in to the temptation of removing plants before identifying their sex. Pruning the taller ones down to size is better than chopping them away if you don't know their sex. You can, if you want, move taller and shorter plants into separate grow rooms, depending on your setup—a method of thinning commonly used for segregating males from females for breeding programs.

There is also the cosmetic aspect to thinning. Thinning your grow makes it look nicer and tidier, and improves your overall yield by preventing potentially good plants from being covered by weaker ones growing much taller. Height and size have nothing to do with potency, but can have some significance with yield.

By the time you have finished your thinning, you should have a uniform grow area with some clones that you can use to grow more bud. Thinning should not be used to make plants bushier. We will cover how to accomplish that later.

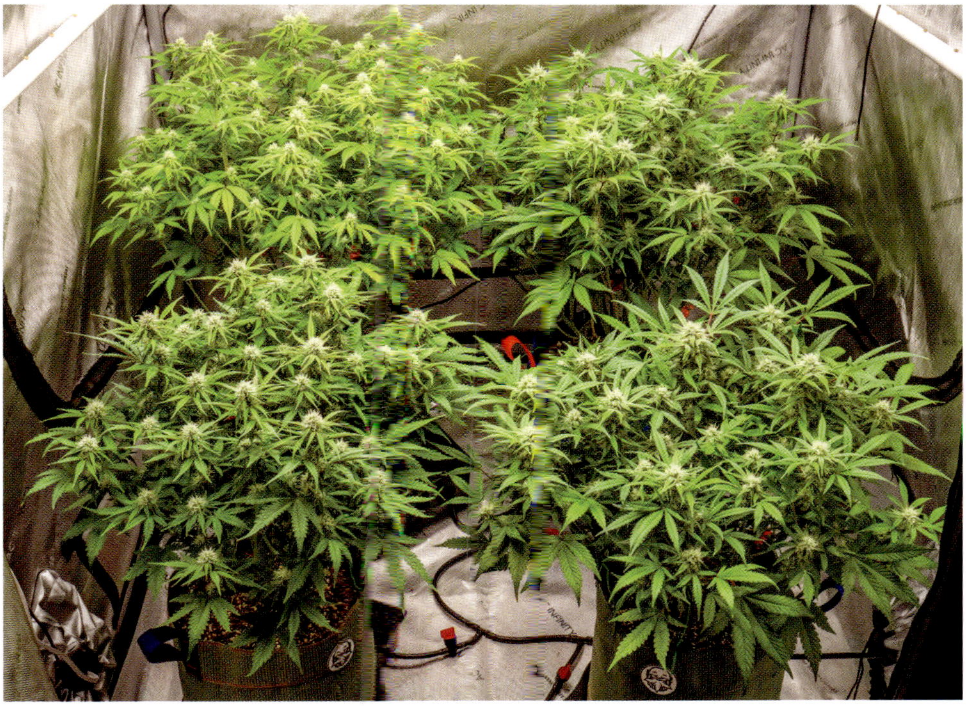

An even canopy is evident in these four plants.

PHOTO: JOE'S CANNA GROWS

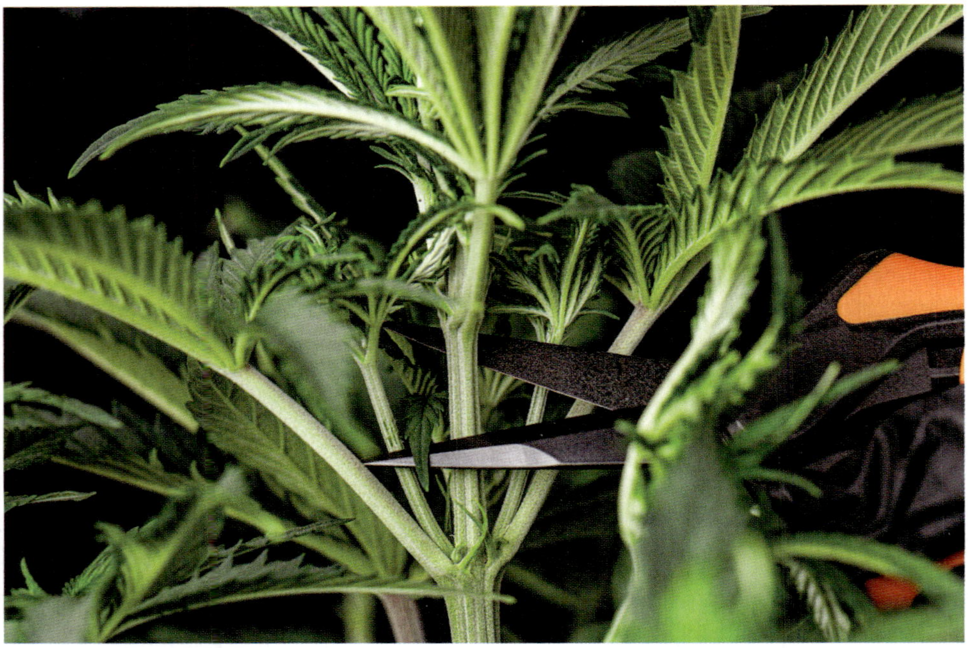

Clipping off the top of the stem results in two top colas growing from that spot.

PHOTO: ROB BRAMHILL

Topping

Topping is the process of splitting the top cola region into two or more colas. You can prune a cannabis plant but leave the top cola to grow. However, topping directly impacts the most significant part of the plant canopy and, arguably, the largest area of bud production. There are a few reasons why topping is recommend, but before we discuss them, let's talk about the timing of topping and what happens afterward.

Topping is all about timing. When you top or prune a plant, it needs to put more time into recovery and vegetative growth. Some cannabis growers will take a pair of clippers to the top of their plant during the third or fourth week of vegetative growth. The top of the plant, just above the last branch formation, is removed by shearing it away at the stem. Then, the main stem splits off in two or more directions, creating a V-shape at the top of your plant. The final result after flowering is two or more top colas instead of one. Some growers have even managed to force a plant to grow more than six top colas. However, topping does not always increase the final yield of the plant, and it may add more vegetative recovery time.

Depending on the strain and the growing environment, a topped plant will likely produce two top colas, each half the size of what the top cola would have been. Like branch production, each strain has a genetically predetermined threshold for bud production that cannot be improved upon . On the other hand, when grown without topping, some plants do not reach their threshold. The strain Blueberry is a good example of this; if you grow Blueberry without topping, you won't achieve maximum bud production from that plant, but you will if you top it. Other strains aren't so flexible, and topping will produce two top colas that share the same volume of bud that a single cola would have produced. So, why top? The answer is in designing your canopy.

Keep in mind that results of the topping method are strain-dependent, and you will need to experiment carefully. If you are starting with a new strain, try topping two out of 10 plants in every grow. You will learn a lot from those two plants. Plants are generally pruned three to four weeks into the vegetative cycle, but can be pruned sooner, later, or more than once. You can shape your plant during this vegetative prune. However, if you continue to prune, you have to spend more time in vegetative growth. Getting some "topping" experience is the only way to learn, but this technique becomes super handy when you understand it.

Pruning during flowering is not advised as the plant will be forced to divert its energy from bud production into branch and leaf production. This results in a slower rate of bud growth. For optimal growth, your pruning must occur well before flowering. Vegetative growth is also necessary before pruning. You also need to leave some leaves when you prune; topping a clone and leaving it leafless will usually cause problems, if not plant death, and you may have to wait weeks before you see a new leaf develop. You can top a plant in addition to pruning for bushes.

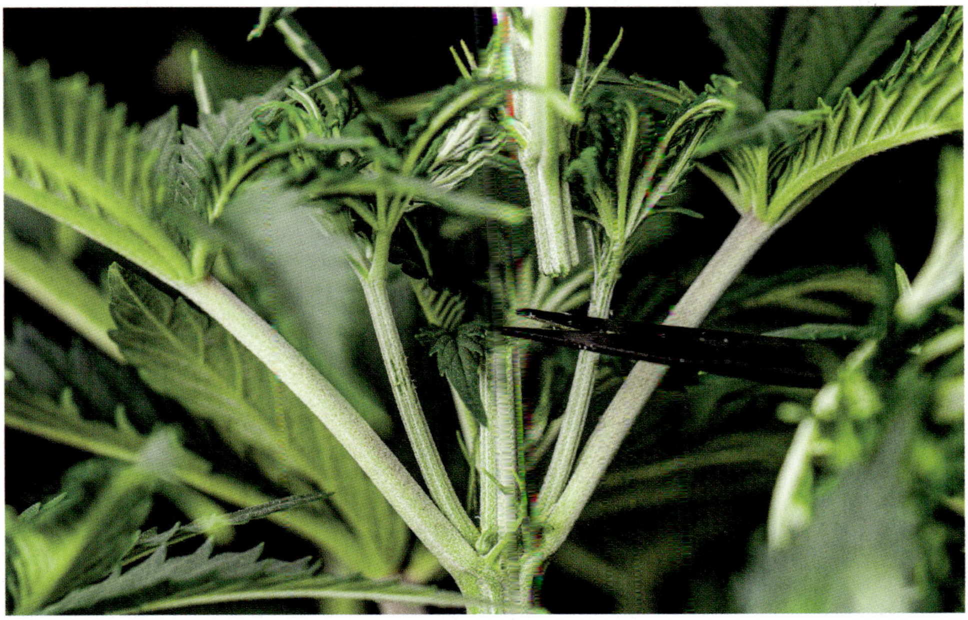

PHOTO: ROB BRAMHILL

You can also clone the clipped-away part. Notice this topped plant already has pre-flowering calyx development.

Topping and Training to Control Plant Height

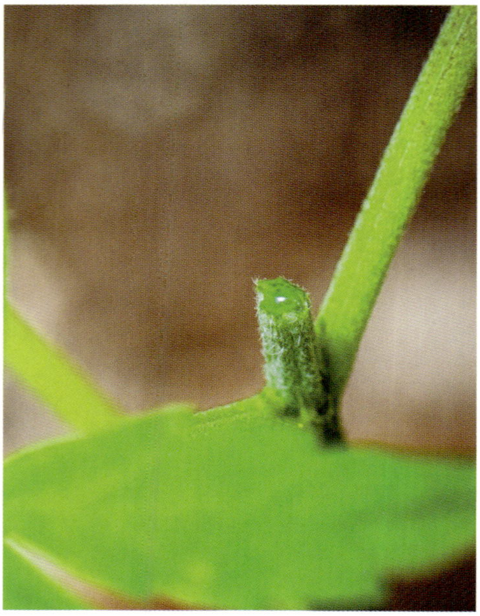

The stem is solid throughout, which is a good sign of health.

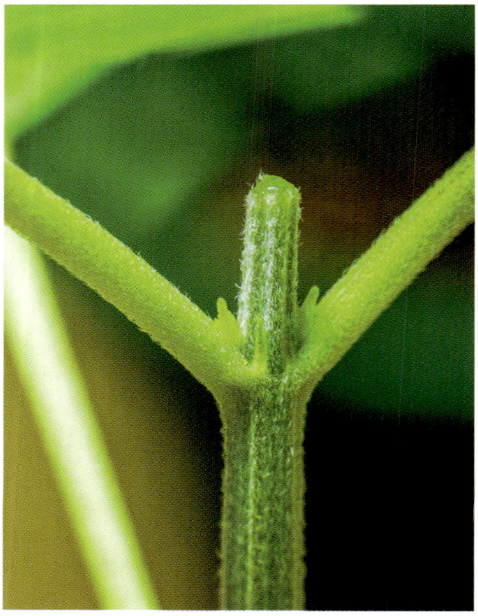

The base of the topped internode has two new sprouts on alternate sides.

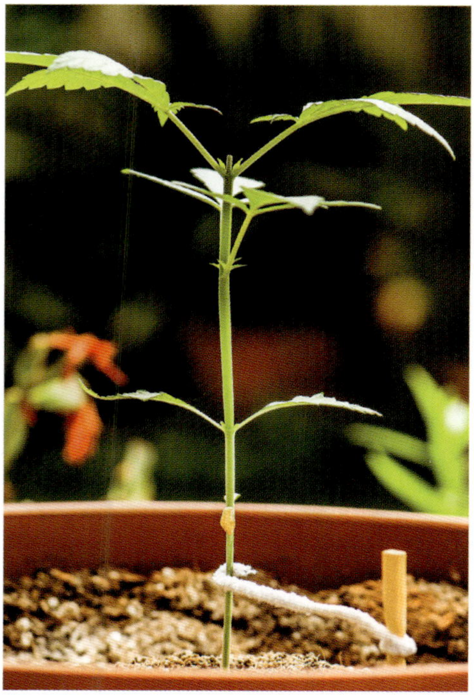

Leaf and stem growth will appear at the base of the topped stem internode.

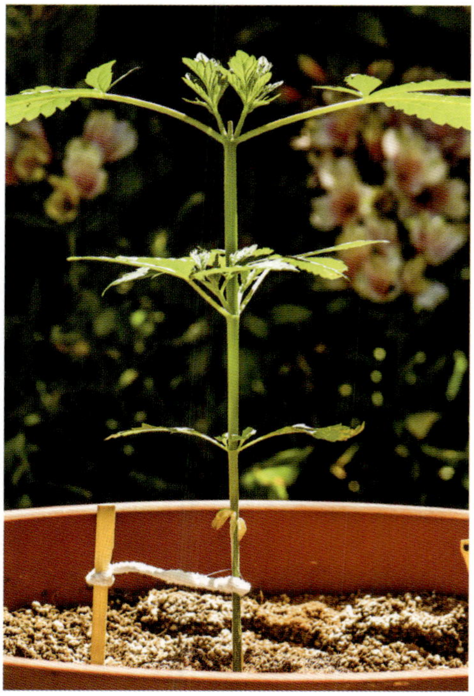

The two new sprouts form two new branches, like two main stems.

PHOTOS: ERIC PALMER

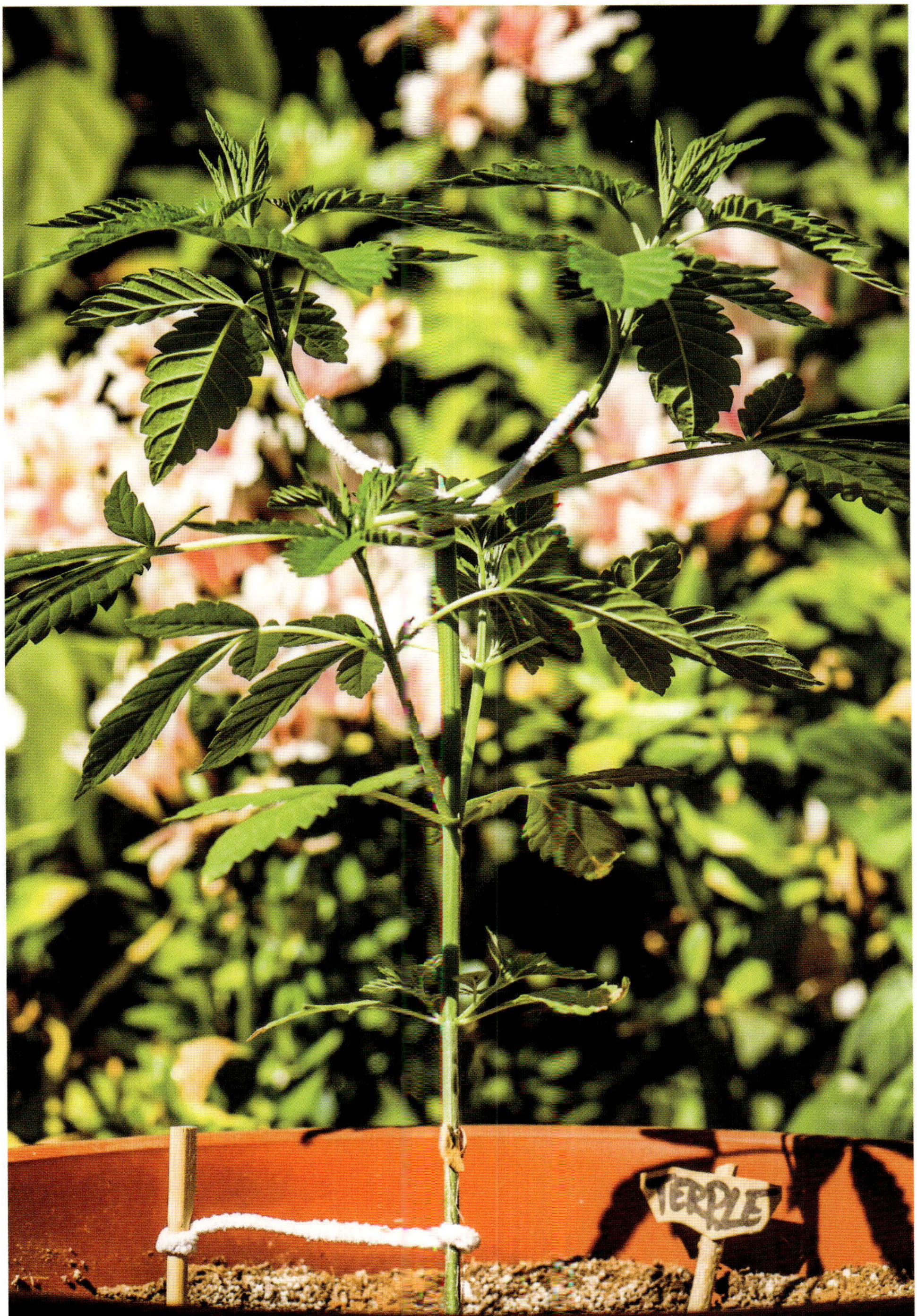

Topping into two branches will show more characteristics of a top cola on a stem than side branches for this Terple strain.

continues...

Topping and Training to Control Plant Height *continued*

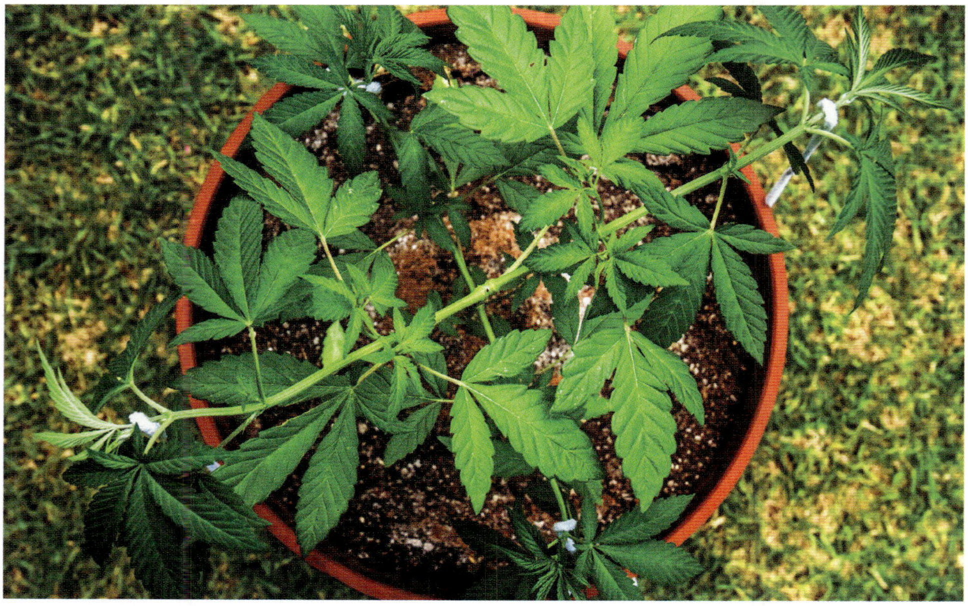

This is an overhead view of how pipe cleaners can be used to shape the height of the topped plant. This is not necessary but an optional way to control branching.

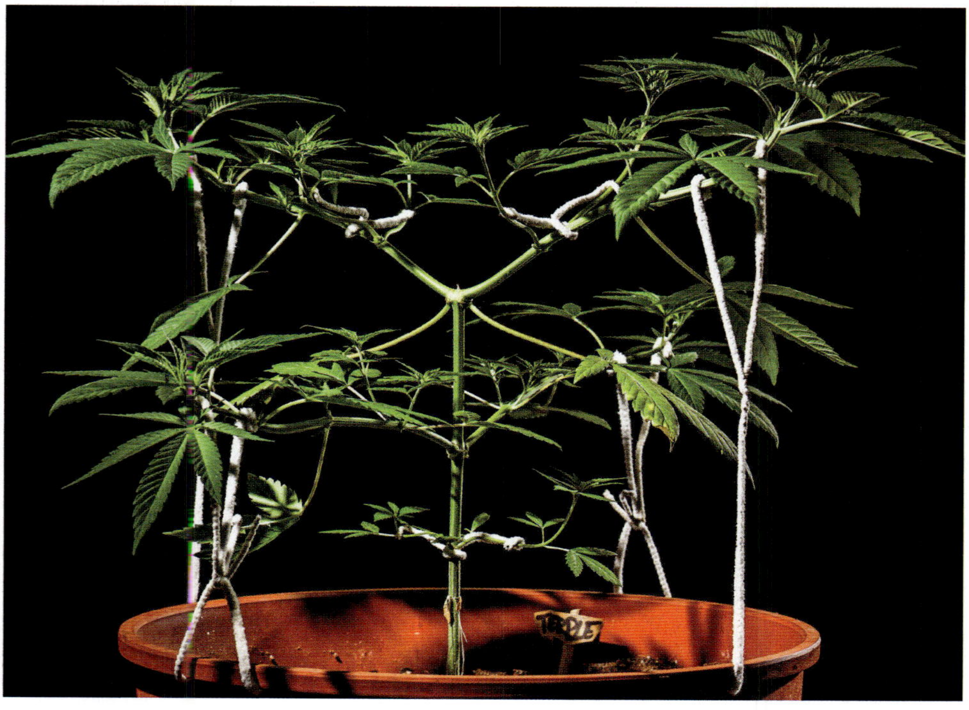

This is a side view of how pipe cleaners can be used to control the height of the topped plant. Some growers prefer to create more space between the topped branches.

PHOTOS: ERIC PALMER

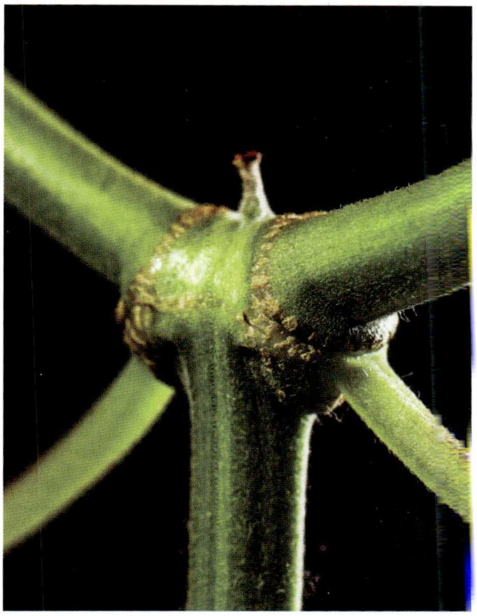

Topped branches are just as thick as the main stem. They will be duplicates of each other.

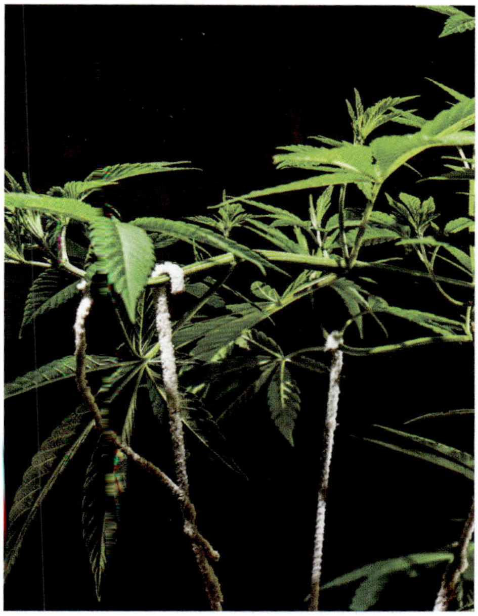

More pipe cleaners are added to tie the plant into a desired shape. This exposes more regions to the light

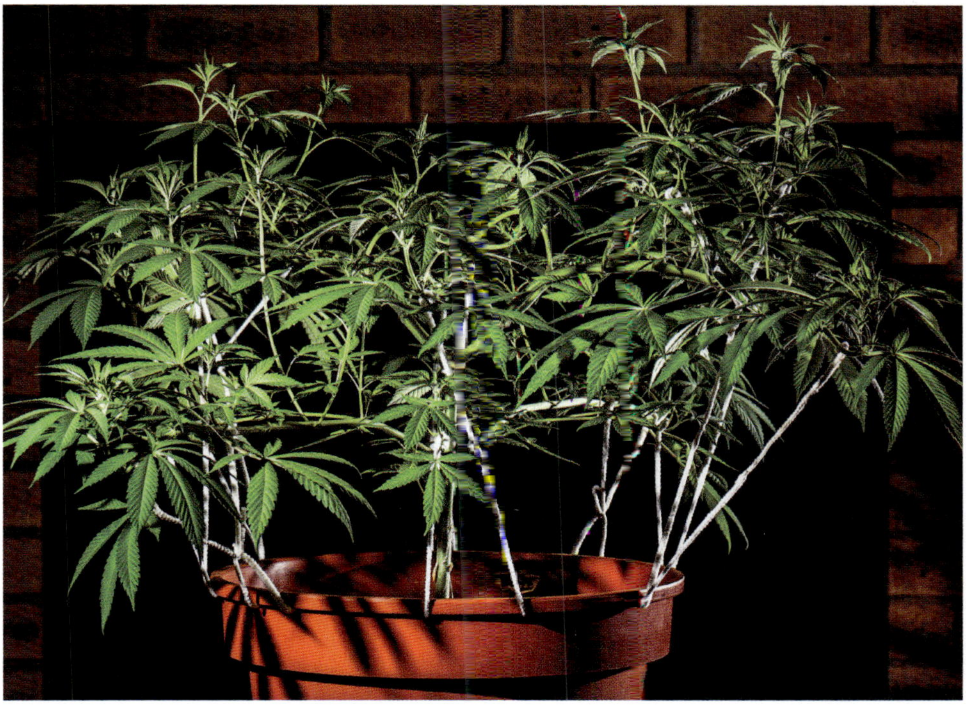

Tying down many branches of the topped plant creates a bushy shape to control height.

continues...

Topping and Training to Control Plant Height *continued*

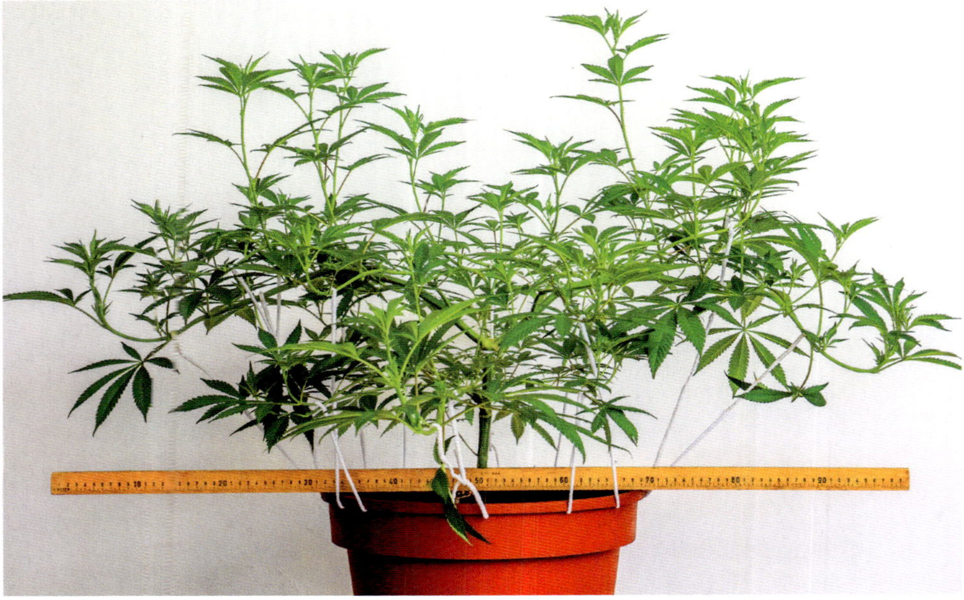

The topped and tied-down plant is now wider than its height. This is perfect for sativa hybrids that are grown indoors.

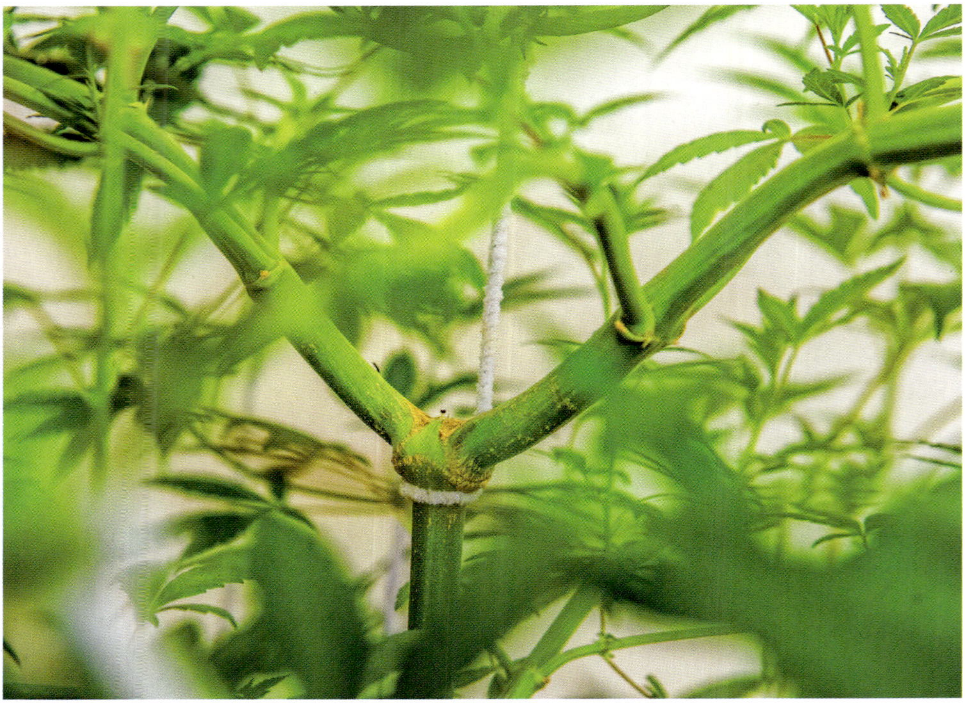

The plant's main stem continues into two pathways of a topped plant. This node region can be tied down with pipe cleaners to shape branches.

PHOTOS: ERIC PALMER

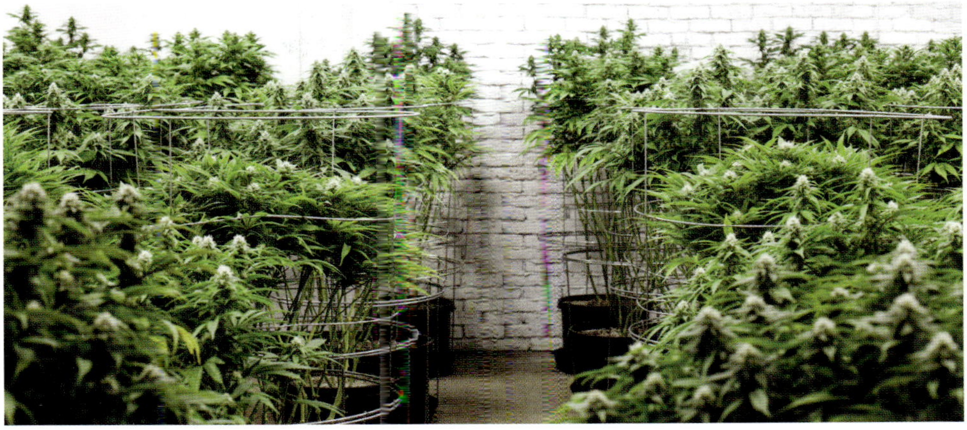

Dealing with lots of branches is best done with a mesh.

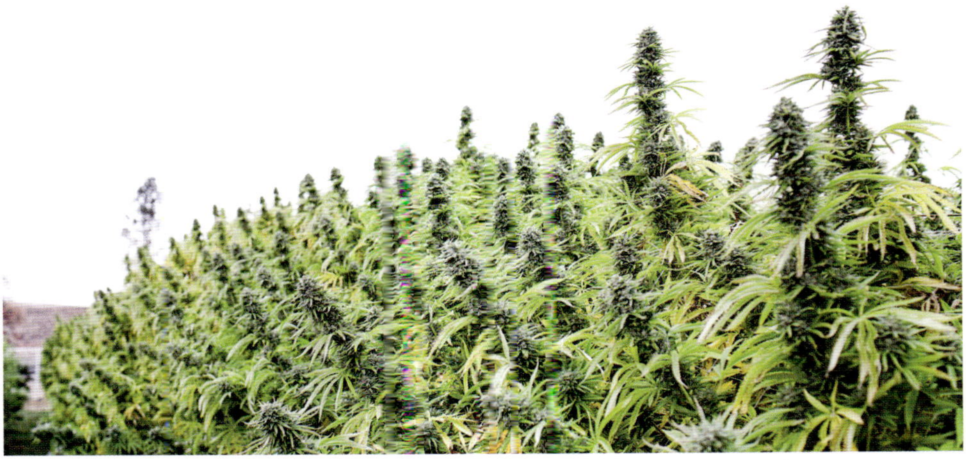

Ten sativa plants and pruning can easily create a massive wall of cannabis colas.

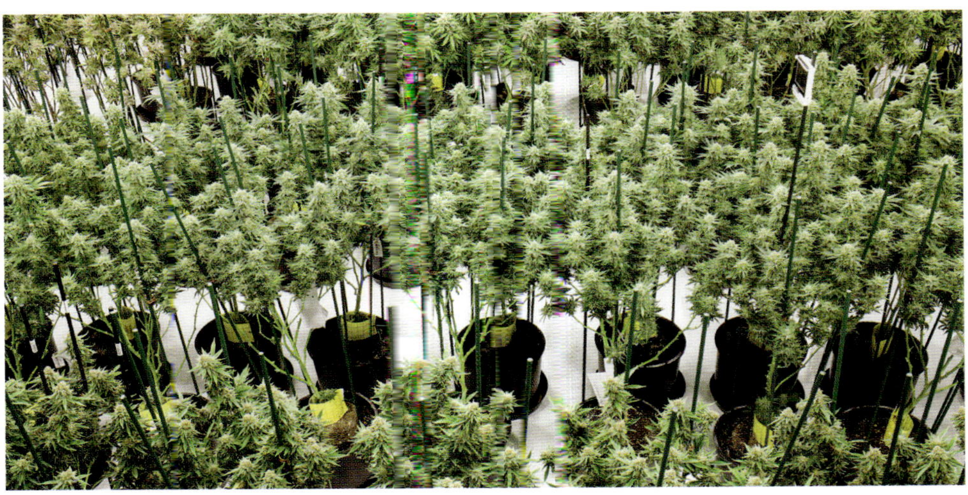

What could have been taller, narrower plants have been pruned into shorter bushes.

PHOTOS: KRISTEN ANGELO

has a junction point or a node that it grew from and that will produce bud during the flowering stages. With the right strain, it is possible to have a single bushy plant that takes up an entire 6 x 6-foot space, and even droops over the sides to completely conceal its pot. Creating cannabis bushes usually requires a few additional weeks of vegetative growth, but you can also use pruning to keep a population of plants shorter. Ultimately, it's your plant to shape how you want.

FIM Technique

There is a topping method called the "FIM" technique which also creates bushy plants and can produce more than two top colas. FIM, which stands for "F*ck I Missed," was allegedly discovered when a grower messed up a topping exercise. At the very top of a cannabis plant, if you push the leaves apart, you should see a tiny bud. This is a leaf bud. If you want to know what a leaf bud looks like, watch how new leaves grow at the top of the plant. The newly forming leaves should be closed in a tight bud that gradually opens up as the plant grows. The key to FIM is to get your slice so that a lower portion of the newly forming leaves is left. If you go down to the stem, you are not doing it correctly. You might not force many branches to grow if you don't go down enough. By slicing this area, you will leave behind a leaf bud that looks like micro-sized fresh lettuce that has been sliced close to the base. It will be fresh, damp, and cleanly cut. Use a pruning clipper to pinch off about 3/4 of that bud, which should result in more than two top colas. You can produce up to eight new top colas in a single FIM clipping.

Super-Cropping Technique

An experimental method of pruning for bushy results is called "super-cropping." Taking a branch between your forefinger and thumb, you should gently crush the branch, causing it to develop multiple branches above the crushed area. Just squeeze lightly until you feel a squish that sounds like a crack, then let go. If it gives easily when crushed, that is the correct side. However, if it is hard to crush and the branch snaps down, you have chosen the wrong side. The tissue damage by crushing the weaker wall promotes branching, just like pruning. New branches will grow just below the damaged areas.

Super-cropping should be carried out during the second or third week of vegetative growth because it can stunt the plant. Super-cropped plants can remain in the vegetative growth stage for twice as long as usual, resulting in a very bushy plant with multiple node regions that should all produce bud. Many growers have thrown super-cropped plants away because they believed they were not flowering correctly. If you super-crop your plants, make sure you have the patience to wait until the process is finished, which is usually about four to six more weeks of vegetative growth. The flowers will spread over the plant up and down the branches at multiple node regions. Super-cropping is experimental and is not recommended for first-time growers. There is some risk of hermaphrodites because of stress. However, this calculated maltreatment forces the plant to use its defense mechanisms and can result in increased resin

Super-Cropping

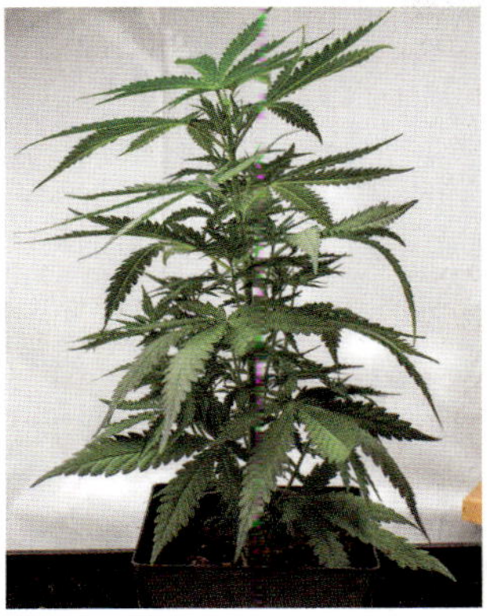

You need the plant to have developed branches.

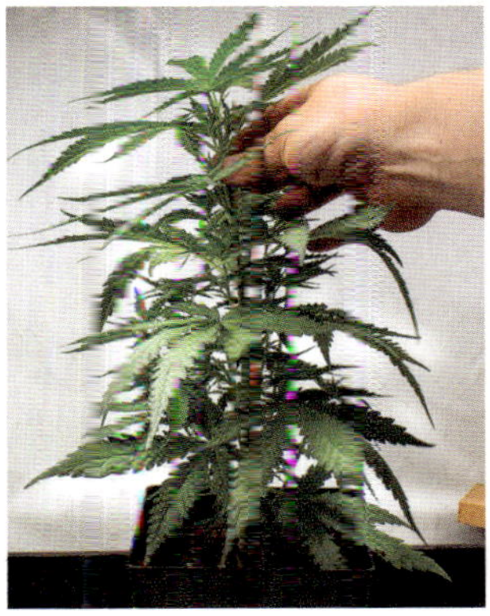

You start with the top.

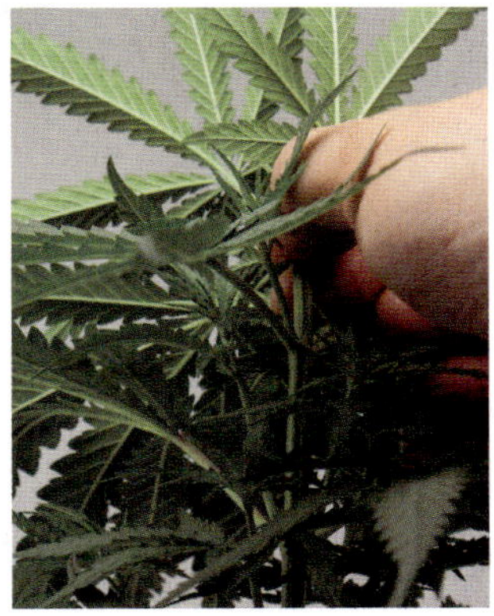

Find a zone above a branching level to super-crop.

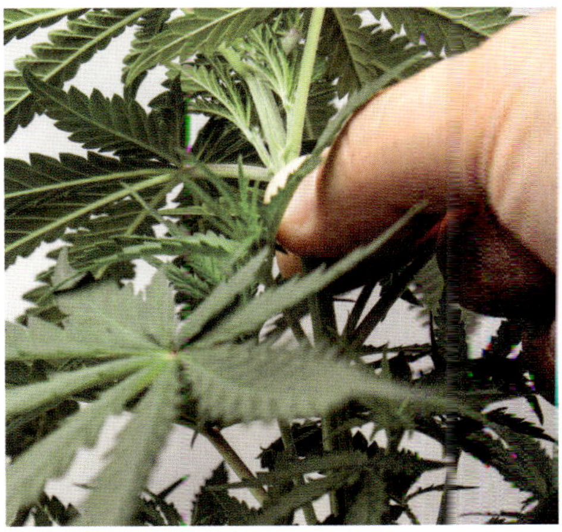

Squeeze gently on it. You will feel it give.

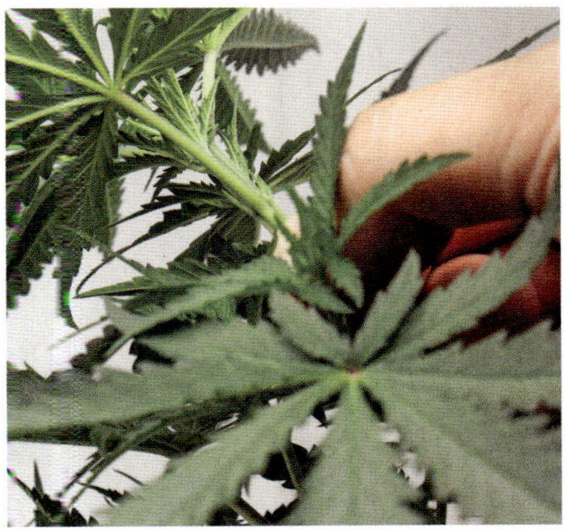

Don't break it off. Just crush it.

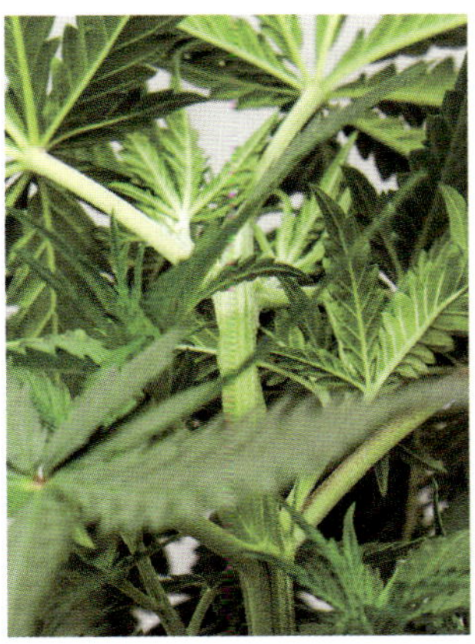

The crushed area acts as if pruned.

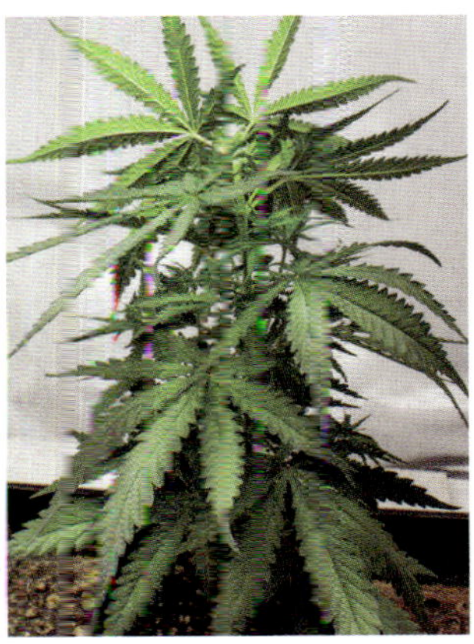

Do this to more branches.

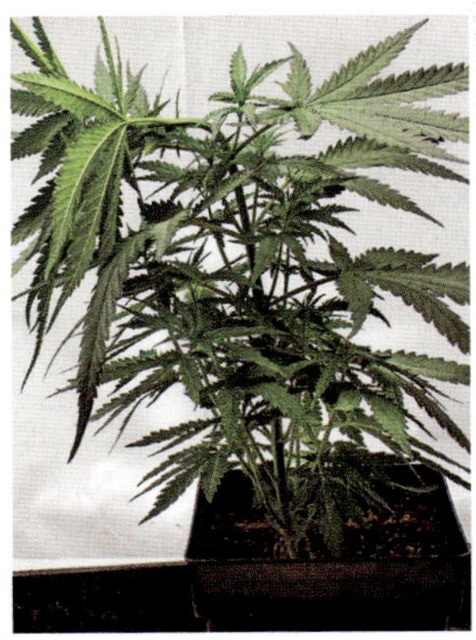

A super-cropped plant will bush more when growing.

PHOTOS: FROM *MARIJUANA DAILY GARDENING* WRITTEN BY HENRY WOODWARD

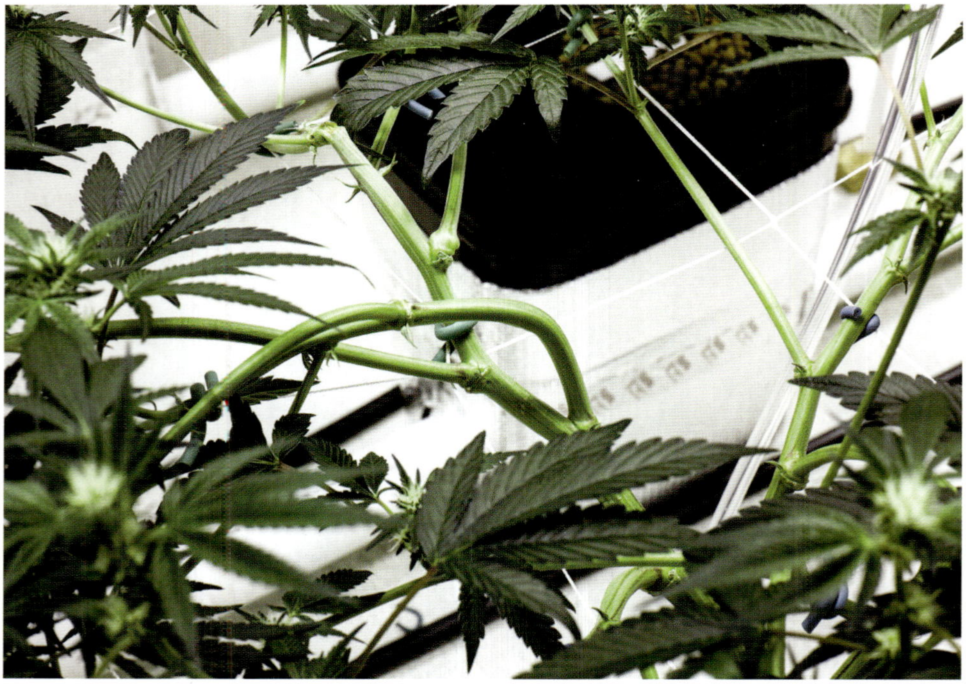

A super-cropped plant with branching developing near the crushed zones.

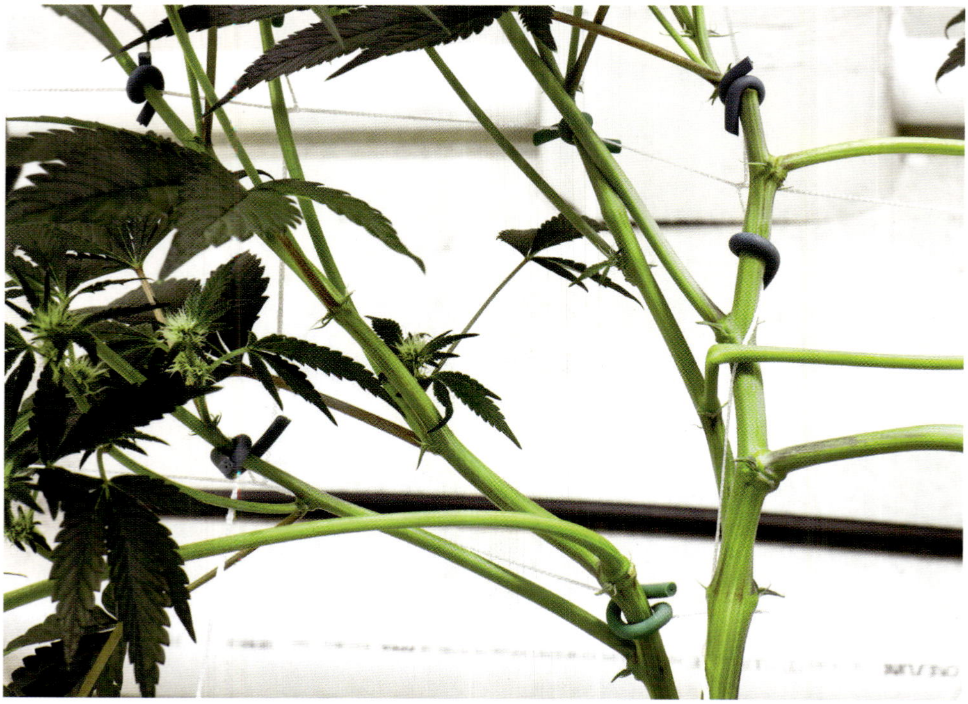

A super-cropped plant may have to be tied up as the branches will eventually get heavy filling with flowers as the broken areas heal.

PHOTOS: KRISTEN ANGELO

production. The procedure is recommended for growers who want to try a different pruning technique to see if it gives better results.

Broken Stem Fixes

In this section, we are mainly talking about breakage, which causes the stem or branch to flop but not fall off entirely. It is not normal for cannabis breaks to be completely clean. It is more likely for the stem to hang with splintered strands of attached fibers around the break. Severed parts are much more likely when predators such as deer are around, as they can chew straight through a stem or branch—but in most cases, you won't remove a branch without a pruning blade. Cannabis is robust. How we fix a break depends on the stage of growth.

Seedling Breaks

A stem can break at any time, from seedling to near harvest time. In the seedling growth stage, you can try fixing a break by taking a short tube, like a paper straw, and cutting it to a height between the soil and the leaf on top. The tube will support the broken seedling. If there is a leaf, it's better to cut the tube lengthwise, open it up, wrap it carefully around the seedling, and push the tube slightly into the soil. If the break is not too severe, the seedling might recover. Seeds can get expensive, so don't bypass this method if you have an accident.

Stem Breaks

A stem break in larger, mature plants is best solved using a hose, so having some

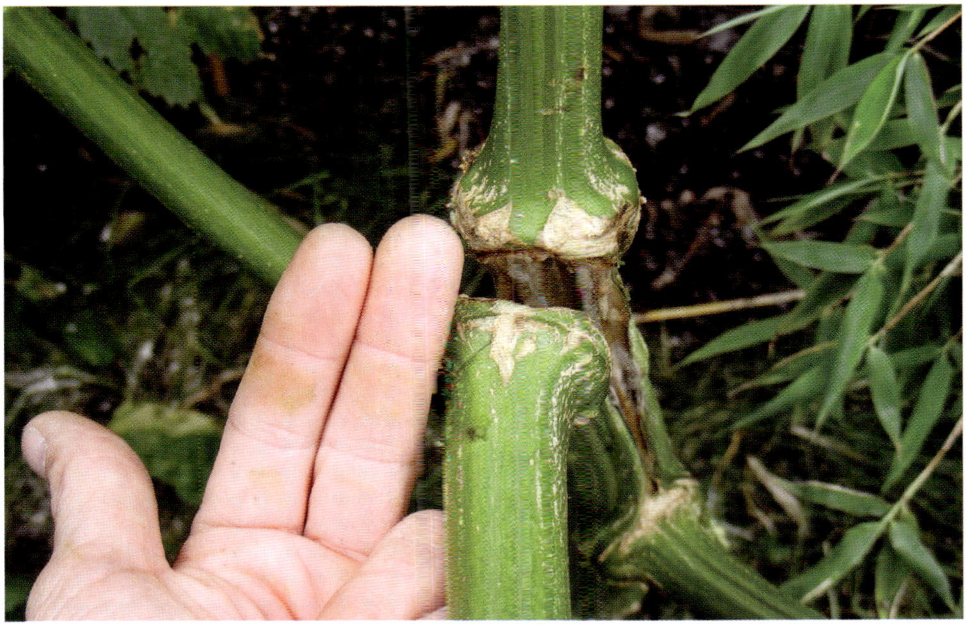

PHOTO: NMS

Flowers get heavy. Here the base has split. This was a topped plant so it's still able to grow.

around can help in an emergency. Hose pipes come in different diameters, so make sure you use one that is not too big or small. As described above, cut a piece of hose to the right size, then cut it lengthwise and wrap it around the break. It is best never to use tape directly on a plant break because it inhibits recovery. Instead, you can use tape on the hose to tighten or loosen it.

This break area will hopefully heal into a sizeable bulbous growth. It will likely behave like it has been pruned or topped, and branching will develop very close to the broken area. Don't remove the tubing until this swelling has stopped growing. The plant will need a few weeks to recover, if it is recoverable.

Breaks and Fungi

Breaks can be susceptible to fungi. If you find fungi development, refer to Chapter 15 for identification and solution. The prognosis is not particularly good for a plant with a break and fungi at the breakage zone because necrosis can set in. If the branch breaks, the branch and leaves may wither, and, at that point, pruning away the entire infected branch is recommended. If you can't amputate because it is too low down in the stem, you must use antifungal treatment or remove the plant entirely to try to slow down the spread of the fungi which will already be present in spores.

Breakage Repair Maintenance

Breakage is not pruning. However, while there is no intent to generate new growth, breakage often forces new growth naturally. You have a choice here: When breakage does occur, you can wait to see what happens with the new growth, or keep pruning it back. That unintended growth may complete with other flowers on its branches and flowering plants, covering an area of bud you want to expose to more light. Furthermore, the break area will still be weak. Depending on the severity and quality of recovery, it might not be a good idea to train that branch. Allowing that branch to undergo too much bud development might not be a good idea, either. The choice then is to give this area special care and attention or remove it. It is not uncommon to find roots trying to grow out from a damaged area, although air outside the break zone will prevent the roots from growing much more. If new branches do not perform well or stay stunted into flowering, you can remove them. On the other hand, if they all seem to grow fine together, leave them be.

Training

We covered training in our discussion about advanced SOG and ScrOG setups. Training means tying down your plant's main stem so that it grows in an S-shaped pattern. Training is mainly used to prevent plants from reaching their natural vertical height without pruning. This technique is of interest to us because it means the plant puts energy into productive growth for optimal results rather than recovery. You can train your plants to bend into other shapes, but the S-shape is the most common.

Low Stress Training with BudHuggers®

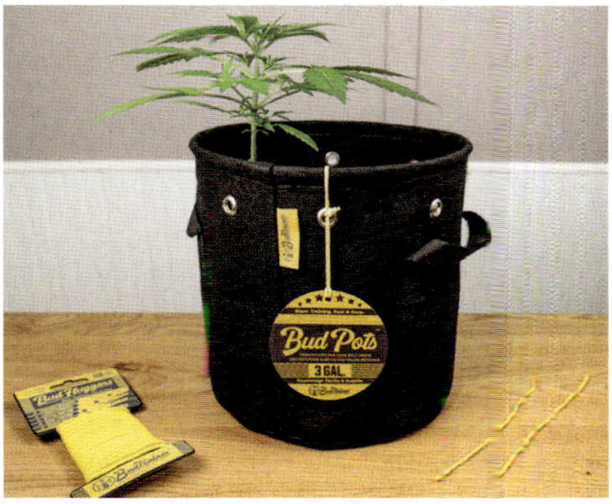

Budpots® have holes around the rim for attaching BudHuggers.

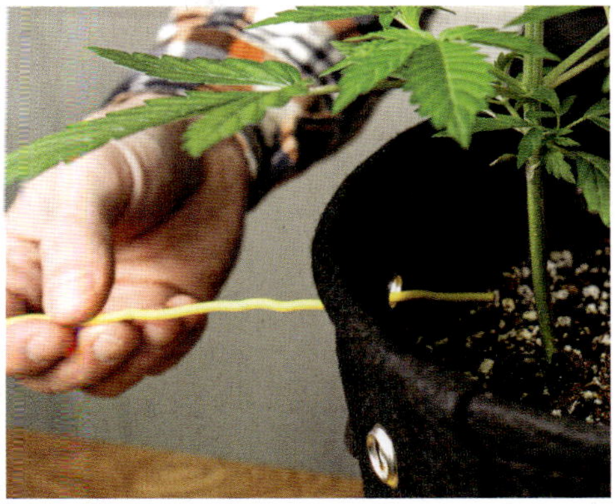

Thread the BudHuggers through the hole, aiming it towards a stem.

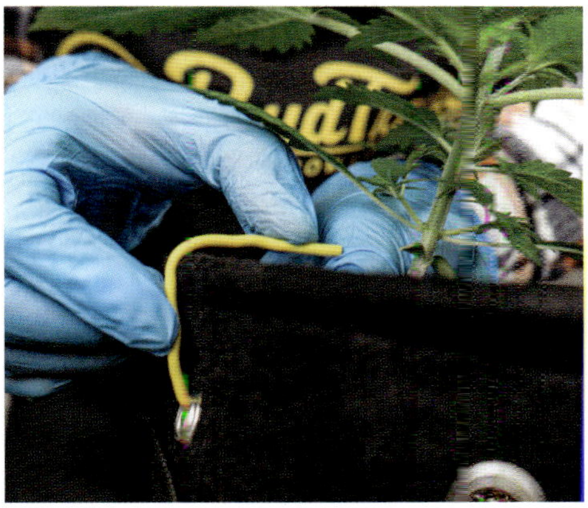

Leave enough room to bend the BudHuggers on the outside.

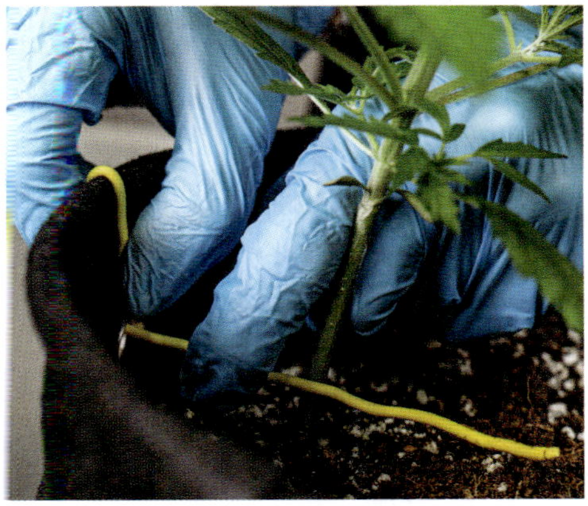

Leave enough room to bend the BudHuggers on the inside as well.

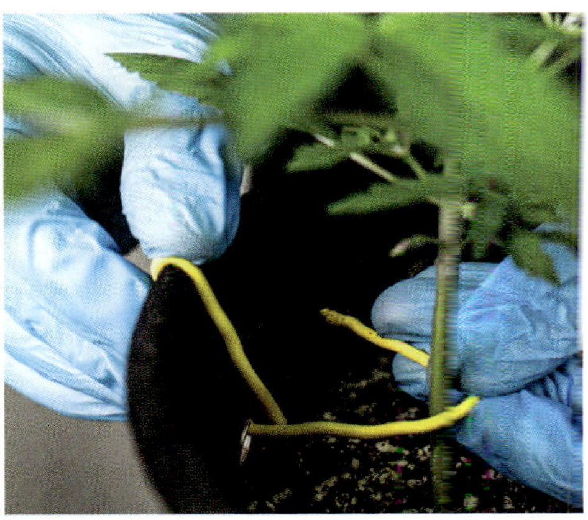

BudHuggers avoid tying the plant and use bending instead.

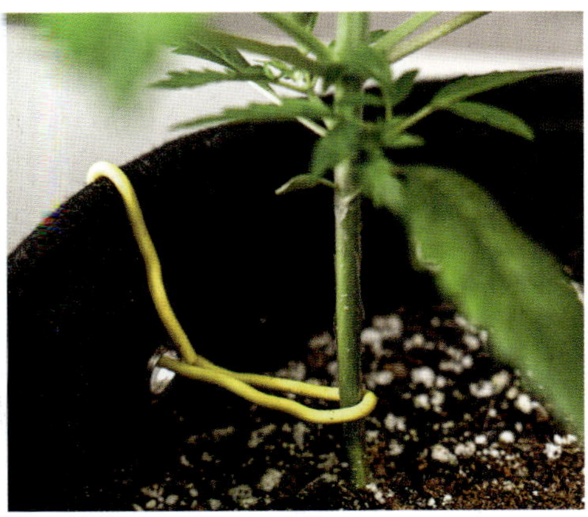

As the stem thickens, the BudHuggers can be adjusted easily. *continues...*

PHOTOS: BUDTRAINER.COM

Low Stress Training with BudHuggers® *continued*

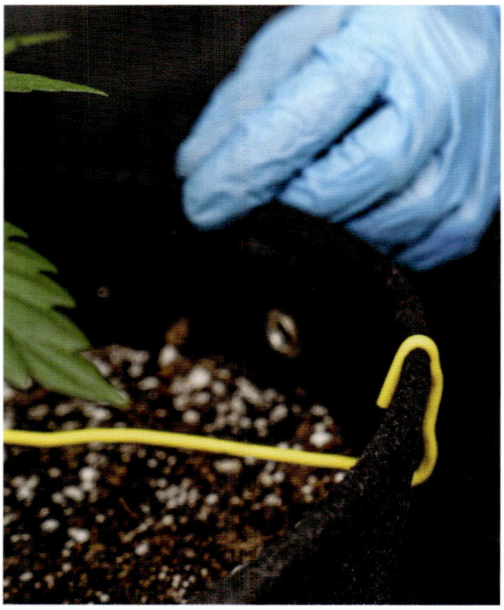

You can also use BudHuggers to train plants in any shape you want. You can bend plants this way.

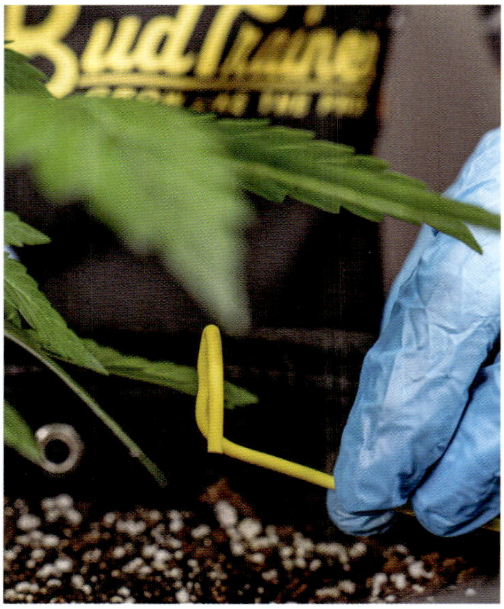

The loop is on the top, so plants can be bent under it. The stem or branch goes under the loop.

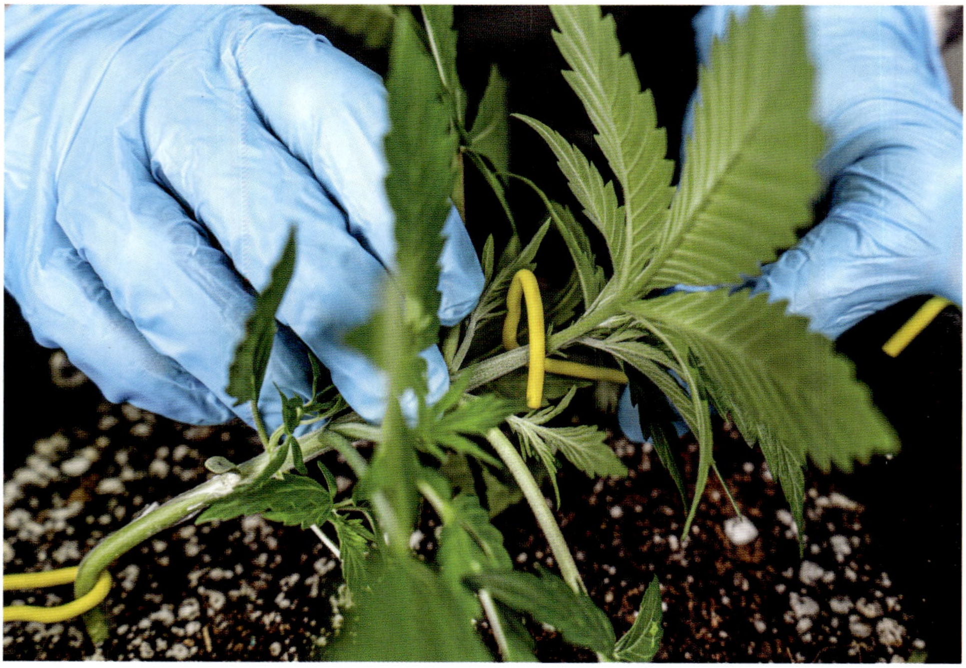

Never force anything with the plant. Notice there is a BudHugger holding the stem. You can adjust the bend over the coming days by moving the upper BudHuggers location or adjusting the Budpot connection.

PHOTOS: BUDTRAINER.COM

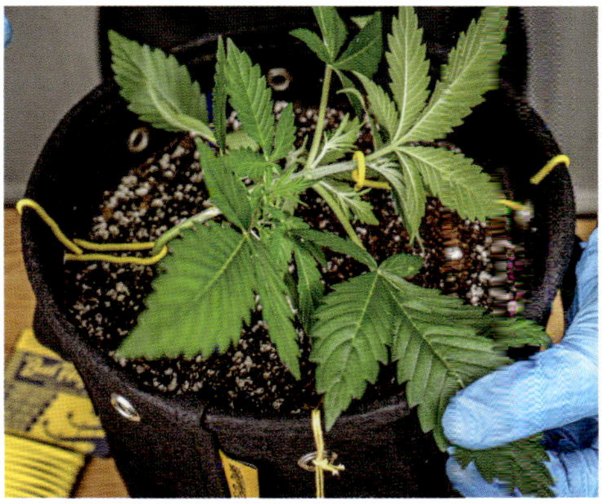

Budpots have many holes around the rim for attaching multiple BudHuggers.

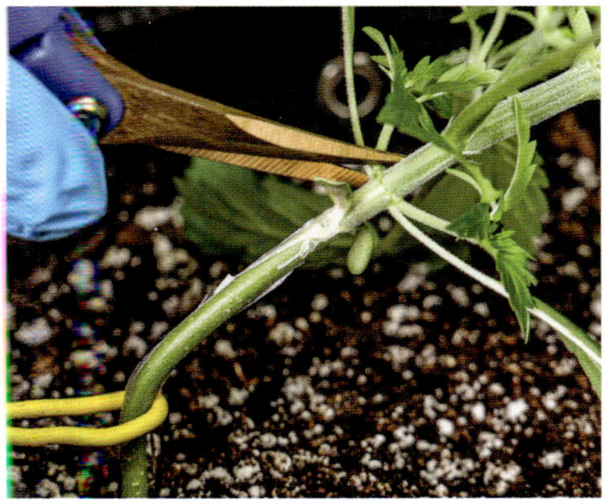

You should prune away leaves that are touching the soil.

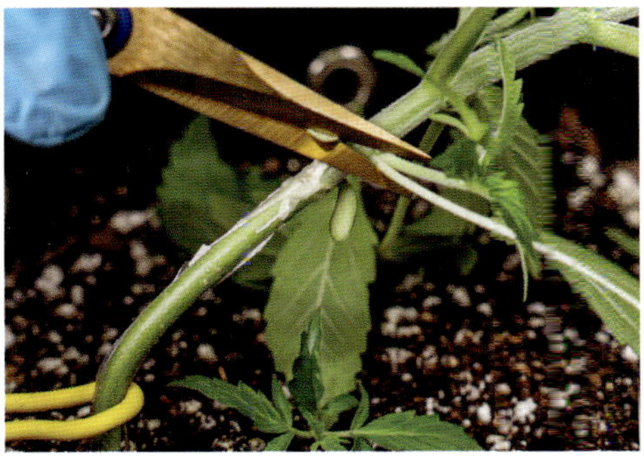

Leaves touching the soil will become necrotic if you don't remove them.

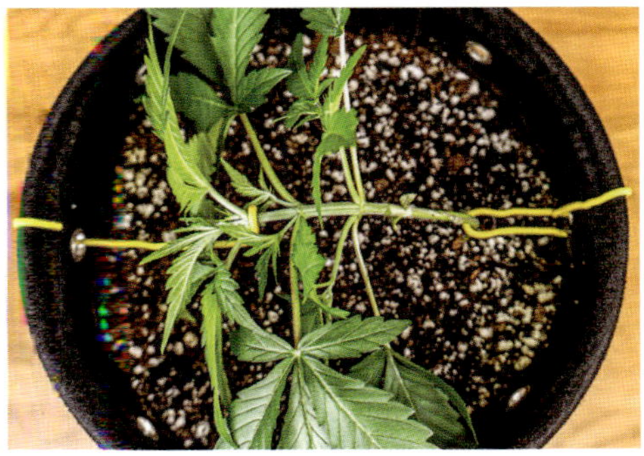

Leaves touching the soil have been removed by pruning them away.

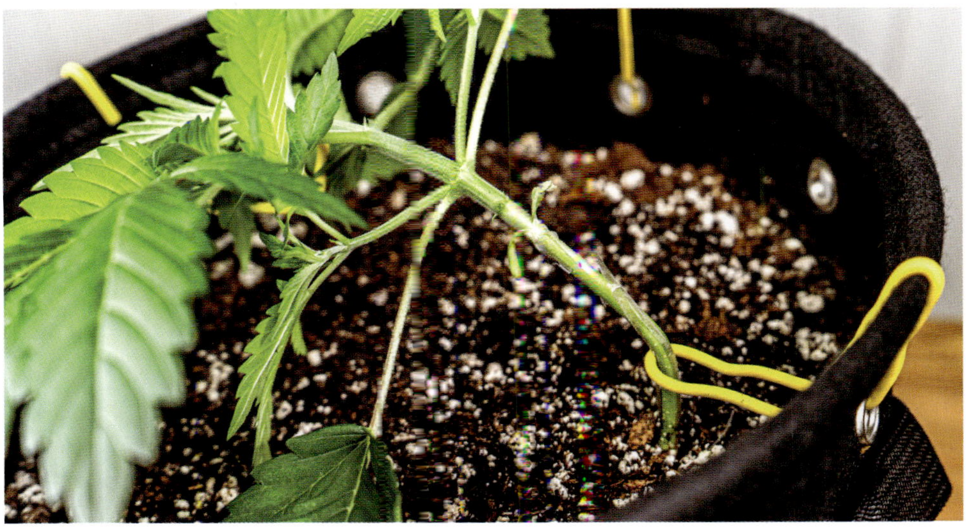

Make sure any bending keeps the upper leaves off the medium. You will need to watch for this as the plant grows.

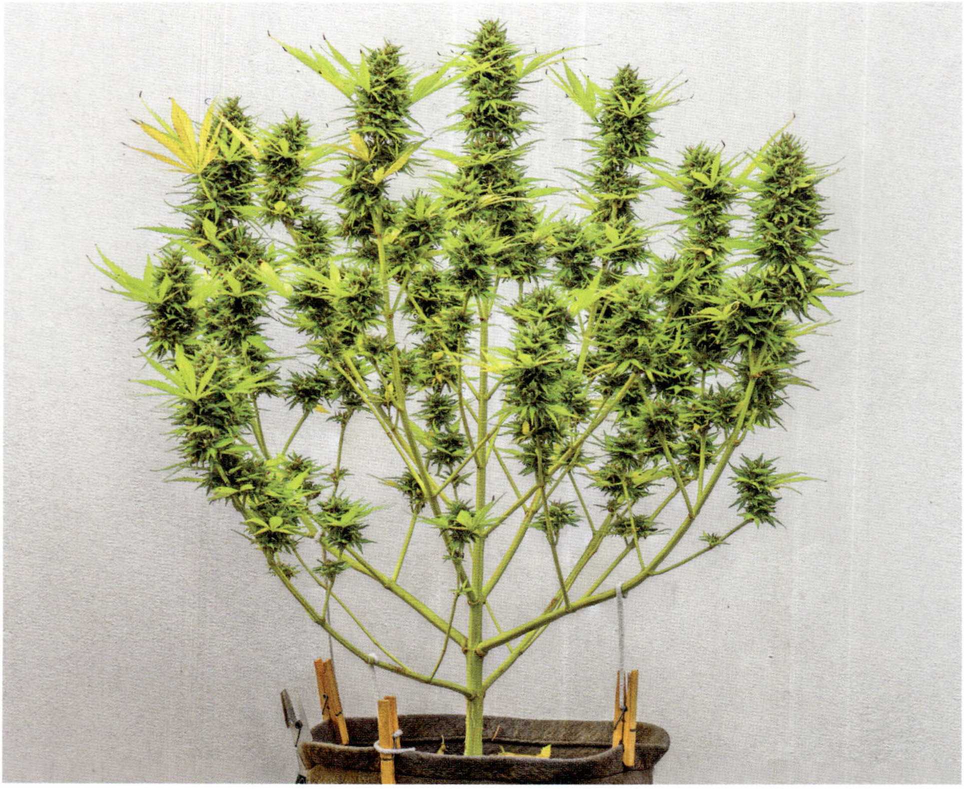

Clothes pegs are handy for extending your training as the plant grows more. This plant has been shaped by tying the side branches down.

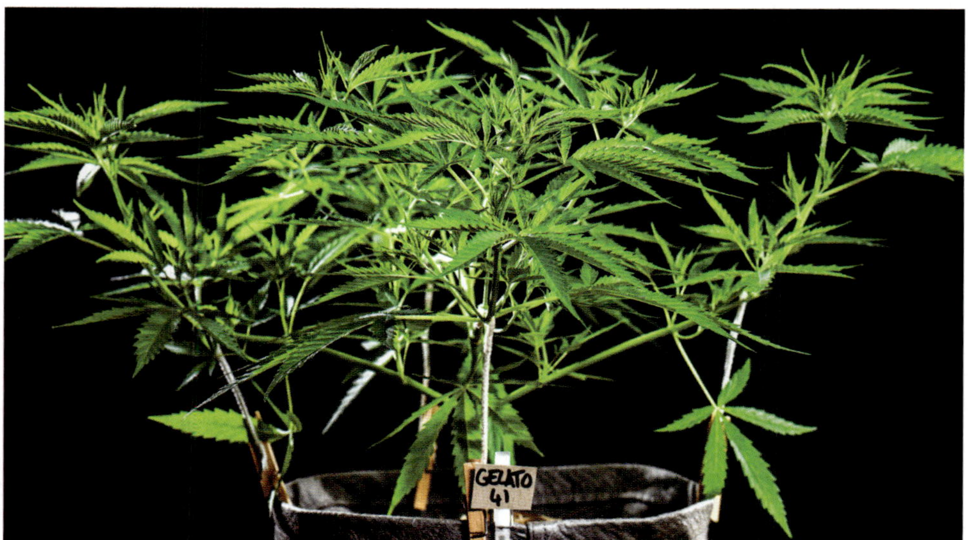

Clothes pegs are especially useful with grow bags because they clip onto the sides very easily. This cannabis plant is being shaped into a bush.

PHOTOS: ERIC PALMER

Training does not stop your plants from growing to their natural potential but instead promotes horizontal instead of vertical growth. Training is helpful if you have restricted grow spaces. You can prune trained plants, but most growers rely on training to achieve optimal results. Training is accomplished by bending the plant over, attaching a line to the stem or branch, and securing the other end to another part of the plant, another plant, or another object. Tightening the line bit by bit over several days allows you to bend your plants without causing excessive stress. Fishing line used to be standard but, for environmental reasons, using biodegradable string from hemp is now preferred, especially if this is done outdoors. If you are growing indoors, some of the lines may be located very close to your lighting, and heat can cause some threads to snap or even burn, especially if you are using high-wattage HIDs—so try to avoid tying near your light. Don't tie your line too tightly around the stem, or you could end up cutting into it and causing plant stress, accidental topping, or even killing it. People have managed to grow plants of all sorts of shapes using this method, from corkscrews to full circles. Some growers even like to grow their plants horizontally during the vegetative growth stage with a 90-degree bend at the base of the plant. Training can improve overall bud production when done correctly with the right strain. ScrOG involves training plants through a mesh screen, and thus maximizes training potential.

Cloning

Cloning replicates an individual biological organism, retaining the same DNA and thus making the clone identical. In nature, this is known as asexual reproduction, or parthenogenesis. Biologists have studied many reproduction systems where individual parts split off and grow into new organisms, such as sea sponge gemmulation or jellyfish strobilation. Regeneration is a mechanism whereby an organism repairs itself. For example, most worms, when split, will regenerate one section while the other dies; however, some can regenerate both sides, such as flatworms and tapeworms. In some cases, regenerated organisms can meet the definition of a clone.

Many organisms can't regenerate complex structures, such as limbs, but some can; salamanders are one example. Plants can often regenerate less complex structures, and a good example is grass, which, when grazed upon, can grow back. Other plants, called runners, stretch below the surface of the soil and produce new plants intermittingly above the surface. Large taproot areas on some plants act as bulbs, producing new shoots that break through the surface as new plants. Tubers, such as potatoes, behave in this way. The designation of an individual plant becomes blurred here. Some annual plants that survive through the seasons do so by expanding underground using these natural vegetative propagative mechanisms. These processes are possible with plants because meristem cells can continuously divide. The damaged area of a plant may try to produce roots after repairing the break, but the air stops the roots from growing.

Preparing a Clone Mother for Cloning

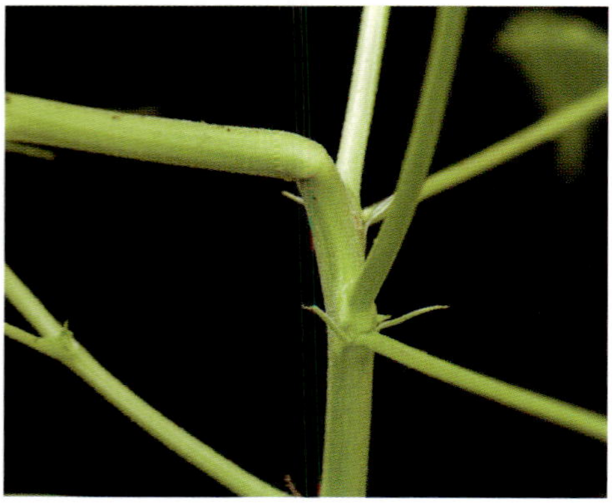

Super-cropping for cloning.

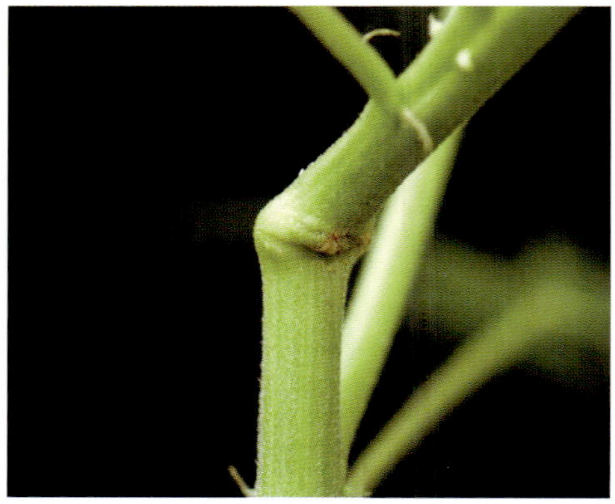

The plant heals while producing more branches.

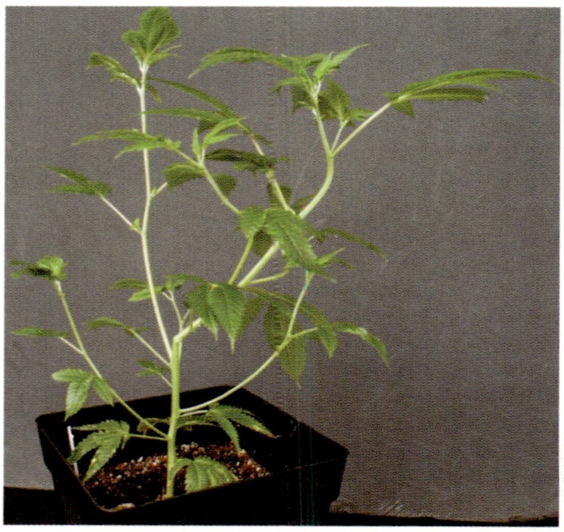

Super-cropping branching.

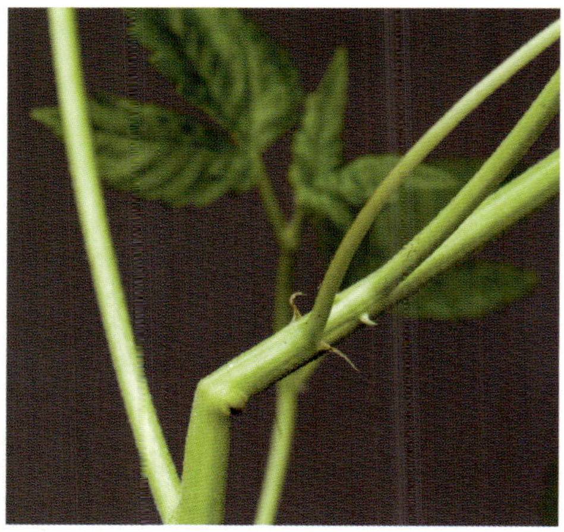

All it takes is to gently crush areas.

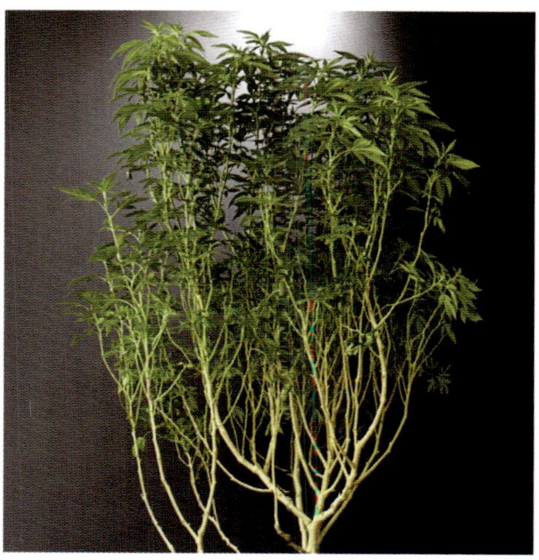

A super-cropped plant is a perfect clone mother.

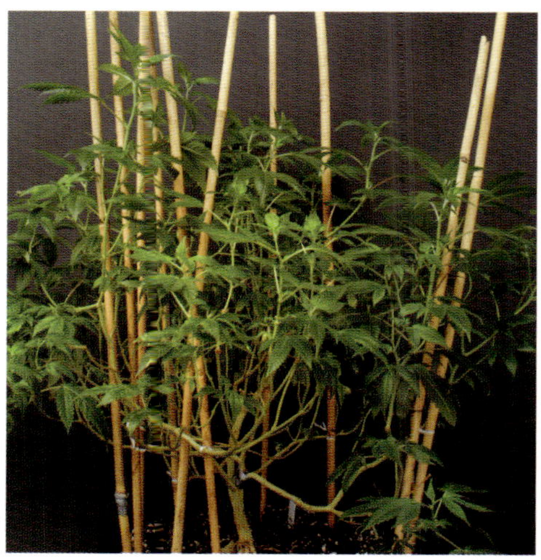

Lots of clones available from a single plant.

PHOTOS: ED BORG

Step-by-step: Cloning 101

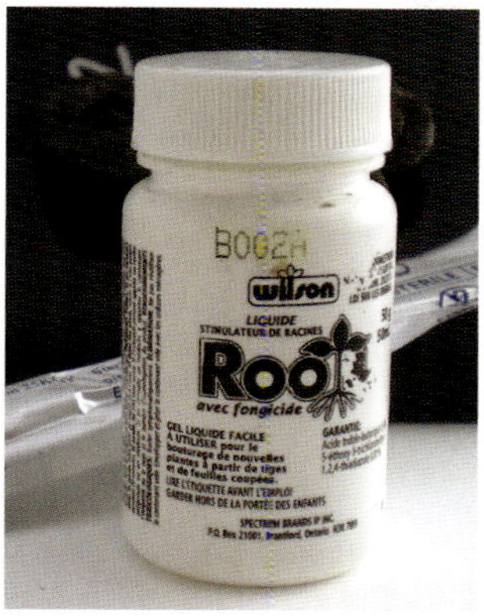

1. Rooting hormones increase success.

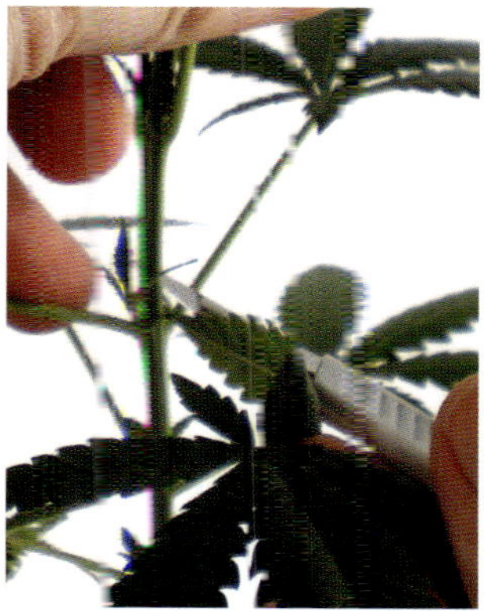

2. Cut one inch below internode.

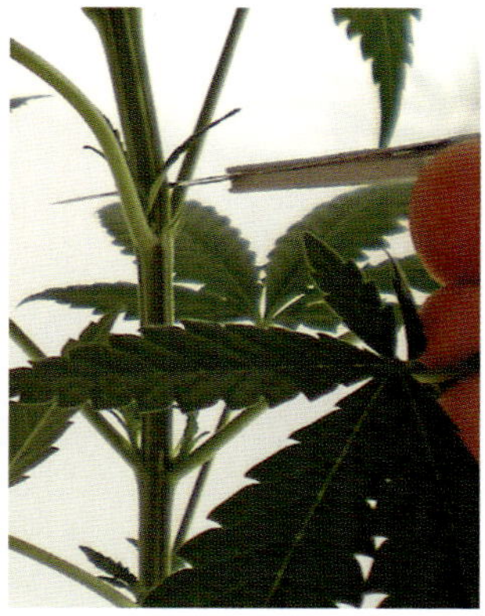

3. Quick clean cut.

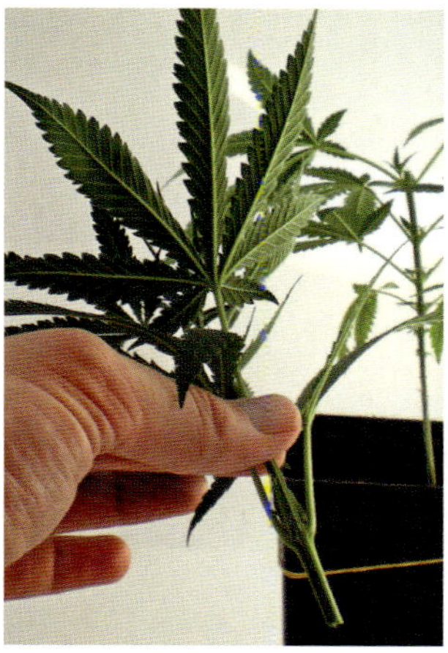

4. Cutting is six inches long.

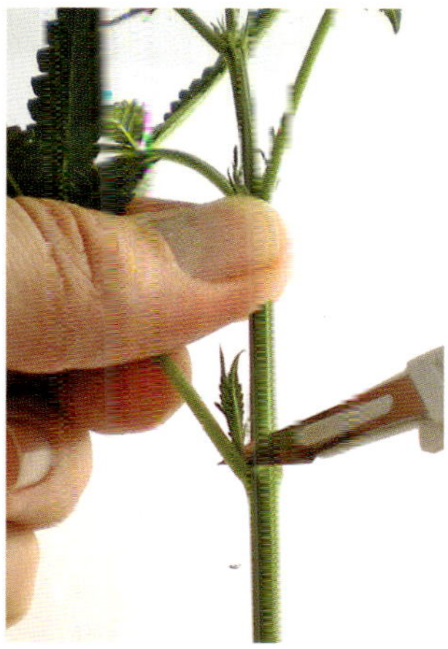

5. Remove lower leaves.

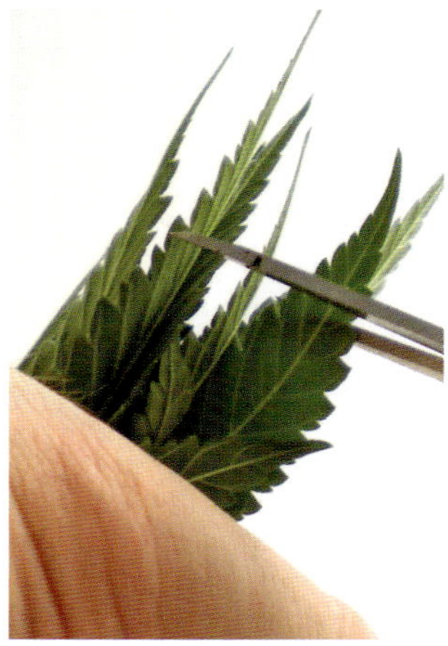

6. Trim extra leaf tissue.

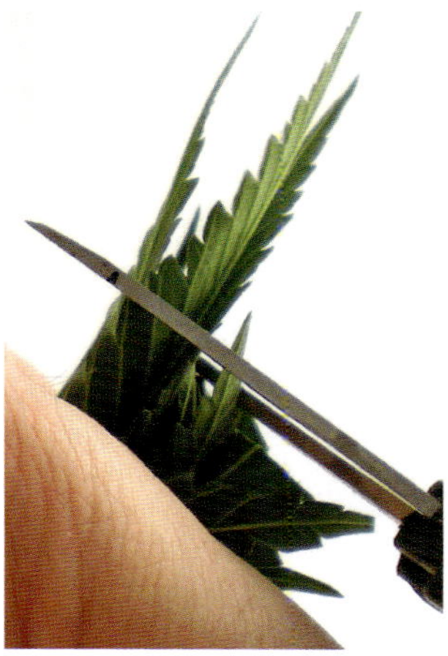

7. Cut off about one third.

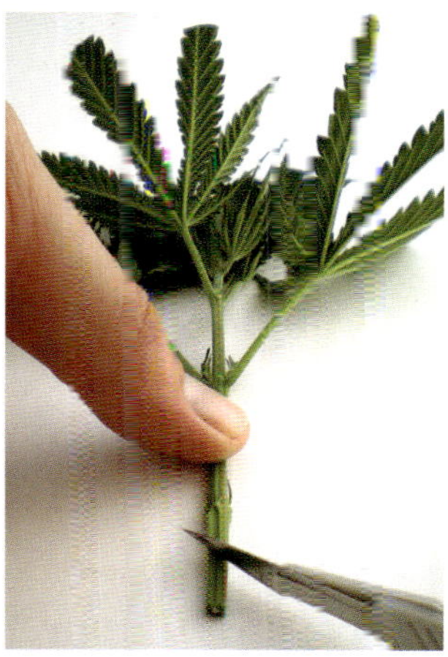

8. Final cut below internode.

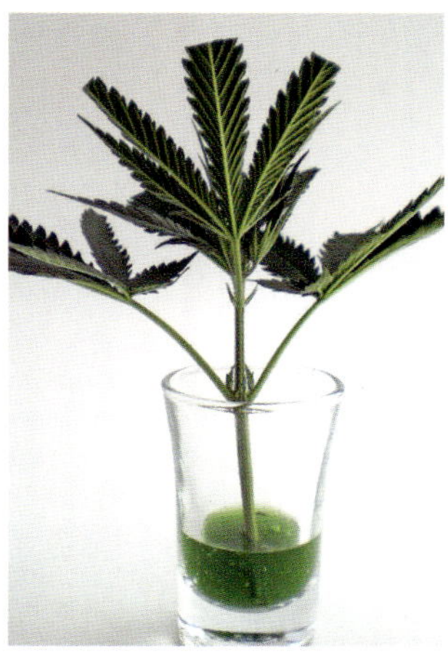

9. Dip in hormones, then plant.

PHOTOS: WEADO

Any cannabis plant can be cloned if it has developed enough node regions in the early stages of vegetative growth. In a large selection of plants from seeds, you may find an excellent mother plant that you wish to keep. You can sustain and keep her genetic profile indefinitely through cloning.[3] Cuttings can be taken from clones in vegetative growth. The best time to get cuttings is when you are pruning. Plants from seed can also be cutting donors but keep in mind that you should label the cuttings to the corresponding plant as they will be clones of that plant only, not another member of the population with variations.

For high success rates, make your cutting above a node with at least two nodes above it and approximately four leaves in total on the clone. Cuttings are typically around three inches in length, but you can take longer and larger ones. Many growers prefer to take smaller cuttings to make shorter clones. You can choose to clone just with a single node and only two leaves, but the four-leaf minimum gives the best results—especially for those new to cloning. Once the cutting has been taken, place it in the growing medium and it should form new roots over the next one to three weeks.

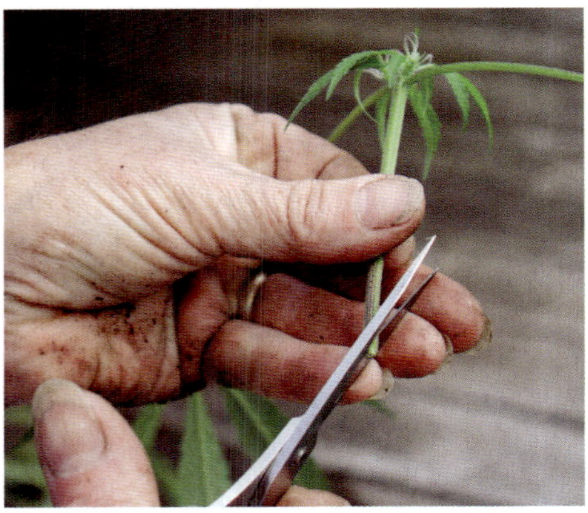

Snip at an angle.

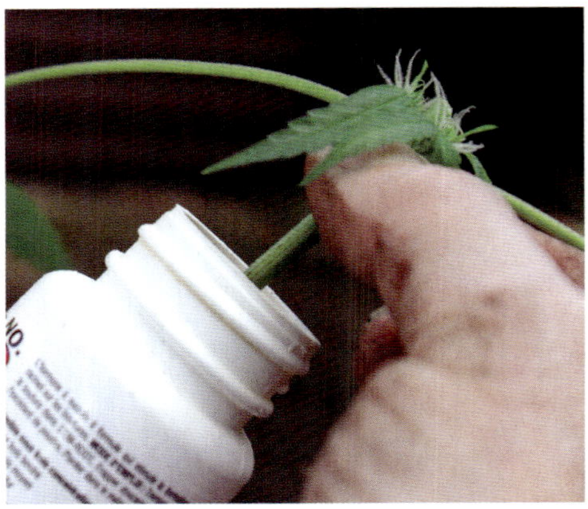

Dip the point into cloning solution.

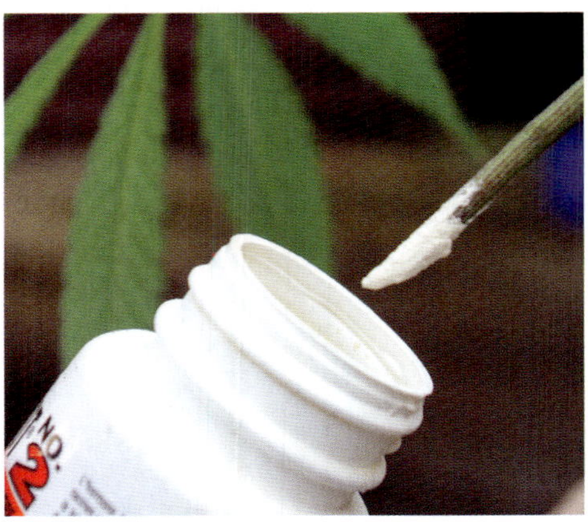

Make sure it is well covered in it.

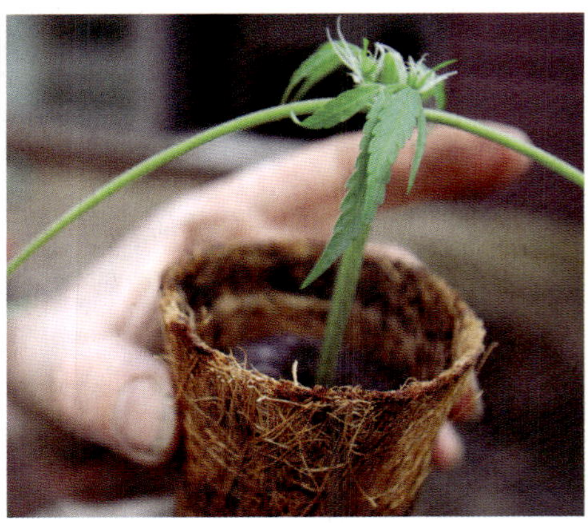

It will sit in its medium nice and steady.

PHOTOS: GCP

Rooting Clones

There are several ways to root a clone, but most use some form of growing medium. The best way to begin is to get some rooting gel to improve success rates. A clone's biggest obstacle is pathogens that can form on the cut zone. The leaf edges, especially those on smaller cuttings, can hang down and easily touch a surface, such as the floor, picking up pathogens that cause the tips to become necrotic. You can prevent this by cutting each blade of the leaf in half, which will still allow the clone to grow. Soil tends to have a lower success rate with clones than Rockwool cubes or other rooting mediums used for cuttings. The medium used for rooting a clone may not be the same as its main growing medium. For example, we may start a clone in Rockwool and later transplant it to soil, either indoors or outdoors. Remember that air pruning forces the roots to search for other areas for nutrients. The volume of air is reduced significantly only once in the growing medium, and the roots will grow beyond the air barrier. Roots need air, but they need it along with nutrients and moisture.

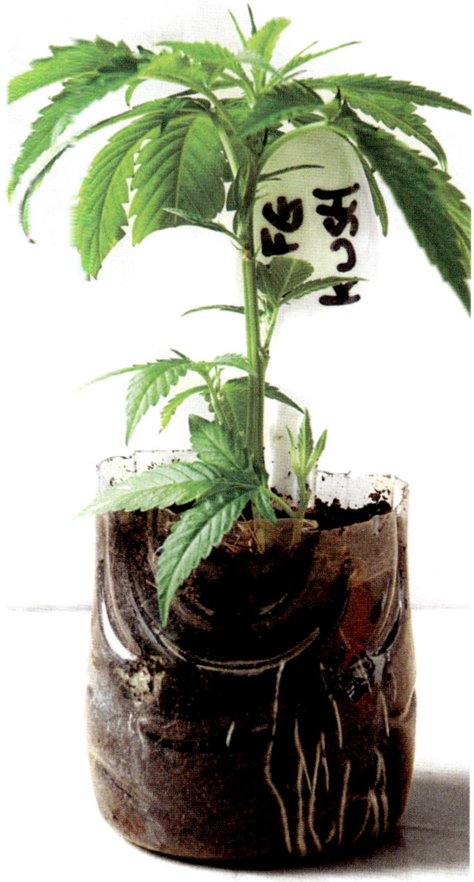

Rooting the clone of an Afghani Kush.

Rooting in Soil

Cloning straight to soil can have a low success rate; its potential success depends on your soil type. Use the wrong soil, and the clone will fail quickly. The best soil for cloning is a standard loam type with an even NPK ratio. Avoid using seedling or cutting soils, as most of these have added hormones and nutrients unsuitable for cannabis or cannabis cuttings. A rooting gel, which contains anti-fungicide compounds and hormones to promote root growth, is recommended to keep pathogens away from the cut zone in the soil.

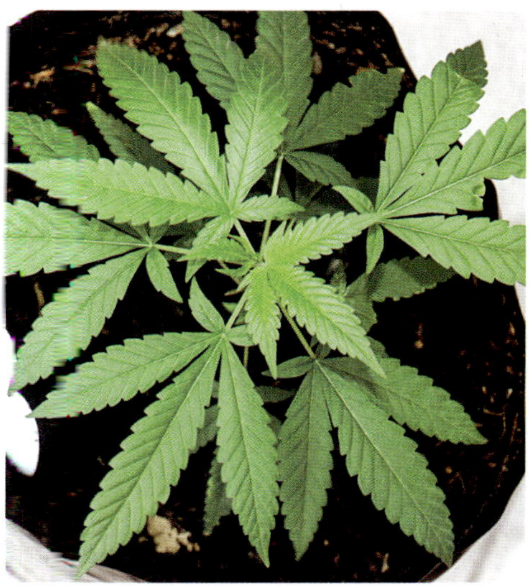

Rooted clones love to produce new leaves.

PHOTOS: ED BORG

Rooting in Water

Cloning in water also has a low success rate because the roots need to breathe once they have developed. If the roots remain submerged in water, the cuttings will eventually die. The cutting must be transferred to another medium, such as soil, Rockwool, or a hydroponic system. This also means that the clone must move through several mediums before finally being transplanted to the main growing environment. Multiple transplants can lead to stress, decreasing the overall success rate.

Rooting in Aeroponics

Some advanced growers like to use an aero-cloning kit that acts like a miniature aeroponic system to propagate clones. However, these systems require a lot of practice before cuttings will root successfully. Once you learn how to use them, you should see higher success rates and be able to move clones into any medium, including soil. While aero-cloning is very sophisticated, it is unnecessary for most growers. You can read more about aeroponics in Chapter 11.

Rooting in Grow Cubes

Rockwool or similar grow cubes provide an easy way to increase your success rate with cloning. In addition, using a rooting gel, such as Clonex, protects against pathogens and promotes root development. Use a clean (or preferably sterile) blade when you make your cut. A disinfectant treatment on your blades helps sterilize them for cutting. There are a few sanitizing products for horticulture use, but even just 70% isopropyl alcohol works fine.

Try to take a piece of a branch approximately three inches between the cut zone and the next node level; if it is longer, the cutting will have difficulty taking in the water and nutrients it needs to grow and produce roots. You are encouraged to snip leaves in half to prevent them from coming into contact with the ground. You can also get more clones into a space by doing this.

Take the cutting and dip the cut area into the rooting solution before placing it into the medium. Fill any gaps in the medium to prevent air from reaching the cut zone, which can stunt root growth.

Clones don't need much light to root. In the past, we tried to avoid using the bigger grow bulbs for cloning as this was a waste of electricity and bulb life. A simple window with some outdoor light was all we needed for the clone to root. Today we use LED lights, as they are cooler to run and, in the long term, more economical. If you plan to clone, you should plan to invest in some LED lighting, which you can read more about in Chapter 7. LED lights are also perfect with grow or clone tents. It makes everything more straightforward to have a clone tent and an LED light on the go, so you always have access to your quality genetics.

Automated Hydro Cloning

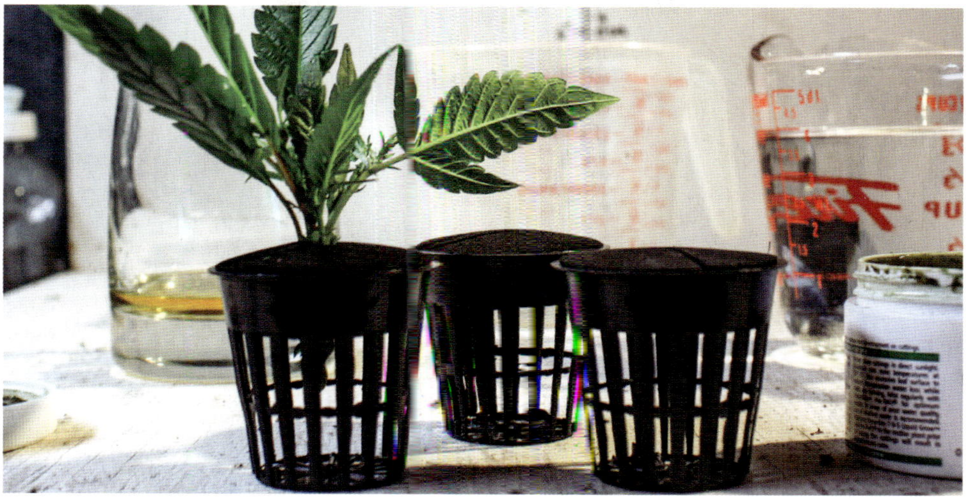

A clipping from a topped plant being hydro-cloned.

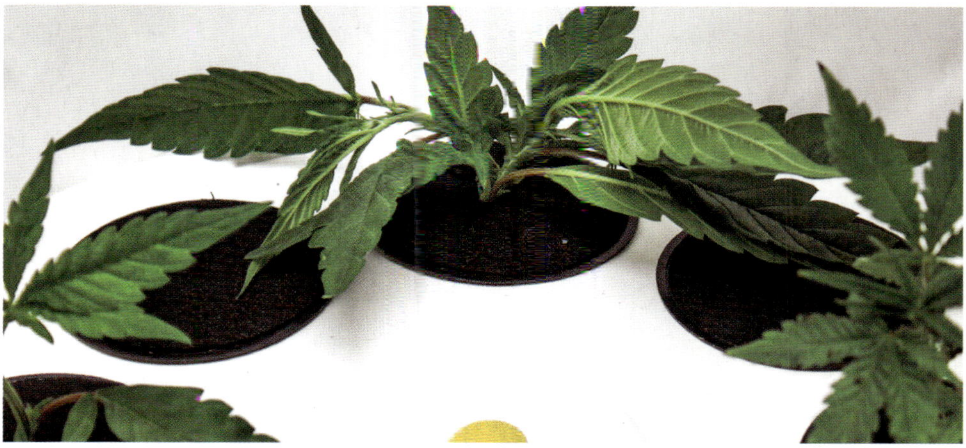

Aero-cloner kits can be used to start roots.

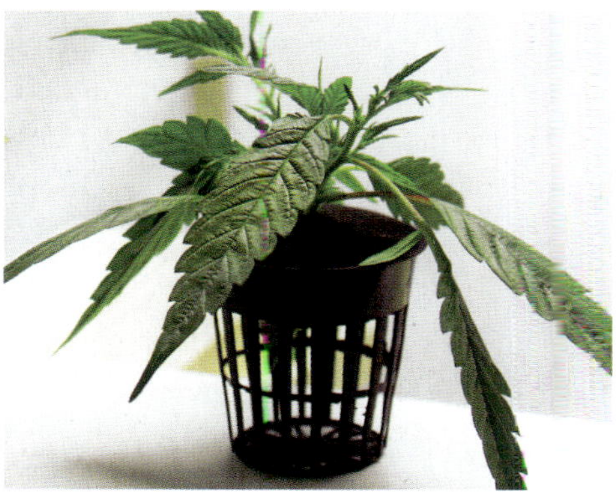

This clone has been growing for a few days.

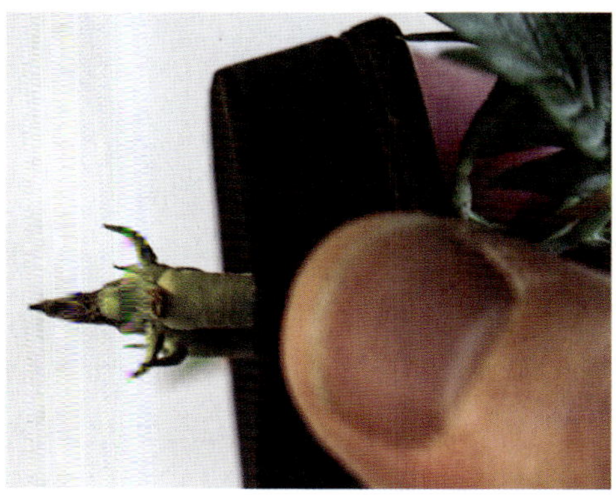

Already the roots are starting to show.

PHOTOS: FROM *MARIJUANA DAILY GARDENING* WRITTEN BY HENRY WOODWARD

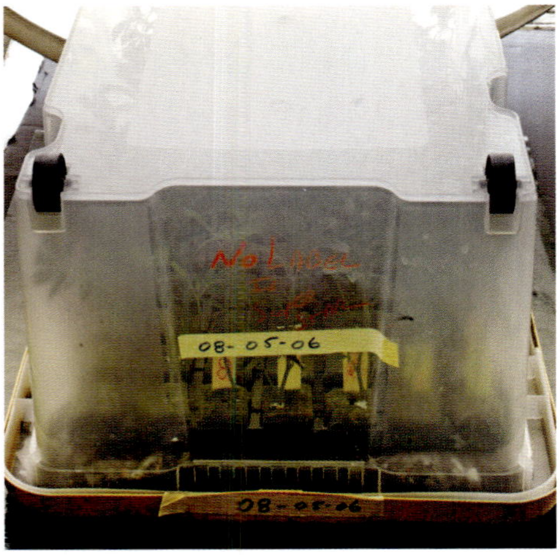

Upside-down container as a propagation kit for humidity.

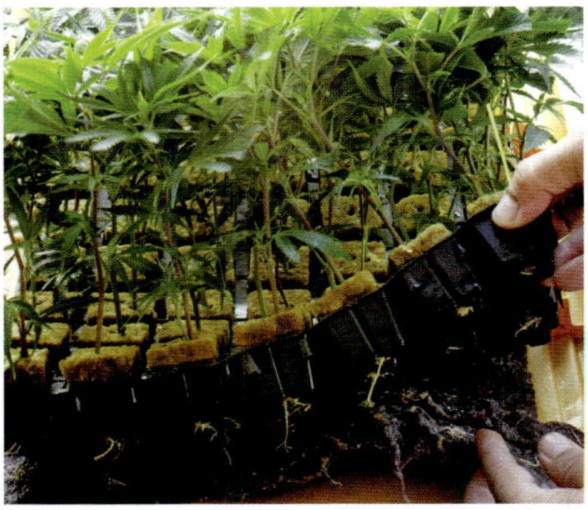

Loaded cube tray is showing roots.

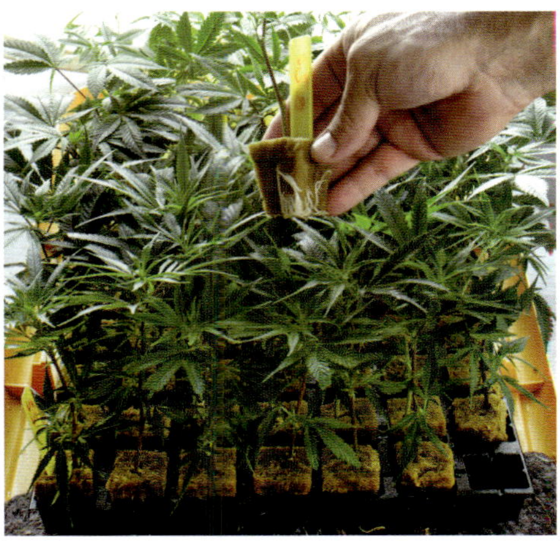

Always label your work.

PHOTOS: ED BORG

If you grow your cutting in small cubes, you can observe the roots' progress. A two-inch square cube is ideal for rooting cuttings. You can cut up larger cubes, but wear a mask if it gets dusty. When the clone takes root in the Rockwool, you will see the roots jut out from the sides of the cube before air pruning prevents them from going further. In most cases, the roots will grow down where the cube base meets the propagation tray. Aeroponic cloning kits make use of air pruning, forcing the roots to grow out of the base of the medium.

If you use bigger cubes, the roots will take longer to grow outside the cube. If you require the clone to be in a larger slab, cut a block to size and cut a zone to insert a smaller cube with roots. This way, you will know that the clone has rooted without waiting weeks for the roots to grow through several centimeters of a grow block. Make sure to cover any openings using pieces of Rockwool after you slot the smaller cube into the bigger one.

The time to move the clone is when its roots have grown outside the rooting medium you selected. However, some LED grow tents allow for the beginning of vegetative growth so that you can leave them there for a little longer. Outdoor growers often wait a while before transferring clones outdoors.

When ready, the clone should be transferred to its new grow medium, whether that is soil, hydroponics, or aeroponics. It is best to go easy on new clones. You don't need to do much work once they are transplanted; avoid starting a full-strength feed or excessive watering. They shouldn't need much food, and we'll address nutrient strengths for clones below. At this point, you have done all you can, and it is time to let nature take its course. The clones need to find their own way in their new home.

After a week or so, you can go ahead with your vegetative growth plans. Of course, there will always need to be some leeway with the time it takes for your plants to start performing as vegetative plants should. They will need to produce more nodes and leaves to get enough light for chemical compound manufacturing and conversion through photosynthesis and other metabolic processes.

A vegetative growth mixture is likely to be too strong for most clones. It is best to gradually achieve the optimal vegetative growth mixture for vegetative growth over several weeks. Chapter 8 describes several ways to figure out what strengths you need. The single best way to find out is to perform experiments.

The usual experiment is done with four clones ready for vegetative growth. You give each clone a different mixture with different nutrient percentages, then, as you incrementally increase the strength, watch how they perform. Using 100% strength solutions with cannabis plants will burn them unless the nutrients are specially made for cannabis. The ideal range for dilutions is between 25–50%. Half of 50% is 25%, and half of 25% is 12.5%, so there are three different strengths for your experiment. When you find which clone responds best, you have a ratio that will work with subsequent clones. You can keep doing these tests until you narrow it down to a more specific ratio. Some people find 12.5% sufficient, while others need to go 50% or more. If you switch nutrient brands, you need to restart the experiment. You will also probably have to restart the experiment if you use a new strain. The experiment is what prevents more extensive failures. The nutrient mixture that works for a few clones should work for all of them.

The grow cube method is still the most successful way of producing clones for most growers. The great thing about cloning is that you can create hundreds of plants from a single mother. Clones also flower more quickly, and the results are predictable because you have already grown the plant from which the clone was taken. For information about obtaining the best results with clones, turn to the SOG and ScrOG growing sections in Chapter 10. Also, look closely at Chapter 11 on hydroponics, which makes use of this technique.

Advanced Plant Care Techniques

We have covered the most common plant care techniques, so let's address some advanced areas of plant care. Experimentation is always recommended, and you can do so before using any of these techniques on your main grow. Learning to clone offers you more chances for experiments and teaches you good practice.

Cloning with Miami Mango

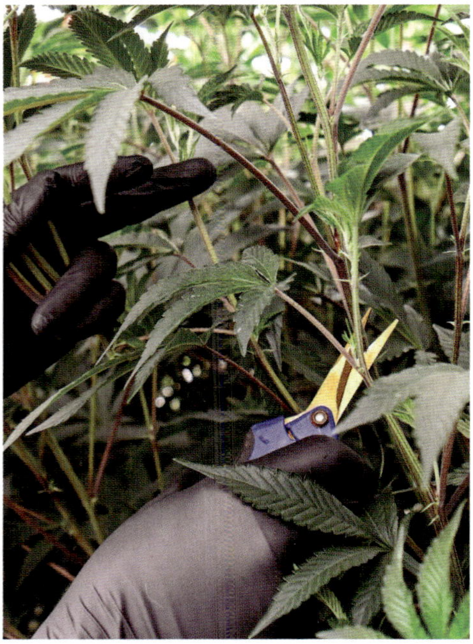

Selecting healthy plants increases your chances for success.

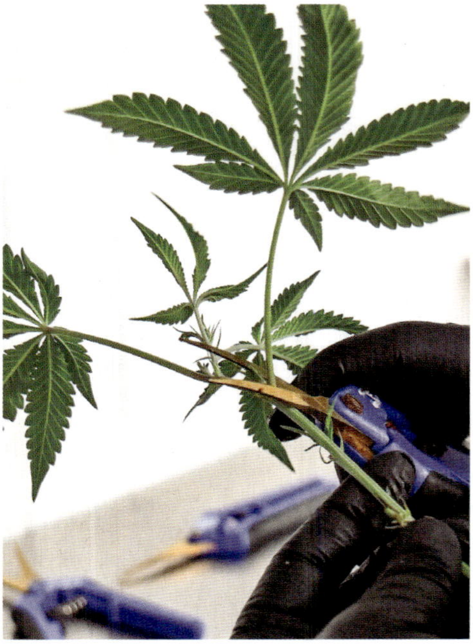

The branch will form the new stem so lower growth is stripped away.

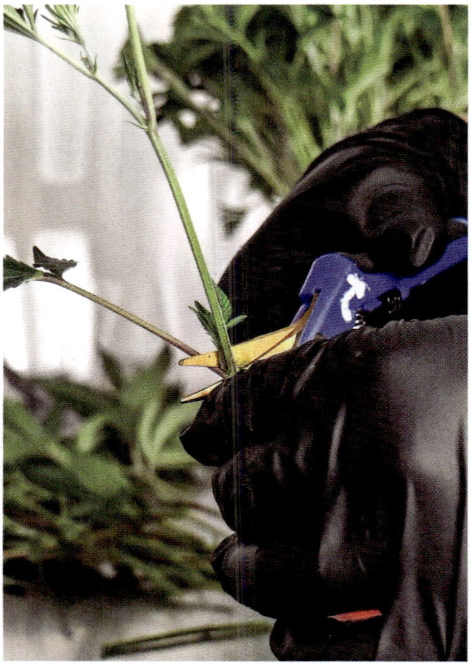

Clip low and leave some length on the branch/stem.

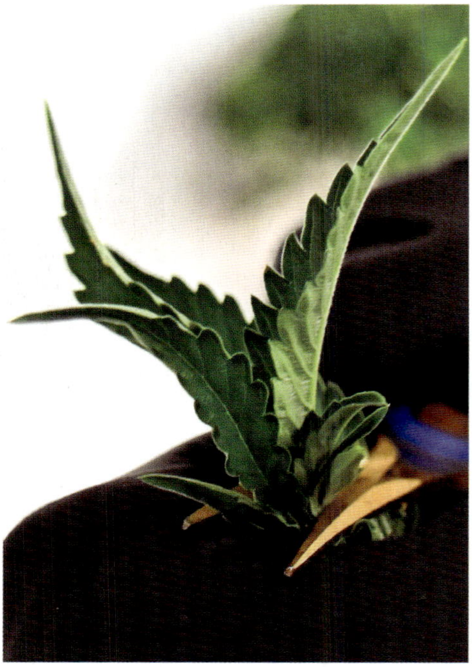

Clip away leaf tips to avoid necrosis while recovering.

PHOTO: MIAMIMANGOCA.COM

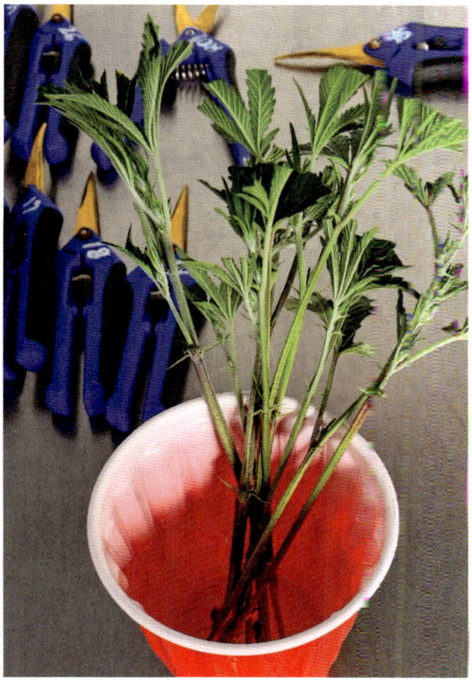

Ensure even lengths and place the cutting in rooting gel.

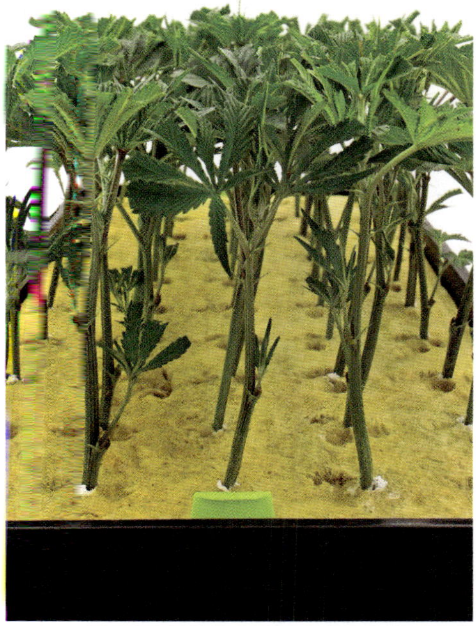

Clipped clones should have an even canopy when rooted.

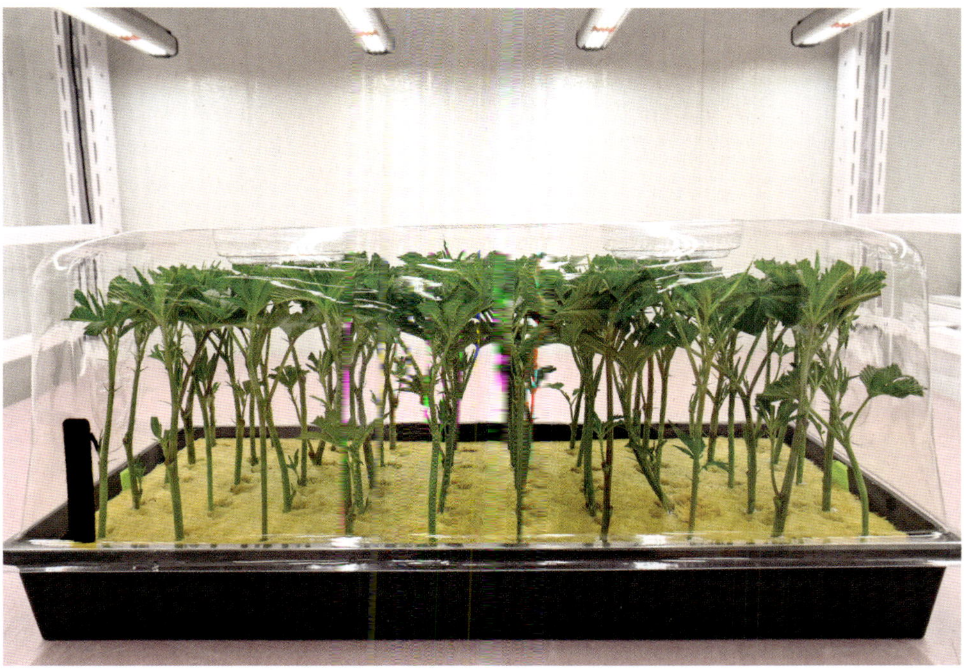

A humidity dome is used with a propagation tray to start the clones. This facility produces 15,000 clones per month!

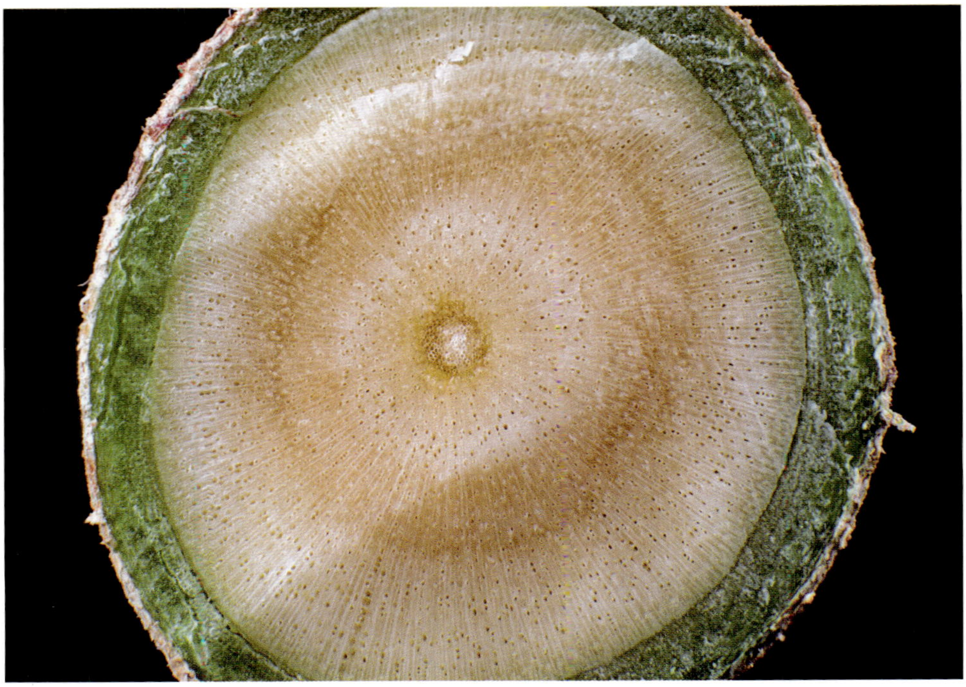

Cannabis plant stems are not hollow. If they are, it may indicate disease. If there is no disease, then it may be genetic.

PHOTO: RUSSELL-HOWLAND PHOTOGRAPHY

Plant Ground Tissue

Before we get into more advanced techniques, we must understand the physiology of the cells in cannabis stems and branches. Think of a stem having two parts: Inner layering and outer layering. The outside is often called bast fibers; this is the substance behind most hemp textiles. The inside is generally called xylem. Under a microscope, you will see that there are more layers.

The primary phloem fibers are formed from procambium, and the secondary phloem fibers are produced by cambium. In developmental biology, these all come from the initiation of cell growth, which forms a thick structural cell wall for plant support.

The area from the cambium to the outside bask of the cannabis plant is called many names, such as phloem, phloem fibers, primary fibers, or epidermis. These names are for convenience rather than an accurate scientific description of all the layers of plant cells. Despite the rigidity of cannabis structure, it is easy to segregate out these layers, which is another reason cannabis is such a farmable textile. You may also work with cell layers in some advanced plant care techniques.

Air-Layer Cloning

Also known as marcotting, air-layering is a combination of grafting and cloning techniques, mainly derived from observing plants behaving as if they were runners. Strawberries are an example of runners, where a long branch-like structure appears to arch away from the plant and go into the ground nearby, producing a new strawberry plant. While many plants do not propagate like this, they sometimes behave as if they do. First, part of a branch topples over, and a broken or cut area touches the ground. Roots grow from the cut zone when it reaches the ground, giving the appearance of a new plant growing as if it were a cutting or a clone. This proves that damaged areas can produce roots which can be rooted and grow. When these damaged areas are separated from the main plant as a clone, they become a truly individual plant.

Grafting joins the main plant, also known as the rootstock, onto parts of genetically compatible plants, or scions, using binding techniques for successful fusion. The connecting of plant tissue is called inosculation, and this happens in nature when plants can become conjoined from abrasions rubbing against each other, causing the outer bark to shave off and the inner vascular cambium tissues between both plants to make contact. Plant repair mechanisms do not recognize differences between genetically compatible plants, and can fuse the plants at these zones during the repair. Manual binding techniques, such as using tape combined with V insert cuts, increase the success rate of a successful bond; because there is limited contact with air, more root growth is produced at the cut zones, but the same principle allows for the propagation of cuttings.

The vital growth regulatory hormones are auxins and cytokinins. Auxins are produced mainly at the top and tips of the plant, flowing down through the rest of the plant, while cytokines are produced at the bottom and travel upwards. These hormones shape the direction of growth, so root development and new shoots depend on the amount and concentration of both. With grafting, the reduced air at the cut zone promotes root development, which we can use in a cloning technique called air-layering.

How to Air-Layer a Clone

To air-layer a clone, you will need:

- Plant
- Razor blade
- Tweezers
- Scissors
- Grow cube
- Rooting hormone (Clonex) gel or powder
- Plastic wrap
- Gardening or rubber gloves

There are a few ways to air-layer, and you can pick the one that works best for you. The following steps work with thinner branches in most cases, but for thicker branches and stems more cutting away might have to be done. In this case, look for the additional steps.

- Find a branch at least 1/8-inch thick with a minimum of two nodes above it.
- Use a razor blade to score a wound at this region, cutting downwards ¼ inch into the branch to meet the phloem.
- Use tweezers to open the slit, but do not break the branch completely.

- Using gloves, apply rooting hormone to the open wound.
- Cut the grow cube down one side and slide it over the break.
- Wrap the area.
- Use an eyedropper to keep the medium wet every day.

After two weeks, your cutting will have roots that will grow into the grow cube. You can then cut away the branch below the roots, leaving you with a clone ready for growth.

If this procedure does not work, it's likely that the slit you made was insufficient, and you need to remove external tissue to promote root production. The outside tissue should be physically removed and not just broken open. This problem occurs often with thicker branches and stems, for which the following technique works best. First, cut around the diameter of the branch or stem below the selected node, and then cut around again somewhere below that. You might see some sap coming out, which carries sugars, water, and hormones. The roots will grow here. Cut a downward slit between the two around-the-branch cuts you just made, allowing you to peel the tissue away from that part and fully expose the inside. The skin you remove is the bast fiber, and the inside layer is the cambium, where cells carry hormones to different parts of the plant. You can rub the cutting tool edge up and down the exposed area of the internode length to gently destroy these carrying vessels. Use this exposed region for rooting hormone treatment, wrapping, and monitoring. Peeling and scraping away the cambium tissue terminates the flow up of some hormones and down that branch. Remember the hormones we discussed earlier: When cytokines no longer interact with the axions that flow down the plant to the air layer zone, it promotes root production at the cut area. Now, we must prevent air from inhibiting root growth.

If you do not wish to use Rockwool, you can make a wrap from the top of a plastic bottle. Cut away the bottle top with enough volume left for the air-layered area to have some substrate, and remove the bottle cap. Cut the bottle down one side so you can wrap it around the cut zone. Technically any substrate can go inside the bottle wrapping, covering the cut area. Mosses and coir brick fibers can dampen the substrate, making it easier to pack. Next, cover the bottle up to create a dark environment. Make sure it's not airtight, as you don't want to create a damp environment for fungi and rot. As long as there are drainage holes and the wrap doesn't allow light to enter, you should see results in four to six weeks. You will need to cut the entire branch away from the plant just below where your Rockwool or wrapping is. When you unpack, you will find roots, which means you have a new clone to use.

Bonsai Clones

Bonsai clones are easy to make but take time. If you succeed, you can put one mother bonsai clone in a grow tent under an LED to provide you with limitless clones. However, you will lose the genetics if the bonsai fails. Two bonsai are better than one, but whatever causes one to fail can quickly cause the rest to fail.

Making Bonsai Clones

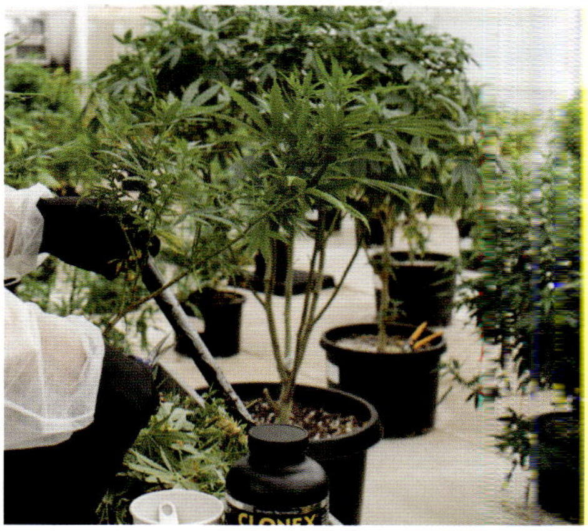

Super short and squat bonsai mom.

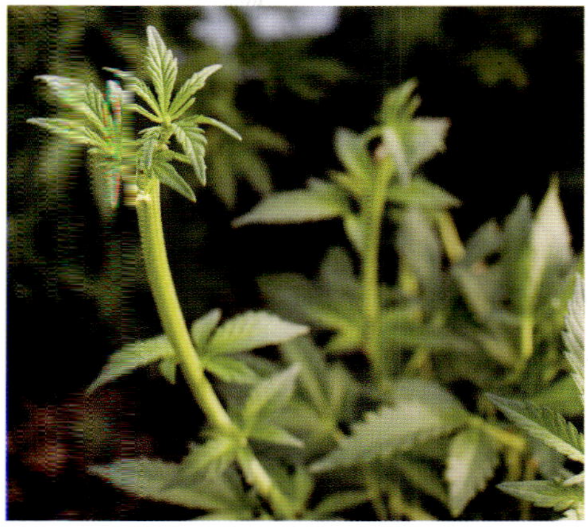

More care is taken with shaping the mother...

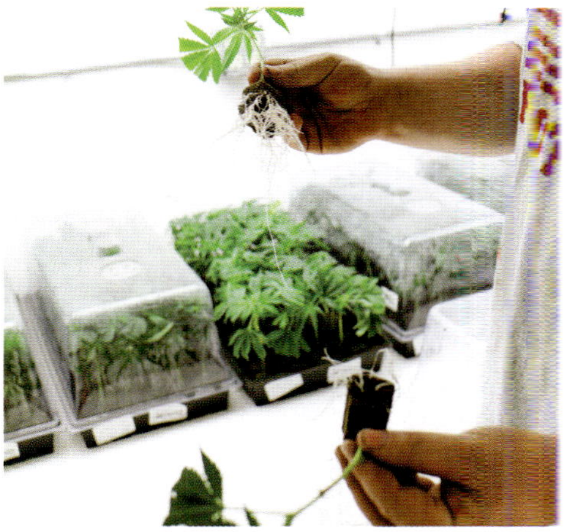

...meaning her clones will look amazing also.

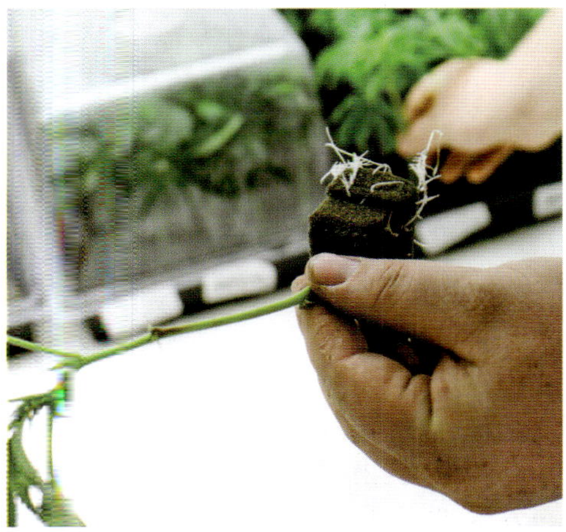

Mother donates top genetics.

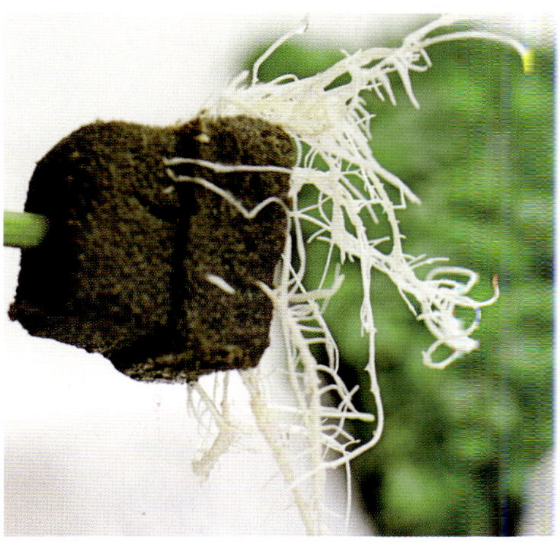

Healthy root growth.

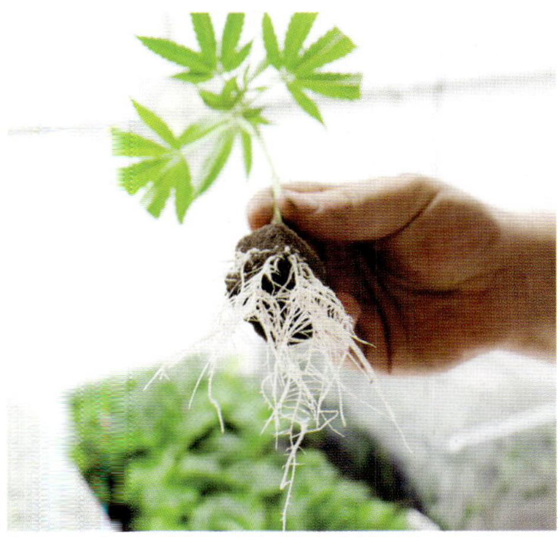

First rate clone. Perfect for hydroponics.

PHOTOS: KRISTEN ANGELO

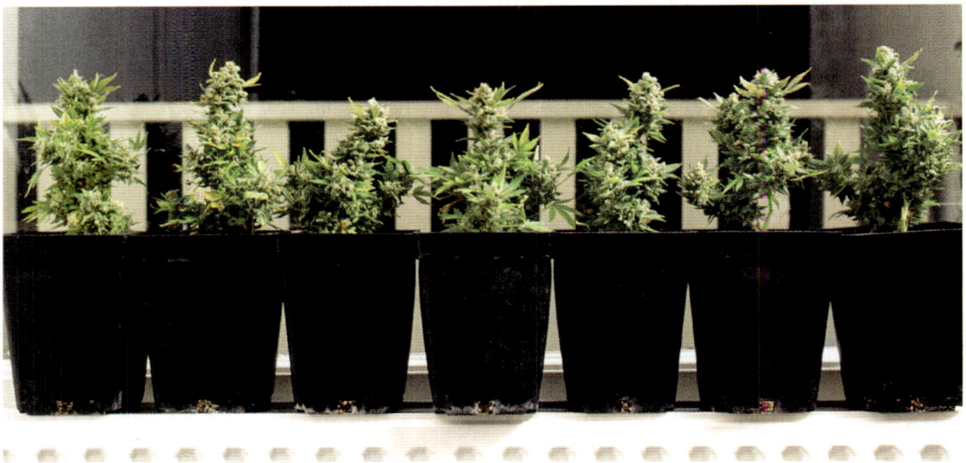

Instead of pruning to keep plants short, consider using genetically short varieties, such as autoflowering strains. Here are seven of them, each no more than 16 inches tall.

First, prepare a cutting using your preferred method and prune the clone using the technique discussed on page 508. The plant should be a short bushy clone with multiple branches so that lots of cuttings can be taken from it. Keep the bonsai short, about 1.5 feet in height, and store it in a clone tent. Diminutive bonsai mother plants can generate at least a hundred clones per year. There is quite a market for them in countries where cannabis clones are legal. Medical users especially like to buy clones from experienced growers because they know that the grower has worked on multiple strains to find a special mother that suits the medical users' needs. Bonsai can also be fun to maintain, and can be presented as an ornamental for show.

Sinsemilla Hermaphrodites

Close inspection of your flowers towards the final weeks of growth is essential to detect the possibility of male flowers. A slight hermaphrodite condition can be treated by clipping away the males to prevent pollination of the females. You must look closely at the female flowers to detect male pollen sacks, which will look like yellow banana shapes in the bud. A small tent may generate a couple of hermaphrodite flowers in the final weeks of flowering. In most cases, the pollen produced is not viable, and should be clipped away as a precaution. Hermaphrodites are a common condition with sinsemilla crops as some plants, in a last-ditch effort to produce seeds, will generate a few male flowers to self-pollinate. We previously covered the genetic theory behind this in Chapter 2.

Reverting to Vegetative Growth

PHOTO: ED BORG

Also known as re-vegging, regeneration, or rejuvenation, this process can be done anywhere between the start of flowering and the end of the plant's peak bloom when it is ready for harvest. Reverting does not work with strains that have autoflowering properties, such as ruderalis or ruderalis hybrids, also known as autoflowering hybrids. If you are able to revert to vegetative growth, your plants probably aren't mostly autoflowering strains; a "mostly" autoflowering hybrid should be autoflowering by definition and bred to lean that way.

Reverting is an attempt to get clones after harvest or to go for a second lower-yield harvest. The results are experimental. To revert a plant to vegetative growth, you first need to change from a flowering photoperiod of 12/12 to a vegetative photoperiod of 24/0 or 18/6. Remove all of the plant's flowers and calyx development by clipping them away from the plant at their base. When your plant is bare of its flowers and calyx development, you can choose to reduce the height of your plant to a stage where it resembles its vegetative growth. Doing this will provide you with clones ready to flower immediately. After a few weeks, your plant will revert to vegetative growth and no longer flower until the 12/12 photoperiod is initiated again. When you are satisfied that your plant has reached a satisfactory level of node production, you can return to a 12/12 photoperiod, and your plant will flower again. Reverting to vegetative growth is a way to harvest more flowers from the same plant.[4] However, it has disadvantages, so cloning is a more practical and quicker method. Reverting to vegetative growth can take up to four weeks, which is time that could have been spent cloning the original plant and growing these clones. Rejuvenated plants tend not to produce the quantities of bud they did during their peak bloom, although it's not impossible for them to do so. Your yield expectations should be set lower than if you were using clones. The growing medium will contain higher levels of phosphorus than nitrogen and potassium. The amount of nitrogen needs to be higher than or equal to the amount of phosphorus and potassium. This can be hard to do without flushing your soil or performing a transplant. Both flushing and transplanting can cause stress, which may lead to sexual dysfunctions in a rejuvenated plant's flowering stage. It is much easier to accomplish this adjustment in a hydroponic system. Finally, rejuvenated plants go through a certain amount of stress due to the photoperiod change, which can induce sexual dysfunction and the hermaphrodite condition.

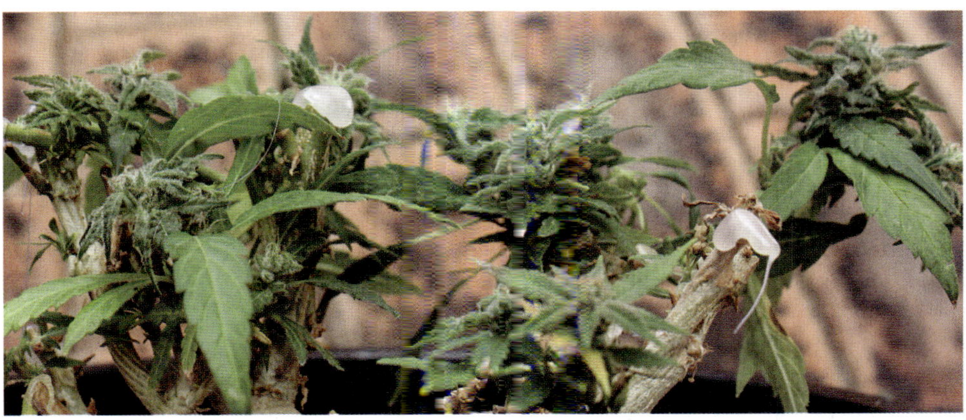

After trimming the buds, a bonsai-like trunk and some baby buds are all that remain. These buds can be regenerated again. Note the white glue sealing the severed branches.

PHOTO: FROM *CANNABIS REGENERATION* WRITTEN BY JB HAZE

JB Haze's Guide To Cannabis Regeneration

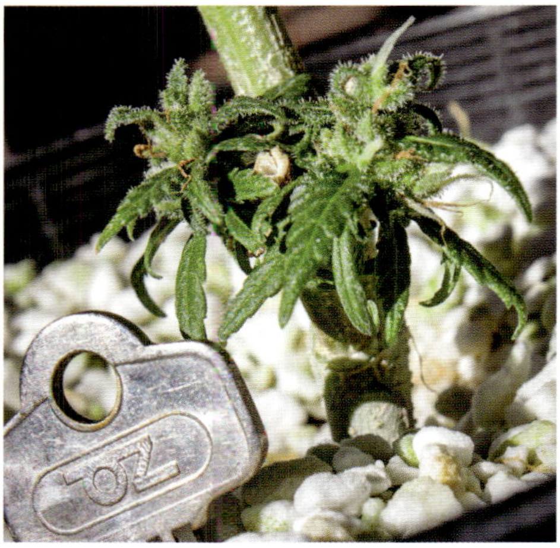

Leave flowers low down on the plant.

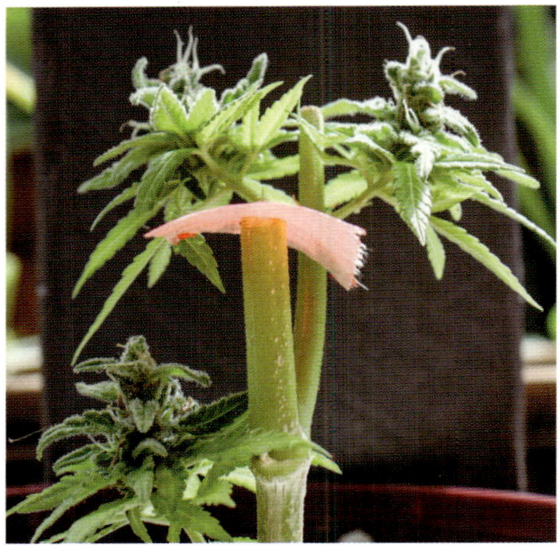

Tape up areas you pruned.

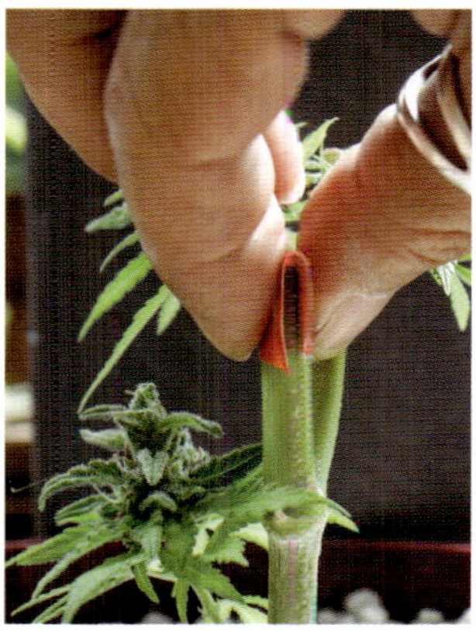

One piece over the top.

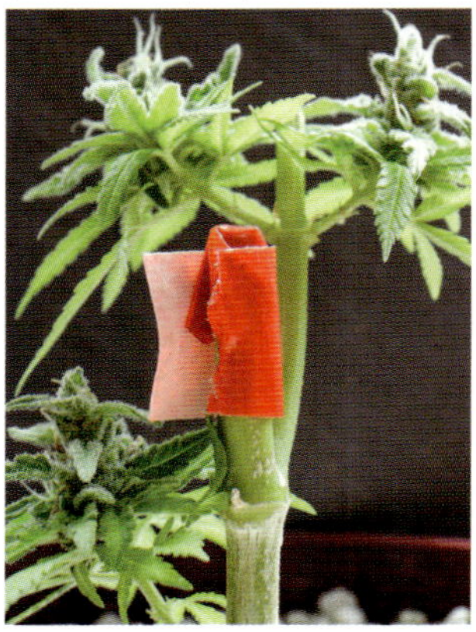

Next piece goes around it.

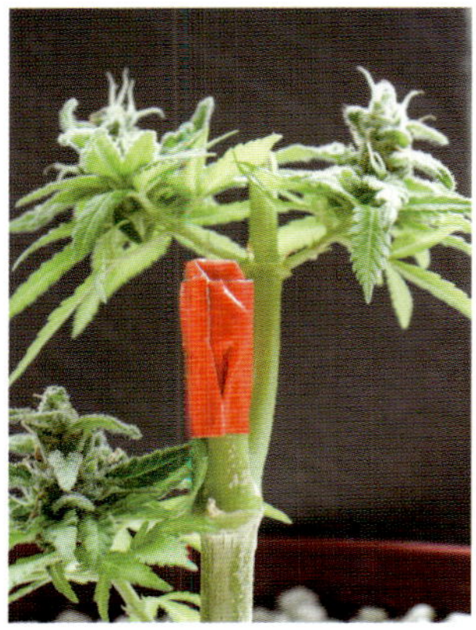

Helps prevent necrosis.

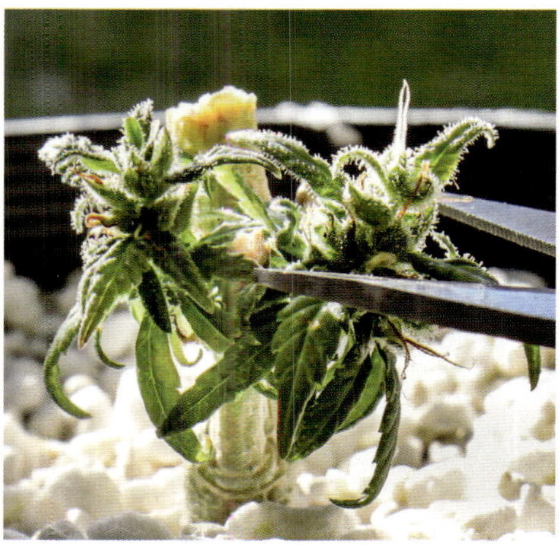

FIM-style clip the buds.

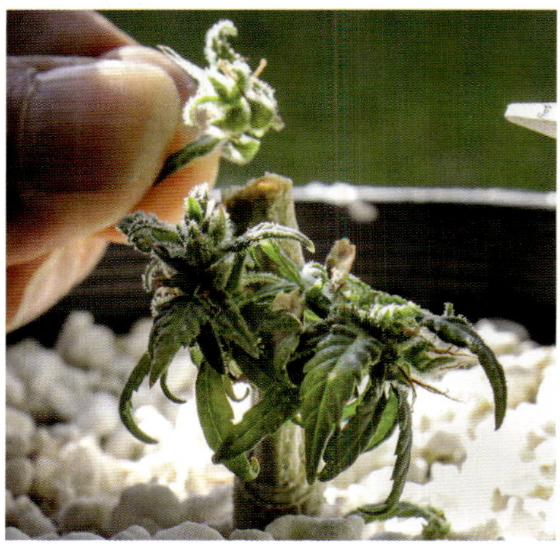

The half-removed buds look like this.

PHOTOS: FROM *CANNABIS REGENERATION* WRITTEN BY JB HAZE

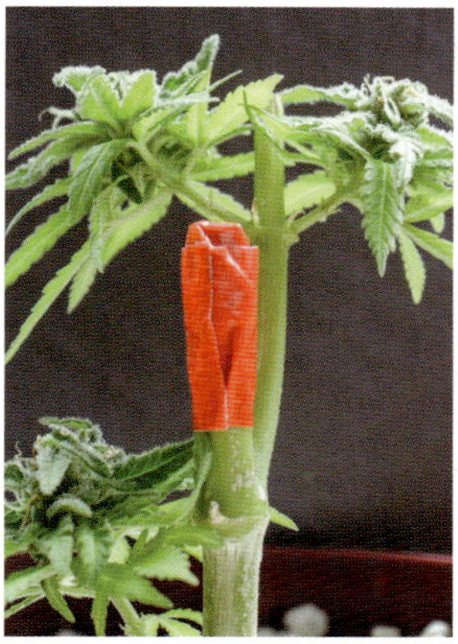

The main stem in this instance has been blocked.

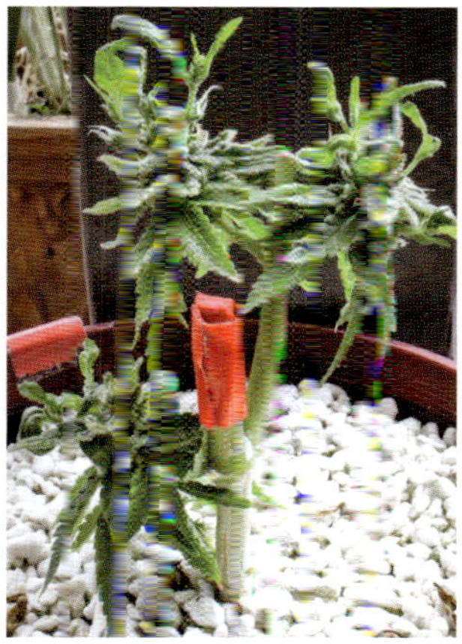

New growth appearing over the coming days.

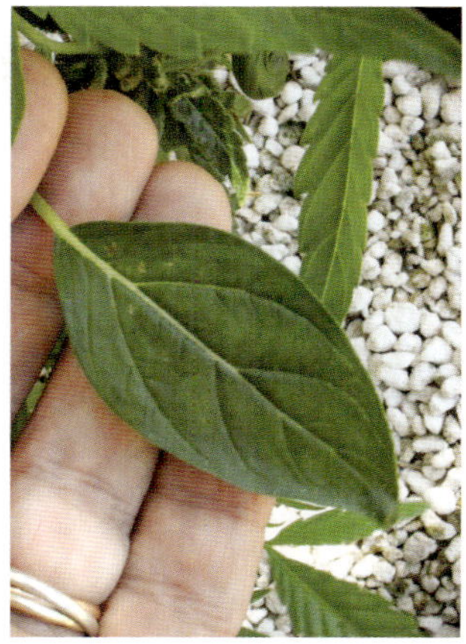

Plant quickly produces single bladed leaf for light.

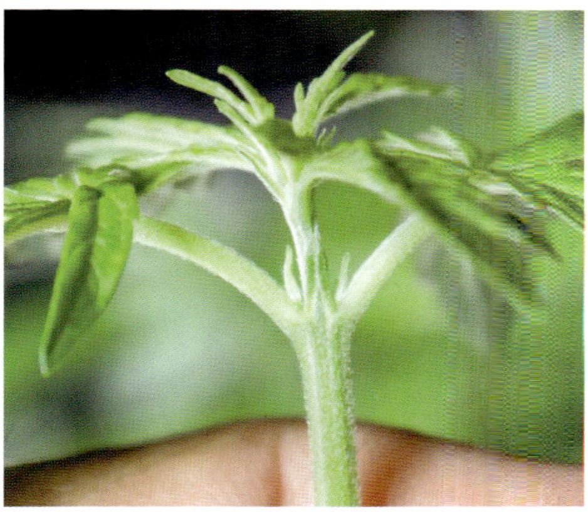

New growth.

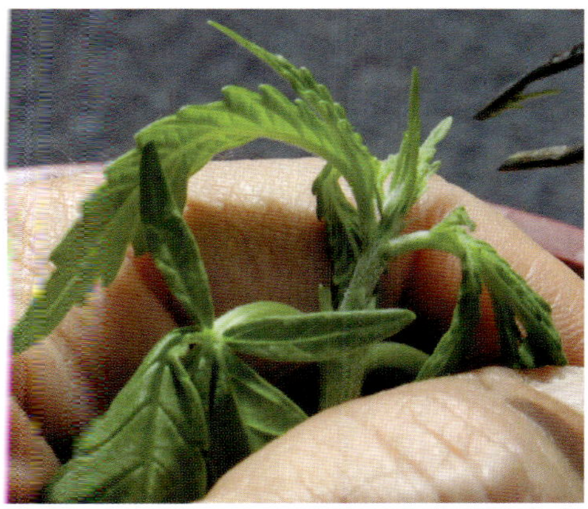

FIM-style works here also.

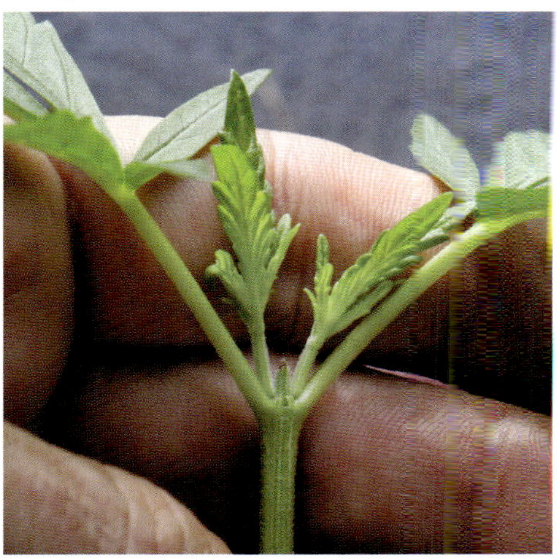

Combining pruning techniques, like topping, to bush the plant.

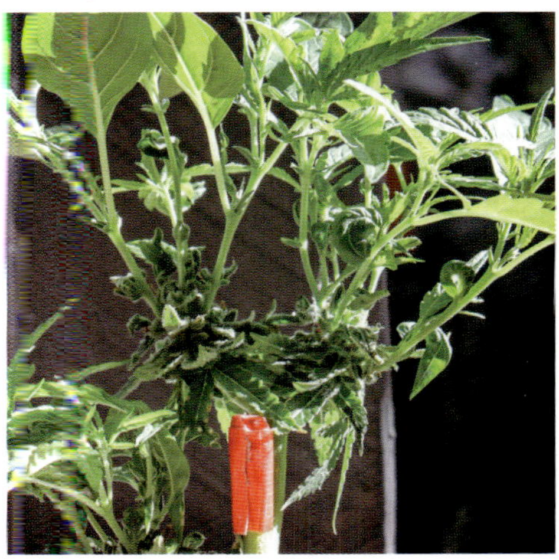

Result is more node regions for bud growth.

ScrOG Cannabis Rejuvenation

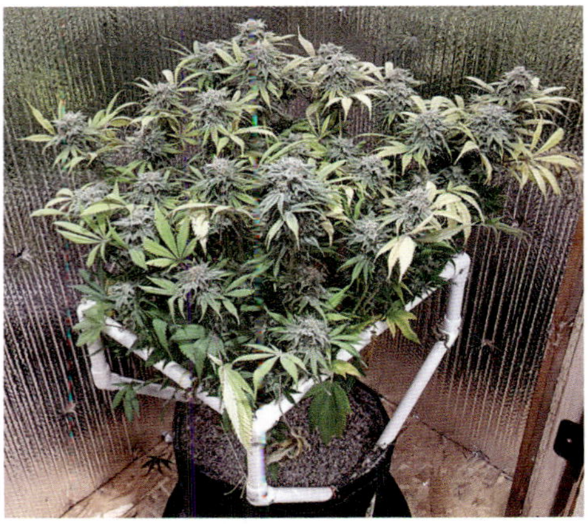
A common question: Yes, you can regrow plants.

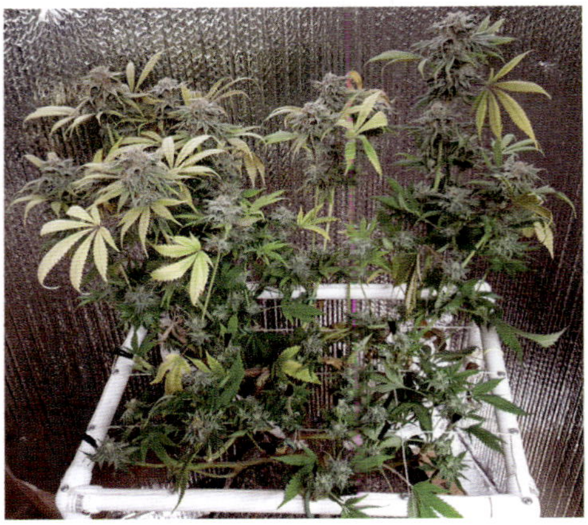
It is best to use heavily pruned plants.

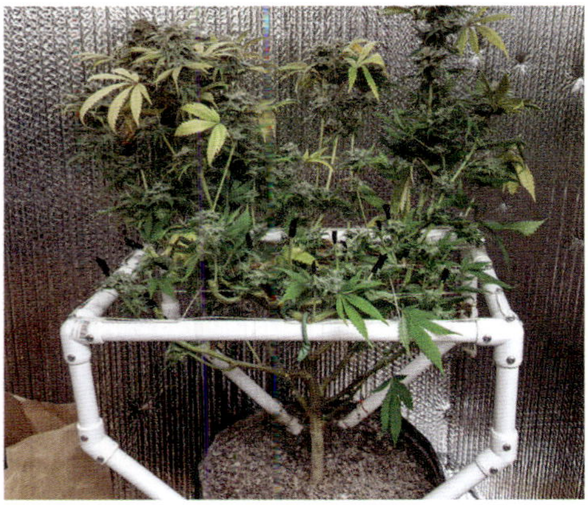
Lots of branches around the mesh area. Keep new flowers.

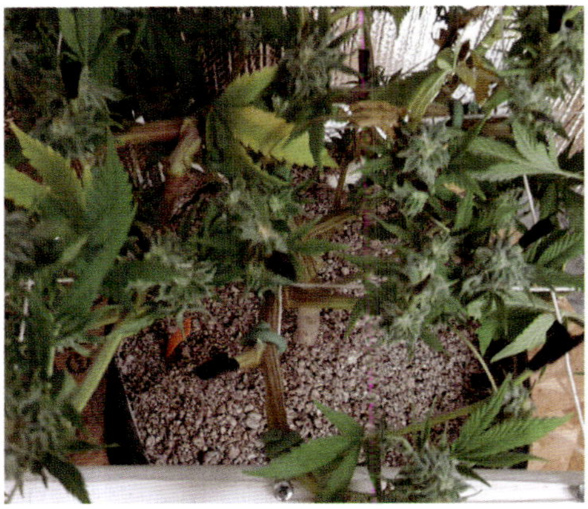
Remove only mature flowers. Prune branches to mesh level.

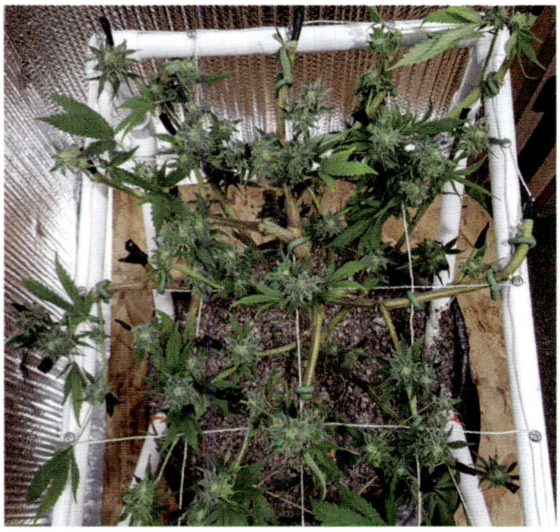
Work branches around the mesh in a new way.

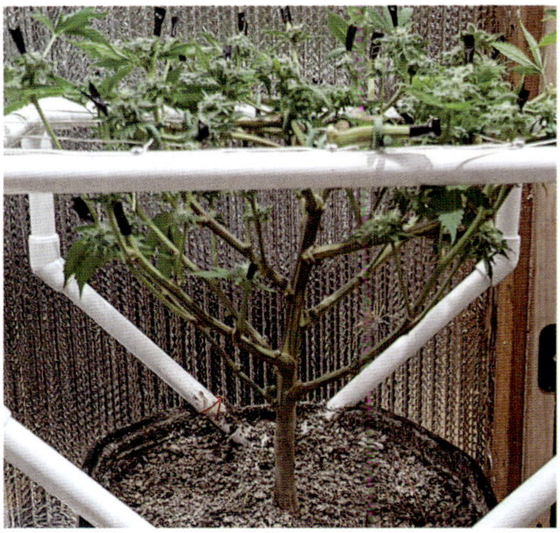
Prune it to taste and tape up cut zones.

PHOTOS: GREEN THOM

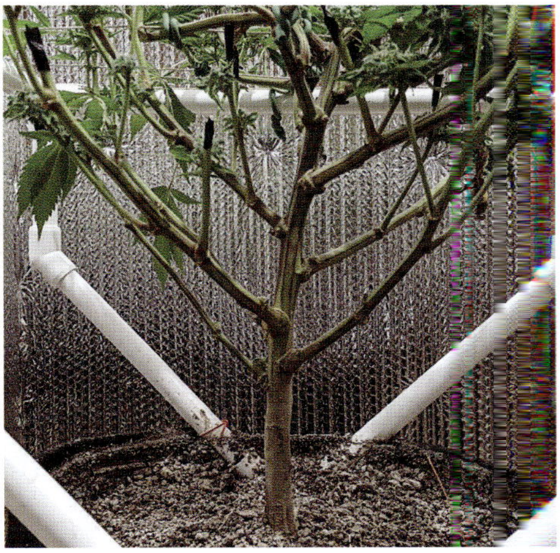

A pruned plant provides more bud sites.

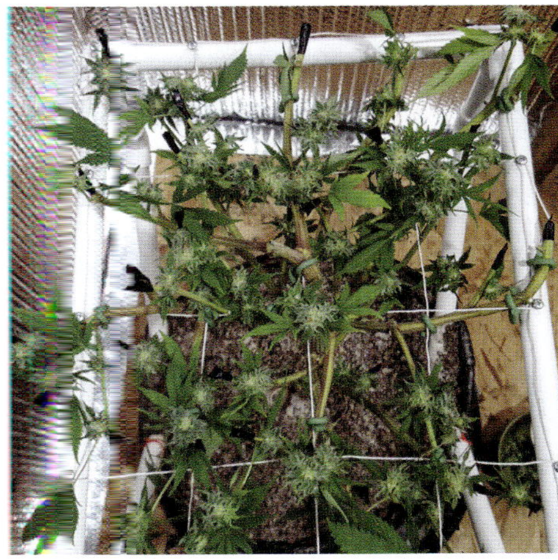

New flowers will become the next harvest.

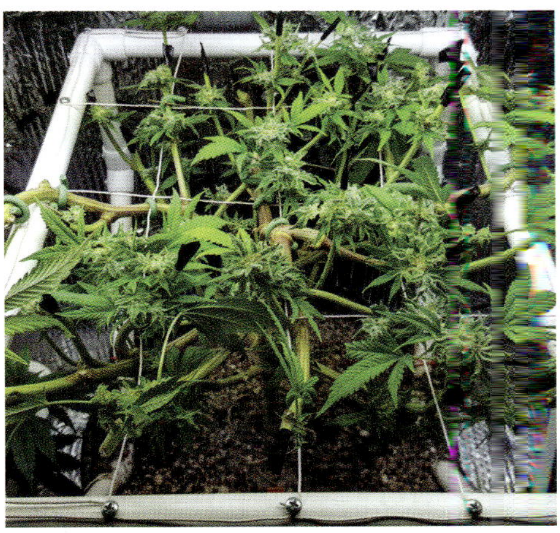

Treat it as you would a ScrOG.

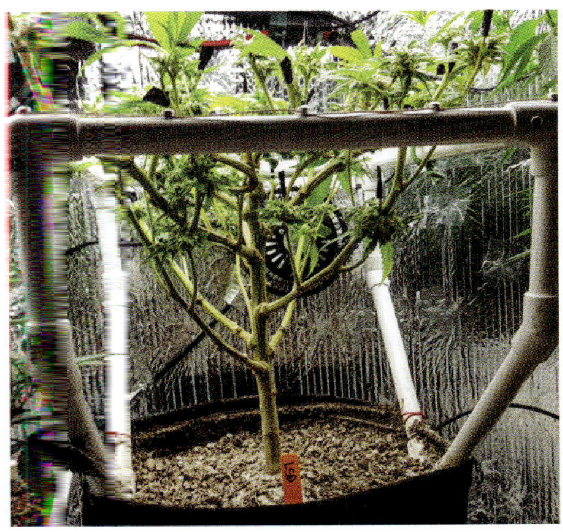

Keep it down.

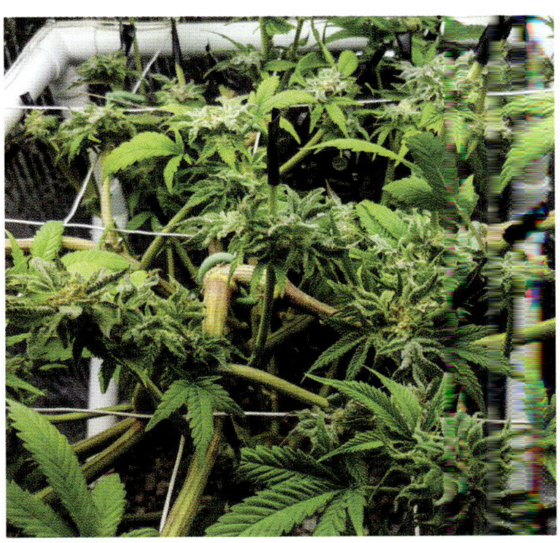

This will become a new canopy of bud.

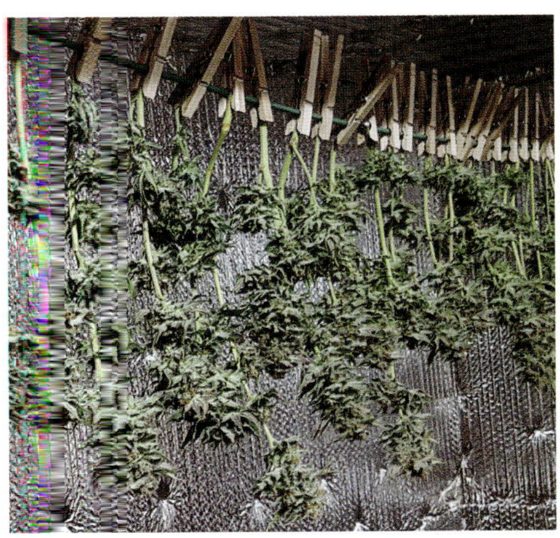

Hang up your harvested mature flowers.

Increasing Your Chances of Females

Previously, growers believed optimal growing conditions would produce more females than males. However, with increasing confidence over the decades, experiments have demonstrated that the sex of cannabis is set genetically in the seed. So why do some growers see more females than males? The explanation is sample bias. If you take 100 seeds, you would have approximately 50/50 chances of getting either a male or female from each seed. However, if you take samples of 10 seeds to make 10 packs, the distribution of 50/50 per pack is only an average; those values can drift in random samples. For example, one pack may have 6 males and 4 females, another 7 males and 3 females, another 8 males and 2 females, and another 8 females and 2 males. A grower may get lucky and end up with several packets of mostly females, while somewhere else, someone has gotten unlucky with more males than females. This is why it is called sample bias; the larger the sample, the more the results resemble a 50/50 split. The smaller the sample, the greater the chance of skewing results away from that 50/50 split.

Feminized Seeds

The best way to increase your chances of females is with feminized seeds, which guarantee a return of only females (no males). Since these seeds will contain no males, pollination should not occur, so you naturally get sinsemilla yields (without seeds), which would otherwise only be possible by removing males. However, feminized plants can still produce hermaphrodites under stressful conditions, and many biological pathways to sexual expression determine if the plant is one sex or a mixture. This means that best practices are still needed for successful results for all female plants.

But how are these miraculous feminized seeds created? The parents of these seeds undergo special treatment: They are stressed with known chemicals that cause pollen production to consist of female chromosomes alone, ensuring that the sexual expression of the seeds is female only. When this pollen, known as 'female pollen', is used with a female plant, the resulting seeds will be female and can be sold as feminized seeds that produce female plants only. Getting feminized seeds helps you use your plants efficiently, as none of their energy will contribute to making males if you don't need the pollen or seeds. For more details, refer to the breeding chapter.

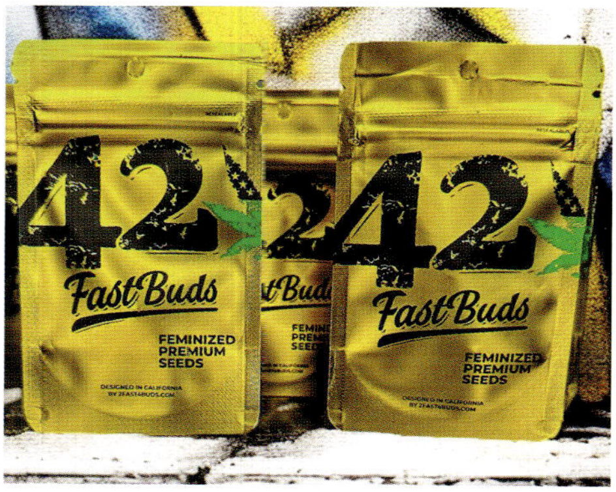

PHOTO: SHOPFREEGROW8.COM

Feminized seeds in packs.

All things being optimal with standard seeds, your sex ratio will be based on samples from a larger population split 50/50 between males and females. Optimizing results will not produce more females but will produce better results. If you want more females from standard seeds, you will need to germinate and grow more.

Secret Sauce Feminized Seeds

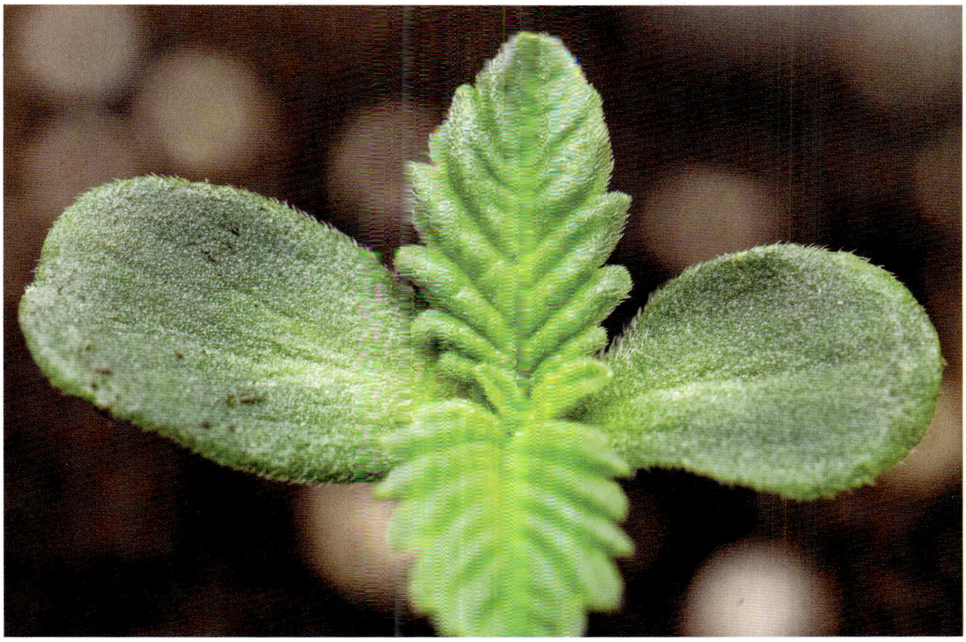

Feminized seeds germinate exactly the same way as standard seeds do. There is no difference in how you grow them either.

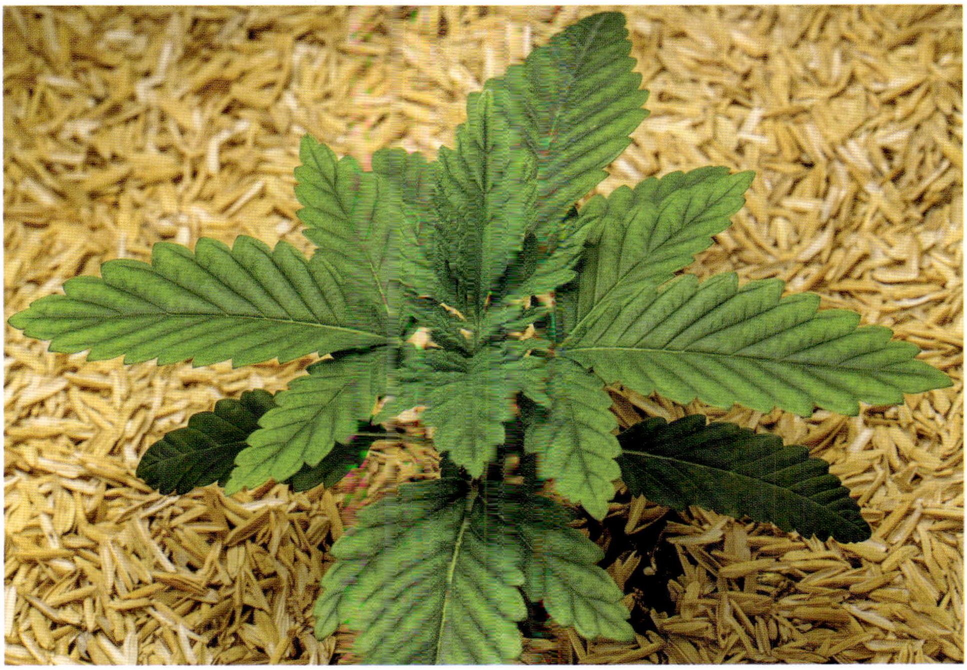

PHOTOS: JOE'S CANNA GROWS

The only difference between standard seeds and feminized ones is that feminized ones always produce only female plants.

continues...

Secret Sauce Feminized Seeds *continued*

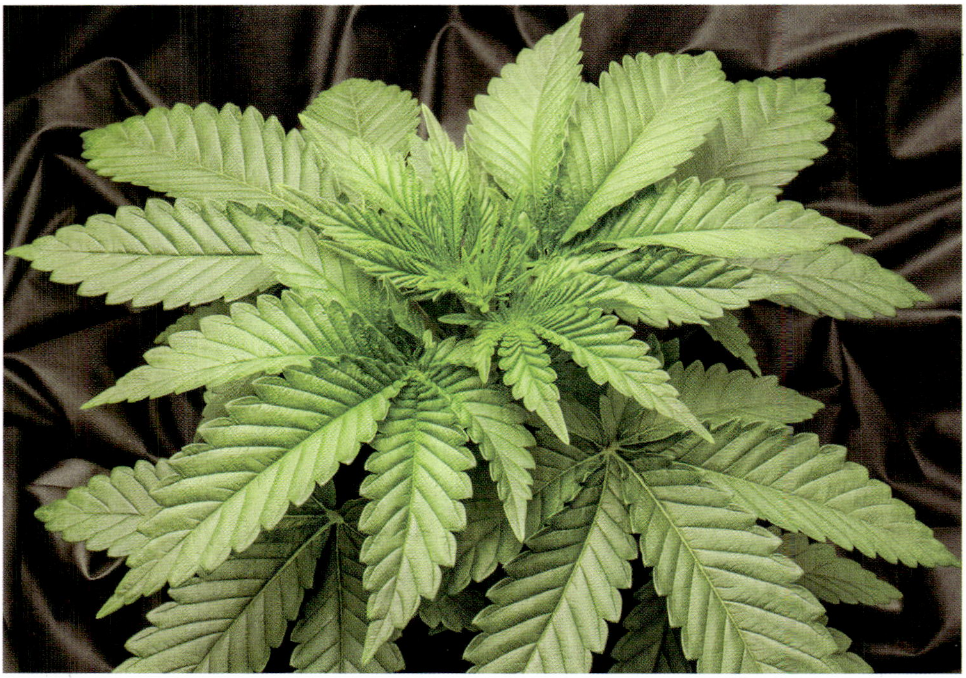

Squat and healthy is exactly how with these beautiful indoor feminized plants should be.

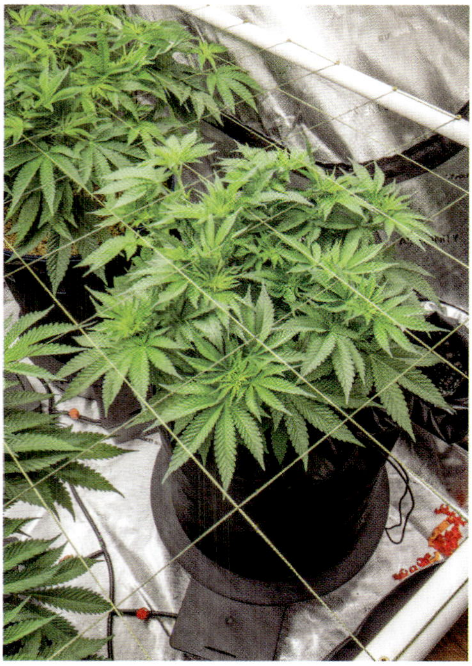

The ScrOG method can also be used with feminized plants.

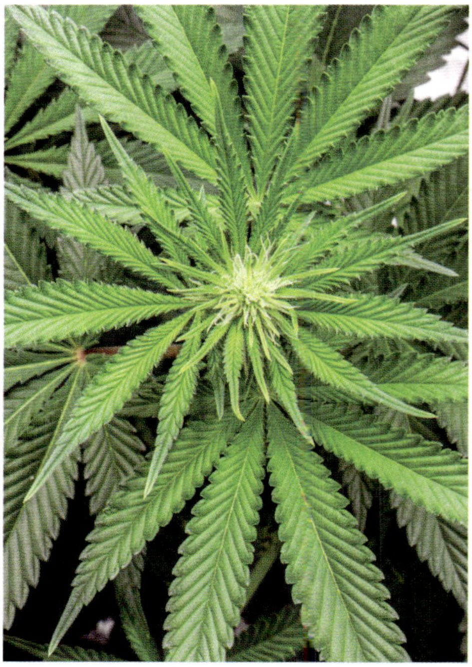

Feminized seeds are an alternative way to get all female plants instead of cloning them.

PHOTOS: JOE'S CANNA GROWS

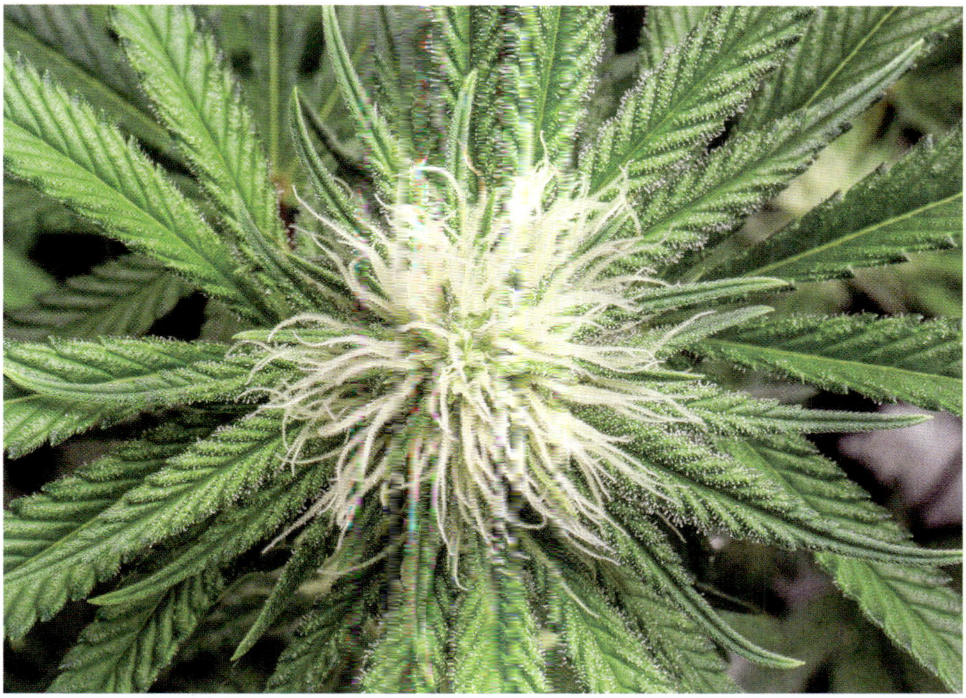

A flowering plant grown from feminized seeds is indistinguishable from one grown from standard seeds or clones.

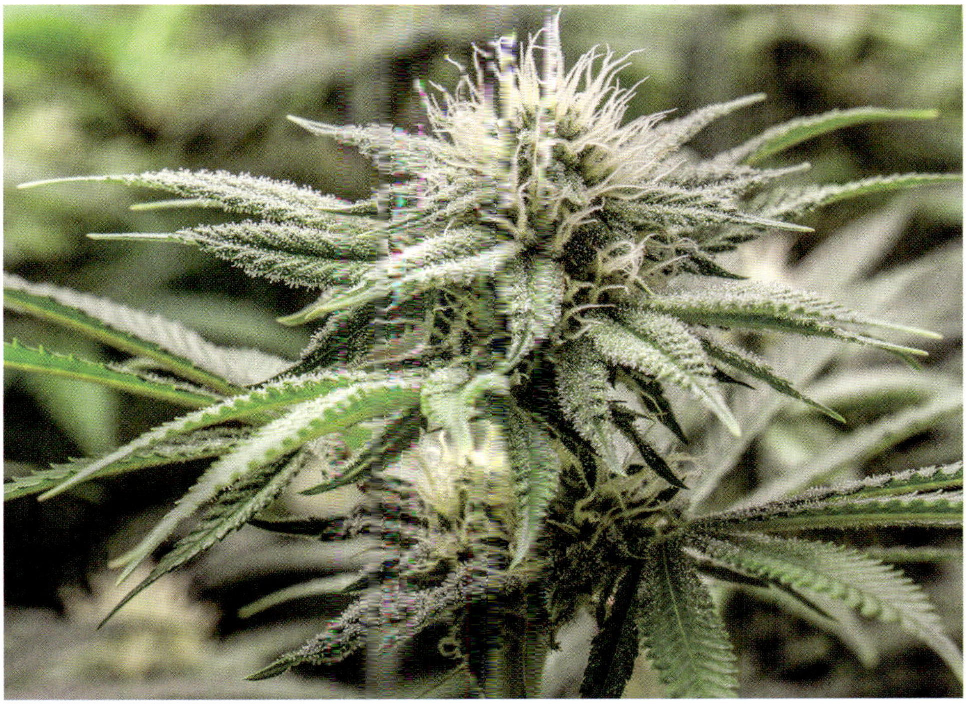

Most standard strains today are offered also in feminized seed format.

continues...

Secret Sauce Feminized Seeds *continued*

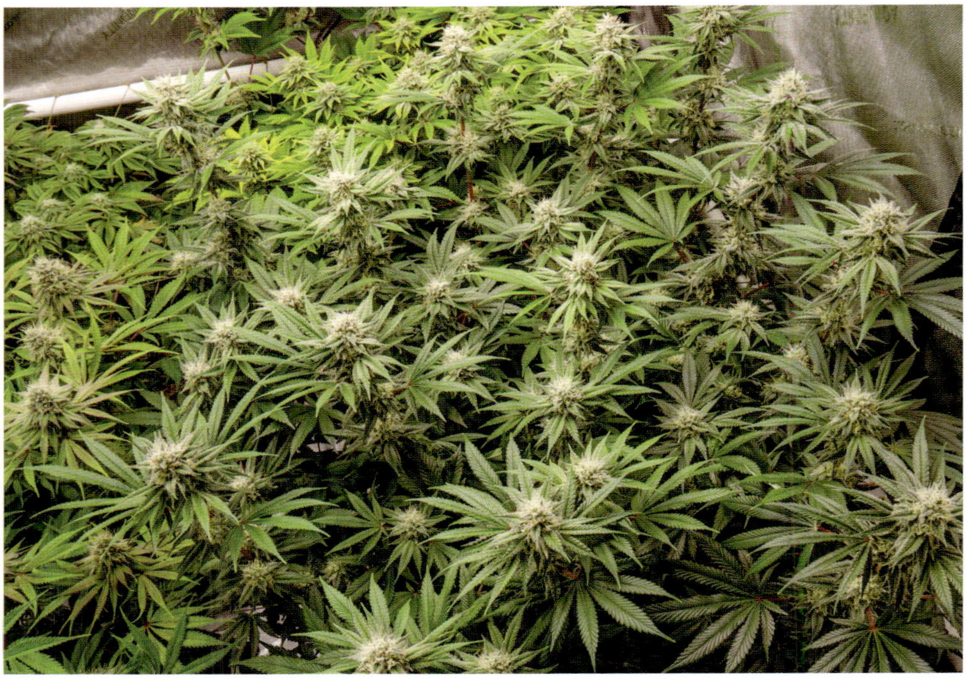

Feminized plants can also be flushed in the final weeks of flowering.

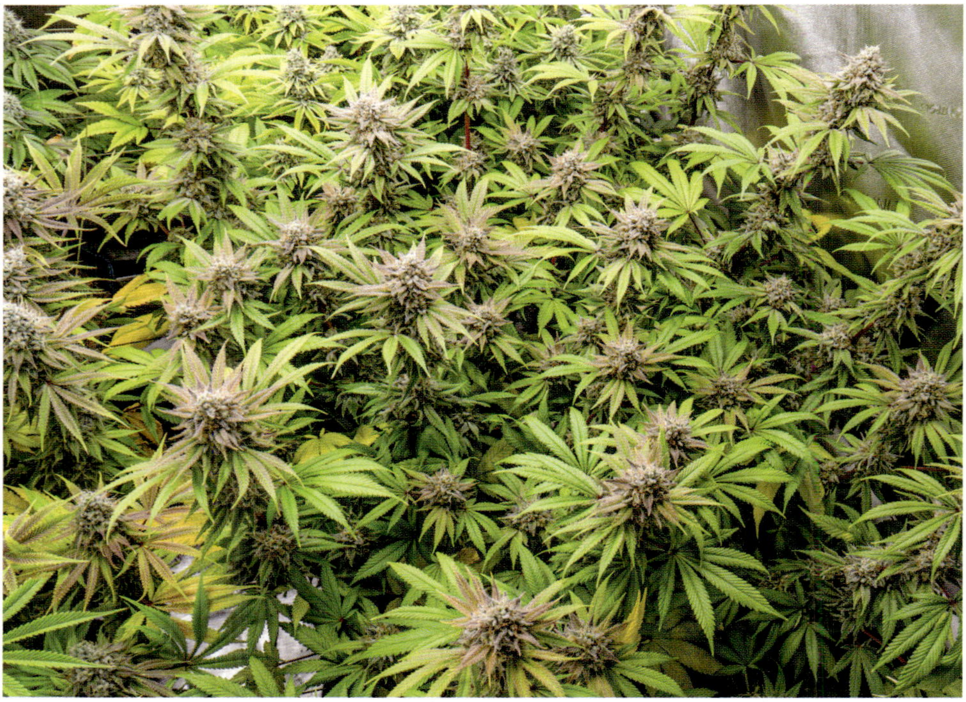

These females have covered every square foot of this garden making this grow very efficient.

PHOTOS: JOE'S CANNA GROWS

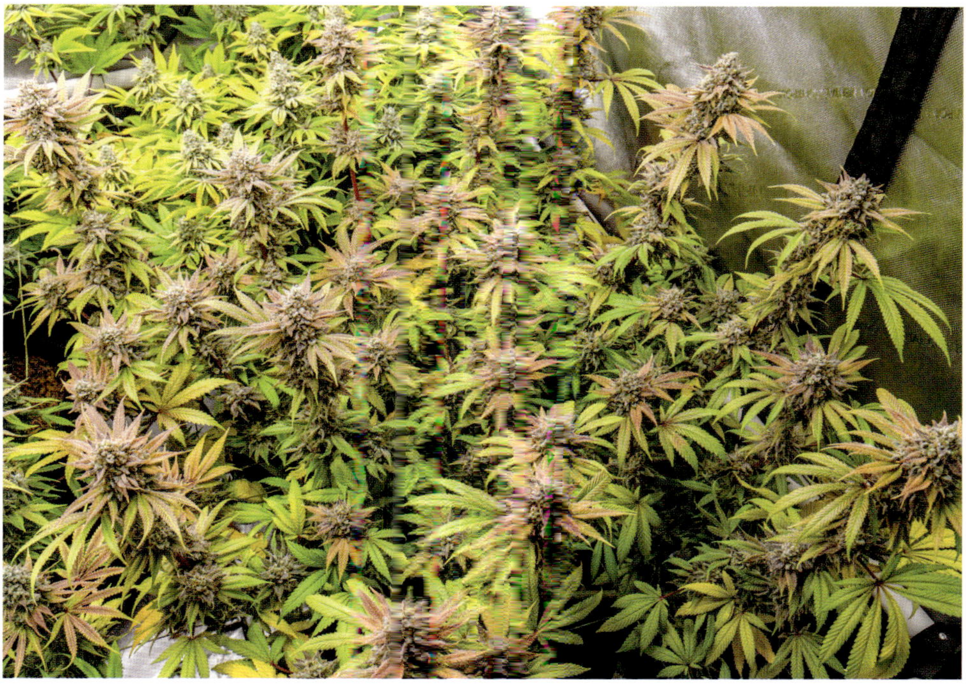

Feminized seeds will always result in a higher number of flowering plants, as standard seeds produce 50% males.

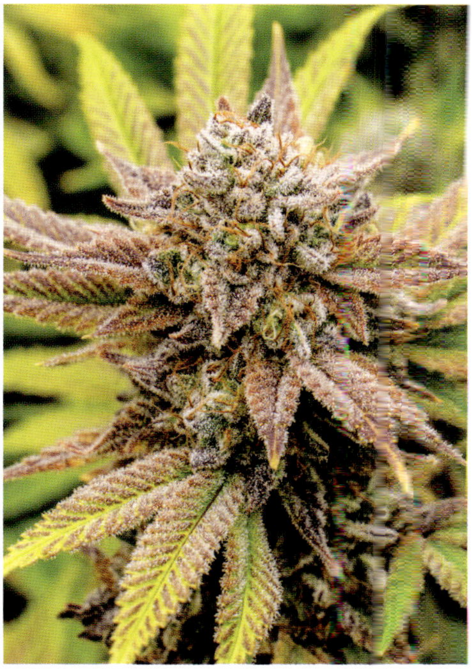

These feminized seeds produced dense buds thick with trichomes.

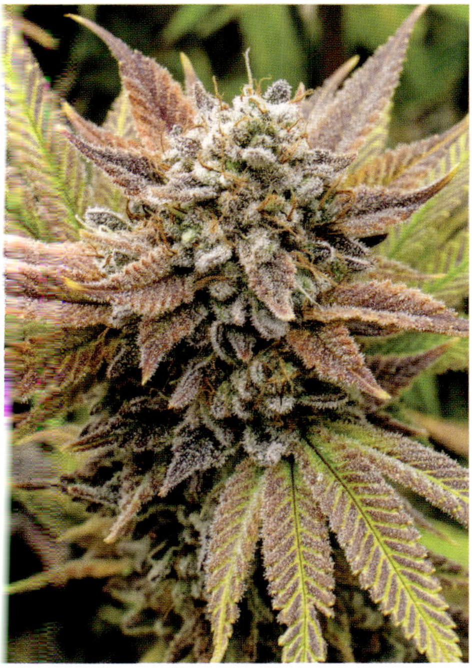

Who wouldn't be happy with such results as these thick buds?

continues...

Secret Sauce Feminized Seeds *continued*

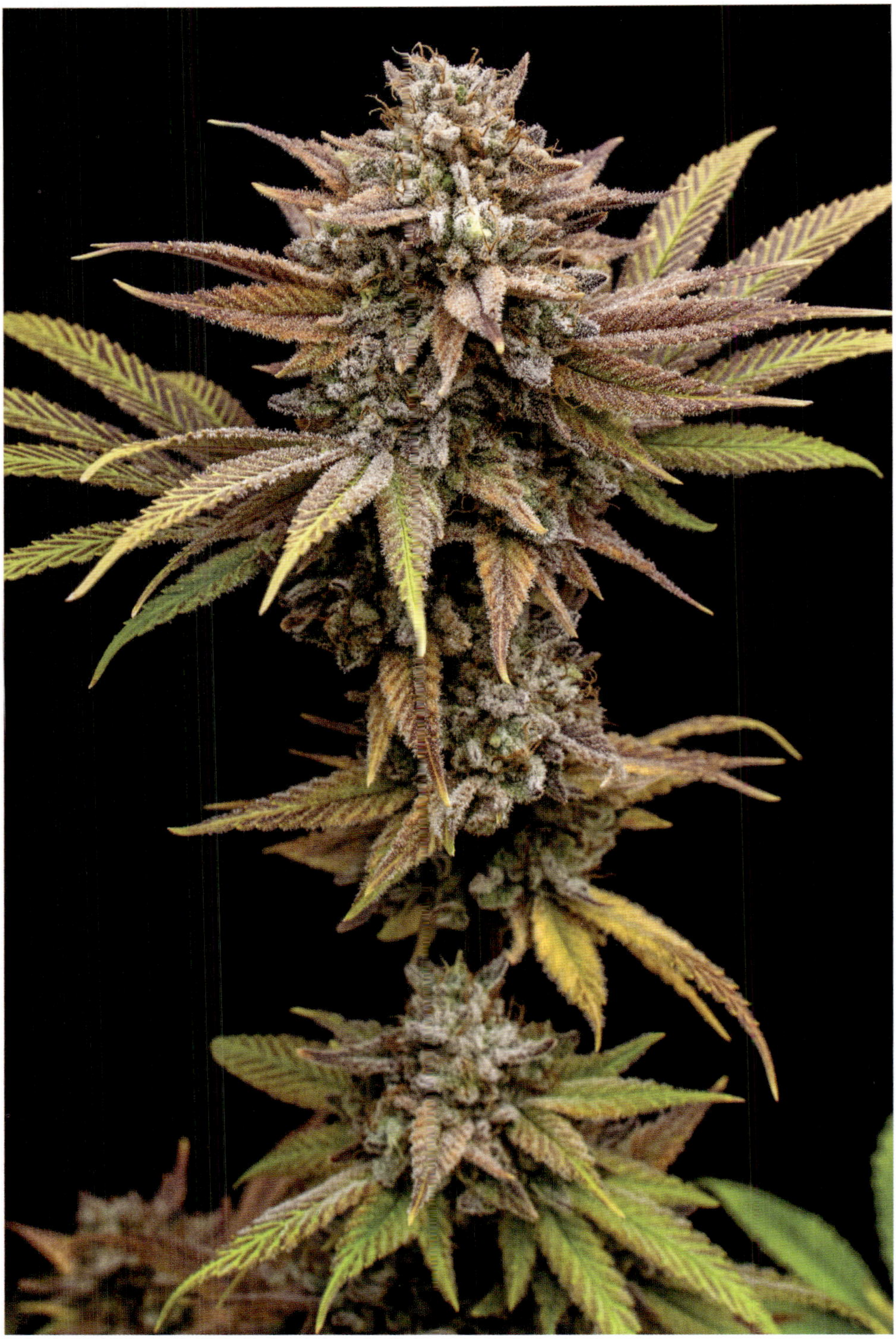

PHOTO: JOE'S CANNA GROWS

This feminized strain was filled with buds between nodes. This is what it is all about.

Optimization

Most growers' main objective is yield, which is the amount of bud your plant will produce by the harvest. However, some growers may prioritize taste before yield. The more you grow, the more you'll understand what your plant needs for optimal results. The two most fundamental factors in producing excellent yields and bud-rich plants are good genetics and optimal lighting. However, high yields may not mean highly potent bud. Potency depends on the strain, genetic cannabinoid compositions, and how well your plant is grown. In addition, different feeding products have some influence over the potency of final yields. For example, some grow bloomers, and advance feeding products containing hormones, may produce more significant amounts of bud but reduce potency or produce a different taste. These changes are due to a trade-off when the plants devote more energy to yield than to the mechanisms developing taste and potency. Learning which feeding products are best requires a degree of experimentation, but experimentation is what growing is all about. The cannabis cultivator must experiment and discover new growing methods through failure. I know plenty of growers who gave up using pot to focus on developing new strains and discovering new ways to increase yield. Cannabis cultivation is a very addictive hobby.

The End of the Grow

At the start of this book, we mentioned that propagation correctly means the stages of cultivation between preparing seeds for germination to harvest. We have now covered all the essential topics of cannabis propagation. At this stage, you should have a fair idea of the following:

- The history of cannabis
- How cannabis is used
- The life cycle of cannabis
- THC, CBD, cannabinoids, potency, and medical use
- Species and strains
- Security issues
- Types of seeds and where to get them
- How to germinate seeds
- Setting up your grow space
- Indoor, outdoor, and guerilla growing
- Hydroponics and advanced grow techniques

With this information, you should feel ready to tackle any challenges with your growth. First, however, you will need to know how to solve problems like pests, fungi, and mold. Chapter 15 focuses on these problems. You can begin to grow now with your current knowledge, but don't skip these chapters. Learning what can go wrong is important in order to identify problems as they arise, which many cultivators fail to do until it is too late. We'll discuss in later chapters what happens after propagation, from harvesting your bud to making hashish, as well as breeding.

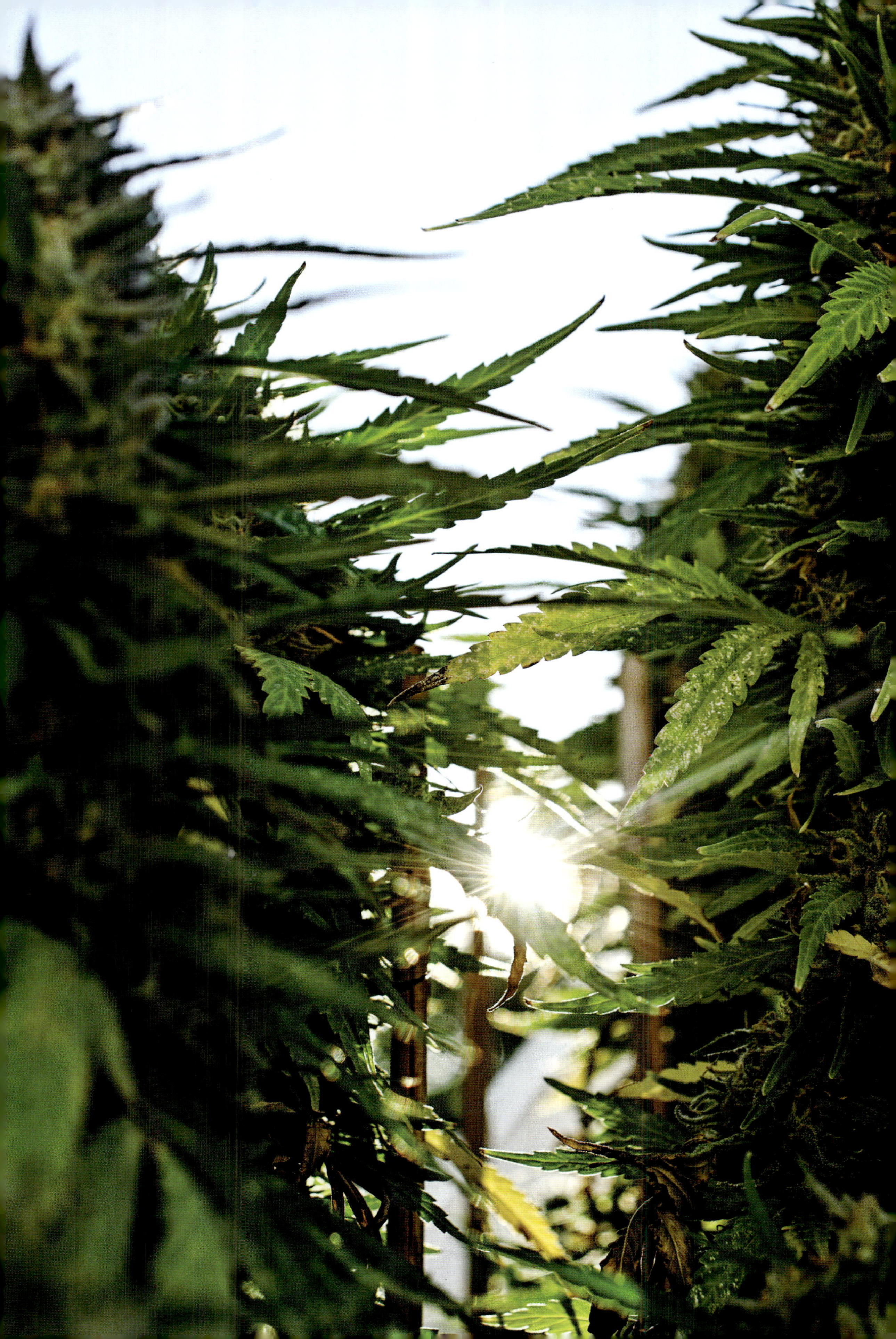

14

Organic Growing

Organic growing is an agricultural practice that embraces an ecosystem service approach, excluding the use of synthetic nutrients, fertilizers, pesticides, hormonal regulators, and artificial genetic modifications. It goes further by avoiding any components that could harm the environment, either directly or indirectly, such as those associated with mining. Organic farming returns natural compounds to the environment from which they are drawn, ensuring a sustainable loop where resources are continually reused, thus leveraging crop surplus, animal waste, compost, natural pest control, and disease management techniques. Any reusable materials are conserved, and waste is minimized through intensive optimization. This self-contained, localized cycle is particularly well-suited for creating organic ecosystems.

Modern organic farming is a scientifically-grounded movement that has significantly influenced agricultural regulations and practices. It has reshaped laws governing commercial farming, particularly those concerning the use of synthetic applications. The urgency of addressing climate change has accelerated the adoption of organic farming principles. When regulated, organic farming leads to government-approved crops that command higher prices due to consumer demand for organic products. The International Federation of Organic Agriculture Movements (IFOAM) sets the global standard for organic agriculture with numerous organic organizations contributing to this framework. Organic products can obtain IFOAM certification, signifying their adherence to organic practices.

To embark on an organic growing journey, you must familiarize yourself with the organic product certifications available in your country to empower you to confidently purchase organic goods, assured of their authenticity. Moreover, should you choose to share your organic products with others, you can actively participate by becoming a member of the organic community. Robust systems of checks and balances have been established for your benefit and the wellbeing of our planet. In the face of the pressing issue of climate change, adhering to organic practices has become an imperative, necessitating the organic path in many agricultural processes.

PHOTO: TRICHOME ART

The carbon cycle plays a pivotal role in organic growing. All organisms, whether large or small, eventually decompose, contributing to this cycle. Living organisms consist primarily of water and carbon, along with numerous other organic chemicals that eventually break down, returning to the ground or the ocean. This decomposition generates primary, secondary, and micronutrients for plants. Animals further the cycle by feeding on plants and redistributing these nutrients as macro and micro molecules. This natural process is gradual rather than rapid, with solid organic materials decomposing more slowly than liquid ones. Consequently, organic growing is often associated with a slow-release nutrient system. Organics can also be available in liquid form for quick or instant nutrient release, depending on the manufacturing process. The environmental friendliness of such products hinges on their production methods; hence the significance of organic certification.

To grasp the intricacies of organic ecosystems, you must understand the concept of upstream and downstream resources. Upstream resources are outsourced goods and energy sources like gas for electricity in local power generators. In contrast, downstream resources are locally produced and used resources. A truly organic ecosystem requires both upstream and downstream components to be environmentally-friendly. Non-eco-friendly upstream energy sources can compromise the overall ecological sustainability of cultivation. Many growers find themselves combining some fossil fuels upstream with entirely organic practices downstream.

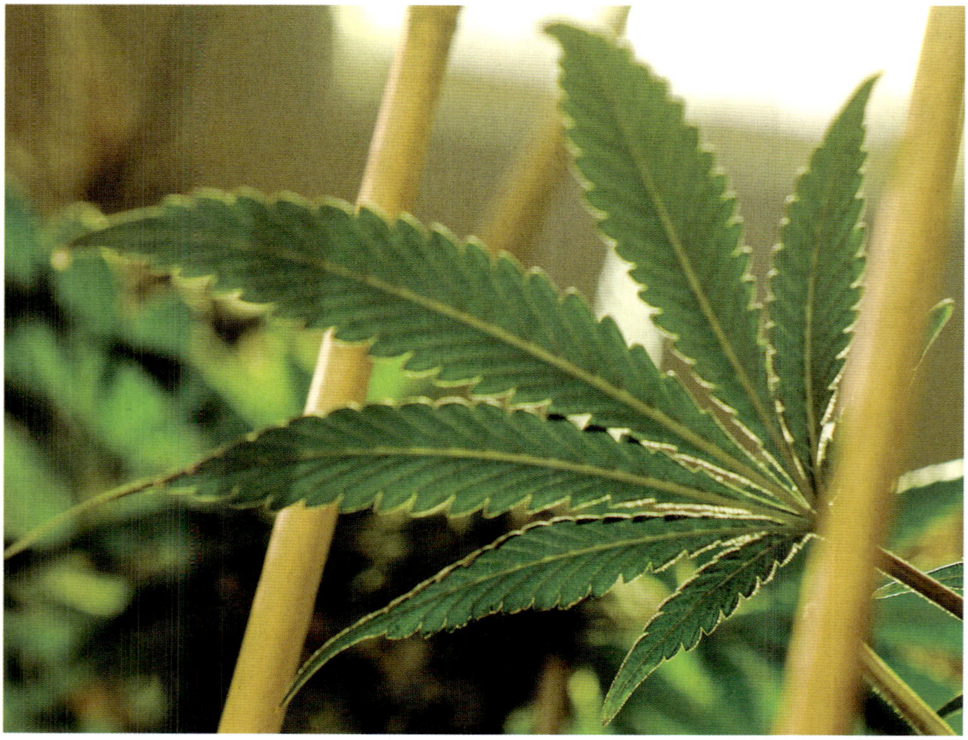

PHOTO: TRICHOME ART

The leaf is the window to studying plant health. The leaf indicates plant wellness or distress. Check your leaf and all will be revealed.

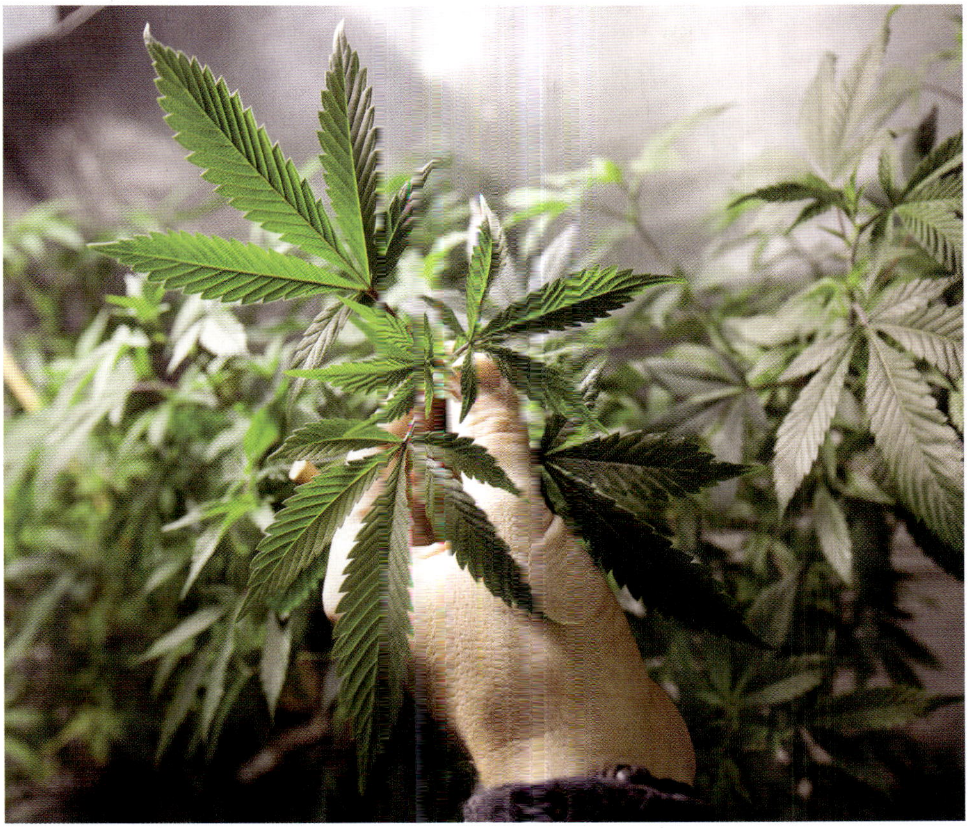

The apical bud at the top of the plant is easy to see by bending the branch. As long as you don't pull too hard this method of checking leaf works fine.

Beyond cannabis cultivation for human consumption, a growing industry is focused on non-edible plant applications, such as wood used for furniture, doors, and frames, or ornamental plants cultivated for their visual appeal and aromatic qualities. These non-edible plants can be treated with various substances to enhance productivity, many of which contain chemicals that are not environmentally-friendly. Although some may incorporate organic components, the final product may not be entirely eco-friendly. In our coverage of nutrients and pesticides, we emphasize the importance of using products specifically intended for food crops and avoiding those labeled for non-edibles. In Chapter 15 on pest control, we explore natural and eco-friendly methods, including the use of pest predators, crop rotation, interplanting, and companion plants.

Synthetic nutrients offer rapid and targeted results, making them fast-acting solutions. However, they can also lead to overfeeding and plant burn if not used judiciously. In contrast, organic nutrients are generally slower to release, except when concentrated in liquid form.

PHOTO: PHILOSOPHER SEEDS

Maintaining the right balance between watering frequency and nutrient application is critical in organic growing. Overwatering can limit aeration in the growing medium, while underwatering can hinder nutrient application. Avoiding direct application from the bottle by diluting nutrients with water is essential to prevent plant burn. Striving for a well-aerated, slightly drier medium is advisable, although novice growers may start with increased watering frequencies and lower nutrient concentrations to prevent burn. Experienced growers, through meticulous record-keeping, can fine-tune the ideal balance. If plants appear to wilt during the light cycle, timely watering is necessary to support their health and growth.

A Brief History of Organic Cultivation

While contemporary organic farming is firmly rooted in a practical movement with a holistic approach benefiting humanity, its origins are diverse, influenced by factors ranging from religion and industrialization to chemical experimentation, wartime efforts, and genetic research. The historical evolution of organic farming theory and practice is intrinsically linked to advances in biochemical engineering during the early 1900s, spurred by the rise of industrialization. Simultaneously, mechanical engineers actively pursued the development of machinery that maximized efficiency while minimizing economic costs—a goal that was extended to include maintaining the health of our environment.

The annals of history contain numerous examples of organic cultivation practices predating the introduction of synthetic alternatives. However, it was during the era of industrialization and advancements in chemical engineering that organic farming theory and practice began to evolve significantly.

In 1924, Rudolf Steiner took a religious approach to advocate for organics, coining the term "biodynamic" in his book *Spiritual Foundations for the Renewal of Agriculture.*[1] This work popularized biodynamic agriculture,[2] although many of its principles are now considered part of mainstream organic farming. Walter James, 4th Baron Northbourne, expanded these ideas by introducing the concept of the "farm as organism"[3] in his 1940 book *Look to the Land,*[4] further fueling the movement's growth. Over time, pseudoscientific elements were gradually eliminated, partly due to World War II, which redirected scientific focus towards chemical engineering, including organic and synthetic experimentation. It was during and after the war that organic farming saw substantial scientific advancements, as salespeople embraced the concept and expanded its consumer base.

In 1972, IFOAM emerged as a central hub for data collection, analysis, and dissemination. IFOAM played a pivotal role in advocating to governments to critically evaluate synthetic alternatives while promoting the expansion of certified organic produce. This approach was effective, and organic agriculture has continued to thrive, driven by growing awareness of climate change and the importance of healthy living.

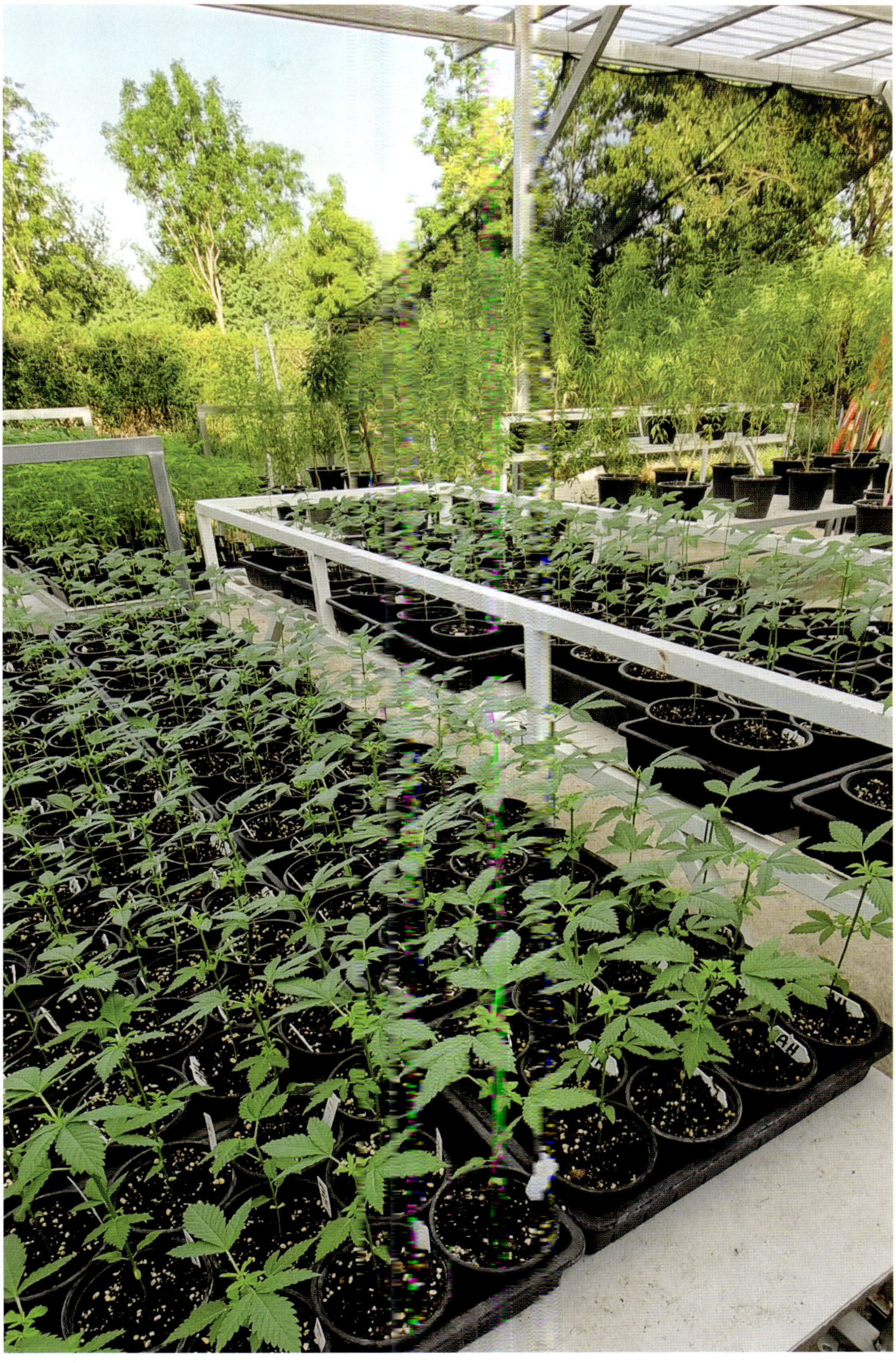

PHOTO: ED BORG

Outdoor sativa-dominant genetics get big fast. This perpetual system has new plants for vegetative growth once the others start flowering

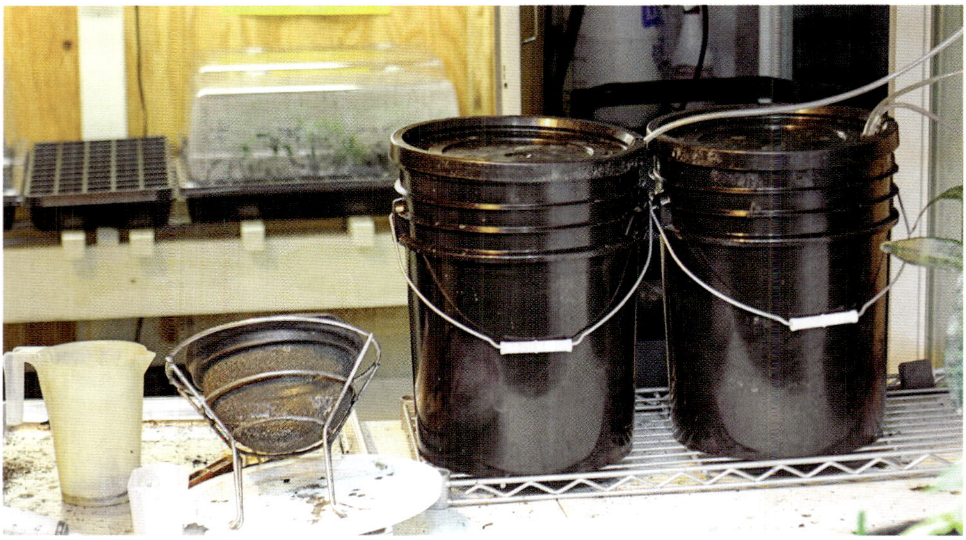

Brewing compost "tea" using aeration with pumps. Plant teas enrich your nutrient program with organic sustenance.

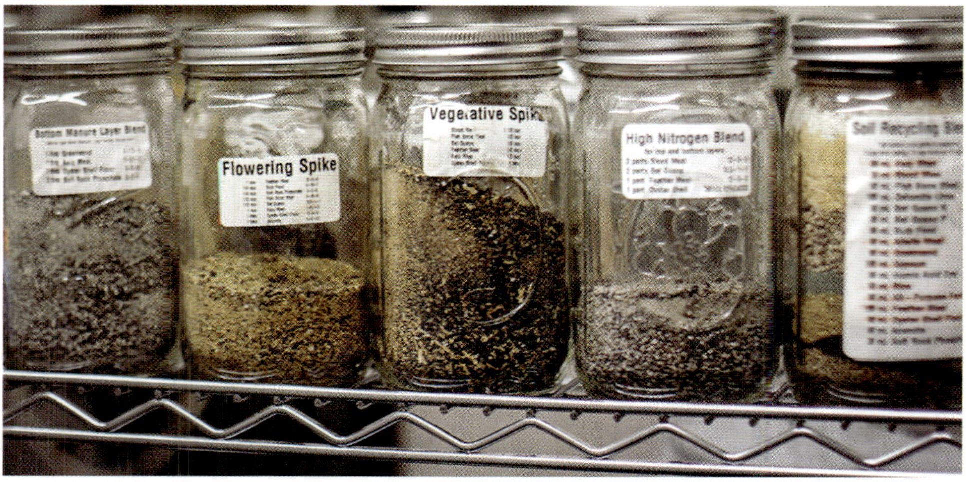

What you once threw away can be kept and processed into organic supplements.

Organic growing relies on natural processing, recycling, time, soil enrichment, and controlled release systems. Natural processing involves blending minerals and organic substances, either separately or together. To combat harmful pests, organic methods prioritize the use of beneficial or friendly organisms. Safety, health, and environmental considerations remain paramount. While artificial growth hormones and enhancers can potentially yield higher results than organics under similar conditions, there is a general scientific consensus that, while organics may not surpass some synthetic supplements in terms of yield, they can certainly match them. Synthetic modification and environmentally unfriendly processing methods can enhance any organic product.

PHOTOS: IAN C.

Nonetheless, organics can compete effectively by adopting environmentally-friendly processes. A 10% lower yield, which may exist in some cases, is a minor compromise when considering the benefits of organic cultivation, including lower energy consumption and pesticide-free practices.

Organic pest and disease control primarily revolve around enhancing genetic integrity through selective breeding. While many organic pesticides are available, not all are environmentally-friendly. Organic pesticides derived from organic materials may still possess properties incompatible with a sustainable environment. It is advisable to choose environmentally-friendly options, which can be identified by the product's certification for keeping those standards. Read up on what certificates are issued in your country for products that meet these requirements.

In 1998, IFOAM took a stance in favor of GMO-free organic agriculture. GMOs, or genetically-modified organisms, raised concerns due to uncertainties about their environmental impact and potential long-term consequences. Although they offer such benefits as pest resistance, high yields, and energy efficiency, instances of problematic GMOs have raised concerns. Proponents argue in favor of stringent criteria for introducing GMOs into the environment. There is a broader consensus that GMOs are intended to improve our world rather than harm it, although concerns about the unknown persist.

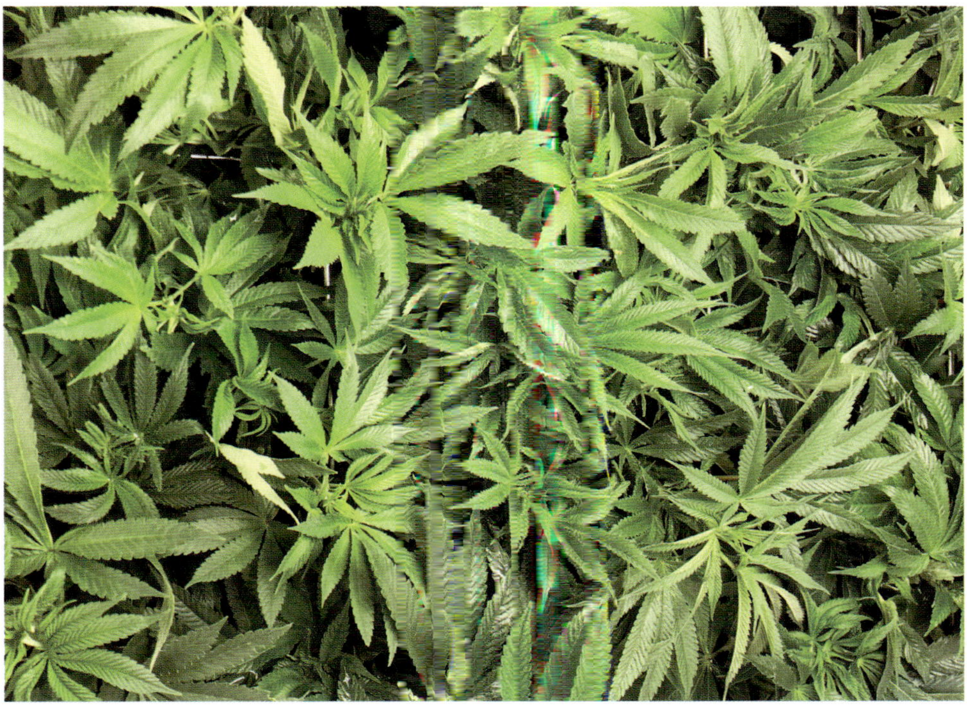

Who says organics can't produce healthiness in abundance? This encouraging lush foliage almost invites swimming through.

PHOTO: NATHAN GUILLARD

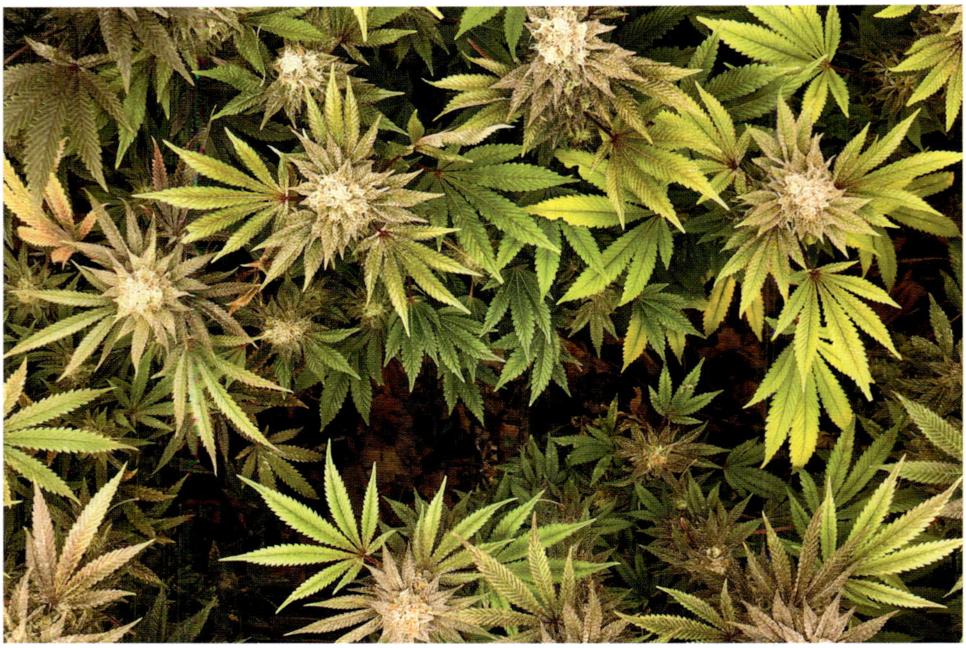

When finishing flowering with organics, much of the leaves will have used up all their nutrient resources.

Organic proponents assert that existing agricultural methods can meet our needs without relying on GMOs. It is essential to recognize that crop genetic codes naturally change over time through natural selection and selective breeding. GMOs, however, can lead to more dramatic genetic alterations not typically observed in nature.

The potential issue of GMOs interacting with non-GMO crops and creating GMO/non-GMO hybrids necessitates careful consideration before GMO crops are released into the environment. This concern has led to the exploration of GMO sterile plant alternatives. Despite these discussions, IFOAM maintains its stance against GMOs. In some situations, addressing problems such as food scarcity in regions with population explosions may require the short-term use of GMOs, even if it means setting aside long-term environmental aspirations.

Organic farming strives to maintain the right balance of nutrient composition while incorporating additional organic chemicals, which can sometimes be necessary. Organic growers acknowledge that organic cultivation, particularly with manure, has the potential to cause water pollution, a concern shared with conventional methods. It is crucial to avoid dumping organics near rivers and using excessive organics close to rivers, as this can lead to pollution and harm river ecosystems. Conventional growers argue that, despite the synthetic supplements they use, there is a lower risk of exposing crops to potential biological hazards. To address the possibility of introducing

PHOTO: NATHAN GUILLARD

unwanted organisms and diseases through organic practices, growers can purify and refine organic matter by heating it in an oven, eliminating pathogens and organisms.

Organic cultivators emphasize the urgent need to transition to organic practices in response to climate change and its challenges. Fossil fuel depletion and pollution further underscore the importance of organic farming. The scientific community is actively addressing the significant role of humankind in contributing to global warming and environmental change.[6] While a level of greenhouse effect is necessary for maintaining habitable zones on Earth (it warms the planet to temperatures that allow for livable environments), excessive carbon dioxide (CO_2) emissions, leading to increased heat retention, can have adverse effects. Rapid changes in temperature can disrupt ecological systems, potentially leading to species extinction in a chain reaction that affects entire ecosystems. Hence, the importance of addressing climate change is underscored by the need to preserve the balance of our planet's ecosystems.

Medical science recommends that governments prioritize and promote organic foods, advocating for organic standards, limiting environmental impact, and encouraging responsible practices. Governments also have plans to transition agricultural lands to organic cultivation exclusively, with the European Union aiming for 20–25% organic farming by 2030. The organic movement continues to garner support, driven by the enthusiasm of organic growers, which fuels research and development within the agricultural sector. Independent organic movements compete with large businesses, exemplifying traditional farming practices that predate the era of synthetics and offering valuable lessons from the past.

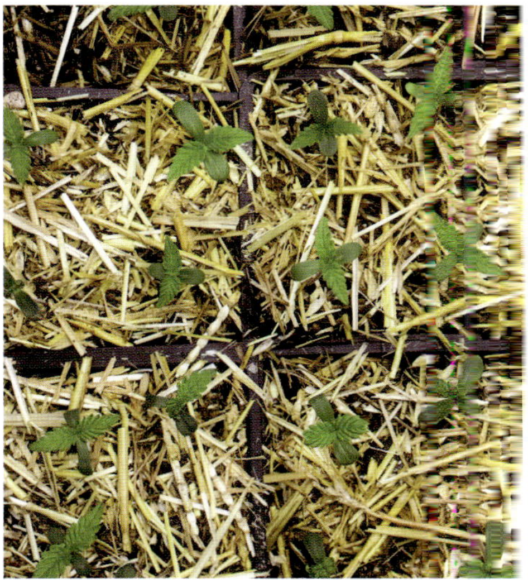

Straw can be used as a mulch to control weeds even at the seedling stage.

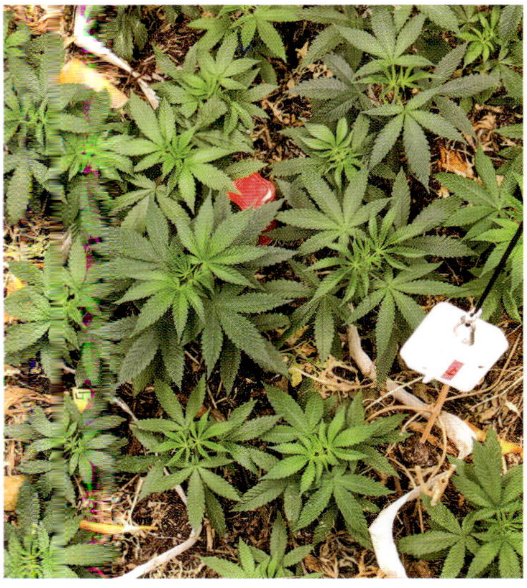

You can take away or add mulch straw wherever you want since you won't be disturbing the medium.

PHOTOS: NATHAN GUILLARD

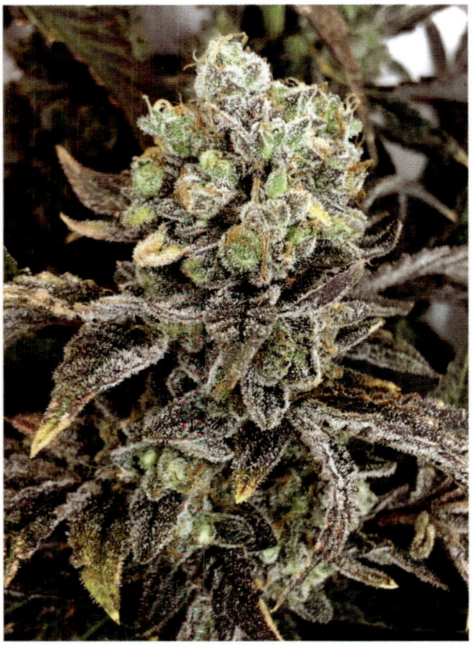

Organic bud appeal is always a treat when you consider how natural it all is.

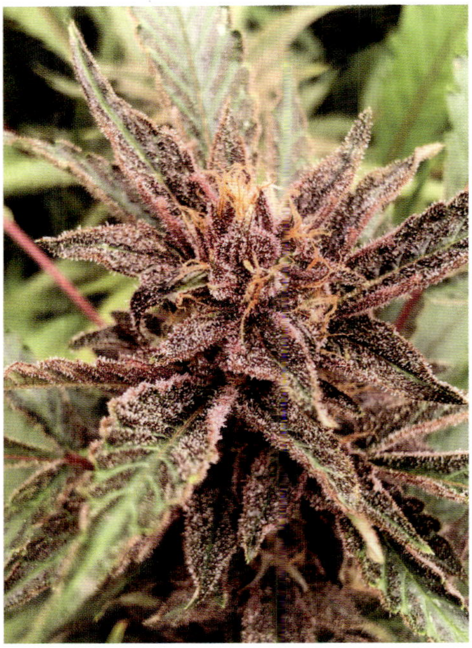

Another advantage is that organics does not depend on strain type.

Let's Get Growing Organically

Embarking on an organic growing journey involves not only discarding all synthetic products but also devising a fundamental strategy to prevent their reintroduction into your garden. When it comes to soil, it's essential to source it organically and treat it accordingly. Additionally, adopting an eco-conscious perspective on waste reduction is crucial; if you can reuse something, don't discard it, but use it once more.

You may come across the term "humus" in discussions or at your local grow shop. Humus refers to organic vegetable compost. The natural process of humification continuously breaks down organic matter in the soil, resulting in a mixture containing carbohydrates, lignin, organic acids, compounds, proteins, resins, starch, sugar, and waxes. Humus is a product of nature and, therefore, considered a form of natural compost. On the other hand, compost is something akin to humus that humans intentionally create.

Organic cultivation can be approached either reactively or proactively. Reactive organic growing involves responding to environmental cues, taking a passive stance, and requiring minimal attention. Proactive organic growers are more actively engaged in their gardens, conducting regular checks and continuously optimizing their cultivation practices. For optimal results, proactive organic growing is the recommended approach.

PHOTOS: NATHAN GUILLARD

Growing Organically Outdoors

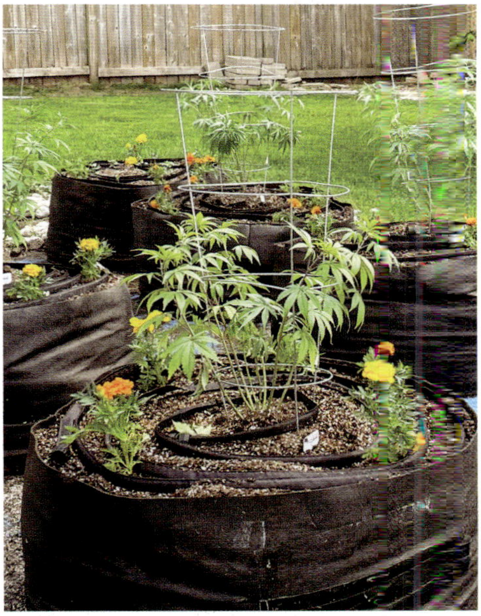

Ornamental marigolds around the plant because they make great companions.

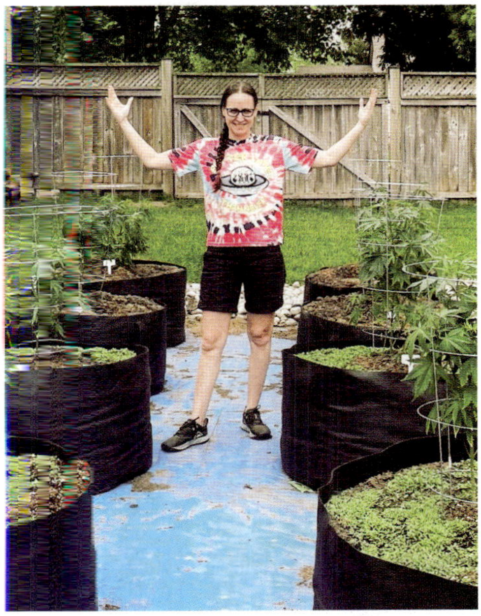

Started indoors for four weeks. Transplanted outdoors, these will grow into large plants.

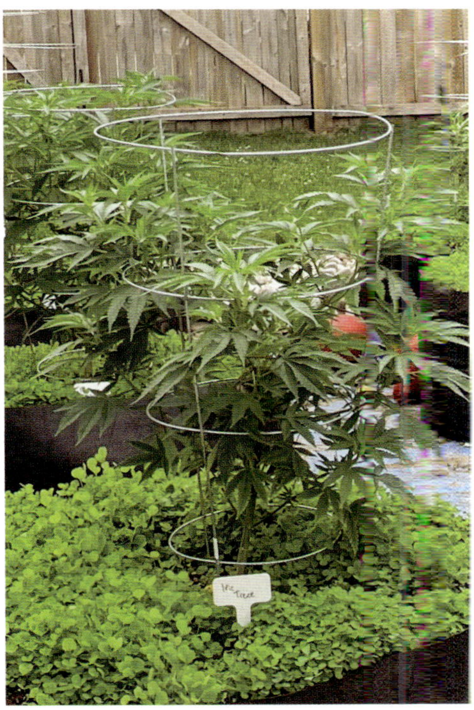

That cool futuristic-looking trellis is a tomato cage. Outdoor plants get very big very fast.

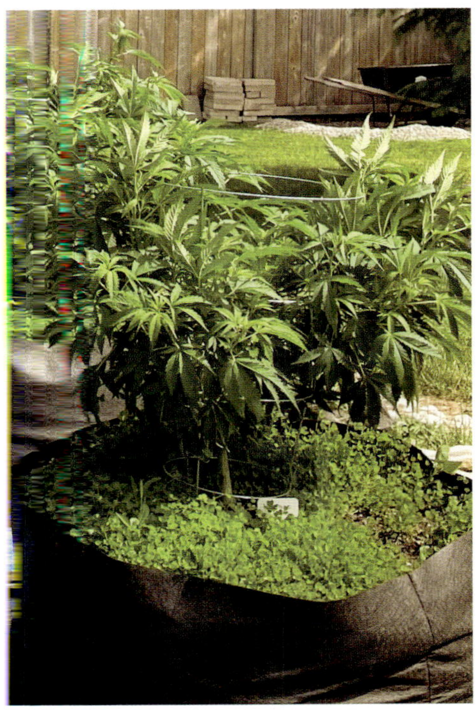

There's plenty of space left for plants with similar nutrient needs.

continues...

PHOTOS: TANYA PETERSEN

Growing Organically Outdoors *continued*

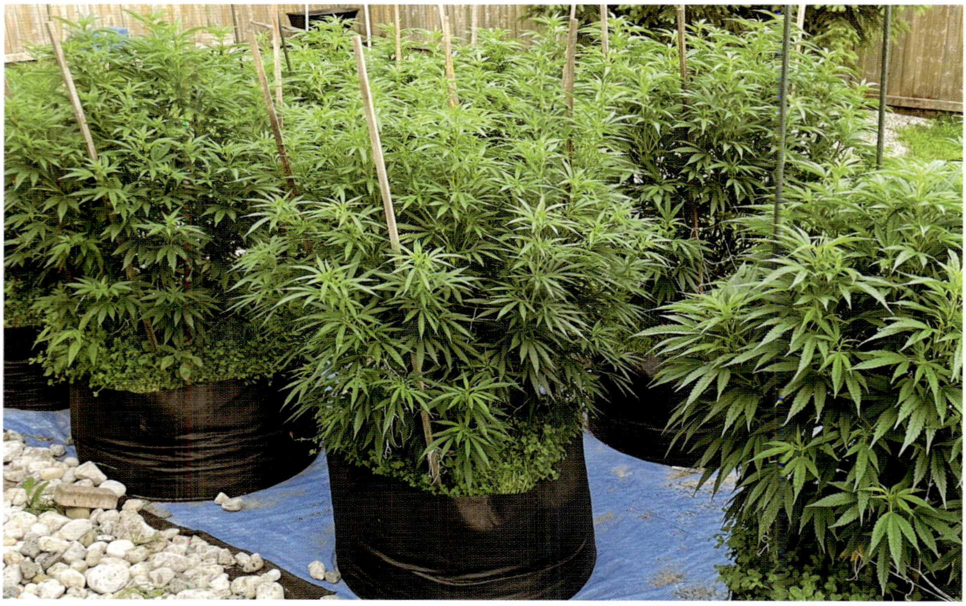

If you do not cover the top of vegetative growth with a net, how do you control the bush?

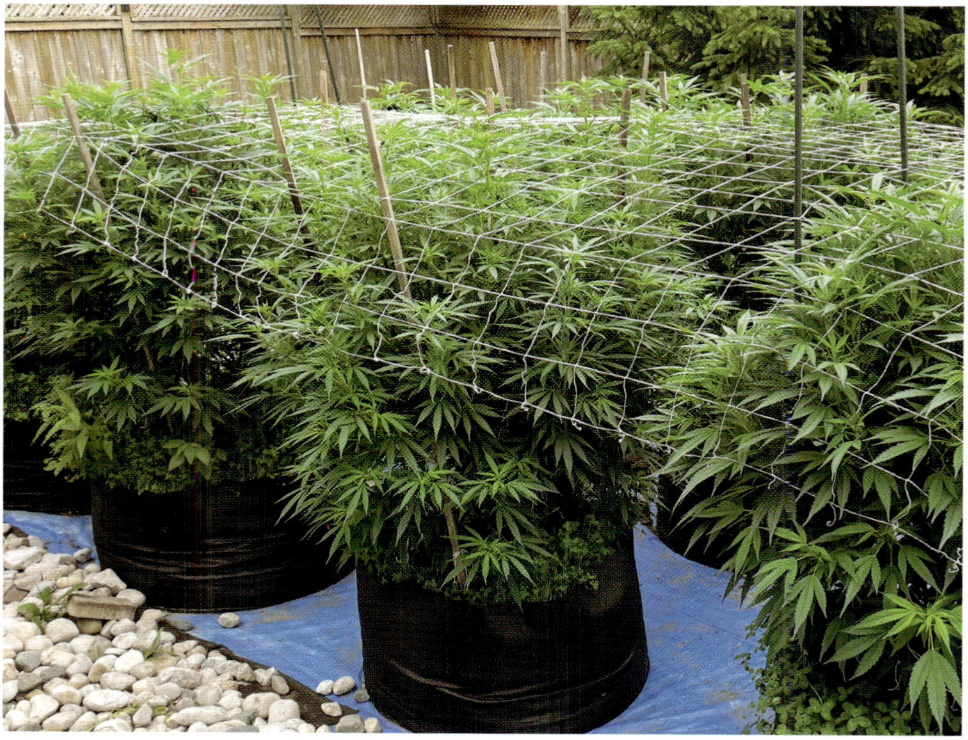

A net across the top is the easiest way to manage any large selection of sativa bush. An even canopy is ideal for this.

PHOTOS: TANYA PETERSEN

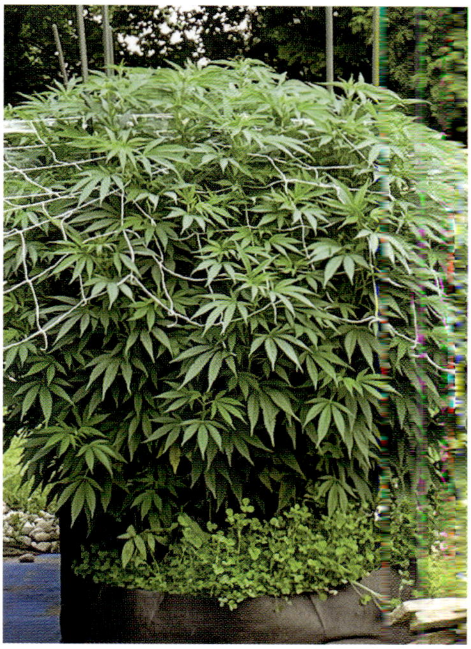

Compost teas encourage rapid growth. This means an additional net is needed on top to keep the plant bushy and upright.

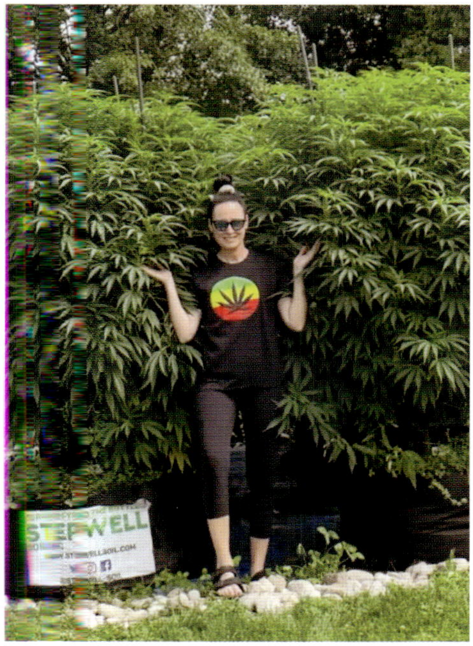

The netting across the top is still there but flowers have covered the top canopy.

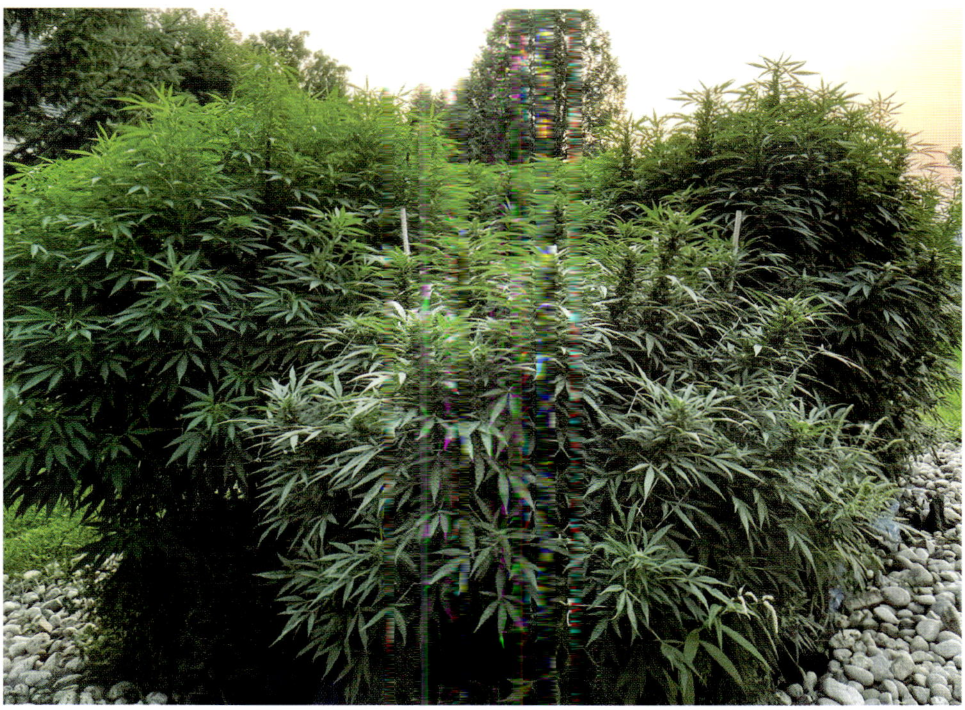

Look closely, and you can see the netting that prevents these plants from keeling over. *continues...*

Growing Organically Outdoors *continued*

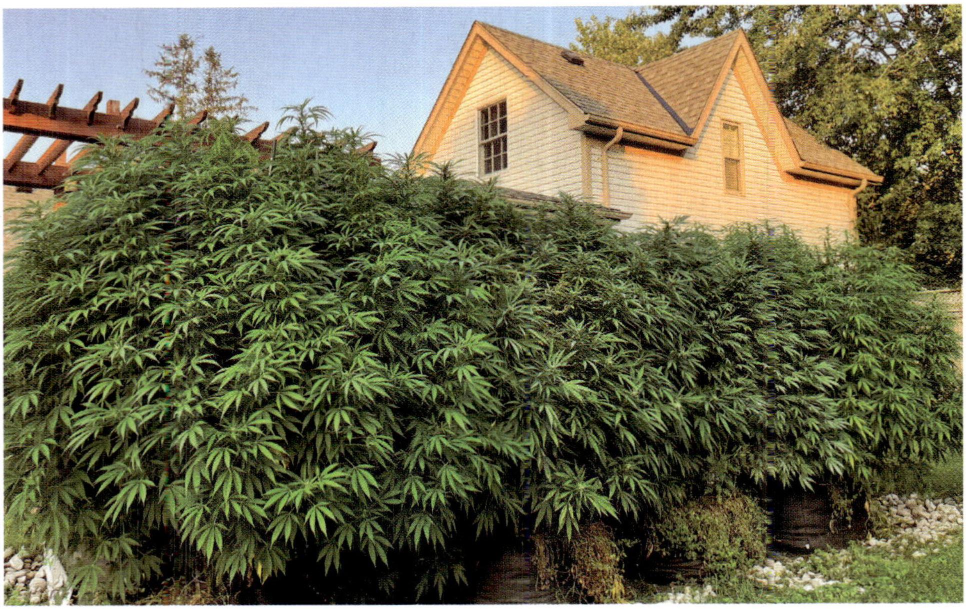

Outdoor sativa will produce the biggest buds you will grow. When using organic supplements, the results are just as impressive. It's genetic.

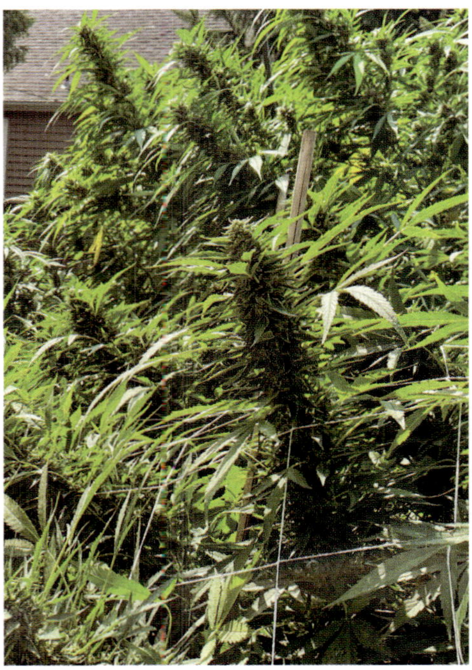

An outdoor sativa side branch can easily compete with the top cola of an indoor plant.

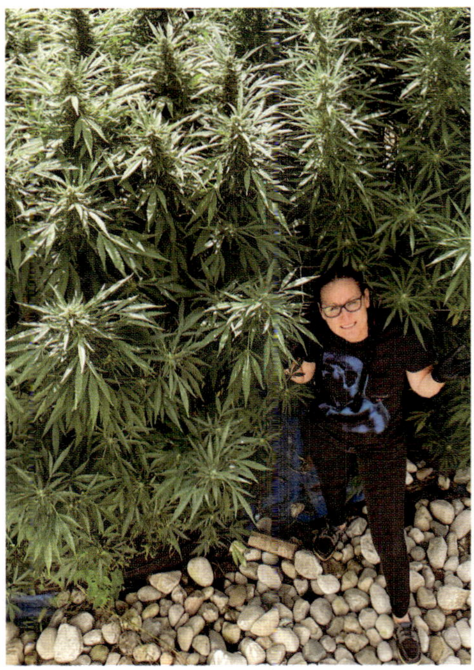

It is easy to mistake all these side branches for individual plants when they are actually the same plant.

PHOTOS: TANYA PETERSEN

Crop Rotation: Nurturing Your Soil

For outdoor growers, the practice of moving patches of crops between growing seasons can significantly benefit soil health and overall cultivation success. Imagine having cannabis in one section, cabbage in another, and carrots in yet another. The key is to cycle them. Different crops have different nutrient requirements, and instead of depleting the same minerals consistently while neglecting others, crop rotation gives each patch the opportunity to naturally replenish what has been used up.

Fallowing, which involves plowing the land but leaving it unseeded and uncultivated, comes into play as well. Incorporating fallowing into your crop rotation cycle, say once every five years, can lead to even greater soil recovery. Both crop rotation and fallowing contribute to maintaining a balanced pH in the soil, promoting its overall health. Nevertheless, it's essential to continue monitoring and adjusting pH levels as well as nutrient content.

By changing the plant species cultivated in a patch, you also disrupt host-pathogen specificity. This means that harmful organisms cannot accumulate rapidly in one area because their host, the plant species, gets rotated out. This aspect of crop rotation significantly aids in pest control. Note that cycling strains of cannabis alone may not yield the same benefits as diversifying with other crops like carrots or cabbages, as the cannabis strains are often too similar to achieve the type of divergence required for effective rotation.

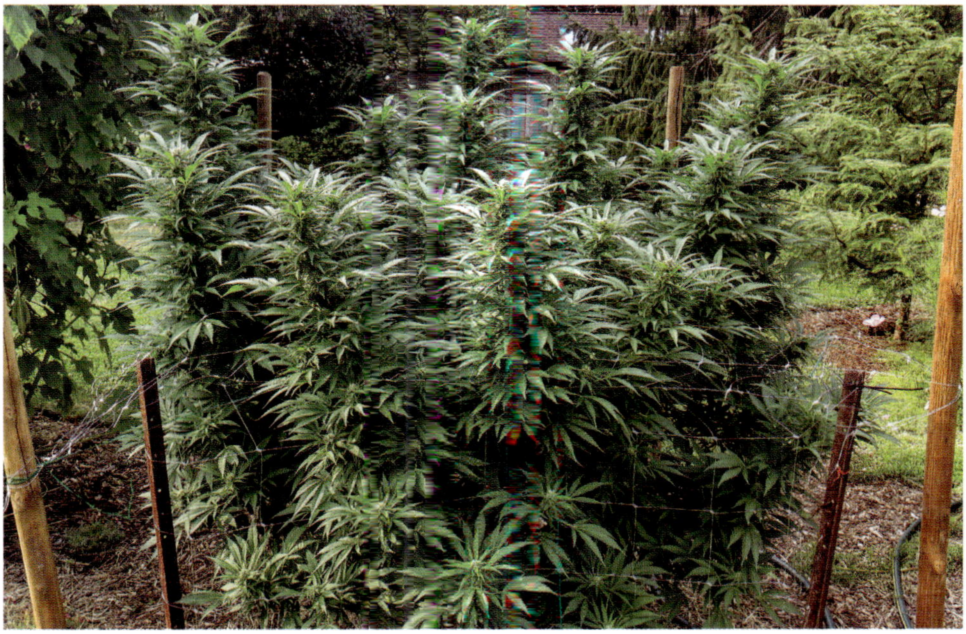

PHOTO: FATHER NATURE, ROBERT BUTTS

An outdoor ScrOG can work fine as long as you have enough netting support to cover the length of these big outdoor genetics.

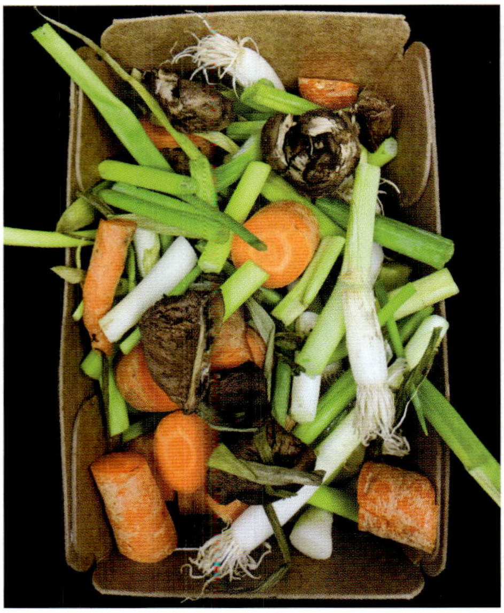

Organic food waste can easily be collected and used for compost.

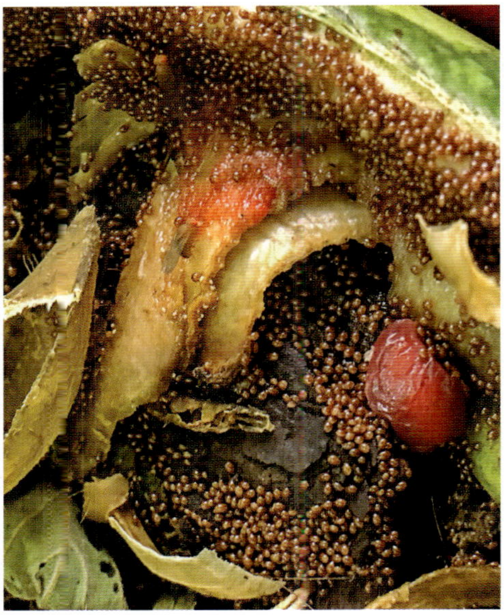

Organic food waste breaks down into clean carbon-based nutrients that plants love to reuse as their main feed.

Compost

Compost plays a pivotal role in organic farming, serving as a fundamental source of organic nutrients. In fact, most organic materials are either compost or are destined to become compost. This valuable resource takes shape through the natural process of aerobic decomposition of organic matter. While this can occur in various environments, including aquatic settings, it typically progresses more slowly in water due to the anaerobic conditions present. To achieve optimal results, your composting efforts should involve aerobic decomposition in dry conditions.

All living things eventually decompose. Since they consume organic matter, the substances they ingest contribute to the organics produced through natural decay or waste materials. Most biological growth either disassembles organic compounds through processes like consumption or waits for them to break down, as in root absorption. These organic components are then reassembled within the organism or used to synthesize new compounds through metabolic processes. While this is a natural and essential process, some synthetic compounds may not be biologically processed in a manner considered healthy, particularly for human consumption. This concern extends to composting as well. For instance, animals that ingest synthetics may produce waste containing compounds related to the use of these synthetic materials, which would not be present otherwise. Although such waste can be treated, it is far easier to avoid introducing these substances into the ecosystem from the outset. Organic growing practices help mitigate these potential issues.

PHOTOS: NATHAN GUILLARD

When it comes to compost, you have two primary options: Crafting your own or purchasing certified compost. Compost can be created from a variety of organic materials, including bark, biodegradable substances, used coffee grounds, grasses, green waste, hay, humus, leaves, manure, microorganisms, mulch, sawdust, straw, wood, wool, and worm compost. All of these materials make excellent organic mulches, enhancing soil health and promoting plant growth. Cardboard and newspaper are sometimes found in compost, but they should be considered mulch materials rather than compost components. They are typically added to allow for proper airflow and serve as a covering layer but decompose more slowly than other organic materials in the compost pile.

Aerobic Decomposition

Aerobic decomposition is a cornerstone of organic farming. It's a natural process that relies on the presence of oxygen to break down organic matter effectively. Nature has its mechanisms for ensuring that air reaches the soil, primarily through the activities of soil-dwelling creatures such as worms and ants, which play a vital role. Worms burrow through the earth, consuming organic matter and excreting nutrient-rich waste. In the process, they aerate and churn the soil, transforming it into the fertile topsoil essential for plant growth. This natural phenomenon ensures that oxygen is readily available in the soil environment, which is crucial for the success of aerobic decomposition.

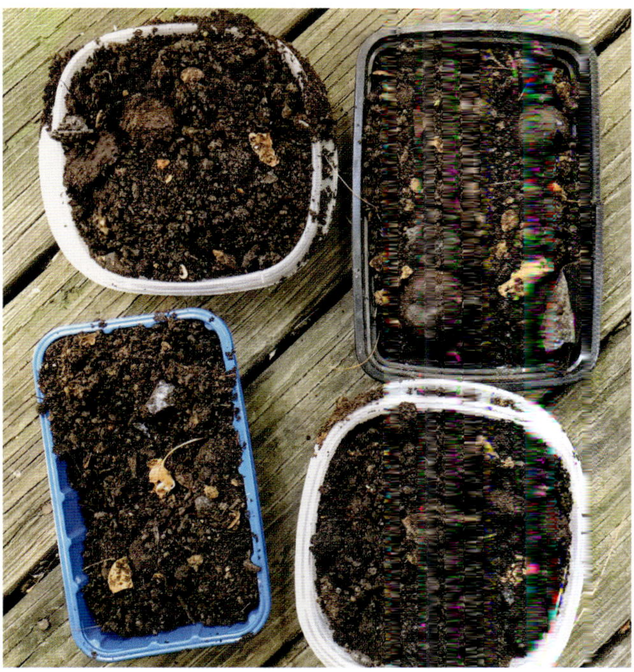

Churning the waste helps introduce oxygen and break down the organics as an aerobic decomposition, resulting in healthy feeds.

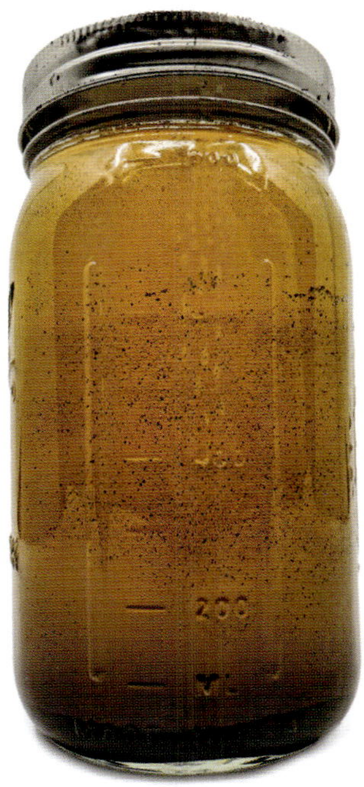

Add water and shake. This compost tea can now be used as an organic feed.

PHOTOS: NATHAN GUILLARD

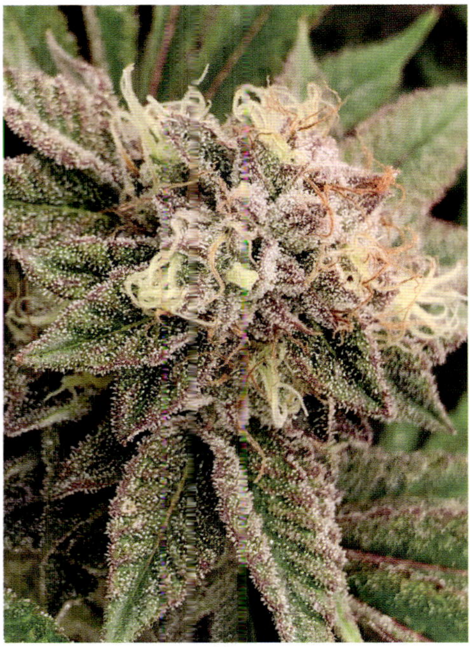

Buds grown organically are indistinguishable from buds that are not.

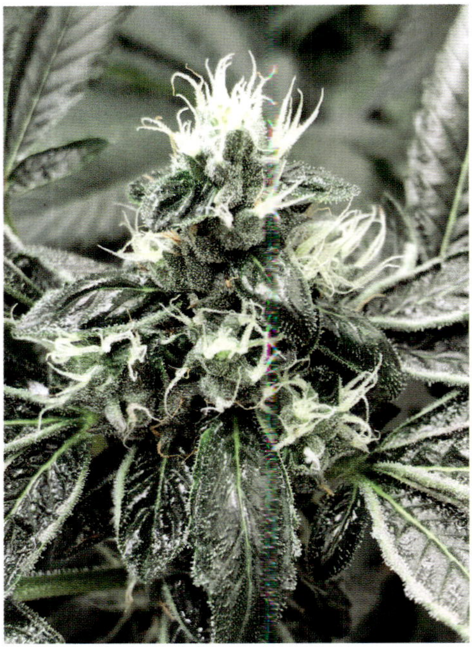

Creamy organic buds on darker dank make this plant quite contrasting.

However, certain conditions can impede aerobic decomposition. For instance, arid environments, coupled with tightly packed compost, can limit the entry of air into the soil, hindering the aerobic decomposition process. On the other end of the spectrum, excessively wet and swampy conditions can also prevent air from reaching the soil. In situations where air is restricted, anaerobic decomposition can occur. While effective in breaking down organic matter, this comes with a significant drawback. It produces a foul, sour-smelling odor, a clear indicator that the compost has undergone anaerobic decomposition, potentially rendering it toxic for plant growth.

Organic cultivators prioritize aerobic decomposition as their preferred method due to its efficiency and the absence of unpleasant odors. This process aligns with the principles of organic farming, emphasizing the creation of nutrient-rich, environmentally-friendly soil to support healthy plant growth.

Organic Composting

In organic farming, composting is a fundamental practice that transforms organic materials into valuable nutrient-rich matter for soil enrichment. To achieve optimal results in composting, organic growers strive to maintain a specific ratio of ingredients, aiming for a mixture of 30 parts carbon to one part nitrogen, commonly referred to as 30:1. This standard in organic composting is known to support efficient decomposition. While it is easier to purchase organic compost with known ratios, many

PHOTOS: NATHAN GUILLARD

growers rely on formulas, experience, and trial-and-error experiments to estimate the appropriate balance. For those seeking precision, it is also possible to have compost samples analyzed, although this can be costly.

The key principle behind maintaining this ratio is to avoid composting ingredients that can introduce toxins into the mix. While a degree of compost toxicity may exist in organic blends, it typically diminishes over time with proper maintenance, including regular aeration of the compost pile.

Carbon-rich organic materials, including leaves gathered during autumn and winter, sawdust, and straw, contribute to the compost's carbon component. Nitrogen-rich organic materials, including used coffee grounds, discarded fruit, manure, various plants, seaweed, and leftover vegetables, contribute to the nitrogen component. Poultry manure, particularly from chickens, is a prime source of nitrogen. A favored nitrogen-rich feed with a composition of 5-1-1 is fish emulsion, highly suitable for stimulating vegetative growth in plants.

Horse manure is recognized for its balanced combination of carbon and nitrogen. Both horse and poultry manure tend to decompose relatively more quickly than that of cattle or sheep. Organic growers are advised to refrain from using dairy products or meat in their compost, as these can attract unwanted pests. If one wishes to incorporate dairy or meat components, it is advisable to consider purchasing organic compost, where these materials have already undergone decomposition, eliminating the risk of attracting pests.

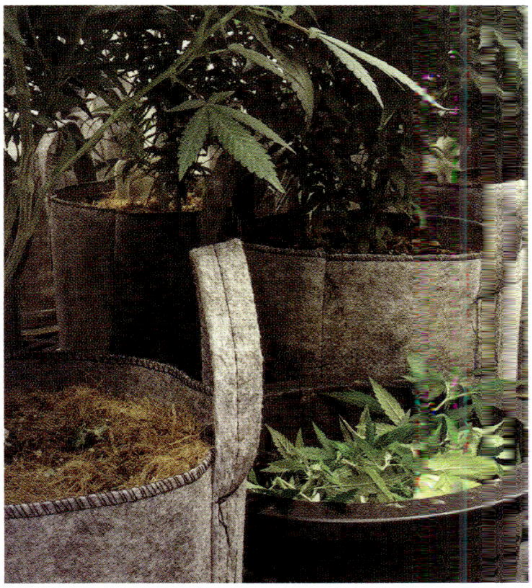

Even the cannabis plant itself, especially leaf trimmings, can be used as compost.

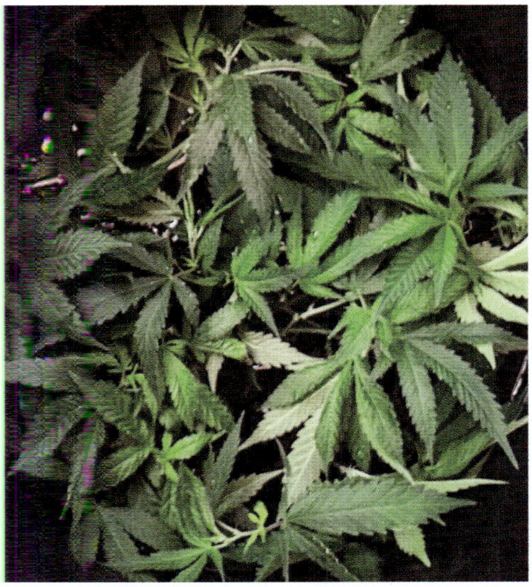

Trimmings should be placed in their own container both for security and composting purposes.

PHOTOS: MONICA GRIFFIN

Compost Bins

Compost bins are invaluable tools in organic gardening. They serve as mini ecosystems where organic materials undergo transformation into nutrient-rich compost. The beauty of compost bins lies in their ability to elevate temperatures significantly, reaching impressive ranges of 122–140°F (50–60°C). If you seek even higher temperatures, you can use insulation wraps to push the boundaries further. This process, often referred to as "active composting," is a testament to nature's incredible ability to break down organic matter efficiently.

Compost that remains below 86°F (30°C), or "cold compost," still contributes to the decomposition process, albeit more slowly. Regardless of the composting method you choose, maintaining a moderate level of moisture is crucial. The compost should possess a dampness resembling that of a wrung-out sponge. If you suspect it is too dry and not breaking down as rapidly as desired, consider adding more water. However, be careful not to overwater and swamp the compost, as excess moisture can hinder the decomposition process.

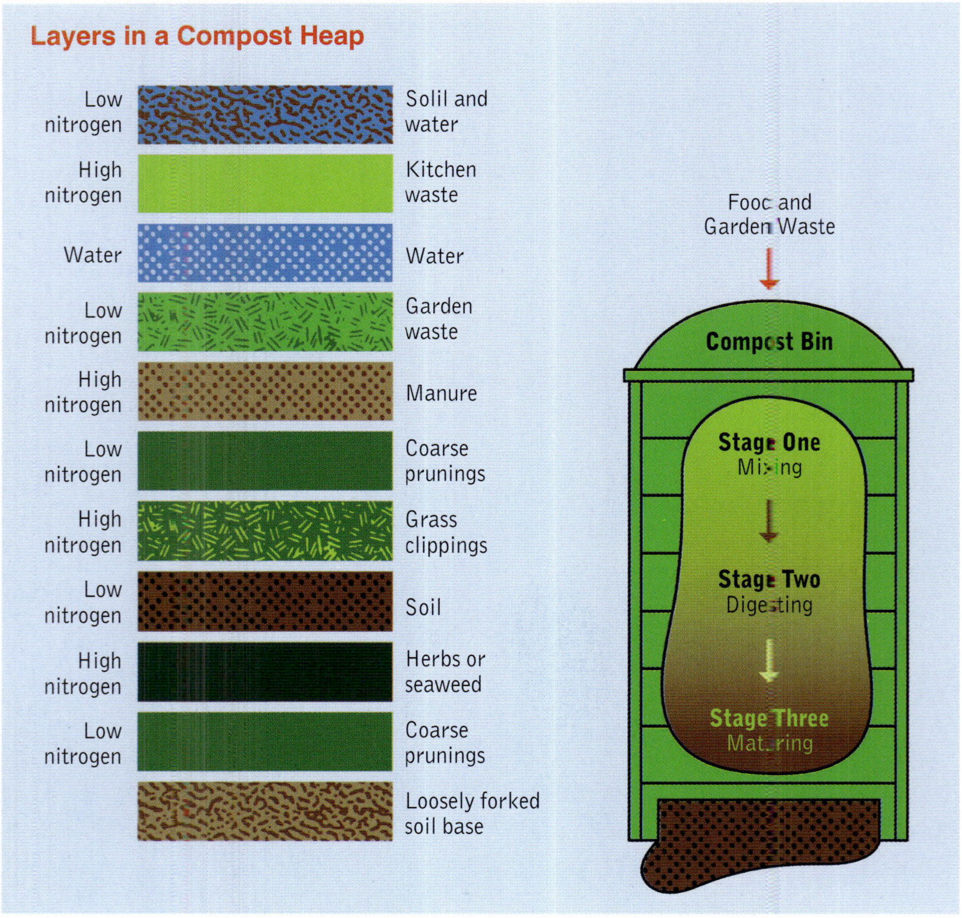

Temperatures in the center of a compost heap can become very high, reaching levels that may be uncomfortable or even harmful if handled directly. Wear gloves when turning or handling compost to protect your hands. A beneficial practice during composting is periodically turning the compost and allowing it to aerate in an open-air environment. This process aids in cooling down excessively hot compost and promotes uniform decomposition. Regular turning also ensures that the compost's internal temperature remains within a manageable range.

It's important to know when your compost is ready for use. Mature compost exhibits several key characteristics. It stops changing color, assuming a rich dark hue. Additionally, it acquires a somewhat brittle texture, signifying its readiness for application. However, foul odors emanating from the compost are an ominous sign, indicating the occurrence of anaerobic decomposition, which can result in the accumulation of potential toxins. The presence of foul smells is often attributed to excessive moisture, suggesting that the compost may have been too wet during the composting process.

Compost bins offer an efficient and sustainable means of converting organic materials into valuable compost for your garden. Understanding the principles of temperature regulation, moisture control, and proper aeration is key to successfully harnessing the benefits of composting. By following these guidelines, you can ensure that your composting efforts yield nutrient-rich compost that enhances the health and vitality of your plants.

Product Compost

Certified organic product compost, readily available in stores, offers organic gardeners a hassle-free solution to enrich their soil. This store-bought compost can be used either independently or in conjunction with a home composting system, providing flexibility and convenience for gardeners. Comparing product compost with your homemade compost allows you to assess its quality and potentially achieve similar results.

One notable feature of store-bought compost is its typically dry state, as damp compost can add extra weight during transportation and occupy more space. However, compost is activated by moisture. Therefore, even if your homemade compost is slightly damp, it remains suitable for use. Compost can exhibit various shades of brown and black, reflecting the diverse organic matter within. Quality compost should exude an earthy aroma, possess a brittle texture, and sift through your fingers when you take a handful.

Compost Leachate

All compost naturally contains residues that can be found in the fluid drained from wet compost. When compost is relatively new, these are often highly nutritional. Through the process of watering, organic nutrients within the compost leachate disperse throughout the growing medium, providing essential sustenance to plants. Compost leachate can be created by rinsing, straining, or crushing compost to release its nutritional fluids.

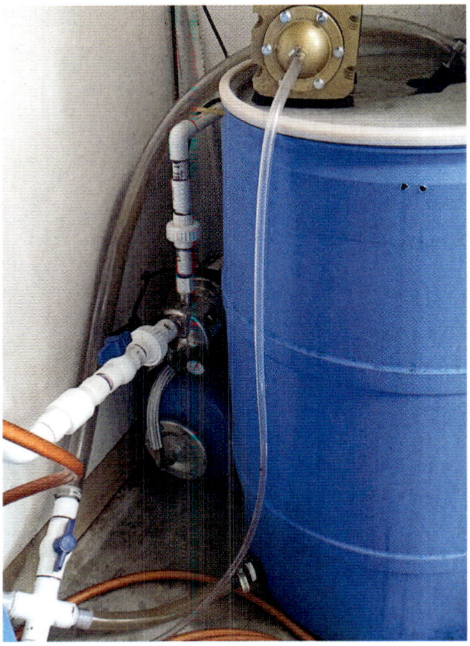

Automated systems pumping leachate around for compost tea making.

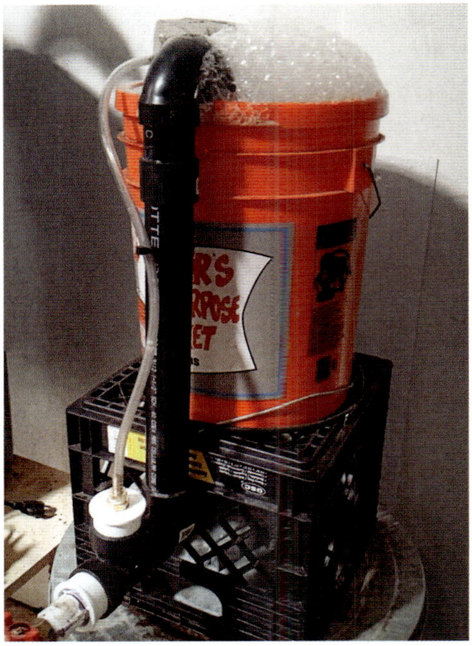

Leachate being aerated with gravity-driven tea dispensing.

However, this traditional method of leachate production differs from modern approaches. Modern methods are more controlled, activate a higher population of beneficial microbes, are easier to manage, generate less mess, and yield higher-quality results.

Some compost bins come with systems designed to capture leachate. If yours lacks such a system, fluids may leak through the lower air openings. This leakage may indicate that the compost is excessively wet, which can be caused by rainfall if the bin is not adequately sheltered. To mitigate this issue, consider reducing the amount of water-retaining organic matter used in the compost.

To make the most of compost leachate, you can create compost tea by infusing water with the nutritional fluids extracted from compost, providing an organic and nutrient-rich boost for your plants.

Compost Tea

Compost tea is a valuable liquid solution that can provide your plants with essential organic nutrients. To prepare compost tea, follow these steps:

Gather Ingredients

Materials for compost tea: De-chlorinated water, compost, unsulfured molasses, an air pump, and distribution equipment for aeration.

PHOTOS: MONICA GRIFFIN

Building an Aeration System

To effectively aerate the mixture, you can purchase a gang valve system at your local aquarium store. This will provide multiple airlines to enhance aeration in the compost tea container. You will also need an aquarium pump and hose to pump air through the gang valve. The shop can assist you in selecting the appropriate valves and hoses.

Dechlorinating

If you don't have access to dechlorinated water, you must dechlorinate your water supply. Bubble the water for at least one hour to encourage chlorine evaporation.

Mixing

Add compost to the dechlorinated water and add about one ounce of unsulfured molasses to stimulate microorganism activity in the mixture.

Aerating

Use the gang valve system and aquarium pump to aerate the compost tea mixture. Allow it to bubble for two to three days while occasionally stirring to ensure proper breakdown.

Straining

Once the compost tea is ready, strain it through a cloth into a watering can or container for convenient application in your garden.

Making Adjustments

If you find that your compost tea is not breaking down as quickly as you like, use less compost and more unsulfured molasses to achieve the desired balance. Experience will guide you in refining the process.

Attending to Chlorine Concerns

If your local water supply contains high levels of chlorine and the tea is not fermenting properly, extend the aeration time or obtain dechlorinated water to ensure microbial health.

Checking Quality

Pay attention to the scent of your compost tea. If it emits a foul odor, something may have gone awry in the process. Reevaluate the quality of your compost and the mixing procedure to address any issues.

You can also ferment compost tea on a basic scale by mixing compost and water in a container for a week. However, this method has a higher failure rate and may result in an unpleasant odor if not carefully managed.

Living Teas Evolved: The Churn
by The Rev

Greetings Earthlings! I'm Rev, the author of *True Living Organics*. I want to introduce you to my True Living Organics (TLO) methodology which is focused on all-natural style growing. In this section, I will teach you how to build and use my creation, the Churn, to increase the health and vitality of your garden.

In TLO, we are able to leverage Mother Nature's strength. Two of nature's many virtues are adaptation and evolution. I often ask myself "What would Mother Nature do?" and from this question, I was able to create the Churn. The Churn is essentially a very concentrated living tea that lives on, and on, and on. The life within this container evolves and adapts to become a powerful, self-sustaining tea. Let me show you what I'm talking about.

Starting Your Churn

The size of your Churn can be determined by the size of your garden. I use a 1-gallon Churn for each of my grow rooms. I normally flower 8 to 10 female plants per room under 400-watt bulbs in 3-gallon containers. If I were using 1,000-watt bulbs, I would need a larger water reservoir and maybe a 2-gallon Churn. Your Churn can be 1 gallon, 5 gallons, or bigger. The main rule of using the Churn is to keep the microbial life

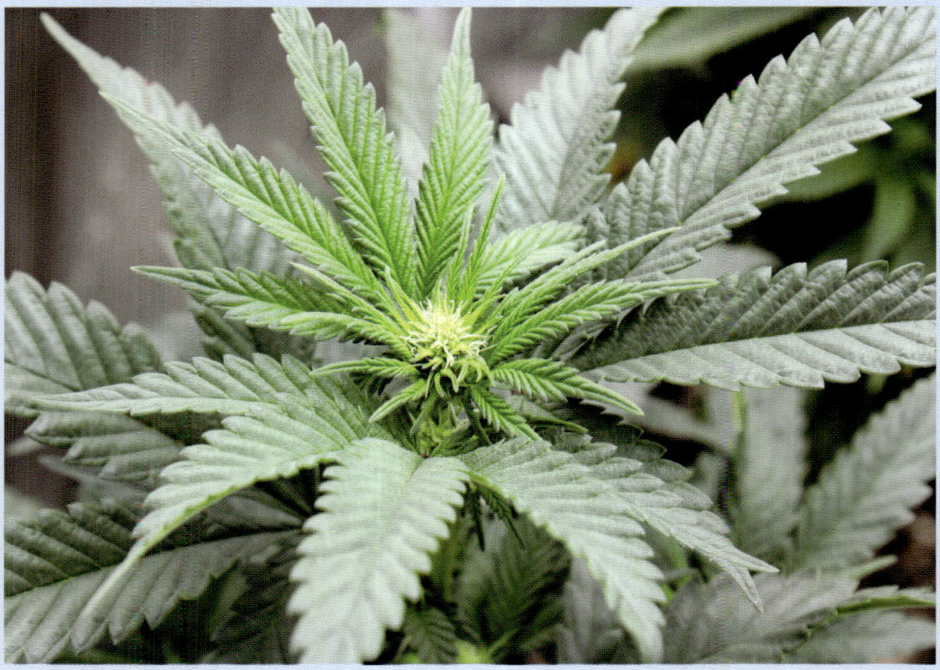

Using the Churn keeps plants healthy and happy.

PHOTOS: THE REV

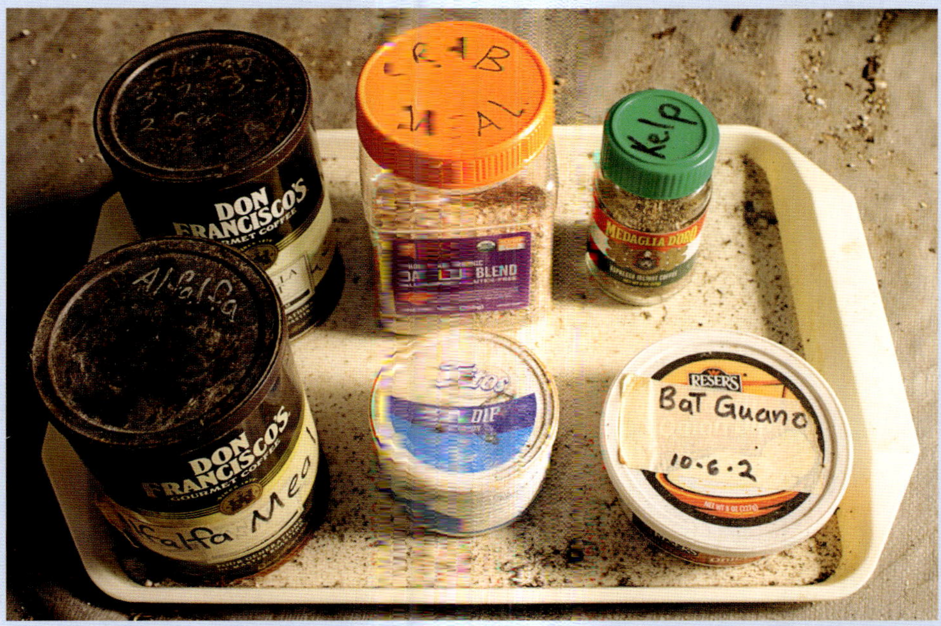

On-hand churn dry additives: Granulated chicken guano, crab meal, kelp meal, alfalfa meal, diatomaceous earth, and bat guano.

evolving. Much like a sourdough starter, saving a small portion of it will allow you to simply refill your Churn with water and let it do its magic. The bacteria in the Churn evolves and doubles in as little as 20 minutes. Completely depleting the Churn of its contents means that all those amazing bacteria will be lost and you will need to restart the process from scratch. I normally refill my Churn with water for 6 weeks. After the 6-week mark, the pH starts to get too high, so I clean it out and restart a new Churn with a bit of the old Churn's water to preserve the microlife.

Rev's Tip: If you are using compost or worm castings in your Churn, you will want to dump out all the Churn's contents and start anew every 3 weeks or so. If you use aquarium water, or mostly minerals, you can go 6 weeks between cleanings. Always save a cup of your old Churn water to add to your new Churn to keep those little microguys evolving.

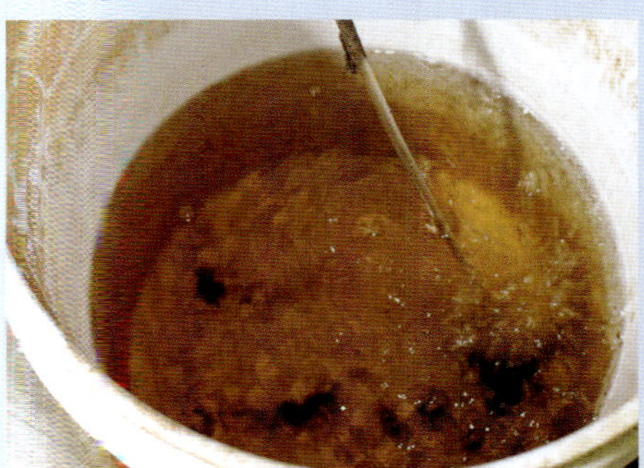

My 5-gallon plant water bucket.

To build the Churn, you need a container such as a gallon pitcher, an aquarium air pump, some airline, an air stone, and your fe

ready to rock. I recommend you keep a reservoir of plant water—dechlorinated groundwater around 50 ppm—in a can, tote, or bucket in your garden. This water should be kept aerated with an air stone. You will also need a Total Dissolved Solids (TDS) meter to measure the parts per million (ppm) levels of your Churn and plant water.

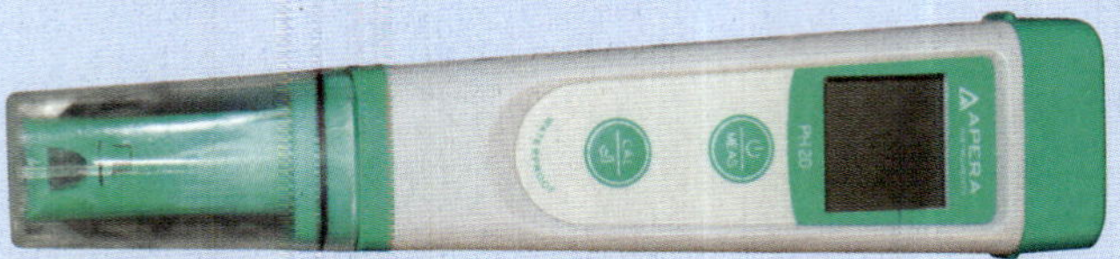

A TDS meter is an essential tool to have when using the churn.

Fill your container, what will soon become your Churn, with some of your dechlorinated groundwater. Add the air stone so it starts bubbling and aerating. Now you're ready to add some stuffs. Here's a little suggested Churn starter:

- 1 gallon dechlorinated groundwater
- 1 heaping tablespoon worm castings, compost, or TLO soil
- 1 tablespoon crab meal or another shellfish meal
- 1 teaspoon kelp and/or alfalfa meal
- 1/8 teaspoon dolomite lime
- 1/8 teaspoon molasses
- 1/4 teaspoon diatomaceous earth (DE), agricultural or food-grade only
- 1/4 teaspoon bat or bird guano, not the high-phosphorus kind

Optionally, if you have a fresh-water fish tank, add about ½ cup of the water—or if you have a stacked worm farm, add about ¼ cup of the liquid leachate from your farm.

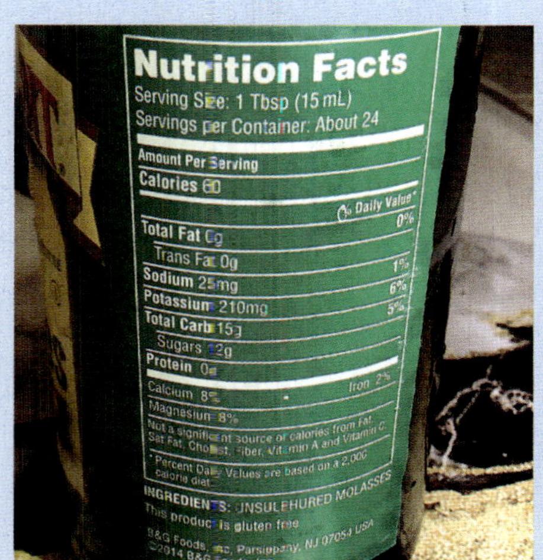

A close look at molasses shows excellent nutrient contents.

There are four things I always add to my Churn: Worm castings, crab meal, alfalfa meal, and dolomite lime. You can keep it just as simple or make it more complex by adding more components, but whatever you do, stay as consistent as possible with your additions. I have run my Churn using just some dolomite lime, adding about ½ cup of fish tank water as my nutrient additions, and that worked out awesome! I still, to this day, add fish tank water to my Churn. But you could run your Churn using just dolomite lime and fish tank water. Or just dolomite lime and worm leachate.

PHOTOS: THE REV

After adding your nutrients to your Churn, you should allow it to bubble away for at least 24 hours, then check the ppm with your TDS meter. When you build the Churn, you are creating a ridiculously concentrated tea that should read well above 100 ppm. As long as the ppm value is over 100, you're all good. It could be 300 ppm, that's fine too. Mine fluctuates between 180 and 280 ppm. This wide variation is okay because we don't directly feed our plants with Churn contents. Instead, Churn water is added to our reservoir of plant water. Lemme 'splain...

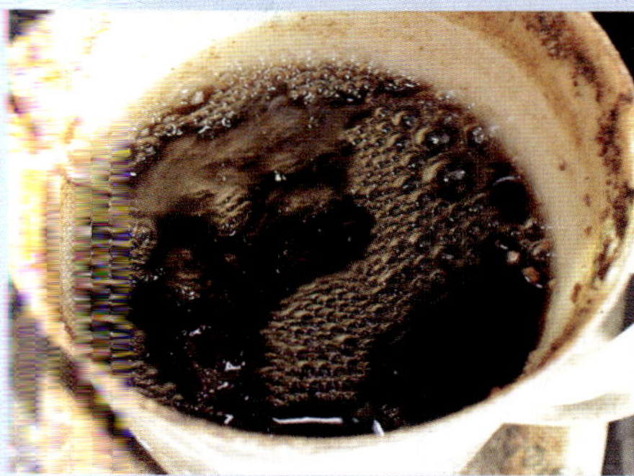

The Churn bubbling away.

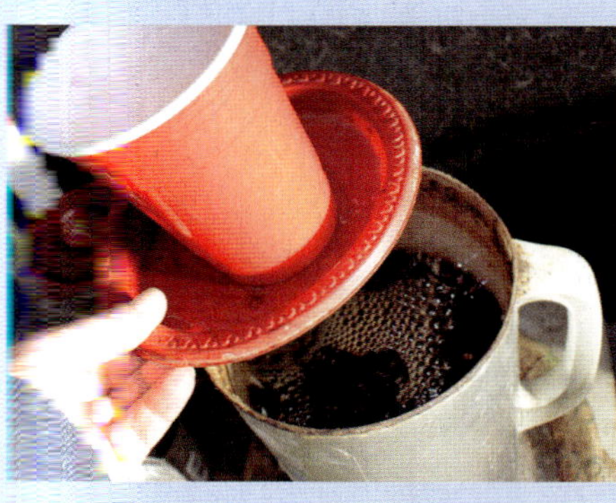

I always have lids for both the Churn and my plant water to keep the humidity in check in the growing rooms.

Your plant water should read 30 to 55 ppm. We want to increase that ppm to around 61 to 65 ppm. We do this by adding small amounts of our Churn water to our plant water reservoir, an ounce at a time. Once you add a single ounce of Churn water to your plant water, read the ppm again and it will give you an idea of how many ounces of Churn you will need to reach your desired ppm value. I usually add about 4 oz. of my Churn water to my 5-gallon reservoir of plant water. You simply do this with every watering up until the last 10 days of flowering. At this time, you back off the Churn additions to fully fade your plants.

Rev's Tip: Fading your plants simply means forcing them to use up all their stored nutrients during the last two weeks of growing for a high-quality final product.

The ppm value of your Churn can vary. If the Churn water is closer to 100 ppm, then it will take more Churn water to raise the ppm of your plant water. Closer to 300 ppm Churn water will take much less to raise plants' water ppm value to desired levels.

Maintaining and Using the Churn

As you use the contents of your Churn, you can just refill it with water, diluting your Churn. I always leave the last 25% of the Churn contents before refilling or refreshing it temporarily between cleanings. This keeps the microlife evolving over time.

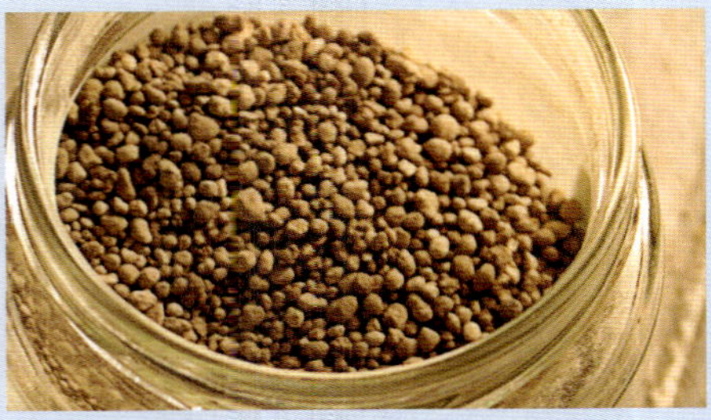

I always add pelletized fast-acting dolomite lime to my Churn for pH goodness.

You can also add additional ingredients along the way when the ppm gets too low. After adding new ingredients, bubble it for at least 24 hours before using it in your plant water. Make sure to keep your additions consistent. This will create a stable environment for the microlife to evolve in. My suggested Churn ingredients represent a good balance of nutrients. You can certainly modify the list of additions, but don't add things like Sul-Po-Mag or rock phosphate. These types of ingredients will dominate the ppm levels of the Churn.

When you are taking water from the Churn to add to your plant water, simply pour it off the top of the Churn. All the particles of the Churn will be settled on the bottom of the container. As your Churn gets older you may notice some not-so-great smells. This is normal, but might indicate that a cleaning should happen soon.

The water you add to your Churn can be dechlorinated groundwater that is under 60 ppm. Alternately, it's fine to use rain, distilled, or reverse osmosis filtered water. You just need to use dolomite lime in your Churn to keep the pH around 7.0. I like using fast-acting prilled/pelletized dolomite lime, but the powdered grade is all good too.

The Churn Summary and Additional Info

Consistency has a lot of power when it comes to leveraging Mother Nature's strengths. Add Churn water to your plant water every time you water and wind down additions as harvest approaches. Keep ppm levels consistent and keep Churn additions consistent. Mother Nature will do the rest.

- I used to run my Churn for years at a time without cleaning it. Recently, I have noticed that the calcium buildup causes the pH to run super high. As a rule of thumb, the more organic matter you add to your Churn, the more often it will need to be cleaned. Always save a little old Churn water to add to the new Churn to keep the microlife evolving.
- Keep a couple of gallons of distilled bottled water (low-ppm water) on hand in case you add a bit too much Churn water to your plant water.
- Make sure to have lids on your Churn and plant water reservoir. This open bubbling water can add to humidity inside your growing room, especially overnight.
- I keep my 5-gallon plant water reservoir evolving like the Churn. I always leave a little bit of plant water in the bucket before refilling. You may get a little algae

PHOTOS: THE REV

in your reservoir, especially if it's in direct light. Not a big deal, all good. This keeps life evolving there.

- I have some special additions I add to my Churn that are totally optional. I add about 1/2 teaspoon of bee pollen and just a few granules of Epsom salt. You can overdose fast on Epsom, so use it carefully! I add the bee pollen every time I add other ingredients. I add Epsom salt about every other, or third time.

So, that's basically all you need to know. If it sounds at all complicated, trust me, it is not. Once you get rolling with it, you get savvy very quickly—especially with regards to how much Churn water to add to hit your targeted ppm for your plant water.

Finally, I want to leave you with a warning. Feeding your plants water that is over 67 ppm will result in overdosing in the long term. Stick to low- to mid-60s. Grab a copy of my latest book, *True Living Organics: Druid's Edition* on Amazon for more information about the Churn and so much more. For some solid genetics born and bred using TLO, visit Kingdom Organic Seeds online. L8r G8rs.

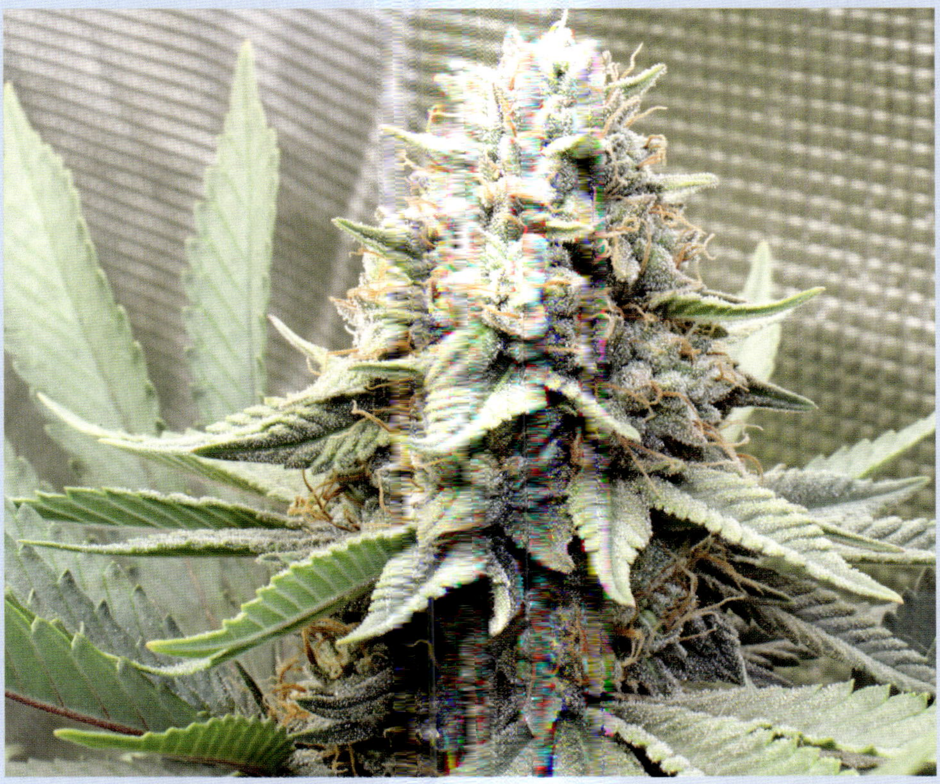

Keeping your Churn ingredients and your plant water ppm consistent works like a dream for highly exotic genetics.

Running an Organic Tent Garden

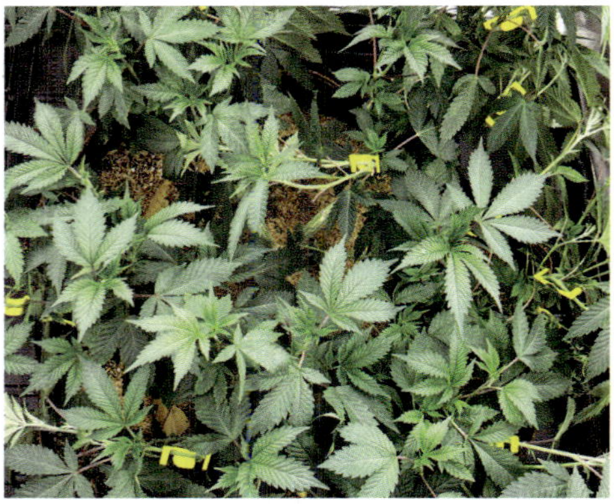

Young plants are trained with some BudHuggers to stay upright.

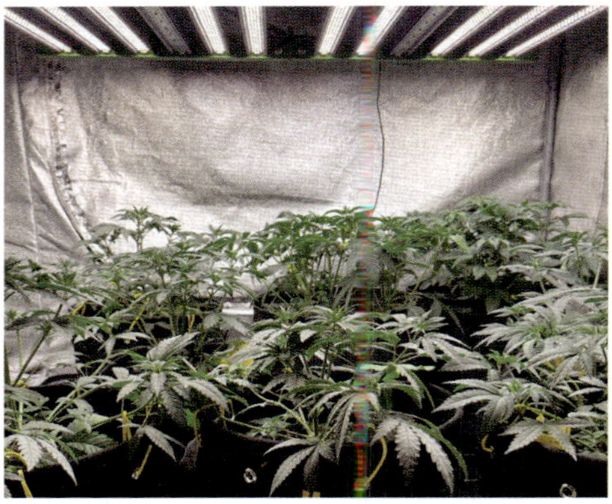

Inside the tent, the light is at its lowest and should be raised as the plants grow.

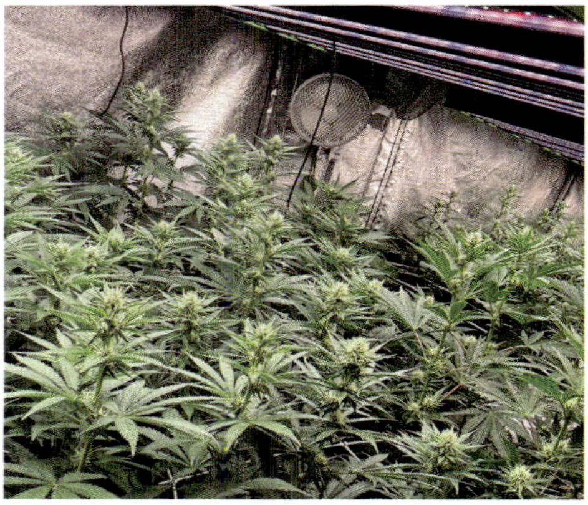

ScrOG + tent is a perfect way to grow this indoor strain.

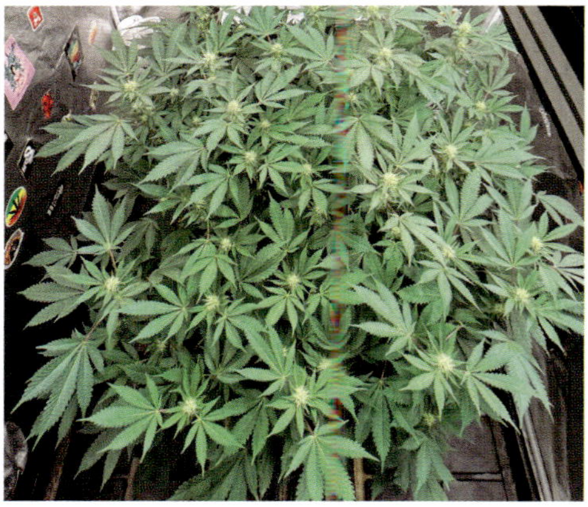

An even canopy is the way to go and best practices produce this.

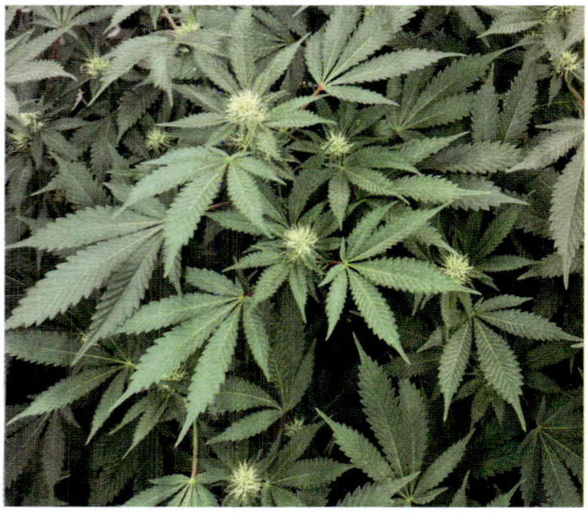

At the start of flowering the canopy will be tight but will spread quickly after.

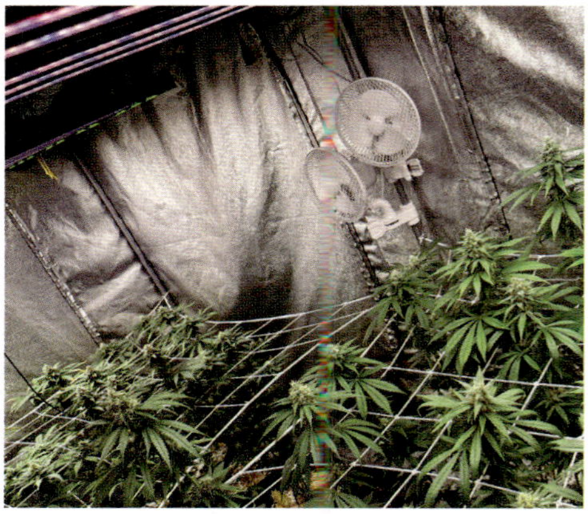

Towards later flowering the spread is evidently controlled by the netting.

PHOTOS: TANYA PETERSEN

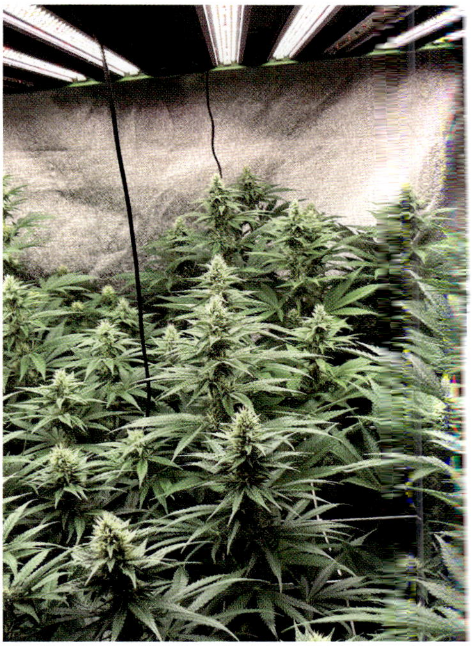

These organic buds just keep growing and growing as long as the environment provides.

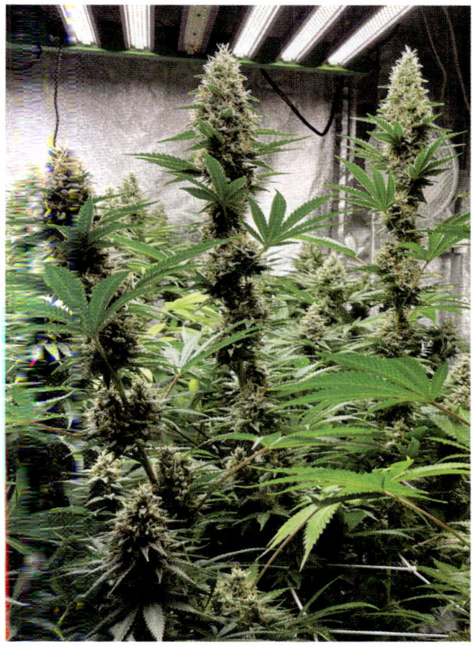

Cannabis won't hold back with how big buds can get under optimal lighting conditions.

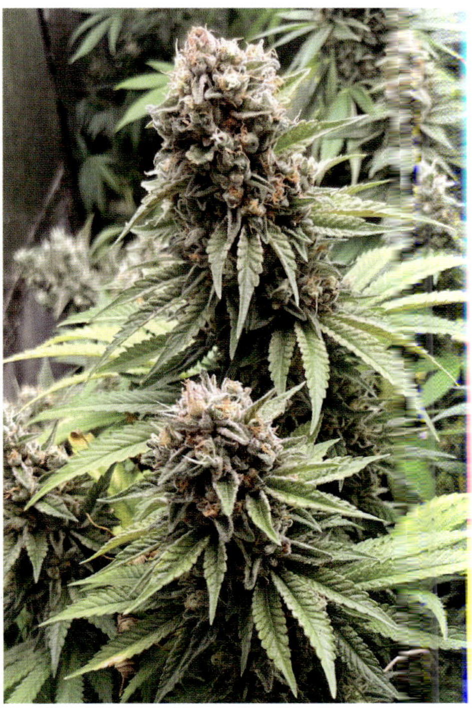

Who says organics can't produce buds just as big and dense as any other process?

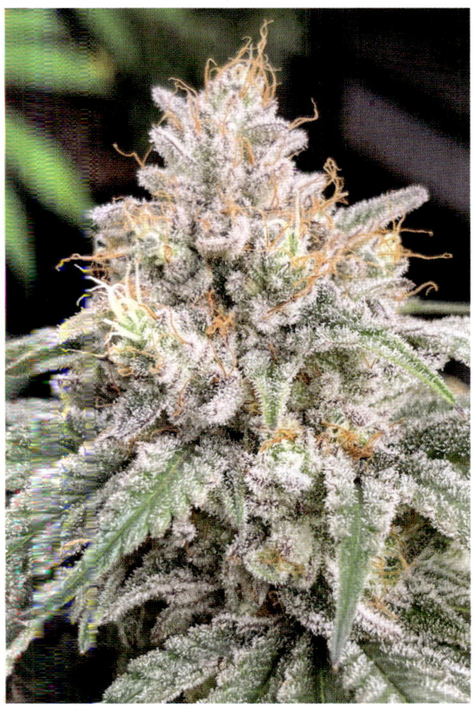

Most grows are close to being organic but just haven't developed an organic plan.

Mulch

Mulch is a versatile and valuable tool in organic gardening, serving multiple functions to enhance your garden's health and productivity. Not only does mulch protect the soil, but it also aligns perfectly with organic principles due to its organic nature.

Mulch is a fundamental component of organic gardening, offering various advantages to improve soil health, water conservation, and pest control. Whether you opt for traditional organic mulches or explore innovative solutions like geotextiles, the choice of mulch plays a pivotal role in the overall success of your organic garden. Stay informed about evolving mulching techniques, as they continue to shape the future of organic cultivation.

Benefits of Mulch

Mulch acts as a protective layer over the soil, preventing erosion, temperature extremes, and exposure to harsh weather conditions. This ensures that your soil remains fertile and retains its structure over time. It serves as an insulator, keeping the soil cooler in hot weather and warmer during colder spells, creating an ideal environment for plant growth. By covering the soil, it minimizes water loss, ensuring that your plants receive a consistent water supply, even during dry periods. Mulch effectively reduces soil erosion caused by heavy rain or wind, particularly crucial for sloped or elevated garden beds. In regions with heavy rainfall, mulch helps to prevent soil compaction and nutrient leaching caused by excessive water exposure.

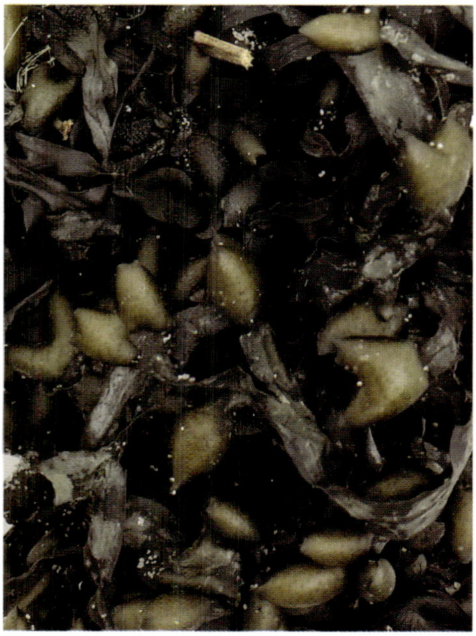

Seaweed foraged from a beach can be used as a mulch as long as it has been washed down with a hose.

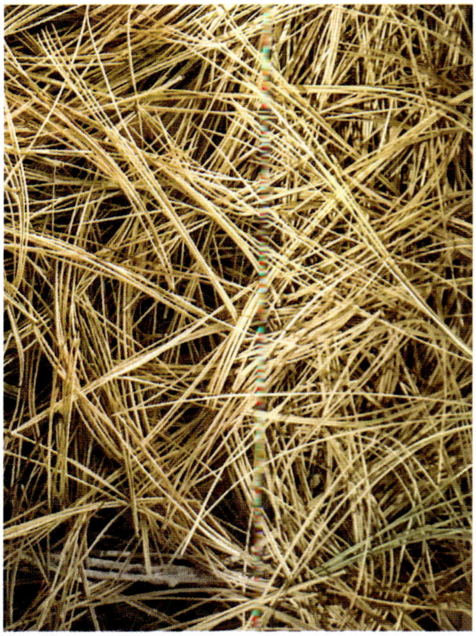

Pine needles are a natural mulch found in nature. They can be foraged, washed, and used as a garden mulch.

PHOTOS: NATHAN GUILLARD

Mulch is also a natural weed suppressant, blocking sunlight from reaching weed seeds and preventing them from germinating, thus eliminating the need for synthetic weed control methods in organic gardening. Root-dwelling insects and other pests are also deterred by the presence of mulch, a barrier to their access to the soil and plant roots.

Managing Mulch

Maintaining the quality of your mulch is essential. Mulch can develop a foul odor if it undergoes anaerobic decomposition. To prevent this, ensure proper aeration by periodically turning or rotating the mulch.

Types of Mulch

Organic mulches include compost, bark, cardboard, grass, hay, leaves, newspaper, sawdust, straw, wood, and even wool. These materials decompose at varying rates, influenced by environmental factors. However, once the benefits of a particular mulch start to diminish due to decomposition, it's advisable to replace it.

While traditional mulch materials are common, innovative solutions like geotextiles are gaining traction. Geotextiles are geotechnical fabrics used for protection and slope stability. These advanced materials can serve as an effective mulch alternative, offering unique benefits like erosion control and barrier protection.

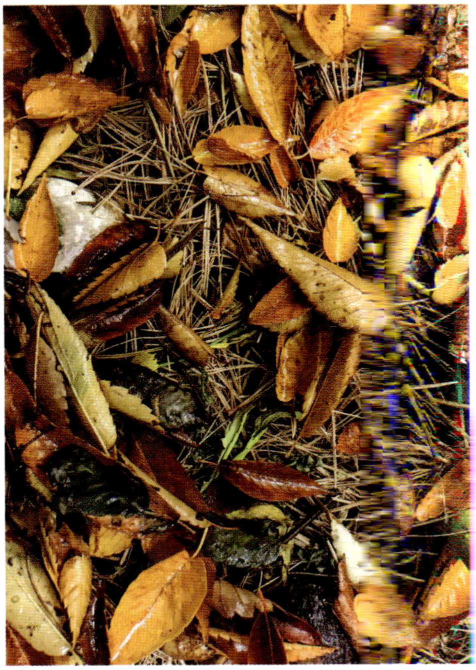

You can mix what you forage into a mixed mulch.

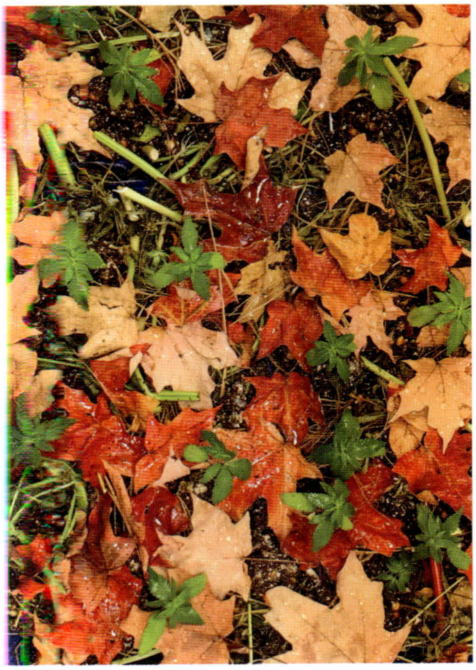

The maple leaf will dry out and crumble but by then it has done its job.

PHOTOS: NATHAN GUILLARD

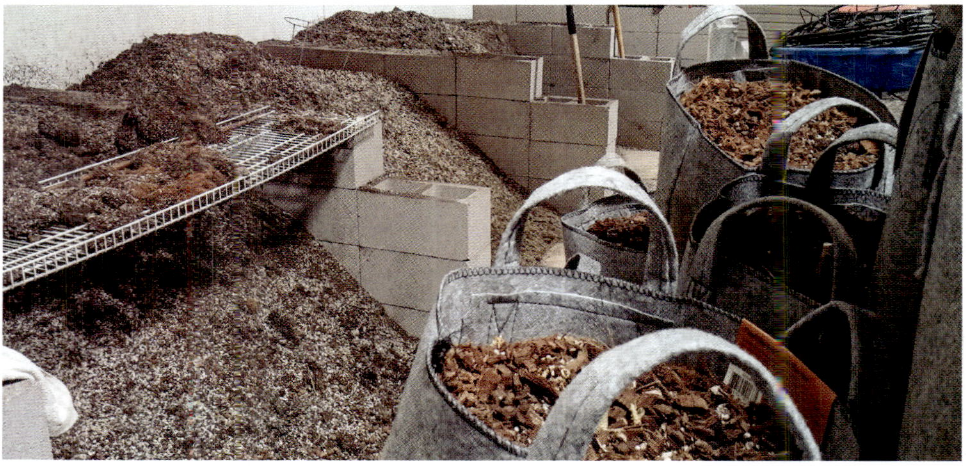

Grow bags with organic substrates mixed from the bulk piles.

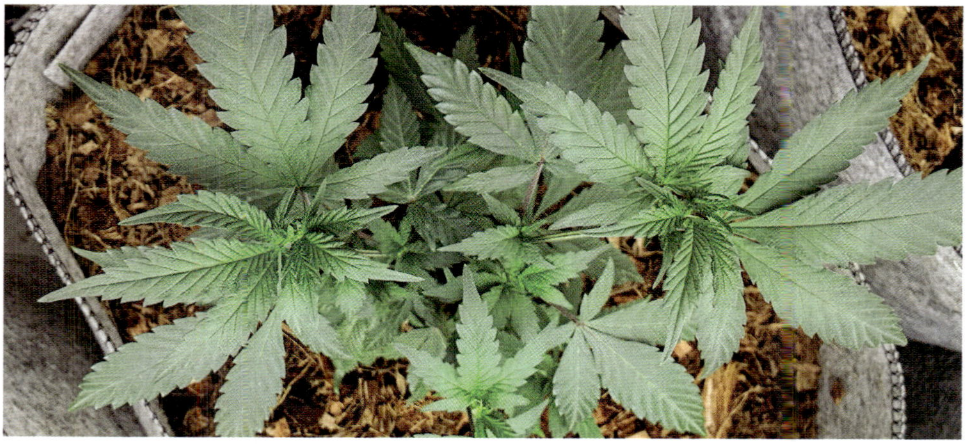

Clones transplanted to the grow bags.

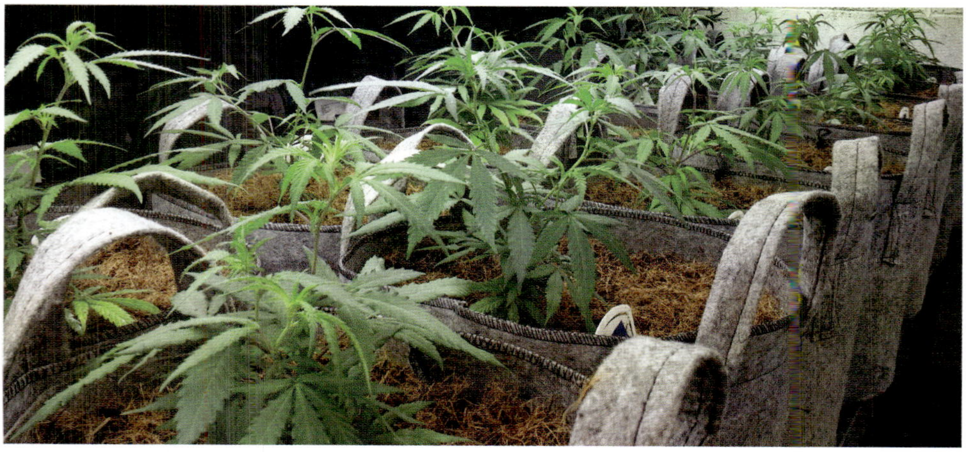

Grow bags transported to the vegetative growth area.

PHOTOS: MONICA GRIFFIN

Vermicomposting

Vermicomposting, or "worm composting," has garnered popularity for both its lack of odor and its nutrient-rich output. This organic gardening technique traces its roots back to the practice of keeping worms in gardens. Farmers, recognizing the value of worms in soil cultivation, have long embraced their role in enhancing soil health. Vermicomposting harnesses the power of these remarkable creatures, resulting in a valuable by-product known as worm castings or humus manure.

Choosing the Right Worms

The two most common worm species used in vermicomposting are the red worm, or red wiggler, *Lumbricus rubellus*, and brandling worm, *Eisenia fetida*. These worms can be acquired from organic stores or fishing bait shops. While finding a natural supplier is an option, it's often more convenient to purchase them from established sources.

Vermicomposting Bins

Vermicomposting bins come in various designs to suit different needs. They are usually constructed from wood, plastic, or stainless steel. Regardless of the bin type, all vermicomposting systems should include adequate airflow and a drainage system. There are primarily two types of vermicomposting bins: Undivided and continuous.

Undivided bins are layered with bedding, organics, and compost. While relatively easy to use, they require manual removal of worms when harvesting vermicompost.

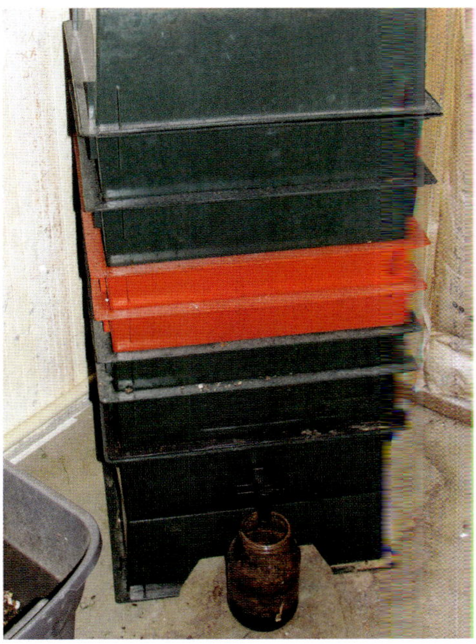

A personal worm farm will create your very own worm castings fertilizer.

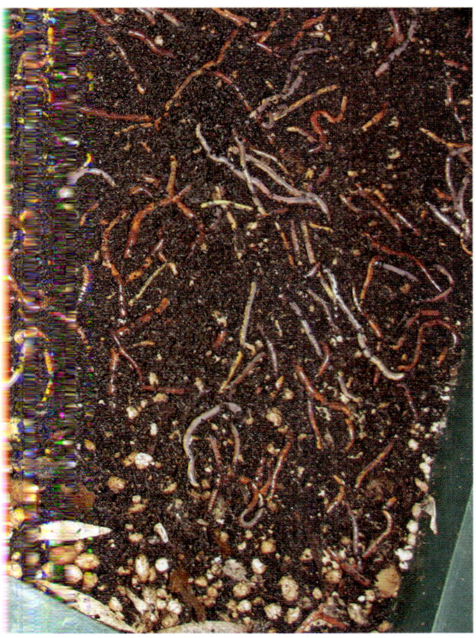

Worm farm showing worms in top tray.

PHOTOS: THE REV

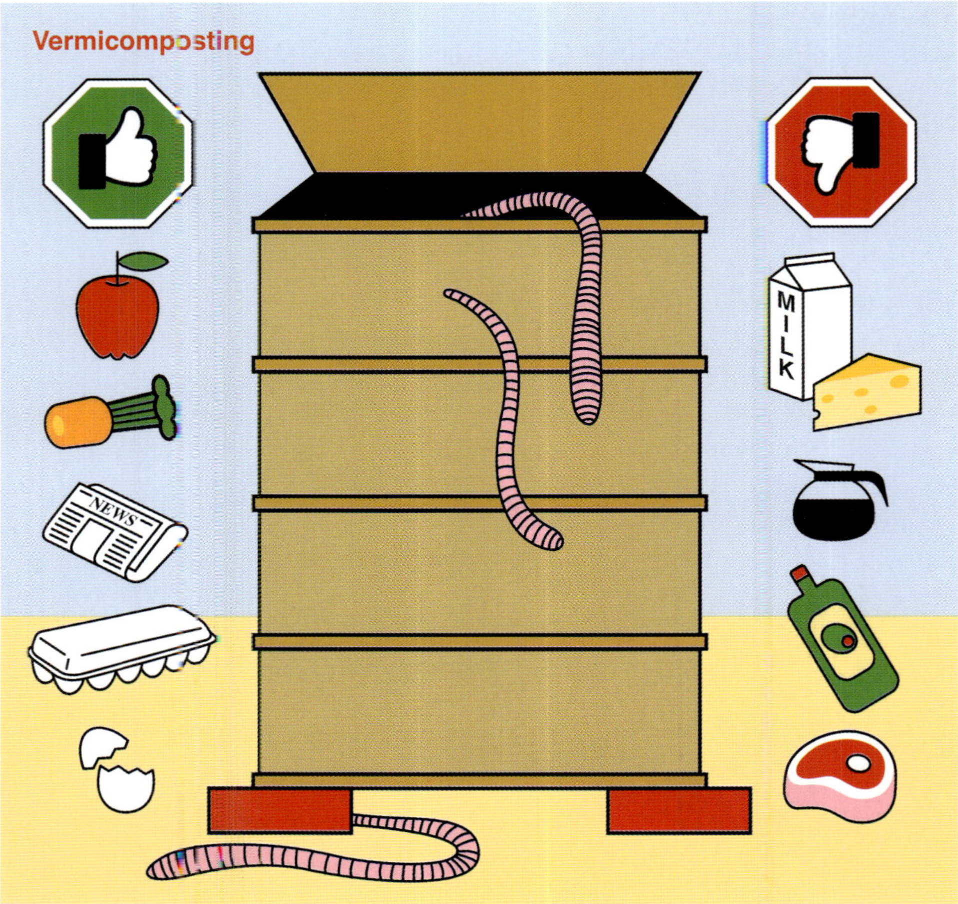

Continuous vermicomposting systems, as the name suggests, provide a continuous supply of vermicompost without the need for manual worm removal. They rely on vertical or horizontal stacking to encourage the worms to migrate toward fresh organic material.

Larger-scale operations often create "windrows," rows or lines of compost where worms remain within the heaps of organic material due to their size and abundant food supply.

Begin your vermicomposting by selecting an appropriate bin and preparing the bedding with such materials as damp newspaper, soil, cardboard, sawdust, moss, or a combination of these. This carbon-rich bedding serves as a foundation for your vermicomposting system and helps manage odors resulting from organic decay. Ensure that the bedding remains adequately damp within your system.

The more worms, the better. Worms can consume organic matter equivalent to half their weight each day. To determine the right number of worms for your system, weigh them and gauge the maximum capacity your bin can handle.

Managing your Bin

Vermicomposting bins thrive at temperatures between 55–80°F (12–27°C). Red wigglers can survive within a broader range, from 40–90°F (4–32°C). Protect your worms from temperatures below 40°F, as this can be fatal. If necessary, bring the bin indoors during colder spells, but ensure that the environment remains suitable for continued vermicomposting.

Properly layer the bedding and organic feeds in your bin. As older organic matter breaks down, add new materials and cover them with fresh bedding. This helps maintain a balanced decomposition rate and prevents rotting of newly added organics. Avoid using fruit skins, especially if they come from non-organic sources, as they may contain pesticide residues that could harm your worms. Maintain a balanced pH level around 7, similar to that in regular organic gardening.

Ensure adequate aeration in your bin to prevent anaerobic conditions. Foul odors may also result from high nitrogen levels, which can be mitigated by adding more carbon-rich materials. Keep flies away from your bin to prevent infestations, and promptly address ant issues if they arise.

Harvesting Vermicompost

When it's time to harvest your vermicompost, sift through the material to separate the valuable worms from the compost you intend to use in your garden. This ensures the continuity of your vermicomposting operation.

Vermicomposting is a powerful and eco-friendly method for enriching your garden's soil with nutrient-rich humus. By providing optimal conditions and proper care for your worm companions, you can harness the benefits of vermicomposting while adhering to organic gardening principles. Worm castings produced through vermicomposting offer a sustainable and natural way to enhance soil fertility, making it a valuable asset in your organic gardening toolkit.

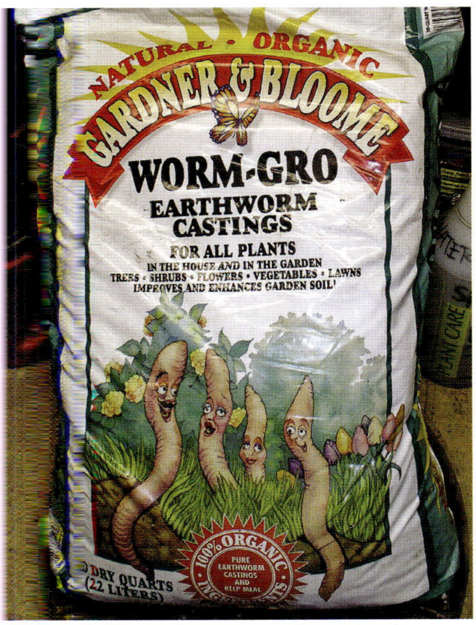

These bagged earthworm casings are of a high quality and great for your soil mix.

PHOTO: THE REV

Coir Blocks

Coco coir blocks, a convenient and efficient solution for cannabis growers, bear a striking resemblance to the wrapped grow slabs used in hydroponics. Coco coir in its

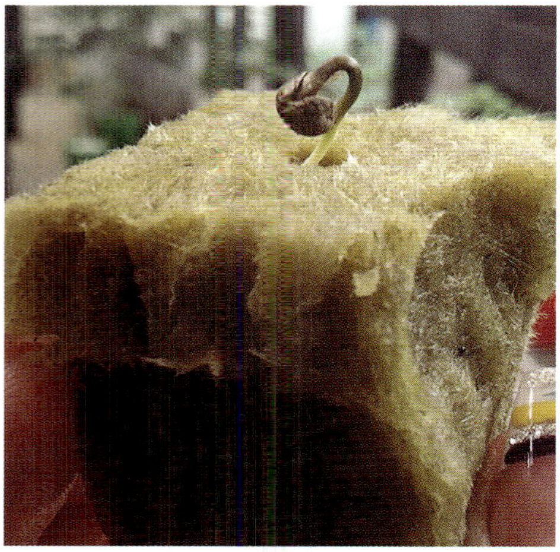

Coir is a fine, organic, puffy, and soil-like substrate. Its pH is neutral.

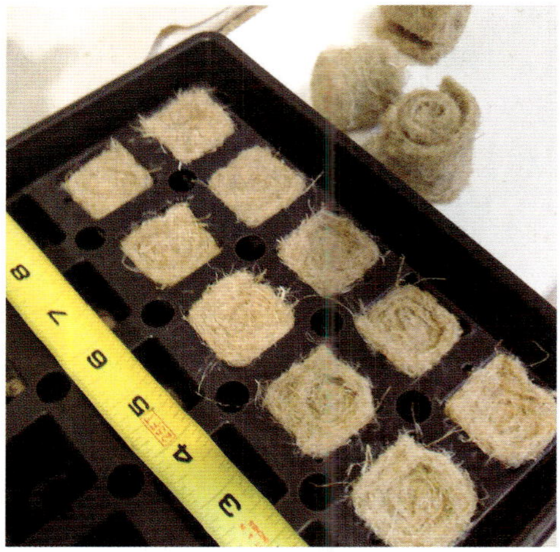

These are hemp fiber-based grow cubes. Totally organic.

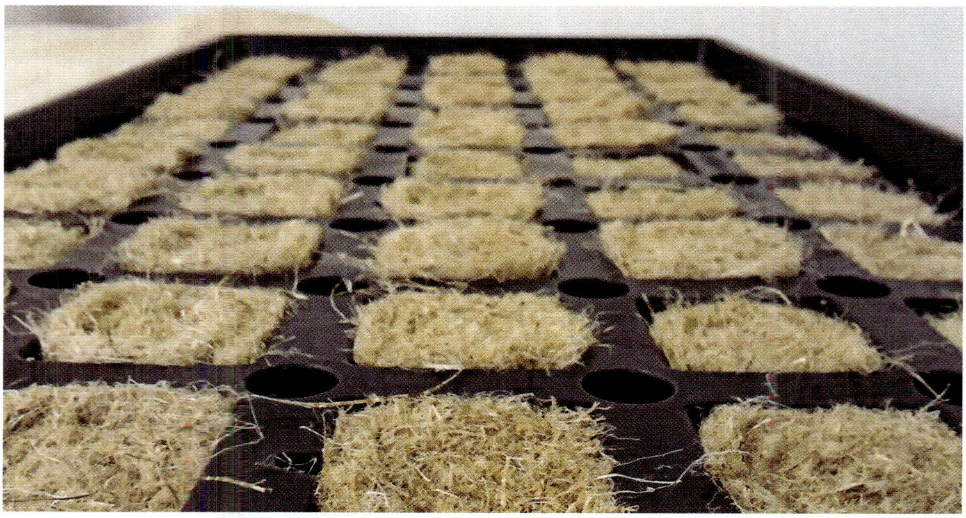

Hemp fiber grow cubes from Hemp Solutions are an organic and canna-friendly way to germinate seeds and grow organically.

PHOTOS: MONICA GRIFFIN (TOP LEFT), HEMP SOLUTIONS (TOP RIGHT AND BOTTOM)

loose form is also available, though blocks offer a distinct advantage in their compact, compressed form that is incredibly easy to store. These blocks, although initially compact, have the remarkable ability to expand into a light, airy, soil-like substrate when introduced to hot water. This quality makes them an indispensable component of cannabis cultivation, ensuring the presence of vital air in the growing medium.

In cannabis cultivation, soil must be well-aerated. Cannabis thrives in soil that allows for adequate air circulation. This is precisely where coir blocks play a pivotal role. When incorporated into the growing medium, they not only provide the necessary aeration but also exhibit a neutral pH level. This neutrality significantly contributes to maintaining an optimal pH balance in the medium, a crucial factor for successful cannabis cultivation.

The utility of coir blocks extends beyond this introduction, as explained in numerous references to their use throughout this book, particularly in Chapters 10 and 11 on indoor and hydroponic cultivation. Their versatility and compatibility with various organic substrates make coir blocks an invaluable resource for cannabis growers seeking an efficient and effective means to enhance their cultivation practices. Whether used as a primary component or in conjunction with other substrates, coir blocks will prove their worth in your pursuit of premium cannabis yields.

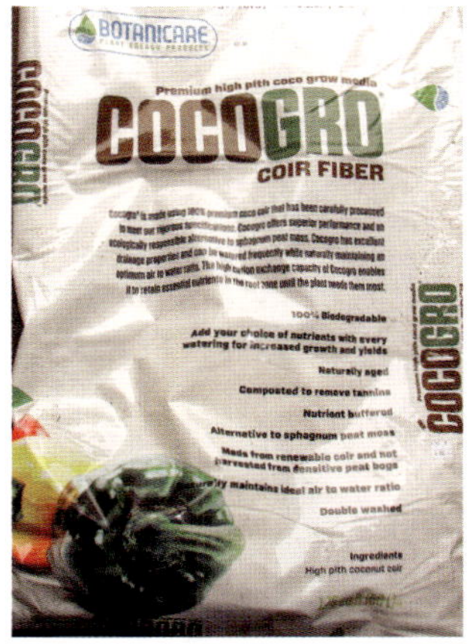

This coconut coir product is great at buffering the pH of your soil mix.

Organic Feeding Products

In organic cannabis cultivation, feeding products range from liquids to semi-solid compounds. Among these offerings, fish, blood, and bone-based granules are particularly favored and find their place in numerous mixtures. While liquid variants are primarily tailored for organic hydroponic growers, their versatility ensures that growers of all types can benefit from their use. Additionally, organic soil stimulants are readily available to complement your feeding regimen and boost microbial activity in the soil.

The organic materials used for feeding products undergo a transformation into smaller molecular stages as they decompose. Throughout this process, nitrogen, among other essential nutrients, exists in various forms. One of the key distinctions in organic feeding products lies in their release mechanisms; some operate on a slow-release basis, while others deliver nutrients more rapidly.

Solid organics represent the slowest form of nutrient release. Granular organics, on the other hand, break down the solid material into smaller particles, allowing for a more evenly distributed release, although it is still relatively slow. These slow-release

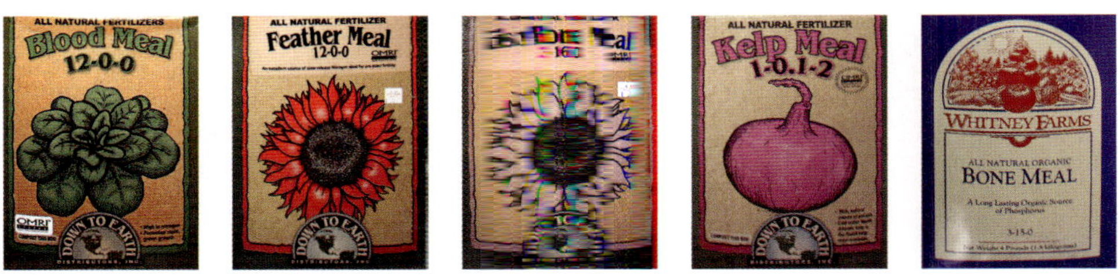

Various organic meals are available at most garden centers. Pay attention to the NPK values to determine what supplement your plants need.

PHOTOS: THE REV

systems offer the advantage of requiring infrequent feeding, reducing the need for regular garden visits. However, they may not be suitable for all growers. For instance, organic hydroponic cultivators typically require a faster release system to meet their plants' nutritional needs. Despite the varying release speeds, the end products provided by slow-release and fast-release systems are the same; the primary distinction lies in the rate of nutrient release.

Modern fast-release systems, typically liquid nutrients that may require additional dilution with water, provide instant feeding. These products are commonly found in the hydroponics section of gardening supply stores, available in single or multi-packs. For detailed mixing instructions, particularly for indoor growing and hydroponics, refer to Chapter 11. Fast-release systems can be effectively integrated with soil-based cultivation. Unlike synthetic nutrient brands, where compound recombination can alter the composition, fast- and slow-release organic systems generally mix without complications. This characteristic minimizes nutrient lockout, a problem frequently encountered when using synthetics, which we discuss further in Chapter 8.

Incorporating fast-release systems into organic cultivation is often beneficial. For example, if you realize that your slow-release nutrient application has been insufficient and your plants require more nutrients immediately, fast-release products offer a solution. Additionally, during the flowering stage, you may need to increase the phosphorus levels in your nutrient regimen, which can be conveniently achieved with fast-release nutrients. Finally, addressing nutrient deficiencies promptly is crucial, and fast-release systems provide an effective means to tackle this issue.

The flexibility of organic feeding products, which includes both slow- and fast-release options, enables you to tailor your nutrient regimen to your specific needs as a cannabis grower. By understanding the nuances of these products and their applications, you can optimize your cultivation practices for superior results.

Vegetative and Flowering Organic Nutrients

In our exploration of organic feeding products for cannabis cultivation, we've discussed the merits of fish emulsion as an excellent source of nutrients for the vegetative stage. However, it's no secret that fish emulsion has a strong unpleasant odor. Hydrolyzed organic fish emulsion, derived from fresh fish subjected to natural enzyme treatments that break them down into a nitrogen-rich nutrient source, tends to produce fewer odors than its non-hydrolyzed counterparts. Many brands now use hydrolysis to reduce the characteristic fishy odor. Interestingly, the use of fish emulsion as an organic nutrient source dates back to the earliest human cultivation practices when people noticed improved plant growth in areas where discarded fish waste accumulated. Today, we can replicate this process on a commercial scale by using natural enzymes to produce fish emulsions from fish waste.

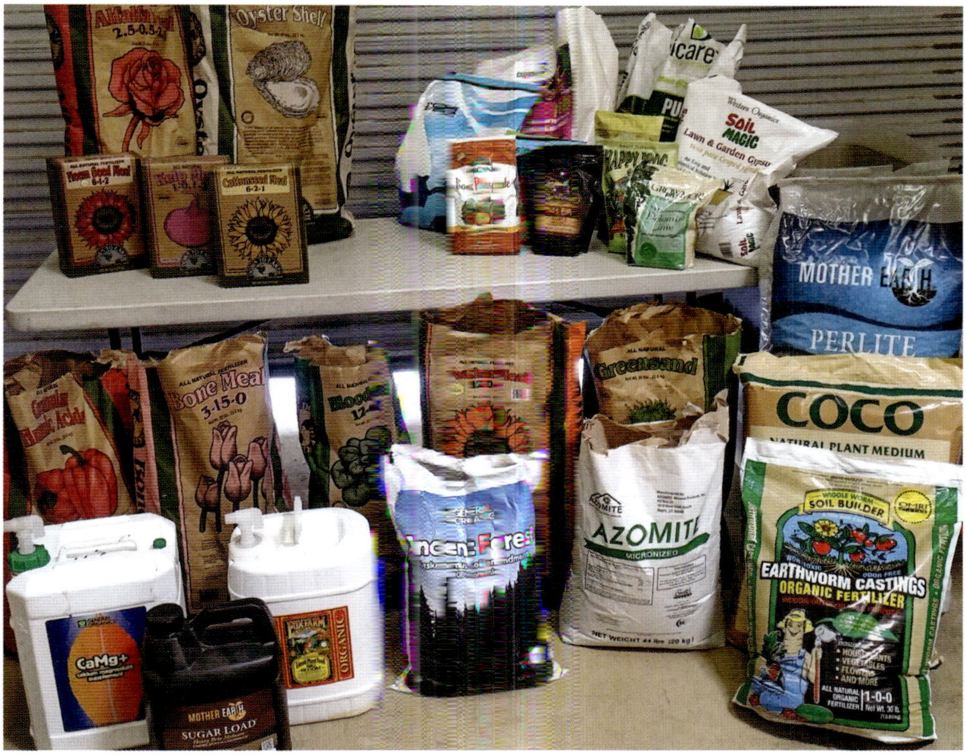

An assortment of commercially-available organic substrates in different sizes and forms.

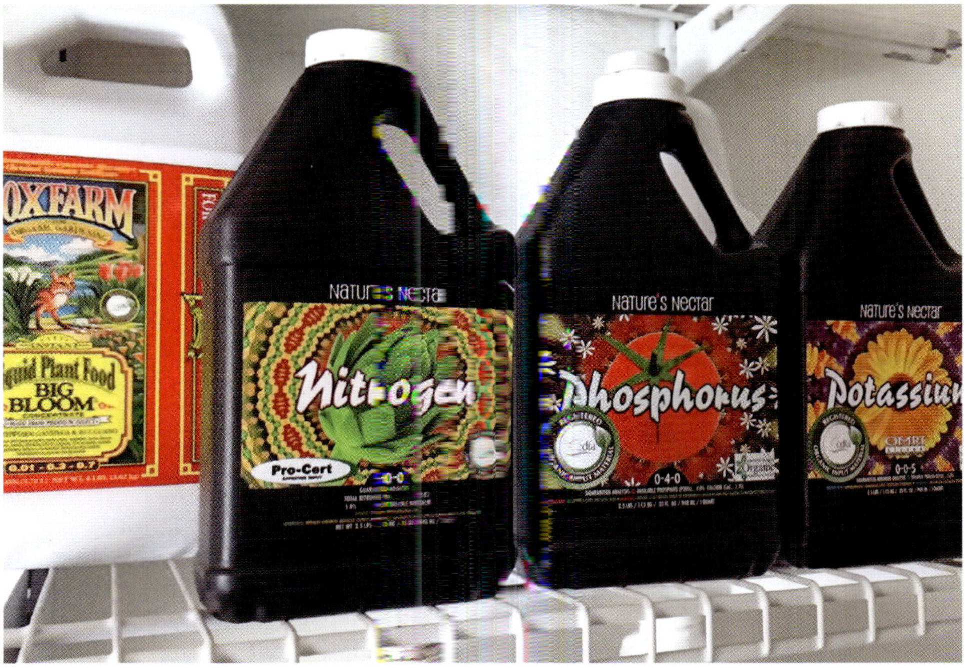

Organic nutrients in liquid form.

PHOTOS: MONICA GRIFFIN

Strong odors are often associated with manure-based products like guano. To avoid these odors, source guano from fresh and properly prepared sources. Fresh organic products have an organic smell, which, although distinct, is not unpleasant. The foul odors typically emerge as these products begin to decompose.

For outdoor growers using smelly organic nutrients, introducing other plants with strong floral aromas to the grow area can masking odor. This strategy helps reduce the impact of cannabis smells on the surrounding environment while potentially enhancing the overall olfactory experience. The balance of aromas depends on which plants emit the most aromatic molecules.

The concentration of phosphorus in your feeding regimen plays a pivotal role in promoting flowering. Many commercial producers label their products as "bloom" nutrients, recognizing that they are primarily used for flowering plants. When selecting organic nutrients for flowering, buy products with higher phosphorus levels. These can include seabird and bat guano products, bone meal mixes with elevated phosphorus content, and acidic mixes featuring higher phosphorus levels. When using these products, be prepared to experiment with pH adjustments using pH-up and pH-down products to maintain a neutral pH.

To introduce organic phosphorus into your flowering medium when it's in a solid state, you have several options: A slow-release top granular layer, a liquid organic instant release, or a combination of both. Sativa strains with longer flowering periods are likely to benefit most from slow-release flowering nutrients. For these strains, applying a top layer of organic granules designed for flowering, which gradually breaks down with each watering, can be an effective approach. Indica strains with shorter flowering periods tend to thrive when provided with instant-release flowering nutrients in liquid form. Hybrid strains can benefit from a combination of both slow and fast-release nutrients. Opting for granular nutrients during flowering can expand your range of organic feeding options, potentially at a lower cost.

As the organic market continues to diversify its product offerings, it's essential to scrutinize the nutrient ratios of organic products. For vegetative growth, aim for equal or higher nitrogen to phosphorus and potassium ratios. During the flowering stage, prioritize higher phosphorus levels in relation to nitrogen and potassium. Depending on the preparation and mixing processes, organic nutrients may be available in both forms. These guidelines provide a standard framework for using organic nutrients effectively in your cannabis cultivation.

Organics and Hydroponic Systems

While hydroponic growers typically opt for fast-release nutrients due to the presence of nutrient-liquid holding tanks, or reservoirs, in their systems, it's entirely possible

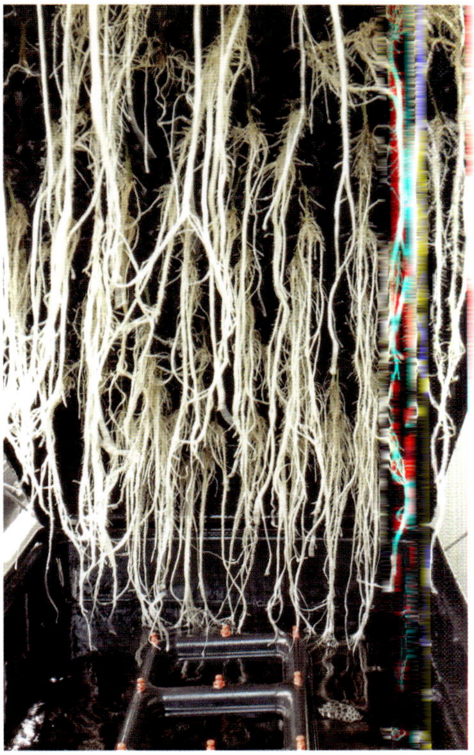

Organic hydroponic healthy root mass.

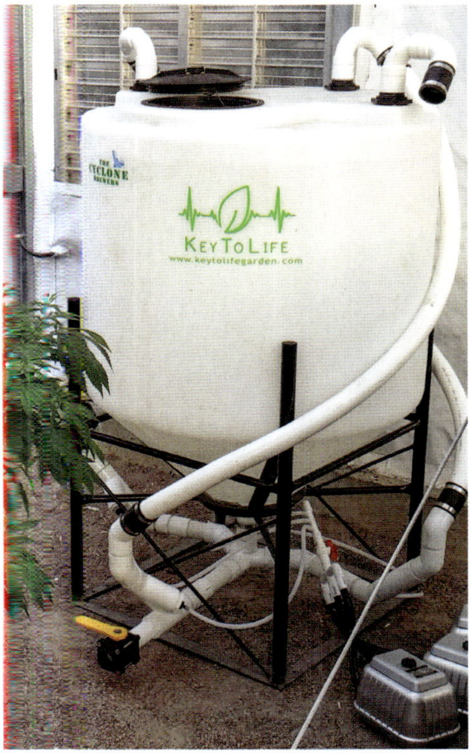

A cyclone brewer that moves water and air around to blend compost tea.

PHOTOS: OPTIMIZE HORTICULTURE CONSULTING (LEFT), KEY TO LIFE (RIGHT)

for hydroponic cultivators to integrate organic nutrients into their practices. One advantage of using multi-pack versions of liquid nutrients is that they offer the flexibility to mix both vegetative and flowering nutrients from the same pack, allowing for customized nutrient blends.

If you're considering combining hydroponics and organic nutrients, check the sections on Nutrient Film Technique (NFT) and Deep Water Culture (DWC) in Chapter 11. These systems are suitable for both beginners and advanced cultivators. A significant advantage of hydroponically grown organic cannabis is the enhanced control over nutrient distribution. For example, hydroponic systems enable growers to halt nutrient flow if needed, whereas soil-based growers might have to transplant their plants out of an overfed soil medium and into a fresh soil pot.

For a more in-depth exploration of hydroponic grow systems and their specific applications, read Chapter 11. Achieving the seemingly incredible feat of "hydroponically-grown organic bud" is indeed within your grasp. This exciting endeavor allows you to harness the best of both worlds, leveraging the precision and control of hydroponics while enjoying the benefits of organic cultivation practices.

Large-Scale Organic Cultivation

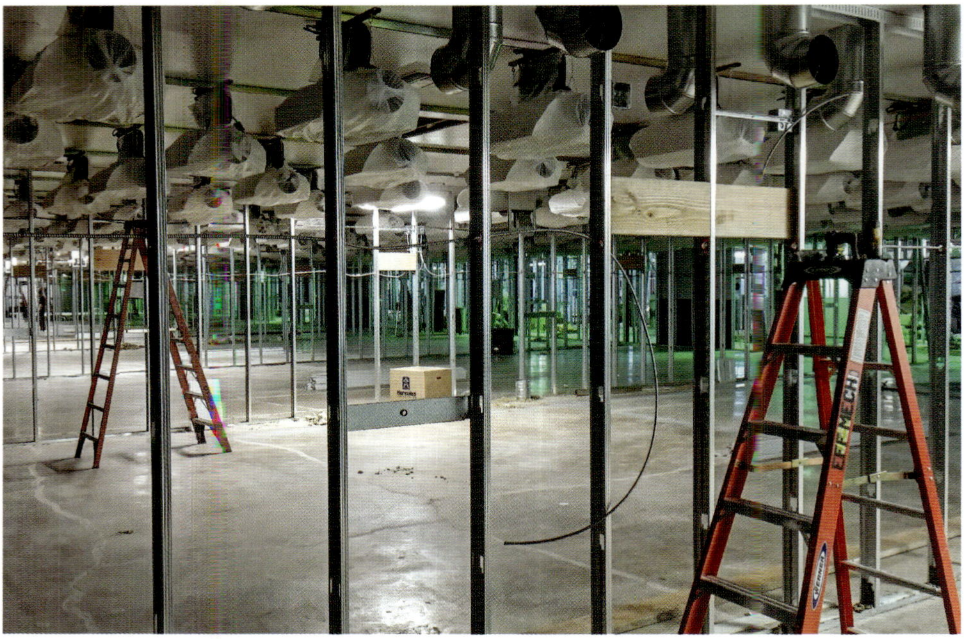

Large-scale grow rooms require extensive ceiling supports while keeping the floor as spacious as possible.

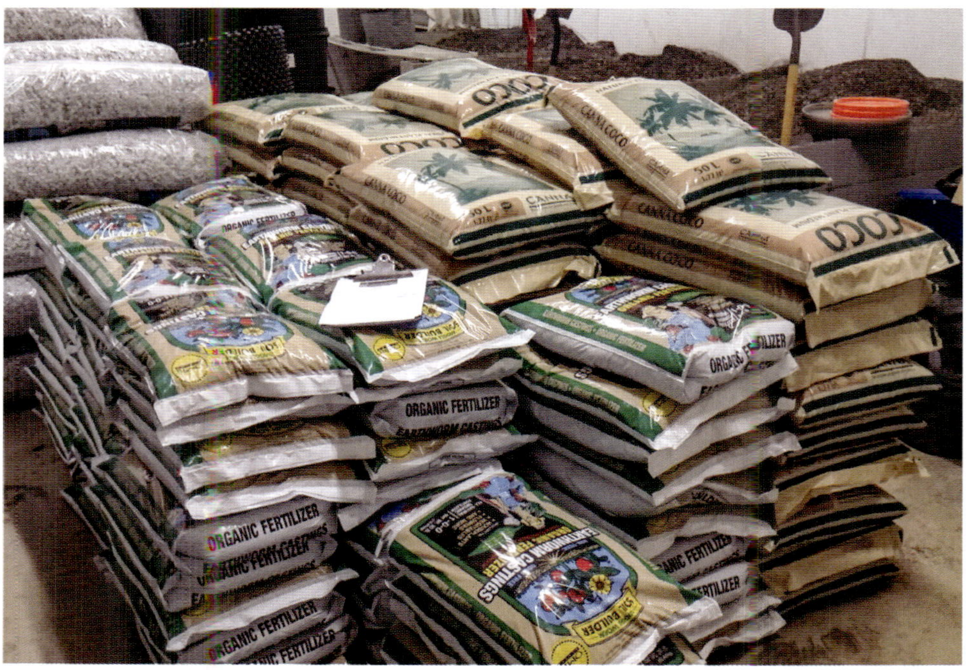

Regardless of whether you are a large-scale grower or a small-scale one,you need a place to store your materials. This is all organic storage.

PHOTOS: MONICA GRIFFIN

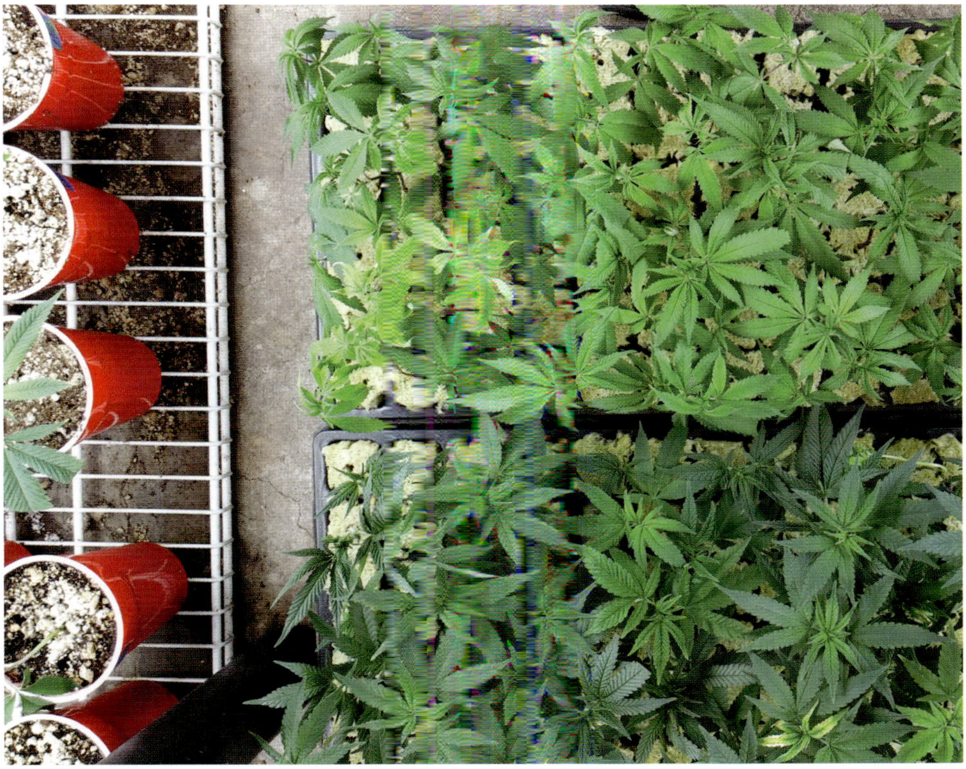

Overhead view of perpetual cloning needed for large-scale cultivation.

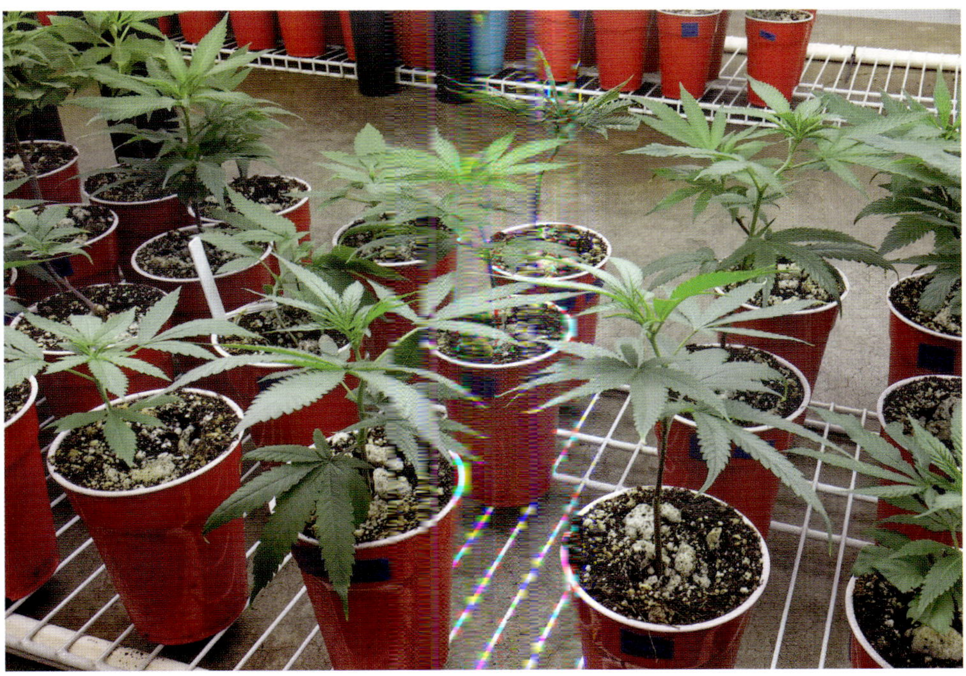

Clones in organic substrate ready to go to the vegetative grow area.

continues...

Large-Scale Organic Cultivation *continued*

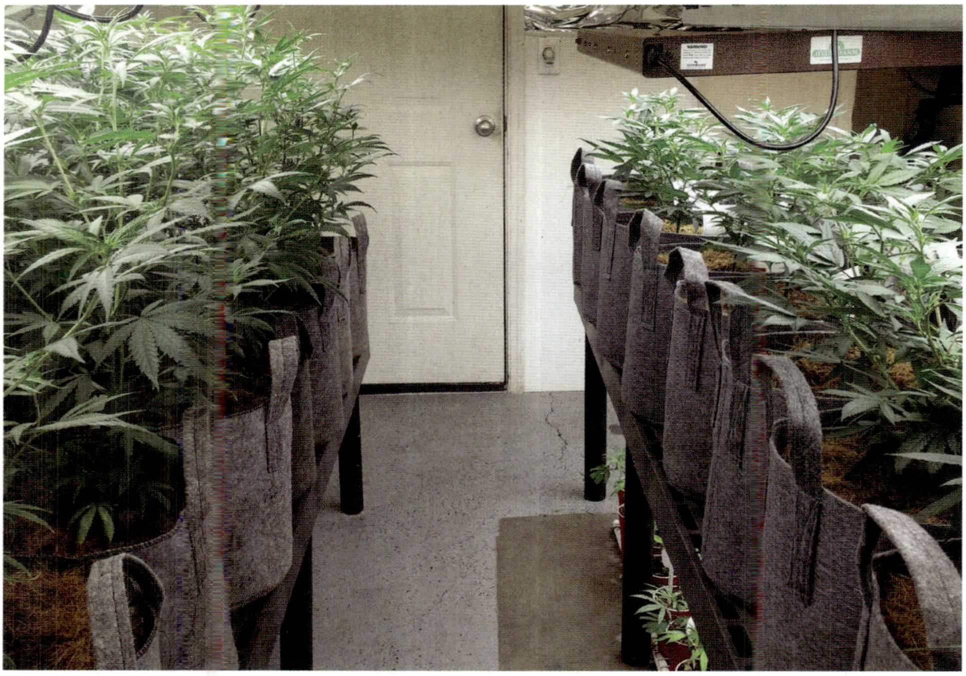

Organic grow bags under LEDs.

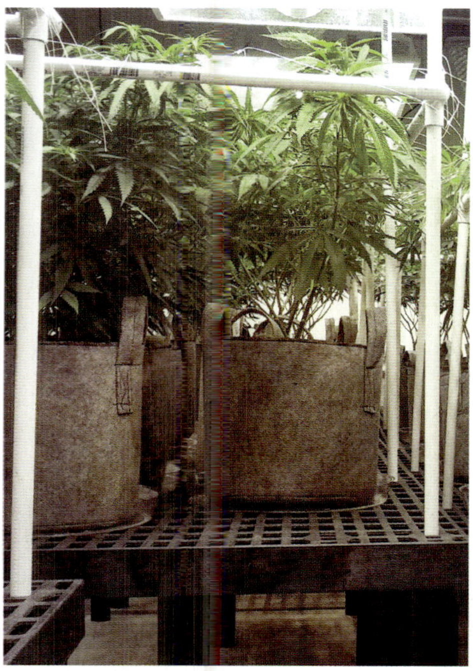

Tables allow for storage/work space under them.

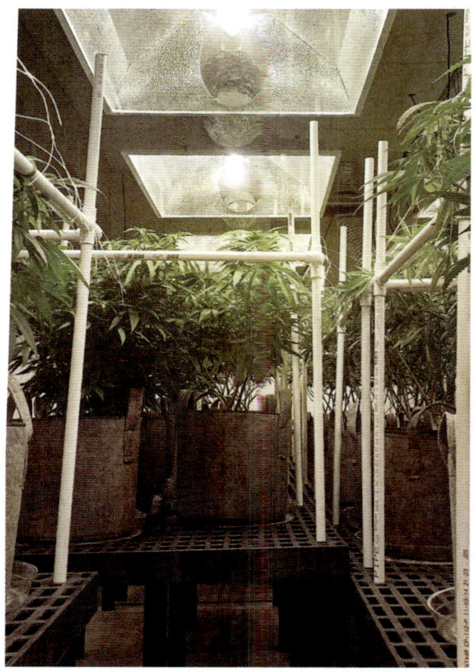

Organic grow bags under HIDs.

PHOTOS: MONICA GRIFFIN

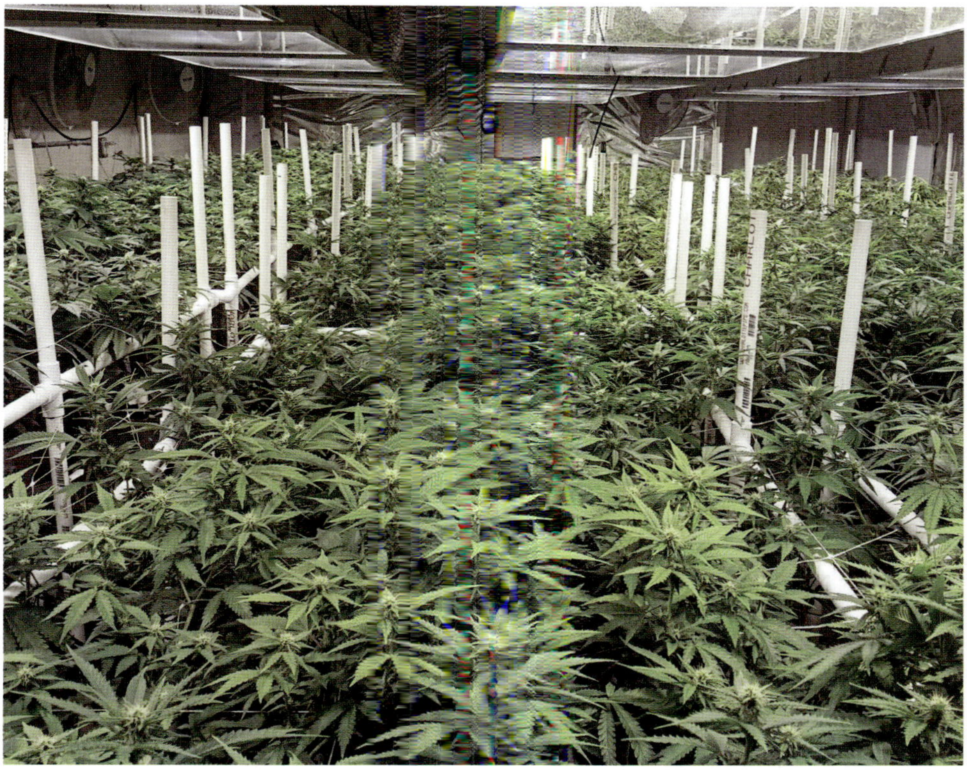

Large-scale organic grow room in the early stages of flowering.

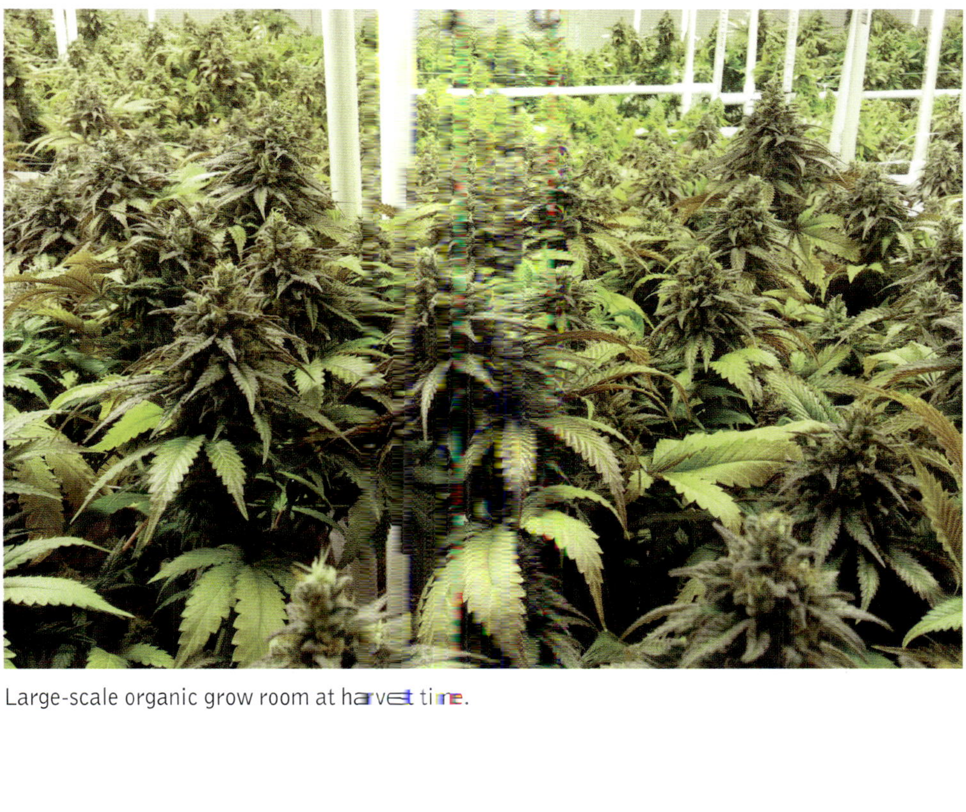

Large-scale organic grow room at harvest time.

Cannabis and Climate Change

The news with regards to cannabis cultivation and climate change is far from encouraging, primarily due to the insufficient use of green energy, energy-efficient equipment, and production optimization within the cannabis industry.[7] There was a time when it was believed that increased cannabis production would benefit the environment. This is because plants cool our atmosphere by using carbon dioxide. With more plants contributing to air purification, organic farming methods, and numerous potential end-product applications, it was assumed that the carbon footprint would be minimal. Unfortunately, the current state of indoor cannabis cultivation is neither environmentally-friendly nor sustainable. This is largely due to its heavy reliance on upstream energy sources like fossil fuels, such as natural gas for electricity, before even factoring in downstream aspects such as packaging and product usage.

The situation bears some similarities to air-conditioned living spaces during sweltering summers. Indoor cannabis cultivation faces similar challenges but on a larger scale, as it involves the regulation of much larger areas. Unless the industry transitions to green energy sources, indoor cannabis cultivation cannot effectively contribute to climate change mitigation. Some growers have taken steps to adopt solar energy solutions, but the ideal conditions for solar power often overlap with outdoor growing conditions, making outdoor cultivation a more economically and environmentally-friendly choice. The issue, however, extends beyond commercial operations to include domestic growers, all of whom collectively contribute to greenhouse gas emissions, pollution, and waste.

While CO_2 supplementation is a concern, the most significant issues revolve around heating, cooling, and humidity control. High-intensity discharge (HID) lights rank next in terms of environmental impact, with transportation and waste disposal contributing more to greenhouse gas emissions than CO_2 supplementation. While office air conditioning, fueled by fossil fuels, poses a similar problem, indoor cannabis environmental control presents a greater challenge due to the much higher energy demands, making it several times more energy-intensive than well-ventilated public buildings like hospitals. When we consider both the commercial and domestic cannabis sectors, it becomes evident that indoor cannabis cultivation significantly contributes to greenhouse gas emissions and environmental issues. The release of CO_2 within the grow room itself is not the main concern; rather, it's the energy-intensive production and storage of CO_2-filled tanks, especially if the energy source is not green. Consequently, there's a pressing need for cost-effective, energy-efficient methods of CO_2 compression if CO_2 supplementation is to be used at all. The equation changes dramatically when the energy source is green, shifting the order of priorities to lighting, transportation, waste management, and CO_2 supplementation as the most significant factors.

Geography plays a crucial role in the challenge. Some regions require far more intensive environmental control due to extreme external temperatures. Even when cooling

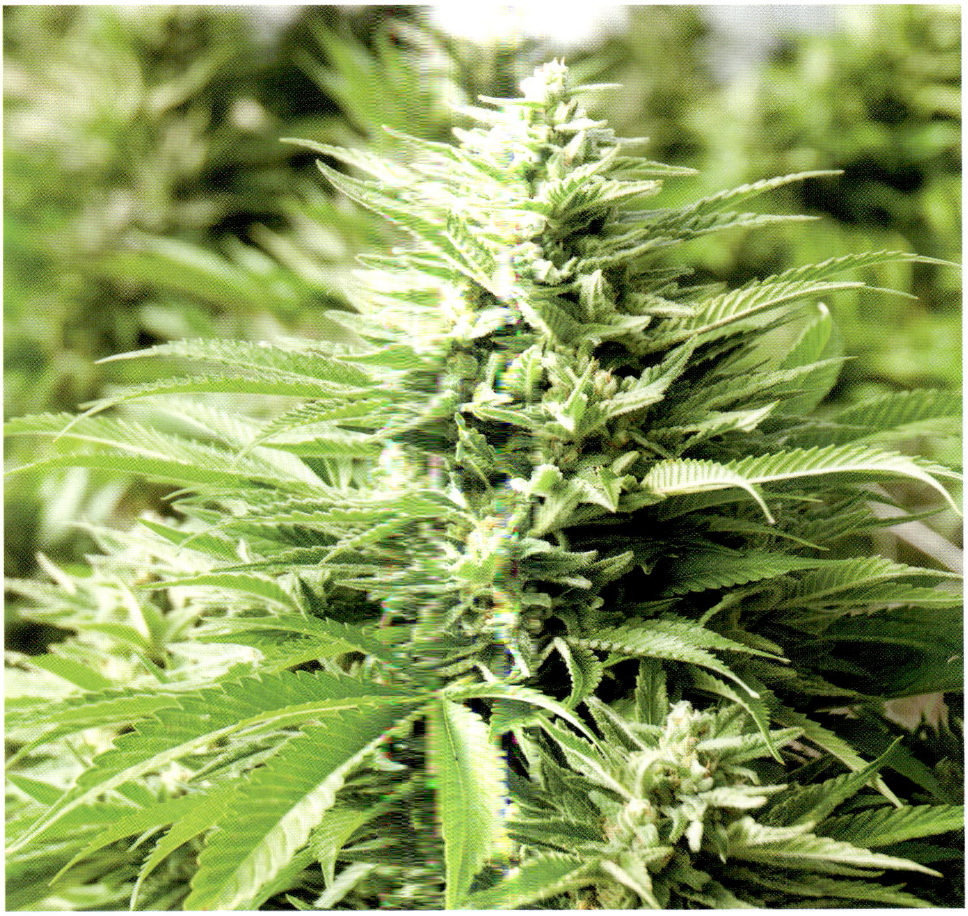

Healthy, lush, green leaves indicate this plant is growing super well.

PHOTO: STONED ROSIE

requirements are minimal, dehumidification alone can significantly contribute to greenhouse emissions. As a result, the adoption of high-efficiency climate control technology becomes imperative. Additionally, optimizing grow room designs is essential to minimize environmental impact.

Switching to energy-efficient LED from HID lights is a step in the right direction, reducing environmental impact, particularly when powered by green energy sources. Where possible, outdoor or greenhouse cultivation should be considered, as it substantially reduces the environmental footprint. It's crucial to advocate for local policies that promote green energy adoption and efficient technology in the cannabis industry. Your support for environmentally-friendly solutions through your votes and choices matters significantly. In the interim, explore options for accessing green energy upstream and take steps to reduce your carbon footprint in cannabis cultivation. Innovators can lead the way by driving positive change within the industry, setting an example for others to follow.

Blackberry: Seed to Harvest

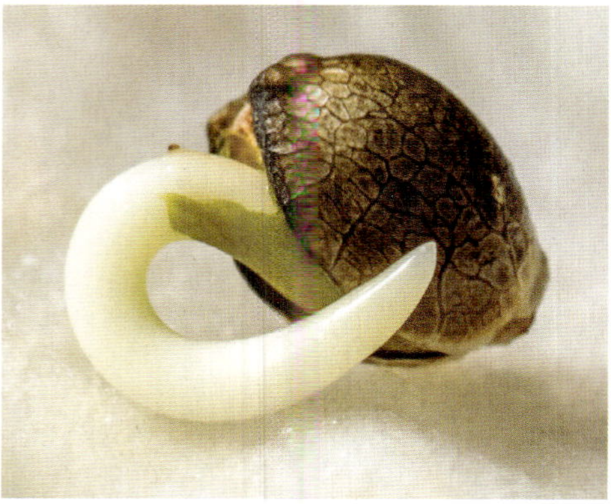

Water germination and towel germination are popular techniques with organics.

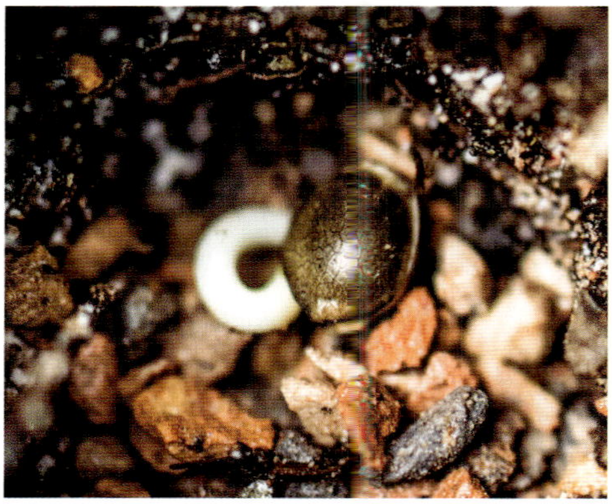

Transplanting seedlings to their new home.

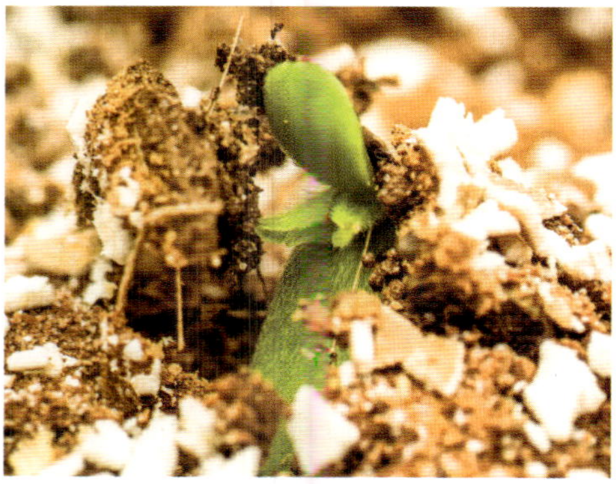

Organic surfaces must be brittle enough for seedlings to push through.

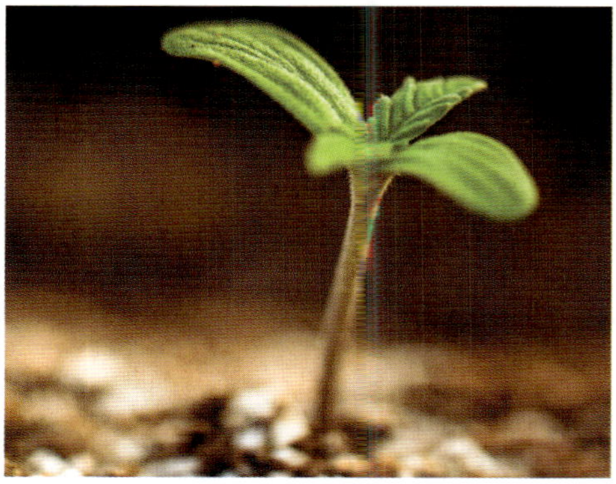

Organic mediums must be dense enough for seedlings to stay upright in.

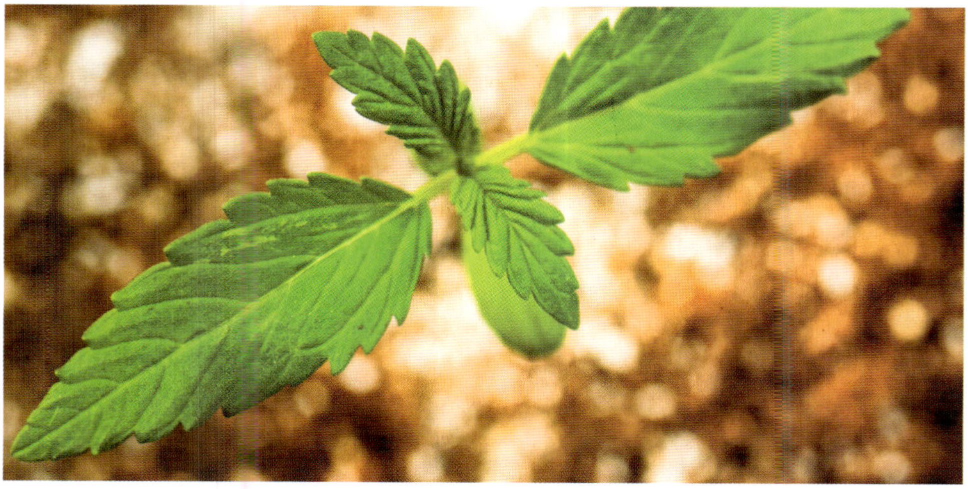

Blackberry strain shows her new healthy sprouts.

PHOTOS: ERIC PALMER

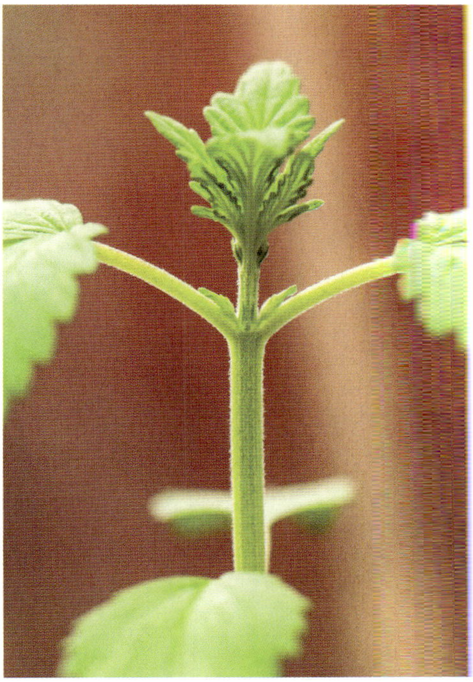

Continuous new healthy growth is what we want to see.

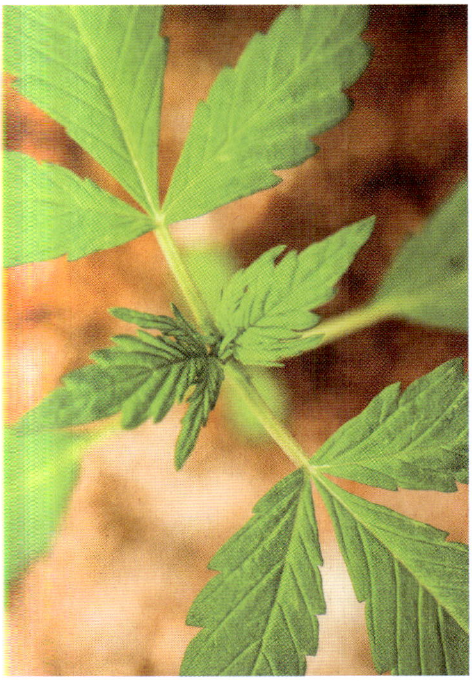

Leaves flat out, receiving light is a sign of good health.

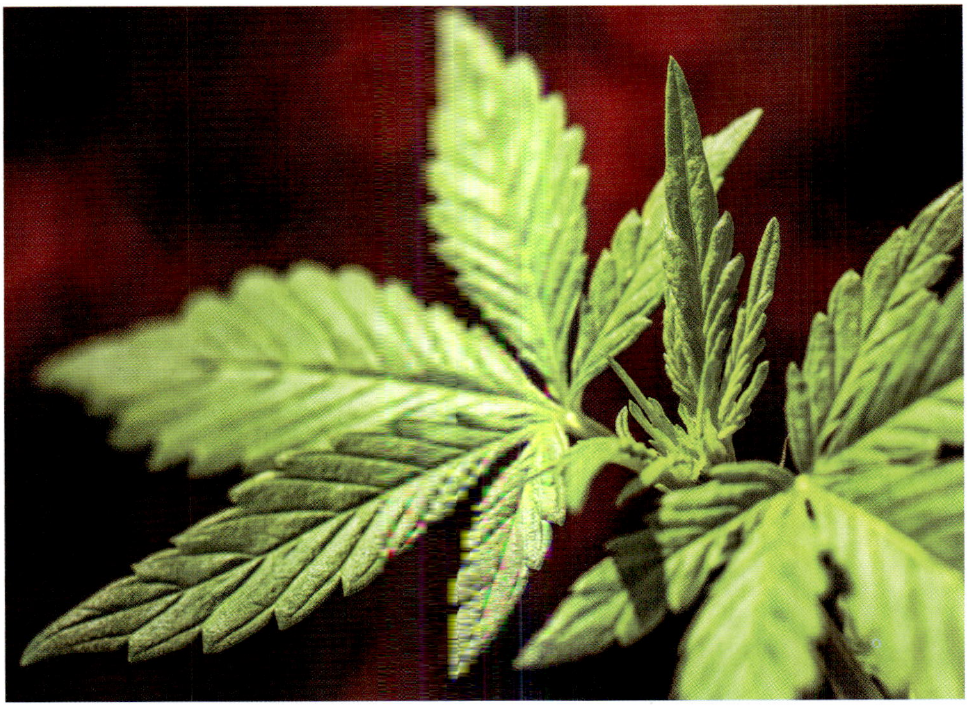

Typical cannabis leaf shape will emerge with time.

continues...

Blackberry: Seed to Harvest *continued*

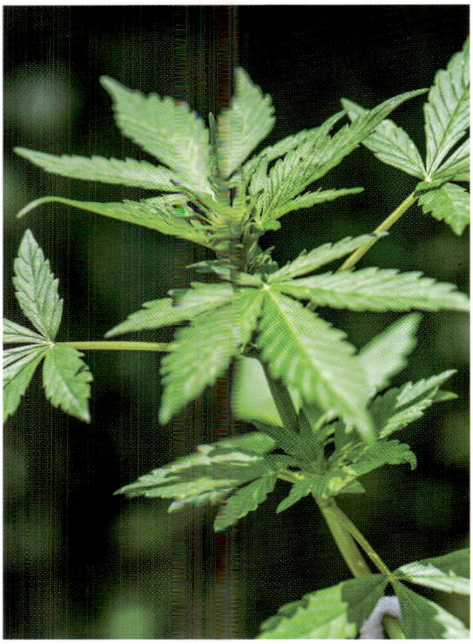

Vegetative growth consists mostly of seeing more of the typical cannabis leaf shape.

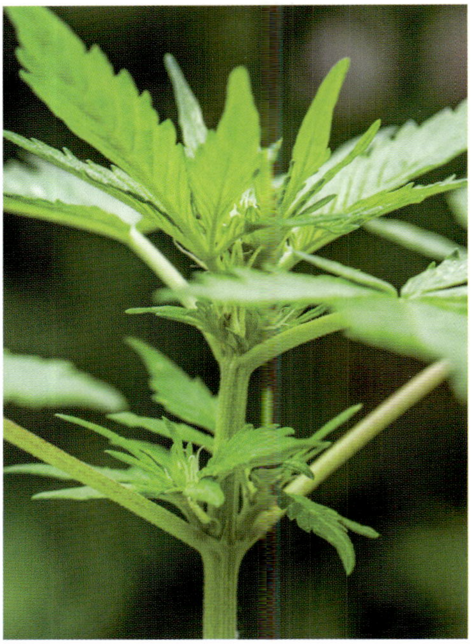

When side branches grow, you can expect pre-flowering to follow.

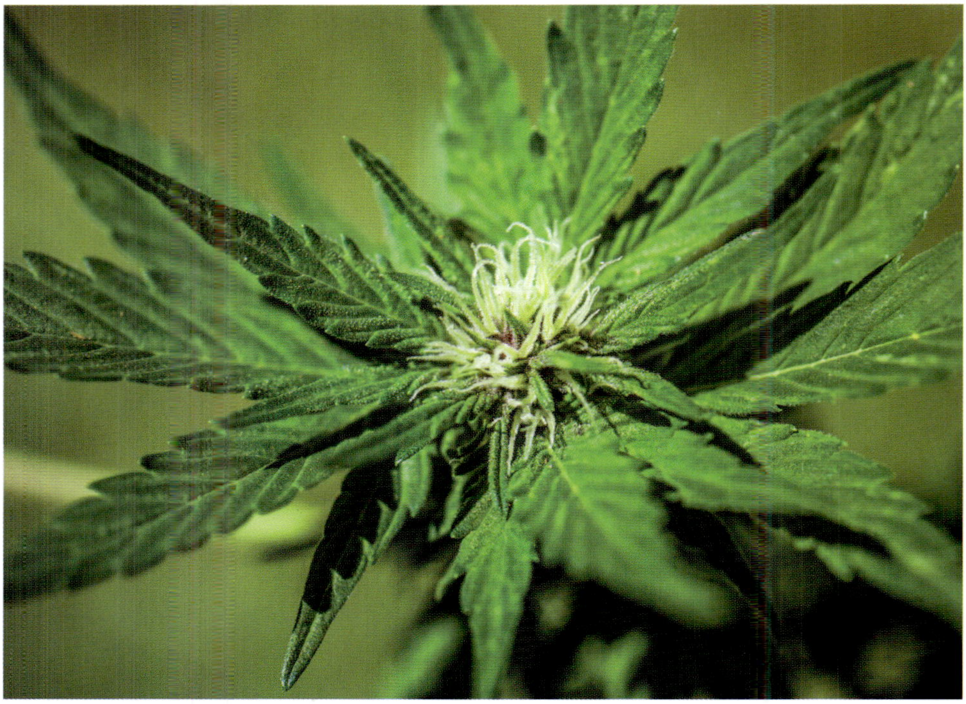

After pre-flowering the flowers are now evident and the plant is in the flowering stage.

PHOTOS: ERIC PALMER

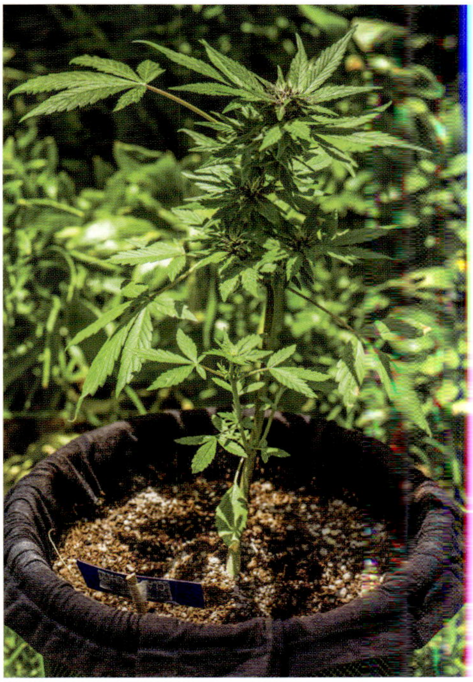

Spin pots with no netting to help tilt her back in the direction you want.

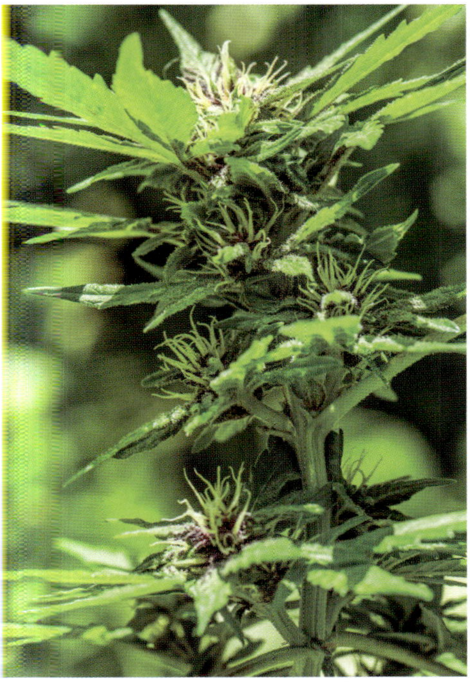

Flowers fill out the internode spacing as the plant bulks up.

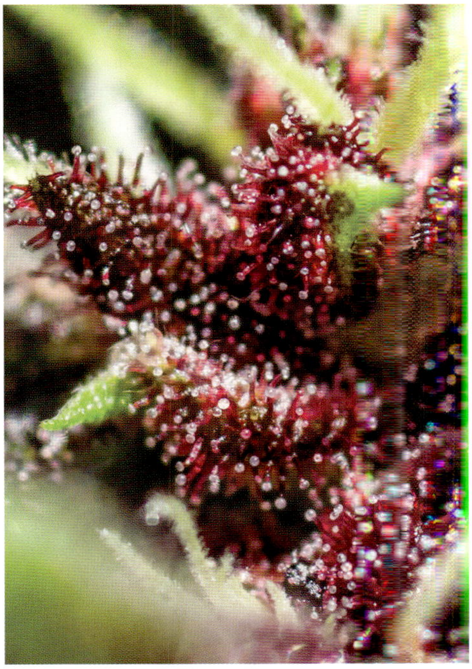

Blackberry gets its name from the deep dark color of its flowers.

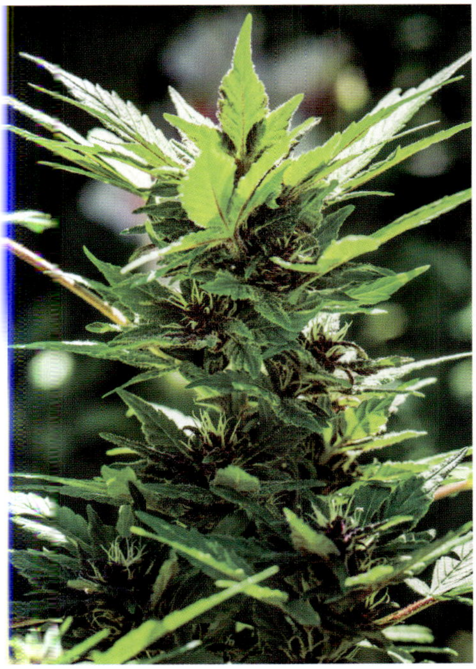

A connoisseur strain is not necessarily a big yielder but still has enough.

continues...

Blackberry: Seed to Harvest *continued*

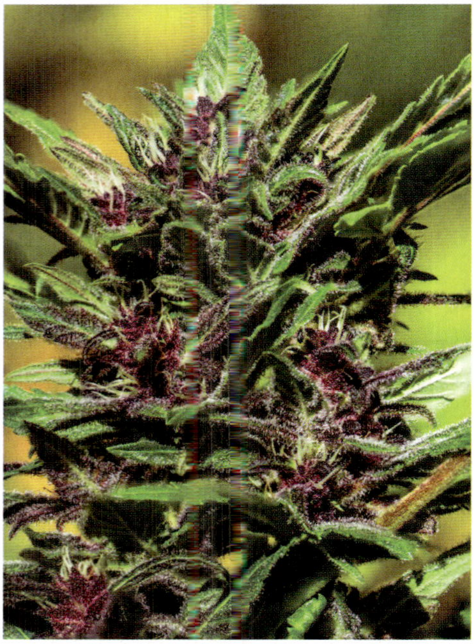

Strains like blackberry speak for themselves. You look at it in awe.

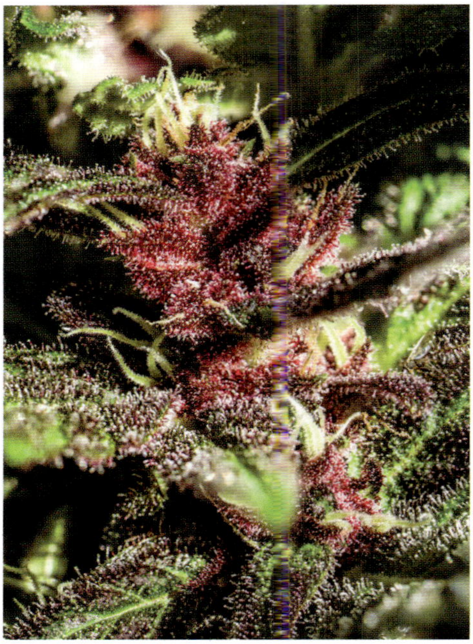

So good that you don't want to use it up.

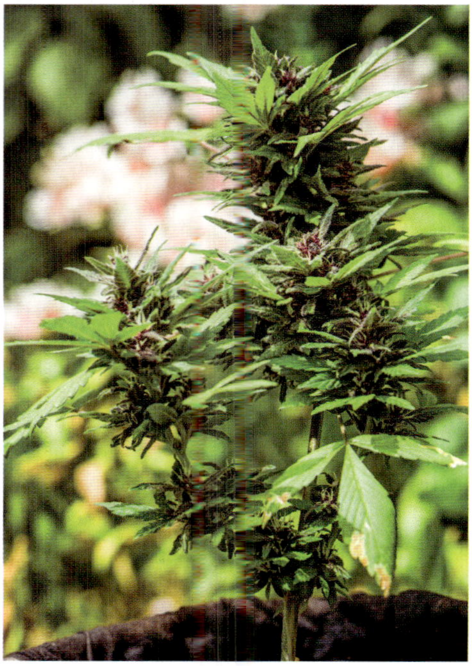

A squat low-yielder might be perfect for what some growers need.

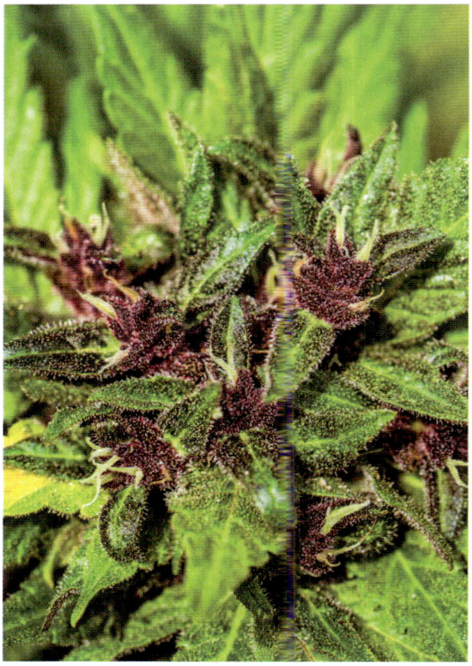

This is a show strain. With microphotography, you can produce stunning results.

PHOTOS: ERIC PALMER

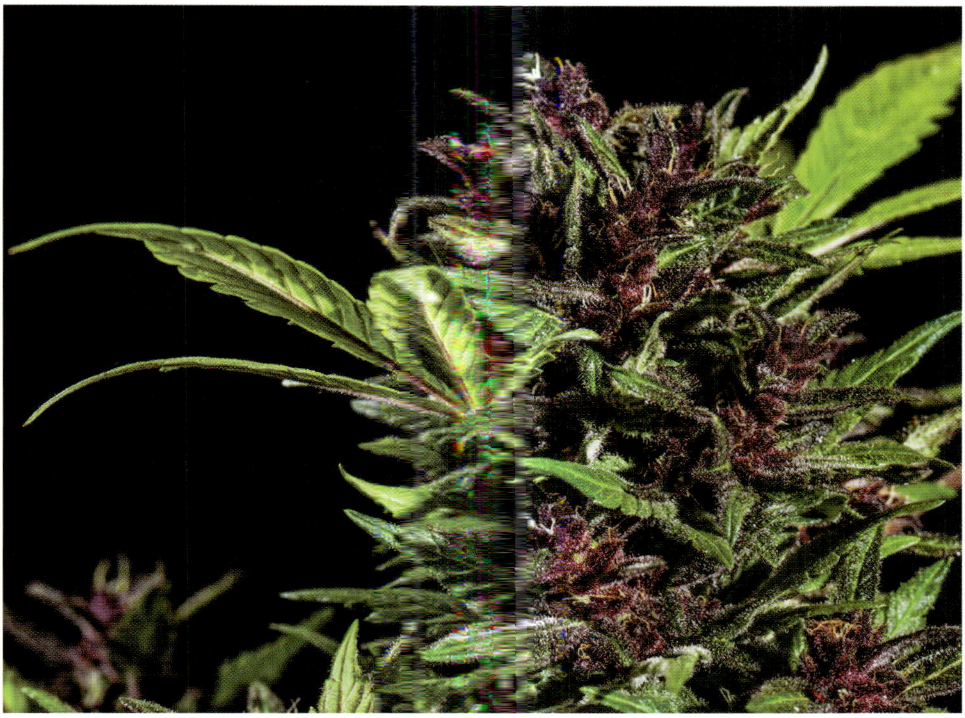

Again, the strain speaks volumes for itself. It looks fantastic.

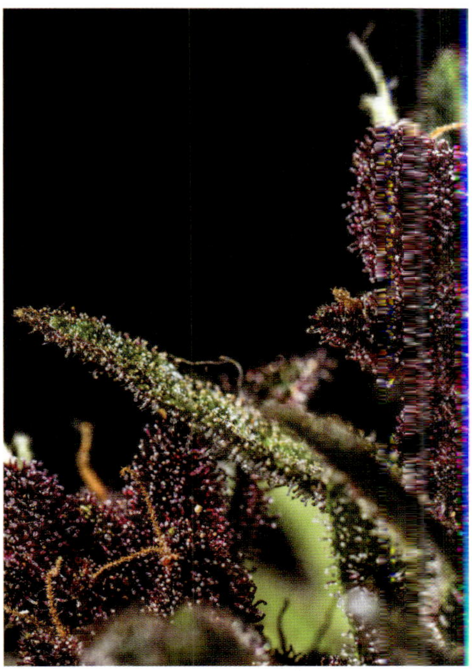

A closeup of the flowers is mind-blowing — how populated the black trichomes get.

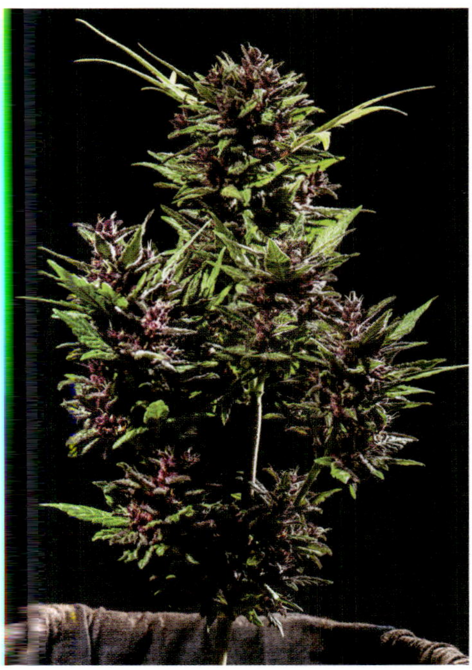

Low yield but big looks.

continues...

Blackberry: Seed to Harvest *continued*

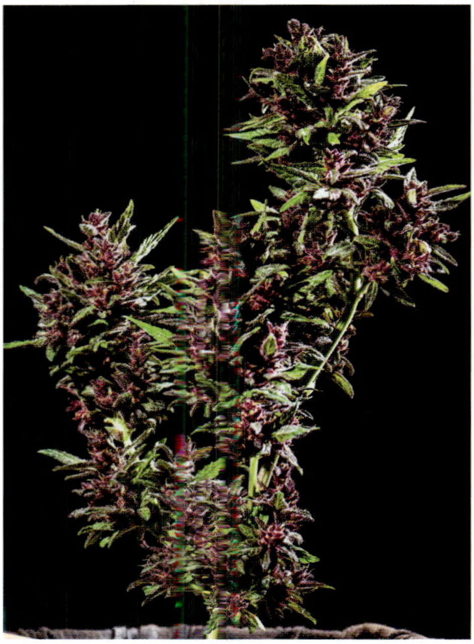

You can remove leaves for the photoshoot.

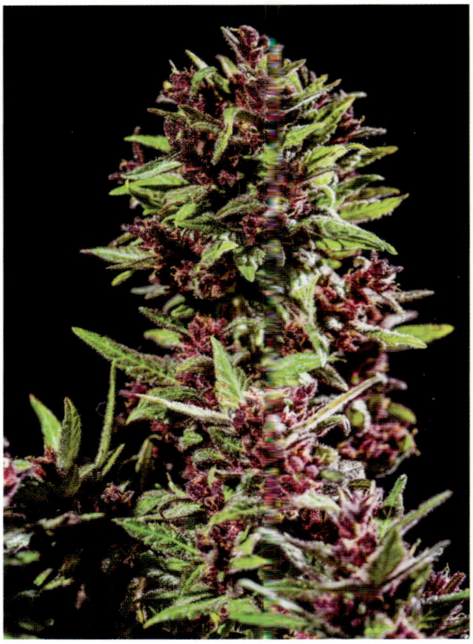

Blackberry stuns even the most seasoned of growers.

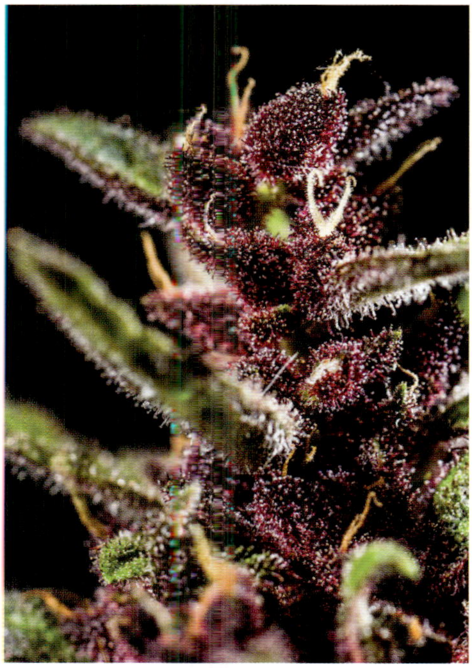

When your bud looks like this it just beats everything else.

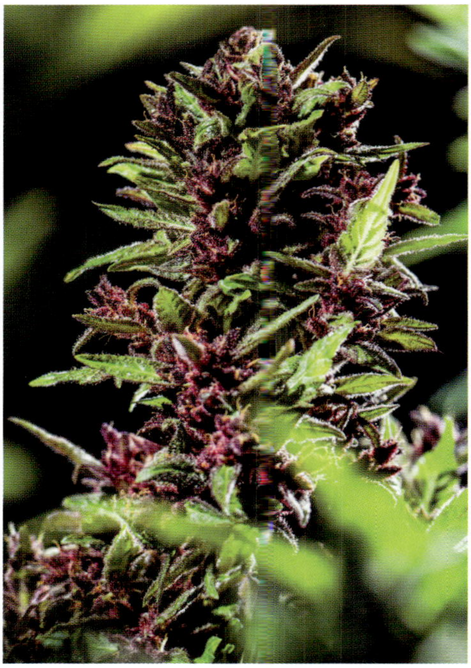

You will need to manicure this plant well when the time comes.

PHOTOS: ERIC PALMER

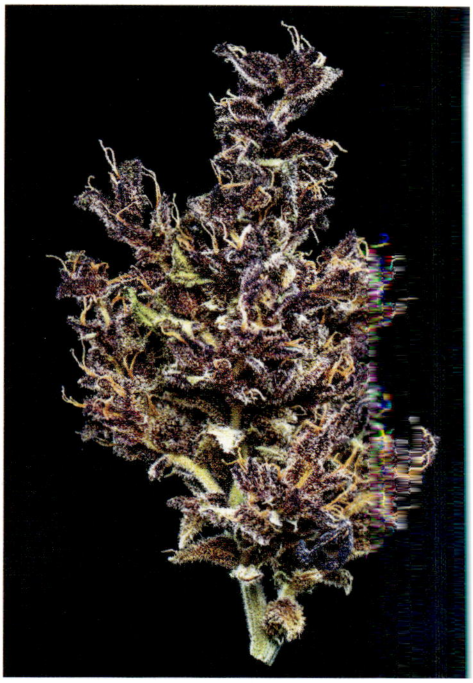

A well-manicured Blackberry bud is stunning to see.

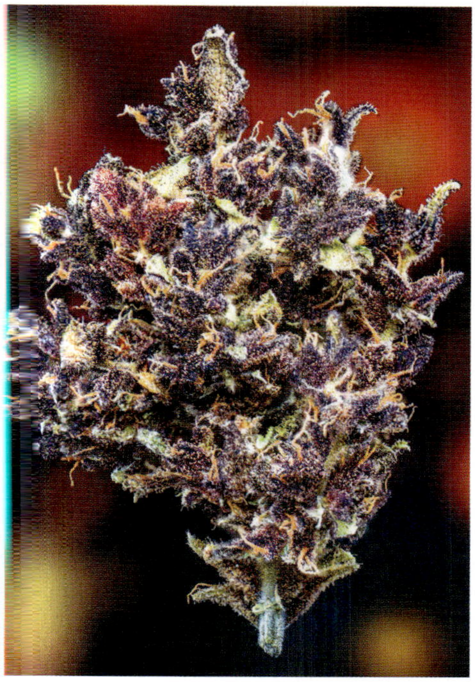

Enjoying the manicuring process is more fun with a pretty strain.

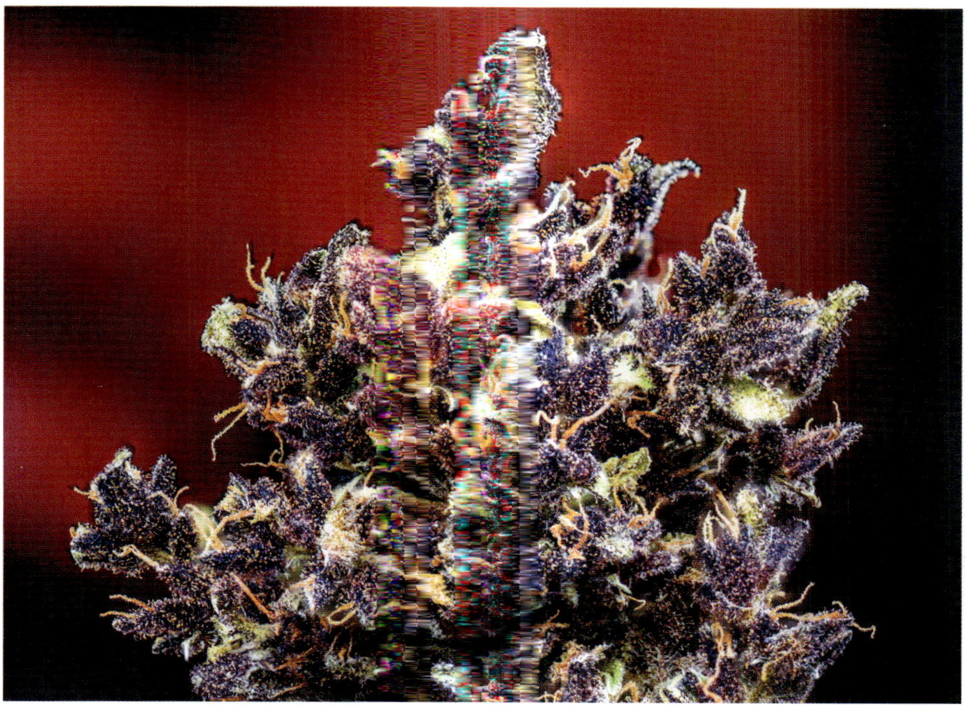

Like a load of blackbirds singing on a bush, Blackberry is a sure winner.

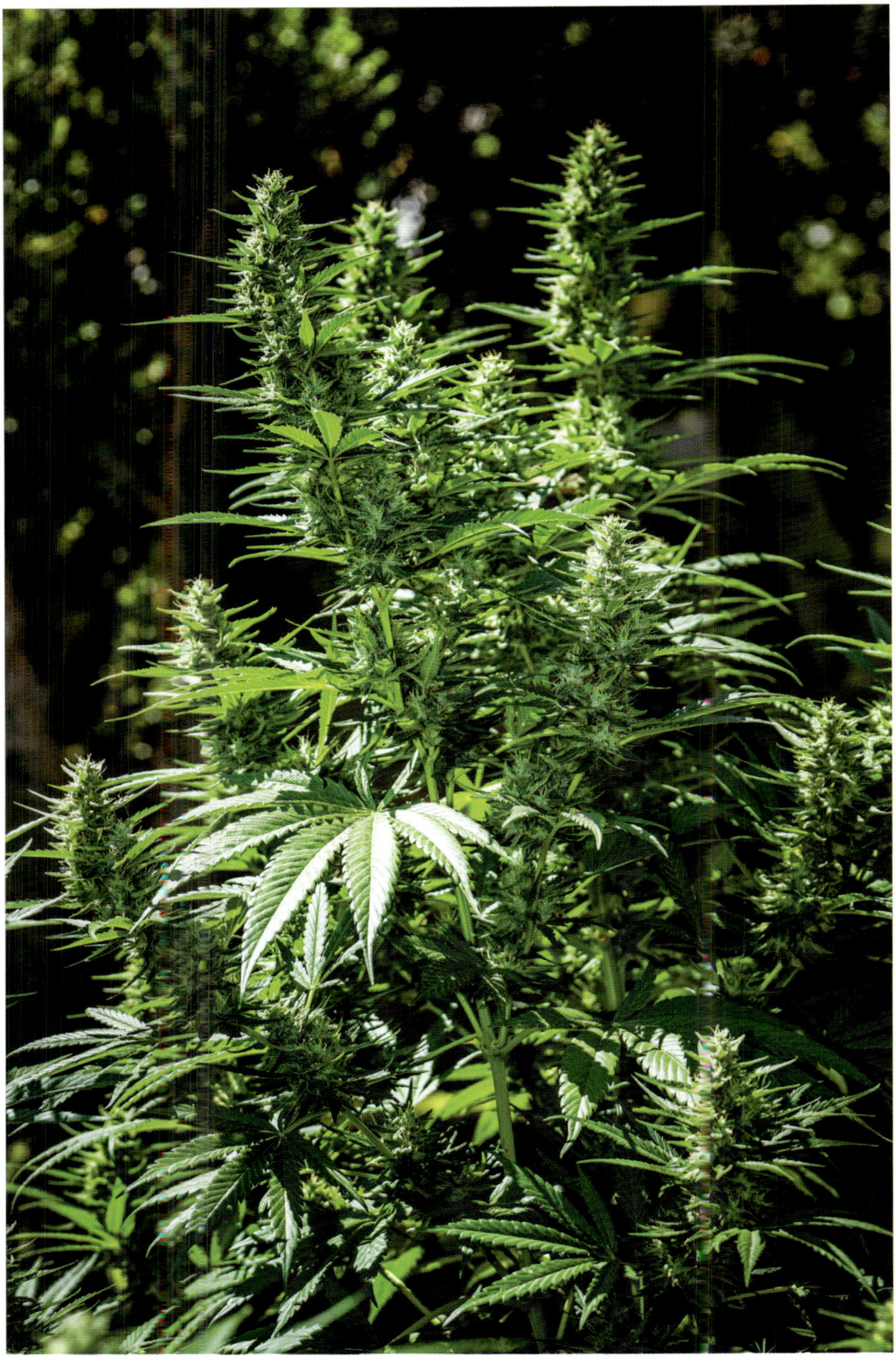

PHOTO: ERIC PALMER

Organic growing is all about organic practices and finding a method that works for your garden. It just takes some thought and planning.

Tips for Successful Organic Growing

Bid Farewell to Synthetics

Begin your organic journey by eliminating all synthetic products from your gardening arsenal. Make a commitment to never purchase them again.

Embrace Conservation

Adopt a sustainable mindset by conserving resources and reducing waste wherever possible. Organic gardening aligns with eco-conscious practices.

Monitor Your Organics

Keep a close eye on your organic materials and their condition. Regularly assess their quality to ensure they remain effective.

Dispose of Toxic Decomposition

Safely dispose of any organic matter that undergoes anaerobic decomposition, as it can potentially become toxic to your plants. Proper disposal is crucial for maintaining a healthy garden.

Take Proactive Garden Care

Take a proactive approach to garden maintenance; get ahead of potential issues before they happen. Regularly tend to your plants and soil, making necessary adjustments to optimize growth and health.

Enhance Your Soil

Consider excavating and replacing existing soil with high-quality organic materials to create a fertile foundation for your plants.

Maintain Adequate Moisture

Organic systems thrive when kept consistently moist. Ensure that your garden receives the appropriate level of hydration to support plant growth.

Control Weeds by Hand

Combat large weeds by hand-pulling them. This manual approach helps maintain a weed-free garden without resorting to synthetic herbicides.

Organize Storage

Store your organic materials separately and in a well-organized manner until you need to use them. This keeps your supplies fresh and readily available.

Sometimes, all it takes is a little more thought about what you are doing to spot the areas where you can make changes for a greener future. Treat your grow as you would the body's temple. Clean, organic cannabis is the way.

Hügelkultur: The Magic of Mounds
by Father Nature

Hügelkultur is a German word meaning "mound culture" or "hill culture". It's an old German and Eastern European regenerative practice of creating sloped mounds by combining wood, topsoil, compost, and organic amendments into the existing soil. Adding these amendments creates a nutrient-rich environment for your plants to thrive in, helping them reach their full potential. Hügelkultur aids in nutrient cycling, water retention, terpene production, and crop sustainability. The amazing thing about mound growing is that the mound provides whatever nutrients the plant requires. The plant tells the biome what is needed through a form of plant exudates, which are fluids such as resin, secreted by the plant. The relationship is symbiotic in nature, and a wonderful experience to be a part of.

There are many ways to construct these mounds. The photo above shows how we designed and built ours. First, the mounds are dug out. Then cured and rotten logs are introduced, along with fish compost and compost tea or EM-1. EM-1 is a microbial inoculant of essential beneficial microorganisms that helps colonize the indigenous microorganisms in your soil. It helps to reduce pathogens, promote nutrient cycling, and accelerate decomposition, improving soil and plant health. These additions aid in the breakdown of the carbon sources to make them more available.

It is important to prep the mounds in advance. We like to make them in the fall in preparation for the following season. If you make your mound in the spring and are planning on planting right away, we suggest charging your biochar. Biochar, which resembles honeycombs under a microscope, is a fantastic carbon source that gets

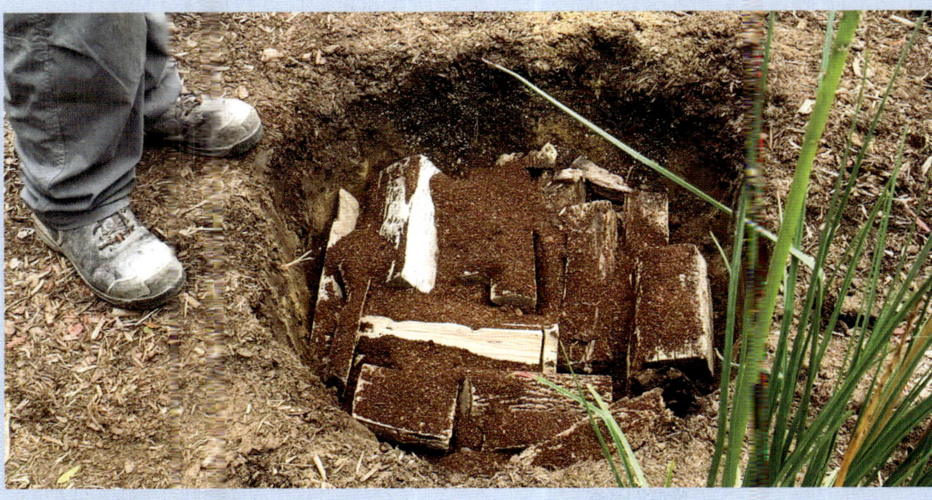

Your dug-out mound will be filled with rotten logs as a starting point.

PHOTOS: FATHER NATURE, ROBERT BUTTS

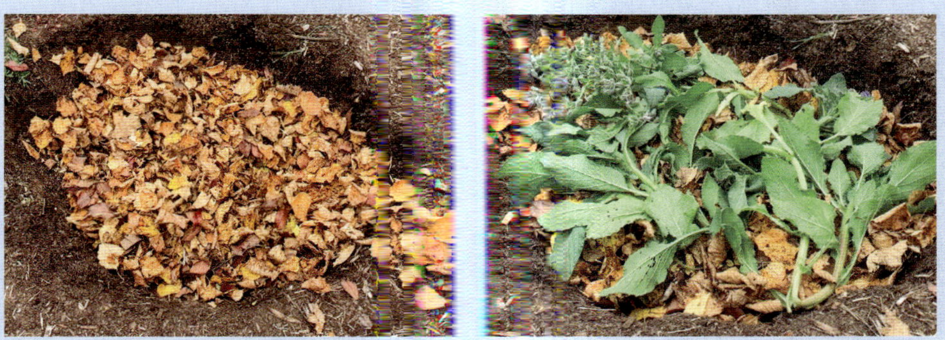

Leaves and greens diversify the microlife in your mound.

colonized by your indigenous microorganisms. Charging your biochar is super easy and can be done with humic acid, fish hydrolysate, EM-1, compost tea, urine, etc. When mixing the amendments into the soil, roughly 5–15% of the total amendments is biochar. We add another layer of compost on top of the mound as well as a layer of mulch. To keep the soil's micro life thriving, we also add EM-1 or compost tea. When constructing your mounds on a hill, create crescent shaped beds so they can collect the water that flows down the slope. With this type of setup, irrigation is usually not required.

The photos above show how we add leaves and greens to our mounds to diversify the microbiology and reduce pathogens. The plant we used here was borage, which has been fed with EM-1 ferment high in silica all season. These plants will deliver nutrients as well as biology to the mound. Compost teas can be used as well.

The soil that has been removed from the pits is combined with regenerative organic amendments. We can then add the mixed soil on top of the logs.

The amendments we used for this mix are:

- Wollastonite
- Huplaso basalt
- Oyster shell
- Flower
- Biochar
- Fish compost
- Earthworm castings
- Leaf compost
- Crab meal
- Alfalfa
- Poultry compost
- Pumice
- Frass
- Trichoderma harzianum
- Bokashi
- Kelp
- Gypsum
- Peat moss

There are many ways to construct these mounds. Instead of mixing all the amendments into the base soil, you can also layer them in the pit and cover it with the soil you dug out. When the wood is stacked into the pit and the mixed soil is added back on top, add organic amendments and compost to the top of the soil to keep the

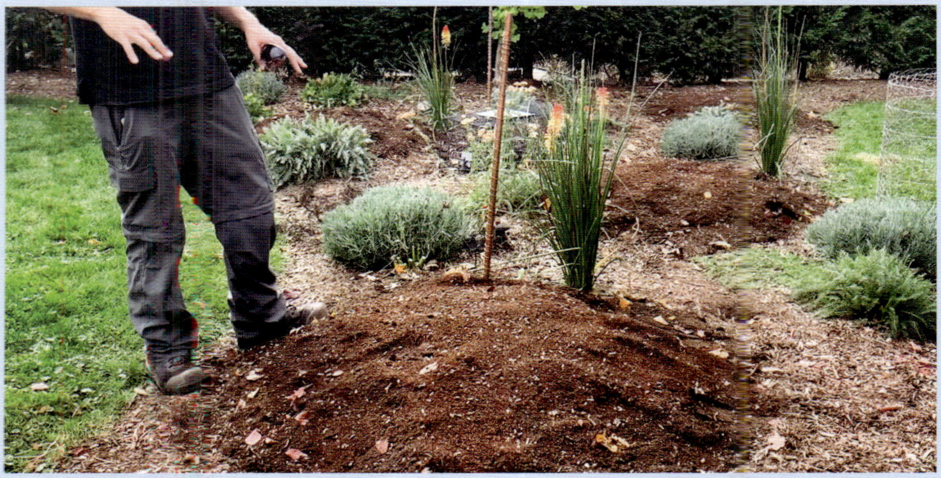

After it has been combined with amendments, the dug-out soil is added back into the pit, on top of the logs.

process evolving. In conjunction with adding compost and nutrient in the spring, add another layer before flowering. This layer should be a combination of earthworm castings, fish compost, bokashi, and organic nutrients.

The photo below shows a mound constructed with a layer of mulch on top. Under this layer is that magical compost top dress, mentioned previously. These mounds will be fed with EM-1 and compost teas all season long. We like to use fermented products when the soil is saturated and compost teas when the soil is a little drier.

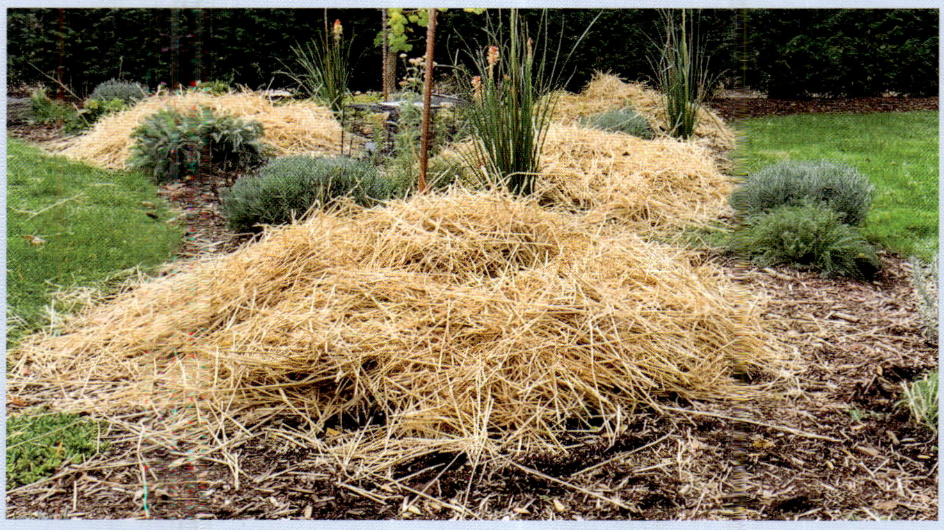

A layer of mulch has been added to the top of this mound.

PHOTOS: FATHER NATURE, ROBERT BUTTS

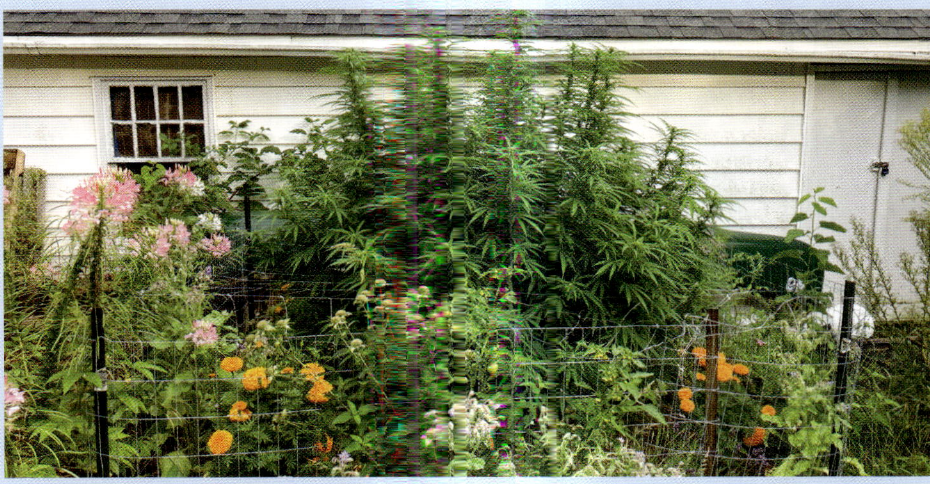

A Pinewarp growing in the rich microlife of a Hügel mound.

This typically means that we use ferments in the spring and fall and compost teas in late spring, early summer, and early fall. The ferments feed the anaerobes while the teas feed the aerobes. We want a good balance of both for this style of growing.

The photo above shows a Pinewarp star that is growing in a Hügel mound prepped three years ago. Each season, we add more compost to that mound to keep the soil fed at all times. Pinewarp varieties have the perfect genetics for this practice, as the plant was bred outside in British Columbia, Canada. This plant is structured to allow airflow. By pruning, we end up with top tier flowers.

These mounds will perform for many, many years. As they mature each season, the microbial properties will evolve and create a richer soil. The more colonies of microorganisms present in your soil, the better your final product will be.

Carbon is the primary food source of these cannabis plants as well as the microorganisms in the soil. This is why we use carbon-based amendments and foliar sprays. As the mound reduces, it makes many forms of nutrients and organic acids available that will play a pivotal role in the health of your garden. Hügel mounds also require less water, as the wood logs retain water.

Utilizing Hügelkutur growing mounds can help you grow in areas that are undesirable. This method is also customizable as the amendments can be adjusted to fit the soil that is used. When growing in mounds, you don't have to worry about things like nutrients leaching out into water sources, soil depletion, erosion or heavy irrigation. Mounds are an environmentally-friendly way to grow.

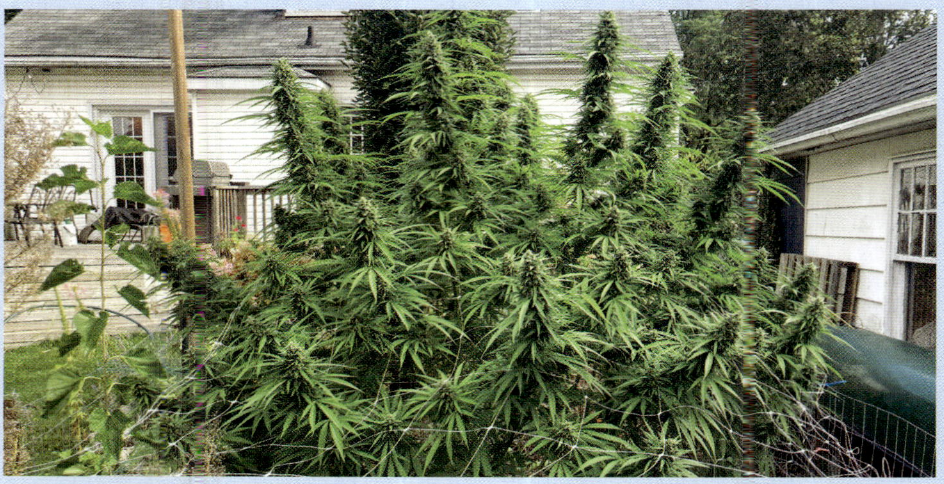

This method has this plant absolutely thriving.

While selecting your cannabis strain, work with an outdoor breeder to ensure that you have the best plant possible for the environment. A lot of indoor genetics are not suitable for outdoor growing unless they have been bred outside for many years. Indoor genetics are very susceptible to molds and insects. It's also best to buy organic seeds and plants grown in soil; if you are using a plant that has been on a hydroponic regimen its entire life, it may struggle in this type of environment. It's not impossible, but we want to select plants that are used to having a relationship with soil. Seeds grown organically in soil are full of microbiology, ready to grow in this environment! Do not use GMO seeds as they do not have the proper root structures to be able to communicate with the rhizosphere, meaning they will not be able to uptake nutrients in a reduced form efficiently.

When sourcing regenerative amendments, make sure that they are low in heavy metals. Not all organic products are suited for organic production. When sourcing our logs, we like to use hardwood species that are cured as well as rotten. We stay away from black walnut and black cherry, as these have toxins that will inhibit the process.

If you are making your own biochar, we recommend utilizing stocks and plant material from previous grows. Cannabis is very conductive and allows for a better caution exchange capacity (CEC) in the soil. The more conductivity, the better the nutrient uptake, nutrient cycling, and communication between the roots and the soil. Conductivity also aids in a decrease of fungal and insect pressure. There are many types of biochar available on the market. When making our biochar, we like to make sure the material is at a moisture level of 5–15%. Usually, leaving your branches for about three or four months will achieve this moisture level.

PHOTOS: FATHER NATURE, ROBERT BUTTS

Throughout the garden, we also like to plant specimens that have symbiotic relationships with cannabis. Many plants such as yarrow, lavender and chamomile will help with terpene production by the way of gas exchange. Both thyme and yarrow encourage the predation of beneficial insects. Marigolds are a cannabis plant's best friends, as they deter insects. The introduction of cover crops is also very beneficial to help build your soil and honor your microbial communities. While there are many options when picking out your cover crops, nitrogen-fixing plants are best.

Hügelkultur is the perfect practice to promote healthy plants with mouthwatering attributes and gorgeous colors. Mound growing truly honors the plant and helps it reach its full potential. Your flowers will have a long shelf life; I have some flowers in storage that are a few years old and still rockin'! Elevated terpene production is a direct result of the diverse biology feeding on all the carbon sources. There is a direct link between carbon and terpene production for all plants, not just cannabis. These mounds will be filled with colonies of beneficial bacteria and fungus, ready to make nutrients available to the plant. This is our favorite way to grow, hands down. Let's honor the plant, the soil, and the people!

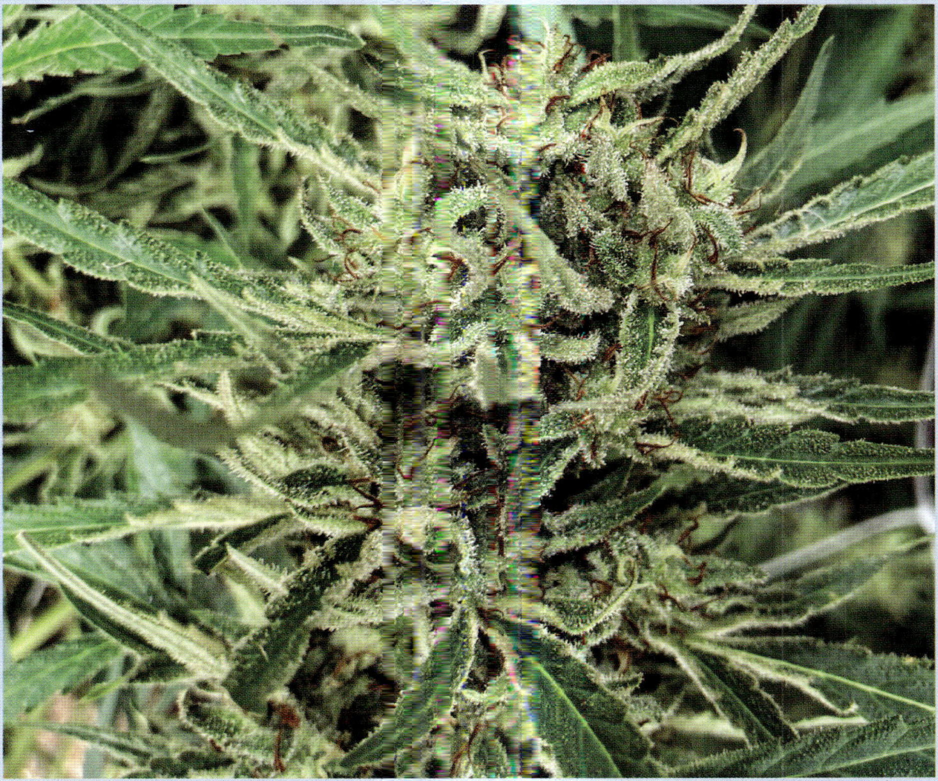

This method will lead to truly mouthwatering bud.

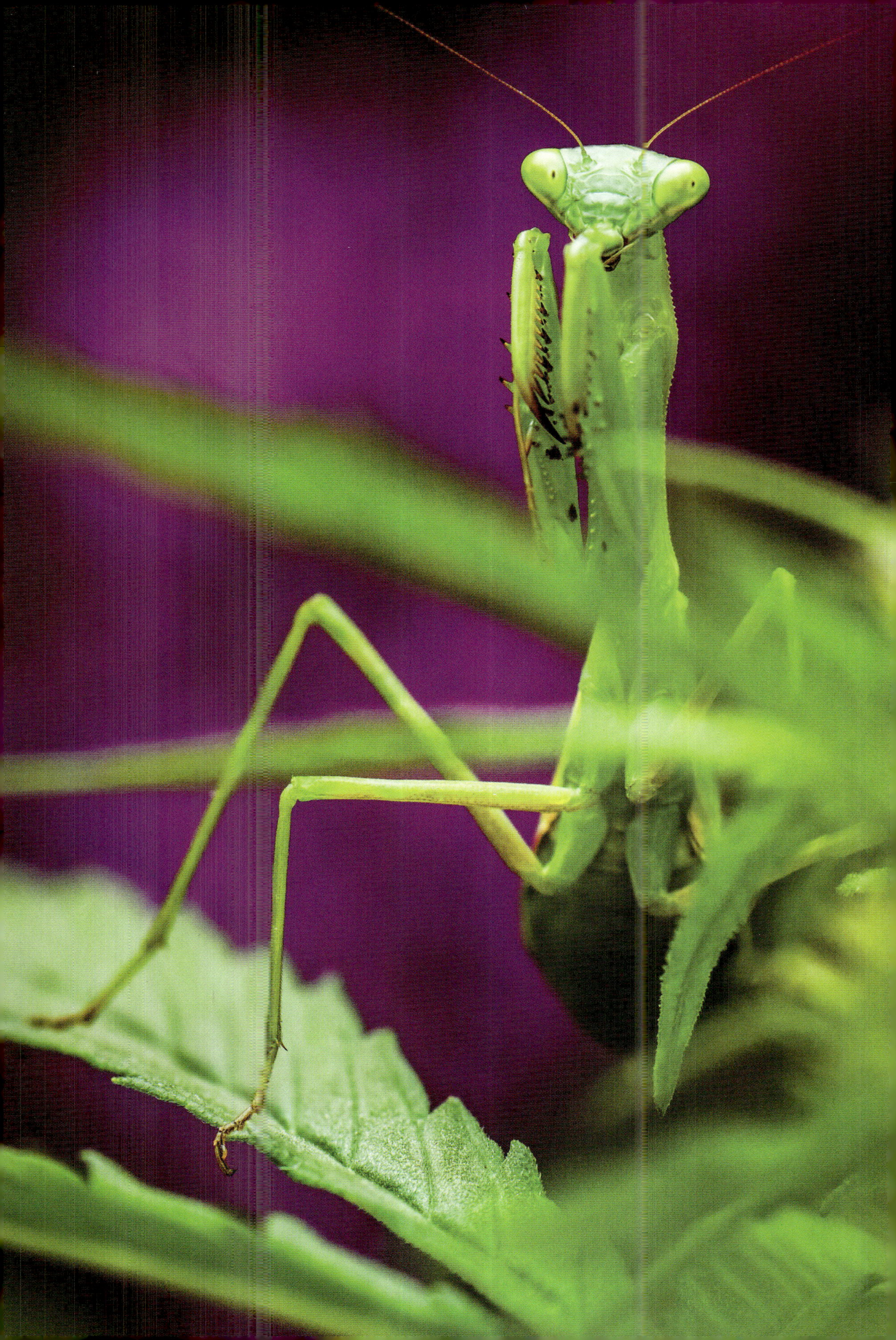

15

Problem Solver

In cannabis cultivation, problems will arise to challenge the quest for optimal results. These issues can range from minor inconveniences, such as pH imbalances, to complex battles against aggressive diseases. Some problems seem to arise randomly, driven by uncontrollable outdoor elements, while others are a direct consequence of our actions. We all encounter issues, whether it's accidentally scorching plants, allowing pH levels to drift too far, or facing unexpected nutrient mix problems. Mistakes are an inevitable part of the learning process for growers, regardless of their level of experience—and it is necessary for us to solve them. It is part of learning. If you were hiring someone to work alongside you in horticulture, you'd prefer an individual who has confronted numerous problems and successfully resolved them over someone lacking such experiences. Each problem you confront is an opportunity to learn and grow as a grower, and these challenges often come with stories to share.

One of the most significant challenges for growers is determining the right type and quantity of nutrients required by their plants. Following closely are issues related to pests, predators, and diseases. These are made more complex because many symptoms associated with nutrient imbalances, pest infestations, predators, and diseases appear quite similar. This chapter aims to provide a comprehensive overview of the problems you might encounter during your cultivation journey and how to identify and effectively address them.

Some experts argue that minor pest attacks can toughen plants. However, excessive stress caused by pest infestations may result in the appearance of hermaphrodite traits and impaired growth. Infestations can also weaken plants, making them more susceptible to pathogenic infections. Breeding strains with pest resistance is vital for outdoor growers, with some strains exhibiting better tolerance to specific local pests. Generally, natural environmental factors like wind should suffice to "harden" your plants.

Pests face more significant barriers in outdoor environments, contending with natural forces and predators. As a result, pest attacks tend to be more frequent and severe indoors, where pests can thrive in the clean and controlled environment. However, outdoor cultivation is not immune to pest issues, and they remain a common concern.

PHOTO: ERIC PALMER

Some pests, such as aphids, thrive in nitrogen-rich environments. Therefore, adjusting your nutrient regimen by reducing nitrogen levels can help combat aphid problems more effectively. This principle also applies to other pests that benefit from nutrient-rich conditions. To address a pest infestation, you may consider delaying your regular feeding schedule, prioritizing the pest issue over plant nutrition. It's essential to act promptly when dealing with pests to minimize any delays in feeding, as prolonged infestations can lead to longer feeding interruptions. Above all, avoid distributing infected plants to prevent the further spread of pests.

Domestic Pets

Pets can pose challenges to your cannabis cultivation efforts. In outdoor gardens, cats can serve as a remarkable defense system against many small predators, making them valuable allies. Yet an outdoor cat can inadvertently introduce unwanted pests into your indoor grow room.

It's essential to keep domestic pets away from your indoor grow room. Indoor pets, such as cats and dogs, have a natural inclination to interact with indoor plants, which can lead to some undesirable consequences. Cats, particularly kittens, may choose the base of cannabis plants as their personal litter box. Puppies and young dogs are prone to play with cannabis plants, often biting their stems.

How pets interact with indoor plants is similar to how they might interact with Christmas trees, especially concerning electricity and lighting. Prioritize your pet's safety over your cultivation efforts. To minimize any risks, always exercise caution when using pesticides and avoid leaving pellets on top of the soil.

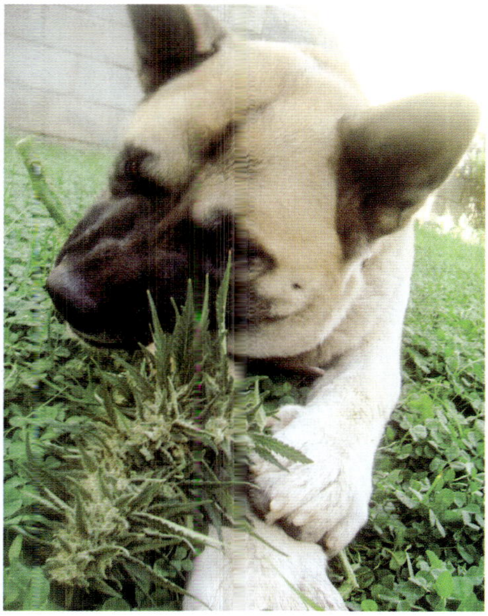

Dogs can dig up and chew plants.

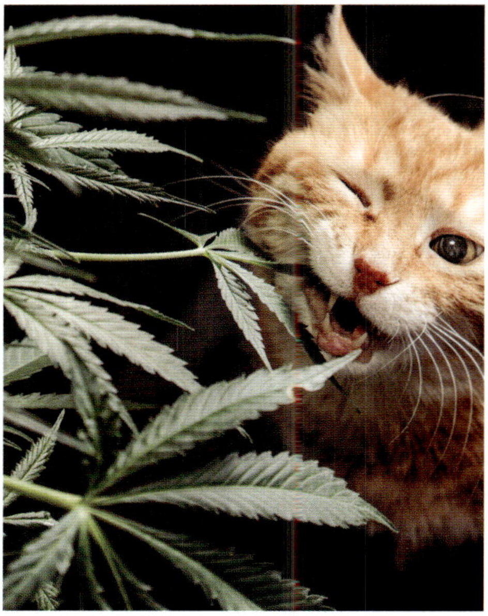

Cats can also topple plants or chew leaves.

PHOTOS: CAÑAMO, CHILE (LEFT), DEEP ROOTS/SHUTTERSTOCK.COM (RIGHT)

Preventing and Dealing with Issues

It is far better to be prepared for issues than having to chase them up. The difference between a problem that is solved and one that persists is often due to prevention techniques. The earlier you catch a problem, the easier it will be to solve. Sometimes, we can only slow down the problem to minimize its spread well before harvest time. There are many things you can consider preparing yourself for issues.

Row Covers and Shade Netting

Row covers and shade netting are transparent tents equipped with piping that can be shaped into tunnels and domes to protect plants from predatory pests, particularly flying ones like grasshoppers. These mesh coverings allow sunlight to penetrate and reach the plants beneath. However, these covers need to be adjusted to accommodate the growth of plants. For this reason, they are typically used during specific stages of growth, especially in the early phases. While they can be helpful, it's generally better to have a crop without these covers, as they block some light and maximizing photosynthesis is crucial. This is one reason why greenhouses are highly favored by outdoor growers.

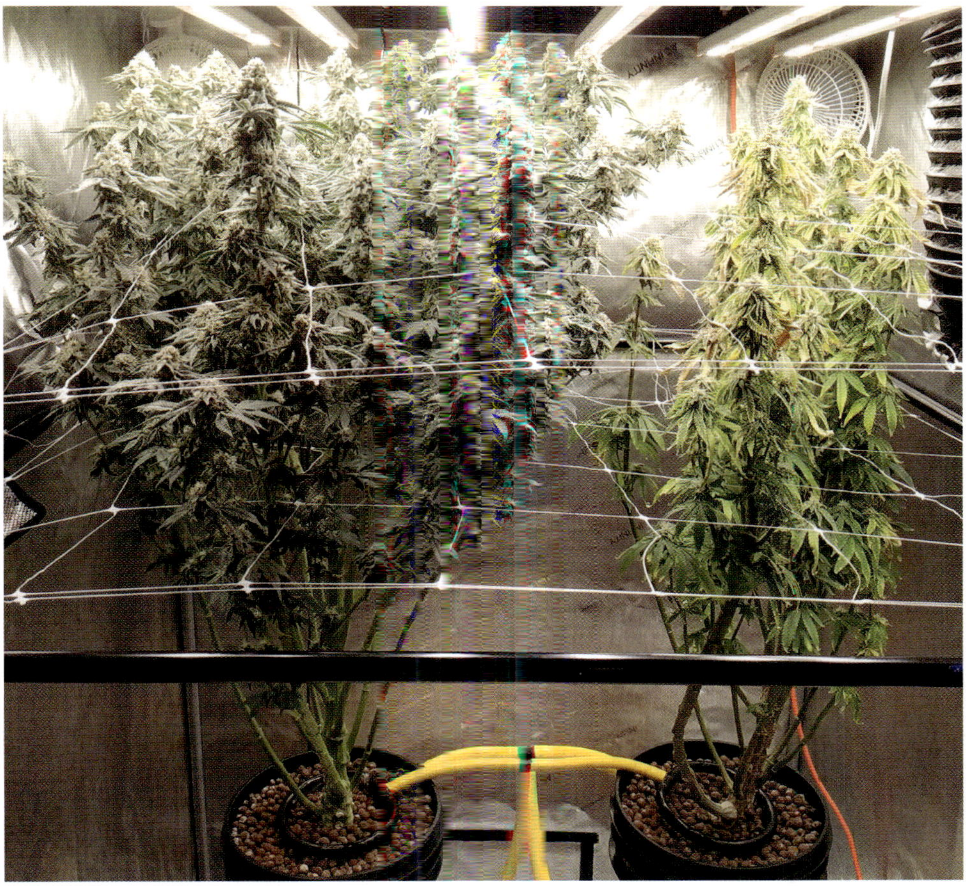

The plant on the left is healthy but the one on the right doesn't seem to be doing so well.

PHOTO: @TREETRUNK422

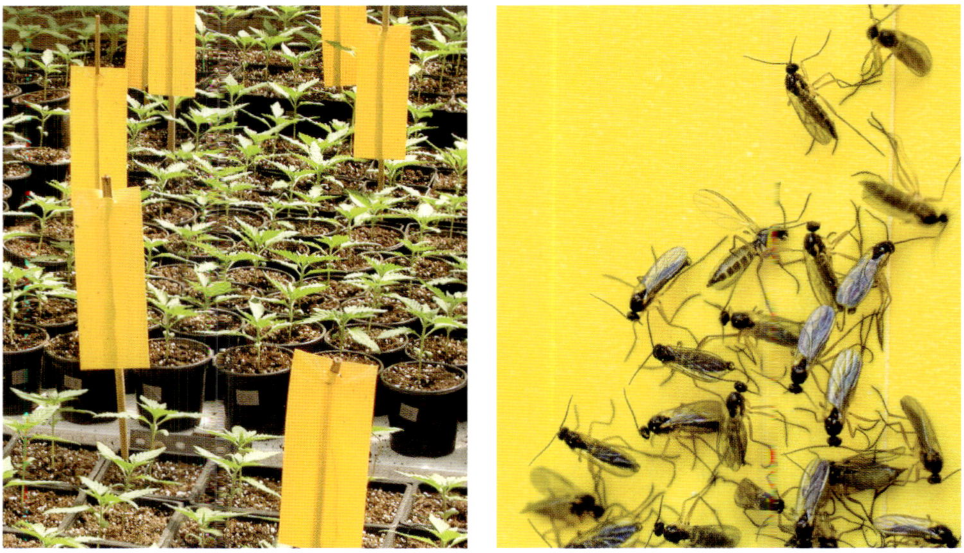

Gnats and other insects can be captured on sticky traps.

PHOTOS: MANDALA SEEDS (LEFT), JULIEK2/SHUTTERSTOCK.COM (RIGHT)

Yellow Insect Tape

Yellow insect tape can be useful for reducing insect populations, but it's not a solution for infestations. Yellow tape does not discriminate between harmful, neutral, and beneficial "pests." For instance, it may trap beneficial ladybirds/lady beetles as readily as harmful gnats. Moreover, yellow tape primarily captures flying insects. Although tape can be part of your pest management strategy, in most cases, additional measures will be necessary to address pest problems.

Water Blasting

Water blasting is a technique used to dislodge insects from plants during the vegetative growth stage. It can be effective in sending some pests on their way or reducing their numbers to more manageable levels for subsequent treatments. Targeted misting with a spray bottle can have a similar effect, serving as a form of "hand-picking" for pest control. Alternative approaches are often more effective for achieving a permanent solution to pest issues rather than merely making them temporarily disappear.

Tool Cleaning and Segregation

If you intend to use one set of tools indoors and outdoors, ensure rigorous and routine cleaning to prevent the accidental introduction of fungi or pests into your indoor space. Clumps of dirt can harbor microscopic larvae and spores, which can develop into fungi. Dirty outdoor tools can inadvertently transport entire ecosystems into your indoor room. Footwear can also be a vector for carrying outdoor contaminants indoors. The cleaner you keep your tools and surroundings, the better your chances of avoiding pest and fungal issues.

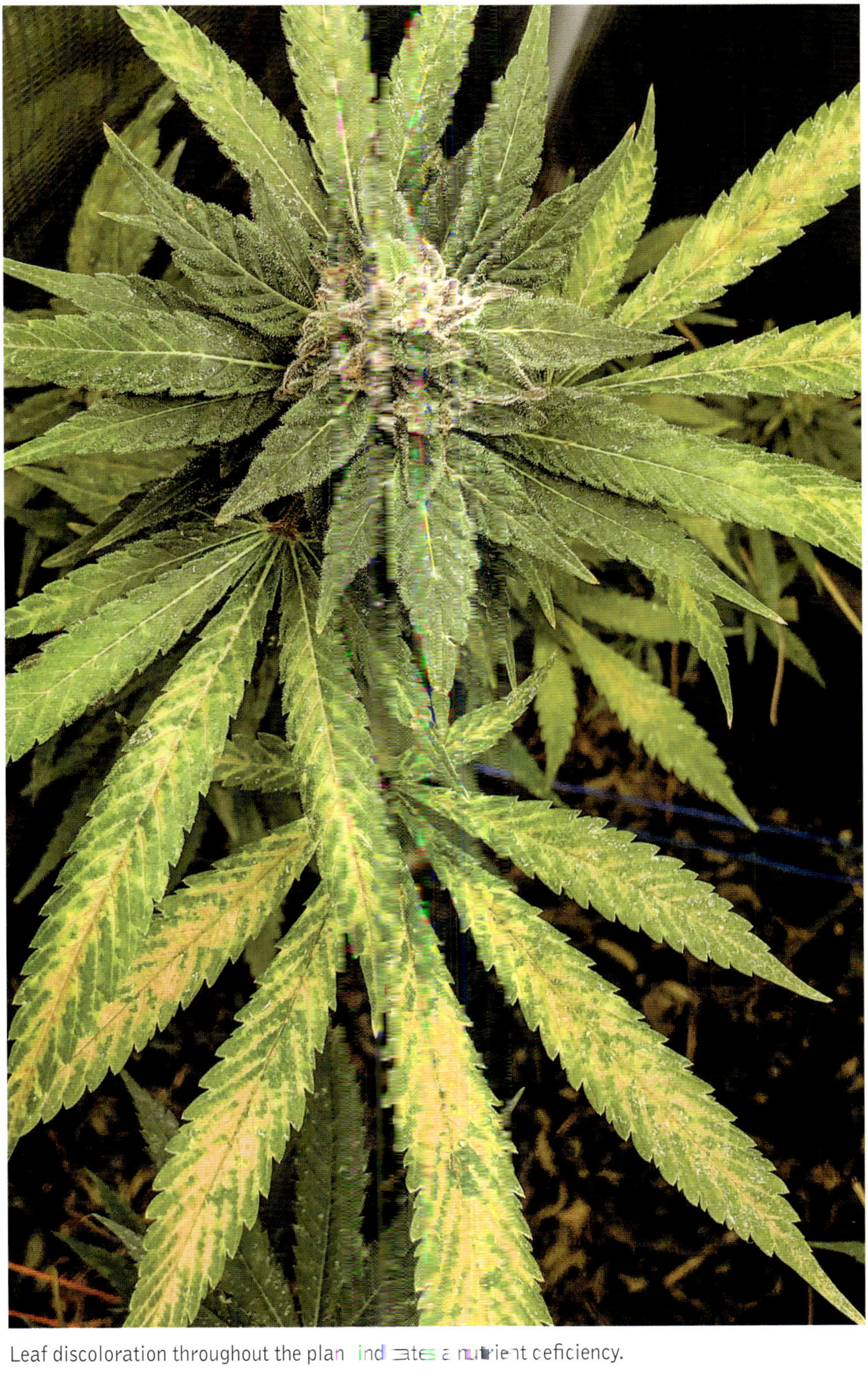

PHOTO: NATHAN GUILLARD

Leaf discoloration throughout the plant indicates a nutrient ceficiency.

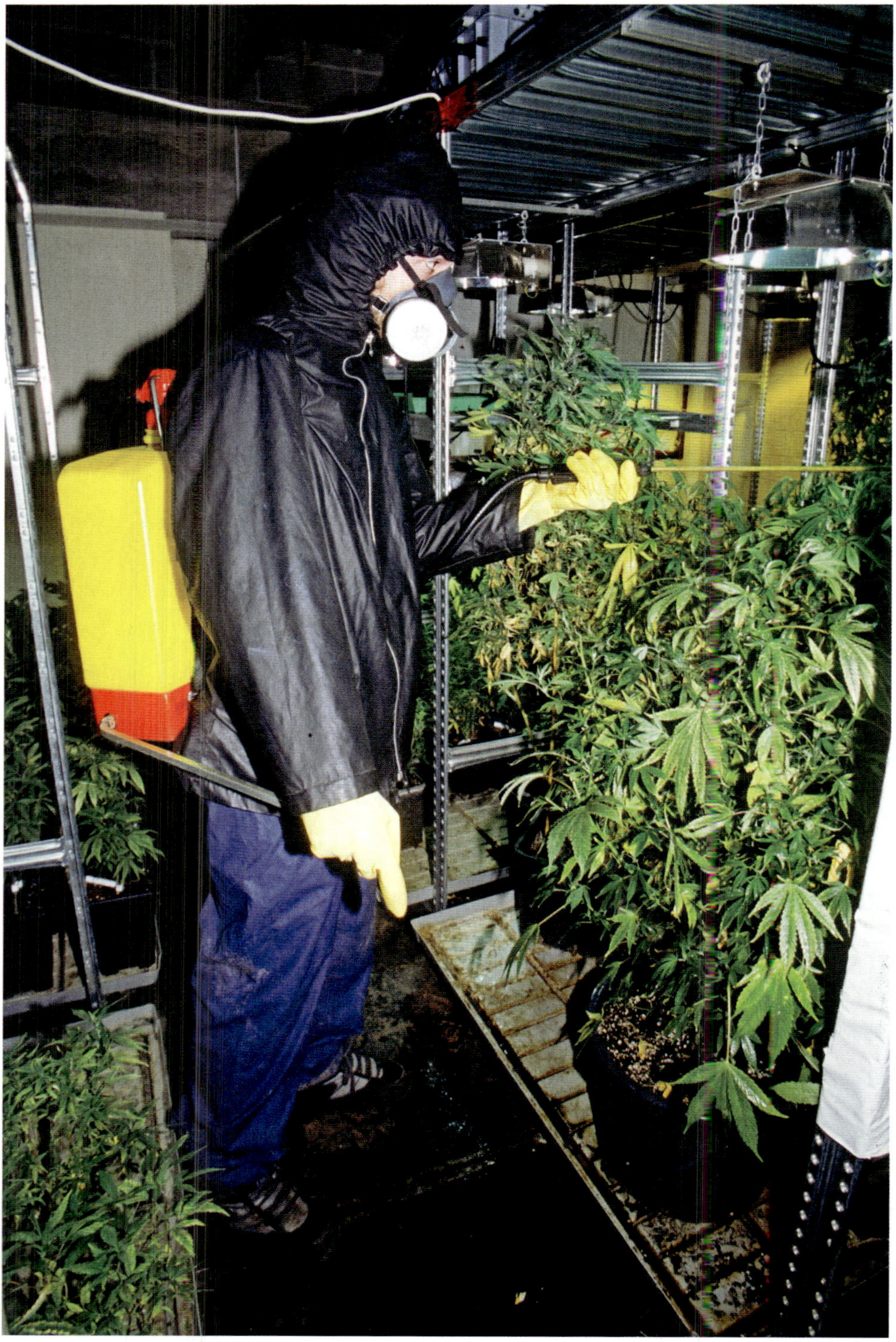

PHOTO: ANDRE GROSSMAN

Resorting to stronger measures to combat a bad pest infestation should only be done in the vegetative growth stage.

Pesticides, Insecticides, Herbicides, and Fungicides

The proper use of pesticides, insecticides, herbicides, and fungicides is of paramount importance in cannabis cultivation. These substances are specifically designed to combat various threats that can undermine the health and growth of your plants.

Pesticides and Insecticides

These are formulated to eliminate or repel pests that might infest your cannabis plants, including a range of insects, mites, and other small creatures that can cause significant harm. It's essential to choose the right pesticide or insecticide and, for new growers, choosing the recommended products in this book is a safer approach. Beware of new or experimental products that may not be suitable for cannabis cultivation.

Herbicides

Herbicides serve a different purpose. Their main function is to control and eradicate unwanted weeds and plants that can compete with your cannabis for resources. However, be cautious when using herbicides, as you risk unintentionally harming your cannabis plants. Instead of using general herbicides, consult updated lists of herbicides suitable for cannabis cultivation, often recommended by agriculture programs.

Fungicides

Fungicides are specifically designed to combat fungi, including molds and mildews, which can pose a significant threat to cannabis crops. Addressing fungi problems is crucial, and new growers can benefit from detailed solutions provided below.

Important Guidelines

Pay close attention to recommendations when working with these substances.

Only Use Repellents and Pesticides for "Food Product Use"

Choose repellents and pesticides that are explicitly marked "Food product use" on their labels. Steer clear of products labeled "Not for food products" or similar. If a pesticide or repellent is not certified as safe for food products, it should not be used on your cannabis plants. If it is designated as safe for food products, you can rest assured that it can be safely used on your cannabis buds.

Read and Follow Product Instructions

Carefully read and follow the product instructions provided with any pesticide, insecticide, herbicide, or fungicide you intend to use. Do not take shortcuts or deviate from the recommended application methods. Adhering to these instructions is essential for both your safety and the health of your plants.

Consider Organic Options

In many cases, pesticides and repellents that are safe for food product use are also organic or derived from natural sources. Choosing organic solutions can be a wise and environmentally-friendly approach.

By adhering to these guidelines and considering the specific needs of your cannabis plants, you can effectively manage and mitigate various threats while maintaining a healthy and thriving crop. This is especially important for novice growers looking to ensure the success of their cultivation efforts.

Pesticides

Pesticides are essential tools for combating various pests that can threaten your cannabis crop. They come in different formats, each designed for specific applications and pests. Understanding the types of pesticides can help you make informed choices when addressing pest-related issues in your grow.

Pellet-type pesticides, typically available in boxes or tubs, contain small pellets around 0.08–0.4 inches (2–10 mm) long. They are used primarily to combat such pests as slugs, snails, and larvae, which consume the pellets and die.

Sprays are available in liquid form or as fine powders that need to be mixed with water before application. Some come with nozzles attached to the bottle, allowing for their direct use without additional mixing. Others require dilution with water before application. These sprays can be effective against a wide range of pests.

Powder pesticides are not designed for spraying directly onto the plant but are added to the medium around the plant's base. They are effective against low-level pests like slugs and snails, creating a barrier to protect your cannabis plants.

Gas pesticides, or pest bombs, are used to fumigate indoor spaces to eliminate pests. They are typically used for clearing areas with pest infestations. Once the pests are eradicated, the room can be cleared of any dead pests.

Microbial-based insecticides are newer, environmentally-friendly pest-control options. They use beneficial microorganisms to combat pests, providing a natural and sustainable solution.

Some active ingredients common in pesticides are acetic acid, *Bacillus thuringiensis*, *Beauveria bassiana*, canola oil, pyrethrins, caprylic acid, capric acid, garlic oils, geraniol, chitosan, *Chromobacterium subtsugae*, cinnamon oil, clove oil, thyme oil, soybean oil, citric acid, *Isaria fumosorosea*, mineral oils, *piperonyl butoxide*, and potassium salts of fatty acids. These ingredients offer various ways to address pests effectively in your grow. It's essential to explore the available treatments to determine which products are suitable for your specific needs.

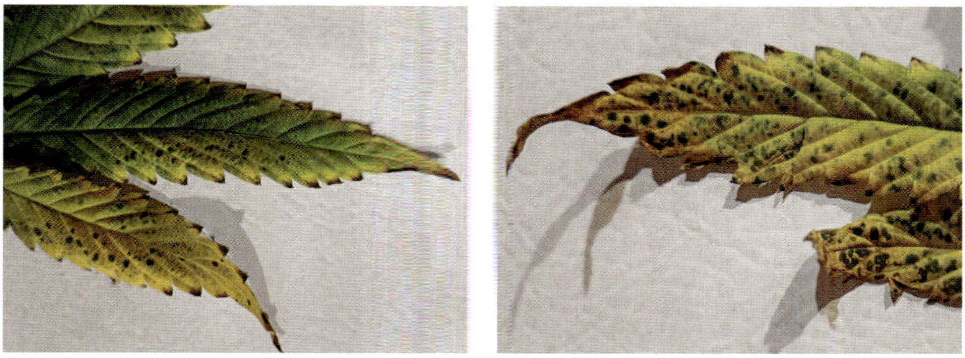

Disorders that look like nutrient deficiencies can sometimes be due to a pest problem instead.

PHOTOS: @TREETRUNK422

Why Cannabis Resin and Soapy Pesticides Don't Mix

Pesticides that are soapy in nature are typically intended for use during the vegetative growth stage of your cannabis plants. Applying a soapy pesticide to a flowering female plant is not advisable for several reasons:

- Soapy pesticides, when applied in large amounts, can inadvertently remove some of the trichomes from the plant, primarily due to the method of application.
- Soaps add water weight to the plant, causing stems and branches to bend. This added weight can slow photosynthesis, negatively impacting growth.
- Soapy residues on leaves and stems can disrupt photosynthesis until the plant dries, further stunting growth.
- The exposure to indoor lights before the plant dries can lead to undesirable chemical reactions and potential burning of the plant.

To avoid these issues, it's crucial to address pest problems during the vegetative stage of your cannabis plants, long before buds and resin production begins. While soapy pesticides may become a last resort, they often come at the cost of reduced yields and quality.

Repeat Targeted Application

In some cases, pesticide manufacturers may recommend repeat applications to effectively combat pests. These can be targeted, which means you treat specific areas of your plants rather than applying the pesticide to the entire crop. This approach offers the advantage of enabling you to use different treatment compounds on different areas of your plants, providing a way to experiment with potential solutions.

Where the pest problem is severe, you might need to combine multiple methods in a single area. However, it's essential to do this sequentially, because the reaction of different compounds, when applied simultaneously, can be unpredictable. This sequential approach also allows you to assess the effectiveness of each method individually and ensure that your pest problem is effectively addressed.

Pest Index

A multitude of pests can adversely affect cannabis, ranging from minor nuisances to severe threats. While our pest index is not exhaustive, it highlights common culprits responsible for most cannabis-related pest problems. It's highly likely that the issue you're facing is covered in this chapter.

Identifying pest attacks can be tricky because their symptoms can mimic those caused by other factors, such as nutrient imbalances, overwatering, underwatering, overfeeding, pH fluctuations, or heat stress. Additionally, not all pests leave visible bite marks. Many of them feed by sucking on plant leaves, flowers, branches, and stems, penetrating the plants with sharp mouthparts to extract plant sap. In some cases, this feeding leads to changes in the plant's leaves or curling, changes also associated with nutrient disorders or overfeeding. Inspect your plants for signs of pests routinely.

Differentiating between a pest attack and non-pest-related plant issues primarily hinges on the presence of the pests themselves. Pest damage varies widely, making it unreliable as a sole indicator of infestation. To confirm the presence of pests, you must actively seek and identify them before implementing eradication measures. A magnifying aid, like a high-quality camera on your phone, is a handy tool for pest identification, often providing better magnification than a traditional magnifying glass.

Familiarizing yourself with the signs of infestations can help you rapidly identify pests in your cannabis grow. Reading through the following descriptions can help you address a wide range of problems, as many treatment approaches are similar for different pests.

In indoor growing environments, responding swiftly to pests is crucial, as they don't face the same natural predators found outdoors. Not all insects are harmful to your garden; some actually prey on the pests you don't want. We'll also introduce you to these "beneficial" insects, so you can recognize and encourage their presence.

For large commercial operations, professional pest scouting and data gathering play a vital role in monitoring field crops, preparing for potential pest threats, and implementing appropriate management strategies. Pest scouts survey areas, gather information on weather conditions and farming history, and engage with experts. They use various methods, including sweep netting and technology, to collect potential pests for identification and control, managing pest issues on an industrial scale.

Honeydew

If you see raindrops or dew-like secretions on your plant leaves, that may be honeydew, the sugary secretion left by insects. Partially "stained" leaves, a result of honeydew, may lead you to suspect nutrient disorders or other issues. The presence of honeydew can make plants more vulnerable to mold fungi. Even if you can identify the fungi, it may take time to recognize honeydew as the issue's cause. Typically, honeydew becomes apparent first, followed thereafter by pest problems and mold. In most cases, identifying pests can be challenging without a magnifying aid. When pests multiply and congregate, they become easier to spot. Honeydew plays a significant role in insect colonies' mutualistic and symbiotic relationships, attracting pests like ants.

Ants

Ants, in the Formicidae family of insects, are known for their cooperative and industrious nature. They can quickly damage cannabis plants by nesting in the substrate, interfering with roots, and consuming leaves. Ants are often associated with bite marks on the edges of leaves and are known to farm aphids, another type of pest. Getting rid of ants can be achieved by various methods, including the use of cinnamon powder, neem oil, boric acid, vinegar, or organic colony-killing pesticides for food plants. In addition, incorporating diatomaceous earth into the soil can create unfavorable conditions for ants. Ants typically continue to use the same point of entry, which once identified, should be treated with pesticides or oils to prevent further intrusion. When dealing with garden colonies, eliminate the ant source and treat the entry points. As always, exercise caution when using pesticides around pets.

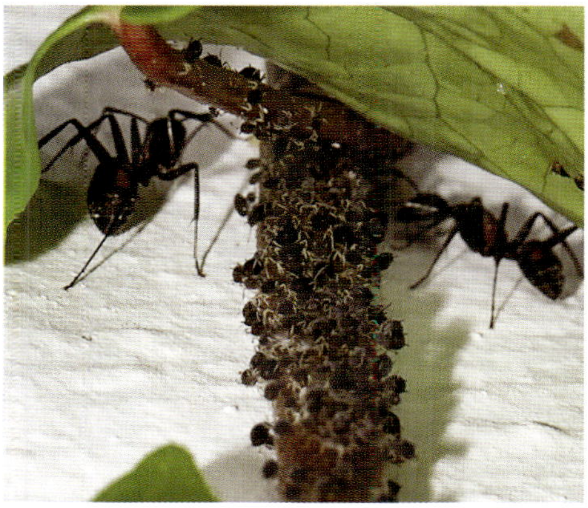
The symbiotic relationship between ants and aphids is a double problem for the grower.

PHOTO: MANDALA SEEDS

Aphids

Aphids, soft-bodied insects in the family Aphididae, are among the most common pests encountered by cannabis growers, both indoors and outdoors. These tiny insects feed primarily on plant juices, extracting sap from the plant's stems, branches, and leaves. Aphids are about 0.12 inches (3 mm) long and come in various colors, with yellow and green being the most prevalent. Some aphids have wings.

Aphids produce a frothy or foamy waste material, honeydew, which is often visible around their feeding areas on the plant. These pests tend to target new growth or the undersides of leaves near the node regions, but they can be found anywhere on the plant. Aphids are frequently accompanied by their offspring, and they reproduce at an incredibly rapid rate, primarily through asexual reproduction, resulting in an all-female population. Some aphids transmit diseases, making their swift elimination a top priority.

Identifying aphids can be challenging since they are tiny and move relatively slowly. For a thorough inspection of your crops, use a magnifying aid. Aphid infestations

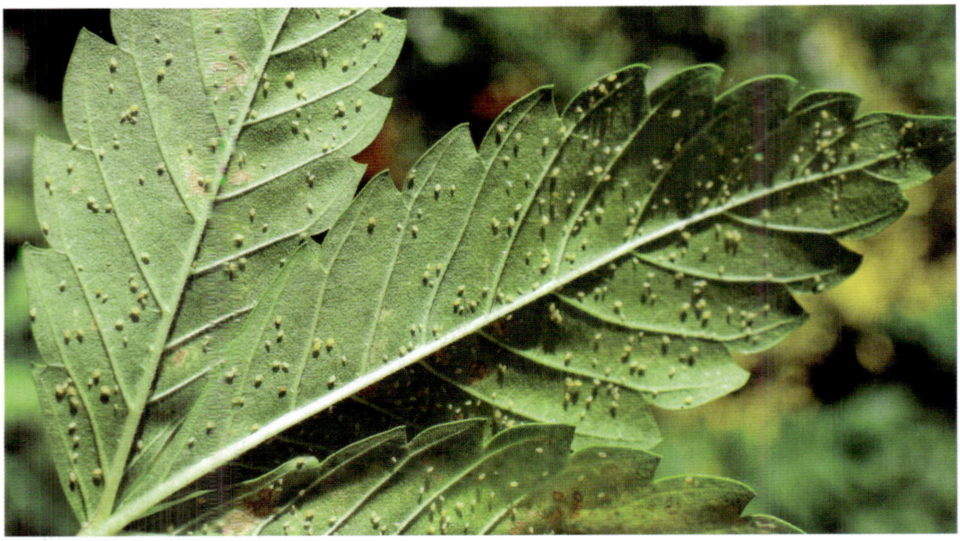

The underside of a leaf can reveal hidden pests feeding on the plant.

can resemble the symptoms of underwatering, leading to leaf wilt. During an aphid attack, you may also observe signs of plant stunting and leaf curl.

Ants collect the honeydew that aphids excrete. Therefore, it's crucial to address any ant infestations before treating an aphid problem.

You can effectively remove aphids from your cultivation space by using a pyrethrum-based insecticide. However, spraying your plants with pyrethrum-based insecticides, especially before the flowering stage, may cause some stress to them and even hinder their growth.

To prevent future aphid issues in an infested room or tent, consider spraying the interior with a pyrethrum-based insecticide. Ensure you cover corners and frames, then allow the area to air out, following any instructions before reintroducing plants into the environment.

For mild aphid problems, focus on spraying only the infected areas of the plant. When aphids affect flowering plants, it can be problematic, as spraying can damage the buds and separate trichome glands from the cannabis flowers. Therefore, try to address aphid problems before the flowering stage. If you've taken preventive measures against aphids before flowering, the chances of an infestation should be minimal, unless aphid-contaminated items are introduced into the grow room.

In addition to pyrethrum-based insecticides, soapy pesticides like Safer's Soap can act as a deterrent to aphids. You can create a solution by mixing dishwashing detergent

PHOTO: PONG PONG/SHUTTERSTOCK.COM

with hot water, which effectively cleans the grow room and pots while suffocating the unwanted aphids. You can also use essential oils such as rosemary, eucalyptus, and peppermint in homemade pesticide solutions to combat aphids. Additionally, introducing ladybugs, natural predators of aphids, into your cultivation space can serve as a biological control method.

Trying to solve infestations on flowering plants is salvaging and far from a regular grow, let alone an optimal grow. Professional growers avoid salvaging because it is better to solve the problem so future grows are cleaner and can be optimized. Do not use soaps and detergents during the flowering period and instead focus on combating the problem before flowering next time. If you do not, the same problem will occur again in the following round. If you must spray during early flowering, only spray the base of the plants, but this is not a global solution to the problem of aphids. You need to tackle the source during vegetative growth. Anything done after that is salvaging.

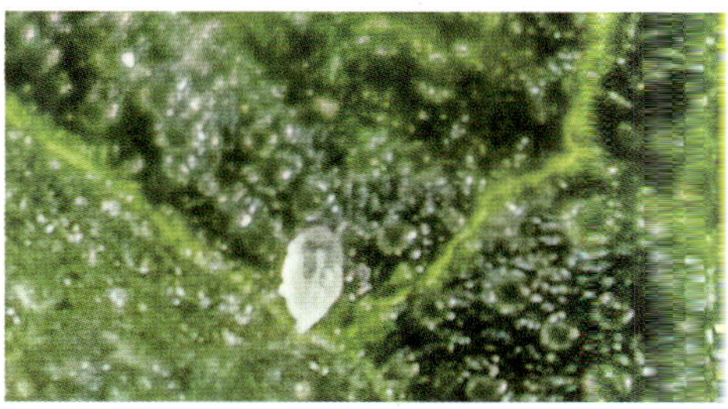

A broad mite is microscopic; you need a magnifying aid to see them.

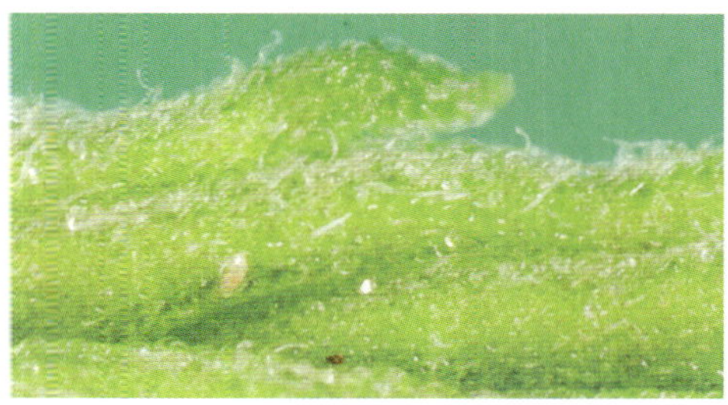

Here, you can see the type of damage done by mites.

Broad mites

Broad mites of the Tarsonemidae family are microscopic, less than 0.2 mm long, and, like mites, cause problems because they feed on the plant. Their damage is consistent with various nutrient disorders and necrosis, so that they may be responsible for these and not a lack of nutrients. They are tiny, yellow or translucent in color, and are found on the underside of leaves. They lay eggs on the leaf and their numbers rapidly increase without treatment or control. The primary chemical control is via insecticides such as miticides, which reduce their numbers and hopefully eliminate them.

Cutworms, Caterpillars, and Larvae

Irregular holes in leaves are indicative of larger pests, often larvae or insects in their early developmental stages. These young insects can be particularly troublesome because of their voracious appetites, as they consume anything green that fits into their tiny mouths. It's truly astonishing to discover the sheer volume of foliage a single caterpillar can devour in a single day. In less than four days, one caterpillar alone can reduce an ounce of cola to mere stem and stalk. These pests are often referred to as "borers" due to their ability to infiltrate any part of the plant. Consequently, they

PHOTOS: DINAFEM SEEDS

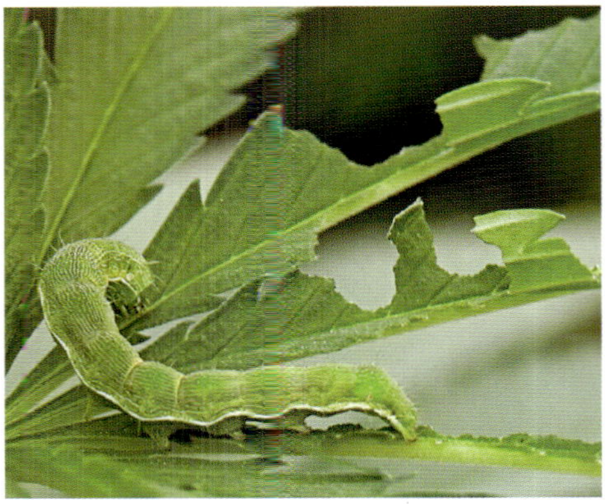

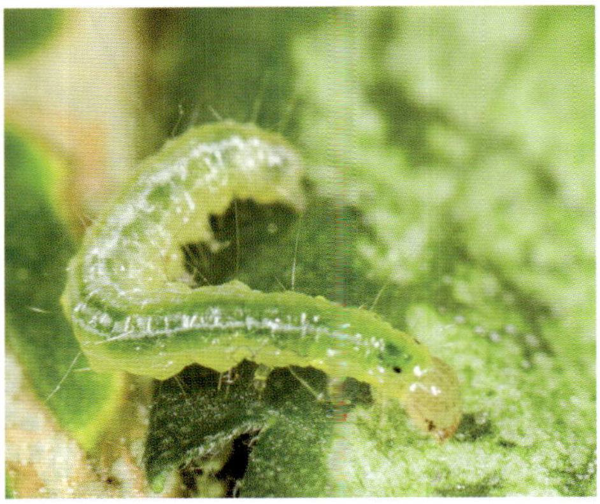

If you see caterpillars/inchworms, then remove them physically. They can finish eating a plant in no time at all.

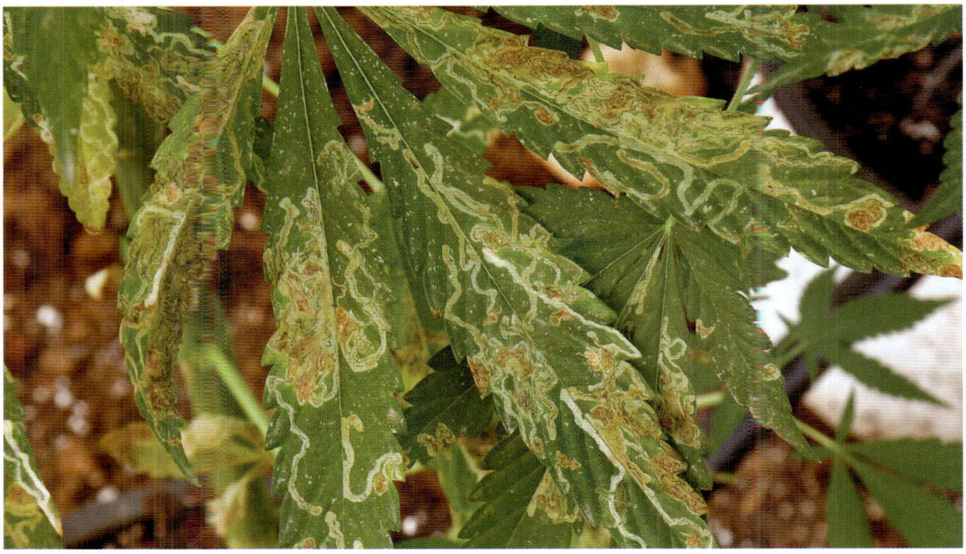

Typical larvae markings on a leaf caused by them burrowing within.

present a significant threat to your crop and should be dealt with promptly. Caterpillars, in particular, have a penchant for consuming young seedlings and fresh growth—and while other pests can also leave holes, these are usually the culprits. Given that some larvae can survive the winter, clear away as much outdoor debris as possible after the harvest to prevent their resurgence in great numbers the following spring.

While removal by hand is an option, the most reliable method for eradicating cutworms, caterpillars, and larvae is to use a repellent designed for these specific pests. Typically, a single product can effectively target all three types. Cutworms can also be physically removed from your cultivation area. Note that they tend to hide at night in a "C" shape in the soil or under cover, such as a piece of wood.

PHOTOS: MANDALA SEEDS

Leaf miners, larvae that feed on leaves and leave distinctive trails behind them, are another concern. Flies also produce larvae, which are sometimes hard to detect directly as they bore within the leaves. However, they often leave characteristic looping patterns on the foliage, which can help identify their presence. When a larva has already tunneled into the plant, external treatments are typically ineffective, although you can try neem oil. Removing the affected leaf can be a starting point, but in severe infestations, you may need to destroy the entire plant to prevent the pest from spreading to other nearby plants when the larvae hatch.

Gnats

Fungus gnats, in the Culicidae family, are a common nuisance around cannabis plants. Often resembling freshly hatched flies or tiny mosquitoes, they tend to feed on cannabis leaves but primarily subsist by siphoning sap from the plant's phloem. While the damage caused by a gnat infestation is similar to the effects of aphids, it is critical to address gnat problems promptly even though they typically inflict less harm.

Fungus gnats can take up residence in the soil, where they target the plant's root system. Excessive watering creates favorable conditions for their larvae to flourish, particularly in the top layer of soil. Therefore, if you encounter gnats, re-evaluate your watering practices, with a focus on improving airflow for enhanced drying. Where overwatering is avoided, the appearance of significant gnat populations is much less likely.

The term "fungus gnats" hints at these insects' reliance on fungi as a vital part of their natural life cycle. These fungi, however, exist in such microscopic quantities that their spores typically float through the air unnoticed as they do not harm cannabis when present in small amounts. Overly moist conditions in the soil create an environment conducive to the proliferation of these minute fungal spores, which can attract gnats, allowing a more extensive fungal tissue to emerge. Since gnats often live on the surface of the soil, you can apply insecticides directly to the soil or use diatomaceous earth to control their populations. You can also use yellow strips to trap gnats, but attach them to cards you securely position in the soil using stakes. If the strips become laden with gnats, be prepared to use more.

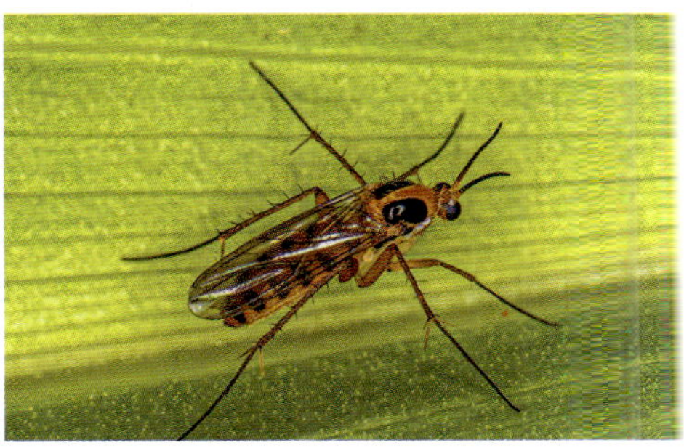

Mosquito-looking insects are likely gnats.

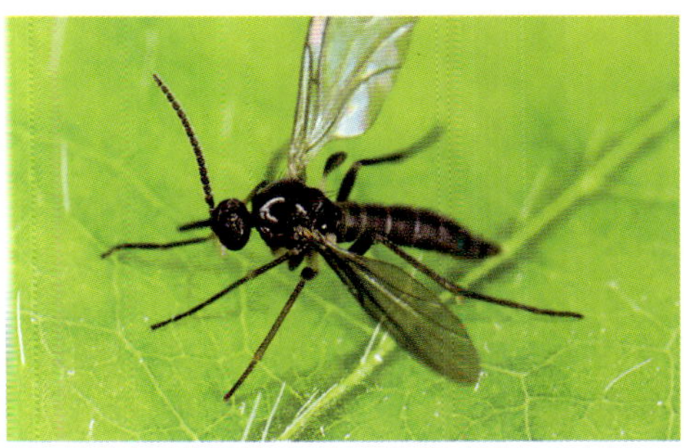

Gnats are winged and can fly from plant to plant.

PHOTOS: VINICIUS R. SOUZA/SHUTTERSTOCK.COM (LEFT), TOMASZ KLEJDYSZ/SHUTTERSTOCK.COM (RIGHT)

Grasshoppers

Grasshoppers, in the Acrididae family, are insects renowned for their remarkable jumping abilities, thanks to their specialized long legs. Some male grasshoppers emit a distinctive high-pitched clicking sound. It's crucial not to confuse unwanted grasshoppers with beneficial praying mantises, which serve as valuable pest controllers. When present as solitary individuals or in small numbers, grasshoppers might create a few holes in leaves and then move on. These minor encounters are relatively easy to deter, and you can treat grasshoppers almost like transient tourists in your garden.

However, when grasshoppers appear in substantial numbers, especially if they have developed wings, they can transition from a minor nuisance to a severe threat. When winged grasshoppers congregate in large quantities, they are often referred to as locusts. Locust swarms are migratory and have a voracious appetite, posing a grave danger to a wide variety of vegetation. They can strip a plant down to its bare stems and branches within a matter of hours. In the face of a severe locust assault, growers might have no option but to salvage cuttings from their affected plants and start anew in a different location. Even pesticide-laden plants are not spared when locusts travel en masse, rendering pesticides generally ineffective against their overwhelming attacks. However, if dealing with smaller grasshopper numbers, the same treatments used for aphids can deter them.

In substantial infestations, the damage caused by grasshoppers can extend beyond leaf holes and include stem breakage. Therefore, if you observe both stem breaks and a multitude of holes, it's plausible that a grasshopper infestation has recently passed through your garden. Droughts and arid conditions in hot weather provide ideal breeding grounds for grasshoppers, so remain vigilant during these periods. In natural

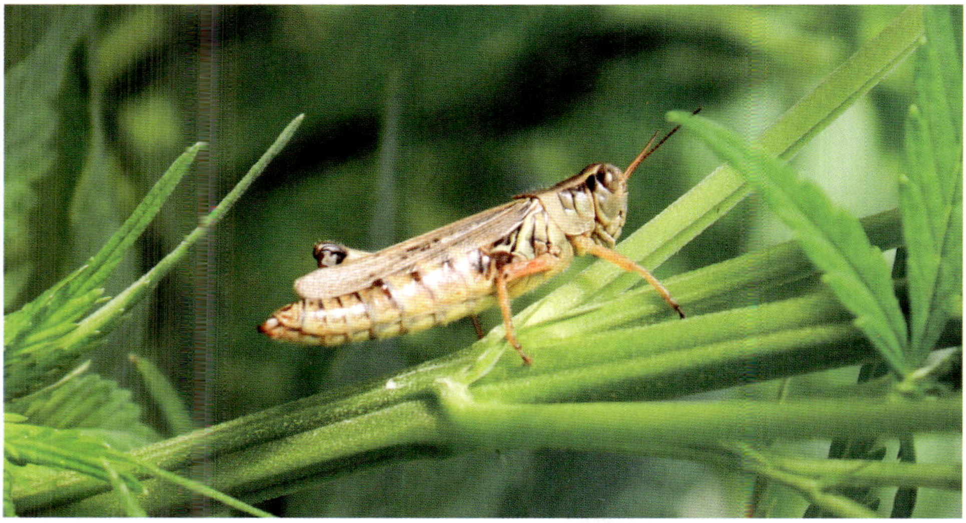

PHOTO: STONED ROSIE

One or two grasshoppers in a grow are okay, but lots are certainly not.

ecosystems, birds play a vital role in controlling grasshopper populations by preying on them. Attracting birds with bird feeders can be a helpful strategy, but remember to remove the feeders if you are planting cannabis seeds, or birds might eat them also. Additionally, for situations where mild, sporadic damage occurs, consider using row nets as a protective measure.

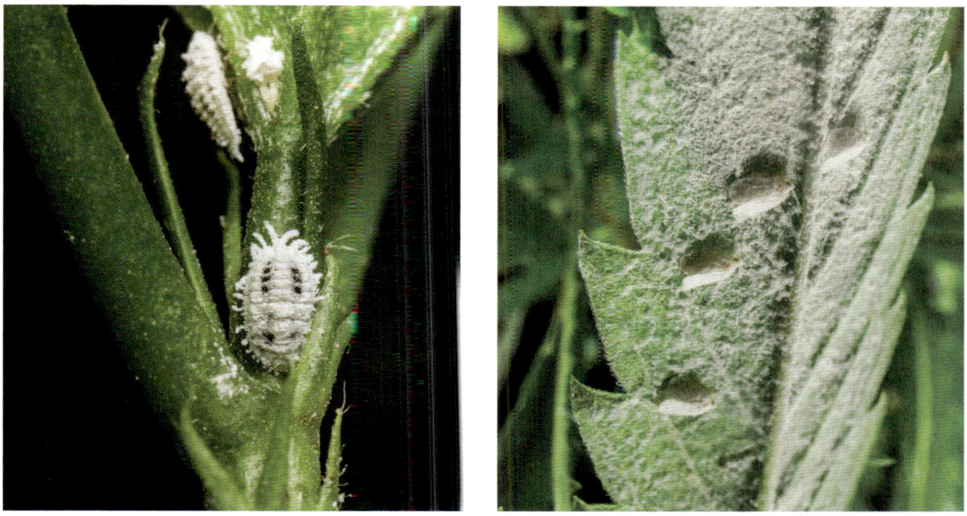

Mealybugs look like pale warts on the plant until you magnify them.

PHOTOS: PRAPHAB LOUILARPPRASERT/SHUTTERSTOCK.COM (LEFT), BARRIOGRAPHY/SHUTTERSTOCK.COM (RIGHT)

Mealybugs

Mealybugs, in the Pseudococcidae family, are often described by growers as "hard aphids" due to a waxy powder that gives their backs a shell-like appearance when viewed under a microscope. Their presence can result in the development of a moldy-looking area on the plant. These pests target plant tissues and feed on the sap from the phloem, which makes their treatment similar to that of aphids. Without the aid of magnification, it's easy to mistake mealybugs for aphids, particularly because they also excrete honeydew. Their honeydew secretions can create conditions conducive to mold fungi growth. However, unlike aphids, mealybugs can be manually removed when present in small numbers.

Some growers have observed that an initial encounter with mealybugs may not be a severe problem but can escalate in subsequent growing cycles. Even a low mealybug count can lead to the laying of eggs and the presence of larvae in hard-to-detect locations. Therefore, it's crucial to take preventive measures once these pests are identified, including thoroughly cleaning the grow room after each harvest to minimize the chances of the next generation hatching. If specific parts of a plant are infested, removing them can help reduce the overall mealybug population. Dealing with an infestation typically involves repeated applications of control methods; remember that you can use multiple strategies in succession for more effective results.

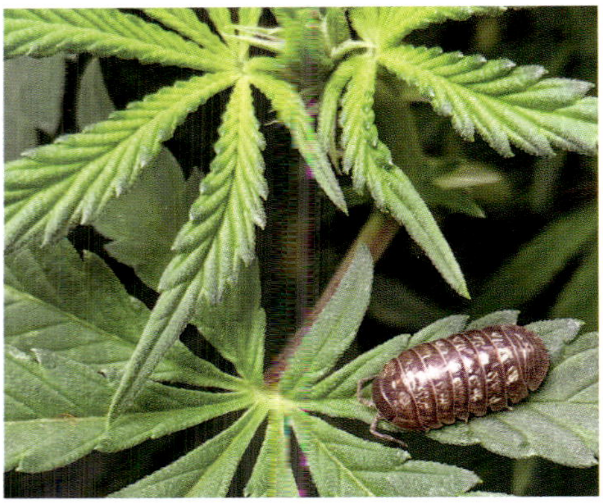

Rollie pollies are larger than mealybugs and can curl up.

Pill Bugs

A commonly found detritivore called rollie pollies feeds on dead and decomposing matter and leaves behind an excretion similar to worm castings. In small numbers, they provide a benefit because they also attack pests; however, they also attack beneficial bugs. In damp conditions, they thrive and, if present in large numbers, will start to consume seedlings and plants, making them a problematic pest. They are easy to trap and reduce in numbers, making them beneficial again.

At night, leave circular slices of orange flat on the soil. In the morning, any nearby pill bugs will have gathered in the soil under the slice and can be scooped out and disposed of far away from your garden. You can repeat this process until the numbers are so low that they no longer attack plants and become beneficial again. If you have a problem with birds or animals taking away your fruit slices, you might try using a small amount of beer in a lid buried at the soil's surface level. This can also attract slugs. Reducing their numbers, not entirely removing them, is the way forward for optimal balanced conditions.

Root aphids

Root aphids of the Aphididae family infest plant roots. They are not as common as above-ground aphids but are just as damaging. If you see insects moving around the roots, leaving honeydew secretions, then they may be root aphids. Any affected plant needs to be quarantined to prevent spread. Biological controls include predatory insects like ladybugs or lacewings; neem oil and insecticides (for root aphids specifically) can be used to drench the soil and kill the unwanted creatures. You may need repeat applications of these, so keep monitoring the roots in case the infestation returns. Identifying these pests as early as possible helps with successful removal.

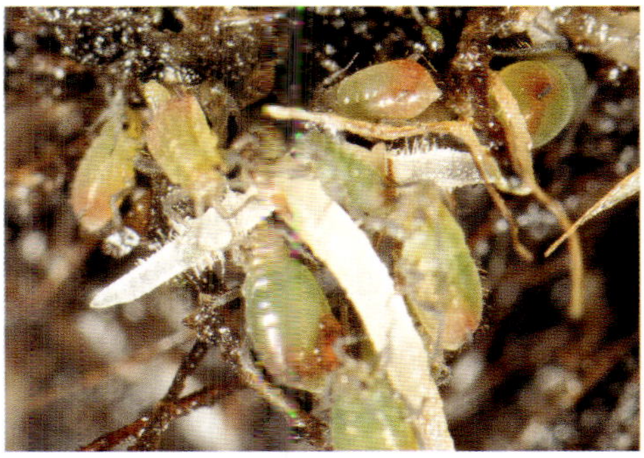

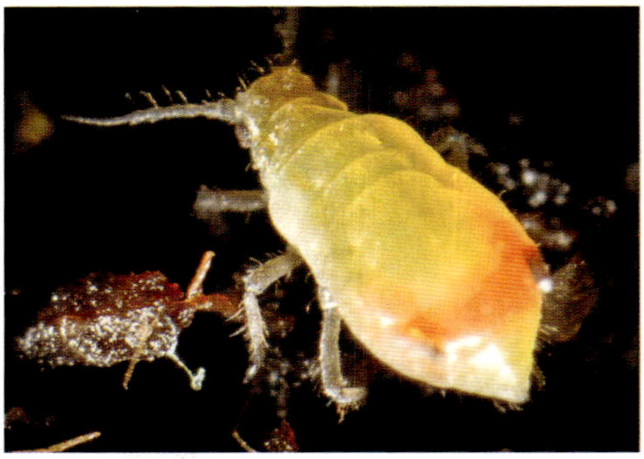

The translucent-looking root aphids are found under the soil.

PHOTOS: NATHAN GUILLARD (TOP), DINAFEM SEEDS (BOTTOM)

Scale

Scale insects, in the superfamily Coccoidea, are closely related to aphids and exhibit various forms, including a cochineal form. They can often be mistaken for mealybugs due to their similar powdery appearance; all of these insects fall under the same order, Homoptera. With thousands of species, mealybugs are the most common type of scale, although they are sometimes not referred to as scale insects because they lack the same solid structure. Some scale species are hermaphroditic, while others are winged males that can fly, although these are rarely seen due to their low numbers and short lifespans.

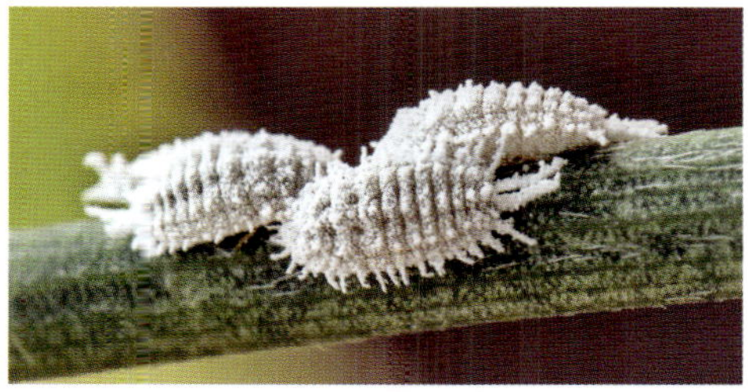

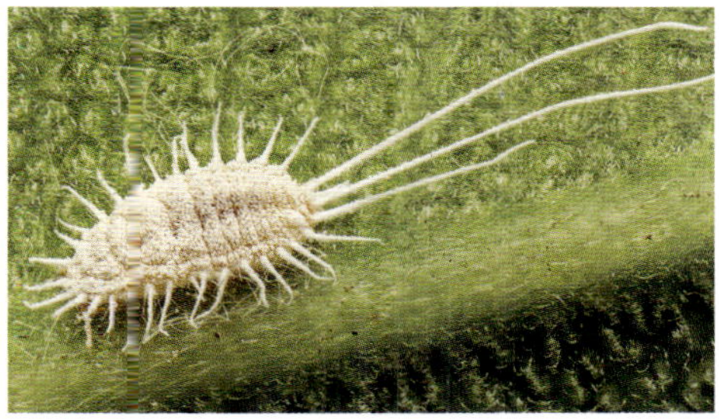

Scale insects are quite similar to mealybugs.

When scale insects are born, they are mobile but eventually solidify, typically on plant branches and stems, where they insert a small, hollow tube into the plant to access its juices. They are also responsible for mold spread. Scale insects can be manually removed from your plants because once they solidify, they tend to remain in one spot on the plant. Another method for dealing with scale is to scrub them off the branches using a scouring pad. It's important to address any ant infestations in your grow room since ants farm scale insects. Eliminate ants before treating a scale problem, following similar treatment methods used for mealybugs or aphids.

Identifying some scale species can be challenging. If you find your plants exhibiting signs of what appears to be a fungal infection or mold, or if they seem to be in distress with symptoms resembling nutrient problems that aren't resolved with nutrient adjustments or fungicides, review any photos you may have taken of the affected areas. It's entirely possible that the underlying issue was a scale infestation that was misidentified.

Seed bugs

Seed bugs are a diverse group of insects of the family Lygaeidae. Many are flat, brown, or gray, and some have wings in the adult phase of their life cycle. This means younger seed bugs will not have wings and appear more like nymphs. These species range from a few millimeters to over a centimeter in length. They use pincers to suck juices from plant

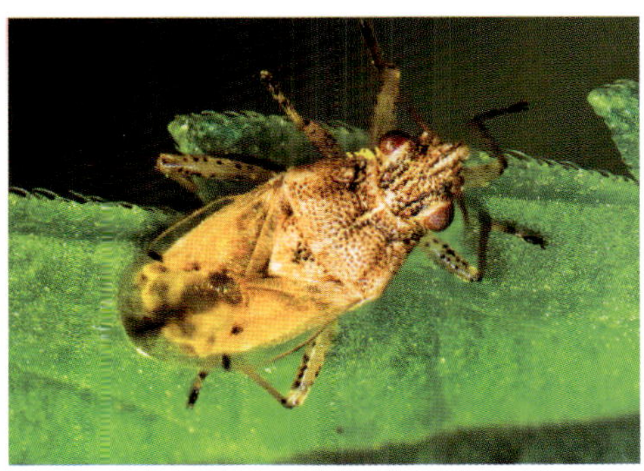

Seed bugs are identified by their flatness.

PHOTOS: ROBERTO MICHEL/SHUTTERSTOCK.COM (TOP), MACROLIFE/SHUTTERSTOCK.COM (MIDDLE), ERIC PALMER (BOTTOM)

tissue. They also feed on seeds, harming breeding programs that expect seeds as the end product. They tend to move away from cold areas, which is why, in the wintertime, they often find grow rooms much more suitable for their new homes.

Slugs and Snails

Slugs and snails, in the class Gastropoda, are characterized by their flattened underside, which they use for movement and which leaves behind slime trails as a telltale sign of their presence. These pests feed on the leaves and stems of plants and can be particularly detrimental to cannabis seedlings. While birds naturally help control their populations, the shells of snails can provide them with protection.

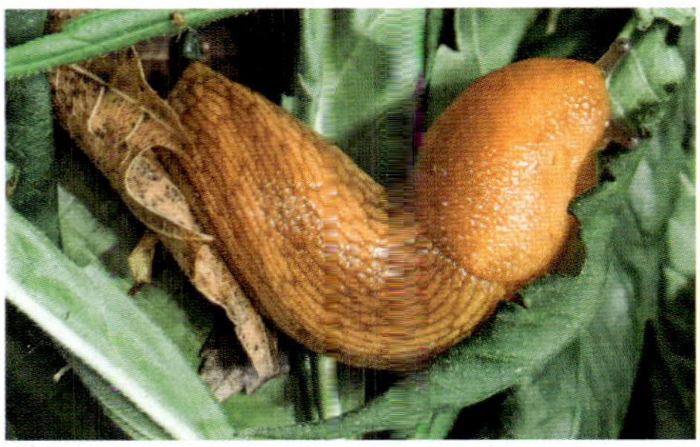

Slugs will eat away at stems and leaves.

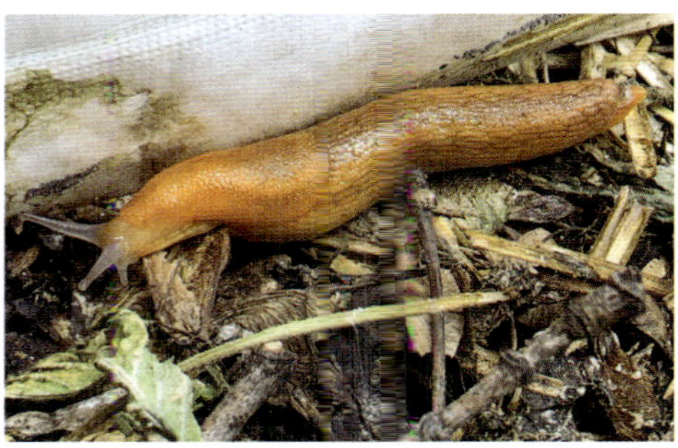

Pick them up and relocate them.

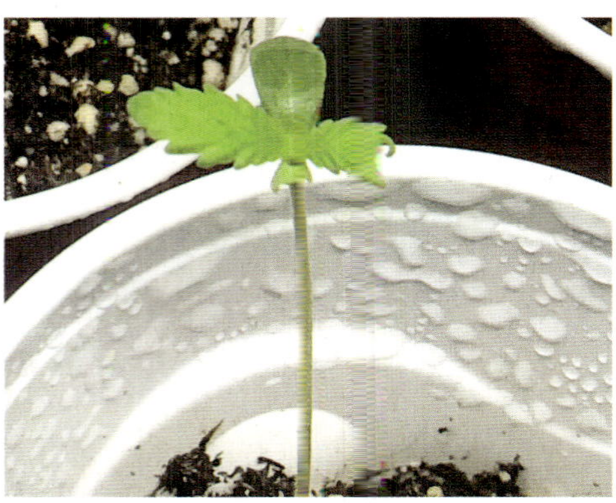

Rodent damage to a seedling.

PHOTOS: NATHAN GUILLARD

To manage slugs and snails, the most effective approach is to manually remove them from your growing area through hand-picking. Alternatively, you can repel or eliminate slugs and snails by using specialized slug and snail pest pellets. You can also spread diatomaceous earth around the growing space to repel them. However, do not use salt around your growing space, as salts can absorb water, disrupt nutrient balances, and increase pH levels. Salt is lethal to snails and slugs and will act as a deterrent but don't use it because the concentration is wrong for your soil (Epsom salts are used for Mg correction only). The most efficient method remains finding and physically relocating them to another area of your garden to prevent further damage.

Small Plant-Eating Animals

Numerous species of small burrowing plant-eating animals can become cannabis pests. The problem arises when these creatures decide to chew through your plants, as they are known to be voracious eaters capable of decimating an entire crop within days. Whether small animals try to consume your cannabis largely depends on your specific location, with lagomorphs (such as rabbits) and rodents being the most common culprits. The primary driving factor behind their choice to target your crop is often the absence of alternative food sources. This may explain why some outdoor crops remain relatively undamaged while others are completely destroyed.

Cats can help control many of these small burrowing plant-eating animals by stalking them, although they may not always catch them. Dogs can also be effective in chasing them away. Another method to deter these creatures is the use of predator urine. Fencing is a viable option, but it's essential to ensure that the pests in question cannot burrow or squeeze through the fence's openings. Human activity, such as regular visits to the growing area, can often scare them away. Greenhouses offer a popular solution if the pest problem becomes particularly severe.

Spider Mites

Spider mites, minuscule pests about half the size of the period at the end of this sentence, are imperceptible to the naked eye. However, they usually congregate in their adult form in clusters on various parts of the cannabis plant. Initially, their presence might make it appear as if your plant has fallen victim to a disease, fungi, mold, dusty spots, or tiny discolored specks. But closer examination, especially if you notice the cluster in motion, can reveal that you're dealing with spider mites.

Under magnification, they look like a curious cross between aphids and spiders.

Spider mites spin webbing around, simplifying their movement between different parts of the plant, such as from leaves to buds. This webbing not only facilitates their rapid traversal but also enables a larger population to inhabit a specific area of the plant. Since spider mites feed on plant juices, leaf wilting is a common symptom of their infestation. As the attack persists, the plants ultimately succumb to the damage, and in flowering, the buds may become enveloped in webbing, rendering them unusable.

Spider mite infestations tend to manifest with remarkable speed. Identifying their minuscule eggs requires a high level of magnification, presenting a challenge because you ideally want to detect and address the issue before the webbing appears, or before a severe infestation takes hold. Upon discovering webbing, especially in flowering, some growers opt to remove the entire affected plant, as they understand that webbing typically signifies numerous eggs primed to hatch, and as the infestation advances, the webbing intensifies, ultimately ruining the flowers and making them unsuitable for consumption. Consequently, one can assume that both eggs and spider mites have infiltrated the buds.

Treating spider mites largely follows the same strategies applied to aphids, although you can buy specialized pesticides designed specifically for their control. During the vegetative growth phase, soaps can be effective in eradicating spider mites, but

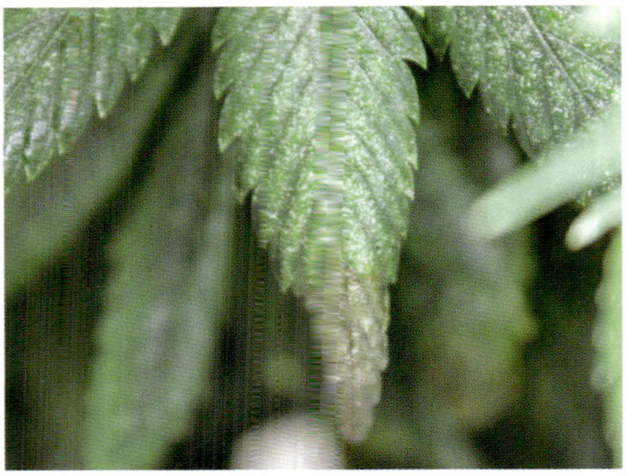

Sometimes you may not see webbing, only the resulting damage. This looks like a nutrient deficiency, but it is not.

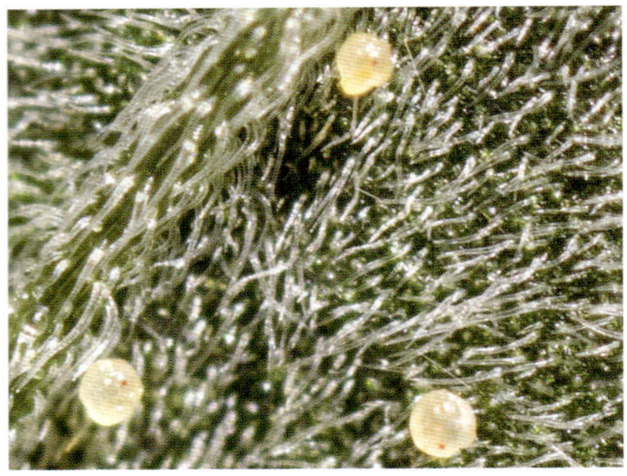

Mite eggs are microscopic translucent bubbles, and you need an aid to see them.

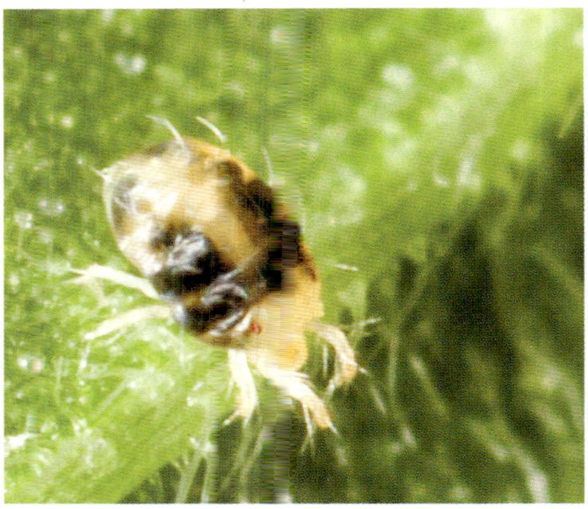

You can see the trichomes and this spider mite at higher magnification.

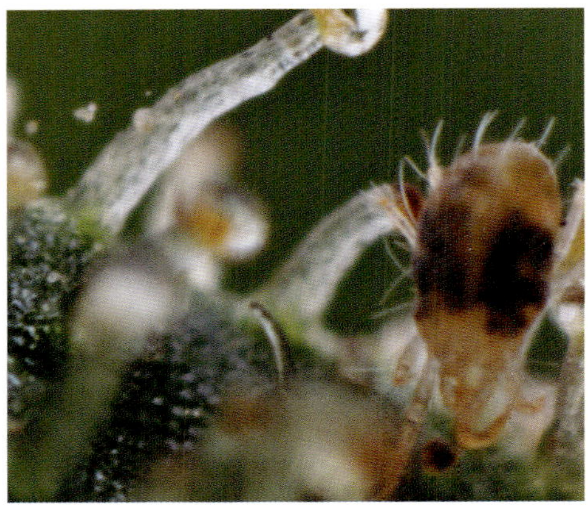

Some mites are so small they are hard to detect even with a magnifying aid.

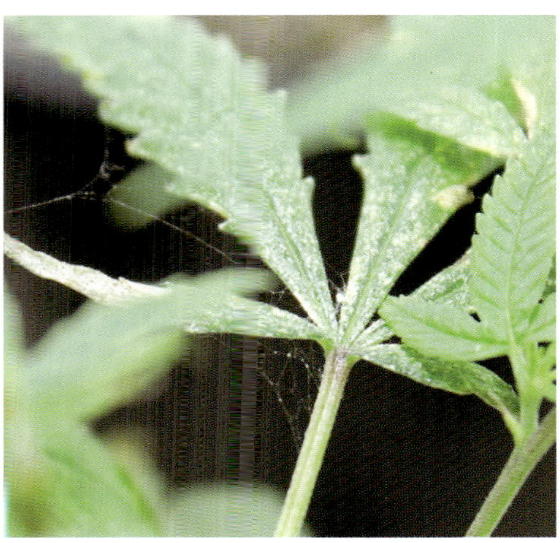

Webbing revealed nearby with the same damage patterns on the leaf.

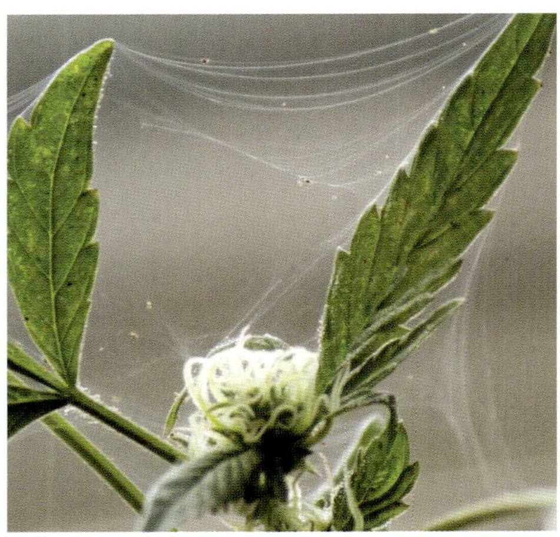

Spider mite webbing can span across multiple leaves.

PHOTOS: TYLER J. MARKWART AND DANIELLE HALLE (TOP AND BOTTOM LEFT), DINAFEM SEEDS (TOP RIGHT AND MIDDLE LEFT), TRICHOME ART (MIDDLE RIGHT), ZENKY PHOTO/SHUTTERSTOCK.COM (BOTTOM RIGHT)

caution is required when using soap on flowering plants. Sticky pest trap tape, while somewhat effective, may not significantly reduce the numbers, as spider mites reproduce at an alarming rate. Lady beetles can also play a crucial role in controlling spider mite infestations through predation.

Even seasoned growers can face formidable challenges when combating spider mites. The outcome greatly depends on the stage at which you detect the infestation. Even with early identification, spider mites can outpace your treatment efforts. Therefore, dealing with spider mites often necessitates multiple applications and the sequential use of various methods. Spider mites unquestionably rank among the most formidable pests that growers can encounter.

Termites

Even though their primary diet doesn't consist of plant matter, termites possess the extraordinary ability to tunnel through a variety of challenging materials, including plants, which renders them highly destructive pests. Although relatively uncommon, when they do infest, they can rapidly gnaw through wood and sever a plant at its stem's base within a matter of days. Termites, in the order Isoptera, are social insects that live in colonies. Their role as cannabis plant pests remains a subject that requires more in-depth research, so stay informed about any recent developments if you encounter this issue.

Termites are notably averse to water. If you happen to overwater the soil surrounding your plants, it may drive them away. However, while overwatering may discourage termites, it also creates conditions conducive to the emergence of gnats, specifically fungus gnats.

The most effective way to deal with termites is to locate their nest and flush it out with water. Identifying the source of the termite infestation is better than directly treating your plants for them. If you can pinpoint the termite source, which might be some distance from your plants, you can use readily available commercial products designed to exterminate termites. However, be aware that most of these products are not intended for plant use or human consumption.

Thrips

Thrips, in the Thysanoptera family, are minuscule insects with pale white or light brown semi-transparent bodies in elongated, slender forms. In their adult stage, thrips develop wings and darken in color. These tiny pests tend to target the flowering parts of cannabis plants, resulting in the disintegration of floral development, giving affected areas a silvery, patchy appearance. Thrips feed on plant juices and deposit their eggs inside the leaves, leading to the development of leaf blotches that may resemble symptoms of other insect attacks or nutrient deficiencies.

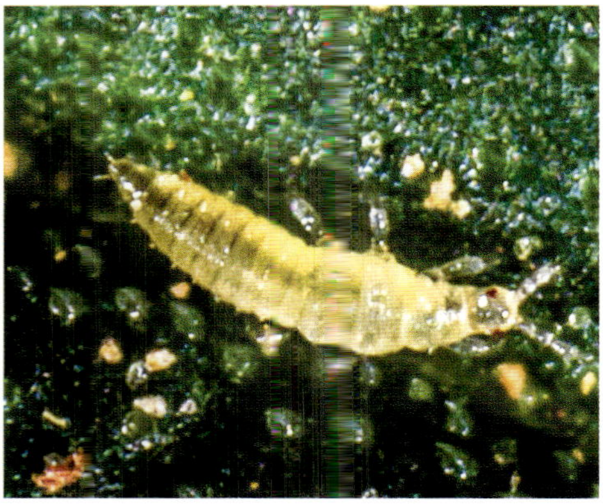

A thrip just after its earlier larvae stage.

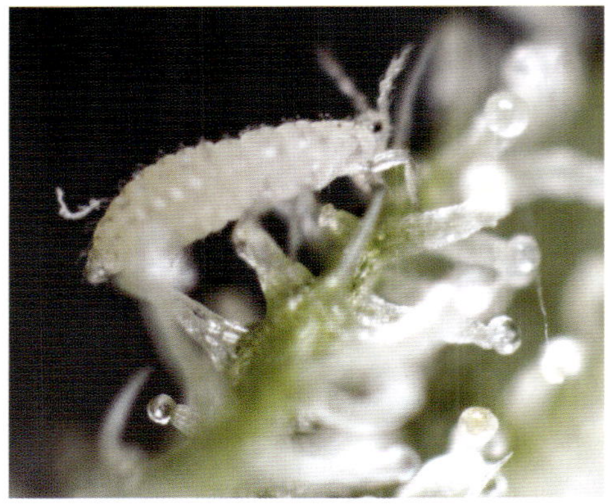

Thrips can be too small to see with the naked eye.

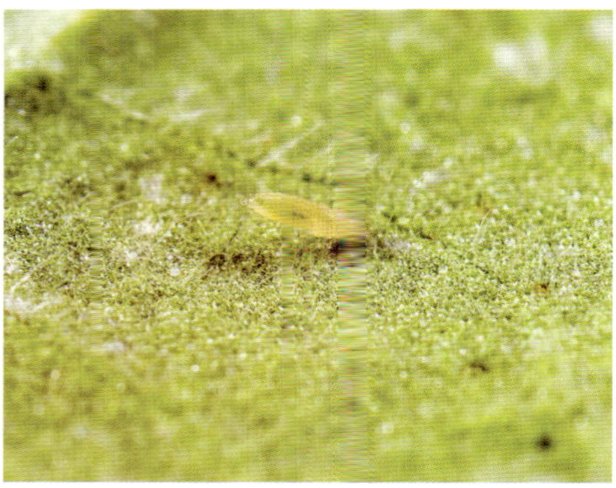

Some thrips can be translucent at this stage.

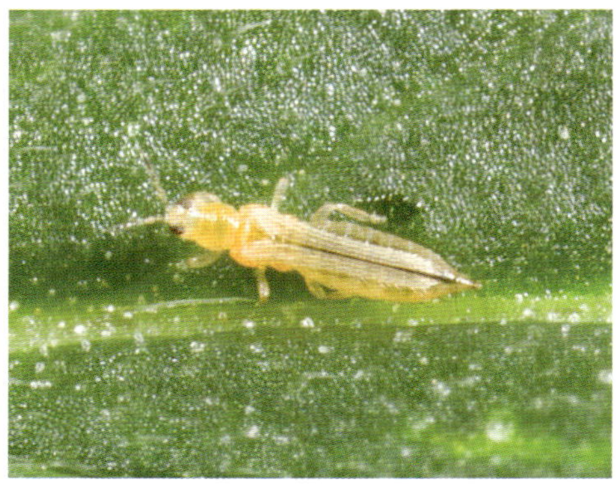

Adults are more insect-like and less translucent.

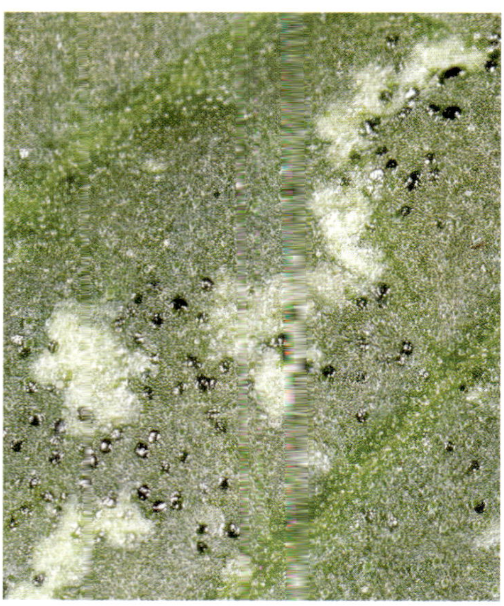

Adult thrips may change to a darker color.

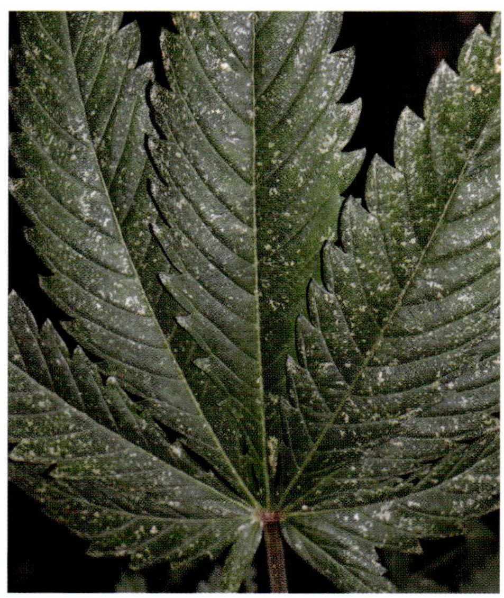

An example of the "silvery" damage caused by thrips.

PHOTOS: ERIC PALMER (TOP LEFT), TRICHOME ART (TOP RIGHT), DINAFEM SEEDS (MIDDLE AND BOTTOM LEFT), MANDALA SEEDS (BOTTOM RIGHT)

Outdoors, thrips tend not to be a persistent issue, as their natural predators, including beetles, ladybirds, lacewings, and mites, help keep their population in check. However, when they do manage to establish themselves in your outdoor garden, they can cause considerable damage. The situation is even more concerning indoors, where they can thrive and reproduce rapidly in higher numbers. The specific type of thrips known to target cannabis is the western flower thrips, *Frankliniella occidentalis*.

To swiftly address thrip infestations, you can use sticky tape or soaps and oils, much like the treatments used for other pests such as aphids. However, you can effectively prevent thrips from infiltrating your growing space by taking such precautions as not introducing outdoor plants into your indoor grow room or subjecting any incoming clones to quarantine checks.

Whitefly

Whiteflies, in the Aleyrodidae family, are typically around 0.16 inches (4 mm) long. There are more than 200 species of these insects, varying in shape, size, and color. One species, in particular, is known for its preference for greenhouse environments, earning it the name "greenhouse whitefly."

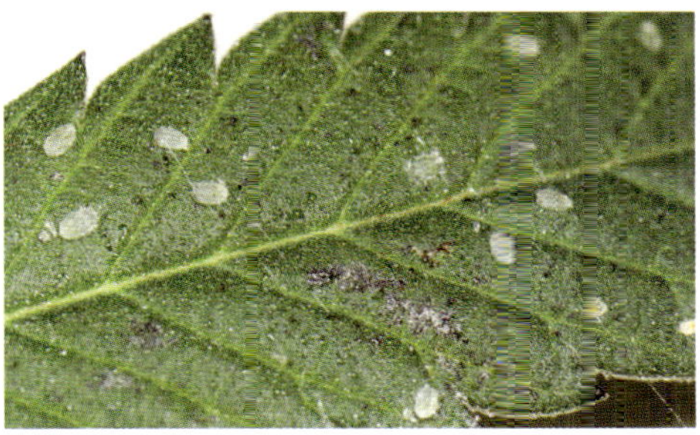

Whitefly larvae are similar to mite larvae but larger.

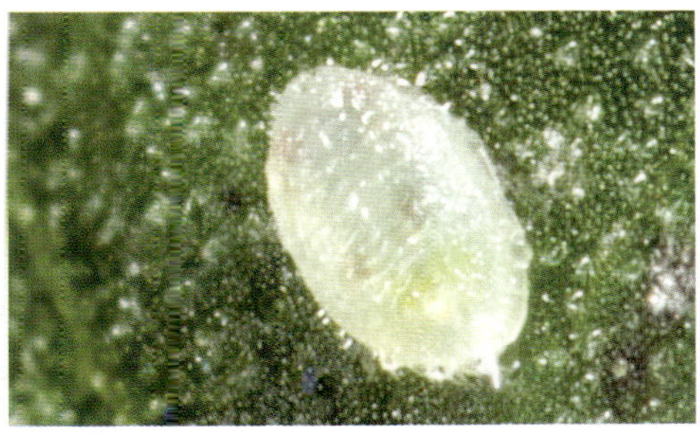

The early stages look like a translucent mealybug.

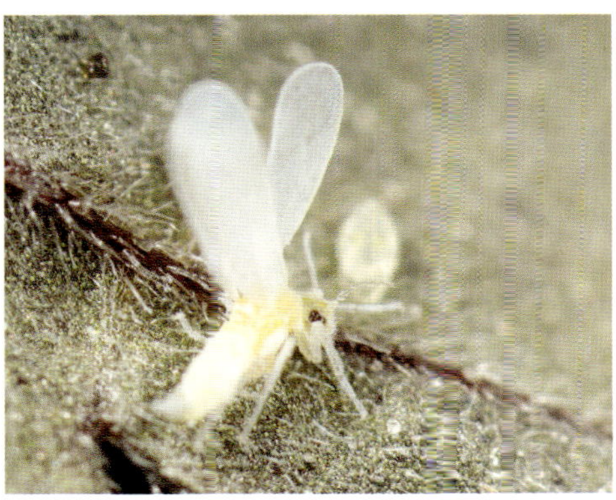

Adult stage produces wings and more fly-like features.

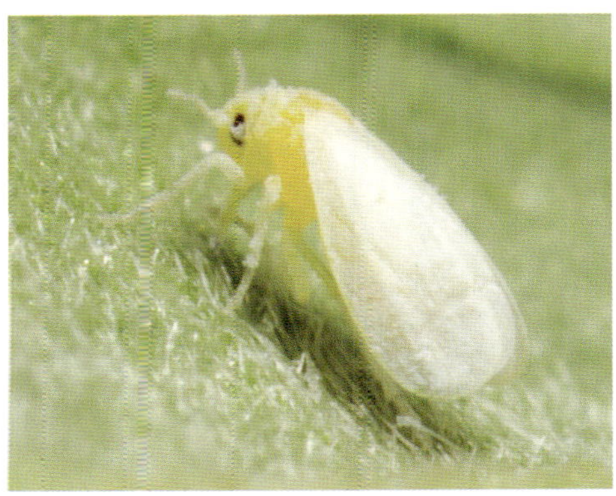

Whiteflies have white wings and a green-yellow body.

PHOTOS: DINAFEM SEEDS

Whiteflies have waxy white wings, which they use for short-distance flying. When your plant is disturbed, you may hear them buzzing before you spot them. Their white color stands out against the green foliage, making them relatively easy to detect. Whiteflies can pose a severe threat to your crop and quickly reduce your plant to a state of ruin. They feed on plant juices and secrete honeydew, a substance that can encourage mold growth in the affected areas.

Early detection of whiteflies is essential, as they lay numerous eggs. Once eggs are present, you must act quickly to combat a full-blown infestation of these flying pests. The methods for dealing with whiteflies are similar to those used against aphids, and products such as Safer's Soap, available in most grow shops, can effectively eliminate them. Other types of soaps and sprays are also suitable for controlling whitefly infestations. Again, try to avoid the use of soap on flowering plants.

Natural predators of whiteflies include spiders, ladybirds, and beetles. Pest tape can also be quite effective in reducing their population. Whiteflies are a common challenge faced by cannabis growers, both indoors and outdoors.

Friendly Pests, Beneficial Pests, and Predators

Often called "friendly pests," these pest predators may initially appear to be plant pests but do not harm your crop. They play a crucial role in naturally controlling many troublesome pests. Beneficial pests can be intentionally bred or purchased to maintain a steady population. For example, lady beetles can reproduce when provided with a consistent food source of aphids and other insects. Many stores now stock pest predators, and you can contact your local agricultural supply store to inquire about their availability. Some companies even offer the option to have predator pests delivered by mail.

Beetles

Ground beetles typically have black, brown, or blueish bodies with wings and solid wing covers on their backs. They are most effective at ground level in eradicating such pests as snails, slugs, cutworms, and harmful insects. These beetles are commonly found in the soil or under debris like rocks and wood. While they are harmless to cannabis, they effectively prey on slower-moving insects.

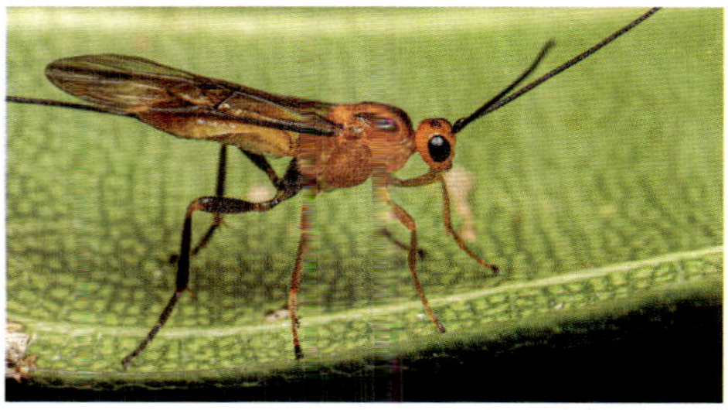

PHOTO: VINICIUS R. SOUZA/SHUTTERSTOCK.COM

Braconid wasps control pests and aid crops.

Braconid Wasps

Braconid wasps, in the order Hymenoptera, lay their eggs in parasitic relationship with unwanted pests like aphids, scale insects, cutworms, and various types of larvae. This parasitism occurs after the wasp injects its eggs into the host pests. For instance, when cutworms are injected, they eventually develop tiny cocoon-like pods on their back and sides. As they mature, braconid wasp larvae consume the host insect from the inside out.

Bugs

Some species of "true" bugs are effective in controlling undesirable pests. True bugs feed by extracting bodily fluids from their prey. Assassin bugs (identified by their red undersides), big-eyed bugs (with large eyes), pirate bugs (featuring checkered black and white or gray and brown patterns), and damsel bugs (characterized by long, large front legs and varying shades of gray, brown, or tan) are some of the most common true bugs you may encounter. Pirate bugs are particularly effective against spider mites and thrips. True bugs are typically over half an inch long and move relatively quickly around your plants.

Earthworms

While not pest predators, earthworms play a vital role in soil health by aerating the soil and depositing essential nutrients such as nitrogen, calcium, phosphorus, and potassium. Worm castings, an organic fertilizer product, are primarily made from earthworm waste material. You can cultivate earthworms to create your organic fertilizer.

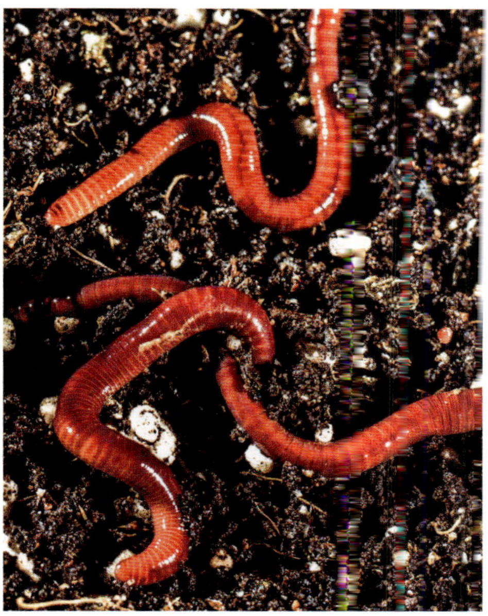

Worms naturally aerate the soil by churning it up. This makes them beneficial.

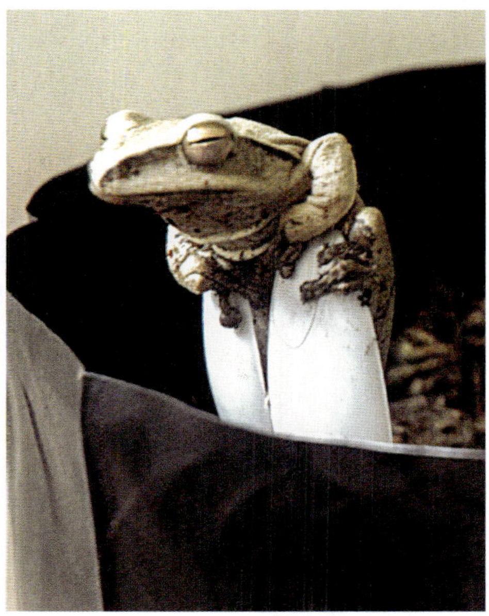

A frog will catch insects and eat them. It is harmless and usually moves on.

PHOTOS: ERIC PALMER (LEFT), ED BORG (RIGHT)

Frogs

Frogs are natural insect predators that consume a wide range of pests. If you have frogs in your garden, they can significantly contribute to pest control. The challenge lies in maintaining an environment that keeps them around.

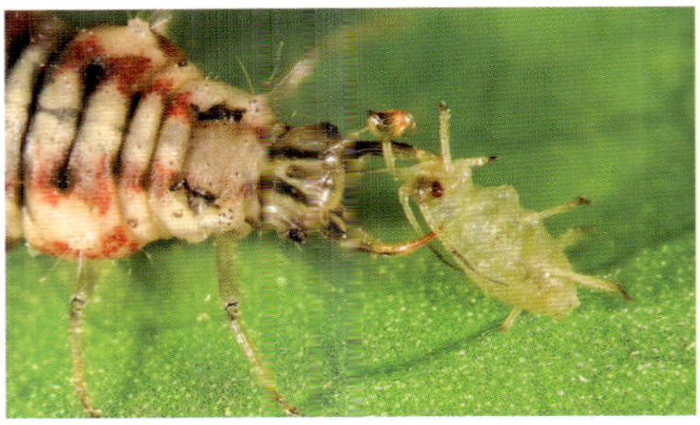

A lacewing larva captures and feeds on an aphid.

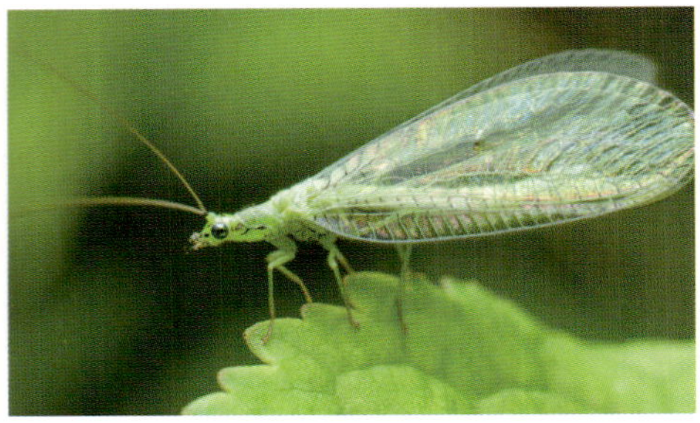

An adult lacewing has translucent wings.

Lacewings

Lacewings feed on aphids and spider mites. They are usually green, have large, semi-transparent wings extending well past their bodies, and sport two long and slender antennae . Lacewings typically reach about 2.5 cm in size and can be easily approached and handled. Be sure not to mistake lacewings for whiteflies, as whiteflies harm your crop, while lacewings target the pests you want to eliminate.

Ladybird Beetles

Also known as "ladybugs," these exceptional pest predators feed on a variety of insects harmful to cannabis. They have a particular appetite for aphids, mealybugs, scales, and spider mites. Ladybirds require a diet of aphids and other insects to lay eggs, and the more they consume, the more eggs they produce. One female ladybug can devour up to 4,000 aphids throughout its lifetime and lay around 2,000 eggs. Ladybirds are the preferred pest predators for cannabis growers.

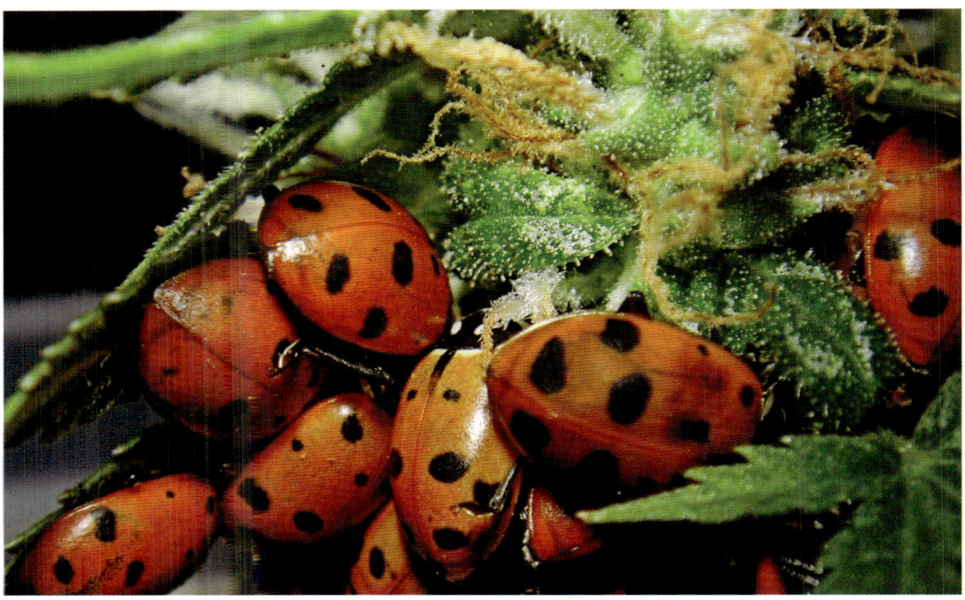

Ladybirds/ladybugs will consume mites and aphids in no time.

PHOTOS: PROTASOV AN/SHUTTERSTOCK.COM (TOP LEFT), ABRAMOFF/SHUTTERSTOCK.COM (TOP RIGHT), KRANE (BOTTOM)

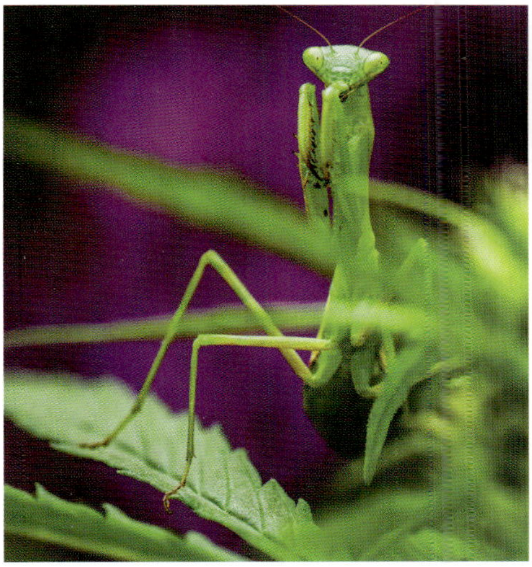

Triangular head and praying front arms identify the mantis.

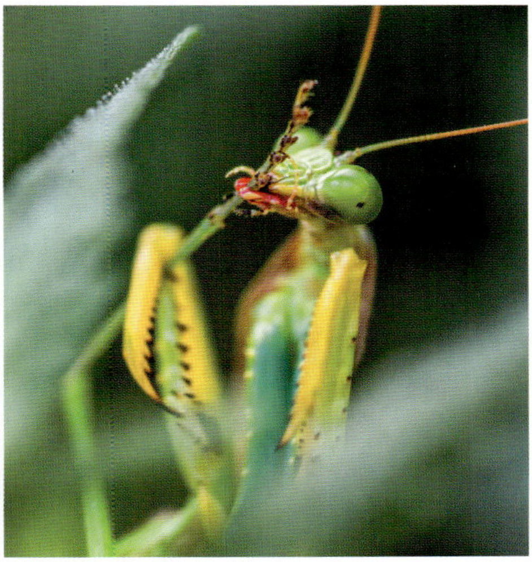

Mantises eat insects in large amounts and keep on going.

Mantises

Praying mantises are voracious consumers that offer protection to your plants while preying on pests. A mantis can cover a lot of ground and work throughout the entire plant. If you find one, leave it in place; however, if you discover multiple mantises, relocate some of them, as they are known to fight and consume each other. Over time, mantises naturally move from plant to plant, controlling pests along the way.

Minute Pirate Bug

Minute pirate bug belongs to the family Anthocoridae. Orius is a genus of minute pirate bugs and also the most well-known species. Although only a few millimeters in size, they attack and feed on many harmful bugs, which makes them beneficial for controlling plant pests. They use their suckers to absorb mites, thrips, and aphids and their eggs. They are popular, beneficial predators with gardeners, and are commercially available for crop pest management.

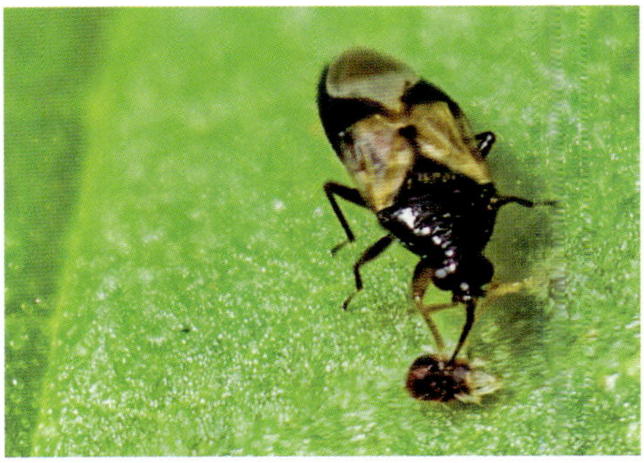

A minute pirate bug feeding on a larva.

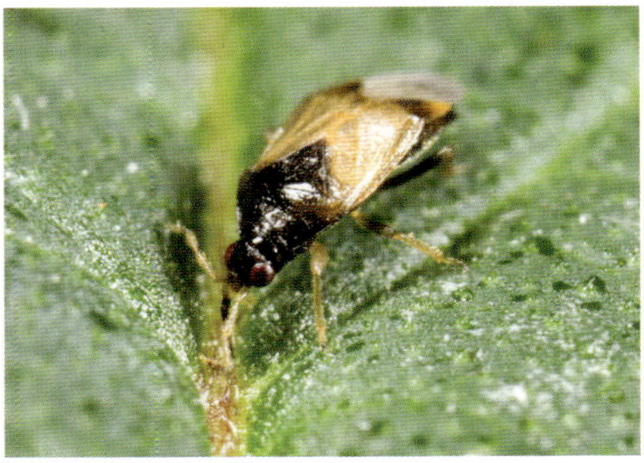

Minute pirate bugs are flat and winged.

PHOTOS: ERIC PALMER (TOP ROW AND BOTTOM LEFT), DINAFEM SEEDS (BOTTOM RIGHT)

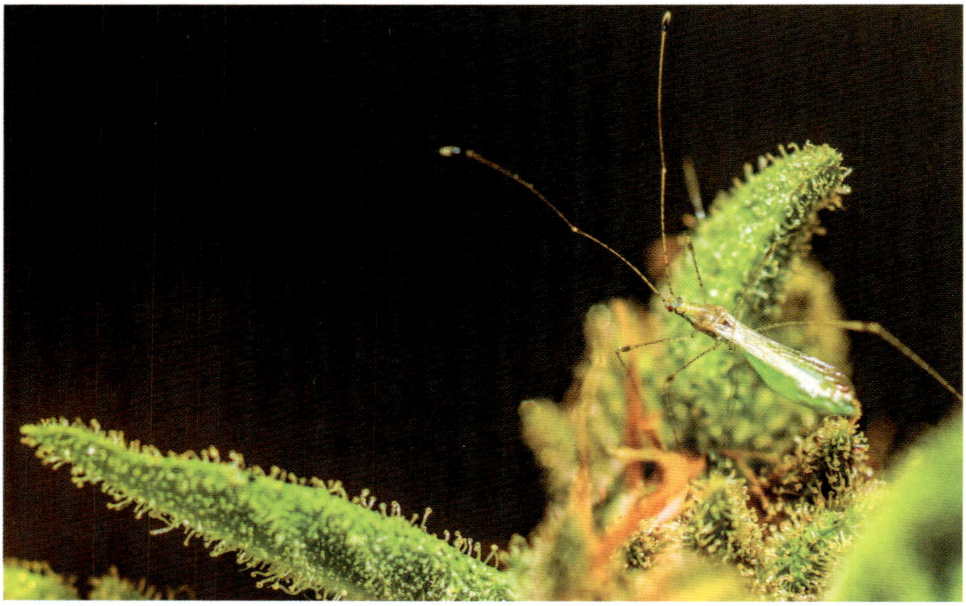

A beneficial pale green assassin bug walks all over cannabis flowers, looking for pests to eat.

Pale Green Assassin Bug

The pale green assassin bug is a beneficial generalist predatory insect belonging to the family Reduviidae. It attacks and feeds on many harmful bugs, including caterpillars and aphids, using suckers that absorb the unwanted pest. Unlike many harmful bugs, they have a visible neck region and spiky legs. These guys bite, so take care when handling them.

Spiders

While most common garden spiders are generally too slow to effectively control common pests, an exception is the Pholcidae family, commonly known as "daddy long legs." These spiders do not spin webs and are unlikely to cover your buds with webbing, as other spiders might. Instead, they roam around your crop and consume nearly any insect they encounter.

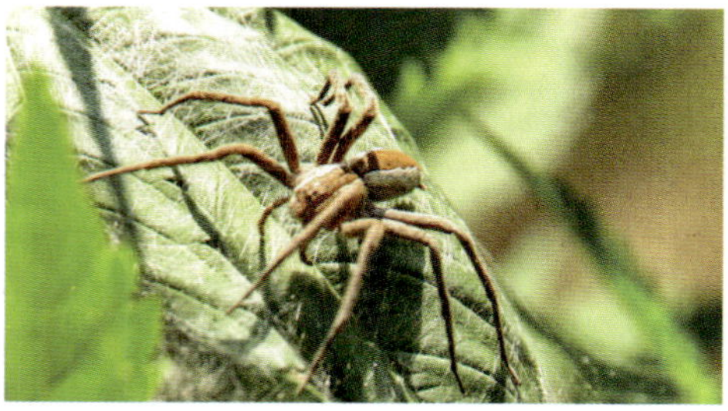

They might make you jump, but they are beneficial and eat pests.

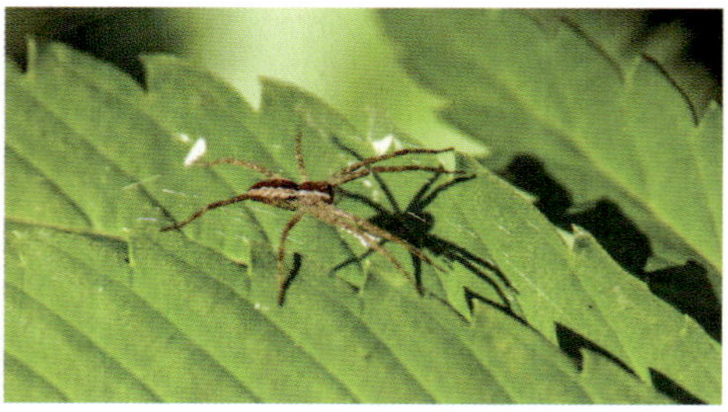

Spiders can cover a lot of ground, meaning they can spread far.

PHOTOS: ERIC PALMER (TOP), DAVID STRANGE (BOTTOM)

Recovering from a Pest Invasion

There are times when pests emerge victorious, regardless of how much you spray or apply control measures. When this happens, it may be necessary to create a clean environment or locate another growing area. This process involves a complete and total removal of your current harvest to prevent reintroducing any pests or diseases into your new crop.

Do not reuse any of the affected plants. If you wish to preserve certain strains by cloning, be very discerning about what you select and implement a thorough quarantine procedure to confirm their freedom from pests. This is particularly important because pest eggs are often minuscule, making them nearly invisible or concealed within a leaf. It cannot be stressed enough that just a few eggs are sufficient for the recurrence of the same pest. In some cases, tiny pests like spider mites can lay their eggs within cuttings and remain undetected during pest inspections because of their inconspicuous nature. While pesticides should have effectively eliminated these pests, certain species, such as powder bugs, lay their eggs inside the stems, resulting in their recurrent presence. If you are unable to eradicate such resilient pests, you may be compelled to discard all your plants and obtain new ones. For breeders, this can be an arduous challenge, as a few resilient bugs can wreak havoc in the grow room, potentially jeopardizing long-term projects. Therefore, breeders must remain vigilant about maintaining a clean grow room.

It is essential never to introduce any item from outside into your grow room without thorough cleaning—especially when it comes to cuttings, which must undergo a rigorous quarantine process to prevent potential pest contamination.

If you are growing indoors, set up a separate small grow room, or several grow tents, to support some cuttings and clones. Take cuttings from the affected plants and transfer them to a clean space. Eventually, you can reintroduce these cuttings to your main grow room to continue cultivating those strains.

Take all of your grow equipment, excluding electrical equipment, to the bathroom for thorough cleaning. Use bleach to clean all equipment and let it soak in a tub filled with water and bleach for a day. Electrical equipment should be cleaned with a cloth.

The number of repeat applications of bleach needed to clean the grow area is typically specified in the instructions, but it is often left to your discretion. More repetitions enhance your chances of preventing a pest recurrence.

When cleaning your grow room, begin with the walls, using bleach if possible. In some cases, you may need to repaint the walls. Cleaning tent canvas is much easier. However, if you use Mylar, it should be replaced after a pest infestation. Do not reuse Mylar, as some pests can attach themselves to it. Don't overlook the corners. Clean out any holes, extraction holes, fittings, pipes, and other areas. Then proceed to clean around the room's perimeter or tent.

After the initial cleaning, consider using pest-killing smoke bombs, available in most grow stores. Follow the instructions carefully and release the smoke bomb in the room. This ensures the elimination of pests, eggs, and larvae. The product labels often recommend reapplication 7 to 10 days after the initial treatment. After the second treatment, clean the room again as before. Repeat the process if necessary. Frequent cleaning increases the effectiveness of pest removal. Fumigation products release chemicals that can be absorbed by the plants' leaf tissue, so refrain from using them when plants are present.

After following these steps, you should have a clean room, free of pests. Dust off the electrical items before returning them to the grow room. Dry the other grow equipment that has been bleached and place it back in the grow room.

Always inspect cuttings for pests. No plants should be reintroduced to the clean grow room until you have taken cuttings from these original cuttings. You will need to cultivate these cuttings for a few weeks and monitor them daily for signs of pests. You may have to use pesticides on the cuttings. Once you are confident that the cuttings are free of pests, take new clones from them. Place these new cuttings in your grow room and closely observe their progress, remaining vigilant for any signs of pests or bugs. If you have followed these steps correctly, you should have eradicated all pests and can safely restart the strain. Cloning twice to ensure the pests are gone may not always be an option, but it can save you from having to go through the process again, especially in cases of severe pest infestations with egg deposition.

Fungi and Molds

Now we turn our attention to mold and fungi. These issues can often arise as by-products of pests that secrete honeydew, serving as a potential vector for the proliferation of fungal spores.

Fungi encompass a variety of microorganisms, diseases, and organisms that thrive by extracting nutrients from plants. This category includes molds, mushrooms, toadstools, rusts, and lichens. Lichens, in particular, lack chlorophyll and grow by acquiring nutrients from plants. Molds, which typically thrive in high-humidity conditions, can usually be controlled by increasing the flow of fresh air into the grow room. Fungicides are effective for eliminating fungi.

Botrytis Fungus

Botrytis fungus, commonly referred to as gray mold, gray blight, or botrytis blight, is the most prevalent fungal issue afflicting cannabis plants. It begins its infestation as

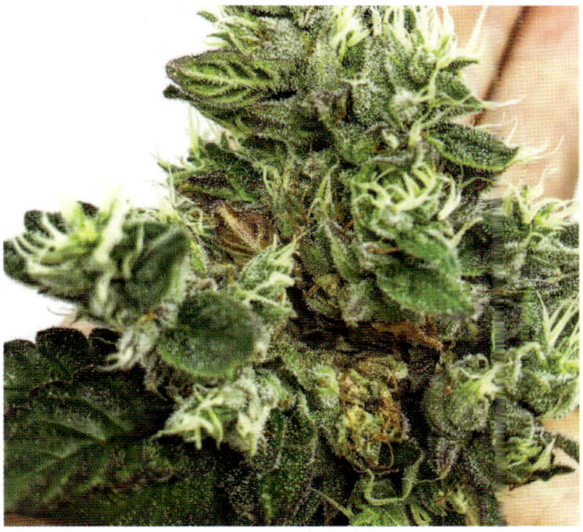

Botrytis-infected flowers starting to rot and looking ill.

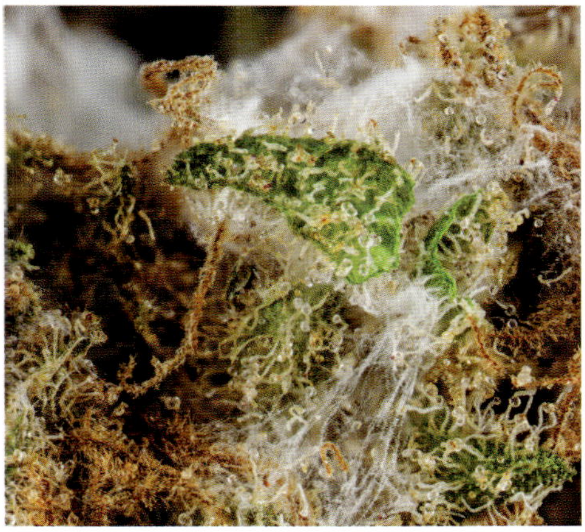

Mold grows like webbing because the fungi filaments are growing.

a white, powder-like growth, gradually transforming into gray as it advances. Note that mold and a pest infestation can sometimes appear deceptively similar due to their dusty appearances. A valuable technique for distinguishing between the two is to observe the affected area for any signs of movement, as pests are typically mobile.

Fungi, including botrytis, release spores that can spread to nearby plants. Because they can lie dormant for extended periods, it is imperative to address botrytis across all nearby plants. Fungus self-propagates through spore dissemination, often evading detection. Notably, these spores do not necessitate a living host to remain viable and can survive in various environments. Consequently, thorough cleaning of the grow room following a botrytis outbreak is essential. Swift resolution of a botrytis problem can prevent the production of spores or keep their numbers so minimal that the issue remains inconspicuous. Fungi are not easily eradicated by manual cleaning, so the affected plant areas typically need to be pruned away.

When searching for fungi, focus on damp areas, such as the growing medium surrounding the plant, as botrytis can thrive wherever it comes into contact with plant nutrients. Fungi are particularly drawn to necrotic plant tissue or other compromised areas of the plant where nutrients are readily available. The fungus then spreads to other parts of the plant, inducing rot. Sections that have been cut during pruning and cloning are particularly vulnerable to botrytis. The presence of moisture and plant damage creates ideal conditions for fungal growth and serves as a prime site for honeydew deposits by pests. These deposits create a perfect environment for the proliferation and spread of fungi. Proper humidity management can help maintain an optimal relative humidity (RH) level, which can either slow down fungal growth or bring it to a halt. In cases of severe fungal issues that require swift resolution, increasing dehumidification may be necessary to prevent the entire crop from being affected.

PHOTOS: TRICHOME ART

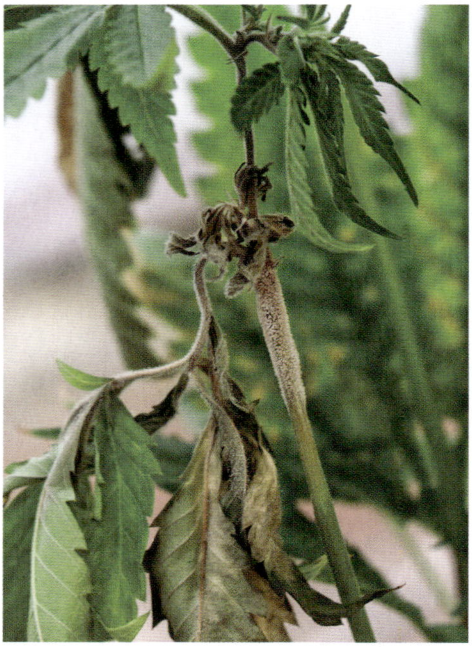

Fusarium is a common type of fungi. There are many more types but they are all very similar in appearance and can be treated the same way.

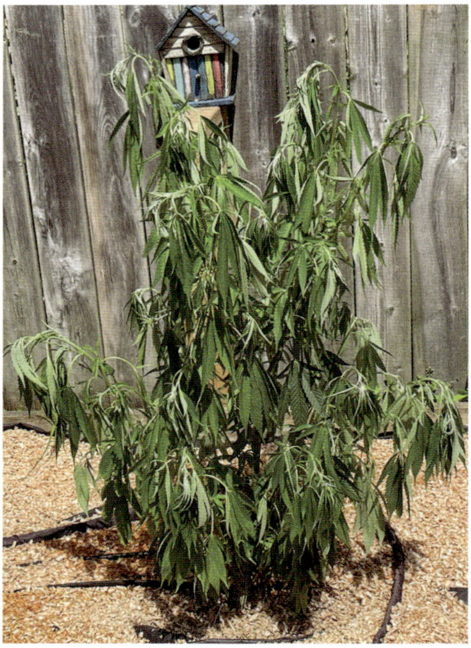

Fungi wilt is like overwatering but with mold on the stems and leaves. This plant won't survive.

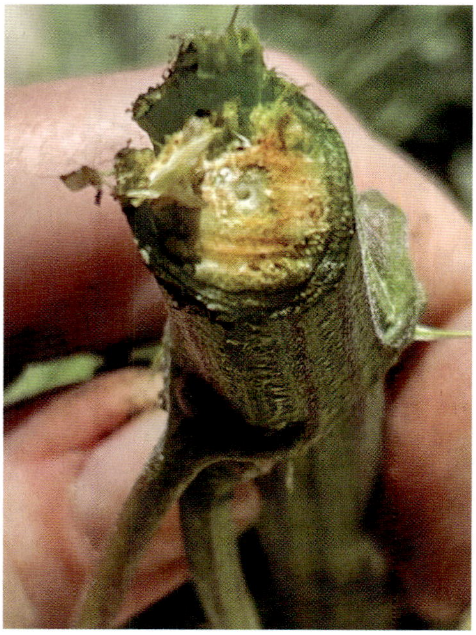

Mold can also rot inside the plant's branches. The fungus is in the middle, spreading out.

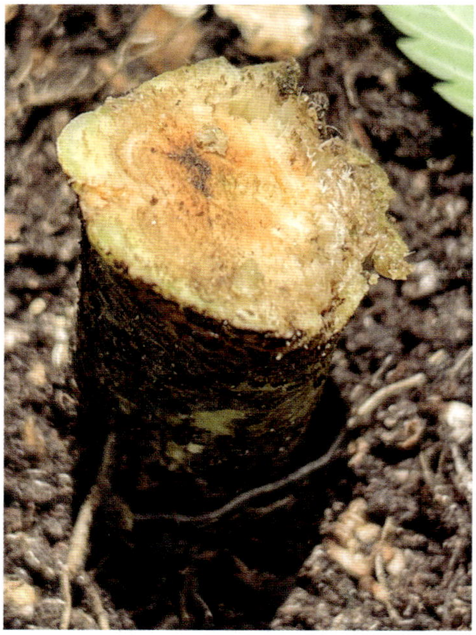

The stem can also suffer a fatal fungi infestation rotting through. This plant will eventually collapse.

PHOTOS: MANDALA SEEDS (TOP LEFT), TANYA PETERSEN (TOP RIGHT AND BOTTOM ROW)

Fusarium

Fusarium is a diverse genus of fungi It is filamentous, making it look like fluffy cotton, and spreads like mold, acting as a plant pathogen. Fusarium causes many problems, including fusarium wilt, root rot, and stem rot. Treating fusarium requires catching it early and applying fungicides. Removing infected plants and ensuring low humidity and good air circulation will prevent it from spreading. To prevent this fungus, thoroughly clean and sterilize your grow equipment. Use fresh soil and avoid overwatering, as fusarium thrives in swampy conditions. Consider selecting strains resistant to fusarium if it is a common disease in your area.

Mold

Managing mold follows a similar approach. Reducing humidity levels may suffice, but if the problem persists, the application of a fungicide to the affected areas becomes essential to prevent rot. As spores tend to settle downward, remove the top layer of soil from the infected plant and discard it. After the harvest, conduct a thorough cleaning of a previously contaminated grow area to prevent further fungal growth during subsequent crop cycles.

To access the most up-to-date list of fungicides recommended for cannabis by agricultural programs, do some research to discover a suitable brand that is both accessible and effective in your region

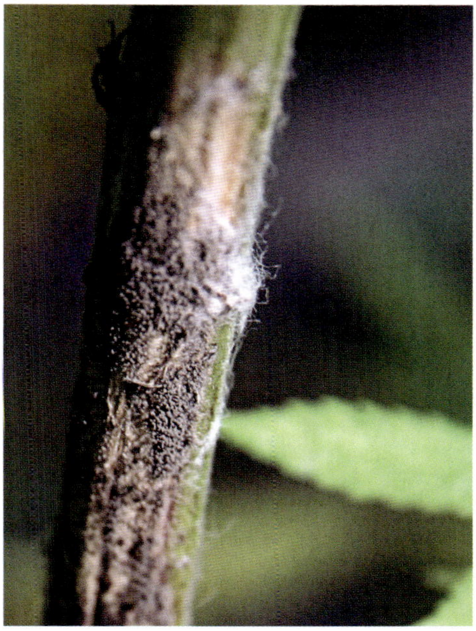

Mold on stem.

Powdery Mildew

Powdery mildew is a common fungal infection that can swiftly infiltrate a crop. As with botrytis and mold, effective prevention is possible through proper ventilation and the maintenance of low humidity levels.

Powdery mildew follows a life cycle that mirrors that of botrytis, beginning with soft white growth that eventually produces spores. Unlike botrytis, powdery mildew retains its soft white appearance without transitioning to gray. While powdery mildew is relatively easier than botrytis to physically remove from plants, it compensates with its rapid spread, often blanketing the plant's leaves in a white film. Furthermore, powdery mildew negatively impacts photosynthesis and results in stunted growth. It can also lead to bud decay. The techniques used to manage botrytis can similarly be used to control powdery mildew.

PHOTO: DAVID STRANGE

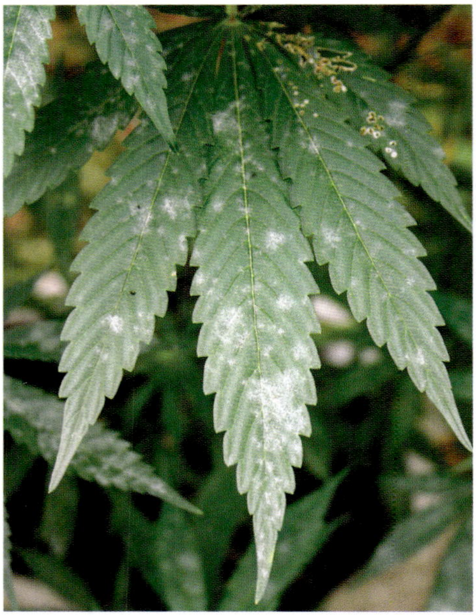

As blotching grows it more resembles fungi. The yellowing near the base is a downy mildew.

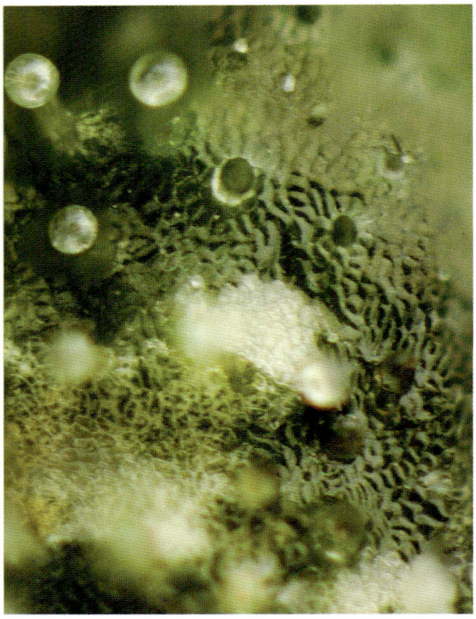

Early stages of powdery mildew spreading between trichomes.

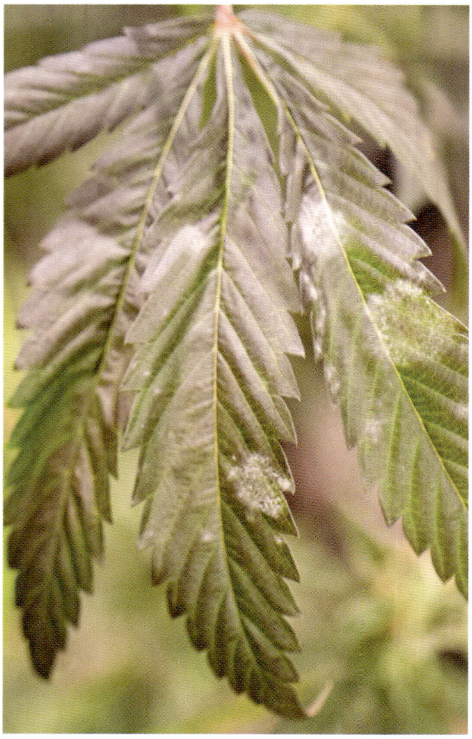

The mid-stage of an attack of powdery mildew; this is visible to the eye.

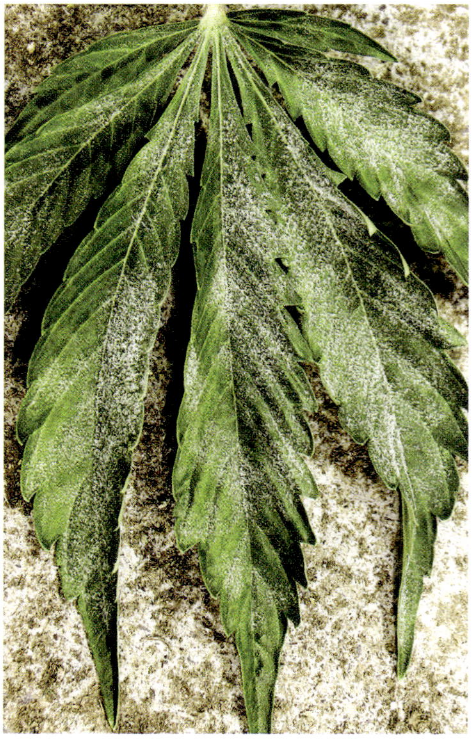

The latter stages of powdery mildew collapsing the leaf structure.

PHOTOS: DAVID STRANGE (TOP LEFT), TRICHOME ART (TOP AND BOTTOM RIGHT), DINAFEM SEEDS (BOTTOM LEFT)

Fungus and mold issues are frequently associated with the presence of pests or directly caused by them. Vigilantly monitor and address pest infestations to mitigate fungal and mold problems, especially those stemming from high humidity and excessive moisture content. Since some of these factors may be uncontrollable outdoors, when outdoor conditions pose insurmountable challenges, moving cultivation indoors offers the advantage of controlled RH levels.

As climate change contributes to higher humidity in some regions, cannabis breeders will need to focus on developing strains with enhanced resistance to fungi and mold. This approach ensures that even in such environments, productivity remains high. Furthermore, cultivating resistant strains allows for the adaptation to other regions experiencing similar challenges, thereby promoting the resilience of the crop in a variety of environmental conditions.

Root Rot

Root rot is a waterborne disease that poses a severe threat to cannabis plant roots. This condition has the potential to lead to the rapid deterioration of a crop, manifesting symptoms that can often be confused with nutrient disorders, overwatering, or underwatering. One of the most prevalent symptoms associated with root rot is wilting. While several variations of root rot exist, they are generally addressed through similar methods.

The primary catalyst for root rot is inadequate water drainage. Root rot thrives in conditions where both water and soil are poorly aerated; this can arise from the choice of growing method as well as the natural composition of the soil. Note that dead roots from previous crops can contribute to the onset of root rot. You can prevent root rot with your selection of suitable soil types and effective water aeration.

Root rot hinders a plant's access to water and essential nutrients by attaching itself to the roots and effectively smothering the plant. It also often results in a rise in pH levels. In hydroponic systems, the root tips may appear burnt—although note that some nutrient products can also discolor the plant roots. In the advanced stages of root rot, the roots look like they are covered in a brown, slimy substance resembling dead algae. Eventually, the base of the plant begins to deteriorate, leading to the plant toppling over. Once a root succumbs to root rot, it remains dead. While the plant can grow new roots, it is unable to regenerate the lost ones. This condition imposes significant stress on the plant, akin to the stress experienced in transplant shock.

Various products on the market are designed to eliminate root rot, some labeled as "root shields," others designated as "root fungicides." However, in the advanced stages of root rot, halting its progression is a formidable challenge. In severe cases, it may become impossible to completely eradicate the root rot, necessitating the cloning

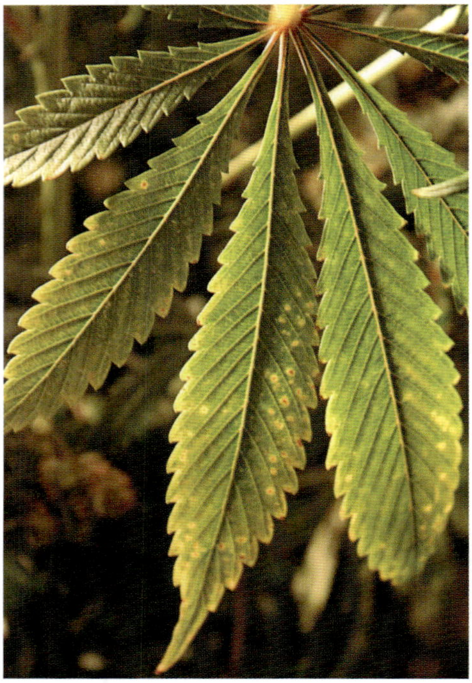

Chlorosis visible on a leaf indicates there is a nutrient problem of some sort.

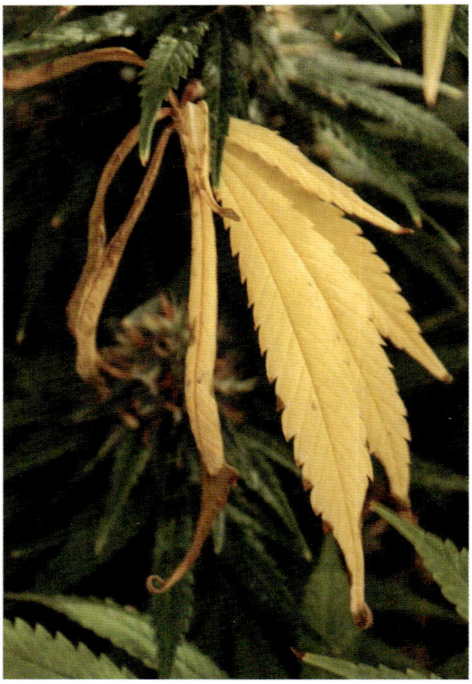

This leaf is completely yellow and dead. Remove it and keep an eye on your plant for other signs of problems.

of the plant to continue its genetic lineage. Recovery from root rot entails enhancing the aeration of the growing medium when feasible, coupled with the application of a root rot fungicide. Lowering the pH below 6.0 can help prevent the spread of root rot. In most instances, it is more prudent to remove severely affected plants to prevent the spread of the disease, especially in outdoor cultivation.

Root rot is significantly exacerbated by overwatering, which highlights the importance of efficient drainage systems, maintaining clean growing equipment, and using rooting gels or powders to reduce the risk of its development. The inclusion of Vitamin B1, or thiamine, can further stimulate root growth and contribute to overall plant health.

Chemical Burns

It is crucial to recognize that certain issues, such as chemical burns, incorrect pH levels, or nutrient disorders, may sometimes be mistakenly attributed to pest attacks.

Plants can experience chemical burns as a result of overfeeding. A plant with a chemical burn looks like a half-smoked joint: Shriveled gray ash at its tip with the burn gradually advancing towards the other end. The affected leaf curls downward and inward, assuming a claw-like shape at its tips.

PHOTOS: DAVID STRANGE

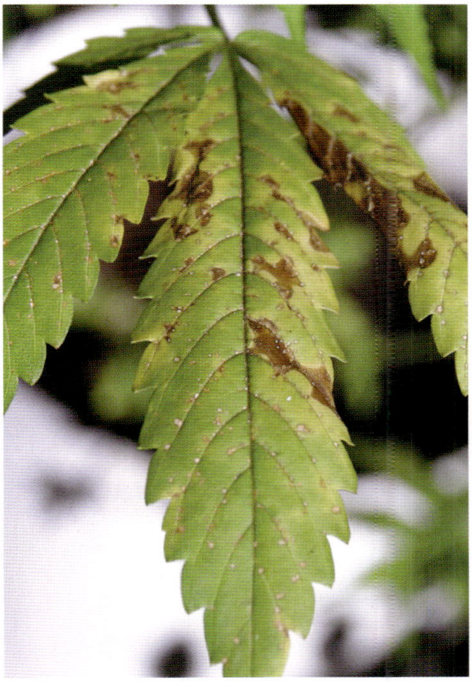

Signs of necrosis on this leaf. Over or under fertilization could cause this. Unhealthy leaves can be caused by a myriad of things.

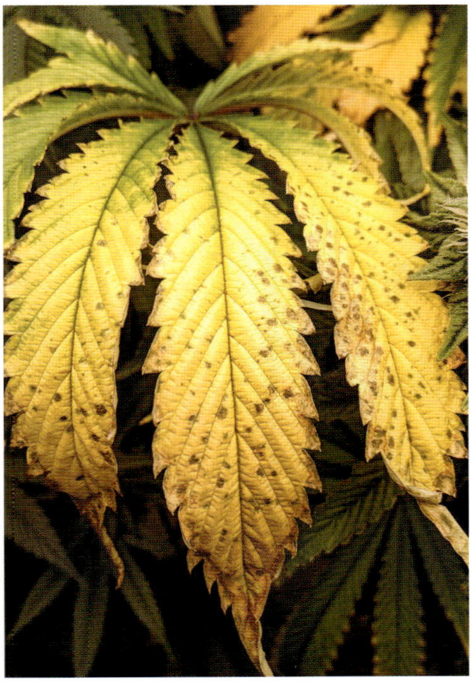

Necrotic tips and discoloration are a sign that the plant's problem is already serious.

Plants possess a vascular system responsible for absorbing water and nutrients, which are then transported to the lower fan leaves and then upward throughout the plant. The evidence of chemical burns often initiates at the tips of the fan leaves, gradually progressing towards the center and upward, leaving behind a brittle residue that disintegrates upon contact, characteristic of a chemical burn. The primary cause of chemical burns is overfeeding, possibly caused by soil with elevated nutrient ratios, using highly concentrated feeding mixtures, or nutrients administered too frequently.

To address chemical burns, refer to Chapter 15. If a solution to what seems like a chemical burn remains elusive, examine the pH level of the growing medium. Notably, pH-related issues can occasionally resemble the symptoms of chemical burns or nutrient deficiencies, and resolving the pH problem may alleviate the situation.

Nutrient Deficiencies

Identifying a nutrient deficiency is the ability to recognize cell collapse in a plant. It is characterized by a gradual loss of firmness in the leaves, resulting in a wilted appearance, typically accompanied by some form of discoloration. Although the affected portion of the plant may wither and die, it is important to distinguish this condition from a chemical burn. The primary distinction between a chemical burn and a nutrient

PHOTOS: DAVID STRANGE (LEFT), @TREETRUNK422 (RIGHT)

Nutrient Deficiencies Guide

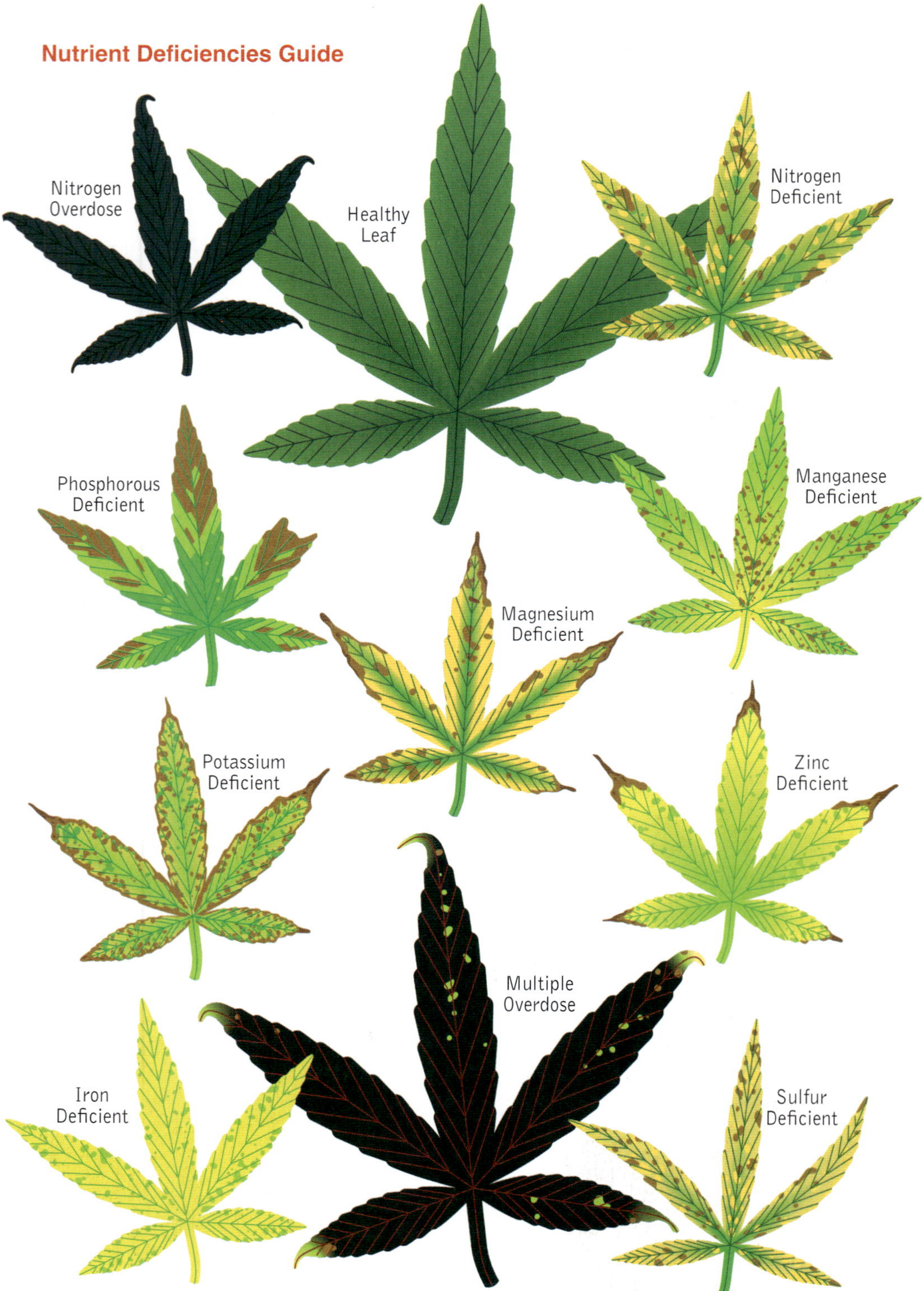

deficiency lies in their appearance. A nutrient deficiency should not resemble a chemical burn, and this distinction is vital for accurate diagnosis. Over time, with experience, you will become adept at differentiating between these two issues.

If you suspect a nutrient deficiency in your plants, check the pH levels, as an incorrect pH can exacerbate nutrient deficiencies. Address any pH-related concerns before embarking on any other corrective measures. If the problem appears to be associated with pH levels, the pH section in Chapter 8 provides comprehensive solutions to rectify such issues.

10 Steps to Saving Your Grow

Here is a concise, step-by-step guide to troubleshooting issues that will help you to identify and resolve problems in your grow. Before proceeding, review all the steps to gain a comprehensive understanding of how to address various issues, starting with the most common and proceeding to less likely scenarios.

Step 1: Begin your examination by closely inspecting your plants for any signs of insects or diseases. It is essential to distinguish between pest issues and nutrient problems, as they can sometimes be mistaken for each other. Look for black dots, indicative of pests, or leaves that appear discolored, dry, and wilted, suggesting a nutrient disorder. Movement on the plant indicates pests.

Pest damage often presents sporadically, affecting isolated areas before moving to others. In contrast, nutrient disorders tend to exhibit a more uniform pattern, affecting the plant linearly, either from bottom to top or top to bottom. This underscores the importance of regular monitoring to detect problems early, as untreated issues tend to become more challenging to resolve over time.

In summary, pest damage is random and sporadic, while nutrient disorders display a more consistent and linear pattern

Step 2: If your plant is in the vegetative growth stage, and you notice yellowing of leaves at the base slowly progressing upward without upward leaf curl, this indicates a need for more nitrogen (N). Similarly, if you observe slow growth, yellow leaves, and signs of wilting during the flowering stage, additional N is required. Nitrogen deficiencies can result in soft stems and pale green leaves, typically affecting older leaf growth first.

Severe nitrogen deficiencies can lead to stunted growth and eventual plant death. On the other hand, if your plant in the flowering stage exhibits a red or dark green/yellow appearance, it likely requires more phosphorus (P). Phosphorus deficiencies can also hinder root development and can cause stems to become either very rigid or weak, depending on the strain.

Step 3: If your plant's leaves exhibit curling, twisting, and yellowing, such symptoms are typically associated with heat stress. It may be that the light is causing burns or there is inadequate air circulation in the grow chamber. To address heat-related problems, refer to the grow room designs in Chapter 8 for solutions.

If these factors are not responsible for the problem, you may have to add magnesium (Mg) to your medium. Epsom salts can be an effective solution. Magnesium issues often begin with the yellowing, then curling upward of leaves, commonly referred to as "praying for magnesium." Necrosis is the eventual outcome of magnesium deficiencies, although a plant can still reach full maturity, albeit with below-average results.

Step 4: If the tips of the leaves turn brown and slightly curl, this is indicative of a potassium (K) deficiency. To rectify this, provide additional potassium to your plants. Potassium deficiencies may also result in red or purple stems, which can either be a genetic trait of the plant or attributed to a cold growing environment. For addressing cold growing environment issues, consult the grow room design section in Chapter 8.

Potassium deficiencies tend to affect new growth before progressing to older leaves. Stems may become soft or brittle, depending on the strain, and in severe cases, the plant may eventually perish.

Step 5: If your plant appears wilted with drooping or curling leaves, this could indicate root rot or a watering issue, which sometimes trigger nutrient-like deficiencies. For solutions to root rot problems, consult Chapter 15.

If these factors are not the true cause, inspect your soil. If your soil or medium is excessively damp or dry, refer to Chapter 8 information on watering practices and related issues and their respective solutions.

Step 6: If the veins of your plant's leaves remain green, but the rest of the leaf turns yellow, this points to an iron (Fe) deficiency. Iron issues generally manifest in new growth areas, which eventually become necrotic and die. To address this problem, supplement your plants with additional iron. While iron is not considered essential for plant growth, failing to address this issue will likely lead to below-average results. Note that iron deficiencies typically do not cause leaf curl initially, but as necrosis spreads, leaves may eventually curl.

Step 7: If your plant's leaves exhibit yellowing along the veins but remain unaffected at the tips without curling or twisting, this indicates a manganese (Mn) deficiency. Adding more manganese to your plants can address this problem. If the issue persists, necrosis may set in, and leaves may begin to curl. While manganese is not a requirement for plants to reach full maturity, the absence of manganese will result in below-average results.

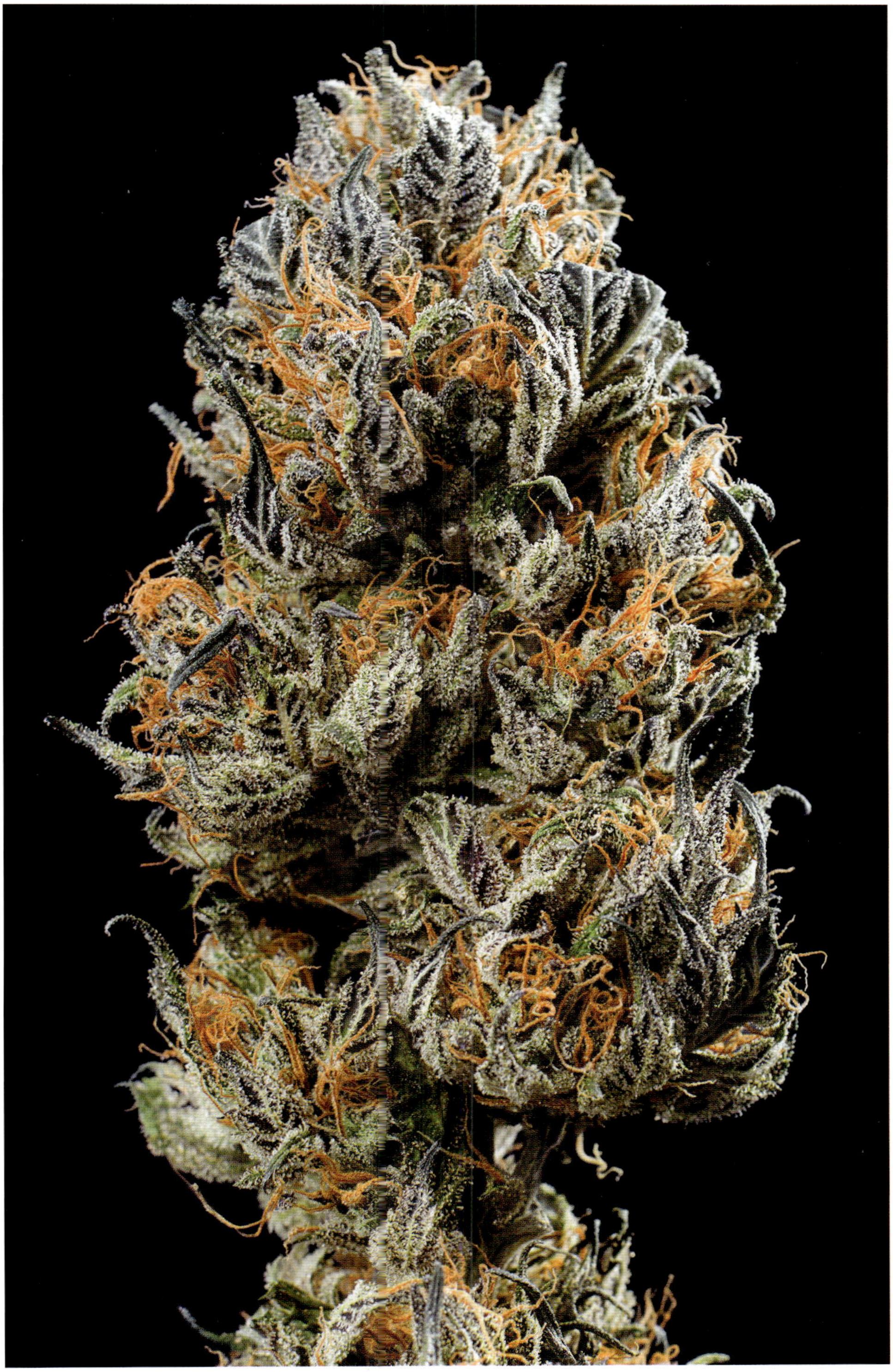

PHOTO: RUSSELL-HOWLAND PHOTOGRAPHY

Healthy buds come about by using best practice and getting to problems as early as you can.

Step 8: If the problem remains unsolved, introduce a secondary and micronutrient formula into your soil. This step should help resolve issues related to calcium (Ca), sulfur (S), copper (Cu), boron (B), zinc (Zn), and molybdenum (Mo) deficiencies. These deficiencies can be challenging to detect, and their symptoms may vary from strain to strain. By incorporating a secondary and micronutrient formula, you should be able to alleviate these problems.

Step 9: If you still haven't resolved the issue, it's time to flush your soil. Refer to the information in the nutrient sections in Chapter 6 and consider switching to a different brand of plant food that includes these elements: Nitrogen (N), phosphorus (P), potassium (K), calcium (Ca), magnesium (Mg), and sulfur (S). You could also add Epsom salts and such micronutrients as iron, boron, chlorine, manganese, copper, zinc, and molybdenum. Try using a nutrient mixture that has been mentioned previously.

Step 10: Your plant may be experiencing a nutrient lockout. If you've correctly followed the previous steps, you may have ruled out this issue. Nevertheless, nutrient lockout can occur when the plant cannot access certain nutrients, possibly the result of the absence of nutrients (deficiency) or a chemical reaction in the medium or solution. These reactions can create toxic substances that block the roots or alter the chemical properties of other nutrients. Factors like pH problems, unsuitable soil types, or the chemical content of treated water can occasionally lead to nutrient lockout. While such occurrences are rare, they may indicate the presence of substances that are incompatible with cannabis plant growth.

When in doubt, transplant your plant into fresh soil or a new hydroponic solution. Certain feeding products may contain active ingredients that do not work well with cannabis, leading to nutrient lockout. In hydroponic systems, you may need to change your nutrient solution. Keep in mind that out-of-date liquid feeding products can precipitate, causing nutrient lockout. Additionally, salt is a compound that can induce nutrient lockout. For resolving these problems, revert to Step 9.

If your plant appears pot-bound, or root-bound, or has outgrown its pot, the root mass reaching its maximum capacity may cause plant stress and issues that mimic nutrient problems. The remedy for this situation is to transplant the plant into a larger pot, following the transplant method described in Chapter 4.

No Cure for Bad Genetics

When all else fails, you may realize you have encountered a "bad seed." Regrettably, the market can be flooded with subpar genetics. Issues associated with poor genetics include mutations, deformities, flowering irregularities, and low germination rates. These genetic shortcomings often manifest as nutrient-related symptoms. In such cases, the only viable solution is to obtain new genetics, ideally from a different breeder. It's essential to communicate the issues you've faced to the seed source, ensuring they are aware of the problems. Some seed banks may discontinue a line due to consistent issues like poor germination rates or unreliable genetics, and your feedback can assist them in addressing such concerns.

Conclusion

By following the advice provided in this book, you can significantly reduce the likelihood of encountering these problems. Even if you do face them, early detection is more likely because of the precautions you've taken. Some people may be disheartened by losing a crop or achieving suboptimal results. However, it's crucial not to give up. What you gain from the experience is invaluable, and overcoming these challenges will provide you with knowledge that those who give up will never attain. Failure doesn't occur when a crop is lost; rather, it arises when a grower doesn't embrace the opportunity to conquer the problem. Remember: You have the potential to overcome these challenges.

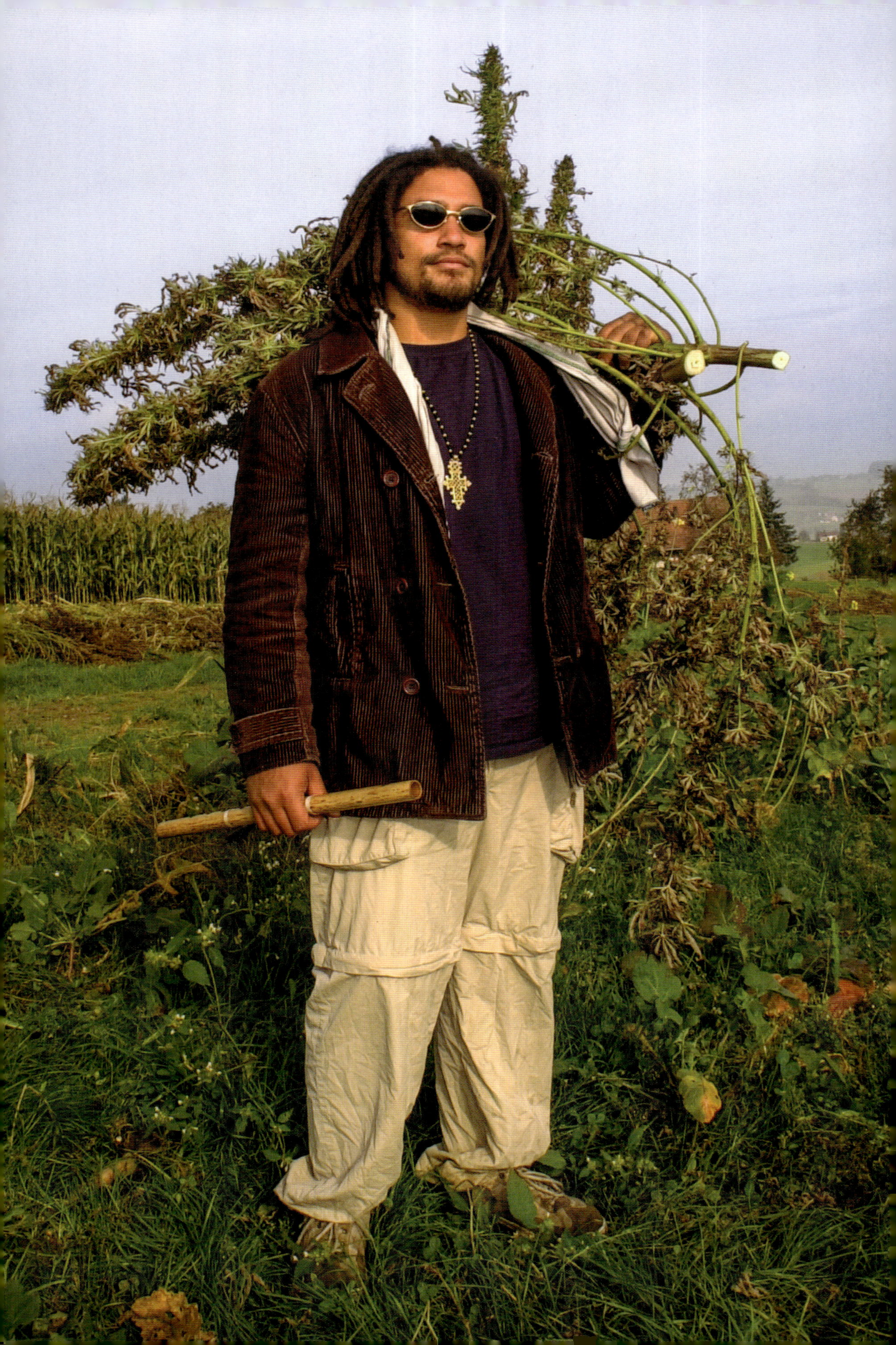

16

Harvesting and Curing Your Cannabis

Harvesting is when you reap the rewards of your efforts. If you followed the breeder's guidelines for flowering time and had a successful cultivation, the fruits of your labor will now establish a consistent supply of top-quality buds.

Before harvesting, read this chapter thoroughly to gain a complete understanding of the process. Planning your handling procedures will help retain more resin for processing instead of unintentionally decorating everything with your valuable cannabinoids. Throughout this process, you should make yourself aware of the distinctive aroma of a fresh harvest to appreciate the changes as the bud cures.

Dealing with Smells

Harvesting can be messy and smelly work. Fresh buds release a potent scent, and resin adheres to surfaces easily. To quickly suppress the smell after chopping down your plants, you will need sealed containers to store your harvested buds. You can wrap cannabis in a canvas spread to transport your harvest over short distances, such as from your grow room to your manicuring space. Canvas spreads made of hemp keep resin from brushing off in large amounts. Packed canvas will smell, however. Many indoor growers sacrifice growing in the flowering room for a few weeks and keep the harvest there to avoid these transportation issues. A carbon filter placed before the exhaust (active extraction fan) can also confine the smell.

Resin Sticks

Resin is very sticky and hard to wash off. After you harvest, your fingers will be covered in resin, which will stain everything from metal and plastic to clothes, furniture, paper, equipment, and even other pieces of bud. Resin on your fingers will destroy everything you touch, including the expensive digital camera you're using to take

PHOTO: ED BORG

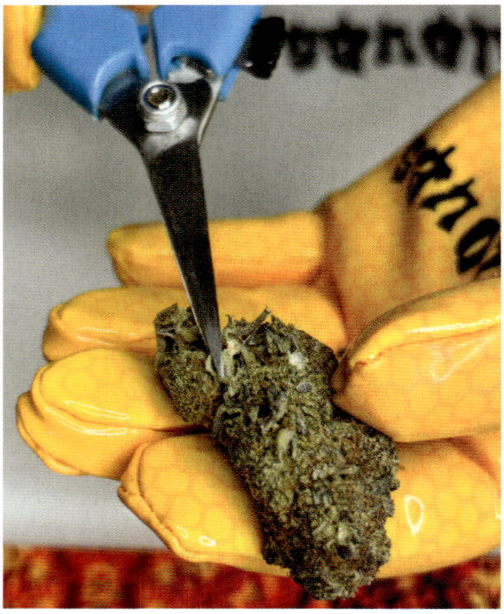

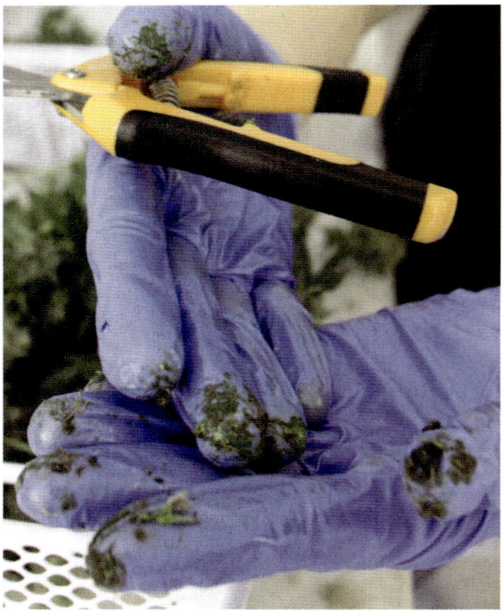

Rubber gloves prevent resin from getting on your hands, making them essential for manicuring.

pictures as you go. You must remove it with alcohol (fast removal) or scrub it off with a metallic cleaning pad. Hot water (slow removal) can work on objects that can be washed, but this method is time-consuming. Your best option to avoid this when harvesting your crop is to wear gloves. Latex gloves are best, as they can be turned inside out and frozen so you can remove usable resin after a few hours.

Label Everything

If you're growing multiple strains, establish a labeling system before harvesting to avoid mixing up your buds. Make sure to keep your buds separate from each other to know which strain you're using when it's time to sample the results of your hard work.

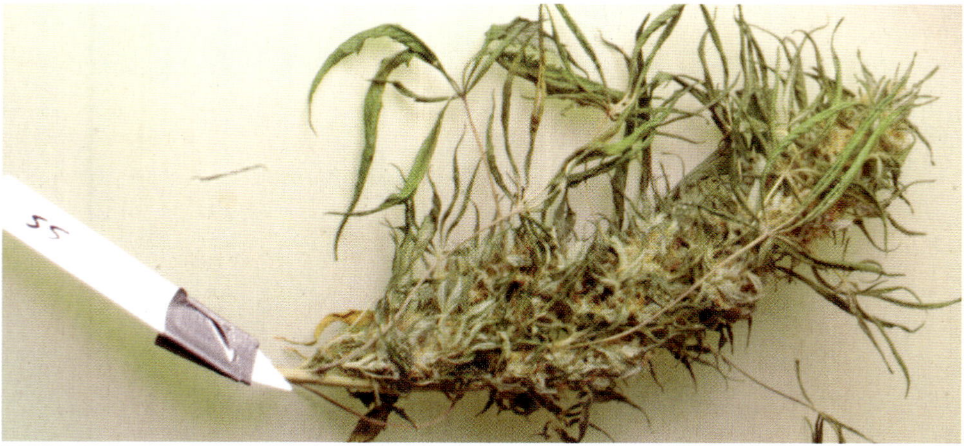

A label is taped to this dried branch of bud so it can be easily identified.

PHOTOS: SILIGLOVES.ORG (TOP RIGHT), PEACE NATURALS / PHOTOGRAPHED BY DAVID STRANGE (TOP RIGHT), ED BORG (BOTTOM)

Quick Bud Samples

Some growers can't resist a quick taste test before their bud is adequately cured. Such samples are typically harsh and may not accurately reflect the final quality of well-cured bud. If you are eager to sample quickly, there are quick drying methods. However, patience during the curing process yields superior results.

Sampling can be useful to help you judge when to harvest the plant in future grows. To speed up the drying process, take a fresh bud sample and put it on a dish. Place it in a microwave on medium power for about two minutes. If the bud does not feel dry and brittle yet, heat it a bit more. Once it feels dry and brittle, you can sample it. The taste will be harsh, and the microwave heat will destroy a good portion of the cannabinoids in the bud, but you will get an idea of the plant's characteristics.

Another way to produce a quick sample is to put some fresh bud onto a sheet of paper, fold the paper, and press the bud down lightly. Place the paper on a working radiator, or in the oven at a low proving temperature (around 100°F/ 38°C) and let the heat dry the bud. When you check your bud later in the day, it should be dry enough to use. You will get similar results if you leave fresh bud to dry for a few days in an airing cupboard.

However, the best method for preparing your harvest is always curing before use.

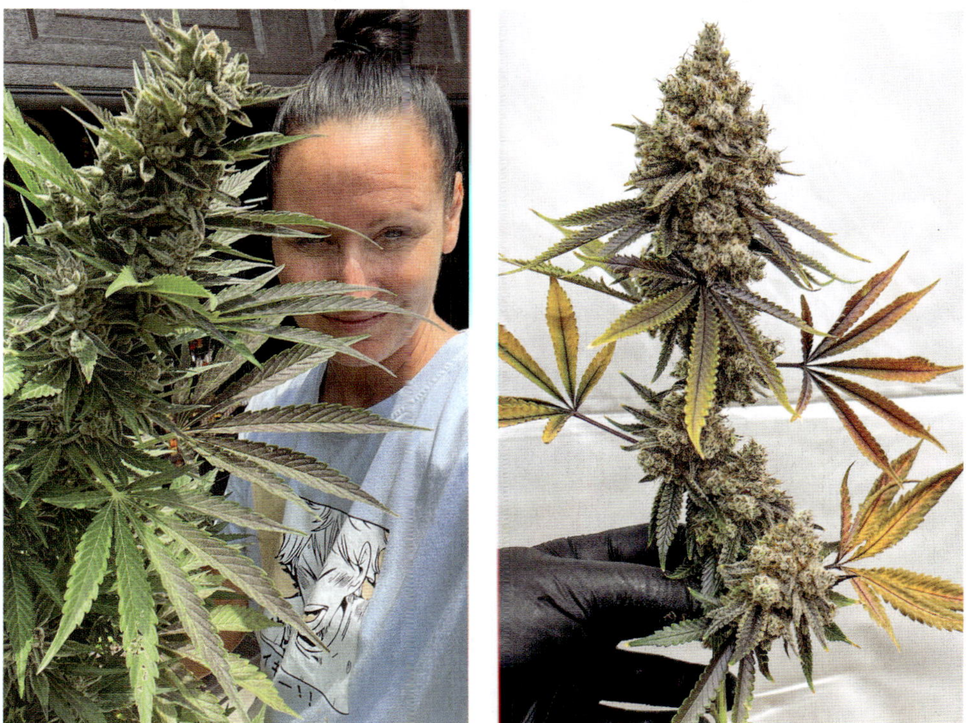

PHOTOS: TANYA PETERSEN (LEFT), TRAVIS HOELLERER @SOFAKINGHIGH (RIGHT)

These freshly selected colas are full of resin-packed flowers and ready for drying

Ready to Harvest

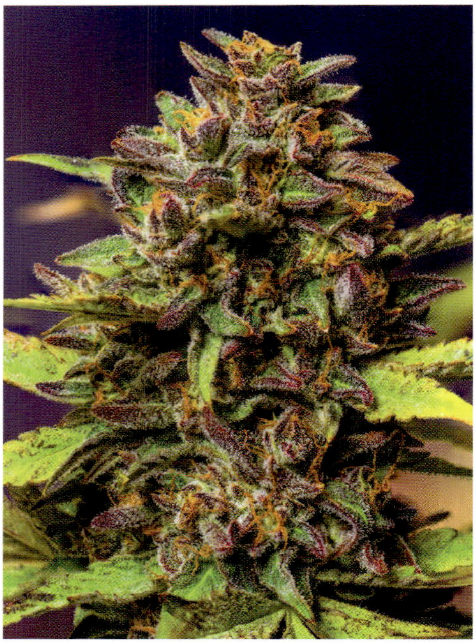
Divine Storm from In House Genetics.

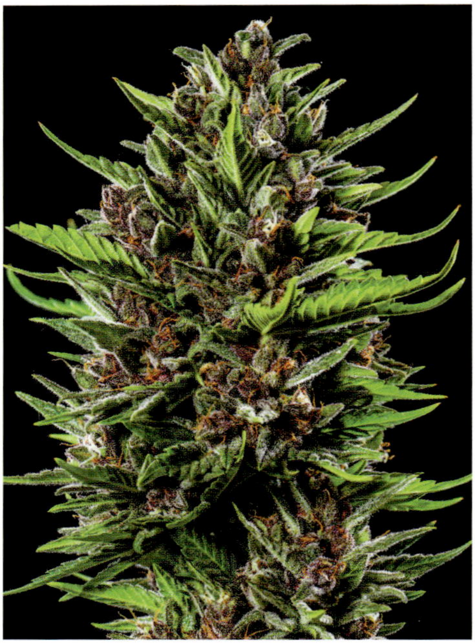
Strawberry Pie from Fast Buds.

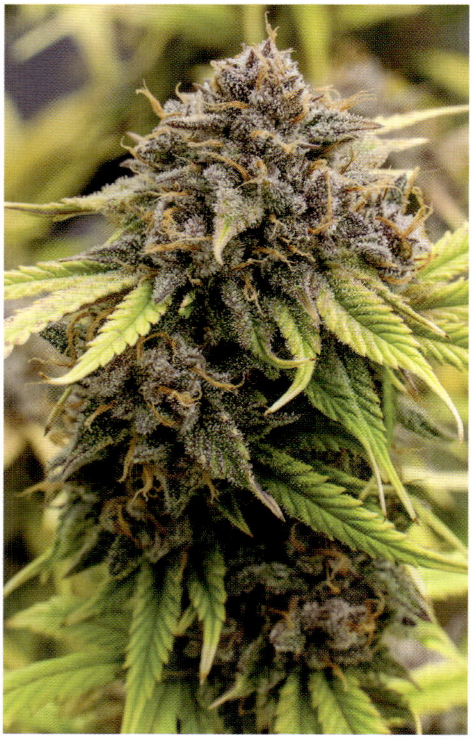
Durbin Twist from Twenty20 Mendocino.

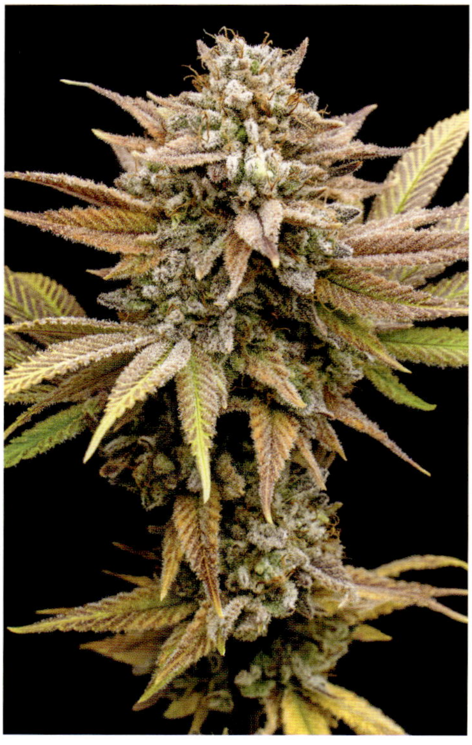
Secret Sauce from Twenty20 Mendocino.

PHOTOS: ERIC PALMER (TOP ROW), JOE'S CANNA GROW (BOTTOM ROW)

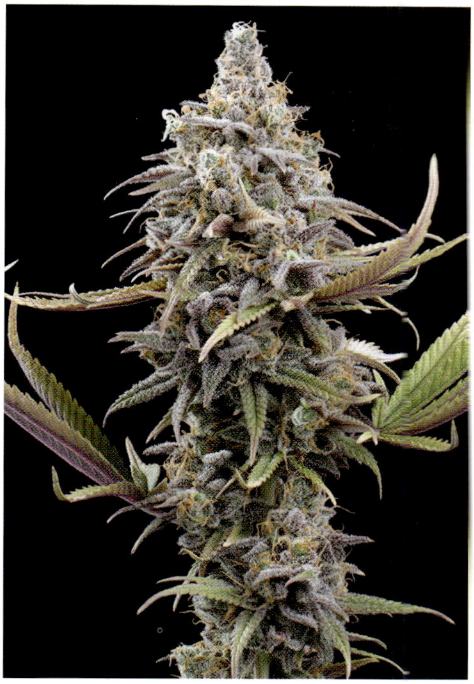

Apollo XX from Brothers Grim.

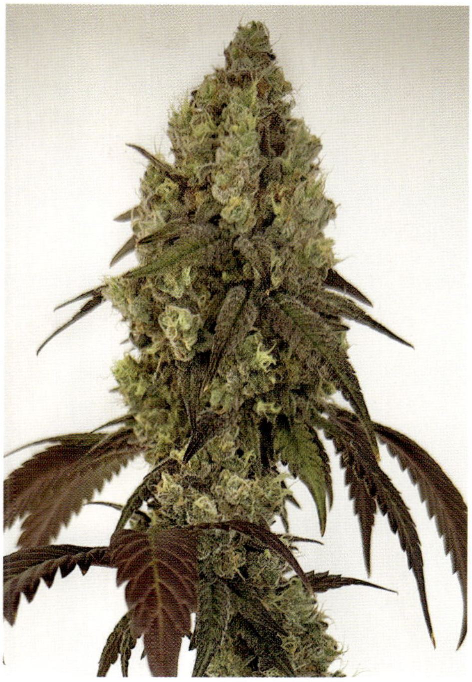

Overtime from Bulletproof Genetics.

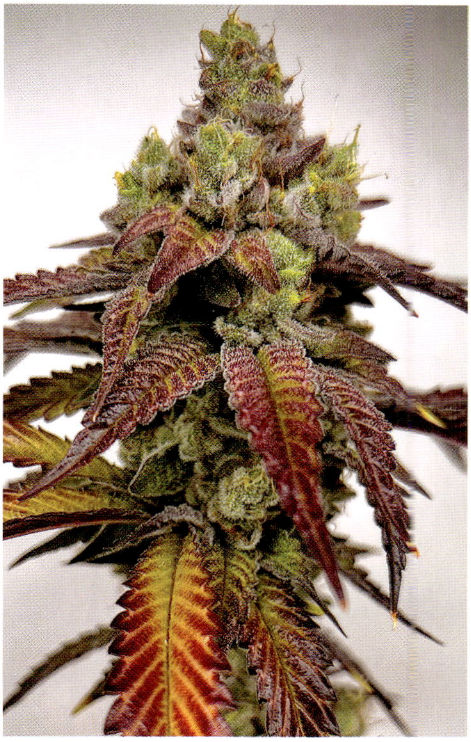

Dream Factory from Exotic Genetics.

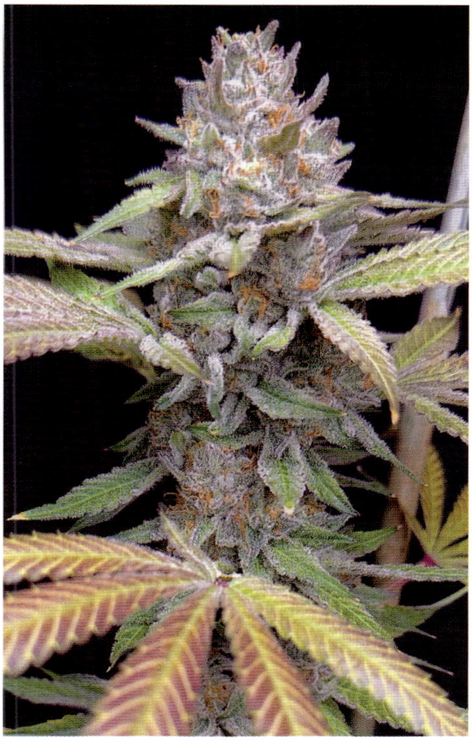

Lemon Cherry Fop from Cookies.

PHOTOS: RUSSELL-HOWLAND PHOTOGRAPHY (TOP LEFT), RYAN GABEY (TOP RIGHT AND BOTTOM ROW)

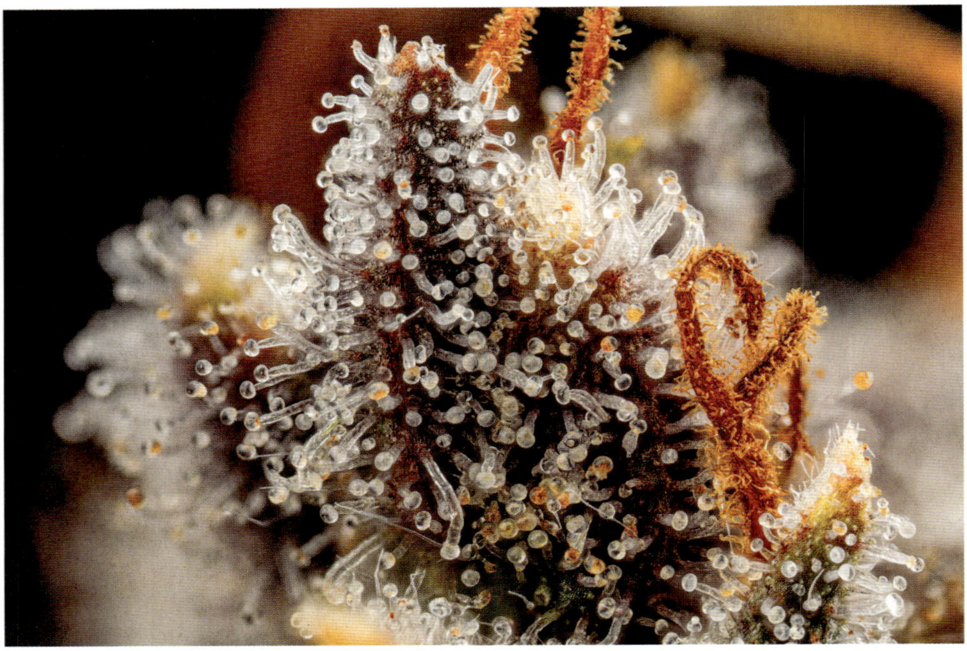
Pistils will take on a dark amber tint when the plant is getting ready for harvest.

Harvest Indicators

Inspect your buds at the end of the flowering stage to determine their ripeness and readiness for harvest. These indicators will help pinpoint the ideal harvesting time, but be aware that not all of them will appear in every strain due to subtle variations:

- About 50–70% of the pistils change color.
- The plants cease the production of trichomes.
- The trichomes stop growing.
- The buds stop growing.
- The fan leaves and lower leaves yellow and naturally fall off.
- The smell has reached its peak.

These indicators stem from both genetic factors and environmental influences and will only be evident in healthy plants receiving all the necessary nutrients. Remember that temperature and unbalanced nutrients can also lead to changes in color.

You can also determine the optimal harvest time by conducting multiple tastings of the same plant. Harvest plants from the same strain at different times and collect and label the bud pieces. If you have only one plant, take samples at various stages of flowering. Dry each sample and store it in a glass jar, noting the number of days the plant was in flower before the sample was taken. Repeat this process every few days until the final harvest. These samples can be tested to determine the strain's optimal

PHOTO: ROB BRAMHILL

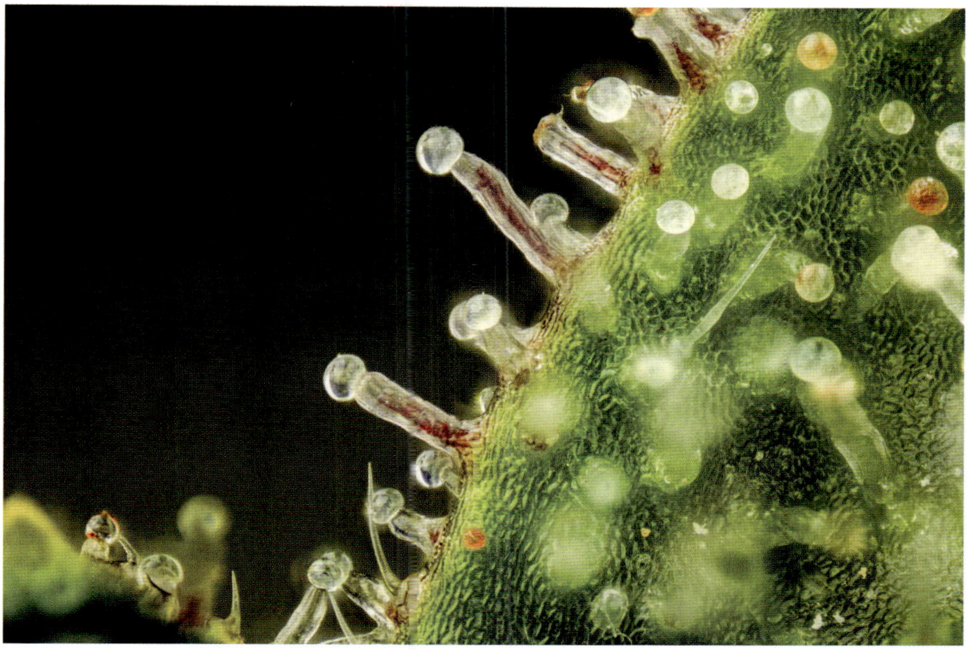

This Cosmic Queen at 10x resolution shows how trichomes are growing on the flowering leaves.

PHOTO: ROB BRAMHILL

harvest time. Label each sample with the exact date and make a note of your preference. The next time you grow the same strain, you'll have a precise harvest schedule down to the day.

The flowering times provided by breeders are generally accurate; however, cultivating a particular strain multiple times will undoubtedly refine your ability to pinpoint the optimal harvest timing.

Expert Harvest Indication

Observation will help you determine when to harvest. You'll need a magnifying aid and some experience. A good phone camera or simple 1.18-inch (30 mm) magnifying glass works well. As the pistils grow out from the calyx, they form resin glands, or trichomes, which gradually change color before shrinking and naturally withering. This alters the appearance of the pistils, causing them to fade and take on a somewhat burnt and dry appearance.

This transformation signifies the end of the blooming period, as trichomes are no longer needed for pollen collection. Resin may accumulate around these trichomes and, while the cannabinoid content is not lost, the resin will slowly convert into different psychoactive cannabinoid compounds. These cannabinoids will transform into other forms of THC and various psychoactive compounds. Exposure to light over time will continue to degrade cannabinoid compounds.

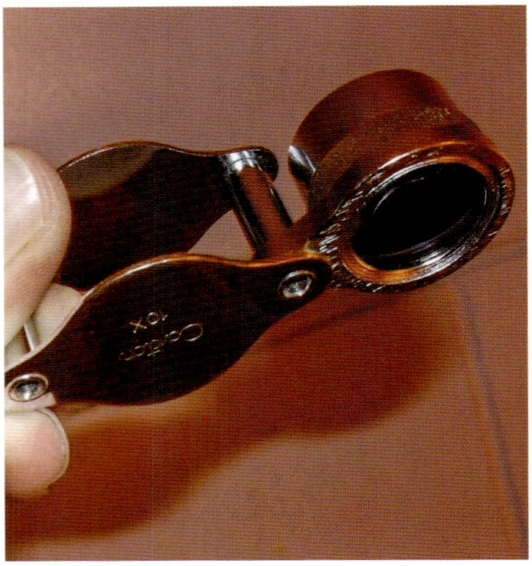
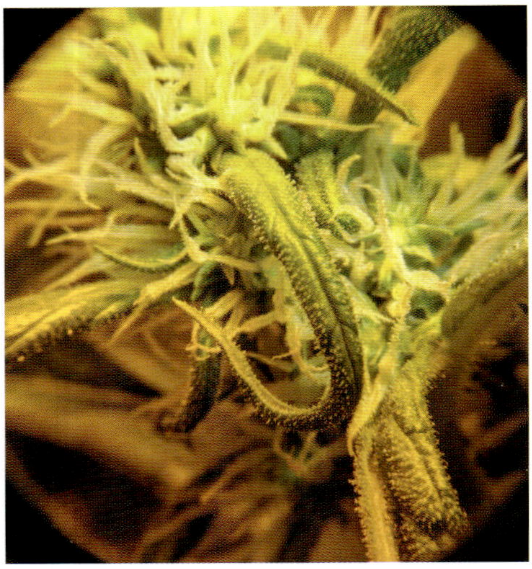

A handheld magnifying glass can help you to investigate the presence of trichomes in your flowers.

It will take up to two weeks before the plant's trichomes and pistils are completely withered. Even then, new trichomes and pistils may develop among the faded ones. This process continues until a change in the photoperiod or cellular breakdown occurs, leading to the plant's natural death, or until the grower intervenes by harvesting.

As the plant reaches its peak bloom, the pistils change color. You can observe this change in the trichomes using a magnifying aid. Check them daily to determine the best time to harvest. Pistils are white and turn to a cream color as they grow. As they turn cream, new white pistils also emerge, and the flower complexion becomes a mix of white and cream. As the flowers mature, the cream-colored pistils turn golden amber. Nearing harvest time, some golden amber pistils will turn orange, red, or brown. At this point, the flower complexion will be a mix of white, cream, golden amber, and brown. Darker colors indicate that the pistils are withering. By harvest time, you will have a low percentage of new pistils, a low percentage of withering ones, and the bulk will be a mature golden. At this stage, any of the significant bud mass on the plant, such as the top cola, may be observed as follows:

1. About 90% of the pistils have reached maturity.
2. Less than 5% of the pistils are withering.
3. Less than 5% of the pistils appear to be in the early stages of growth.

You should determine your harvest time by looking at the pistils that have reached maturity. Compare these to the ones that have passed their peak bloom and harvest the plant just before they reach this stage. This usually corresponds with the flowering time given by the breeder. For a plant with an unknown flowering time, you can use this expert method to predict when to harvest.

PHOTOS: LUKE SPARROW

Trichomes and Pistils

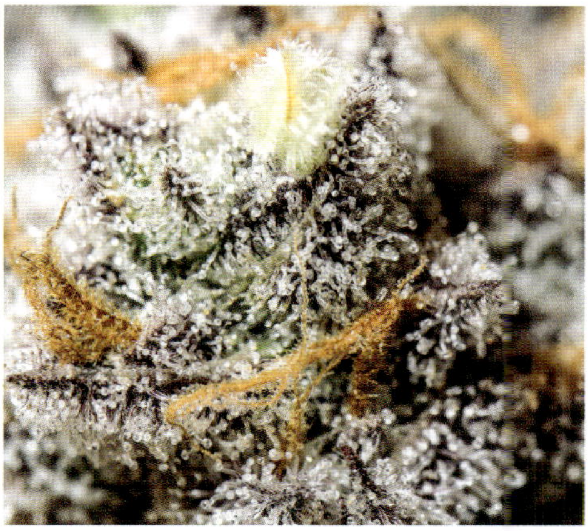

Trichomes covering calyx and pistils.

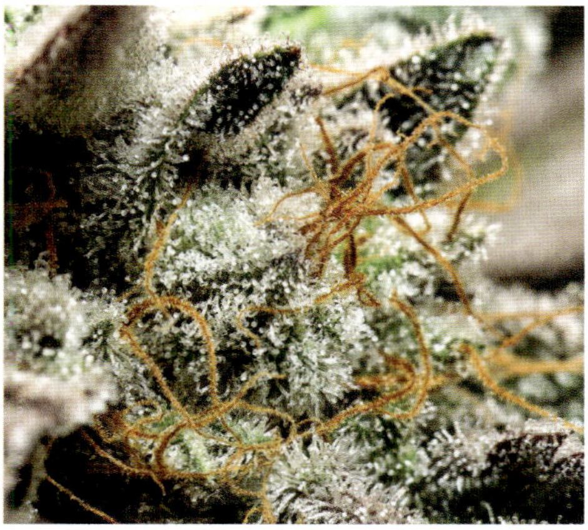

Pistils have noticeably changed to amber.

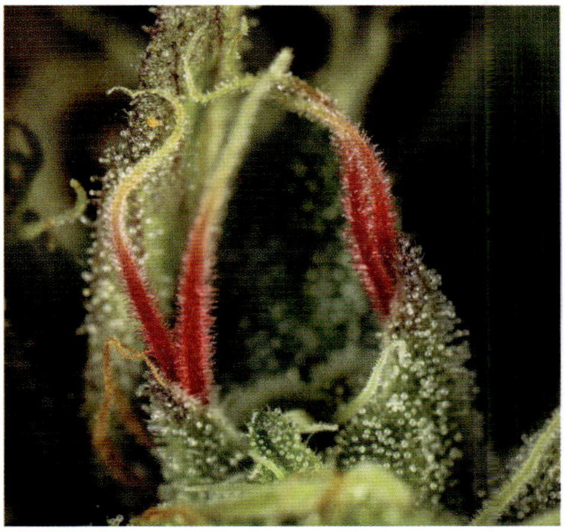

Pistils in the process of changing colors.

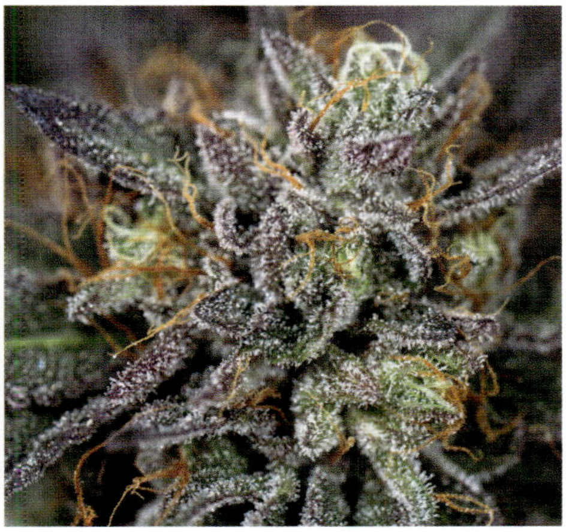

Purple strains are popular for their floral displays.

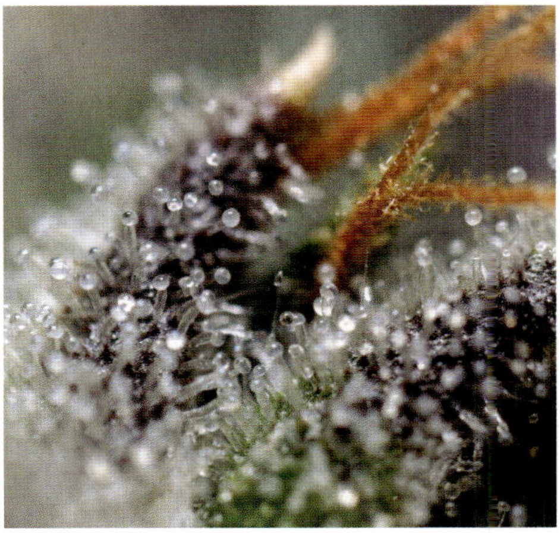

Darker purple/black bud.

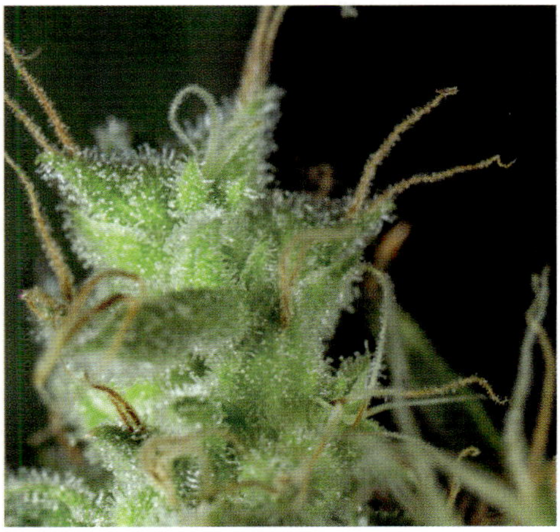

Lighter green/yellow bud.

PHOTOS: DANKSHIRE PHOTOGRAPHY (TOP ROW), BUBBLEMAN (MIDDLE AND BOTTOM ROW)

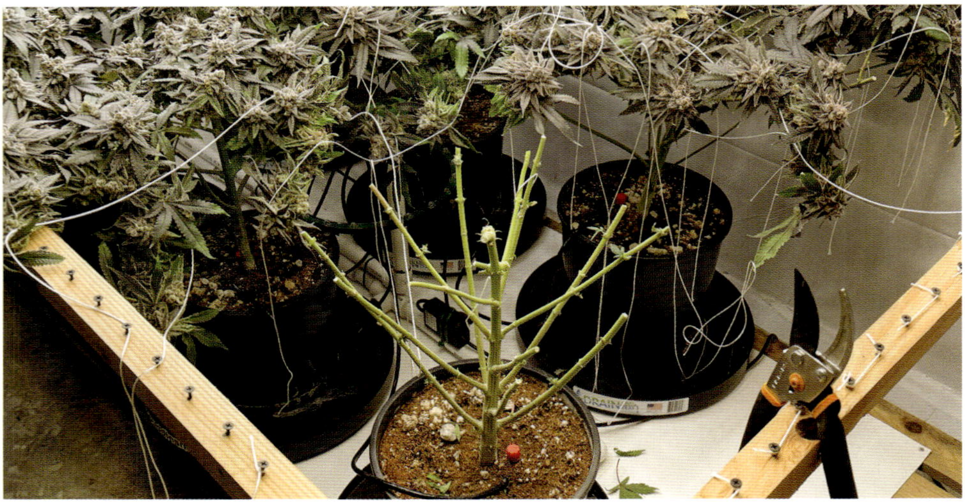

When harvesting, you don't have to pull the whole plant up with its roots. You cut away into manageable parts, such as branches and then main stem.

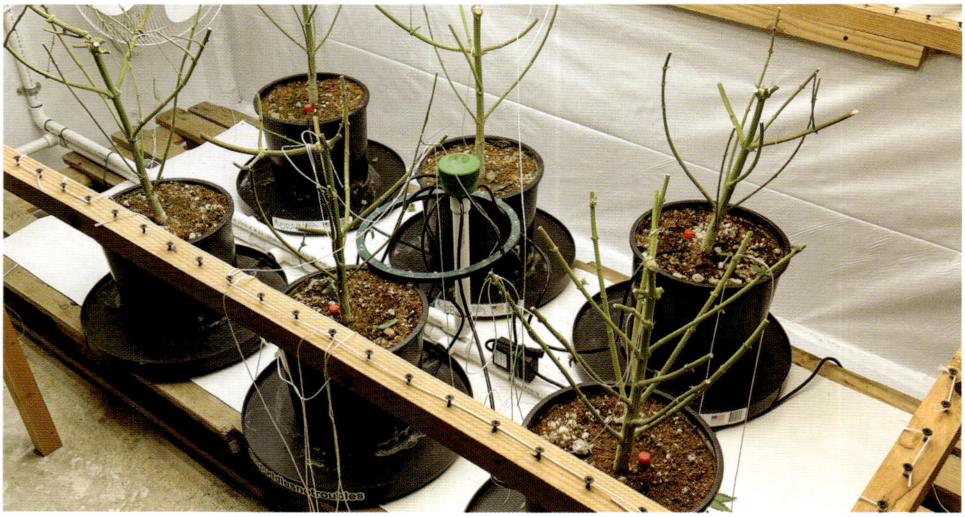

What remains of a ScrOG harvest: Just the stumps of branches and a stem in the growing medium.

PHOTOS: TRAVIS HOELLERER @SOFAKINGHIGH

Do not remove fan leaves, even if wilting occurs. Snip away necrotic parts, especially if the leaves come into contact with the ground, but let the leaves fall away naturally. Fan leaves contain sugars needed for the plant to maintain its health, including that of the floral clusters. Remove fan leaves only when necrosis has spread so much that you cannot simply snip away the affected parts of the leaf.

This process is all about carefully observing trichome color changes over time. Allowing the trichomes to grow past their peak or harvesting them early will affect the final product's cannabinoid ratios.

Trichomes at Harvest

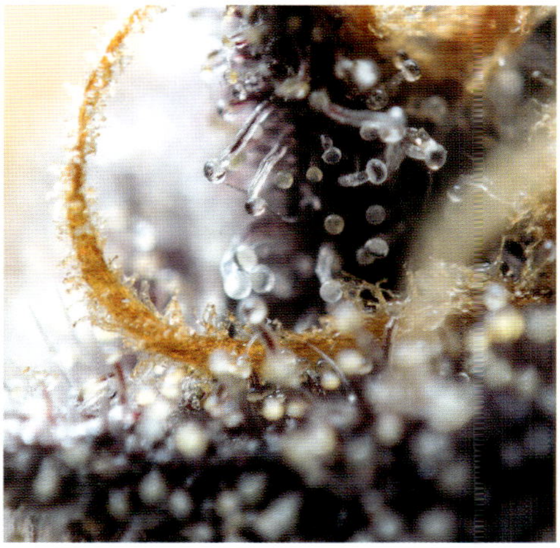

Naturally beautiful.

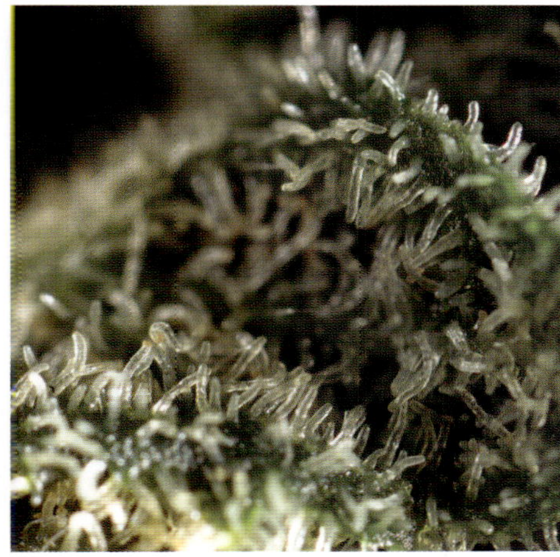

Each trichome packs cannabinoids.

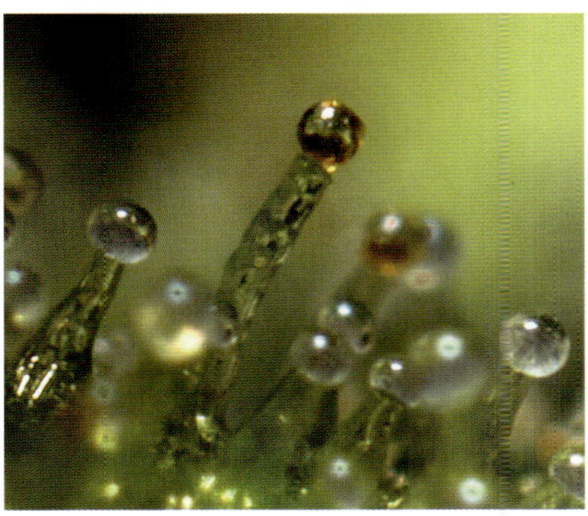

Bulbous head of the trichome.

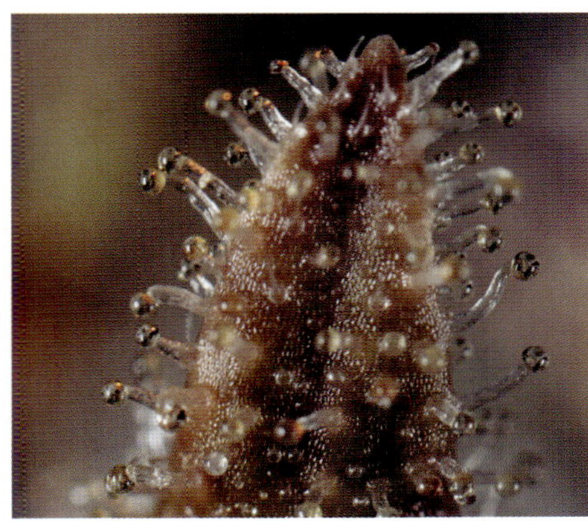

All these heads are still intact.

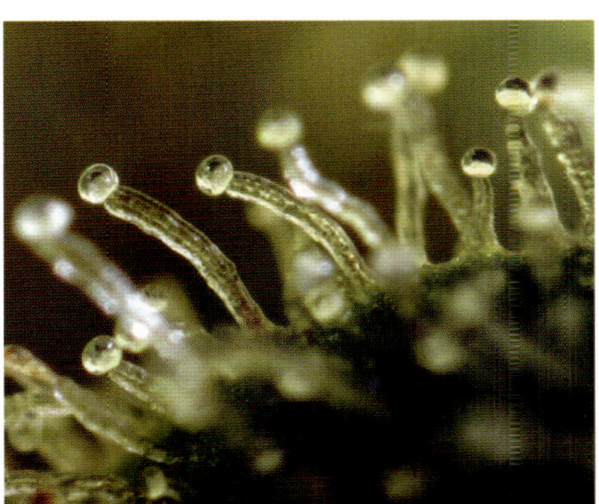

While many might burst, intact is what you want to see.

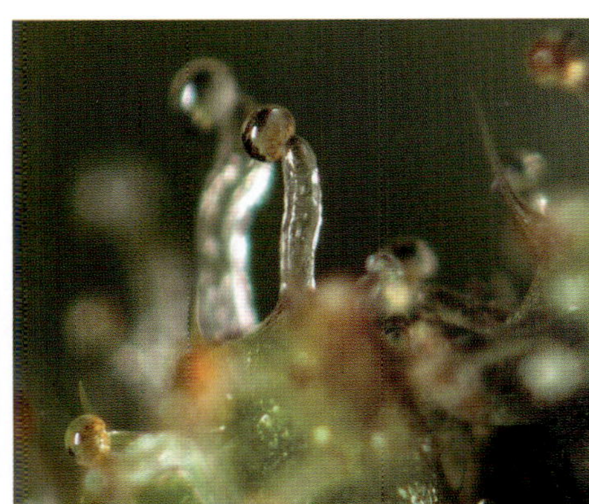

Healthy trichomes are your goal.

PHOTOS: DANKSHIRE PHOTOGRAPHY (TOP LEFT AND MIDDLE LEFT), BUBBLEMAN (ALL OTHERS)

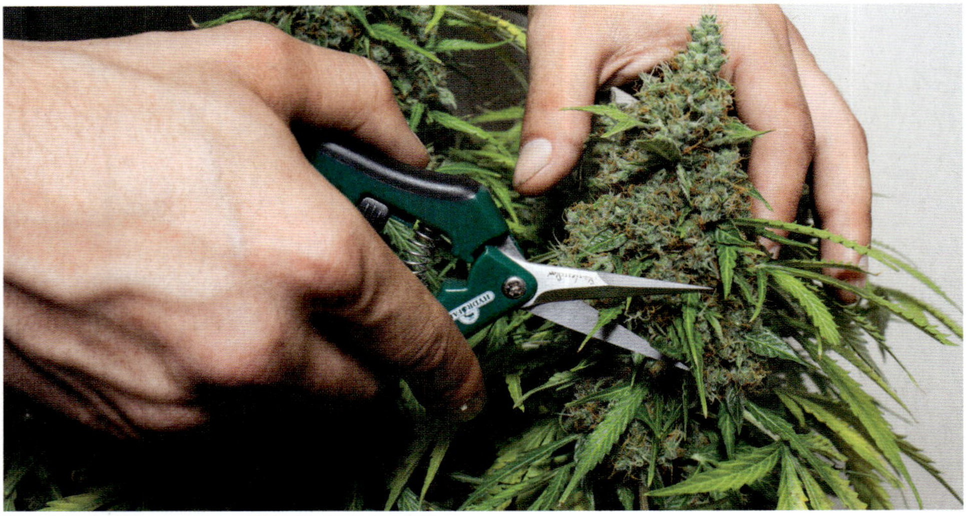

A quick preliminary trim can be done to remove the more obvious leaves from a cola before hanging it up to dry.

PHOTO: DAVID GRAU FOTOGRAFIA

Harvesting for Cerebral or Body Effects

The timing of your harvest plays a crucial role in influencing the effects of your cannabis. Harvesting a plant before its peak will result in a higher cannabinoid content, which induces a more cerebral effect, whereas harvesting after the peak will result in a body-stone. This means that, irrespective of whether you are cultivating indica or sativa strains, you have the power to shape the effects of your buds by strategically choosing when to harvest.

A window of a few days to a week on either side of the peak time is sufficient to achieve the desired effects. For example, indica plants typically deliver a more substantial body effect, so harvesting earlier can introduce some cerebral effects, while harvesting later intensifies the body effects.

Sativa strains are known for their pronounced cerebral effects. Harvesting earlier can enhance these effects while diminishing the body-stone. If harvested later, the body effects are heightened, but some of the more cerebral aspects may be sacrificed. Use sampling and labeling to pinpoint the optimal harvest date for your preferences.

Humidity Management in the Final Week

Some growers opt to maximize dehumidification in the last week before harvest. The balance is shifted from not too humid or dry to very dry. This intentionally stresses the plant, compelling it to generate new trichomes and enhance the size of existing ones. It also has the potential to boost cannabinoid content, a phenomenon when plants experience stress during the late flowering stage. This approach could be an intriguing experiment for seasoned growers seeking to optimize their harvest. To implement this strategy, try to max your dehumidifiers 24 hours before the planned harvest. This reduction in humidity serves an additional purpose: It helps prevent mold, but new mold growth is likely mitigated in the final week of growth anyway, if you get this far without it.

Humidity also plays a significant role during the curing process, and some growers use a dehumidifier to dry harvested plants more quickly. Managing humidity levels meticulously throughout these stages contributes to the overall quality and preservation of the harvested crop.

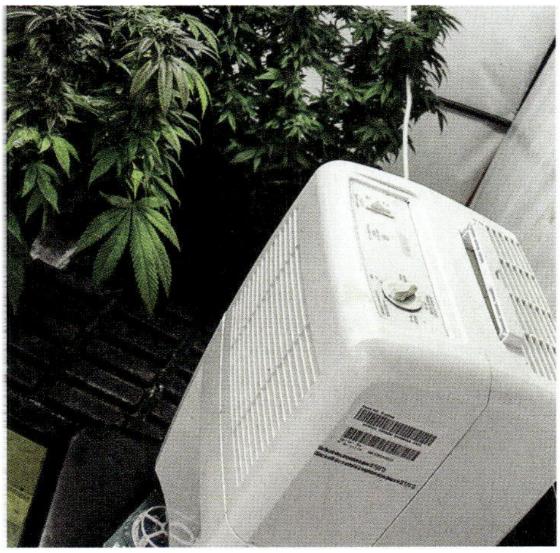

Dehumidifiers help dry the harvest more quickly.

PHOTO: STONED ROSIE

Harvest Flushing: To Flush or Not to Flush

Flushing is more commonly associated with hydroponic systems than with soil. The fundamental idea is to eliminate leftover nutrients and give the plants only clean water during the final week or two of flowering, essentially providing a cleansing period. The absence of additional nutrients will stop the plant from making other compounds, such as starch or sugar, that you don't want present in your flowers. The biochemical pathways behind their production will slow down significantly with flushing.

The effectiveness of flushing is a matter of debate. Plants store minerals during growth and gradually use the stored nutrients during the process of photosynthesis, so it remains uncertain how much unwanted material is actually removed.

Flushing entails placing your plants into a nutrient-deficient environment. The plant may then use up its stored nutrients, resulting in fewer unwanted compounds, or it may be forced to experience a slight deficiency that may impact the final product.

During flowering, the plant directs a significant amount of energy towards biochemical processes that heavily rely on phosphorus. Removing phosphorus from the system can affect these processes unless the plant's nutrient stores are sufficient. A lack of phosphorus results in the plant seeking the nutrient in the growing medium, encouraging root growth over bud growth. Growers who flush believe the taste makes this worthwhile despite the lower quantity.

This is why perforated pots are preferred and why hydroponics makes things much easier for this process. The idea is to overwater and then quickly recover. You want to clear nutrients out and then dry the medium so the overwatering doesn't become a problem. All setups are different; some plants can be moved to a drainage point, while

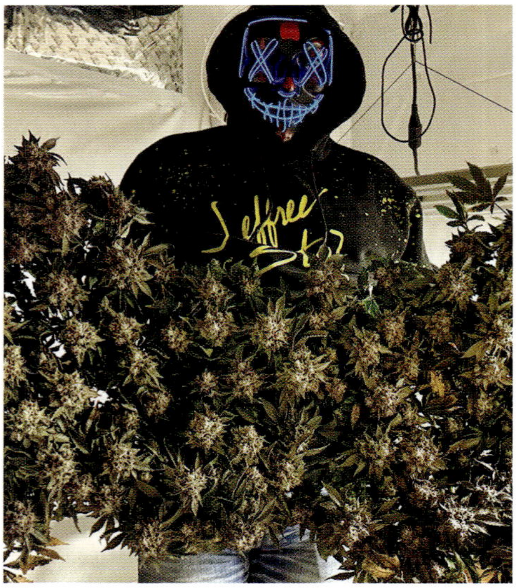

Arms full of freshly harvested bud for drying.

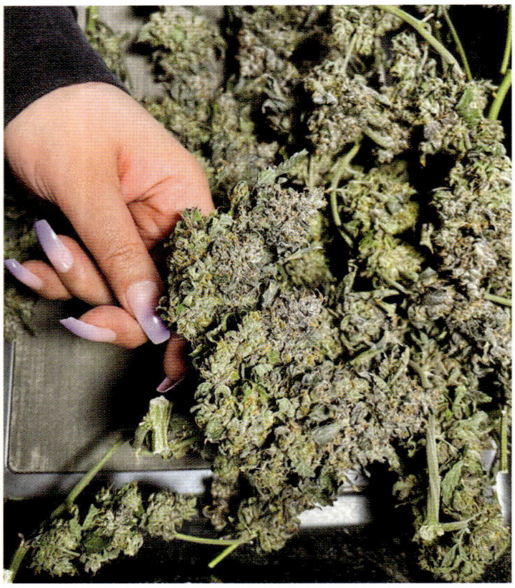

Snapping bud from dry stems should result in an audible cracking sound.

others will have drainage for spills that can be used for flushing. Pour a generous amount of water onto the medium, using a tap, hose, or watering can. Allow the liquid to flow out from the bottom of the pot, paying attention to the color of the runoff. Repeat this process until the liquid is clear, indicating it is probably mostly just the water left. If soil is used, it will become muddy during this process, with some mud being carried away with the water. Promptly move your plant to a warm, dry location and wait for the soil to dry out. You can use a fan on the soil and a dehumidifier. This is important, to help the soil and the plant recover quickly.

Flushing, like transplanting, can shock a plant, which may stunt it and negatively affect the overall yield. Flushing the plant when it has produced 90% of its final yield may divert its remaining energy into resin production instead of the last 10% of yield. Some growers prefer this increased resin production, while others believe that curing well results in full yield and resin potential.

Some users claim that flushed bud tastes better and is less harsh. Many growers choose to skip flushing and concentrate on curing to eliminate unwanted compounds and produce a final product that is flavorful and smooth. Hydroponic growers can derive the most benefits from flushing. Follow the emergency flush section in Chapter 8 to do a pre-harvest flush.

Ultimately, flushing is a personal choice. Experimenting with a single plant or a small number of plants will help you assess the results and determine whether flushing is right for you.

PHOTOS: TRAVIS HOELLERER @SOFAKINGHIGH

Dark Period Harvesting

It is better to harvest at the end of the dark period, specifically during the last hour of a 12/12 cycle, or just before sunrise for outdoor plants, because the metabolic processing of chemicals slows down in the absence of light. Thus, during this final hour of darkness, there is a minimal flow of nutrients or unwanted compounds towards the flowers, and harvesting the plant around this time minimizes the presence of unwanted compounds in the bud. You can introduce light as you harvest, so you can see what you are doing. Additional reduction of these compounds can be achieved through meticulous manicuring and, most importantly, through the curing process. Curing your bud is the most effective method for degrading harsh compounds. To preserve the integrity of your harvest, wrap the harvested plants in canvas, or preferably hemp, to shield them from light.

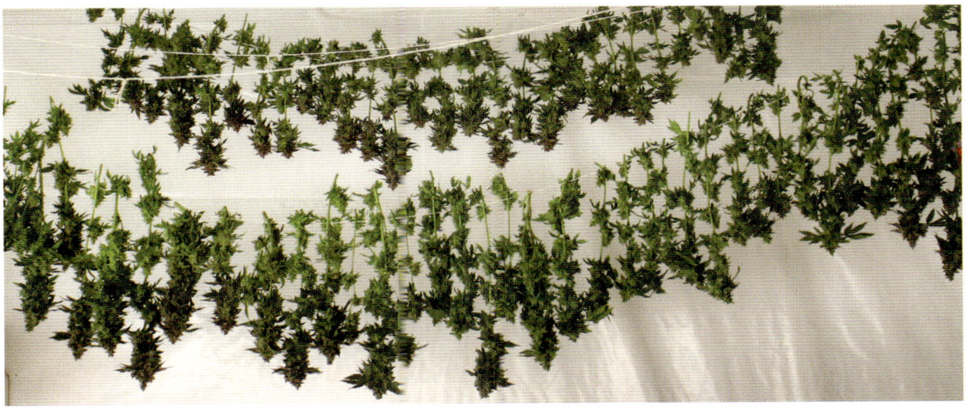

The cannabis plant's natural branching allows many places to hang the harvest upside down on a drying line.

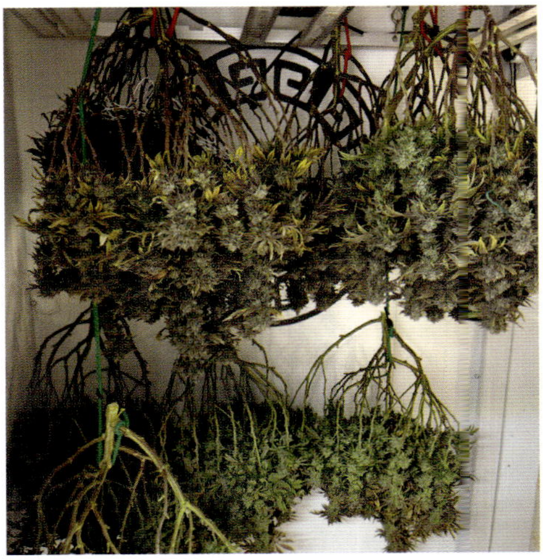

Whole plants can be hung upside down, but smaller sections allow for more airflow.

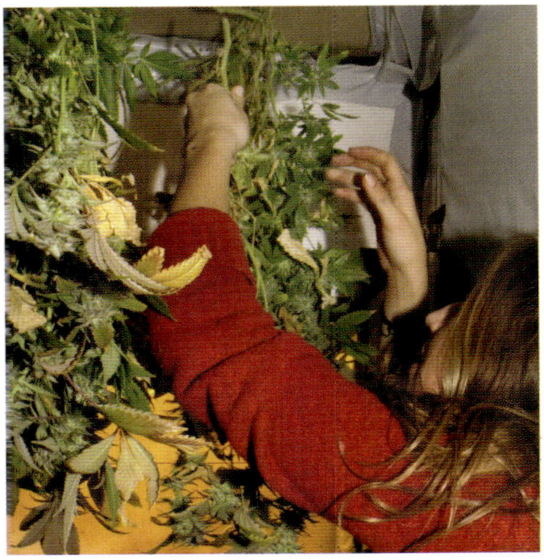

Check the plants occasionally to find out how dry they are getting.

PHOTOS: TRAVIS HOELLERER @SOFAKINGHIGH (TOP), PRESTON BJORNSON (BOTTOM LEFT), ED BORG (BOTTOM RIGHT)

Cannabinoid Stability

Studies on the stability of cannabinoids under light have been conducted since the 1970s. Light is essential for photosynthesis, and UV light can stimulate flowering growth. However, light loses its benefits after harvesting and can even degrade the plant over time. Prolonged light exposure results in molecular changes that diminish both the quantity and quality of THC in your harvested buds. Although dispensaries may display buds under lights, their stored cannabis is likely in darkness to maintain quality. A lightproof room is the best option for drying as it's crucial to avoid prolonged direct light exposure during drying. A lightproof drying room can also serve as your flowering room.

The stability of cannabinoids under temperature has been similarly studied. THC activation through heating, or decarboxylation, is a common practice. Harvested buds contain many cannabinoids, but THCA (tetrahydrocannabinolic acid) and CBDA (cannabidiolic acid) are our focus. They must undergo decarboxylation to become THC and CBD. The temperature of cannabinoids in storage should be considered: Specifically what temperatures produce instability and degradation in cannabinoids. How long will cannabinoids stay stable at certain temperatures? Does the form of cannabis matter in terms of degradation?

Degradation occurs gradually on a molecular level, but noticeable differences emerge over time, detectable within a year when stored at 40°F (4°C) and exposed to light. Darkness slows down degradation but doesn't halt the process entirely. Hashish or solid forms degrade more slowly than extracts like oils. Although quick turnover between storage and decarboxylation may help, adhering to best practices ensures optimal quality. Ongoing research in this field continuously updates our understanding, promising more insights in future.

Indica Harvest

Indica plants typically stand 1–4 feet (30.5–122 cm) tall. When harvesting your indica plant, cut it at the base and carefully lift it. The weight will amaze you. Do not let it touch the ground, to prevent unwanted dirt or dust on the buds. If transportation is necessary, use canvas (hemp).

Hang the harvested plant upside down in a cool, well-ventilated room devoid of light. The curing process benefits from a cool, dark environment. Hanging the plant upside down facilitates natural separation of stems and branches, creating space for air to circulate around the freshly harvested flowers. You can clip away branches and hang them separately if the plant is too large.

The best temperature for drying is 60–75°F (15.5–24°C). If you use a humidifier, aim for a relative humidity (RH) of around 55%. You can go lower but not at the expense of adequate airflow, which should take precedence.

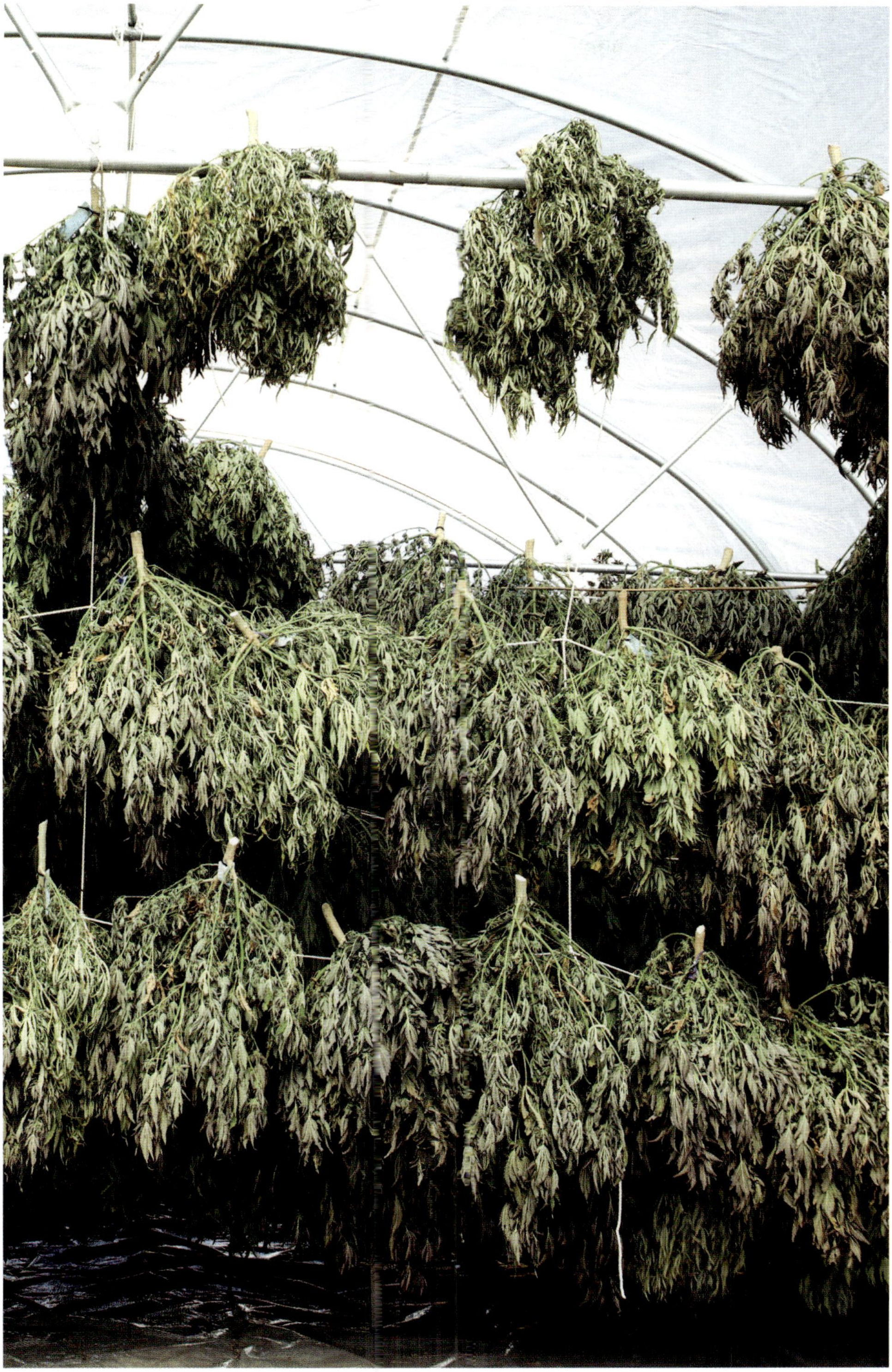

PHOTO: ANDRE GROSSMAN

Having enough space to dry the harvest may be more of an issue than you think. Plan for it.

Strain Variation at Harvest

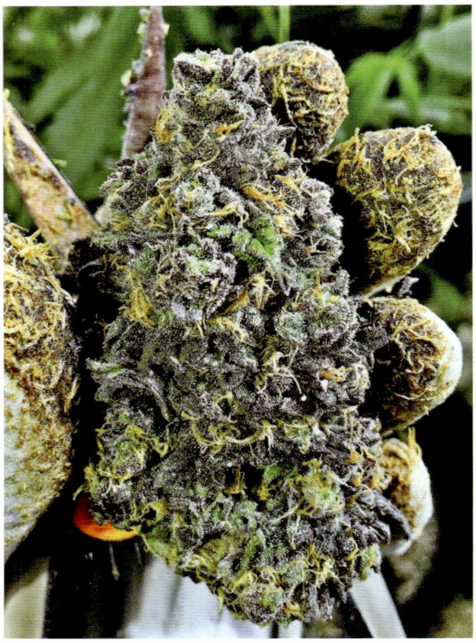

Grand Daddy Purple.

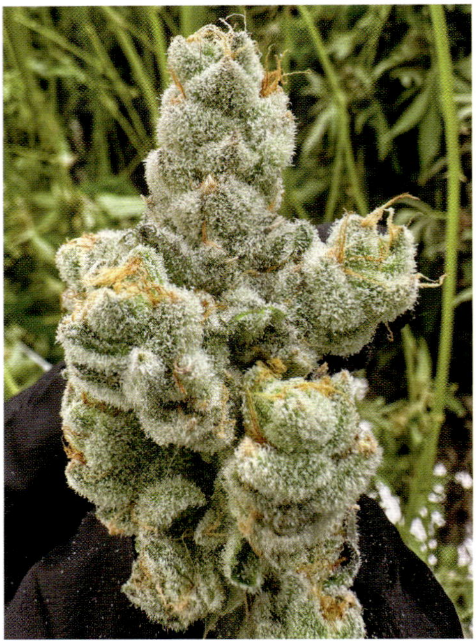

Cereal Milk.

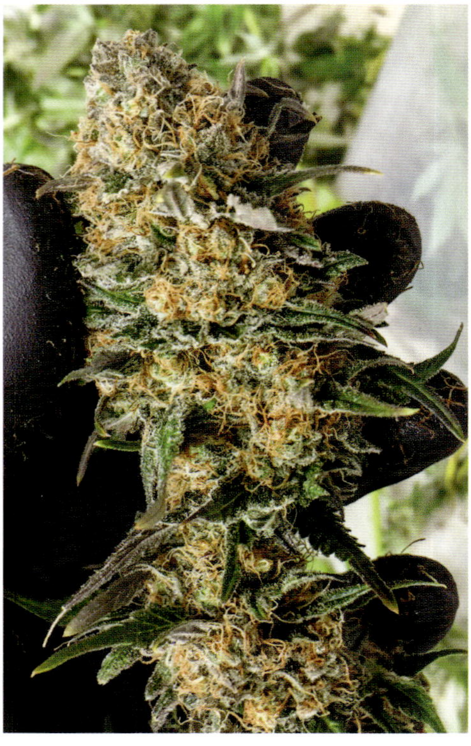

Liberty Haze.

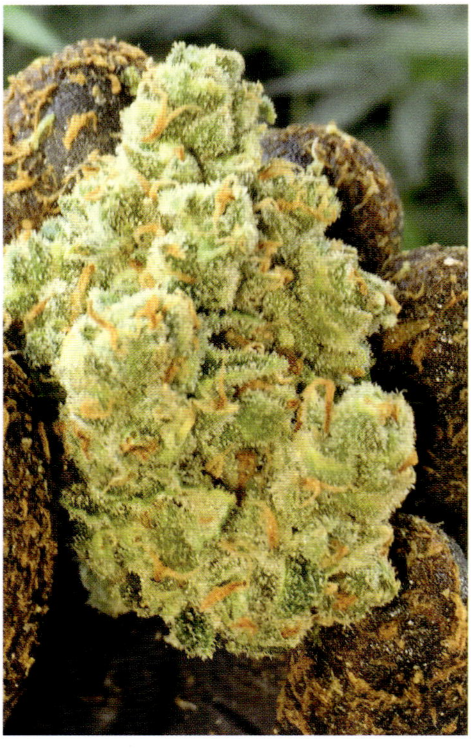

Jack Herer.

PHOTOS: HIP2THECROP

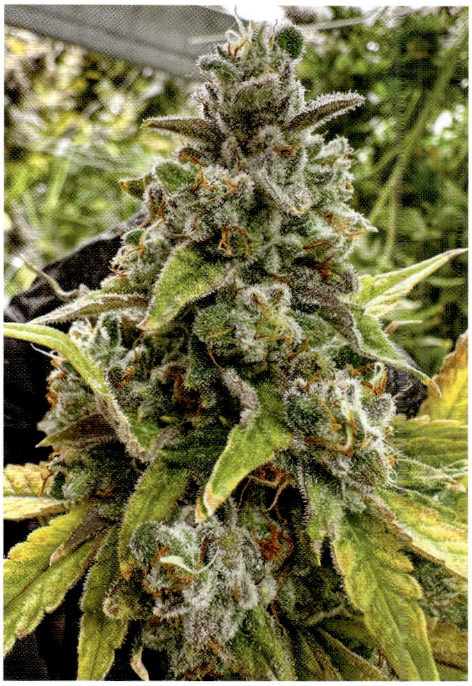

Over Power.

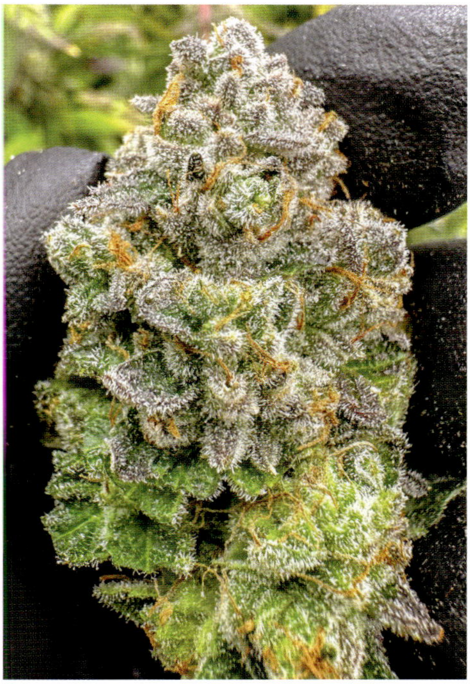

Ice Cream Cake.

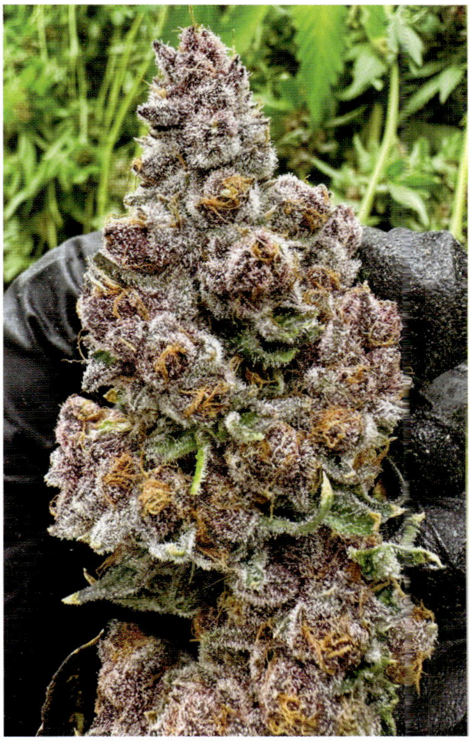

Trop Cherry.

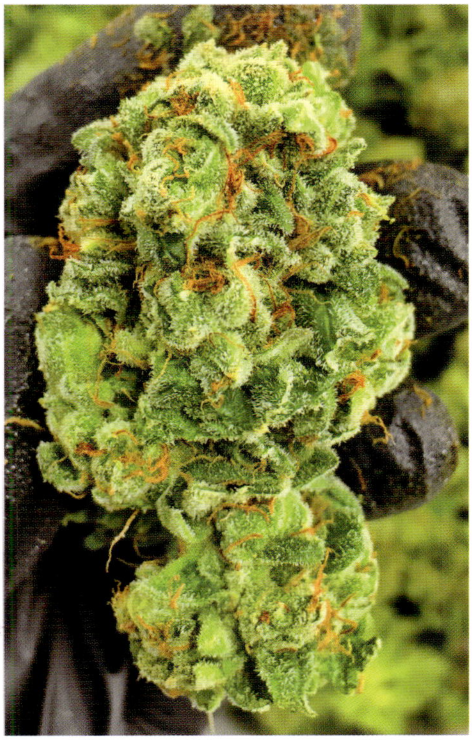

Tangie.

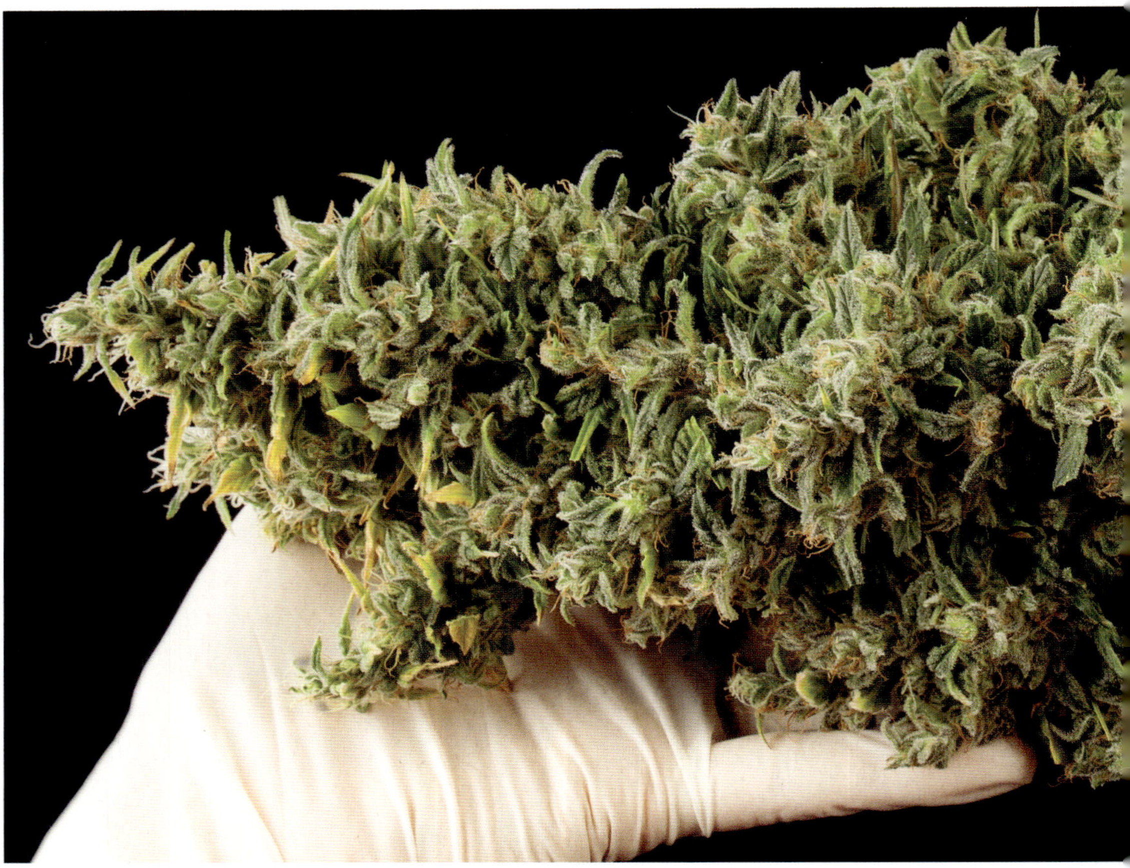

Delivering the baby. Some top colas can be as thick as a bottle of soda.

PHOTO: TROPICAL SEEDS

Many growers hang the plant by its lowest branches along with the fan leaves. You can tie a hemp line to the walls of your drying area to secure the lowest branch over the line and allow your buds to hang upside down. This method eliminates the need for clips. You can use coat hangers as a more economical option though they require more space.

Sativa Harvest

The harvesting process for sativa tends to be more labor-intensive than for indica. Outdoor growers favor sativa plants, which are known for reaching heights of up to 12 feet (365 cm) and producing over 20 oz. (570 g) of bud each. Some sativa varieties can even yield more than 2 pounds (1 kg) of bud per plant, making the harvest of these sizable plants more challenging.

When harvesting sativa plants, use a hemp canvas spread for carrying them. Cut the plant at the base and lay it on the canvas, then roll it up and tightly tie it for transport. If you have multiple plants, you may need more than one spread. Some plants might

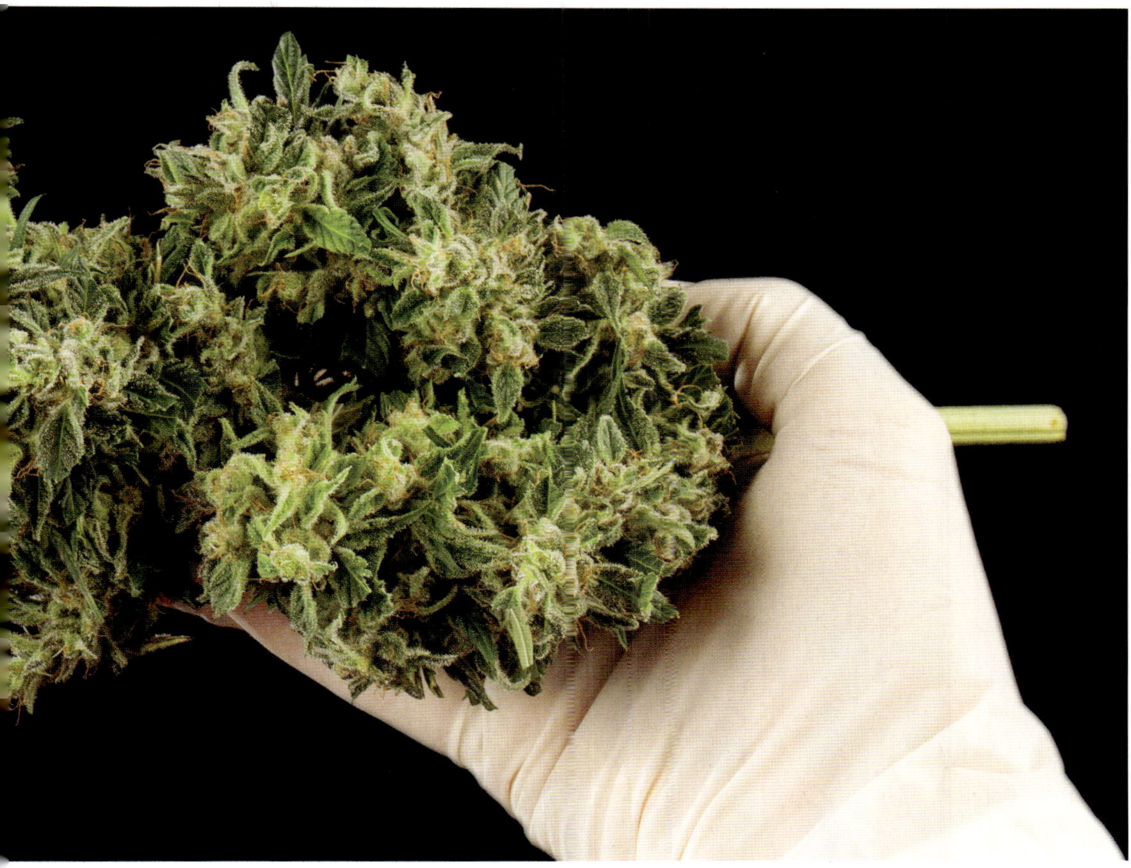

require chopping for easier transport. If you do cut branches away, label them for identification. Avoid dragging resinous plants along the ground as they will accumulate dirt.

Harvesting allows you to access and see parts of the plants usually concealed by their branching, a perspective not available during the growth phase.

Preliminary Manicuring

This initial manicuring technique is designed to help make the drying process easier by removing the bulk of the leaves. With a pair of clippers, remove as many fan leaves as possible from the base near the stem. Then remove the secondary leaves and set them aside in a separate pile. Last, pick off the trim leaves, the smaller leaves surrounding the bud, usually covered in resin, that can be easily separated from the bud. The trim you want to remove is the leaf on the shortest visible branching. Leave the hard-to-reach trim areas untouched for now. Preserve the integrity of the buds; the trim should come away easily without pulling the bud with it. If there is no visible branch on the trim area you are trying to remove, avoid disturbing it, as the bud will not come off as neatly or effortlessly. Due to resin adhesiveness, it usually pulls some bud on a branch next to it. Since that connecting bud is still fixed to another branch, you are ripping, not cutting the flowers away. Any buds that break away during the manicuring process can be placed on a tray, set aside, and labeled for future identification. Keep the area clean by sweeping the ground, or use a hemp canvas to catch any falling buds.

Most growers compost the fan leaves and the secondary leaves, which contain minimal amounts of trichomes and negligible cannabinoids. Middle and trim leaves contain more cannabinoids, especially trim leaves. One can end up with water-extracted bubble hash from just a few plant remains from preliminary manicuring.

Drying Times

Once you've done your preliminary manicure and hung the plants to dry, allow them to remain in this state until a branch easily breaks between your fingers, producing a snapping sound, indicating that the branch is adequately dry. This process typically takes around two to three weeks, depending on humidity, although certain strains may require up to four weeks before the branches snap as desired. If you prefer more moist buds, you can process your results earlier, but this technique is a tried and tested way to gauge when they are ready to cure. We will talk about excess drying later in this chapter.

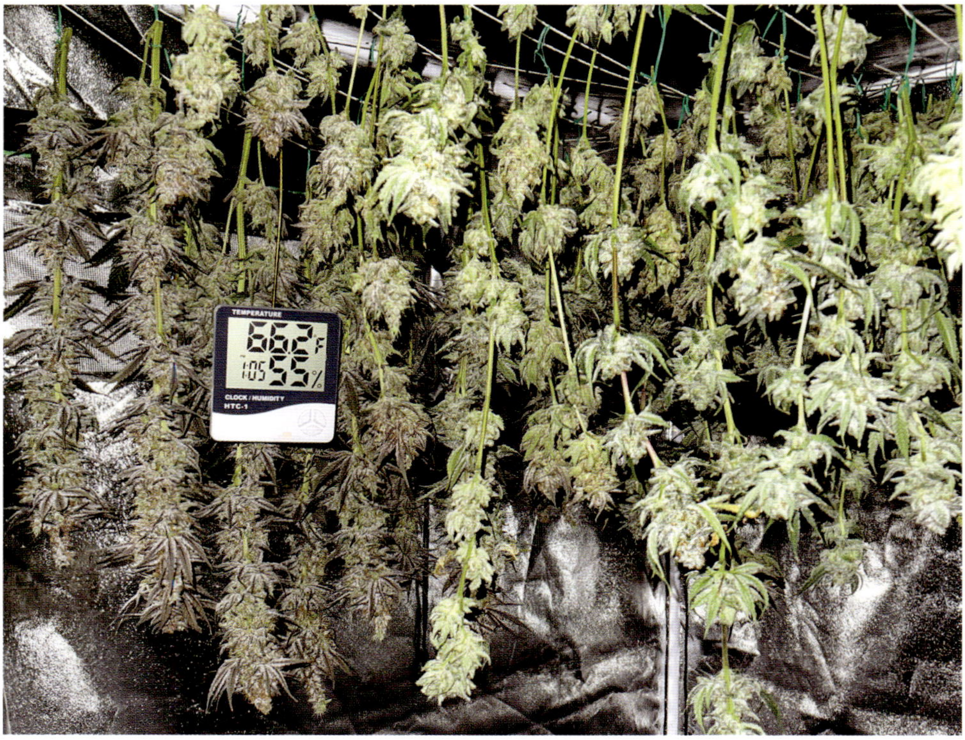

PHOTO: TRAVIS HOELLERER @SOFAKINGHIGH

You can almost hear the snapping sound of these dried branches.

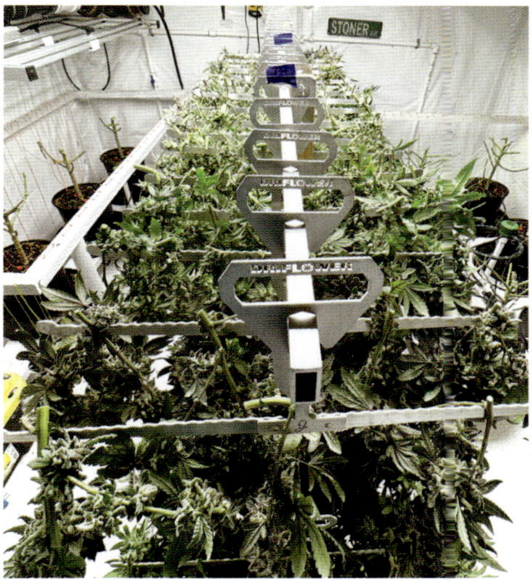

DriFlower hanging solutions. Professional-grade hangers.

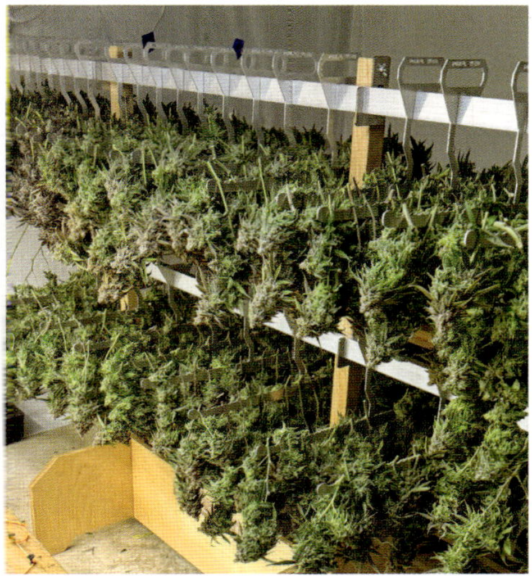

DriFlower hangers looking uniform and neat.

Avoid letting your plants dry out completely. They should not crumble in your hands before manicuring and should still feel slightly moist with some density when squeezed. The primary goal of drying is to remove water. The bud's weight will significantly decrease, dropping to below 30% of its original harvested weight.

Labeling Trays

Prepare all trays with labels before transferring your harvest to the manicuring space. This is especially helpful if you'll be dealing with small trim pieces. Label containers with the strain name so that, as you snip off these trim pieces, you can easily drop them into the corresponding containers. If you're working with only one strain, label each area according to the step, especially if more than one person is helping with the manicuring process, so the rounds don't get mixed up. If you have more than one strain, each strain has its own area with steps, or you work each strain in succession, never having more than one strain worked on at any one time. Once strains get mixed up in these smaller portions, it can be hard to segregate them back out again.

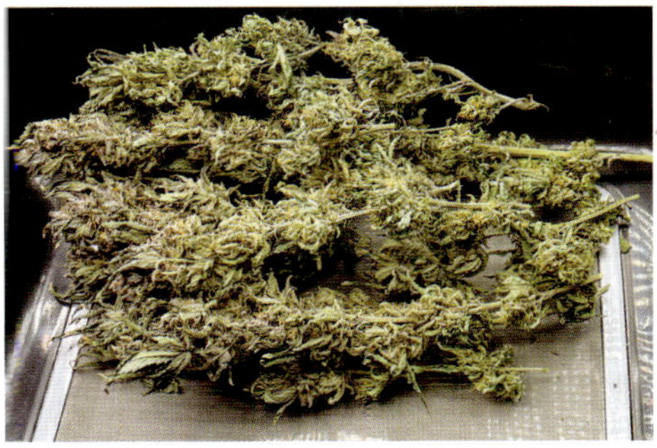

Preparing to spread out the dried harvest.

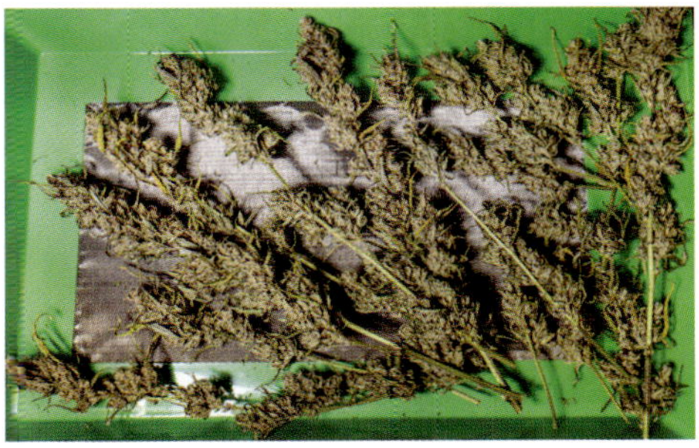

A spread-out dried harvest.

PHOTOS: TRAVIS HOELLERER @SOFAKINGHIGH (TOP ROW AND BOTTOM LEFT), PRESTON BJORNSON (RIGHT)

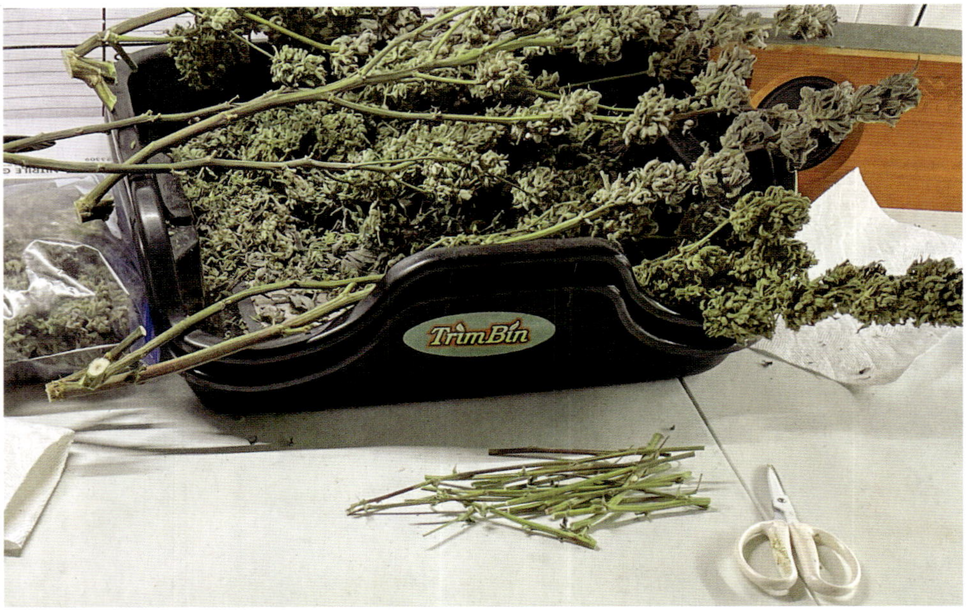

Preparing for manicuring with small scissors and cloth to work on.

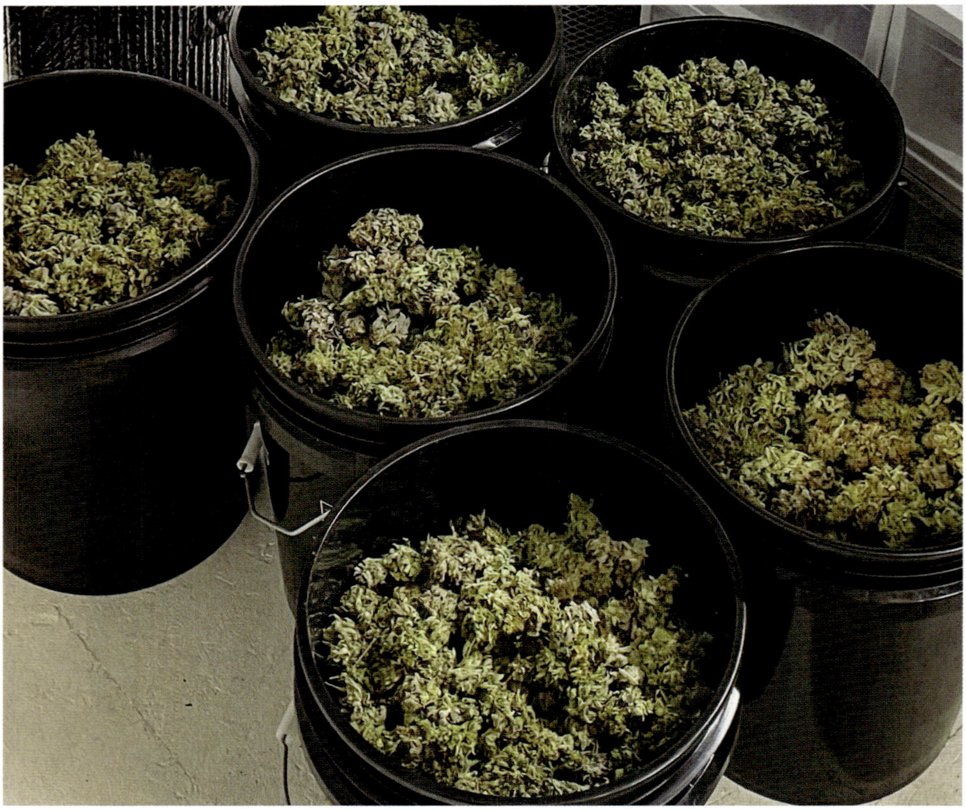

Buckets of nuggets from round one of manicuring.

PHOTOS: PRESTON BJORNSON

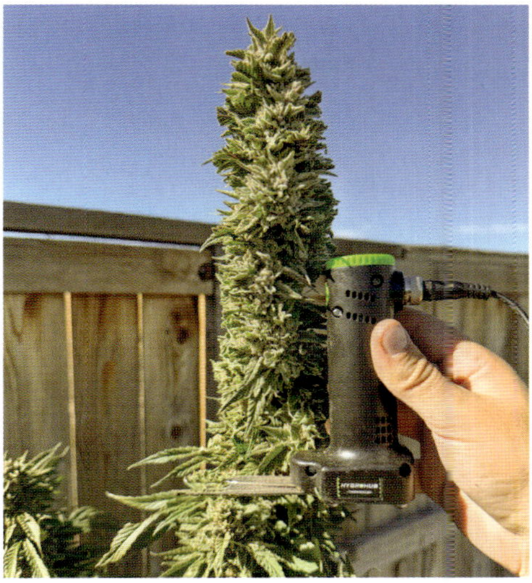

An electric mini trimmer can help speed up the work.

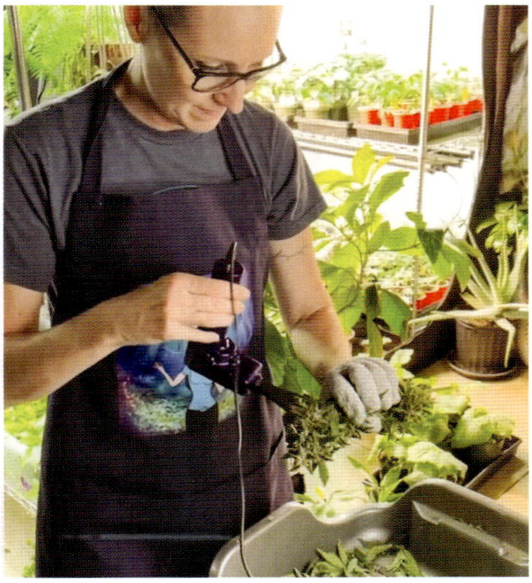

It's easier than manual cutting if you have a lot to trim.

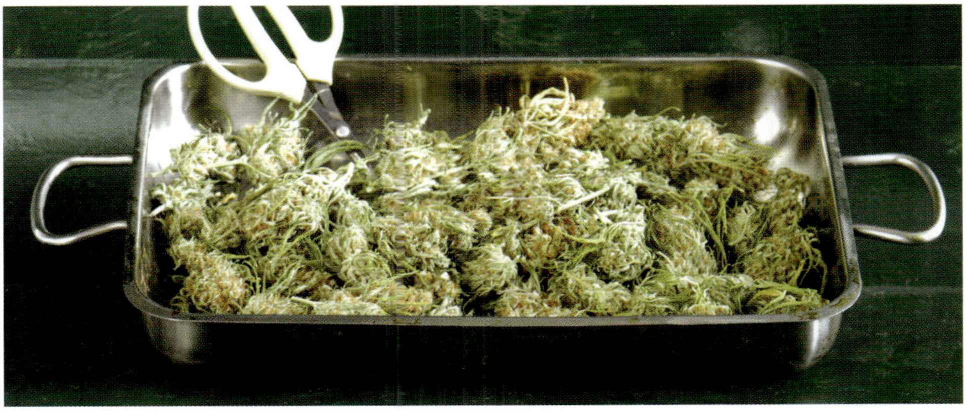

This tray of buds is ready for a round of manicuring.

PHOTOS: TRAVIS HOELLERER @SOFAKINGHIGH (TOP LEFT), TANYA PETERSEN (TOP RIGHT) ED BORG (BOTTOM)

Manicuring

Manicuring is a crucial step in preparing your bud for curing, to distinguish the best from the rest. You will need trays, canvas spreads, sharp scissors, and rubbing alcohol. Because manicuring is time-consuming, some growers like to set up music, podcasts, or audiobooks in their work station. The process can leave your fingers covered in resin, so ensure you have everything you need beforehand, including food, drinks, and a vaporizer. If you opt to use latex gloves, you can place them inside out in the freezer after use and hand-roll the hardened resin.

Take as much of your hanging bud as possible and pile it on the canvas. Try to keep the strains separate and label each heap. It is easy to get buds mixed up during the manicuring process. Wrap the canvas over your bud to avoid light degrading the THC levels.

Industrial Cannabis Harvesters

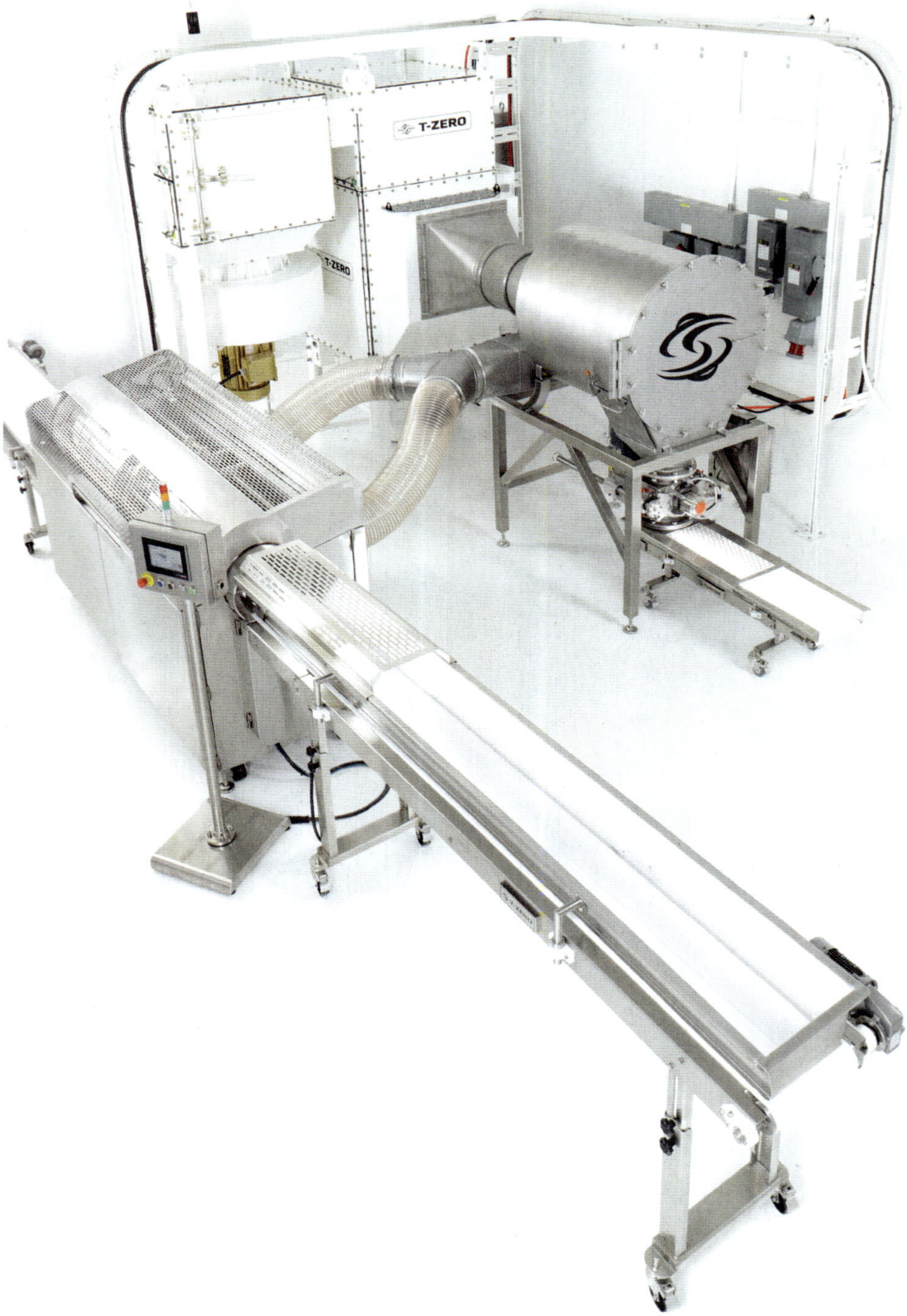

PHOTOS: TWISTERTRIMMER.COM

Large industrial trimmers are efficient, adaptable, and built for significant returns, processing many pounds of bud per hour.

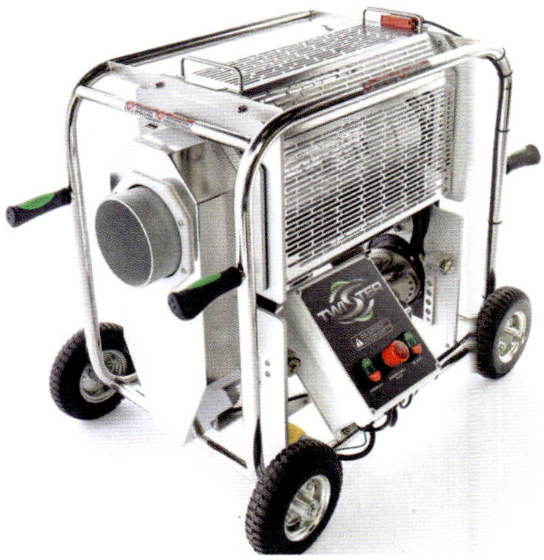

The Twister T2 is designed for high-volume trimming.

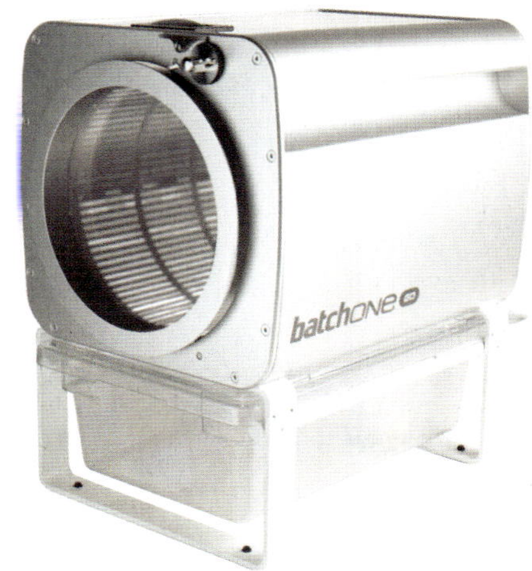

Achieving the tightest batch style trim with Twister BatchOne.

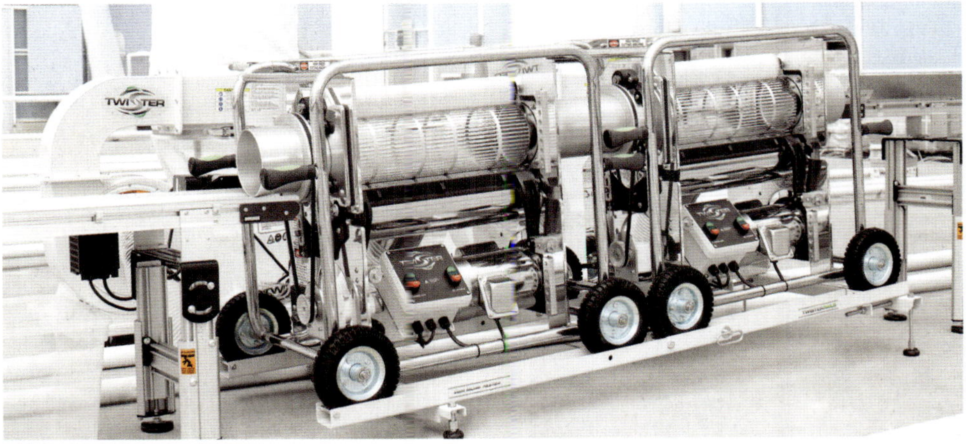

Twister technology can be linked back-to-back to increase productivity.

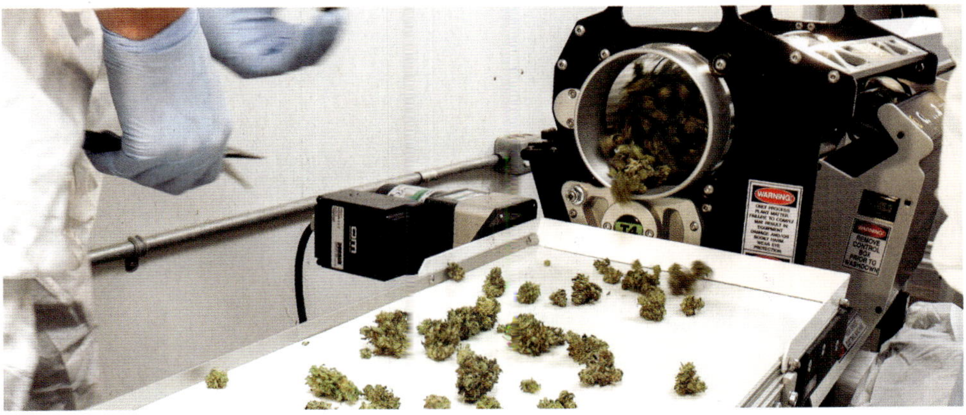

Industrial trimming technology using tumblers and conveyors: The Twister T4.

Side Branch Trimming

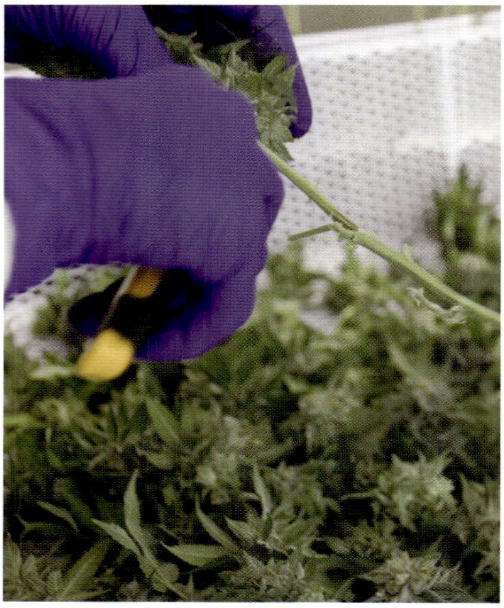

Some growers like to remove smaller bits of bud from their plants and work with these separately to the larger colas.

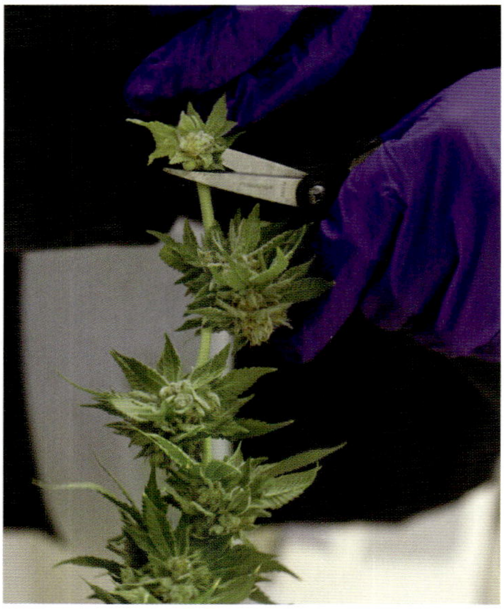

It's easy to clip these away from branches at their base.

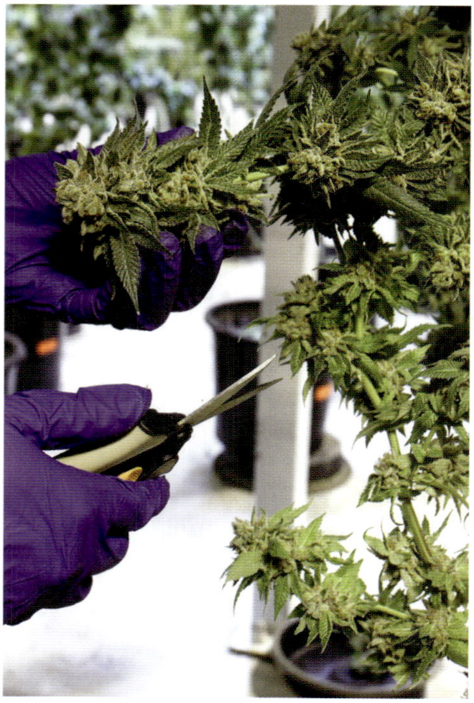

Side branching medium-sized colas can also go in.

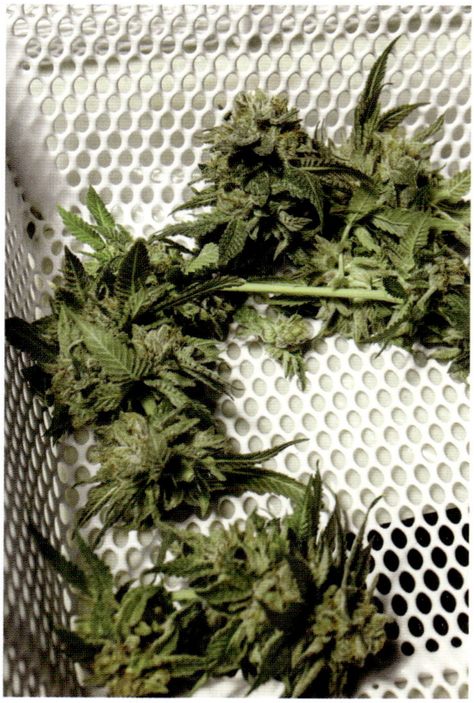

Place them into a labeled basket as you work along.

PHOTOS: PEACE NATURALS / PHOTOGRAPHED BY DAVID STRANGE

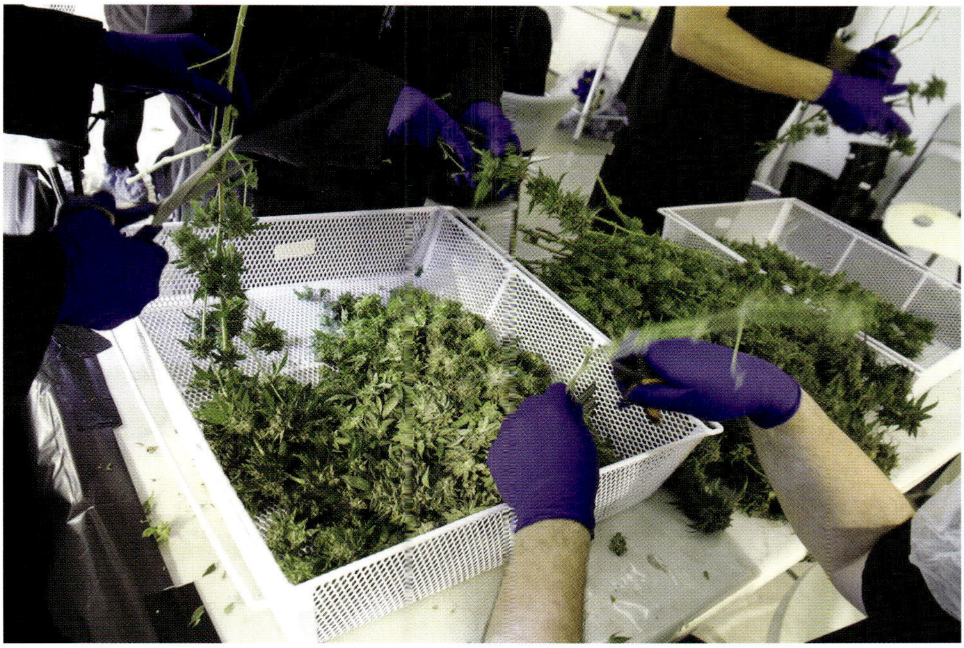

Working from a source basket, bud on branches are removed for pre-manicuring. The baskets have airholes for drying in storage.

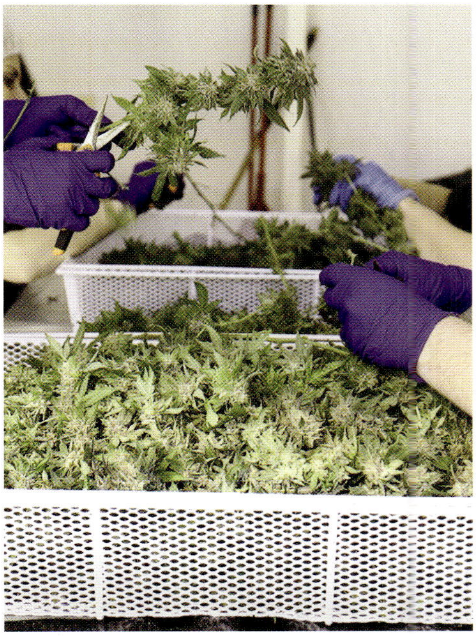

Bud is removed from the branch and placed into a basket that is filling up fast.

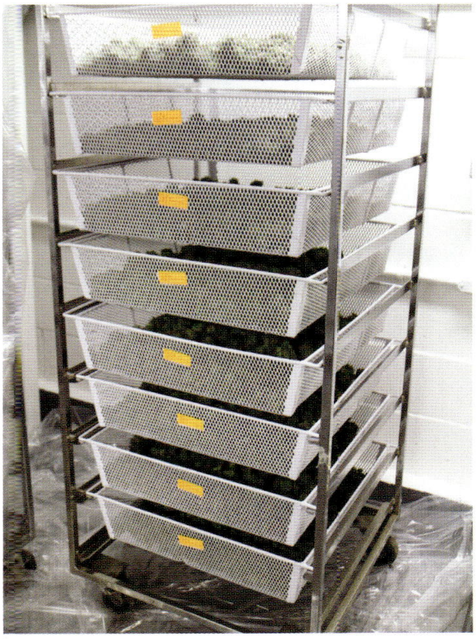

These labeled baskets are racked up on a trolley and moved to the dark room for drying. Buds can be manually moved around each day to get fresh air.

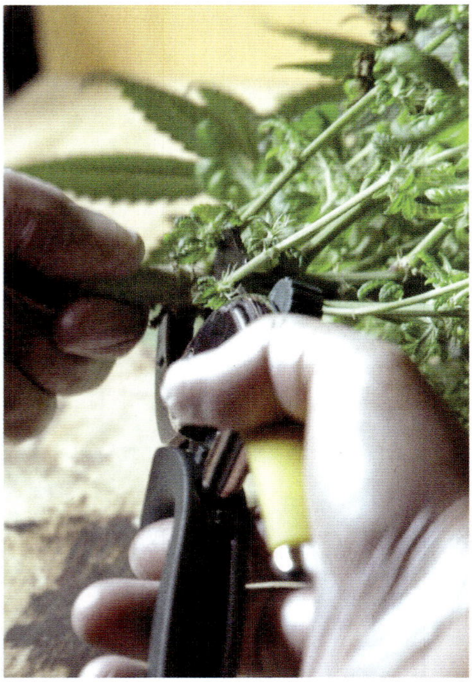

Separate each branch by clipping them away.

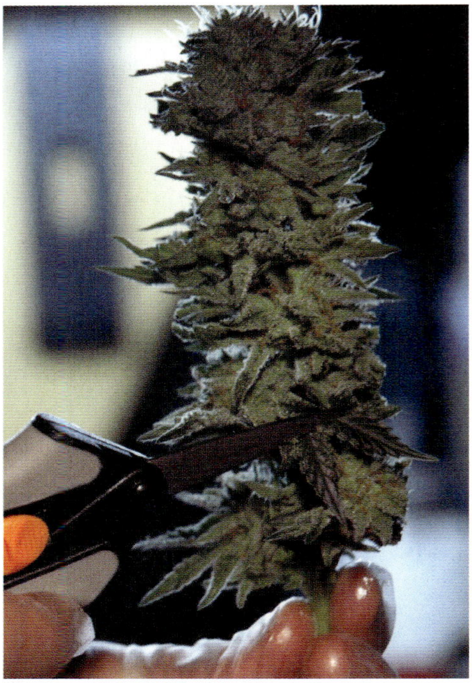

Remove the largest leaf trim first.

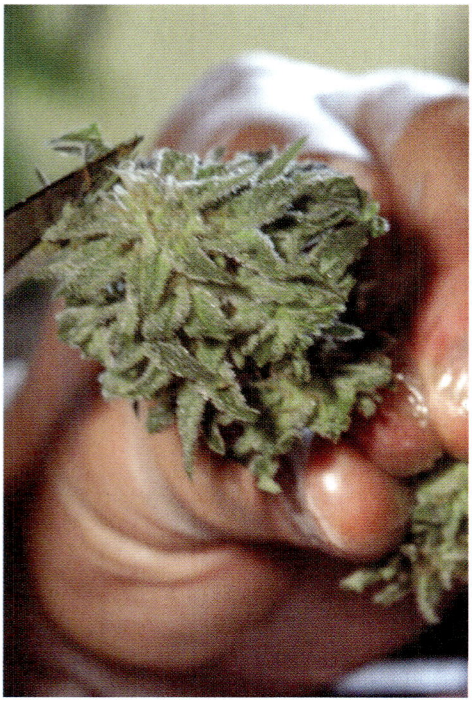

Twist around slowly removing trim to leave only bud.

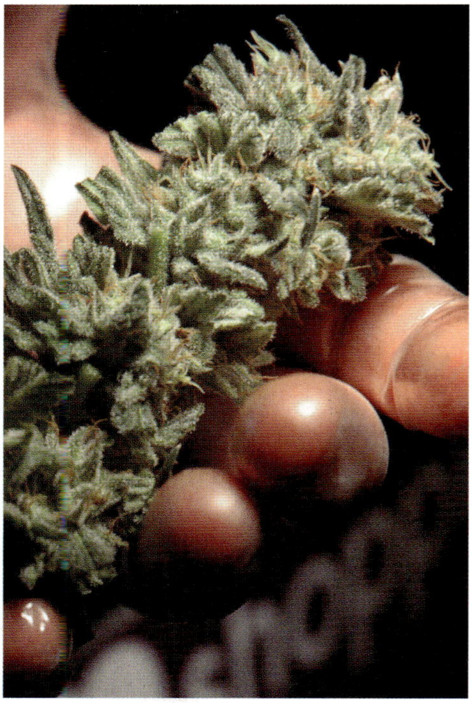

How much you want to trim depends on your taste.

PHOTOS: STONED ROSIE

First Round Manicuring

Separate your first plant out from the heap and, with your fingers, remove as many branches and leaves as possible. They should break away easily. Remove any trim you missed during the preliminary manicure. Next, chop the remaining branches into convenient, workable sizes for handheld manicuring. Repeat this process with all the other plants until you fill your tray with the first round of hand-manicured plants.

Second Round Manicuring

Pick up your first bud piece and clip away as much of the branch or stem as possible. You should be able to separate the leaf from the bud by snipping the leaf at the base. Avoid snipping flowers. The stems of the leaves are covered in trichomes, so hang on to these leaves; they are very high-quality trim.

Repeat this process until you have removed as much of the leaf as possible. If you cannot reach the leaf base without disturbing the surrounding bud, snip away as much of the leaf as close to the bud as possible and then label the trim separately.

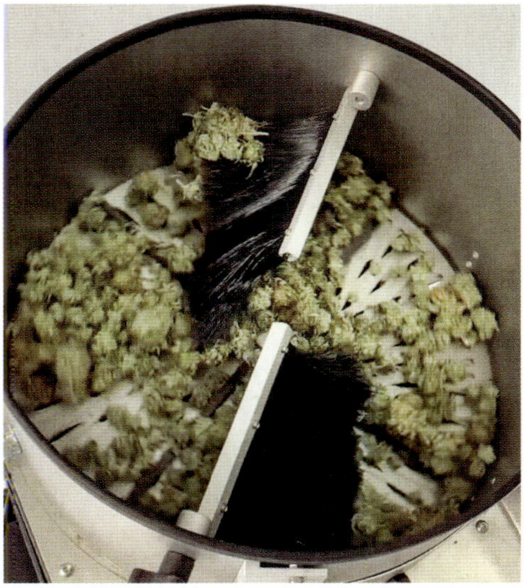

Trimpro Drypro in action, manicuring buds.

Rotate the plant by the stem to access the other side of the bud. This movement is the quickest way to access all of the leaf sites on the plant. To avoid removing the pistils, use the tips of the scissors when you snip so that the blades do not go past the piece you want to cut. Repeat this process with every piece of bud and you will eventually end up with manicured pieces of bud ready for curing.

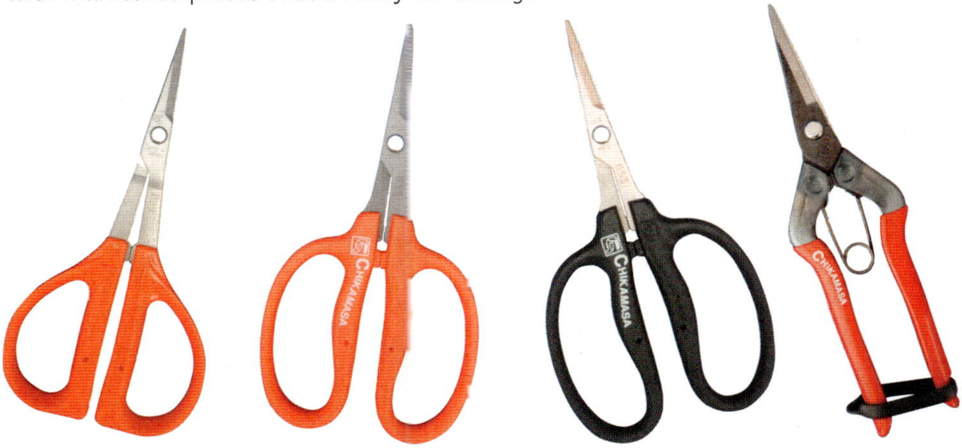

Clippers of different types. All have the same short-styled blades that are perfect for manicuring.

PHOTOS: TRIMPRO.COM (TOP), CHIKAMASA (BOTTOM)

Precision Trimming

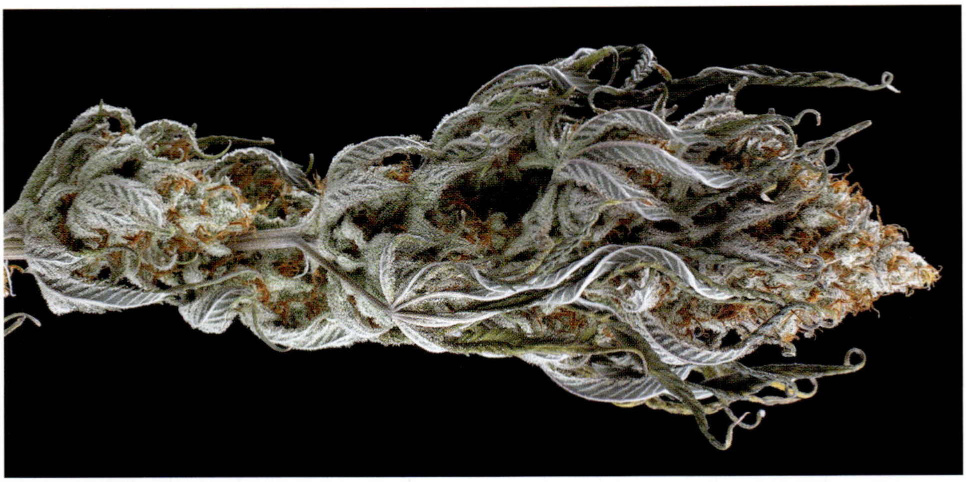

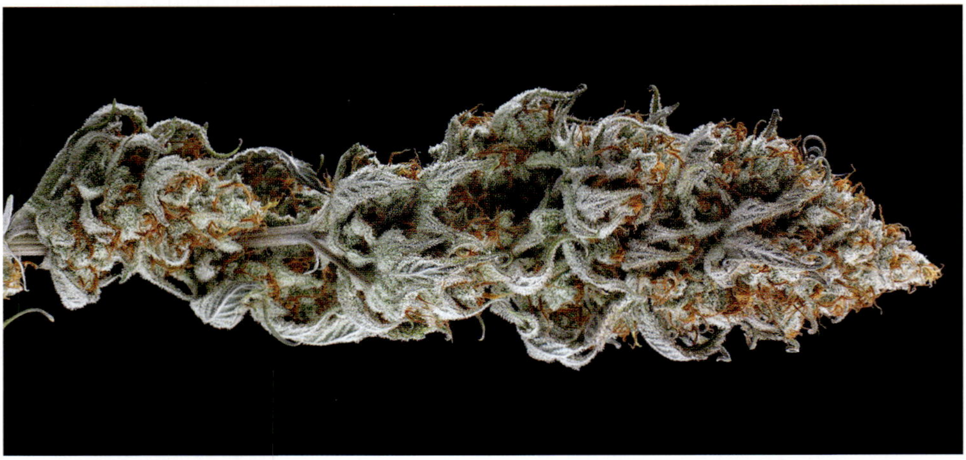

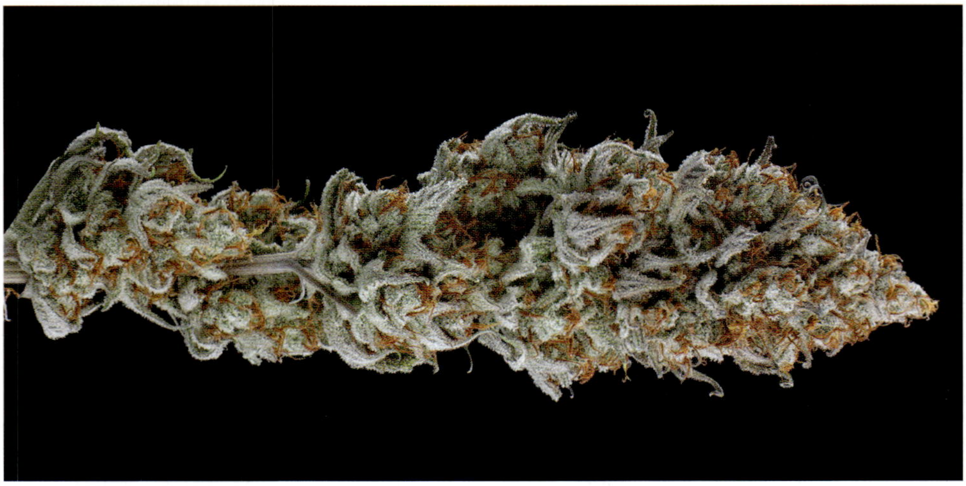

PHOTOS: RUSSELL-HOWLAND PHOTOGRAPHY

From unmanicured to manicured in a few steps, revealing all the bud colors underneath.

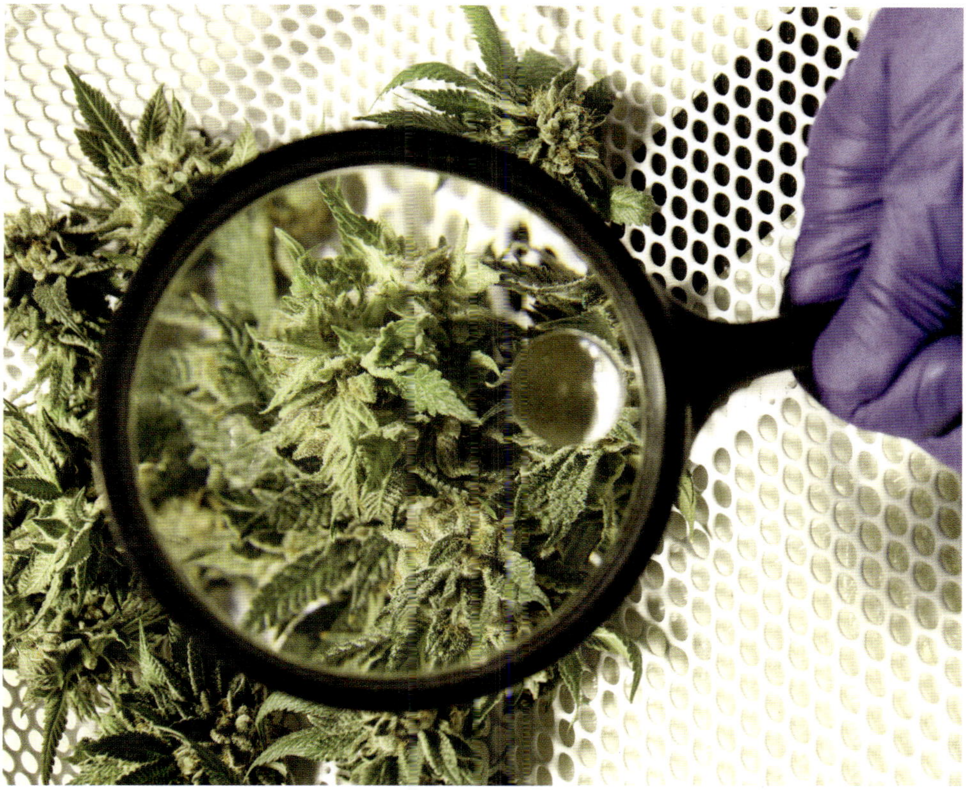

If you want to know if trim is worth processing you need to examine it for trichomes with a magnifying aid. If you can see trichomes on the trim then hash-making extractions are the way to go with it.

PHOTO: PEACE NATURALS / PHOTOGRAPHED BY DAVID STRANGE

Manicuring for Weight or Quality

How much you remove depends on the quality of manicured bud you want to end up with. The method above produces the best-quality manicured bud from your harvest, but the weight of the overall product will be reduced.

A dried bud with the trim leaves will be of medium quality but will weigh more than the best-quality manicured bud. Most in the cannabis community would prefer a smaller amount of higher-quality bud. However, it is your choice whether to manicure your bud for maximum weight or quality.

Several leaf piles will remain after preliminary and intensive manicuring. Some people compost this leftover matter; others make hash from it. Most leaves will be too harsh to vaporize directly but do contain some cannabinoids. Use a magnifying aid to help you distinguish the leaves with high trichome content for hash-making, especially if you plan to use the cold-water extraction technique using bubble bags described in Chapter 18. Make sure you don't get resin on these items, as it will be hard to wash off.

Professional Trimming

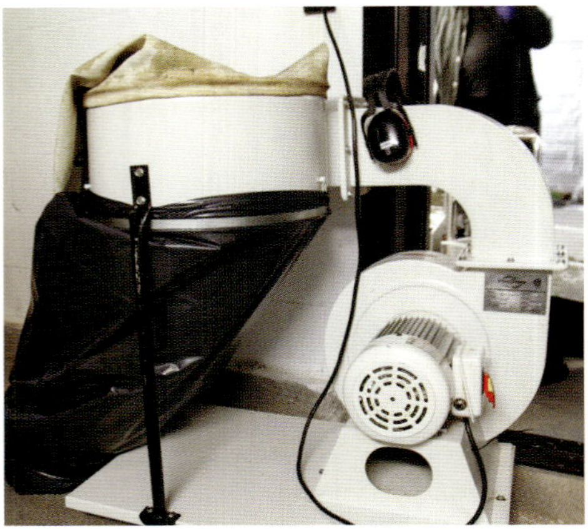

Trimming technology makes bulk work easier.

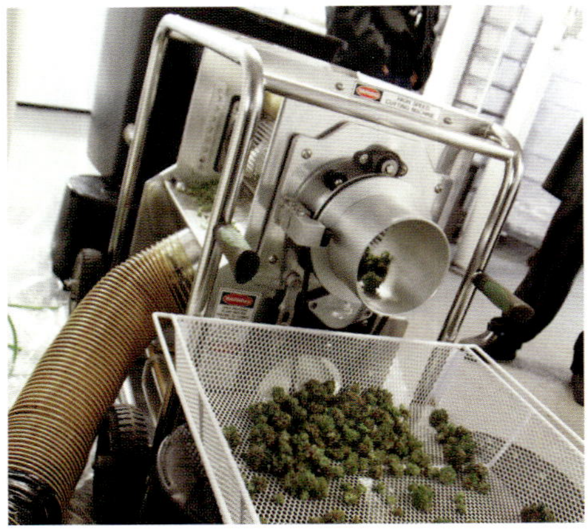

The trimmer outputs into a basket.

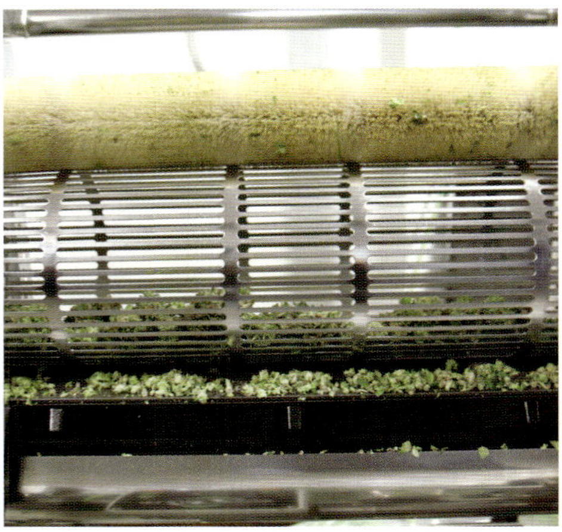

The tumbler spins, trimming buds.

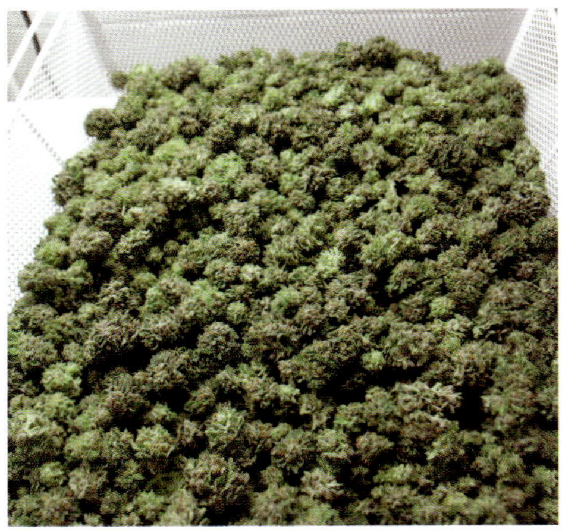

Trimmed bud mounts up in the basket.

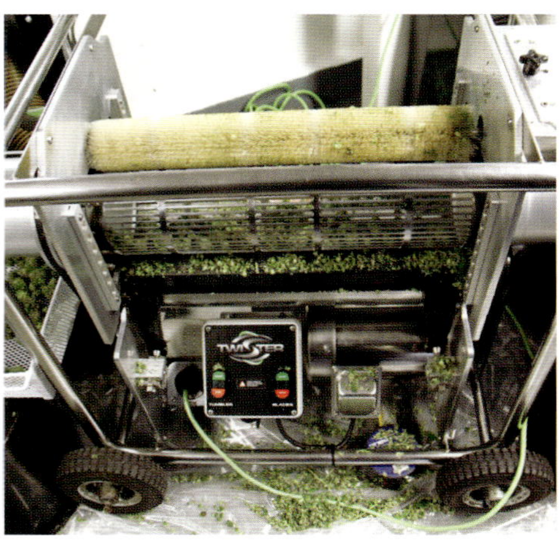

A lot of excess trim falls through the tumbler.

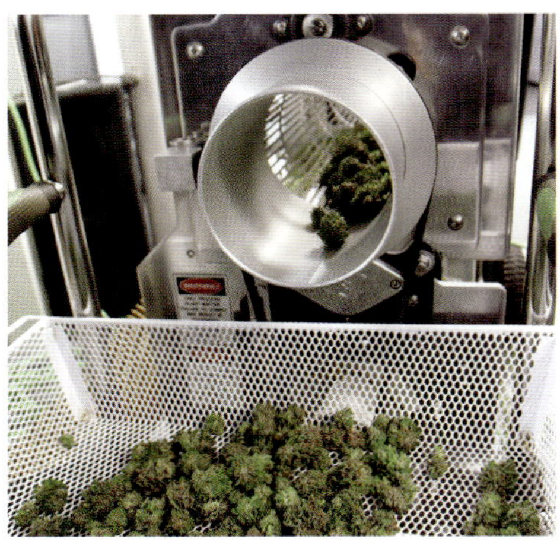

The process is quick and effective.

PHOTOS: PEACE NATURALS / PHOTOGRAPHED BY DAVID STRANGE

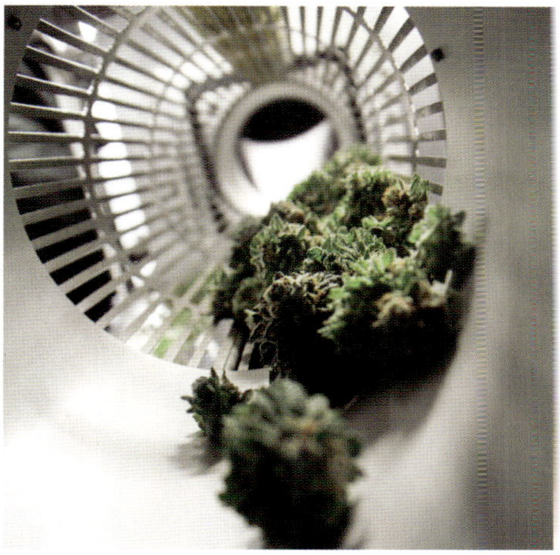

Inside the Twister T4 tumbler.

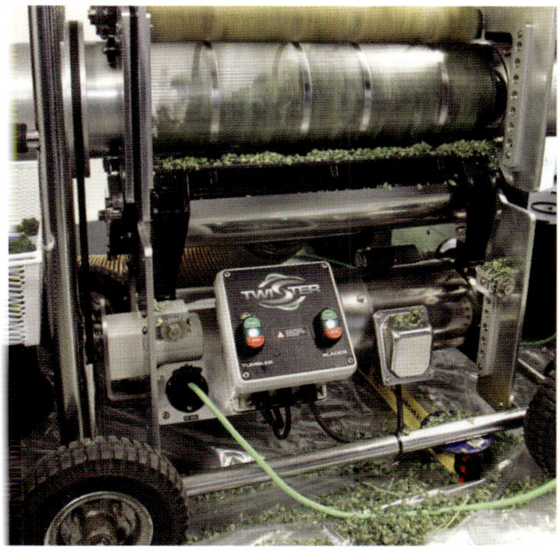

It rotates quickly to allow for the finest manicure.

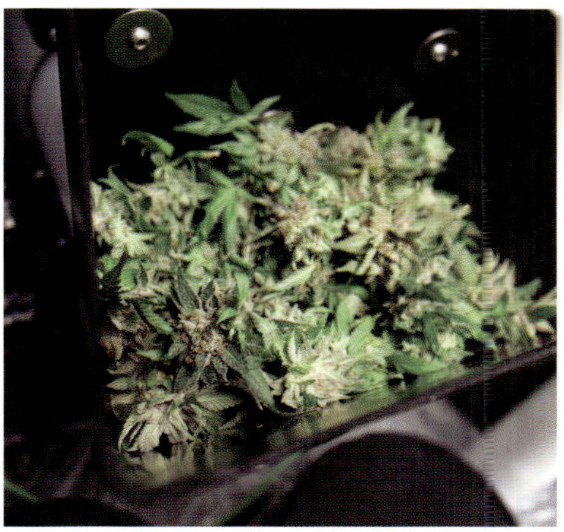

More bud is added in.

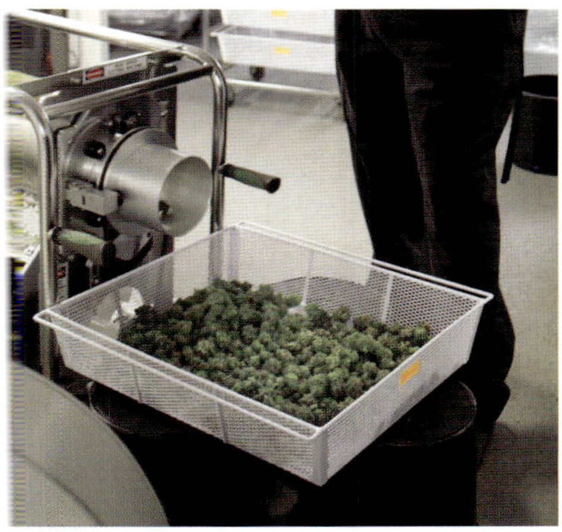

This would take hours to do manually.

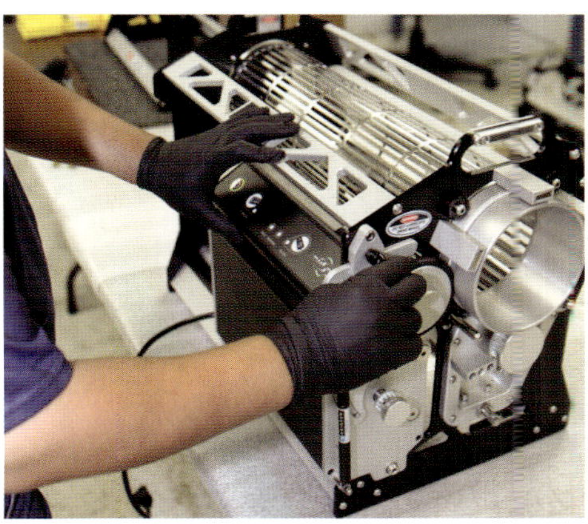

Easy to assemble and disassemble.

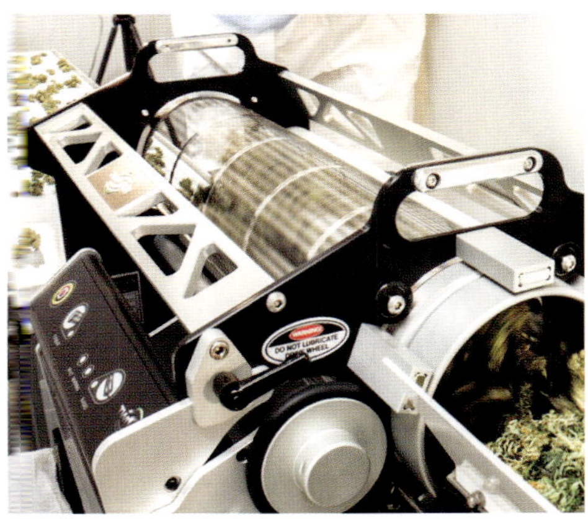

Conveyor belt out back instead of directly into a basket.

PHOTOS: PEACE NATURALS / PHOTOGRAPHED BY DAVID STRANGE (TOP AND MIDDLE ROW), TWISTERTRIMMER.COM (BOTTOM ROW)

Cured Bud

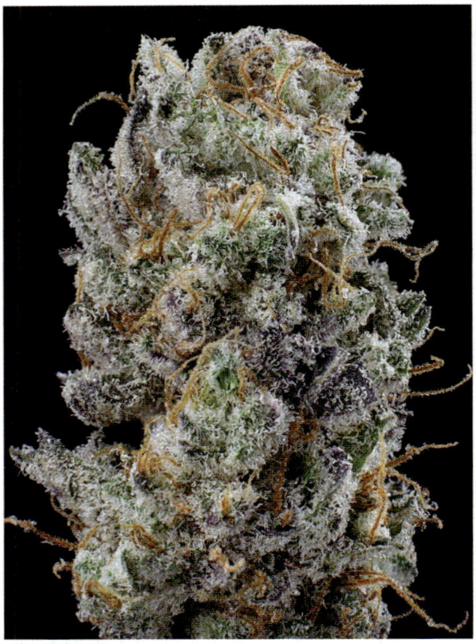

Singapore Sling from Tiki Madman.

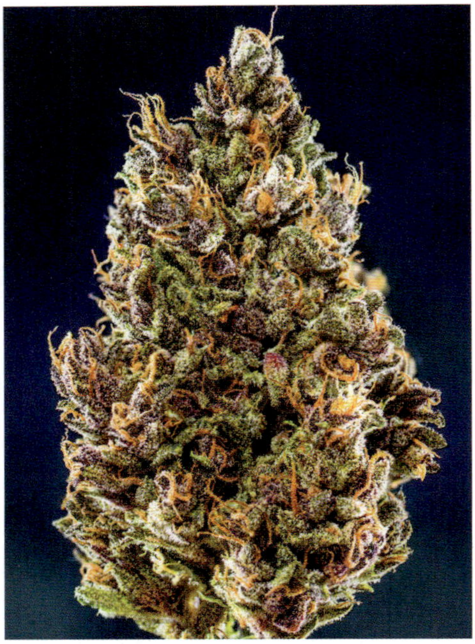

Strawberry Pie from Fast Buds.

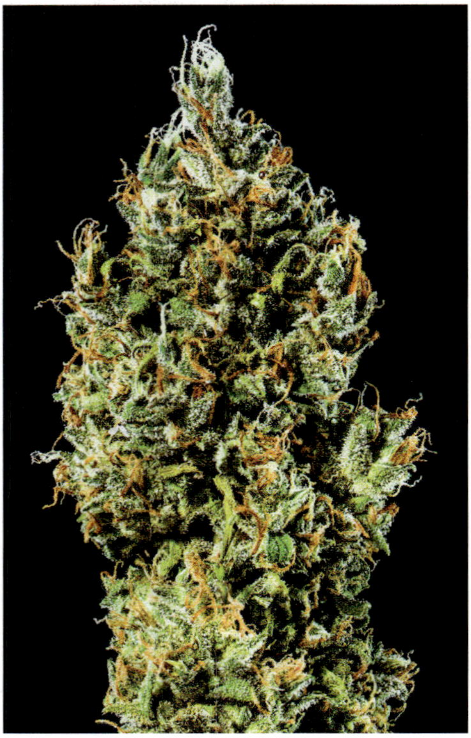

Tangie'Matic Auto from Fast Buds.

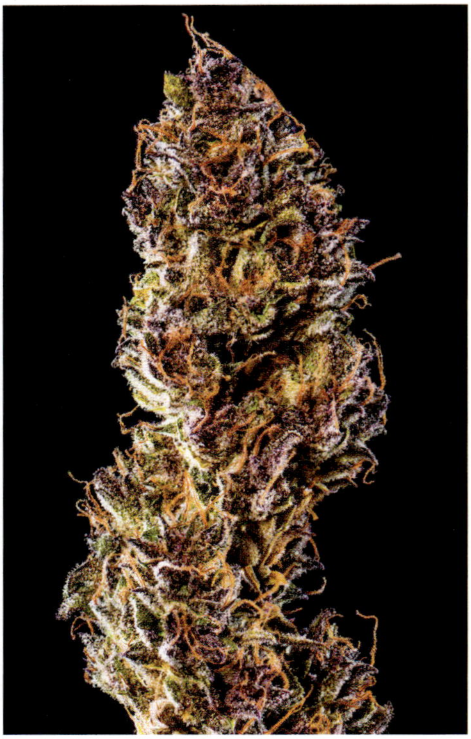

Tropsanto from Oni Seeds bred by Harry Palms.

PHOTOS: RUSSELL-HOWLAND PHOTOGRAPHY (TOP LEFT), ERIC PALMER (ALL OTHERS)

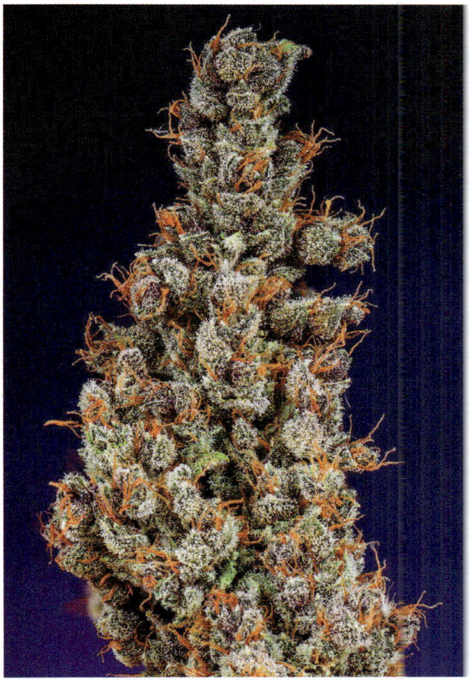

Tropicana Cookies Auto from Fast Buds.

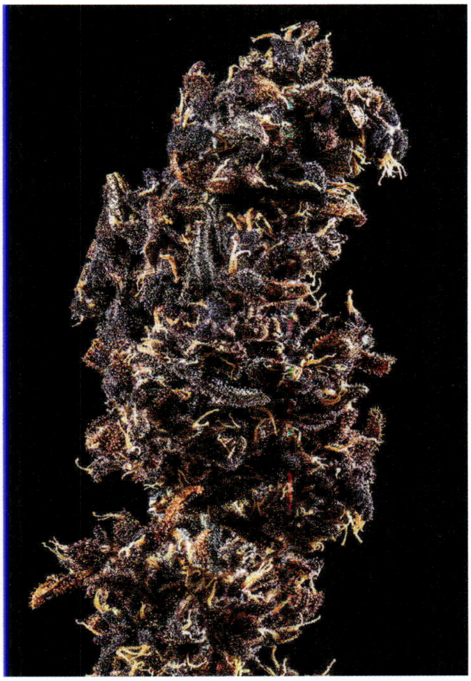

Devil Cream Auto from Sweet Seeds.

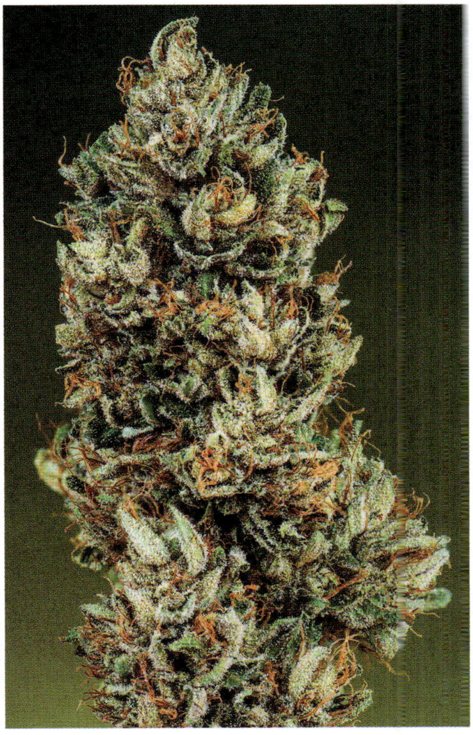

Bubba Island Kush from Dutch Passion.

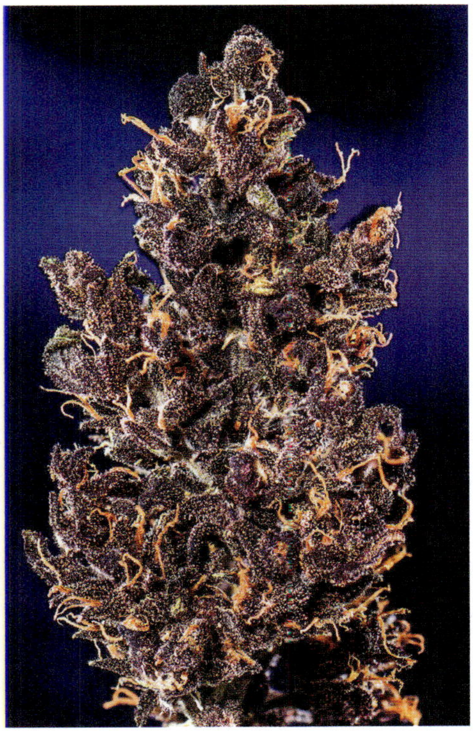

Purple Punch from Seedstockers.

PHOTOS: ERIC PALMER

Bud Storage

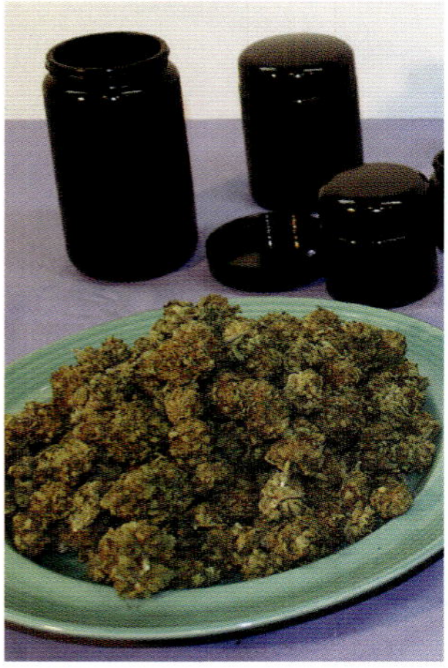

Organize dried buds.

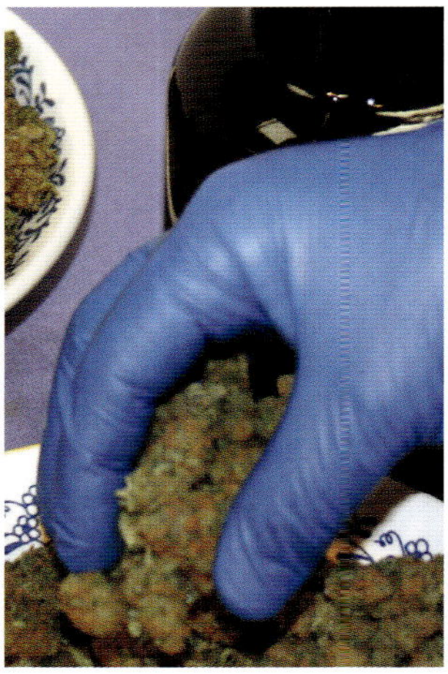

Wear gloves.

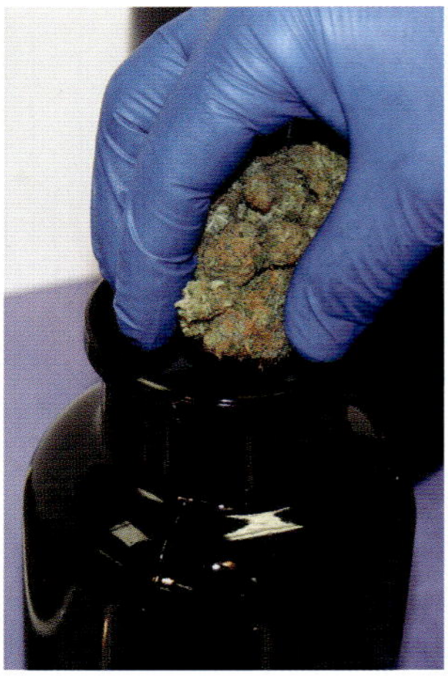

Carefully place bud in jar.

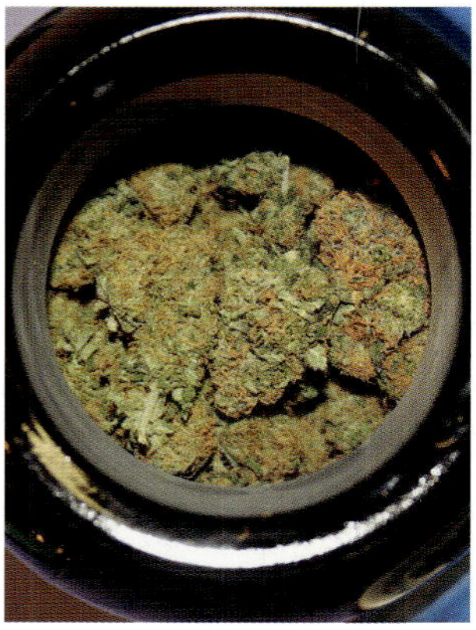

Leave room for air.

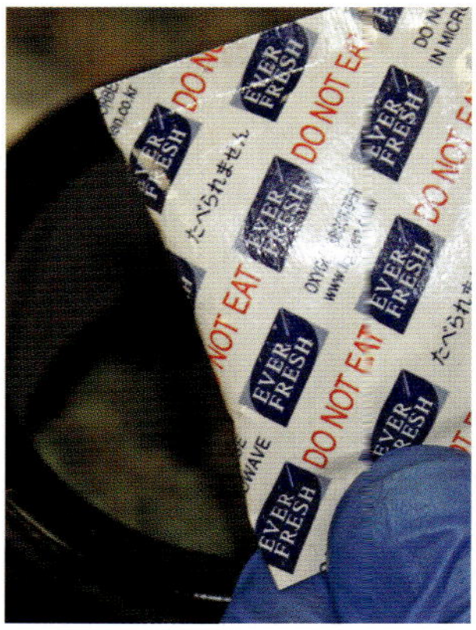

Insert Oxygen Absorber

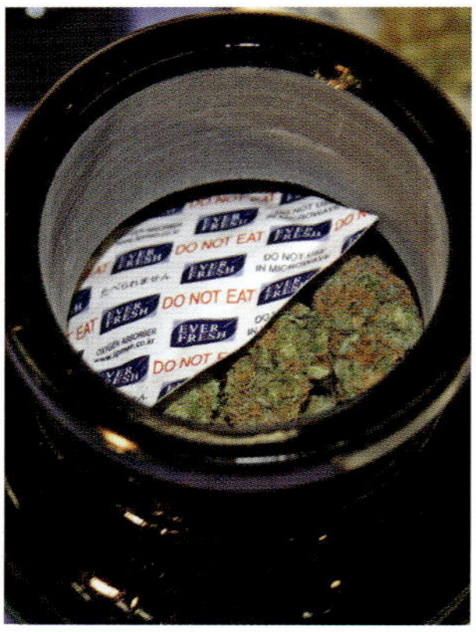

Place gently on top of bud.

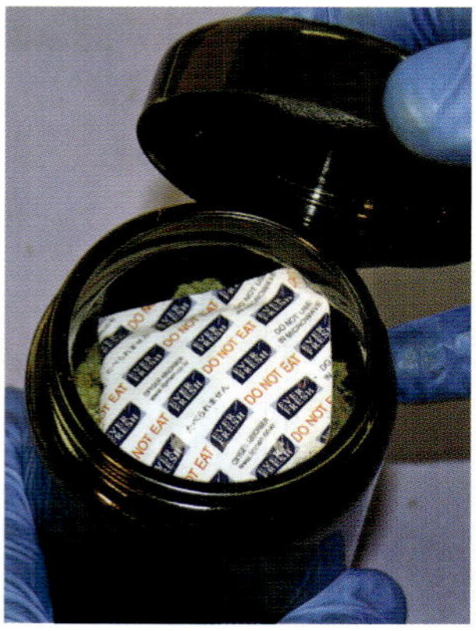

Close lid gently on MM Jar.

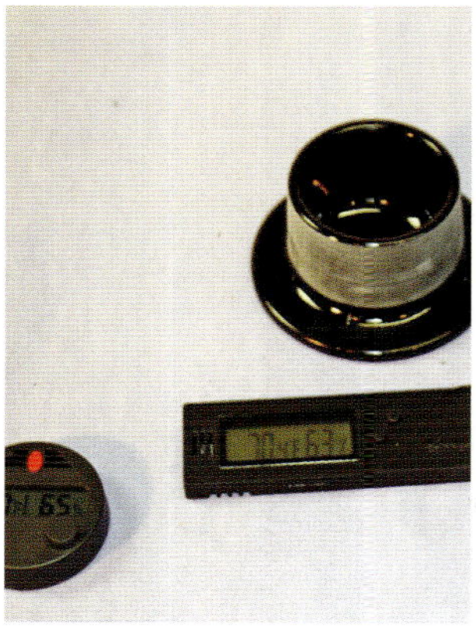

Monitor temperature ard humidity.

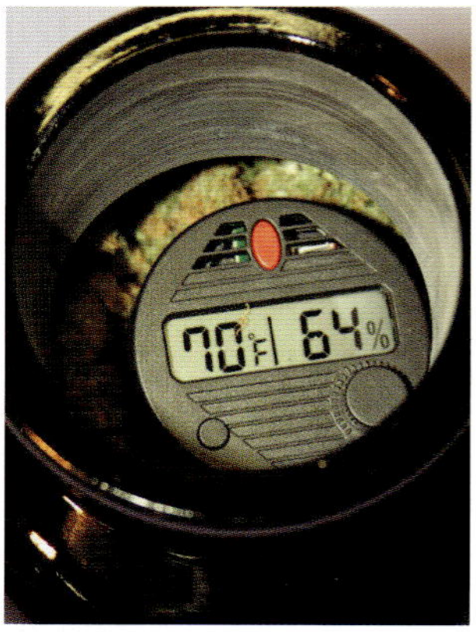

Perfect temp and moisture levels.

PHOTOS: MM JARS

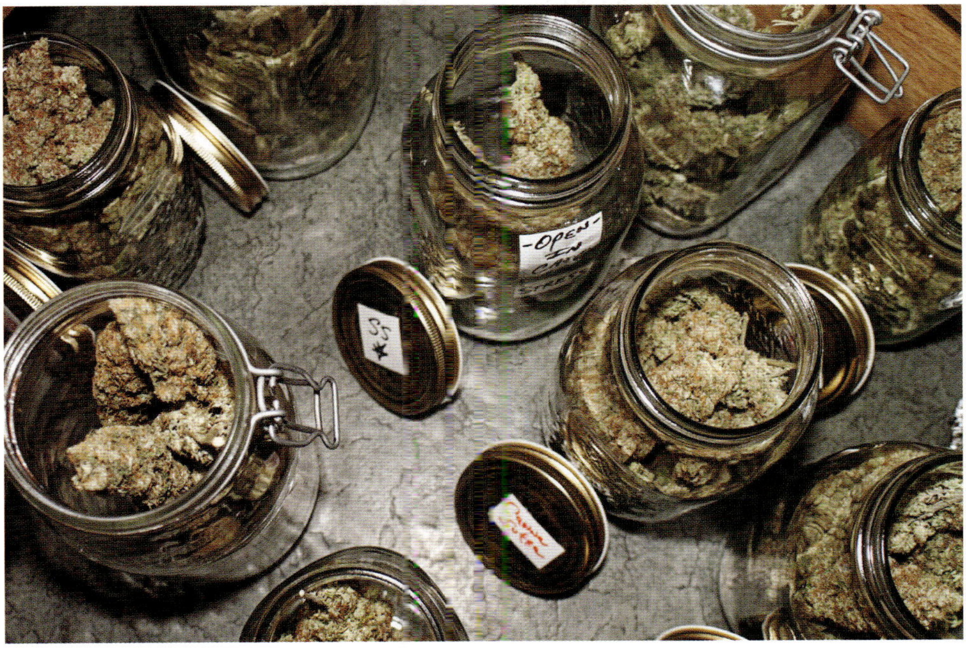

When the buds are dry enough you will begin the curing stage by canning them.

PHOTO: ED BORG

Curing

The next step is to can and cure your buds. Canning is a great way to maximize the potential of your bud. All you need are cans with removable lids. Select cans with large brims that allow your whole hand to fit inside. The wider the brim, the better. Make sure you label the cans well. Glass jars are transparent, and while light in the latter stages of curing doesn't impact cannabinoid changes as much as temperature, there can still be cellular photosynthetic activity in the early stages, so store them in the dark. As time passes cell death will stop photosynthesis. Harvesting bud doesn't automatically stop photosynthesis on that part. If it did, clones would not be possible.

If you've hung your plants upside down and dried them for three weeks, you can subtract that time from the canning period. If the planned canning period is the minimal three weeks then go an extra week drying or canning. Although you can have usable bud two weeks after harvest, waiting for four or more weeks for the bud to cure will result in a higher quality bud. Sampling is the best way to judge the optimal timing. Patience is essential and will be rewarded with the best-quality bud.

At this time, preparation may also be required for projects like water bubble hash extraction. The remaining branches and stems may contain THC, but only in small quantities. Smaller stems on which pistils are found can be used to experiment with water extraction. See Chapter 18. You can compost larger stems and other organic material you won't be using. See Chapter 14.

Place the can in a cool, dark room or cupboard. Open the lid for around six hours every day, and then seal it again. Move the bud around daily or every couple of days during the first few weeks. This popular and effective curing technique results in great-tasting bud. Let the bud cure for three to four weeks before sampling. Bud cured with the canning method is at its highest quality during this stage. Beyond this point, THC cannabinoids change composition and lose potency as degradation occurs. While other curing processes exist, canning is an effective and affordable option.

Canning also induces sweating in the bud, which enhances decarboxylation while causing the bud to retain its smell and flavor. Continue to air out the buds after curing. By opening and closing the can at different intervals, you can control how damp or dry your bud becomes. Open the cans for ten minutes twice each day to make them

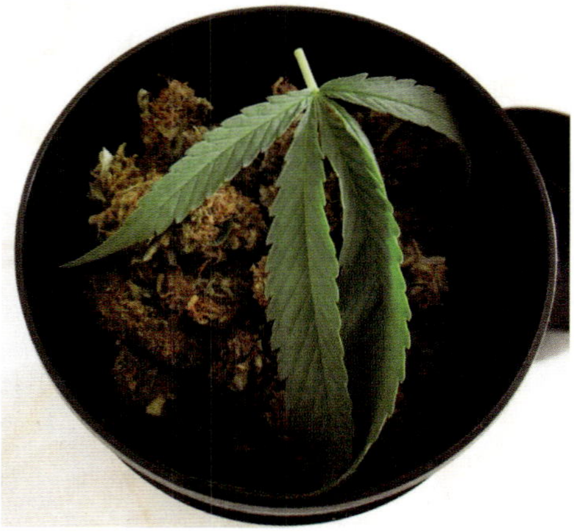

An open can of cured bud.

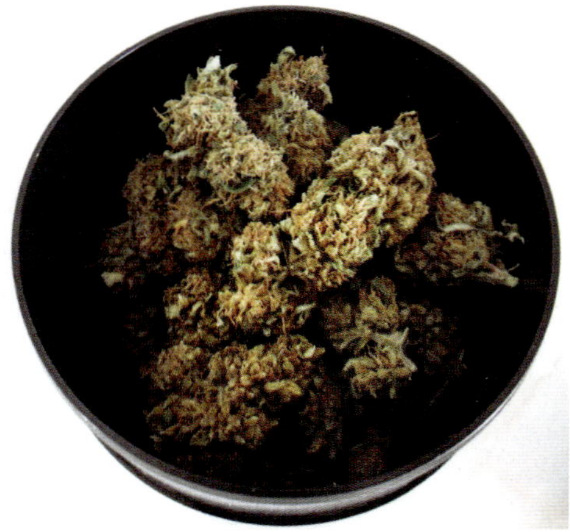

Give your canned buds some air each day.

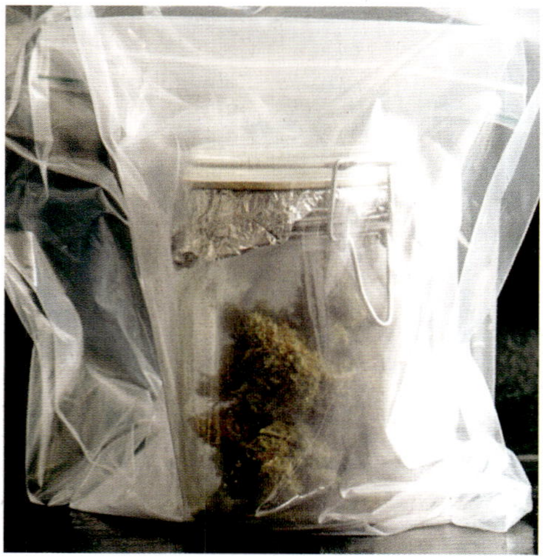

You might want to pack them to contain smells.

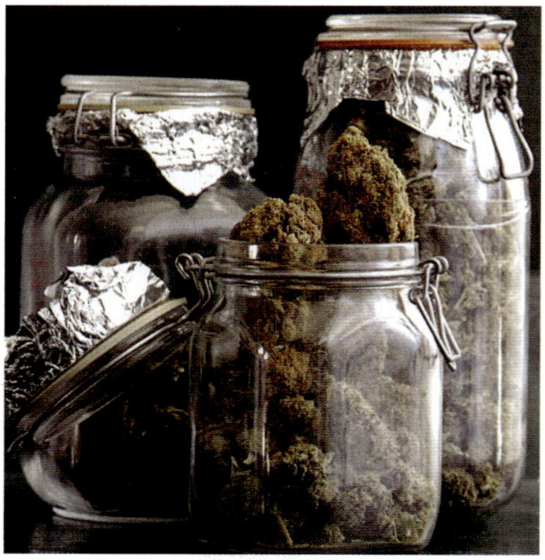

An open jar will usually smell quite pungent. First-class results.

PHOTOS: ED BORG

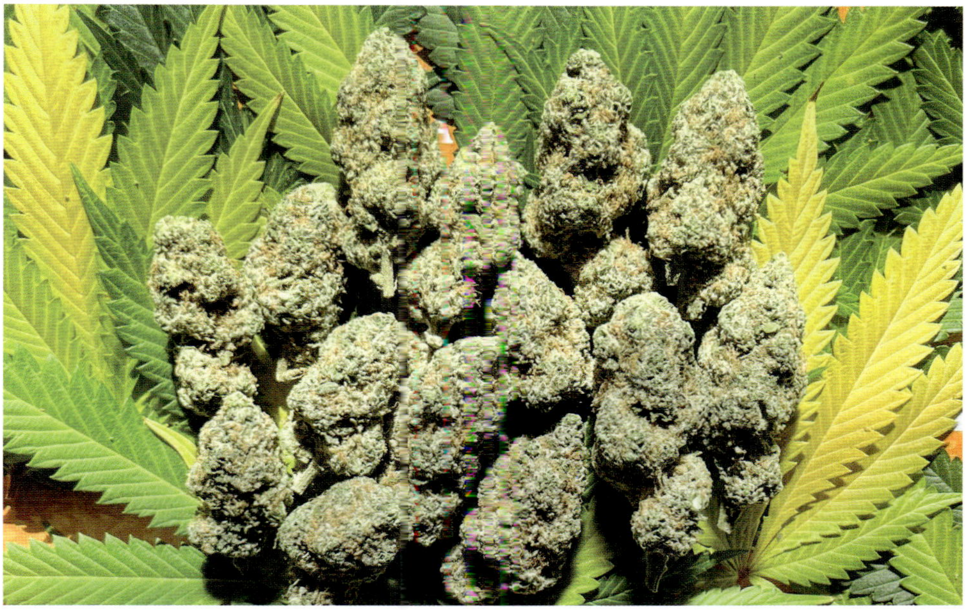

Nugs, dense and dry, revealing their final weight.

dry quicker. If they are too dry, you can add bud of the same strain from a moist can to exchange their moisture. Mold problems arise when old buds are transferred between cans. You can use slices of apple, orange, or other fruit to bring back moisture. They will also add their aroma and taste to the buds.

Drying your bud removes moisture which makes THC easier to vaporize and thus more psychoactive. Applying heat also removes water but will affect the overall cannabinoid content of the bud. Do not press the bud or pack it tightly during curing, as the bunching of THC particles makes them harder to vaporize.

Most of all, curing helps to break down chlorophyll, which contains magnesium. Magnesium is responsible for the sharp and harsh taste in the back of your throat when you vaporize fresh bud. Magnesium flashes like a sparkler when it burns.

Labeling is everything. When placing a piece of bud into a can, label each one with the date. Use older bud before newer bud.

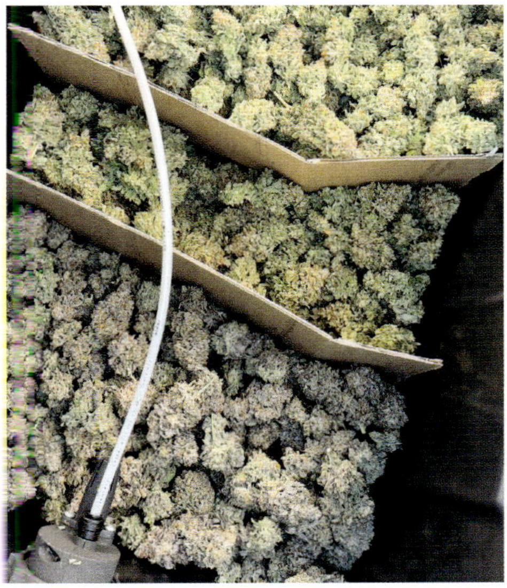

A box full of these dense and dry nugs.

PHOTOS: TANYA PETERSEN (TOP), TRAVIS HOELLERER @SOFAKINGHIGH (BOTTOM)

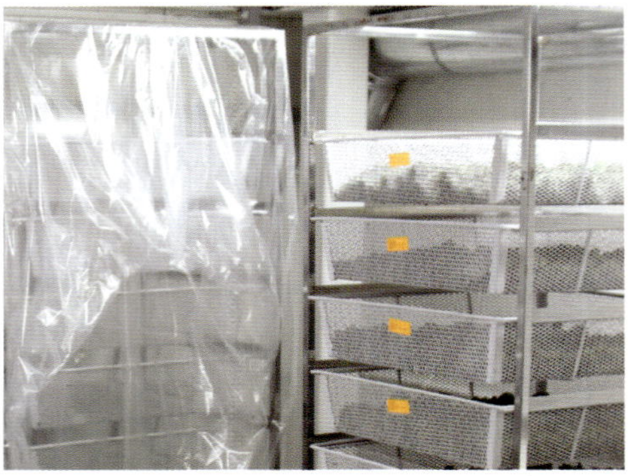

Screens can prevent some mold spores from settling on harvested bud.

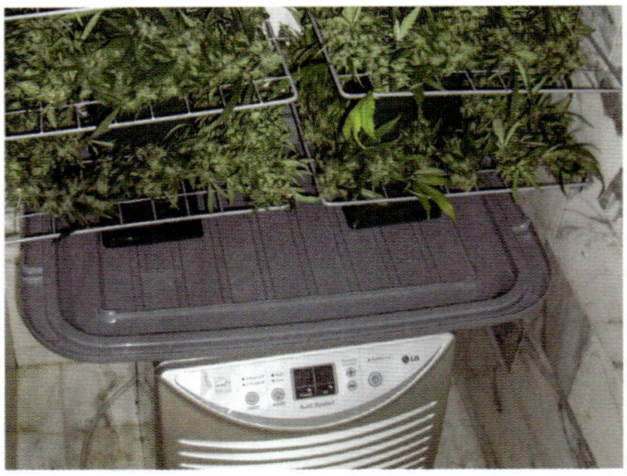

A dehumidifier prevents moist conditions from occurring.

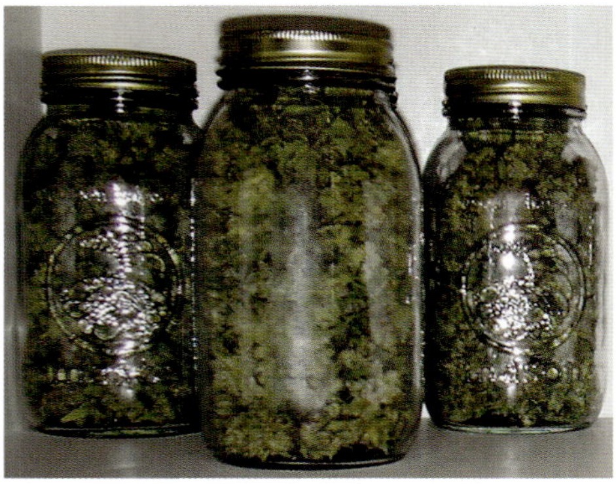

Top middle jar is fogging up with moisture, which means it needs fresh air fast.

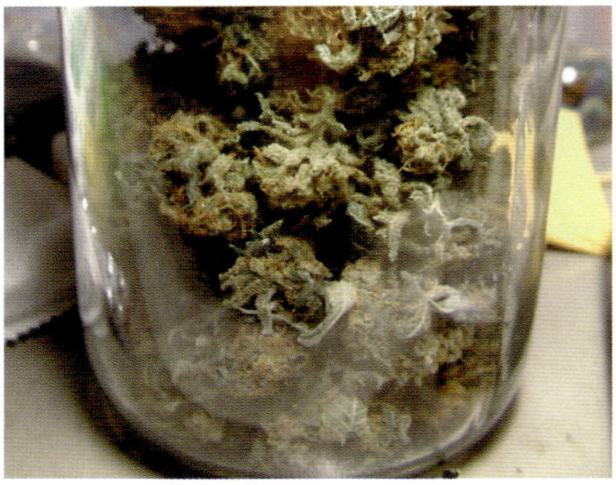

The bottom right of this jar is fogging and moist. You need fresh air and a dry jar.

PHOTOS: PEACE NATURALS / PHOTOGRAPHED BY DAVID STRANGE (TOP LEFT), MEDICINAL CLONES/CANNANETICS (TOP RIGHT AND BOTTOM ROW)

Mold

Throughout this book, we have covered methods to prevent mold through the design of grow rooms and the use of fungicides. Mold, a type of fungus, has microscopic spores that are present in the air. It thrives on the moisture and nutrients found in various substances like food, flowers, and decaying organic matter. The spores grow hyphae, white or gray fluff similar to webbing. If you're unsure what mold looks like, boil some tomato soup, let it cool to room temperature, pour it into a small plastic container, and put some clear plastic wrap on top, but don't vacuum seal it. There should be a layer of air between the film and the soup's surface. Leave it in the light for a few days. Blotches will appear on the surface. Since the soup was boiled, most pathogens were eliminated, meaning that the blotching is coming from another source: Spores in the air, captured as we put the film on, using the soup's nutrients to grow and produce more spores. That is mold.

Regularly cleaning a grow room is essential to eliminate as much mold as possible. Using intake filters helps prevent most mold spores from getting in, and any spores that enter are usually ventilated out. Flowers harvested in clean grow rooms are relatively safe from mold spores. Outdoor grows are more challenging as they are subject to environmental factors. Mold decays buds. Just like moldy food, moldy bud should be thrown out immediately, as it is unsafe for human consumption.

Besides checking your flowering plants for mold, check your cured bud. Unless your curing cupboard has a HEPA filter, spores in the air will likely settle on the bud during occasional breathing periods. These spores may grow and thrive, leading to nutrient absorption and bud decay.

HEPA filters are one solution to preventing mold growth while the cans breathe. For most growers, the simpler solution is to use the bud before spores can grow. Mold can occur at any time and will occur eventually. Even in the best conditions, six- to eight-month-old bud can get moldy. When you consider this, as well as the degradation of cannabinoids and potency over time, you'll understand why people avoid aged bud.

The rate at which mold grows depends on nutrients, water sources, and temperature. You can't prevent herbs from containing mold-friendly nutrients, but you can decrease the RH with a dehumidifier and the temperature with ventilation. Avoid keeping bud sealed up in stale air. Check them regularly for signs of mold. That means opening the bud slightly with tweezers and looking between the nodes. Use a magnifying aid if the mold is difficult to see, but the naked eye can usually spot hyphae. The moment you find any, throw it away. Fire may burn up the mold, but spores can still be released as it happens. Some cannabis won't be burned, such as with edibles and vapes. If you are constantly seeing mold, you must clean your curing area and cans and consider a HEPA filter for airflow screening.

You can freeze bud for long-term storage for up to one year, but this can cause several problems. Freezing separates trichomes from the flowers, so most frozen bud ends up being good enough only for use as kief for hash processing. Bud doesn't taste as good after a long time in storage and can spoil if not vacuum-sealed. If you want good-tasting, fresh bud, aim for perpetual harvests.

Hemp

Cannabis plants offer more than just flowers. Hemp is cultivated globally from the bast fibers present in all cannabis plants to create textiles.

Mechanical Hemp Harvesting

Mechanical harvesting, though primarily used for processing the bast fibers of a hemp plant, can also be applied to cannabis. The six layers of a plant stem pertinent to growers are the epidermis, cortex, bast fibers, phloem, xylem, and the pith at the core. The bast fiber, situated between the cortex and phloem, is used to produce textiles. Proper processing of bast fibers involves retting.

Traditional Hemp Harvest

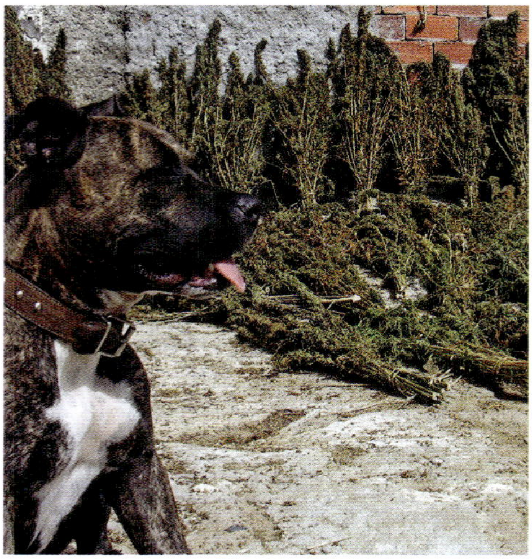
Natural bacteria in the environment helps degrade pectines in the stem.

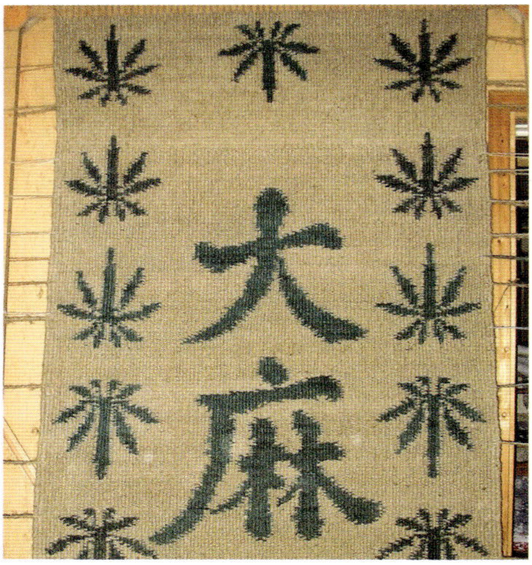

Hemp textile.

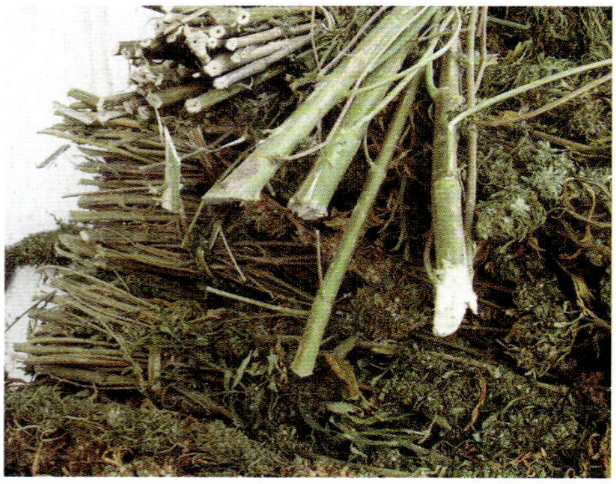
The best fiber is the layer between the cortex and phloem.

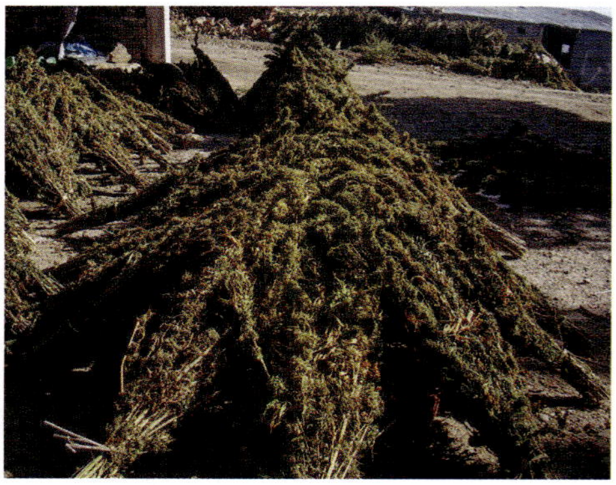
Hemp being retted.

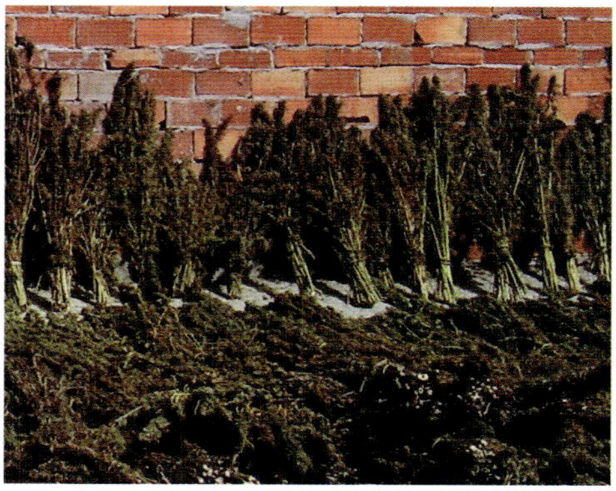
Harvested plants are turned over periodically.

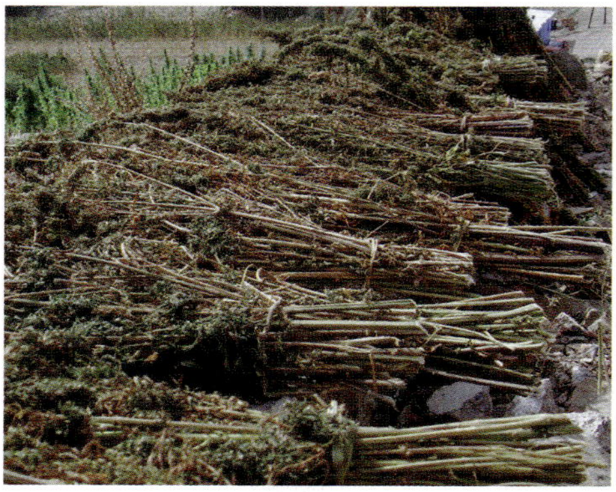
Turning over is done by pivoting in rows.

PHOTOS: PAULO FERREIRA

Retting

Retting separates the bast fibers from the stalk so that a biodegradable process occurs within the harvest. The traditional method of retting is to leave the plants outside on the ground after harvesting and periodically flip them. The plants are turned daily to expose each side to the elements. This is sometimes called swathing the harvest. Natural bacteria in the environment degrade pectins in the stem and branches. Many hemp farmers leave a considerable distance between the plants, typically equaling the projected height between furrows, so the plant can fall into this empty space when it is cut down. The result is long stretches of plants lying on their sides that can be turned over from left to right and from right to left again by machines in a process called windrowing. This takes two to three weeks in order for plants to be well retted.

Plants are also retted in water, usually in a water tank or river. However, this is more difficult as you need to accurately judge when the retting is finished, or the quality of the fiber will be affected. Under-retting will make the fibers hard to separate while over-retting will weaken the fibers. Retting in water takes one to two weeks. On an industrial scale, it is done in large vats, and the water is refreshed after a few hours of initial placement to remove waste material. The leached hemp liquid can be used as a fertilizer. Once this leaching is finished, the hemp is stored for a few days to a week before it is ready. Depending on the fiber quality you need, you can use both water and dry retting over a longer period.

Larger plots can use mechanical turners for windrowed hemp turning. Windrowed hemp can then be stacked using a baler. The hemp can be cut into pieces with rotary blades or discs/bars with blades at various heights. One advantage to this is getting the seeded heads along with fiber rather than focusing on one or the other. The woody core of the stem can be removed after peeling the fibers off. This decorticating can be done during the retting process.

The next steps depend on what you want to do with your hemp fibers, and there are many things you can do with hemp in an eco-friendly world. The fibers are processed into yarn, using physical manual labor, machines, or chemical treatment to make them fleecy and soft.

Additional treatments, such as ligand removal, can make them even softer. The yarn is then made into clothing. Anything that cotton can do, hemp can do better. Some uses of hemp don't require processing to be softer. Hemp is also used in solid biocomposites, such as in car doors. Some modern eco-friendly cars are built from hemp. Seeds from hemp can even be used in hemp oils. Cannabis is more than just its flowers. It has many other ecological uses that all cannabis cultivators should try to become familiar with. Cannabis growers should also support the hemp cause by actively buying hemp products, and even possibly making hemp themselves.

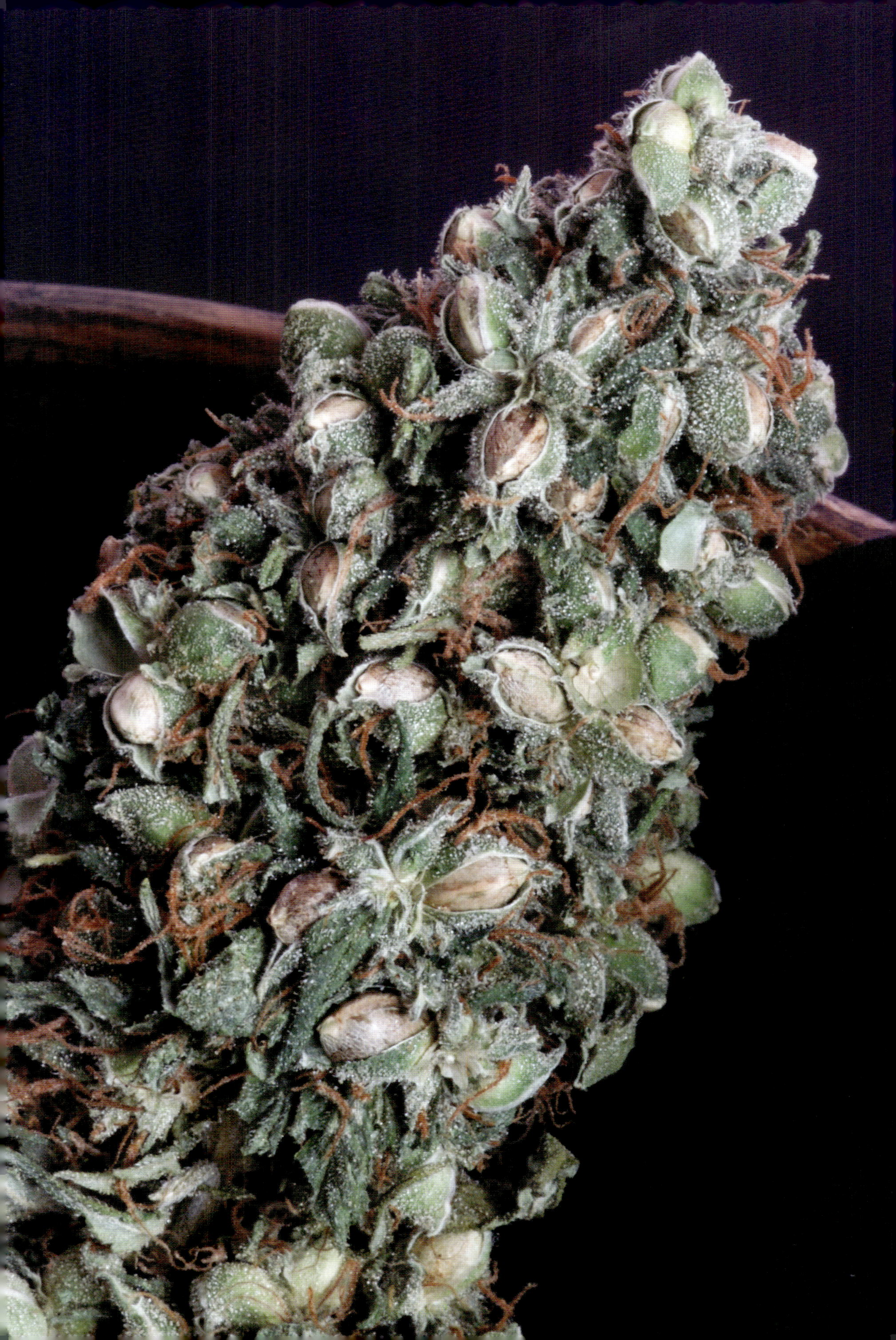

17

How to Breed Cannabis

To continue growing a cannabis strain you enjoy, cloning is your best option. Cannabis breeds are typically sold as seeds, involving the reproduction of both male and female plants through human selection. However, there's also a market for select clones from hybrids that exhibit new characteristics absent in the parent plants. While clones are acceptable, it's preferable to have the strain in seed format for distribution and storage. Although a select clone from a hybrid cross can be bred to produce seeds, the process involves many generations and trait selection.

Female plants produce seeds when pollinated with male pollen. This does not mean that by purchasing any pack of seeds, you can 'breed' males and females by collecting any seeds the plants produce, because you're allowing males to pollinate females randomly, not selectively. Nature takes its course, and it's natural selection at work, not breeding selection. Also, using this method won't fully replicate the strain unless the two parent plants come from the same inbred line (IBL).[1] In stable plants with minimal variation, allowing males and females to interact and produce seeds freely can yield plants very similar to their parents. In contrast, plants with more variation, such as hybrids, will produce offspring with greater variation, meaning you won't replicate the parent plants as closely. This variation can lead to different outcomes—better, worse, or the same. What's considered better or worse depends on the environment and personal preference. For breeders, better or worse is often subjective concerning taste, smell, and color, but it can also be objective, like resistance to mold. Is it more desirable to have higher potency or higher yields? That's personal choice and encompasses much of what the breeding market focuses on, including medical strains bred for specific cannabinoid contents and ratios. There's also an overlap between recreational and medical strains.

PHOTO: ED BORG

Allowing stable males and females (IBLs from the same breeder and strain) to breed should result in seeds that inherit most of the parents' characteristics. Starting with 10 seeds, you can expand to over 100 seeds, creating a germplasm that you can store

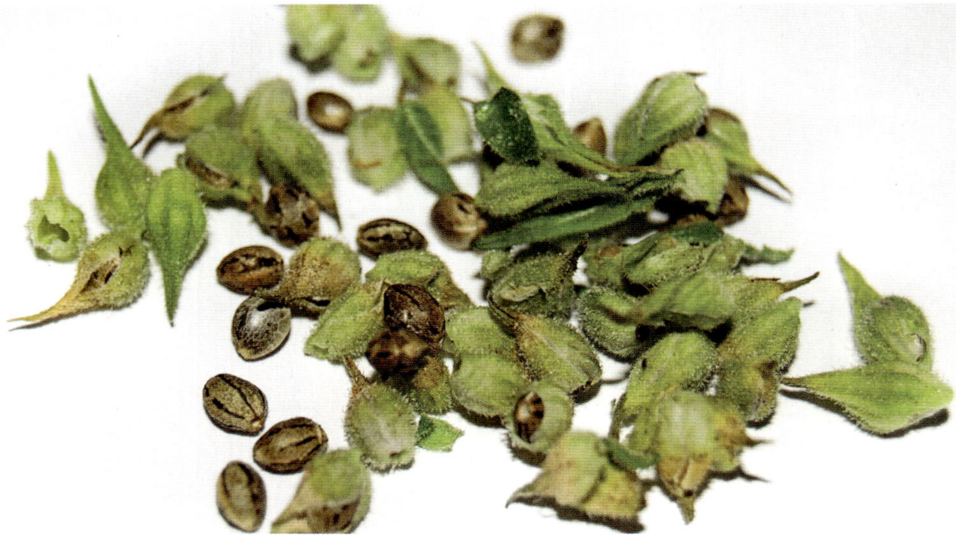

Harvested seeds have gray and black striations when the fresh green seed cases are off the bract. Seed breeders will spend days peeling the green seed casings off and preparing the seeds for sale and further breeding projects.

PHOTO: CH9 FEMALE SEEDS

or pass on. The germplasm serves as your resource for your genetics. If you want to create a plant with characteristics from two different strains, breeding from seed is your only option, as cloning rarely retains the males. This is the key difference between cultivation for product and cultivation for breeding: Breeders cultivate and clone both male and female populations.

This chapter introduces basic breeding procedures and then delves into advanced techniques, including breeding a true strain and backcrossing; if you want to produce seeds from two strains, this chapter is for you.

Making Seeds

How easy is it to produce seeds? First, it is important to maintain healthy plants and a stable growing environment. When your male plants release their pollen in your grow room, they will pollinate the female flowers. If you want to limit the number of seeds produced, you can reduce the number of male plants. With active ventilation, pollen will disperse throughout the grow area via the airflow. Less pollen means fewer seeds, but even a minuscule amount of pollen is sufficient for each seed. A single male plant can pollinate numerous females. However, it's crucial for males and females to flower simultaneously. If males release their pollen too early, there won't be much available for the females. This can occur when crossing indica with sativa plants, as the later-flowering sativa female may not synchronize with the earlier-flowering indica male. Breeders often collect pollen first and then apply it directly to their females using a brush, making this a non-issue.

Collecting and Pollen Storage

Collecting and storing pollen requires different processes for indoor and outdoor cultivation. When collecting pollen indoors, it's essential to turn off extraction, intake, or general fans during male flowering. These fans can disperse pollen throughout the grow area, reducing the amount available for collection. Even a tiny amount of pollen is sufficient per seed, and a single male plant can pollinate multiple females. However, for successful pollination, males and females must flower simultaneously. Turning off fans may result in temperature issues, but LED lighting, which produces less heat, is becoming popular for male cultivation.

During the male flowering phase, LEDs are kept on for a 12/12 photoperiod, while fans are turned off. This allows males to release their pollen, which can be easily collected for storage or future use. It's also feasible to clone males and produce pollen under LEDs in small grow tents. Unlike female flowers, male pollen production doesn't require high light intensity. However, this doesn't mean that males don't need any light or photoperiod adjustment. Maintaining the 12/12 photoperiod during flowering is their natural state, as photosynthesis is still essential for pollen production. Without light,

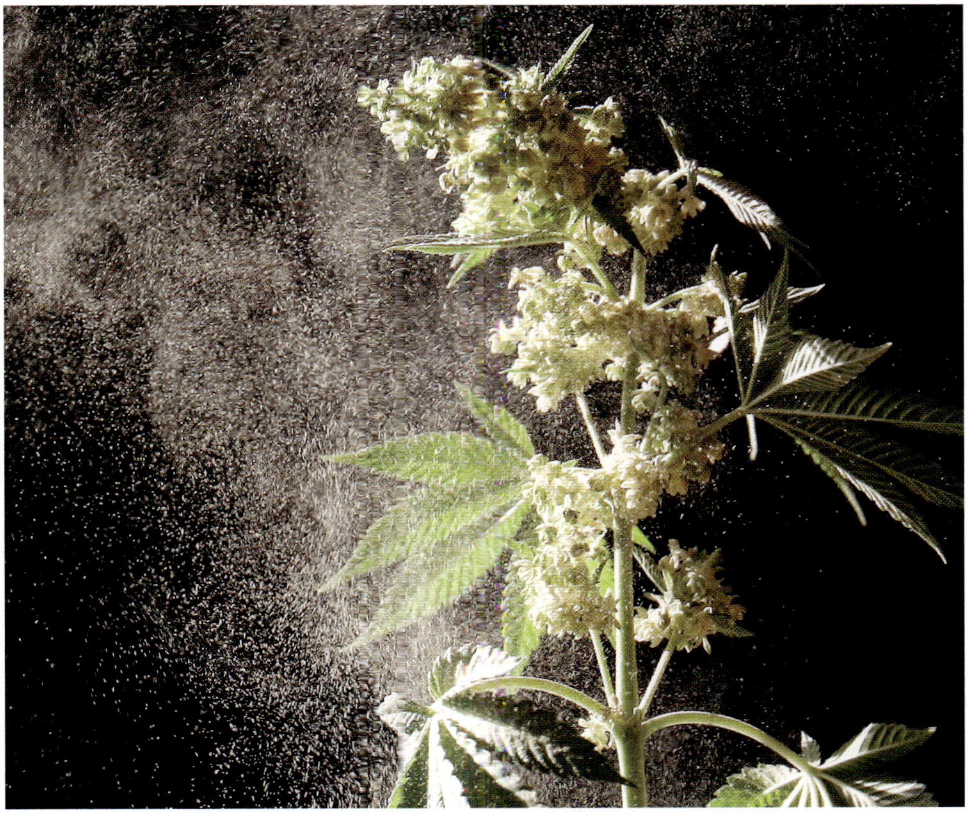

Fans or wind will blow pollen from a male plant everywhere and negate attempts to grow a sinsemilla female crop. However, this pollen is valuable for breeding and is necessary to make seeds.

PHOTO: ANNIBALESEEDSHOP.COM

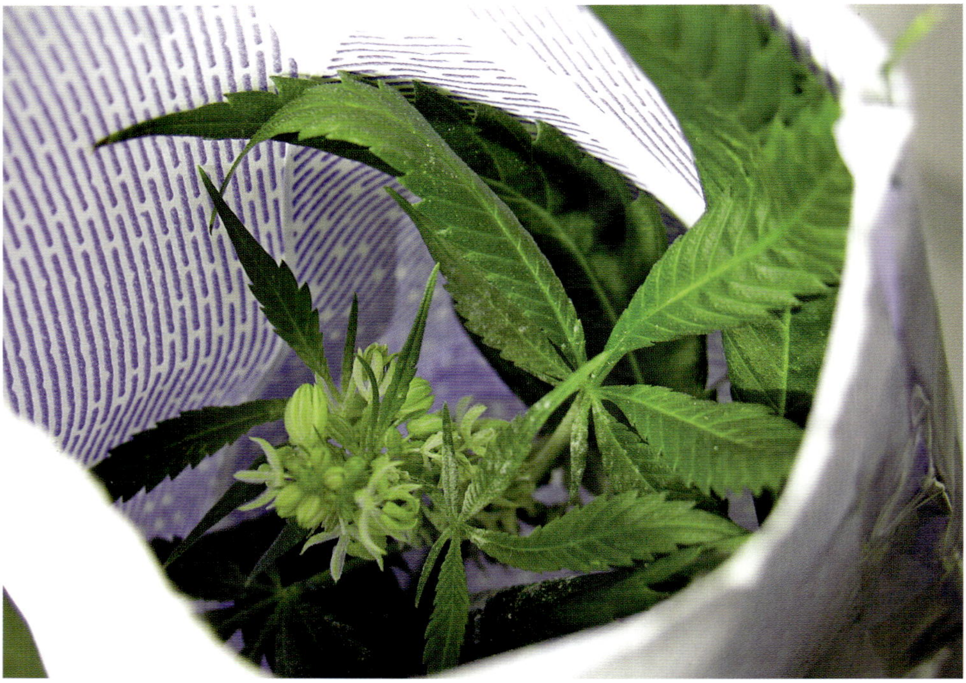

You can collect po len by placing a flowering branch into an envelope with the side cut away.

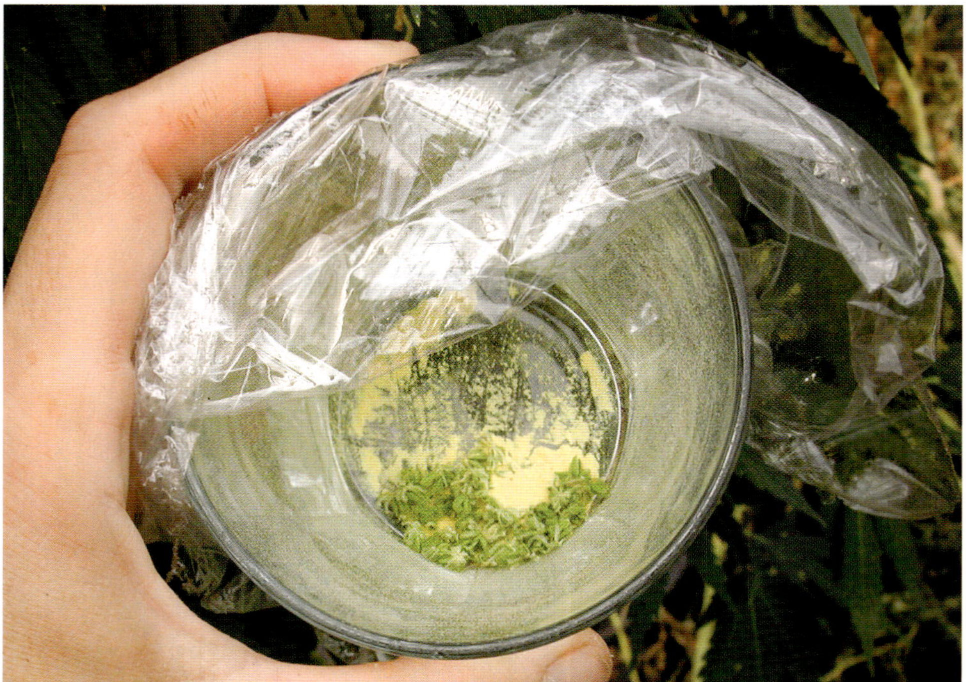

You can also tap the flowers into a container such as a plastic beaker and place cellophane on top to seal it when finished.

PHOTOS: DAVID STRANGE (TOP), MANDALA SEEDS (BOTTOM)

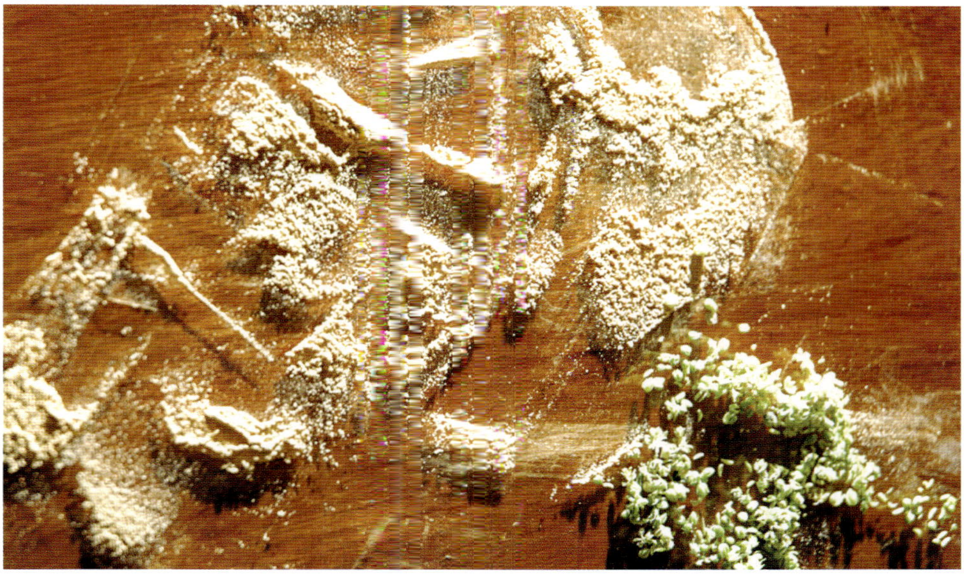

You can't underestimate how much pollen can come out of one flower. All of this pollen came from the flower parts in the lower right of this picture

PHOTO: ED BORG

photosynthesis ceases, and the plant enters a state of stress. In some cases, the plant may even release non-viable, or immature, pollen in a desperate attempt to reproduce before succumbing to the lack of light. The ability to partition male pollen production into small cloning tents under LEDs is one of the innovative possibilities that LED lighting has introduced to cannabis cultivation.

Outdoor pollen collection presents unique challenges due to uncontrollable wind factors. However, in a closed greenhouse during the flowering period, if the environment remains calm, you can use the indoor pollen collection method.

If wind is an issue, bagging is the more effective choice.

To use the bagging method, tie small pouches around most of the male flowering parts. Ziplock bags are ideal for collecting pollen. It's not necessary to seal the bags tightly around the stems; instead, tie them on loosely, allowing some essential airflow to prevent mold. The branches and leaves will naturally secure the bags in place as you slip them on, and a string can further secure the bags around the male flowers. You will be able to see the pollen accumulating inside the bag. If you don't have clear bags or prefer brown bagging, expose one flowering part of a branch. When this part starts releasing pollen, it's likely that others will follow suit, collecting pollen into your bags. Sometimes these releases are only minutes apart, making it necessary to closely monitor the male flowering stage. The key is to attach the bags just before the pollen drops and leave them in place. When the branch releases pollen or you observe

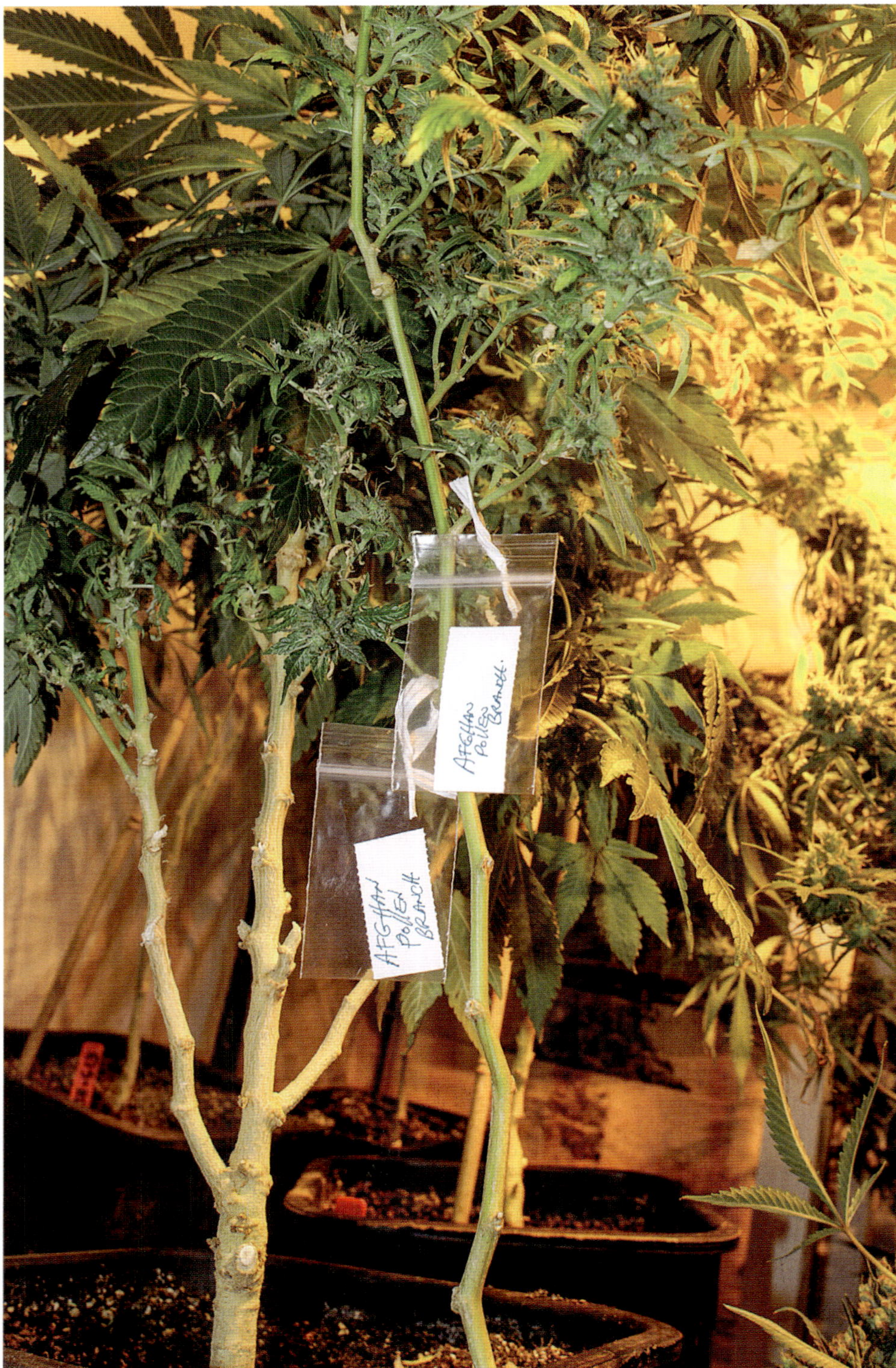

PHOTO: ED BORG

Transparent bags with labels are attached to male flowers when they are mature enough.

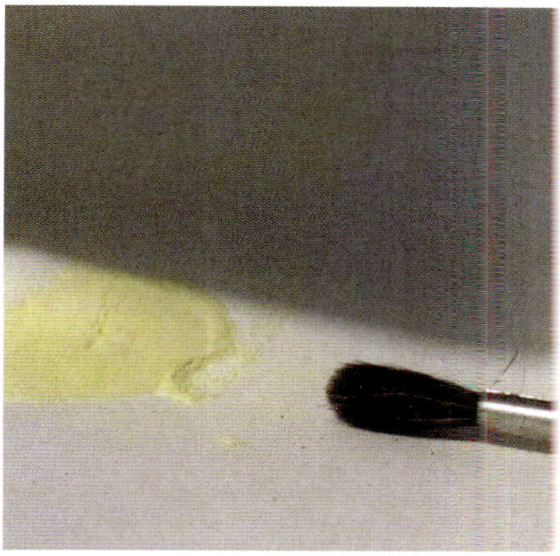

A clean brush is ideal for putting pollen on females.

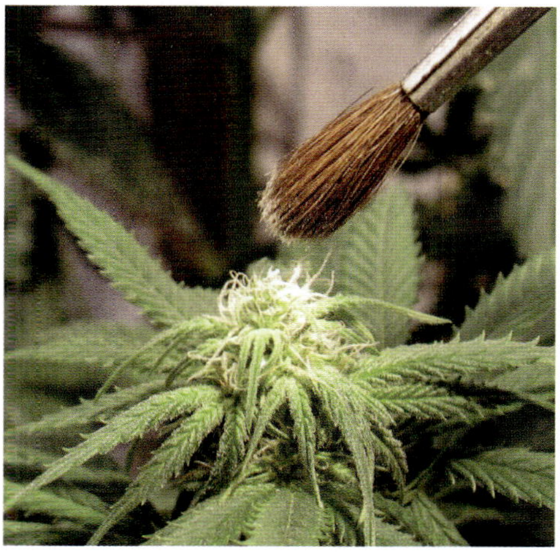

After dipping the brush into the pollen, paint it onto the female flowers.

pollen accumulating in your pouch, you should be able to collect a significant amount. It's not necessary to perforate the bags if you introduce them just before pollen is released. However, it's crucial to remove the bags promptly after pollen collection to prevent condensation and moisture buildup, which can make pollen collection more challenging and introduce mold. This method allows you to collect all the pollen a male plant can produce.

If there is no wind, collecting pollen after it falls from the pods onto the leaves below is a simple process that doesn't require bagging. Pollen can be collected using a sheet of paper inserted between the stem and supported by the leaves on the branches. The paper can capture a substantial amount of pollen and can easily funnel it into a jar for storage. You can place paper on multiple branch levels of the plant. While this method may not capture all the pollen, it can collect enough for your intended project.

You can also sieve a male flower to gather the particles, which will include pollen. This is a useful method when dealing with situations where minimal pollen was produced or when it was dispersed by the wind.

Breeders typically transfer the collected pollen into a labeled collection jar, indicating the source plant. This pollen can then be applied with a brush to female flowers for pollination or stored for future use. Film canisters or white plastic medical pill containers are suitable for this. While pollen can be stored in the freezer for up to 18 months, it's best used within six months of collection, as there is a good chance that, like seeds, they will not be viable after a long time—although some particles and a few seeds could be. In short, it's not something we can depend on. Most breeders go through cycles of collection, storage, and use shortly after.

PHOTOS: KAYA

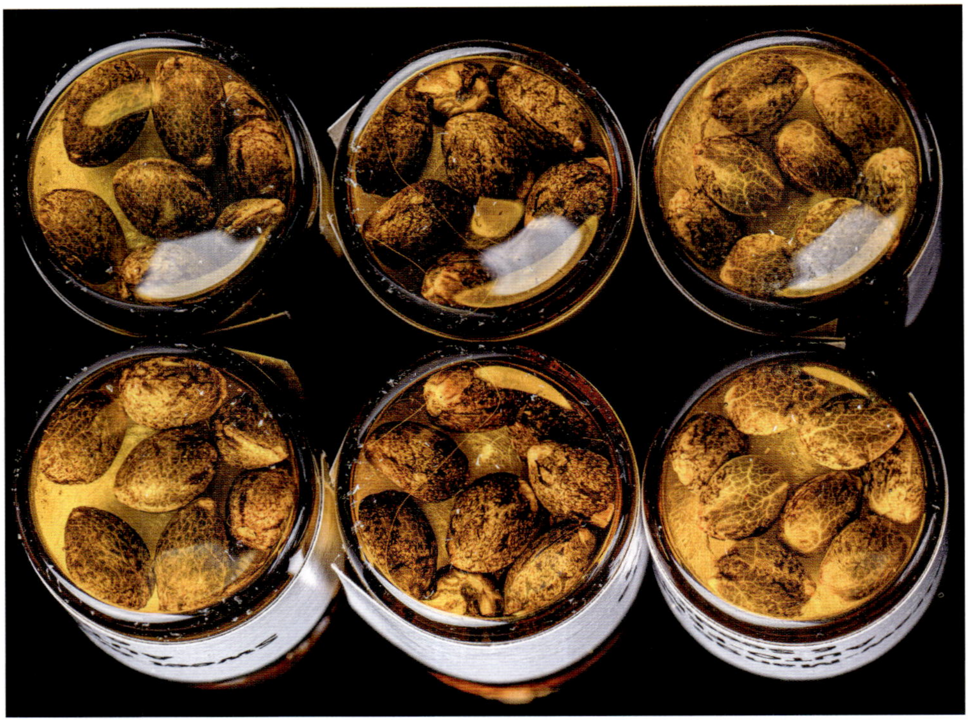

Store seeds in a small plastic container. You can also reuse plastic Tic Tac boxes.

Creating and Storing Seeds

If you have pollinated your plants, you will find seeds in the buds at the end of the flowering stage. These seeds should appear gray, tan, or dark brown. They may also have stripes, bands, or colored markings. If the seeds are pale cream or white, they are likely not viable, indicating premature harvesting. It's essential to wait until the end of the flowering period to harvest your seeds. If you harvest seeds too early from one plant, wait for the others to finish flowering before collecting seeds. To pinpoint the ideal seed maturity, consider taking samples daily rather than harvesting all at once. This method helps ensure that your seeds are ready for collection.

Collecting seeds from dry, cured buds is more straightforward than from freshly harvested plants. You can simply shake them out once the buds are dried. However, if the buds are very sticky, the seeds might be mixed with the bud material, making it challenging to separate them from the sticky calyx pods. Do not squeeze the calyx directly, as this can damage the seeds inside. Instead, gently tease the seeds out from the calyx with your fingers. If you prefer not to keep the bud material, you can brush a flowering branch containing seeds against some fabric or a sieve to release the seeds from their calyx pods, then separate the seeds from other flowering materials in the catching tray. Some machines are available for separating seeds from flowers on a larger scale, most using vibrations to free the seeds from the flowers, as sieving can be

PHOTO: ROB BRAMHILL

more destructive. These range from small units resembling saucepans to larger farm machinery. While they are not cheap, they can significantly reduce the time required for processing bulk loads. However, most growers do collect seeds manually.

If you plan to use the seeds after two years, store them in an airtight container and place it in the freezer. For seeds for use within the next two years, a standard film canister or a similar container will suffice. Keep this container away from heat and direct light, and prevent it from becoming damp, as moisture can spoil your seeds. Containers stored in the freezer should remain sealed until you are ready to use the seeds. When you decide to use them, allow the seeds to thaw at room temperature for at least 12 hours. Note that most growers do not depend on frozen seeds, but prefer shorter turnaround times by producing fresh seeds using fresh pollen in each cycle.

Simple Breeding

Your breeding approach will depend on your ultimate goals. Do you aim to develop a completely new strain, produce seeds that closely resemble the parent plants, or simply cross two plants to create a straightforward hybrid strain? Answering these fundamental questions should guide your decisions before you embark on a breeding project. The following section explores the basic concept of producing seeds that resemble the parents.

Continuing a Strain through Seeds

Let's say you've invested $120 in Amnesia Haze seeds and want to multiply your supply without introducing traits from other strains. This is a straightforward process. Ensure that the male and female plants you intend to breed come from the same strain batch—that is Amnesia Haze all from the same breeder. If you were to use Amnesia Haze seeds from different breeders, you would likely encounter significant variations, because most breeders create their own versions of popular strains. To maintain consistency, always use the same strain from the same breeder. If your grow room contains only Amnesia Haze seeds from one breeder, you can work with groups of males and females. By applying the pollen-gathering and application methods discussed earlier, you'll produce more Amnesia Haze seeds. Unless your strain is an IBL or derived from a highly stable pure lineage, you may lose some of the original parent plants' characteristics in the process. The stability of the strain you use as the source will directly influence the level of variation you can expect. This does not make you a breeder, as you are merely producing seeds from the same strain with the potential for some variation while obtaining free seeds. This approach simply allows you to share seeds of the same strain with others and avoid repurchasing seeds from that particular strain.

To understand this concept, consider the difference between digital and analog. When you digitally copy a file, you maintain the integrity of the source material. In contrast, analog copying involves a process that loses information because it relies on electrical signals, which are waves that replicate based on their closest counterparts rather than binary code. It's somewhat like having a list of possible things it could be and then copying from this "could be" list. The analog copying mechanism aims to identify the signal and replicate it, introducing subtle variations between the original signal and the duplicated form. This results in variations between tapes copied from one to another, leading to a loss of original data and the introduction of alternatives that alter the sound, or degradation of the source material. If stable strains are analogous to digital copying, then unstable strains, such as new hybrids, are akin to analog copying because there's a significant amount of variation for the copying mechanism to select from.

However, just as a skilled sound engineer can remaster a recording to enhance its quality, a breeder can work with the traits of plants to engineer the desired characteristics. Breeding is a form of engineering, whereas copying is merely duplicating. Breeders operate within an analog-like reproduction system but can carefully select and manipulate traits to achieve the desired outcome. They can mix the original traits with new ones in the parts they are refining, similar to how a sound engineer combines the original sound with new elements during remastering. Breeders obtain these traits from the source material or introduce new traits from external sources, such as another plant. They can select specific aspects of the source material and combine them with selections from new material. By repeating this process, they eventually attain the desired traits in a plant. Then, it's time to see if their strain can achieve platinum status in the world of cannabis cultivation.

Making a Simple Hybrid

Creating a simple hybrid is a straightforward process. Take a male plant from one strain and a female plant from another, say Big Bud and Skunk. The outcome will be a hybrid called Big Bud × Skunk, but there will be variations among the offspring. Some plants will predominantly display Big Bud traits, while others will lean more towards Skunk. Genes not expressed by either of the parents may also emerge in the offspring. However, if your goal is to breed for specific traits, aiming to eliminate variations and ultimately produce uniform plants or even an IBL, you need a fundamental understanding of plant genetics. True breeding goes beyond simply copying or randomly hybridizing plants.

Introduction to Plant Genetics

Sound engineers obtain their sound either from the source material or new material. In breeding, this translates to genes, specifically cannabis plant genes. The source material contains genes that are expressed, as well as some that remain hidden. Genetic recombination, or sexual recombination, is the process responsible for generating variation. It occurs when, during the cell division process of meiosis, different parents reproduce, resulting in the reshuffling and passing on of new genetic material. This process can reveal traits that weren't evident in the parents, particularly when there is a wide range of genetic diversity to choose from. When we successfully bring out new

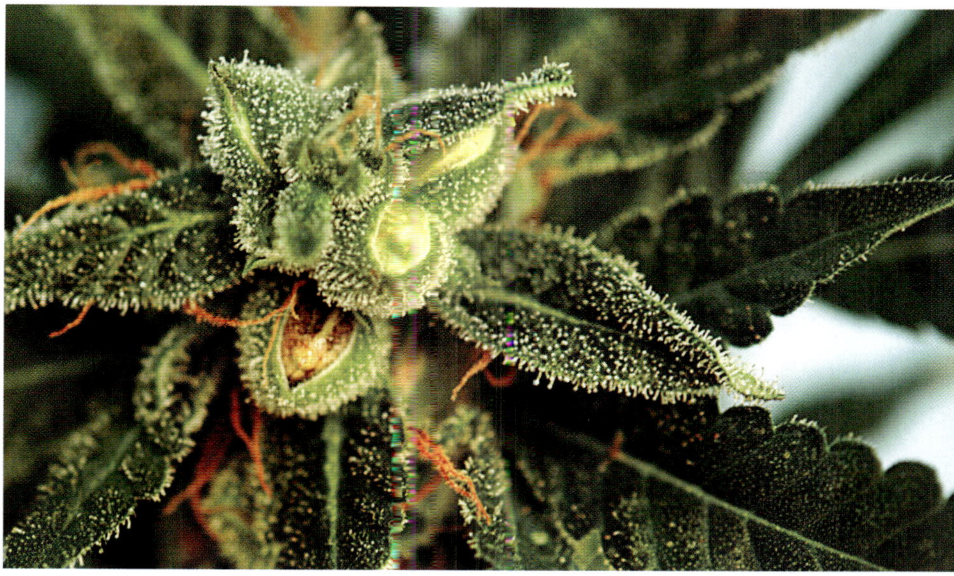

The swollen calyx has formed a seed and is now splitting open to release it. Breeders will collect these seeds a day before they drop.

PHOTO: ED BORG

genetic material, select for it, and stabilize it within a population, we've effectively bred for that trait, whether it be quantity, quality, color, smell, taste, harvesting time, or more. As long as we've incorporated it as a standard feature in our strain, people growing our seeds should observe this trait in the majority of the population. Mutation serves as another source of new genetic information. While most mutations are neutral, some can be harmful, or deleterious, but on occasion, we encounter beneficial mutations that we can selectively breed for.

Dominant/Recessive and Genetic Notation

Assume that the dominant allele B carries the hereditary trait for big bud, while the recessive allele b carries the hereditary trait for small bud. Because B is dominant, a plant with a Bb genotype will consistently produce big bud. In this case, B dominates over b. To display a recessive gene in the phenotype, both genes in the gene pair must be recessive. Therefore, a plant with either a BB or Bb gene combination will always yield big bud, while only a plant with the bb gene combination will produce small bud. This fundamental principle forms the basis of all breeding activities and is commonly referred to as the law of inheritance, established by Gregor Mendel.

The next concepts to understand are those of variation and stability. These are opposites and mutually exclusive. Yet, comprehending what contributes to variability and stability enables you to exercise control over both. This involves creating new traits through variability, subsequently stabilizing them for consumer use. In essence, we aim to harness variability for selection and then achieve trait stability through breeding.

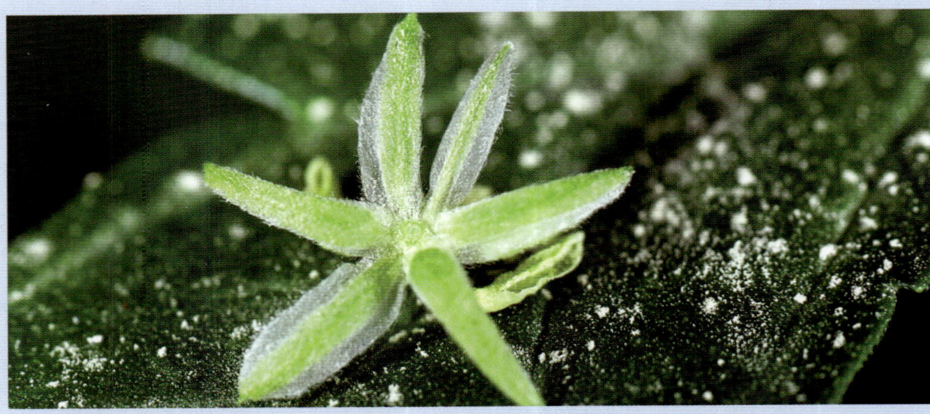

A macro-image of an open male flowering structure surrounded by pollen grains all over the leaf.

PHOTO: KALIMAN SEEDS

A Genetics Glossary

Genetics can initially be a bit challenging to grasp, so let's begin by explaining a few fundamental concepts and key terminology.

Chromosome

This is a threadlike structure of nucleic acids and proteins found in the cell nuclei of higher organisms, carrying a set of linked genes, usually in pairs.

Genes

Genes are the units of heredity passed from parent to offspring, typically as part of a chromosome. Genes control or determine specific characteristics in offspring, such as leaf color, stem structure, texture, smell, and potency. Genes can interact with the environment, resulting in changes to their expression. For example, a gene responsible for pistil production may exhibit different quantities under different environmental conditions. This gene's expression is referred to as the phenotype.

Phenotype

The phenotype comprises all the observable features of your plant, including its color, smell, and taste.

Genotype

The genotype is the genetic makeup of your plant, as distinguished from its phenotype. It characterizes how your plant looks internally, summarizing all the genetic information it carries and passes on to its offspring.

Gene Pairs

Life is made up of a pattern of genes, akin to the two sides of a zipper. One side is inherited from the female parent, the other from the male parent. Each gene occupies a specific locus, or position, on the chain, controlling information about the eventual characteristics of the plant. Gene pairs are usually denoted by pairs of letters, like BB, Bb, Pp, or pp. Capital letters represent dominant genes, while lowercase letters represent recessive genes. For instance, B might represent Big Bud, while b could stand for small bud. You can assign any letter to any trait or gene pair when designing your breeding program.

Locus

A locus is a position on a chromosome where a specific gene pair is located (see Gene Pairs).

Allele

Alleles are alternative forms of a gene. For example, the gene responsible for purple bud color may have two forms or alleles, one for purple and one for dark red.

Homozygous

Homozygous describes a plant with identical alleles at one or more genetic loci; it is not a heterozygote (see below) and breeds true. Your plant is homozygous for a particular trait when it carries the same gene twice in the corresponding gene pair, indicating both genes in the pair are identical. This is key to achieving stable genetics.

Heterozygous

Heterozygous refers to a plant with different alleles at one or more genetic loci. When the genes in the responsible gene pair are dissimilar or unequal, your plant is considered heterozygous for a specific trait. This is why hybrids exhibit significant variation.

Dominant

Dominant genes or alleles are expressed even when inherited from only one parent. They control a hereditary trait, appearing in an individual to the exclusion of its counterpart when both alleles are present. Only one dominant allele in the gene pair is required to determine your plant's genotype and expressed phenotype.

Recessive

Recessive genes, alleles, or traits are perceptibly expressed only in homozygotes and are masked in heterozygotes by a dominant allele or trait. A gene is considered recessive when its effect cannot be observed in your plant's phenotype when only one allele is present. The same allele must be present twice in the gene pair for it to be expressed in your plant's phenotype.

Understanding genetic notation will help clarify these concepts further.

The Hardy-Weinberg Model of Genetic Equilibrium (... and how to break it)

To understand plant breeding fully, it's essential to grasp the basics of the Hardy-Weinberg law. Consider questions such as these:

"If purple bud color is a dominant trait, why do some offspring of my purple bud strain have green buds?"

"I've been selecting indica mothers and cross-breeding them with mostly indica male plants, but I still have some sativa leaves. Why?"

A grasp of the Hardy-Weinberg law and an awareness of the factors that disrupt genetic equilibrium, causing it to break, can provide quick answers to these inquiries.

The first question often stems from a common misconception that the dominant allele of a trait will always be the most prevalent—that is, it will always have the highest frequency in a population—while the recessive allele will consistently have the lowest frequency. However, this is not always the case. A dominant trait may not necessarily become widespread throughout an entire population, nor will a recessive trait always fade away.

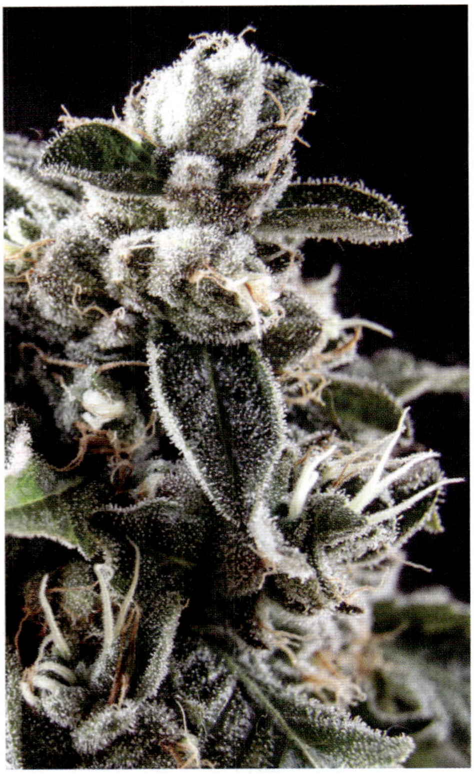

PHOTO: ANNIBALESEEDSHOP.COM

Modern strains are developed through strategic planning to get the most from the plant's genetic strengths.

Gene frequencies can exist in both high and low ratios, regardless of the allele's visible expression. They can also change under certain conditions, leading to variations in plant characteristics. Such changes in gene frequencies over time are responsible for the emergence of different plant traits, driven by selective pressures and natural selection, ultimately resulting in evolution, the process of descent with modifications.

A genetic population consists of individuals of the same species or strain inhabiting a specific area, and these individuals must be capable of interbreeding. Consequently, they share a common set of genes, referred to as the gene pool. The gene pool encompasses all the alleles for various traits within the entire population. For evolution to occur—a process that may give rise to new plant species, strains, or traits—certain gene frequencies within the gene pool must undergo change. Gene frequency pertains to how often a specific allele for a particular trait appears in relation to the total number of alleles for that trait within the population. It is calculated by dividing the number of a particular allele by the total number of alleles in the gene pool. When breeders aim to establish specific traits in a strain they are developing, these concepts become crucial for making those traits prevalent in the population. A strain's description typically includes these standardized features, ensuring that growers can expect those traits to manifest consistently.

Genetic Equilibrium Theory and Application

The Hardy-Weinberg model of genetic equilibrium describes a hypothetical situation in which there is no change, or evolution, in the gene pool. However, sexually reproducing organisms do introduce variation, change, and evolve. While genetic stasis might occur in a lab with clones or under certain circumstances, it is not the norm. Factors that break equilibrium are of interest to us for acquiring new traits to work with. However, returning to equilibrium is necessary to release a strain whose traits are stable across the population. Thus, understanding equilibrium theory is central to comprehending breeding.

Assign the letter "p" to the frequency of the dominant allele B and the letter "q" to the frequency of the recessive allele b. We know that the sum of all the alleles must equal 100 percent, so:

$$p + q = 100\%$$

This can also be expressed as:

$$p + q = 1$$

There is a formula for all the possible random combinations of members in a population like this. It would always equal:

$$p^2 + 2pq + q^2$$

Where:
p = frequency of the dominant allele in a population
q = frequency of the recessive allele in a population
p^2 = percentage of homozygous dominant individuals
q^2 = percentage of heterozygous recessive individuals
$2pq$ = percentage of heterozygous individuals

Now, consider a population of 1,000 Black Domina cannabis plants, where 360 plants emit a skunky smell, while the remaining 640 plants emit a fruity smell. If you assume that the skunky smell is a recessive genotype "vv" based on information from the seed bank, you can use the formula to answer specific questions.

According to the Hardy-Weinberg law, what is the vv genotype frequency? Since 360 out of the 1,000 plants have the vv genotype, the frequency of vv in this population of Black Domina is 36%.

According to the Hardy-Weinberg law, what is the vv allele frequency? The frequency of the vv allele is 36%. As q^2 represents the percentage of homozygous recessive individuals, and q is the frequency of the recessive allele in a population, the following must also be true:

$q^2 = 0.36$

$(q \times q) = 0.36$

$q = 0.6$

Thus, the frequency of the v allele is 60%.

According to the Hardy-Weinberg law, what is the V allele frequency? Since $q = 0.6$, we can solve for p.

$p + q = 1$

$p + 0.6 = 1$

$p = 1 - 0.6$

$p = 0.4$

The frequency of the V allele is 40%.

According to the Hardy-Weinberg law, what is the frequency of the VV and Vv genotypes? Given what we know:

$VV = p^2$

$V = 0.4 = p$

$(p \times p) = p^2$

$(0.4 \times 0.4) = p^2$

$0.16 = p^2$

$VV = 0.16$

The frequency of the genotype VV is 16%.

$VV = 0.16$

$vv = 0.36$

$VV + Vv + vv = 1$

$0.16 + Vv + 0.36 = 1$

$0.52 + Vv = 1$

$Vv = 1 - 0.52$

$Vv = 0.48$ or 48%

These calculations demonstrate how, with limited information, we can answer various questions about the genetic composition of a population using this formula. Furthermore, knowing one part of the equation allows us to calculate the other.

The frequencies of V and v (represented as p and q) will remain unchanged from generation to generation, provided the following five conditions hold true:

1. The population is sufficiently large.
2. No mutations occur.
3. No genetic exchange occurs with outside populations.
4. There are no mating preferences: for example, VV males do not prefer vv females by nature.
5. Natural selection does not favor any specific gene.

While these conditions may contribute to maintaining a stable population, they are not conducive to generating variation except in larger populations. To address this, let's explore the requirements for each condition:

Stable	Variation
Large population	Large population
No mutations	Mutations
No mating preferences	No mating preference
No outside genetic exchange	Outside genetic exchange
No natural selection	No natural selection

The Hardy-Weinberg law dictates that the sum of all alleles in a population should total 100%, even though individual alleles may appear in different proportions. We now delve into situations that can disrupt the law of equilibrium.

1. Populations and Genetic Drift

Large populations are essential for both stability and variation because smaller gene pools with fewer members are more likely to face imminent extinction. When there is only one population in a species, it becomes endangered due to its limited gene pool. Smaller gene pools heighten the risk of inbreeding, as mating between close relatives can occur, increasing the prevalence of deleterious genes. Also, genes that are commonly expressed may exit the small gene pool rapidly, as they are less likely to be passed on. All of these factors contribute to instability. Therefore, to maintain stability, large populations are vital.

Large populations are also crucial for fostering genetic variation. Variety, essential for the process of selection, is more readily found in larger populations. For instance, in larger populations, the likelihood of a plant with more desirable properties than others in its gene pool is higher than in smaller populations. The more options available, the better the chances of finding the desired traits.

Genetic Drift

In small populations, equilibrium is more easily disrupted because even a slight change in allele numbers can lead to a significant shift in genetic frequencies. By chance alone, specific traits can be eliminated from the population, and the frequencies of alleles can drift towards either higher or lower values. Genetic drift represents an evolutionary force that can alter a population and underscores the fact that equilibrium cannot persist indefinitely.

2. Mutation

A mutation is a change in genetic material that can lead to heritable variations in offspring. Mutations occur naturally and involve DNA error correction mechanisms that sometimes do not faithfully replicate genetic information as they should. This can result in the duplication and inversion of genes. To illustrate, imagine there was a gene responsible for a single eye. If this gene undergoes duplication and inversion, it would create a mirror image of a single eye, effectively forming a pair of eyes instead of one. The concept of biological bilateral symmetry can be traced back to such duplication and inversion mutations. Visualize any creature in your mind and imagine duplicating and inverting one side of it to produce a mirrored effect. This process can be repeated, giving rise to multiple appendages or features in an organism, as seen in starfish.

Mutations can generate new traits that were not previously present in a population. While these mutations are not desirable in stable populations, they are actively sought after in variable populations as a source of new genetic variation for selection. The mutated genetic code of a plant can be passed on to its offspring, making mutations heritable. This effect is akin to the introduction of foreign genetic material into a population through migration. Various factors can induce mutations. Essentially, a mutation arises when DNA repair processes fail at the cellular level, so anything that disrupts it can lead to a mutation.

3. Gene Migration

Over time, a population can reach a state of equilibrium, which remains stable as long as no external genetic material enters. When new genetic material is introduced from another population—a process known as introgression—it can lead to the emergence of new traits in the original population, causing a shift in equilibrium. This is precisely what hybridization accomplishes and why it is actively pursued, as it provides a source of new genetic material for selection. Stable populations must take measures to prevent the influx of new genetic information from external sources.

4. Natural Selection

Natural selection is the result of three factors working together: Struggle for survival, variation, and reproduction. It leads to the emergence of traits that are better adapted to the environment through nature's selective process. This is akin to breeding for a trait, but in natural selection, the trait arises because it offers a survival advantage to individuals in a population, increasing the likelihood of it being passed on.

Breeders deliberately select and attempt to stabilize traits within a population manually, while nature achieves this through natural selection. However, as breeders, we can select for traits that nature wouldn't necessarily favor. For instance, many domesticated plant varieties wouldn't thrive in the wild because they've been bred for specific, controlled environments by growers.

The environment and other factors can influence certain plants to produce more or fewer offspring. Some plants may possess traits that make them more susceptible to disease, resulting in fewer of their offspring surviving in a disease-exposed population. Others may produce more seeds or exhibit stronger immunity, leading to a greater number of their offspring surviving and contributing to the genetic makeup of the population. Disease resistance is essentially natural selection at work, and the breeder is merely allowing nature to take its course for a desired trait. This isn't manual selection but rather a natural trait humans wish to preserve. Cannabis breeders often retain many regular traits, as the plant still bears resemblance to its wild counterparts due to the genetic closeness between them. These traits have evolved over a long period.

Natural selection isn't always conducive to stability, as it can favor less desirable traits, potentially reducing variation within a population. Moreover, breeding itself acts against natural selection.

Nonrandom Mating

Nonrandom mating, a subset of natural selection, plays a significant role in influencing gene pools. External or internal factors can disrupt random mating in a population. For instance, differences in flowering times can lead to early-maturing females gathering pollen from early-maturing males, thereby excluding late-flowering females from contributing to future generations. This nonrandom mating can also be seen as a form of sexual selection within natural selection, where specific male or female preferences can further shape the gene pool by favoring certain traits.

Natural selection results in changes in gene pool frequencies, which can disrupt equilibrium. While we've discussed the equation $p^2 + 2pq + q^2$ and its use in calculating various frequencies, breeders often rely on simpler calculations. We now understand the factors that can disrupt equilibrium, as well as the distinction between breeding for stability and cultivating for variation.

Earlier, we posed this question: "I have been selecting indica mothers and cross-breeding them with mostly indica male plants, but I have some sativa leaves. Why?" The answer lies in the fact that if it's labeled as "mostly," it isn't purely one type by default.

It could contain elements of both sativa and indica. Additionally, outside genetics may have been introduced into the breeding program. Since the male plants are mostly indica and not pure indica, we'd expect to see a mix of sativa and indica characteristics in the offspring, including the presence of sativa leaf traits.

The Test Cross

You might be wondering how you can determine if a trait, such as bud color, is homozygous dominant (BB), heterozygous (Bb), or homozygous recessive (bb).

If you've obtained seeds or a clone, you may have been told that a trait, like potency, is homozygous dominant, heterozygous, or homozygous recessive. However, it's crucial to confirm this, especially if you plan to use these traits in future breeding. To do so, you'll need to perform a test cross.

Determining a plant's phenotype is relatively straightforward, as you can observe its characteristics, such as appearance, smell, texture, or taste. However, determining its genotype isn't something you can deduce through simple observation, but requires measurement and calculation.

In general, there are three possible genotypes for each plant trait. For instance, if golden bud is dominant and silver bud is recessive, the potential genotypes are:

1. homozygous dominant: BB = golden bud
2. heterozygous: Bb = golden bud
3. homozygous recessive: bb = silver bud

The golden and silver bud colors are the phenotypes. BB, Bb, and bb denote the genotypes. In this example, Bb would appear golden and not silver because B is the dominant allele. You can assign from any two traits (gold or silver) one for these three designations.

In a mostly sativa plant like a Skunk variety, the leaves are typically pale green. However, within this Skunk population, you might spot a few plants with dark green leaves, which suggests that the leaf color trait in this Skunk strain isn't "true-breeding," but likely heterozygous. True-breeding traits are either homozygous dominant or homozygous recessive. Thus, some of the pale-green leaf Skunks are probably homozygous dominant.

The pale-green trait cannot be homozygous recessive, nor can the dark-green leaf trait be heterozygous. A completely homozygous recessive population bb wouldn't have the allele B for homozygous dominant BB or heterozygous expression Bb. So, in a population that's entirely homozygous recessive bb for a trait, you won't find traits for heterozygous Bb or homozygous dominant BB versions of that trait. If a population is

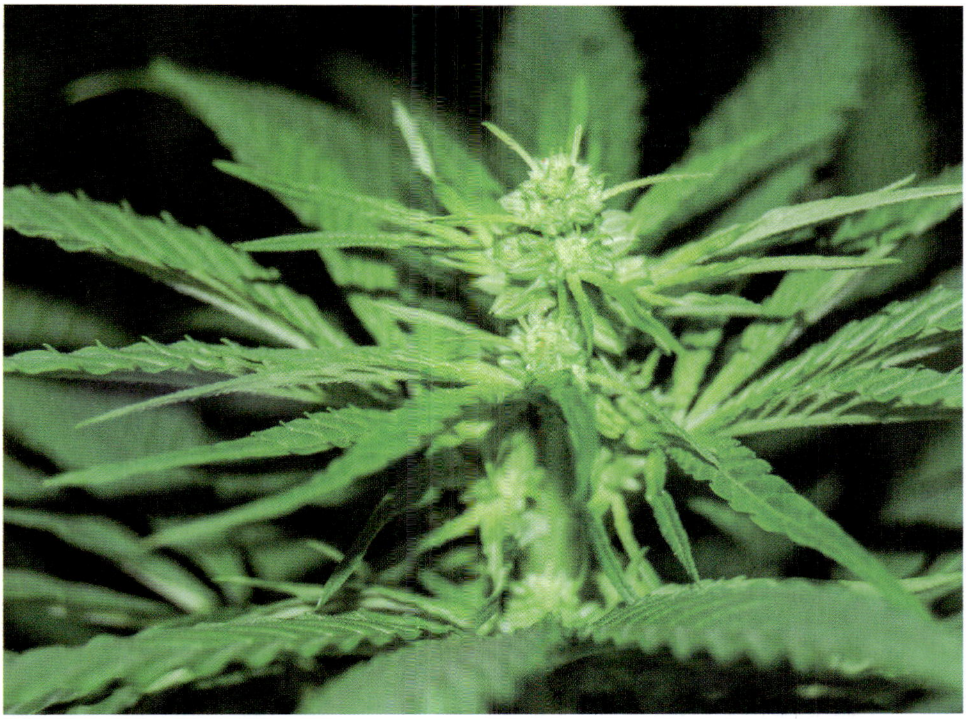

Female plant reversed, producing opposite flowers for breeding.

PHOTO: CH9 FEMALE SEEDS

entirely homozygous for a trait BB or bb,[2] that specific trait can be considered stable, true-breeding, or breeds true. On the other hand, if a population is heterozygous for a trait Bb, that characteristic is deemed unstable, non-true-breeding, or won't breed true.

When another trait can't exist in a bb population for that trait, bb is considered true-breeding. If there's any variation in the trait, and the Hardy-Weinberg equilibrium hasn't been disrupted, the trait is likely heterozygous. In our Skunk example, the presence of only a few dark-green leaves indicates that dark-green leaves are homozygous recessive bb, while pale-green leaves are heterozygous Bb and could be homozygous dominant BB.

If most plants have golden buds, it implies that the golden bud color is a dominant trait. If only a few plants have silver buds, it suggests that the silver trait is recessive. You already know that the only genotype producing the recessive trait is homozygous recessive bb. So, if a plant exhibits a recessive trait in its phenotype, its genotype must be homozygous recessive. A plant displaying a recessive trait in its phenotype always has a homozygous recessive genotype. However, this leaves another question unanswered. Are the golden bud or pale-green leaf color traits homozygous dominant BB or heterozygous Bb? You can't be entirely certain until you conduct a test cross.

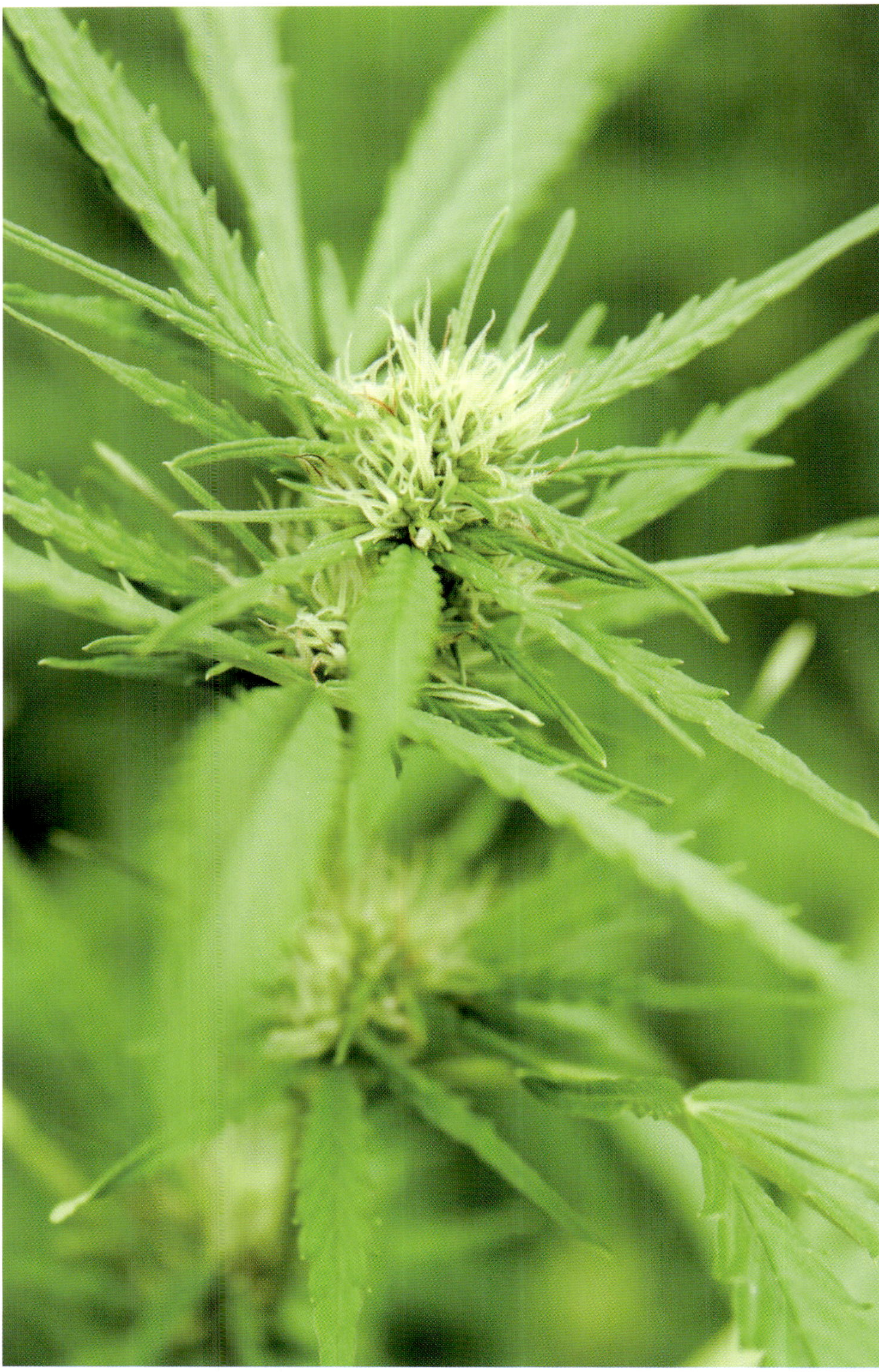

PHOTO: ROB BRAMHILL

You can breed a strain for fixed traits of smell, taste, and appearance.

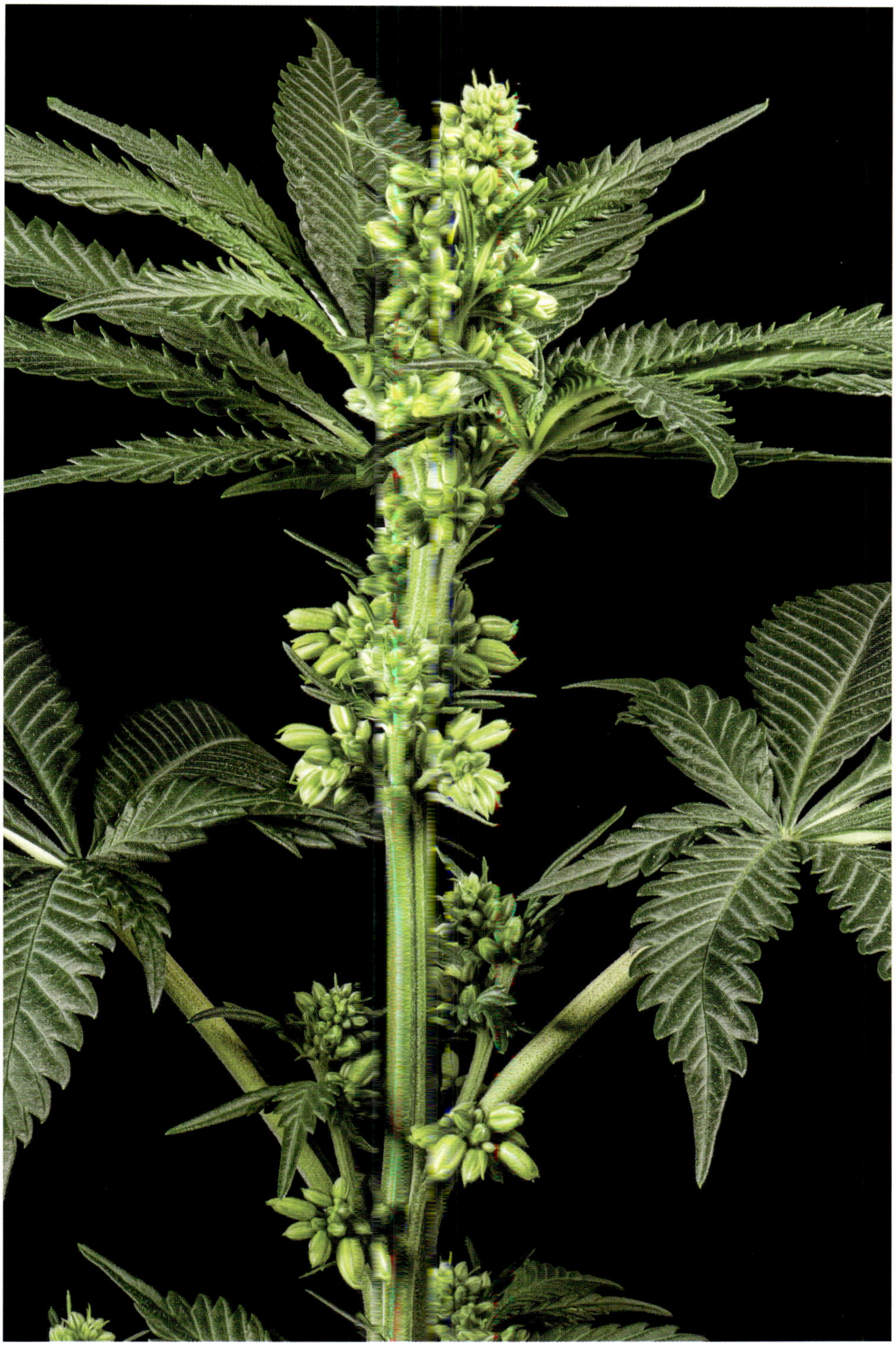

Many cannabis male flowers start to appear in the flowering phase, which coincides with the female plants' earliest flowering phase. Pollination will occur unless sexes are segregated.

PHOTO: ROB BRAMHILL

We've answered essential questions related to trait selection. Armed with some information from population inspection and the equilibrium formula, we now need to determine if some traits are homozygous dominant BB or heterozygous Bb so that we can map the genes on paper without genetic analysis. This knowledge enabled breeders to work with plants before DNA analysis, although DNA sequencing can be helpful now. They can do this because they understand the principles of genetic inheritance, and now, you do too.

A test cross involves breeding a plant with an unknown dominant genotype BB or Bb with a homozygous recessive bb plant for the same trait. Importantly, for the test to work, you need another cannabis plant of the opposite sex that is homozygous recessive bb for the same trait. Keep in mind that once you have a clone with that trait and other homozygous recessives, you can continue using that clone line for other breeding projects during this analysis phase. This discovery is crucial for solving many breeding problems.

This brings us to a significant rule: If any offspring from a test cross display the recessive trait, the parent with the dominant trait must be heterozygous, not homozygous.

This information reveals your genotypes, paving the way for selection and stability. Perform a test cross for each trait you want to manage, and you'll be breeding effectively, shaping a cannabis plant into your desired strain. In our example, the unknown genotype is either BB or Bb, and the silver bud genotype is bb. We'll apply this information in Punnett squares.

	b	b
B	1	2
?	3	4

These calculations apply to two parents that will breed. Picture one parent at the top and another on the left side. There are four fields in the Punnett square to be filled. They are labeled 1-4 for clarity. So, with the known genotype at the top and the unknown at the bottom left, we proceed to fill in the four fields.

	b	b
B	Bb	Bb
?	?b	?b

The first row (fields 1 and 2) produces Bb (field 1) and Bb (field 2) offspring, all exhibiting the dominant golden bud trait. The second row (fields 3 and 4) yields ?b and ?b, which can be either Bb or bb offspring. This leads to offspring with more golden bud Bb or silver bud bb. The first outcome (where ? = B) results in golden bud Bb offspring; the second outcome (where ? = b) leads to silver bud bb offspring. Let's calculate the frequencies:

Outcome 1, where ? = B:
Bb + Bb + Bb + Bb = 4Bb
100% golden bud

Outcome 2, where ? = b:
Bb + Bb + bb + bb = 2 Bb + 2bb
50% golden bud and 50% silver bud

Recap:
Homozygous dominant: BB = golden bud
Heterozygous: Bb = golden bud
Homozygous recessive: bb = silver bud

Remember, to determine the identity of B?, we used another cannabis plant of the opposite sex that was homozygous recessive (bb) for the same trait. Outcome 2 reveals that both parents must have at least one b trait each to produce silver bud in the offspring's phenotype. If any silver bud offspring are produced, the mystery parent (B?) must be heterozygous (Bb), not homozygous dominant (BB).

Thus, when a golden bud parent is crossed with a silver bud parent and produces only golden bud offspring, it means the golden bud parent must be homozygous dominant for that trait. If any silver bud offspring appear, it indicates that the golden bud parent is heterozygous for the trait. Understanding this allows breeders to take control of genes, making it more than just the basics but a core aspect of breeding. These are central tenants and give you the assurances you need when growing large populations for breeding.

To summarize, the steps for conducting a test cross to determine the genotype of a plant exhibiting a dominant trait are:

1. Always cross the plant with the dominant trait with a plant displaying the recessive trait.
2. If any offspring display the recessive trait, the plant with the dominant trait must have a heterozygous genotype.
3. If all offspring exhibit the dominant trait, the plant with the dominant trait must have a homozygous dominant genotype.

The main reasons for conducting a test cross are:

1. When breeding plants, you want to perpetuate a specific trait, such as height, flavor, aroma, and more.
2. To perpetuate that trait accurately, you need to know whether it is homozygous dominant, heterozygous, or homozygous recessive.
3. You can confidently determine this through a test cross rather than relying solely on expensive genetic research technologies.

Note that working with a large population as a breeder increases the reliability of results: The more plants you work with, the more dependable the outcomes. Small populations can skew results.

Identifying a plant with a homozygous recessive trait for the test cross isn't as challenging as it may seem. It might take a few test crosses to find the right ratios falling into place. Fill out Punnett squares and explore all possible crosses from BB, Bb, and bb, as only these three states can exist. You will need to cross:

BB with BB
BB with Bb
BB with bb
Bb with Bb
bb with bb

BB with BB can result only in BB, and bb with bb can result only in bb. Therefore, explore BB with Bb, BB with bb, and Bb with Bb. Keep in mind that the dominant trait is expressed. Try filling in these squares:

BB with Bb

	B	b
B		
B		

BB with bb

	b	b
B		
B		

Bb with Bb

	B	b
B		
b		

We know BB × BB will result only in BB, but BB × Bb is intriguing because even though b is present in the offspring, they will resemble a BB population because the b is not expressed in this generation, as in the heterozygous Bb. For BB × Bb, some will be BB, and some Bb, but none will be bb. However, crosses between those Bb offspring × Bb offspring can eventually produce the bb trait, something that can't be obtained if the parents are homozygous for that trait. So, additional crosses of a test cross can help determine if you have homozygous or heterozygous traits and identify the homozygous recessive. The ratios and additional test crosses provide confidence in accepting whether a trait is recessive or not. Once it is identified, you can breed that trait true.

This methodology empowers breeders to master genetic control, enabling them to craft cannabis strains with precision.

Hardy-Weinberg Equilibrium Part 2

You might wonder how you can breed for multiple traits like taste, smell, vigor, and color. For this, you need to delve deeper into the Hardy-Weinberg law of genetic equilibrium. If you've already tackled the previous Punnett square questions, the following concepts should be easier to grasp.

Now, what will the offspring look like if you cross two heterozygous plants (Bb) for a particular trait? Using Punnett squares can help you determine the phenotypes, genotypes, and gene frequencies of the offspring.

	B	b
B	BB	Bb
b	Bb	bb*

*Pay special attention to this offspring and compare it with the parents.

In this scenario, the resulting offspring will look like this:

1 BB: 25% of the offspring will be homozygous for the dominant allele BB.
2 Bb: 50% will be heterozygous, resembling their parents Bb.
1 bb: 25% will be homozygous for the recessive allele bb.

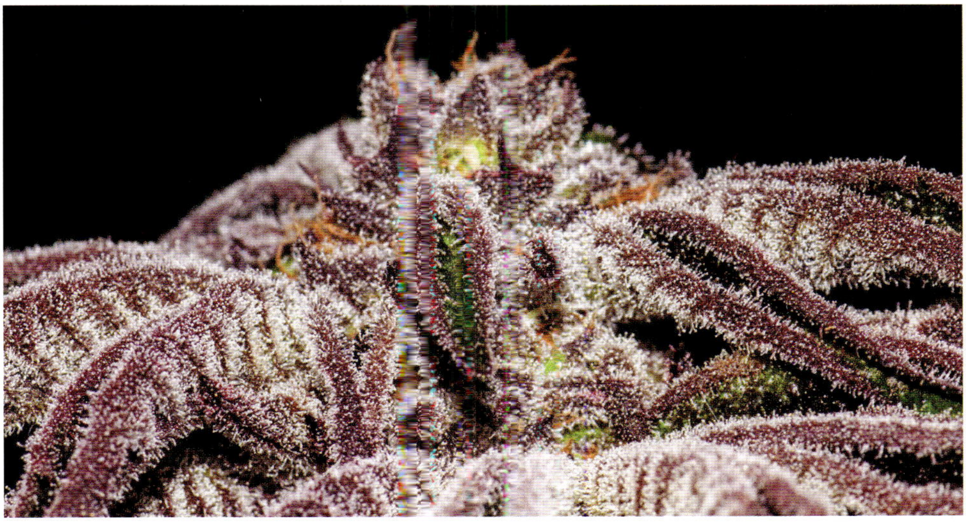

PHOTO: ALPINE SEEDS

Purple leaves and flowers covered in trichomes give the plant an original look compared to regular green.

Note that, unlike their parents, both Bb, 25% of the offspring will express the recessive phenotype bb. Thus, two parents displaying the golden bud phenotype but being heterozygous (Bb) for that trait will yield offspring exhibiting the recessive silver bud trait. This emergence of a hidden trait from seemingly nowhere occurs due to specific gene combinations.

Understanding how recessive and dominant traits pass down through phenotypes and genotypes is crucial for predicting the outcome of a cross and locking down desirable traits in future generations.

When you're breeding a strain, how can you ensure the retention of desired traits throughout the process? This is where the test cross comes into play. Suppose you're producing seeds from a strain obtained from a seed bank. How can you ensure that the offspring will showcase the preferred characteristics? If the trait you want to perpetuate is homozygous dominant BB in both parent plants, there's no way to generate a recessive genotype for that trait in the offspring. This is illustrated in the following Punnett square:

	B	B
B	BB	BB
B	BB	BB

In this case, the recessive trait cannot manifest. Similarly, if both parents possess the recessive trait, they cannot produce the dominant trait, as shown here:

	b	b
b	bb	bb
b	bb	bb

To ensure the faithful propagation of a trait, you must determine whether it is homozygous, heterozygous, or homozygous recessive. Understanding these genetic principles gives you control over outcomes. This is significantly more valuable than blind guessing. This predictive ability allows you to expect the results before they occur. A breeder's calculated predictions align with the grower's expectations.

Mendel's Pea Plant Experiments

Gregor Mendel (1822–1884), an Austrian-Czech-German monk, made groundbreaking discoveries in the field of genetics through his plant breeding experiments in Brno, Moravia (now Czechia). Mendel's observations centered on two distinct types of pea plants that consistently produced uniform results when bred within their respective gene pools but not when crossed with each other. The traits he studied were:

Pea Plant #1	Pea Plant #2
Smooth pods	Wrinkled pods
Green seeds	Yellow seeds
White flowers	Purple flowers
Tall plants	Short plants

Can these traits vary or are they interchangeable? Record keeping is everything to finding out. Mendel noted that offspring inherited the same traits as the parent plants when bred within their respective populations. Because there was no variation within each strain, Mendel inferred that both strains were homozygous for these traits. Given that the pea plants belonged to the same species, Mendel conjectured that either smooth or wrinkled pods were recessive. Representing these traits as SS for smooth pods and ss for wrinkled pods, he ruled out Ss because no traits from the other strain appeared in offspring when bred within their gene pools.

We illustrate this with two basic Punnett squares: SS represents pea plant #1 with the smooth pod trait, and ss represents pea plant #2 with wrinkled pods.

Pea plant #1 results:

	S	S
S	SS	SS
S	SS	SS

All offspring will be SS.

Pea plant #2 results:

	s	s
s	ss	ss
s	ss	ss

All offspring will be ss.

When in doubt, a Punnett square can provide clarity. It's essential to double-check your work, a standard practice in mathematics.

1st Hybrid Cross (The F1 generation)

Mendel conducted his initial hybrid cross between the two strains, resulting in all smooth pods, as seen in the following chart:

F1 cross	s	
S	Ss	Ss
S	Ss	Ss

Until this point, Mendel was uncertain about which trait was recessive or dominant. However, since all pods were smooth, he concluded with certainty that pea plant #1 carried the dominant genotype for smooth pods, while pea plant #2 harbored the recessive genotype for wrinkled pods. This revelation allowed Mendel to determine whether a particular pod trait in future test crosses was homozygous or heterozygous because he had identified the recessive trait (ss).

2nd Hybrid Cross (The F2 generation)

The F1 cross produced offspring that were all Ss. When Mendel crossed these offspring, he obtained these results:

F2 cross	S	s
S	SS	Ss
s	Ss	ss*

*Note the appearance of this offspring and compare it to the parent plants.

In this scenario, Mendel had mated two heterozygous pea plants Ss for a pod trait. The resulting offspring comprised:

25% homozygous for the dominant allele SS
50% heterozygous, resembling their parents Ss
25% homozygous for the recessive allele ss

In his initial cross to create the hybrid plant, Mendel did not have recessive traits for pod shape. However, by crossing the heterozygous offspring, he ended up with some displaying the homozygous recessive trait, some exhibiting the homozygous dominant trait, and others maintaining the heterozygous trait. In breeding terminology, his first cross between the plants is known as the F1 cross or F1 generation, while the subsequent breeding of those offspring is referred to as the F2 cross or F2 generation. Breeders use this important terminology to describe a test population.

Since Mendel had Ss, ss, and SS to work with, Punnett squares could be used to determine traits in the next generation of offspring. Comparing the results with established ratios helped him piece together the puzzle of inheritance patterns.

More on Gene Frequencies

When two heterozygous parents are crossed, the frequency ratio of the alleles will be 50% each. Remember that the genotype can be Ss, SS, or ss, but the alleles are either S or s.

	S	s
S	SS	Ss
s	Ss	ss

Here, we observe S S S S alleles (4 × S) and s s s s alleles (4 × s). This demonstrates that the frequency of the S allele is 50%, and the frequency of the s allele is also 50%. Now, let's see if you can calculate the frequencies of the S and s alleles in the following crosses.

Cross 1

	S	s
S		
S		

Cross 2

	s	s
S		
s		

In these crosses, you can determine the allele frequencies by examining the resulting genotypes.

How to True Breed

Breeding cannabis strains revolves around managing gene frequencies. Reputable breeders who sell strains through seed banks aim for uniformity in growth, indicating that they've worked to stabilize specific genes, resulting in homozygous genotypes for those traits.

Say a breeder has two strains, Master Kush and Silver Haze, with certain preferred traits denoted by asterisks (*).

Master Kush	**Silver Haze**
Dark-green leaf	Pale-green leaf *
Hashy smell *	Fruity smell
White flowers	Silver flowers *
Short plants *	Tall plants

The breeder intends to create a homozygous plant for four specific traits—pale-green leaf, hashy smell, silver flowers, short plants—and name it "Silver Kush,"

To achieve this, the breeder must find the genotype for each desired trait in the ideal Silver Kush strain. This involves working out the genotype of each parent strain for that same trait. As there are four traits in focus, and each trait has two alleles (one from each parent), there are eight alleles that constitute the genotypes for these phenotypes and must be calculated.

Let's start with the pale-green leaf trait of Silver Haze. The breeder will grow numerous

Silver Haze plants and observe if any display leaf colors other than pale-green. If not, the breeder can assume the trait is either homozygous dominant (SS) or recessive (ss). If other leaf colors do appear, the trait is likely heterozygous (Ss) and must be stabilized through selective breeding.

Now, consider the parents:

Scenario 1

	S	S
S	SS	SS
S	SS	SS

If both parents are SS, there would be no variation in the population for this trait. It would already be locked down and breed true without variations.

Scenario 2

	S	s
S	SS	Ss
S	SS	Ss

With one SS parent and one Ss parent, the breeder would produce a 50:50 population, one group being homozygous SS and the other heterozygous Ss.

Scenario 3

	S	s
S	SS	Ss
s	Ss	Ss

If both parents were Ss, the breeder would have 25% SS, 50% Ss, and 25% ss. Even though gene frequencies can be predicted, the breeder will not know with certainty whether the pale-green leaf trait is dominant or recessive until after a test cross. By conducting several test crosses, the breeder can isolate the SS or ss plants and eliminate any Ss from the group. Once the genotype has been isolated and the population reduced to contain only plants with the same genotype, the breeding program can begin in earnest. Accurate record-keeping is crucial in controlling gene frequencies. Therefore, it's vital to use Punnett squares to map out genotypes and label plants accordingly.

Suppose you run a seed bank company named "Pale-Green Leaf Only, But Everything Else Is Not Uniform Ltd.". Customers often seek strains that replicate past winners of the Cannabis Cup or exhibit specific characteristics. To meet these demands, you must isolate all the desired traits while maintaining other desirable characteristics.

The number of tests required to determine any given genotype isn't fixed. You may need to work with a variety of plants to achieve your goal.

The next step in a breeding program is to lock down other traits within that population. This can be challenging because while you're working to stabilize one trait, you must avoid eliminating other desirable traits or accidentally locking down unwanted traits. If unwanted traits are inadvertently locked down or desired traits are eliminated, you'll need to work diligently through multiple cross-tests to re-establish the desired traits.

Eventually, through precise selection and record-keeping, you'll develop a plant that breeds true for all the features you desire. Essentially, you will have a genetic map of your cannabis plants and the genetic source material for those genes.

Successful breeders typically focus on the primary phenotypes that set their plant apart and contribute to its high quality, rather than attempting to map all traits at once. True-breeding strains are developed gradually, one step at a time. Well-known true-breeding strains like Skunk#1 and Afghani#1 took 20 years to create. While not every project will take that long, 20 years equates to 20 cannabis growing cycles, which isn't extensive in the context of the plant's history. Indoor cultivation and cloning can expedite the process, ensuring seeds are planted as soon as possible, unlike in nature where winter freezing delays germination. Additionally, some experiments may require only clones, eliminating the need for full flowering to identify specific traits. Breeders often use labels like Mk1, Mk2, and Mk3 to track long-term projects.

Ultimately, you'll have your Silver Kush strain with the four genotypes you aimed to preserve. Variations may still exist in the population, such as plants with purple stems or varying potency. By continually selecting for desired traits, you can theoretically manipulate the strain to become true-breeding for all traits. However, achieving a 100% true-breeding strain for every phenotype is improbable, and is referred to as a perfect IBL. If you can stabilize 90% of the plant's phenotypes in a population, you can claim your plant as an IBL.

The key to the true-breeding technique is finding a donor plant, one with a true-breeding trait, preferably homozygous dominant, which you aim to incorporate into your project plant. The more traits you stabilize as homozygous dominant, the better your chances of creating an IBL. This doesn't mean the entire genetic line will be true-breeding for every trait, but rather that the strain displays uniform growth for a high percentage of phenotypes.

Additional advanced breeding techniques can help you either reduce or promote specific traits in a population. These techniques may not result in true-breeding for the selected traits but can enhance uniformity in the population for those traits.

Advanced Breeding Techniques

Linkage

Some traits may be linked, making their separation within your breeding choices difficult. If you discover that a trait you desire is connected to another trait you don't, you may need to select which one is more important to you. For instance, you may find that the purple-colored bud you love is linked to the light leaf color you're not so fond of. In such cases, be prepared to shift your focus to another trait if your initial results are inconclusive. Take your time and revisit the issue later for further attempts.

Simple Backcrossing

Backcrossing isn't a method of breeding per se; it's a technique used in breeding. Blindly backcrossing without a clear strategy does little more than increase the likelihood of inheriting recessive deleterious genes without overall improvement. When understood and executed correctly, backcrossing becomes a valuable tool for breeders.

In our initial cross between the Master Kush and Silver Haze plants, resulting in the F1 hybrid generation, let's suppose both plants are homozygous for leaf color. Silver Haze has pale green leaves, and Master Kush has dark green leaves. However, we don't yet know whether the leaf color trait is SS or ss. We can only determine this by observing the offspring.

F1 hybrid cross	s	s
S	Ss	Ss
S	Ss	Ss

This F1 cross produces hybrid seeds, and since S is dominant over s, it will reveal which color is more dominant and which parent it originated from. In this example, the overall results are pale green, indicating that the pale-green allele is dominant over the dark green.

S = Silver Haze pale-green leaf trait is dominant
s = Master Kush dark-green leaf trait is recessive

Because no variations occurred in the population, both parents were homozygous for that trait. However, all the offspring are heterozygous. This is where we can use a shortcut to manipulate the gene pool for that population. We can use clones from the parent plant SS in our cross with the Ss offspring. This technique is known as backcrossing. If our parent is female, we'll need to use males from the Ss selection in our backcross, and vice versa.

F2 backcross	S	s
S	SS	Ss
S	SS	Ss

Our first backcross will result in 50% homozygous SS offspring and 50% heterozygous offspring Ss for that trait. All the offspring will exhibit the pale-green leaf trait. If we didn't backcross and simply used the heterozygous offspring for the breeding program, we would have ended up with 25% homozygous dominant SS, 50% heterozygous Ss, and 25% homozygous recessive ss.

F2 hybrid cross without backcrossing	S	s
S	SS	Ss
s	Ss	ss

Backcrossing significantly helps in controlling the frequencies of a specific trait in the offspring. For example, the F2 hybrid cross produced some plants with the dark-green leaf trait, while the F2 backcross did not.

Now, we perform our second backcross (F3) using the same original parent, kept alive through cloning. Backcrossing for a second time is often referred to as squaring. Since we're dealing with only two types of offspring, Ss and SS, we will either replicate the results of the F2 backcross...

F3 backcross with heterozygote	S	s
S	SS	Ss
S	SS	Ss

...or successfully lock down the desired trait as follows:

F3 backcross with homozygote	S	S
S	SS	SS
S	SS	SS

In the F3 backcross with the homozygote, all the offspring are homozygous dominant SS, ensuring they breed true for that trait. These offspring result from squaring and can never produce the ss traits because the SS trait is now stable and true-breeding. The F3 backcross with the heterozygote generates half Ss offspring. If we breed these Ss offspring with each other, we can potentially produce the ss trait. However, this line would not be stable.

Classic Skunk Breeding

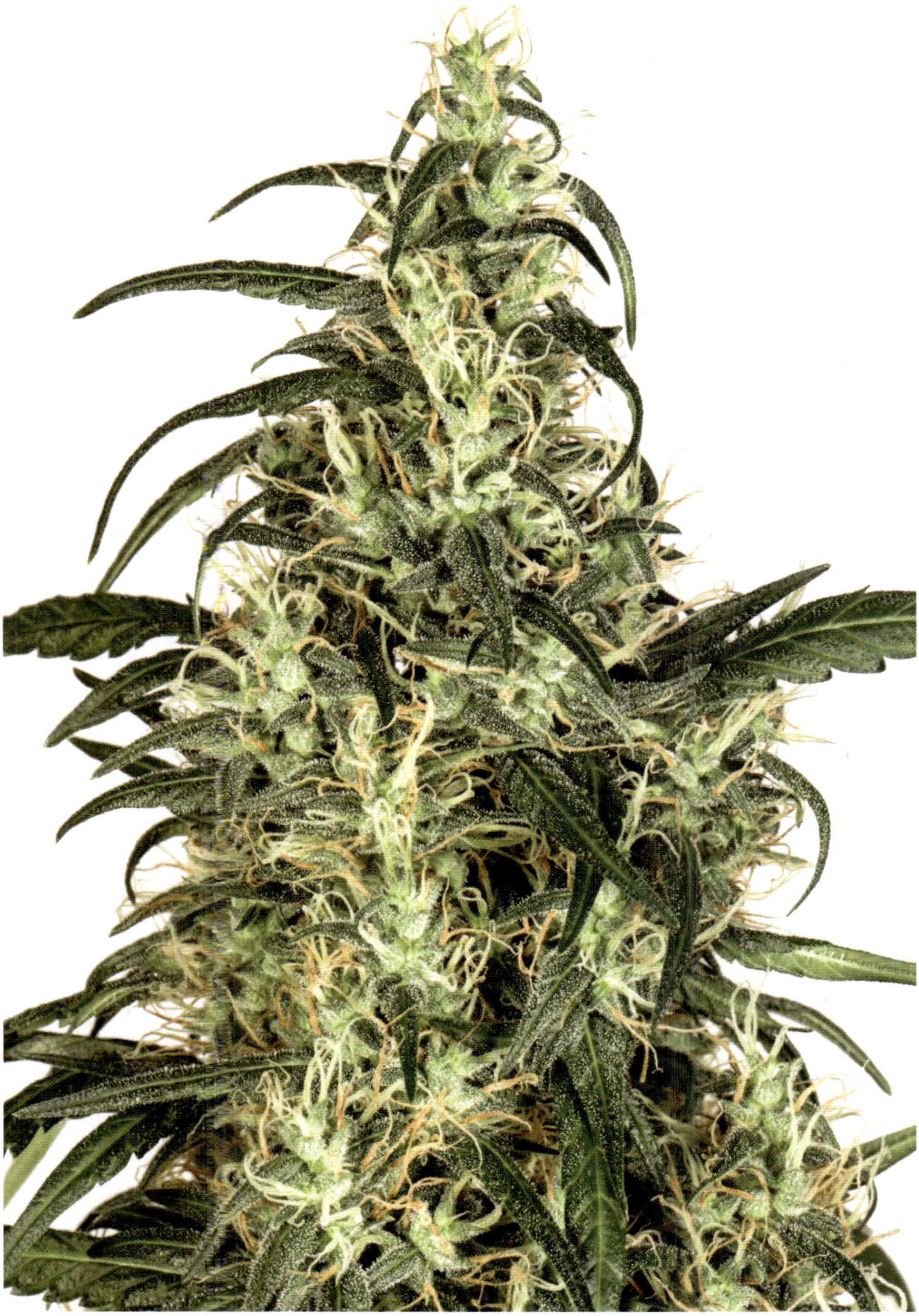

PHOTO: DUTCH PASSION

Skunk #1 from Dutch Passion: A great hybrid for beginner growers that leans towards 75% sativa and 25% indica with nearly 40 years of stabilized breeding.

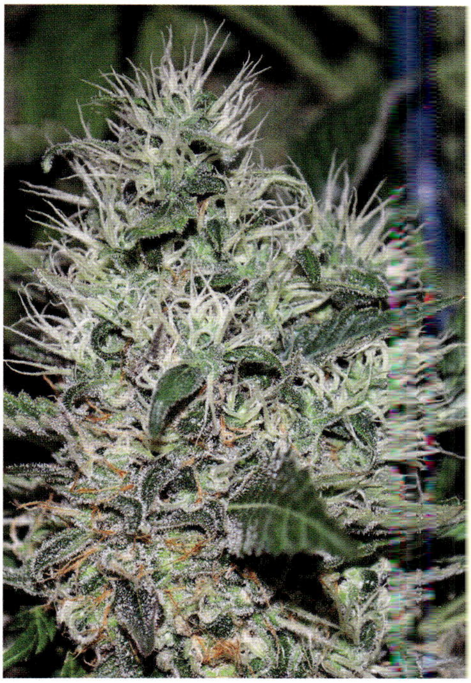

Tahoe Gold 1968 Skunk #1 x 1975 Hindu Kush.

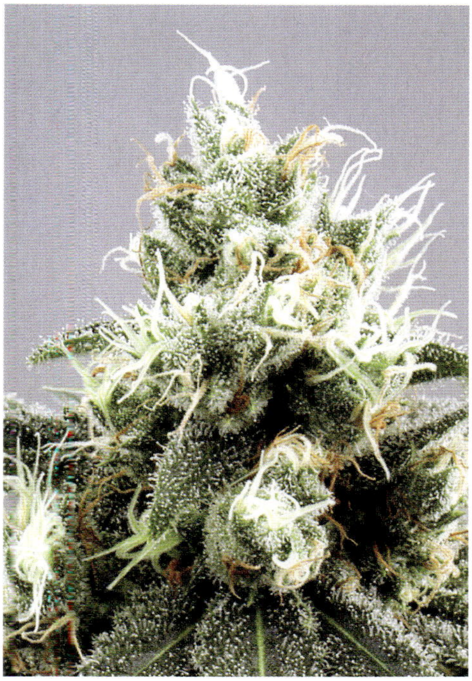

Intense Skunk Unknown Skunk x Afghani Hash.

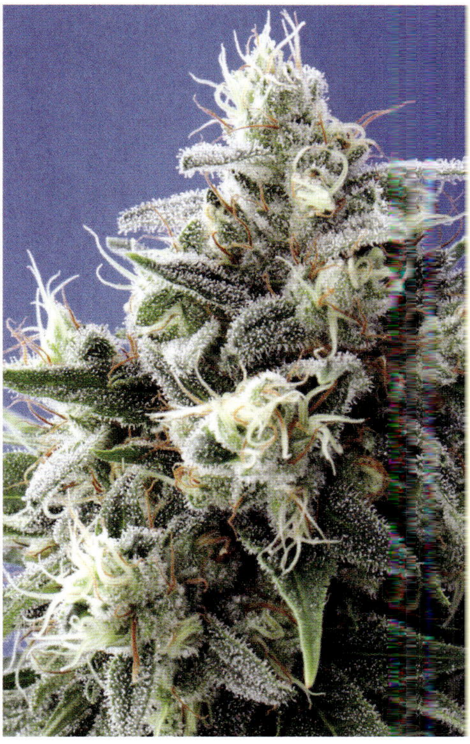

Kick Ass Big White Skunk x Nepali.

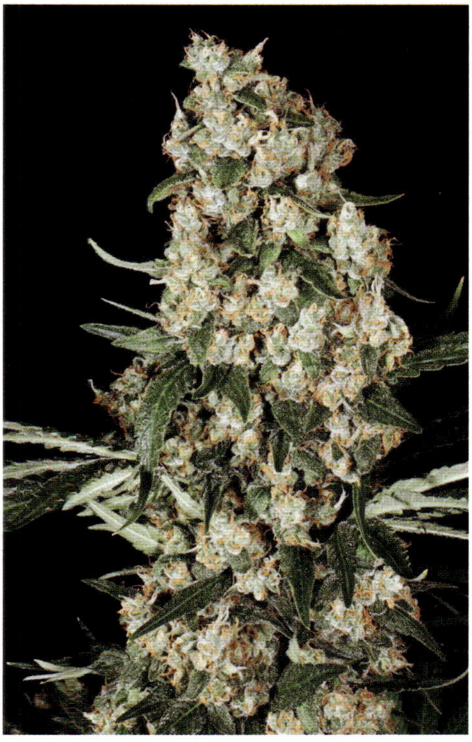

Wappa Special Skunk x Afghani.

PHOTOS: MASTER THAI SEEDS (TOP LEFT), SJAMAAN.COM (TOP RIGHT), DR. GROW'S FEM SEEDS (BOTTOM LEFT), PARADISE-SEEDS.COM (BOTTOM RIGHT)

Classic Haze Breeding

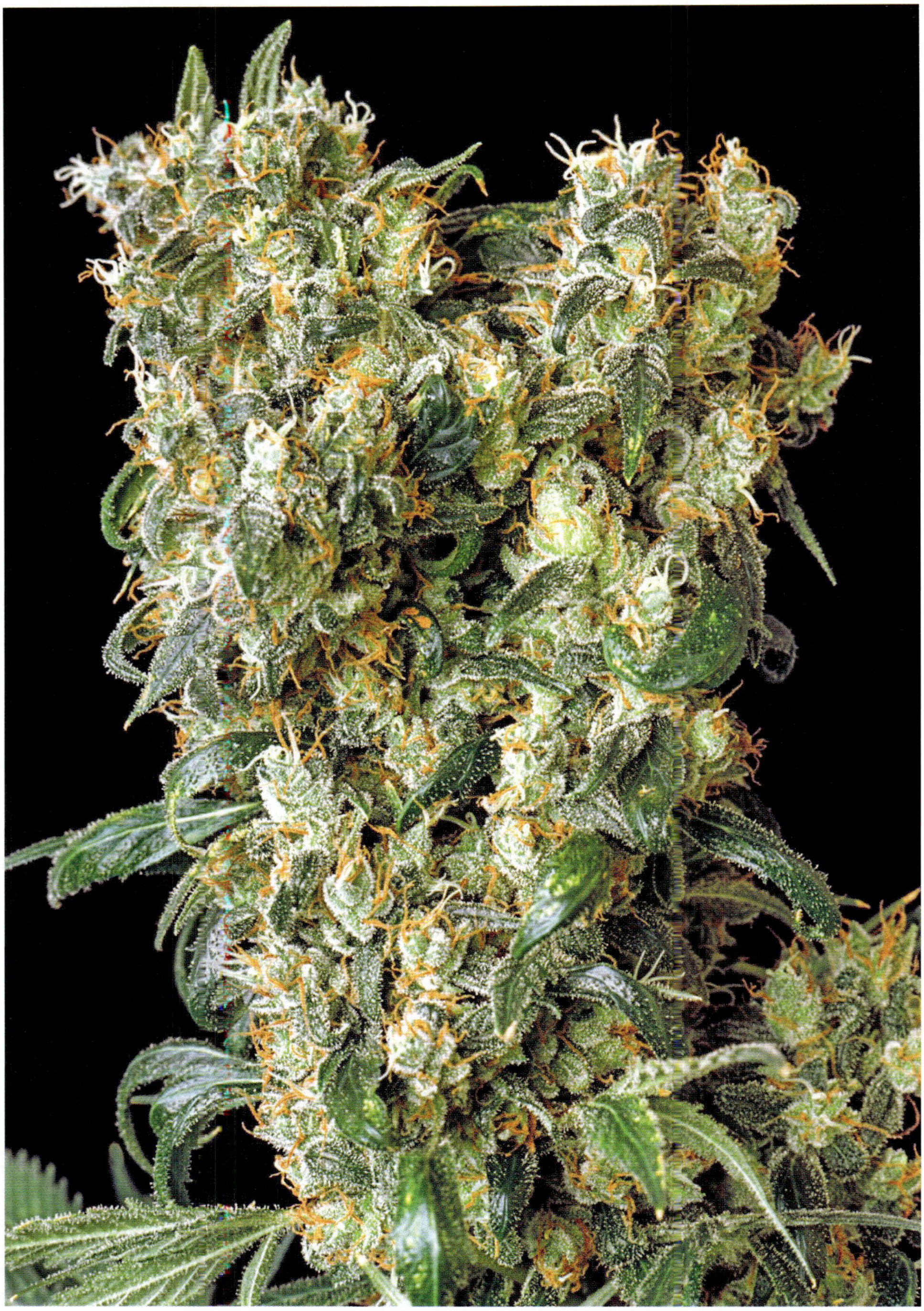

PHOTO: ED BORG

The main cola top was pruned which caused two top colas to grow. Whether they produce more flowers than a single cola depends on the strain. It is usually coequal, and the total amount is shared between colas.

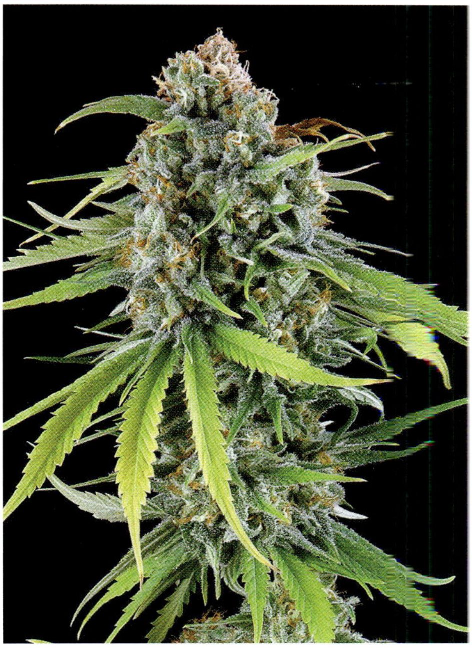

Royal Haze by Dinafem Seeds. Haze #2 x (Skunk x Northern Light).

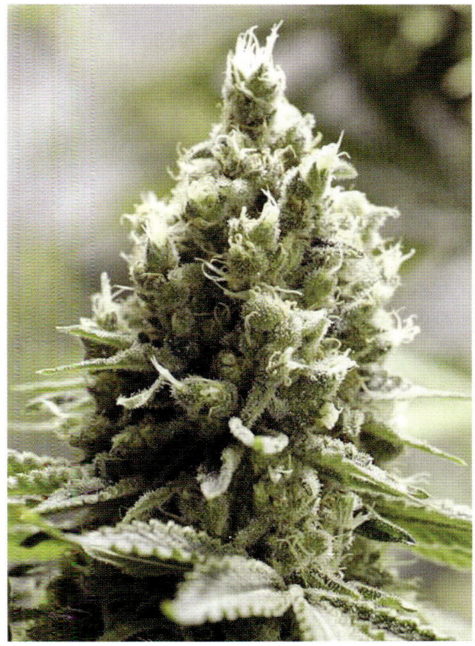

Critical Haze Amnesia Haze x Critical Mass.

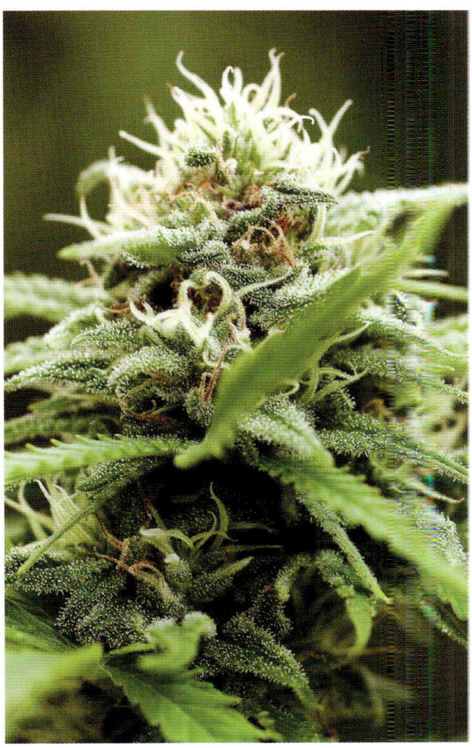

Royal Moby Haze x White Widow.

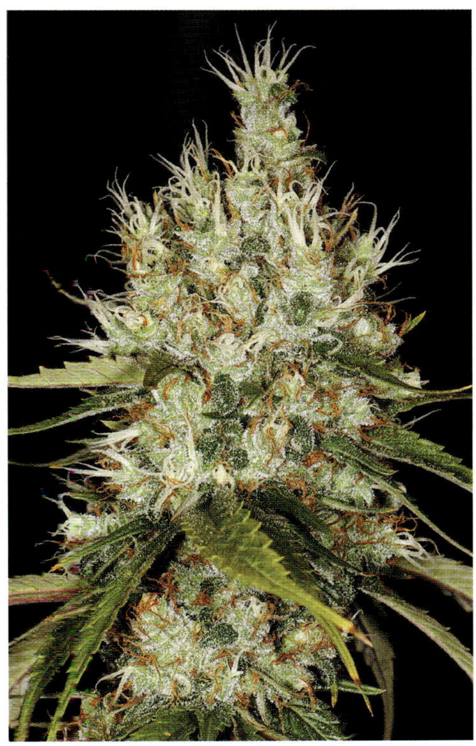

Thai Lights Thai Haze x Atomic Northern Lights.

PHOTOS: DINAFEM SEEDS (TOP LEFT), RESINSEEDS.NET (TOP RIGHT), ROYALQUEENSEEDS.COM (BOTTOM LEFT), DR. ATOMIC SEEDBANK (BOTTOM RIGHT)

Classic Northern Lights Breeding

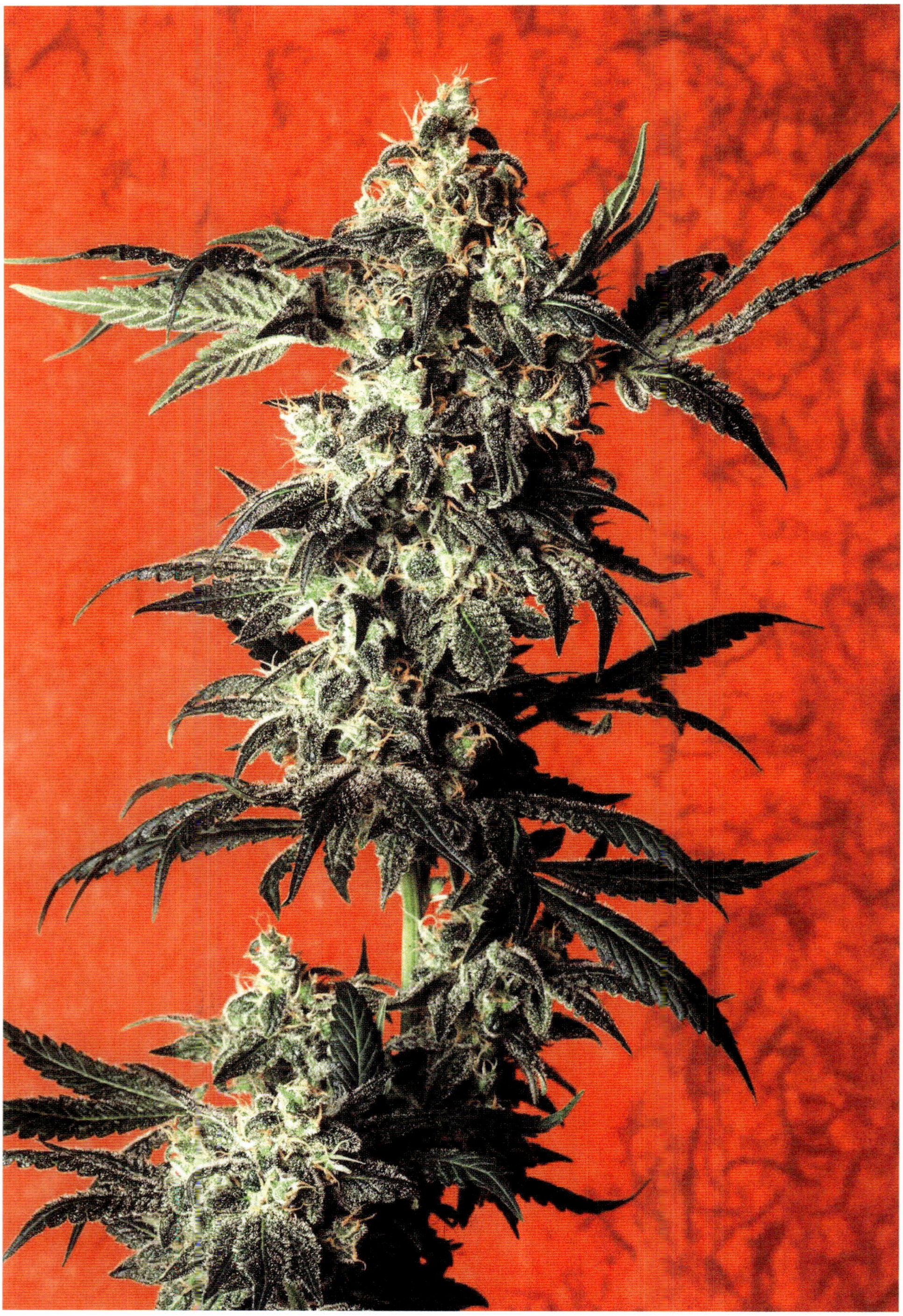

PHOTO: ED BORG

Northern Lights is one of the most popular strains of cannabis to hit North America and Europe. This strain is considered one of the easiest to grow and use for hybridizing.

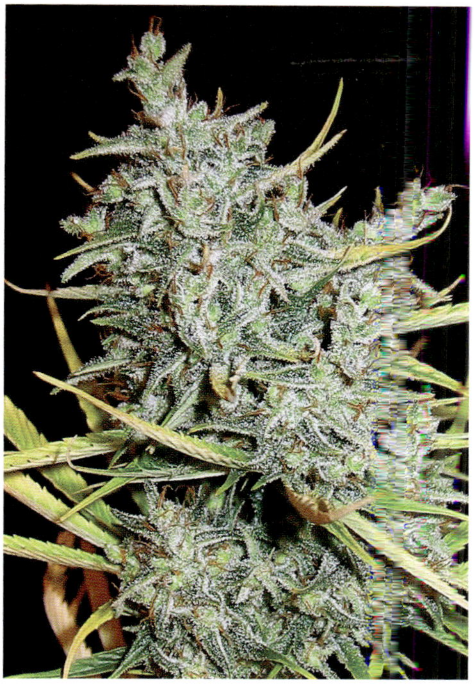

(Mango Haze Northern Lights #5 x Haze) x (Skunk x Haze).

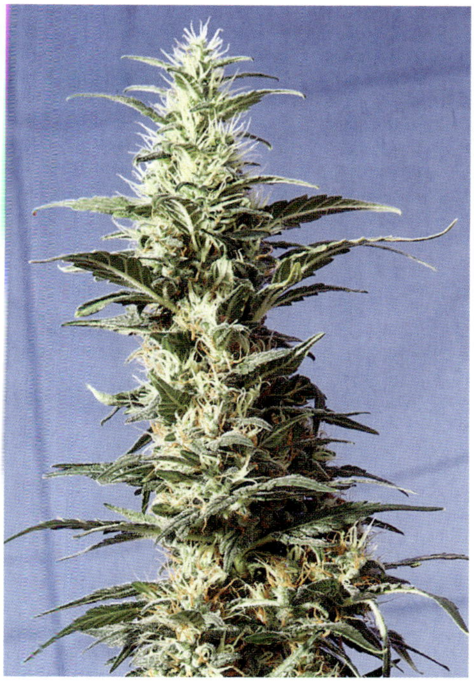

Snow White Northern Lights x White Widow x Cinderella 99.

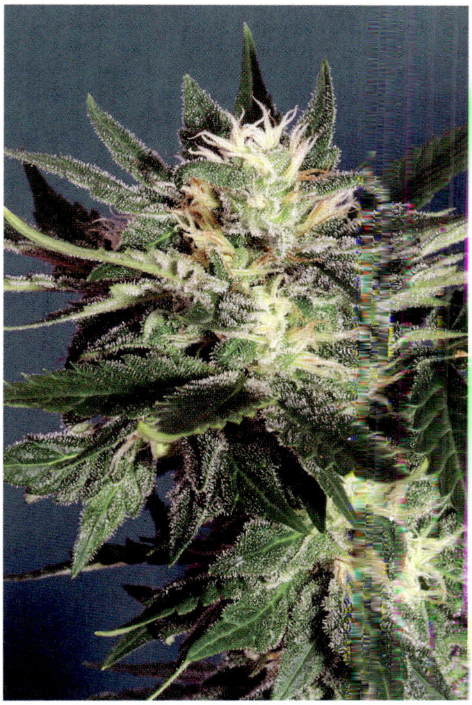

Top 69 Northern Lights Hybrid x Ruderalis.

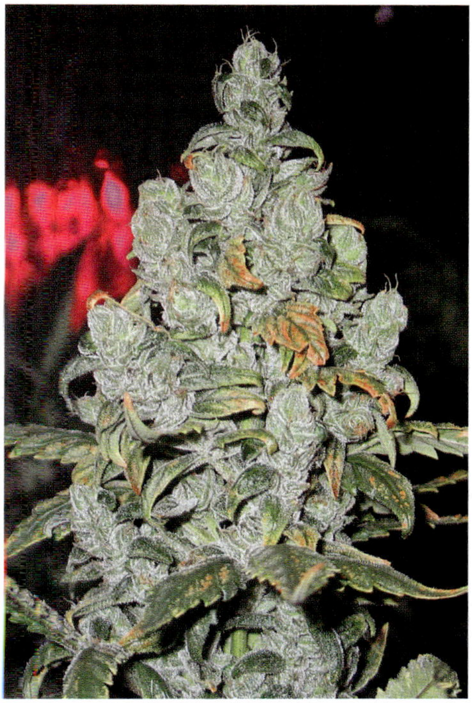

Zindica NL x G13 x AK-47 x Jamaican.

PHOTOS: MRNICE.NL (TOP LEFT), SPLIFFSEEDS.NL (TOP RIGHT), ADVANVEDSEEDS.COM (BOTTOM LEFT), BUMBOKLOT SEEDS (BOTTOM RIGHT)

Classic Kush Breeding

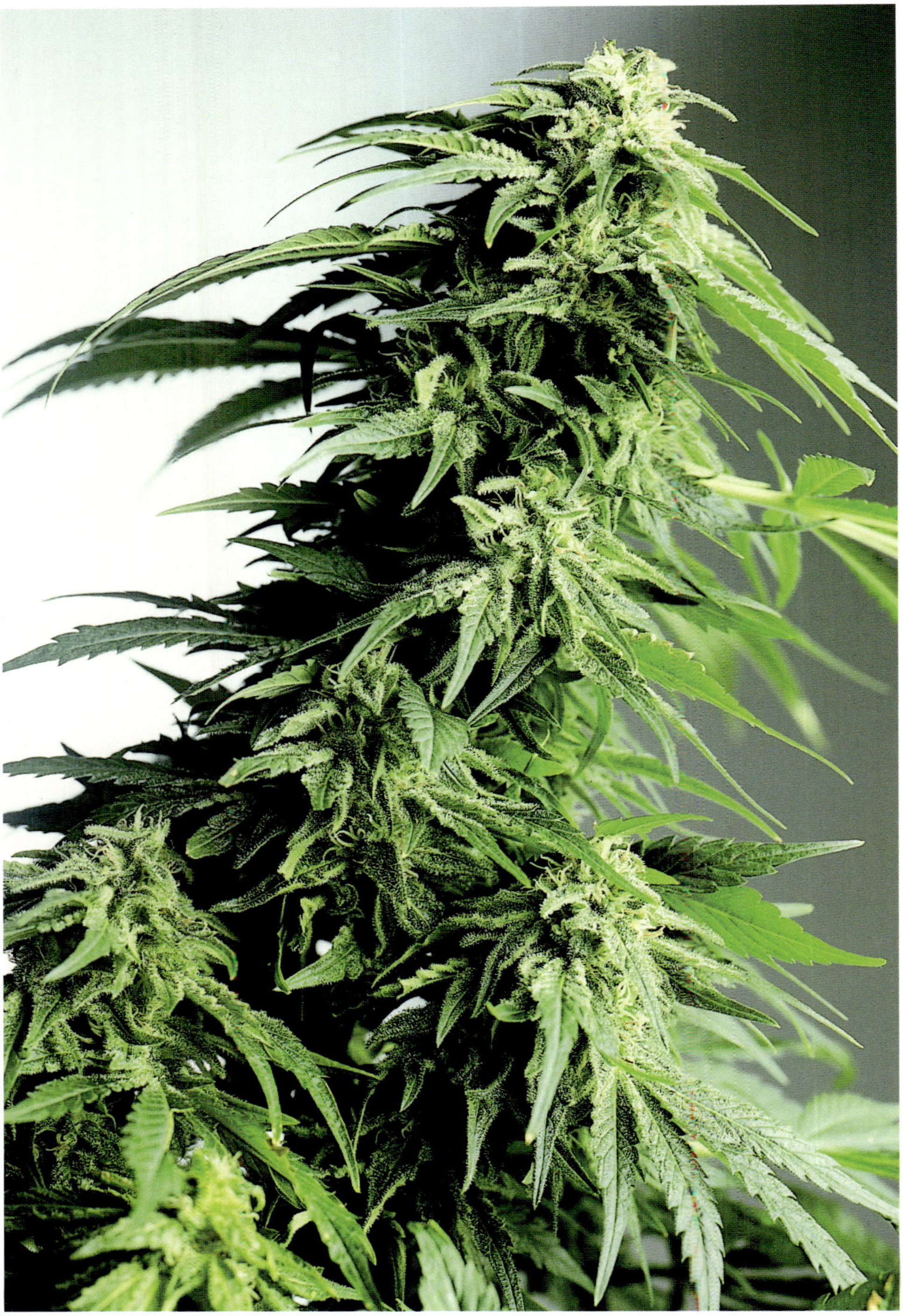

PHOTO: SENSISEEDS.COM

Kush is one of the most popular strains to hybridize because of its pure indica genes. If you have a plant with too many sativa traits for your liking, crossing with a Kush is the way to go.

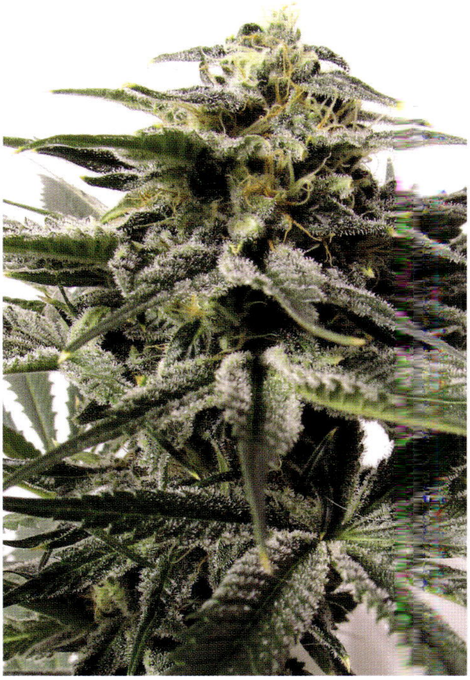

Nevil's SuperKush Kanga's Kush x Jim Ortega's Kush.

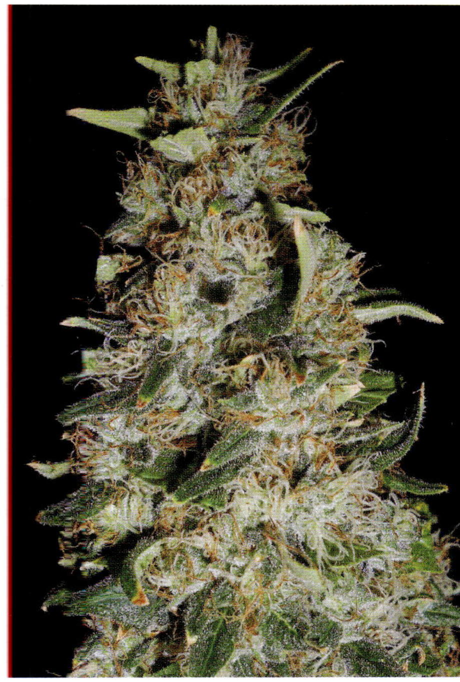

Kush #1 Hindu Kush x Afghani #1.

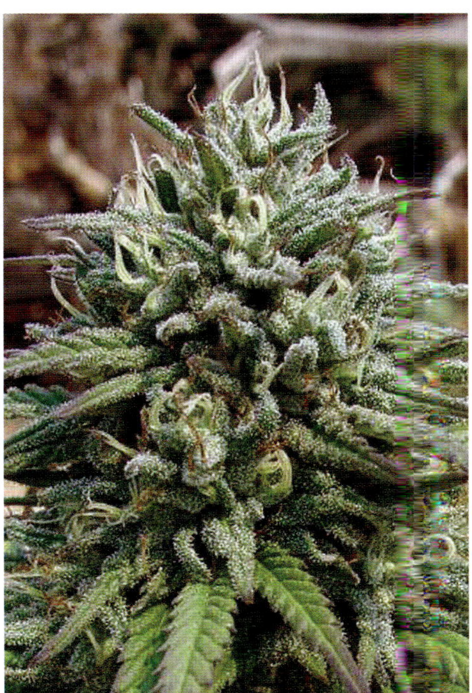

Kandy Kush OG Kush x Trainwreck.

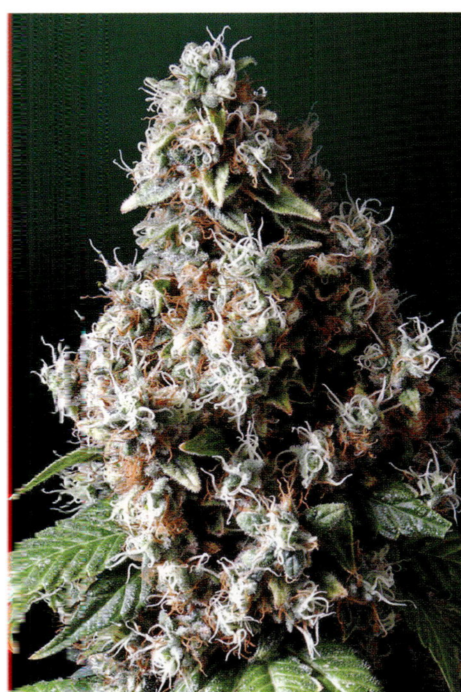

Double Kush Kushage x Afghan Kush.

PHOTOS: MARK HEINRICH (TOP LEFT), TREETOWNSEEDS.COM (TOP RIGHT), DNAGENETICS.COM (BOTTOM LEFT), DELTA9LABS.COM (BOTTOM RIGHT)

How to Establish a Clone Mother

The most effective way to establish a clone mother is by cultivating a substantial population of plants from the same strain. If the strain is an IBL, you will typically observe minimal variation among the plants. However, identifying a suitable clone mother from an IBL strain can pose a challenge. IBLs are deliberately created to produce a population of seed-grown plants that exhibit remarkable uniformity. The process of finding a clone mother from such strains usually stems from a well-planned breeding program, often involving generations like the F3 backcross with the homozygote, where all plants closely resemble the clone mother cherished by the breeder, one they aim to introduce to others.

The optimal approach to creating a clone mother is to carefully select one from a large population of F1 hybrid plants. Should you fail to find a suitable clone mother within the F1 generation, you may consider allowing random mating to occur, and then assess whether the F2 generation yields a candidate. If your search for the clone mother remains unsuccessful in the F2 generation, either expand the size of your plant population or explore different parental pairings to establish a new F1 population.

Note that the quality of a clone mother is inherently tied to the environment in which she is cultivated. This plays a crucial role in determining how the genetic makeup, the genotype, of a plant manifests itself in its physical characteristics, phenotype. Although indoor plants can adapt to outdoor conditions and vice versa, the expressed phenotype can undergo alterations due to variations in the growing environment. This is precisely why breeders often stress the importance of cultivating their strains in the recommended environmental conditions.

Environmental factors have a substantial influence on the expression of genes. For instance, if you observe a purple stem on your plant, you might question whether it's due to a specific genetic trait, nutrient deficiency, or exposure to cold temperatures. These types of inquiries should guide your understanding of how genes interact with their environment and how best to manage them for desired outcomes.

Exploring Autoflowering Hybrids

The emergence of ruderalis hybrids represents a significant development in cannabis cultivation. A primary driving force for their creation was the demand for outdoor strains that exhibit rapid flowering characteristics. These hybrids do not need the near-tropical conditions typically associated with the cultivation of more exotic strains in outdoor settings. The fusion of popular indica and sativa strains with ruderalis genetics has given rise to a new category of cannabis plants known as autoflowering hybrids. This unique combination offers distinct advantages for growers seeking efficient outdoor cultivation options.

Ruderalis does not follow strict light regimes, but automatically switches from vegetative

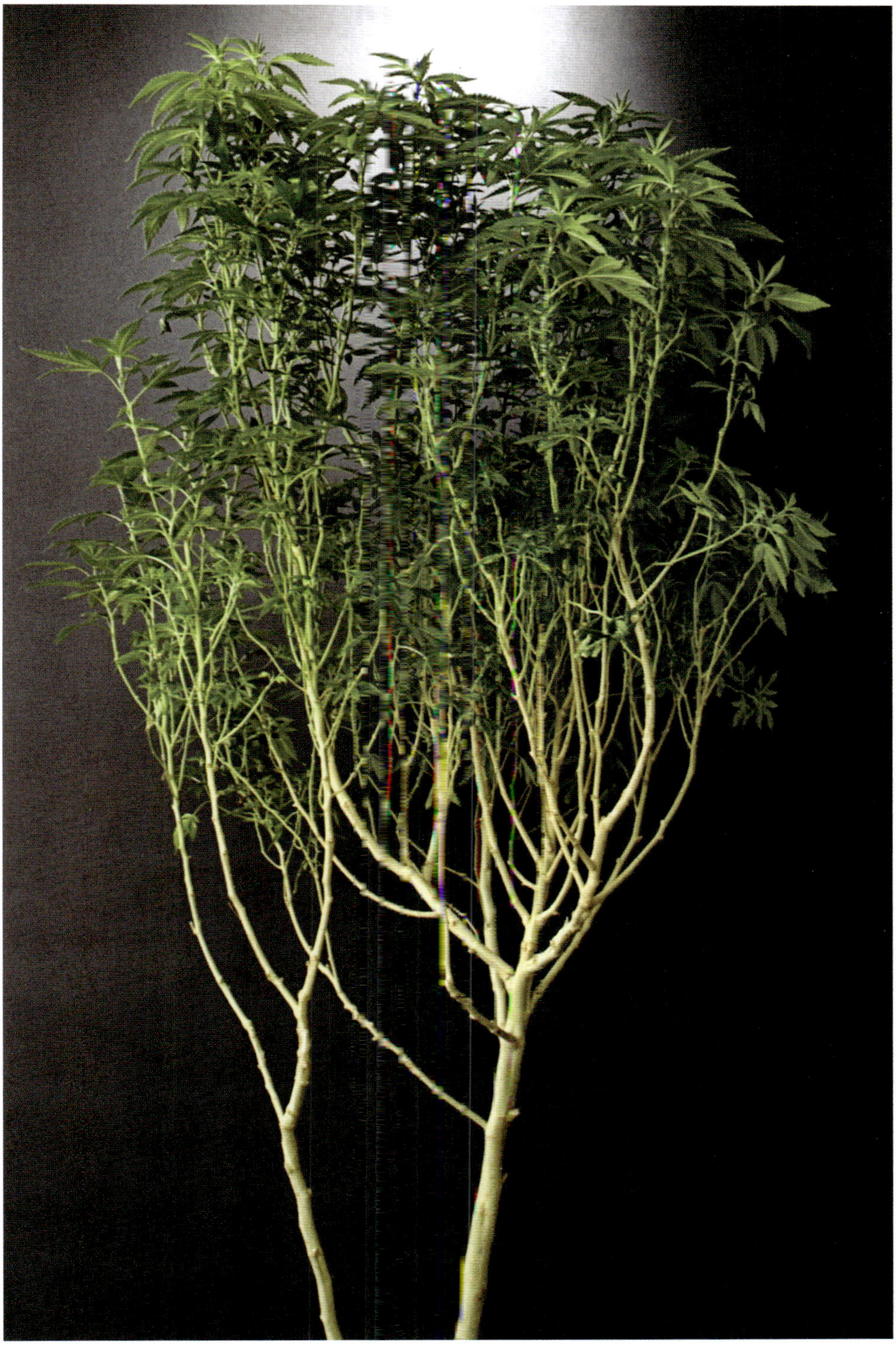

PHOTO: ED BORG

This clone mother is kept in circulation for up to six months. Bending of the branches allows for more shoots to grow out which enables the grower to take many cuttings each week.

to flowering. Flowering is entirely genetically triggered at the end of vegetative growth, irrespective of the photoperiod. This is generally not optimal for cultivators who prefer total control over their flowering times; however, there are instances where you do not have total control. A common problem is when the outdoor location does not have the time needed for the strain to finish flowering before the night frosts start. You could select a strain with less flowering time, but that would be a different strain. Ruderalis autoflowering genetics can be bred with regular strains to create a plant that goes into flowering based on age (time), and not the photoperiod (environment). These are called autoflowering hybrids. The growth time from seed to finish is 7 to 10 weeks, with height between 60 to 100 cm. The speed and size make concealment of this plant easier. Many growers have gone for these smaller hybrids that take up far less real estate and deliver results quickly. However, these traits depend on the breeder, so reading the strain description is essential. Some autoflowering hybrids can be much higher in CBD than THC, for example.

Imagine taking any familiar strain and appending "× ruderalis" to its name or prefixing it with "autoflowering". For instance, you might encounter strains like Skunk#1 × ruderalis or Autoflowering Skunk#1 in the market. These hybrids have garnered considerable attention due to their compelling autoflowering attributes. They stand as a viable alternative, particularly in regions where traditional indica or sativa strains may not thrive optimally in outdoor conditions. This adaptability has contributed to the increasing popularity of autoflowering strains, thereby expanding the horizons of the breeding market.

The appeal of autoflowering hybrids lies in their ability to mature and flower swiftly, regardless of the daylight hours. Unlike photoperiod strains, which require specific light cycles to trigger flowering, autoflowering varieties follow a predetermined genetic timetable. This trait makes them well-suited for outdoor cultivation in various environments, including those with conditions less favorable for traditional strains. Consequently, growers have a compelling reason to explore and embrace autoflowering strains as a valuable addition to their repertoire.

Ruderalis is considered a vigorous plant, despite being generally shorter than indica and appearing weedy, verging on wild, with leaves that develop fewer blades than traditional indica and sativa do. Most pure ruderalis are relatively low in cannabinoids, with higher CBD than THC. A breeder can start by obtaining these landrace ruderalis genetics or getting seeds from a source that has already done some selecting to find the better plants to make seeds with. This means some of the work of removing the less vigorous individuals and their genes has been done. It will take you a few generations if you do it yourself. Another other way to start is with ruderalis, which has already undergone some hybridization. This means you will introduce a regular strain hybridized with ruderalis into a breeding project.

The goal of your autoflowering hybrid breeding pair will be to maintain the preferred traits of the other strain as well as the ruderalis automatic flowering traits. Why can't we just take the gene for autoflowering and put it into regular strains? At the time of writing, it would require genetic sequencing, testing, and gene editing. So, for now, it is the same hybridizing and breeding techniques we have already covered, except for cloning, which is an issue.

Ruderalis clones flower according to age. Taking a cutting and making a clone does not restart the clock. The clone will flower regardless of the photoperiod. You can't stop it. However, you can pollinate clones and make seeds. You can't grow any respectable plant from that clone, as you can with regular strains that can revert to vegetative growth with 24/0. This makes breeding with it more difficult, but not impossible. You may not be able to secure every trait you want because test crossing is more challenging, but you can have an automatic hybrid with quite a few desirable features. So, clones will always be suboptimal, and in terms of results from seed, the ruderalis hybrid will never produce quite the same quantity of cannabinoid levels as their photoperiod-responsive counterparts. It all amounts to lowering expectations for the advantages you get in return.

In summary, the advent of autoflowering hybrids has brought forth a versatile and resilient category of cannabis plants that cater to the needs of outdoor cultivators in diverse regions. By combining the genetics of beloved indica and sativa strains with ruderalis, breeders have unlocked new possibilities for cannabis enthusiasts, further diversifying the offerings within the cannabis breeding market.

Understanding Feminized Seeds

Cannabis sexual expression is complex and multifaceted. However, we encourage growers to begin their journey with standard seeds rather than immediately resorting to feminized seeds. This approach might seem challenging at first, as standard seeds introduce variability with both male and female plants. However, we firmly believe that this initial experience provides invaluable insights and knowledge.

By working with standard seeds, you gain a deeper understanding of the male-to-female ratios and the intricacies of cannabis plant development. This knowledge forms the foundation upon which you can build your expertise. The effort you put into cultivating and managing standard seeds will ultimately reward you with the satisfaction of producing sinsemilla females, achieved through your dedicated efforts. After mastering this fundamental aspect of cannabis cultivation, you can confidently explore the use of feminized seeds.

The journey of cannabis sexual development follows various intricate pathways. Sexual expression itself is a multistage process governed by a complex interplay of over 10,000 genes. These genes orchestrate phytohormone signaling, floral growth, and various

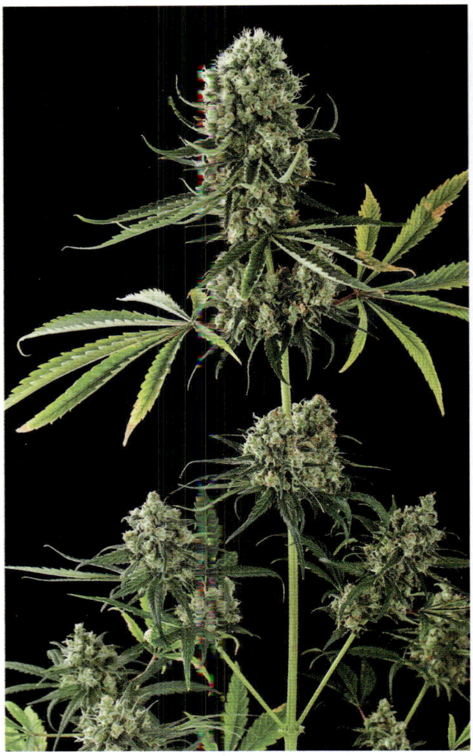

Connoisseur strains like Critical Jack may have obvious gaps in the internodes. They are bred for a certain flowering trait such as taste or potency.

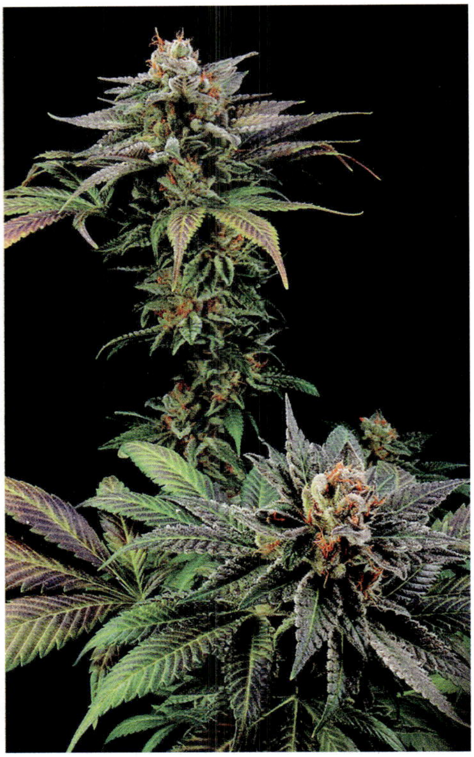

Other strains like Blue Widow may be aiming for color over other traits. This trait is fixed in the population by breeding it true.

metabolic processes. Among these, the plant hormone ethylene plays a pivotal role, as it directly influences sex determination-related genes. Ethylene promotes the development of female plants, while its inhibitors have the opposite effect, promoting males.

Beyond the plant's internal processes, external substances can be introduced to interact with these multistage pathways and influence sexual expression. Historically, substances such as silver thiosulfate (STS) and colloidal silver have been used successfully to promote male flower production, with their pollen remaining viable. Gibberellic acid (GA) has been considered as a potential promoter of maleness, but experimental results suggest it may not stimulate male flowers.

STS and colloidal silver are effective because both contain silver ions that inhibit ethylene production, thereby favoring male development. Notably, these substances do not appear to affect other aspects of the plant, such as its height or growth rate. However, it is crucial to apply STS uniformly to the entire plant, avoiding targeted applications with high concentrations, which can adversely affect specific areas and

PHOTOS: DINAFEM SEEDS

lead to necrosis. Note that different strains may exhibit varying degrees of resistance to this treatment.

Untreated females can also be pollinated with pollen from treated females. Since both parents are XX (female), there is no possibility of XY (male) offspring emerging from this process. This is often referred to as using 'female pollen.' By generating and nurturing these seeds, you'll observe that they exclusively produce feminized seeds, as both parents are XX. While treatment does not seem to produce any noticeable differences other than male flowers, there is a possibility of a linked trait shift towards cannabinoid ratios favoring CBD.

It is important to note that when using regular male pollen on female plants, self-pollination can still occur due to undetected male hermaphrodite flowers unless removed. You need to ensure the females are indeed females and not hermaphrodites.

Feminized seeds are produced through a fascinating process that involves influencing the plant's sexual expression. Starting with standard seeds and understanding the complexities of cannabis sexual development is a crucial step in becoming a proficient grower before you venture into the realm of feminized seeds. This journey not only enhances your skills but also deepens your appreciation of the intricate world of cannabis cultivation.

Concluding Thoughts on Breeding

Cannabis breeding is marked by experimentation that yields new hybrids. From these hybrids, stabilized strains emerge as the ultimate achievement. Quality always surpasses quantity in this endeavor. Breeding is not a sprint but a marathon, demanding dedication over the long term. Sadly, many aspiring breeders abandon their efforts prematurely, constrained by limitations in time, space, and finances. While they may have gathered theoretical knowledge about breeding in a short period, practical experience remains elusive.

Embarking on cannabis breeding necessitates a firm foundation. Be prepared to invest multiple growing cycles to grasp the fundamentals. Breeding is, above all, an exercise in discernment. Don't hesitate to acknowledge when your efforts yield nothing worthy of continuation. Even the most accomplished breeders have navigated through numerous populations before identifying a plant that truly stands out.

The motivations for breeding your own cannabis strain are diverse. Seek originality in your breeding projects, as it often leads to the most remarkable outcomes. If the insights shared in this chapter have piqued your interest and you're eager to delve deeper, read *The Cannabis Breeder's Bible* for an even more comprehensive understanding of the art and science of cannabis breeding.

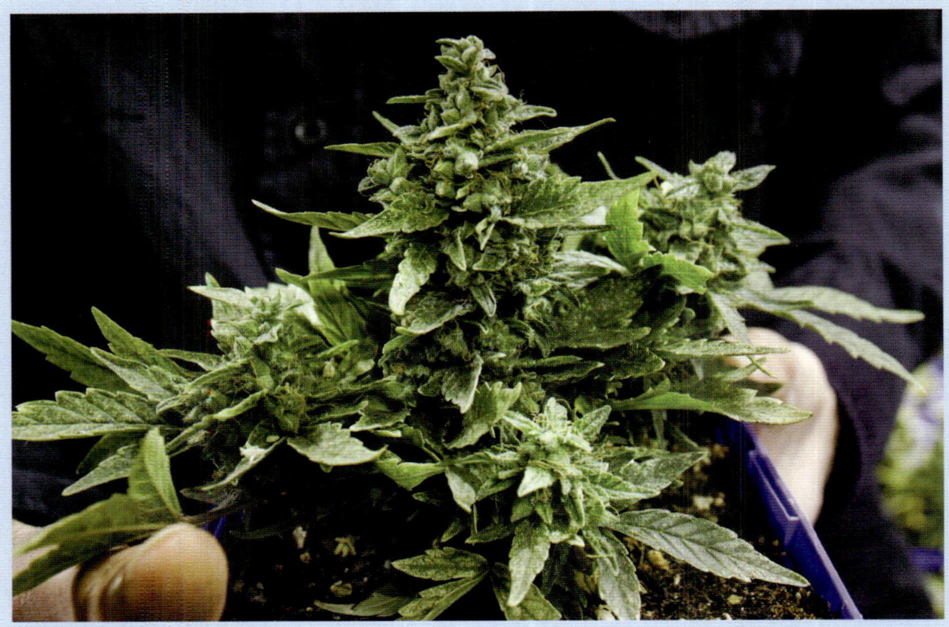

The original Lowryder plants were dank but tiny.

Lore of the Lowryder
by David Strange

Most growers dream of having their own strain, a variety created by them, for them; something to call their very own. A grower's ideal strain would be one that combines their favorite characteristics from growth to smoke and comes with the bragging rights of a job well done—and friends well stoned. However, when it comes to the breeding section in a grow book, most growers become a little intimidated. While much of a grow book can seem straightforward, all of a sudden the breeding section can feel as if that science class you skipped in school has come to bite you in the ass. It can also make breeding seem like something that's only for those growing on a grand scale.

The dream of breeding your very own strain need not be unrealistic. Don't go losing your drive to create the ultimate plant—even if you feel slightly dumbfounded by all that stuff that looks like math. Legends can come from humble beginnings. If you need proof, look no further than Lowryder.

The story of the Lowryder variety—and the subsequent autoflowering craze that stemmed from it—involves previously unknown actors and their rise from obscurity. It's a story of happiness and frustration, setbacks and leaps forward, but most of all, it's a story that came from those aforementioned humble beginnings.

PHOTOS: DAVID STRANGE

Lowryder started a revolution in growing, and like most other strains, it began with a box of seeds and limited resources but a devotion to the making of something truly unique. While the Lowryder journey arguably started when the first plant did its own thing and started to flower automatically indoors, to understand just how incredible Lowryder's history is, a little backstory is necessary.

The first step on any breeding journey is to create an F1 strain: A hybrid of two plants. This, quite simply, involves pollinating one variety with the pollen from another. It's the simplest and most direct way to breed a different and somewhat customized version of a strain that you already like. The two strains that you breed together are known as the "parent" plants, and the better your selection of parent plants, the better the result. The F1 generation tends to be a fairly stable combination of both parents. It also has what is referred to as "hybrid vigor." You'll see many flowers at the garden center labeled F1 because of the marketability of plants with hybrid vigor. This is where the Lowryder story began: Looking for speed from one variety and strength from another.

In the mid to late 90s, seed banks were providing solid genetics but most of them were working out of Amsterdam. In Canada, the most prized genetics were still what I'd refer to as "hand-me-downs." The genetics of a plant that showed itself to have redeeming qualities were shared amongst a circle of friends and/or like-minded growers. This is how the Joint Doctor procured what was to become Lowryder. Referred to

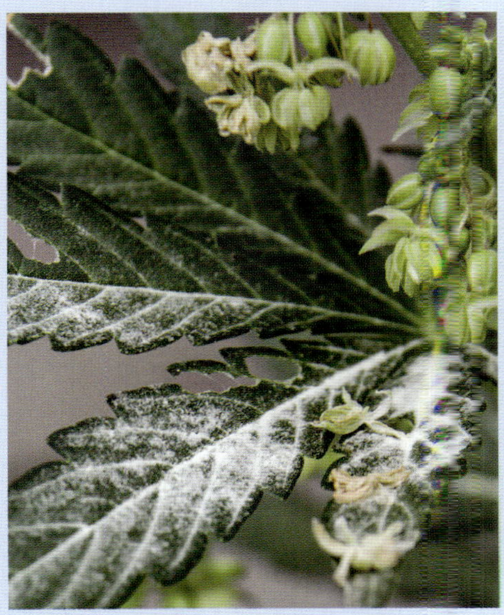

Leaves are heavily dusted with pollen on this Lowryder male.

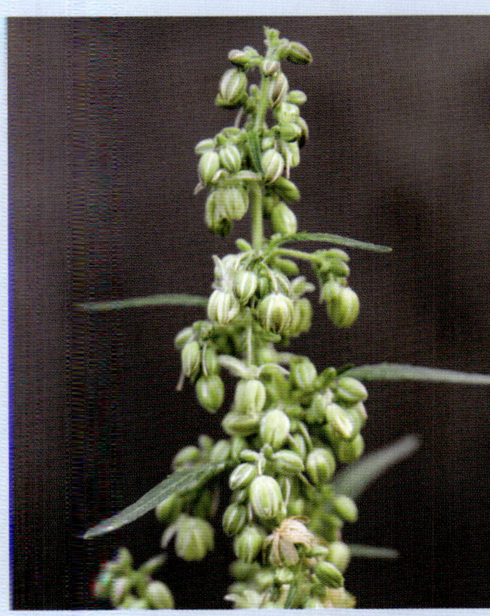

These male flowers have begun to open and are ready to meet the ladies.

as "Mexican ruderalis" by its owner, this set of genetics was pretty mysterious. Ruderalis was known to be of Russian decent. Was this a Mexican variety crossed with a ruderalis? Was it even Mexican—or even ruderalis? This question is never likely to be answered. The Joint Doctor had to content himself with growing the strain, and when he did, he noted that it finished really early outdoors. However, it was untested in an indoor environment. With his curiosity piqued, the Joint Doctor made the decision to cross his new genetics with one of the hardest hitting and most reliable indoor varieties in his arsenal: Northern Lights #2. The product of these two plants was then combined with a William's Wonder plant, to create another F1. At this point, the autoflowering characteristic had yet to show itself. In the midst of his project, the Joint Doctor moved to the prairies of Canada, and in order to create seeds to transport with him, he bred an F2 version of this speedy three-way cross, packed up all his growing equipment, and headed north.

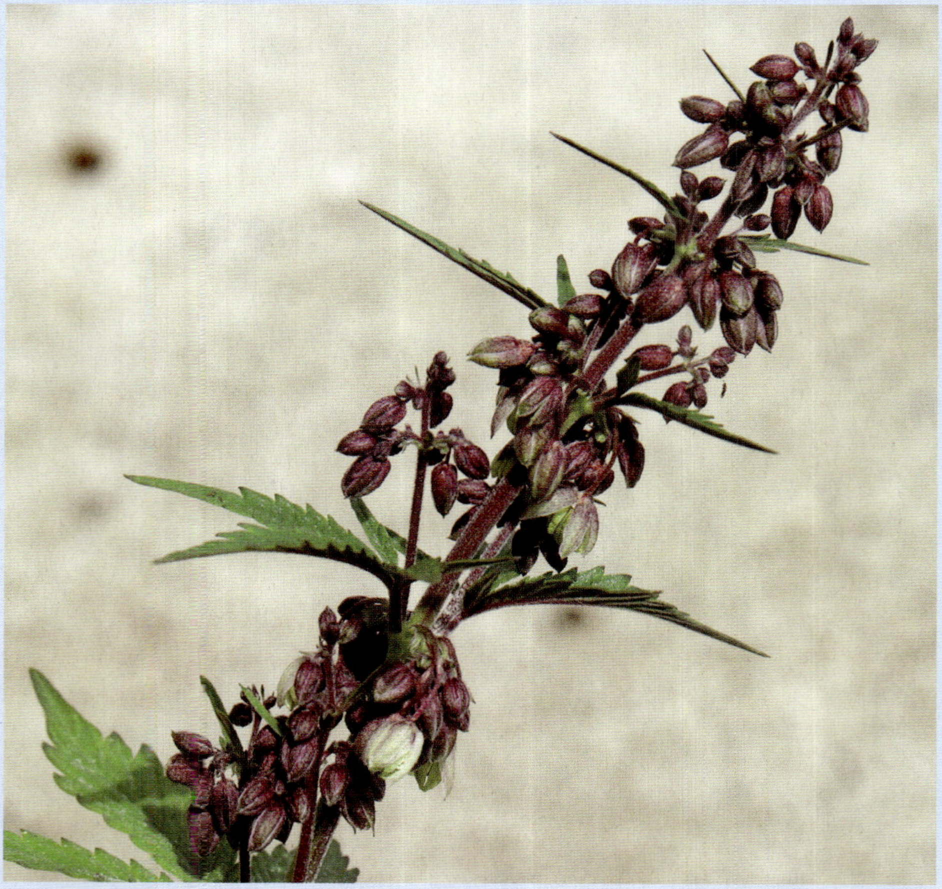

Yep, those are purple male flowers. The power of breeding is only limited by your imagination and time.

PHOTOS: DAVID STRANGE

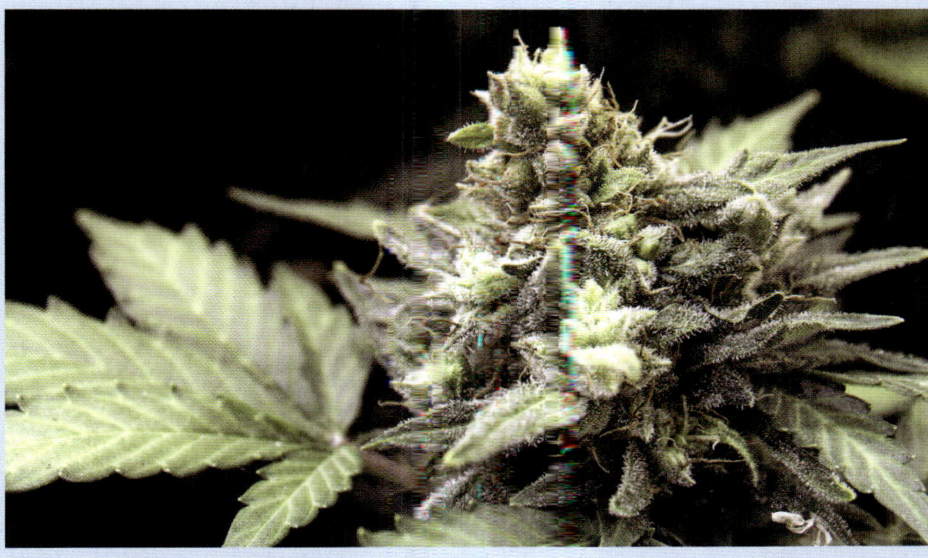

This cola is bursting with some of the first Betty Boo seeds.

This is where I met the Joint Doctor. We had both just moved to the middle of nowhere, far from the center of the cannabis world. As fellow collectors of high-grade and intriguing seeds, we decided to run a cycle together in my basement room. The idea was that we would see them side by side, then swap or crossbreed the best of our beans. My grow space at that time was only a small thing: A 12 x 12-foot room with 5,400-watt HPS lights. That was all the gear that could be procured at the time. Despite these incongruous conditions, we filled my basement with ten of our favorite varieties, five of each, and sitting quietly in the corner, not making a fuss, was the strain that would become known as the Lowryder.

Much has since been made of Lowryder's autoflowering trait, but back then, we didn't even know it existed. The thing about the autoflowering trait is that it's a recessive gene so it does not show itself in the F1 generation. The moral here is this: You may have a truly magical plant on your hands, but the most incredible characteristics in your newly created F1 may not have even shown themselves yet. This is what we learned from breeding Lowryder.

Our grow room had been in the vegetative stage on a 24-hour light cycle, for a few weeks before our tiny plants in the corner began to show signs of flowering. This was truly an oddity but certainly stirred our curiosity. As I stared at this ugly duckling, the Joint Doctor asked:

"What the hell should we do with these weirdos?"

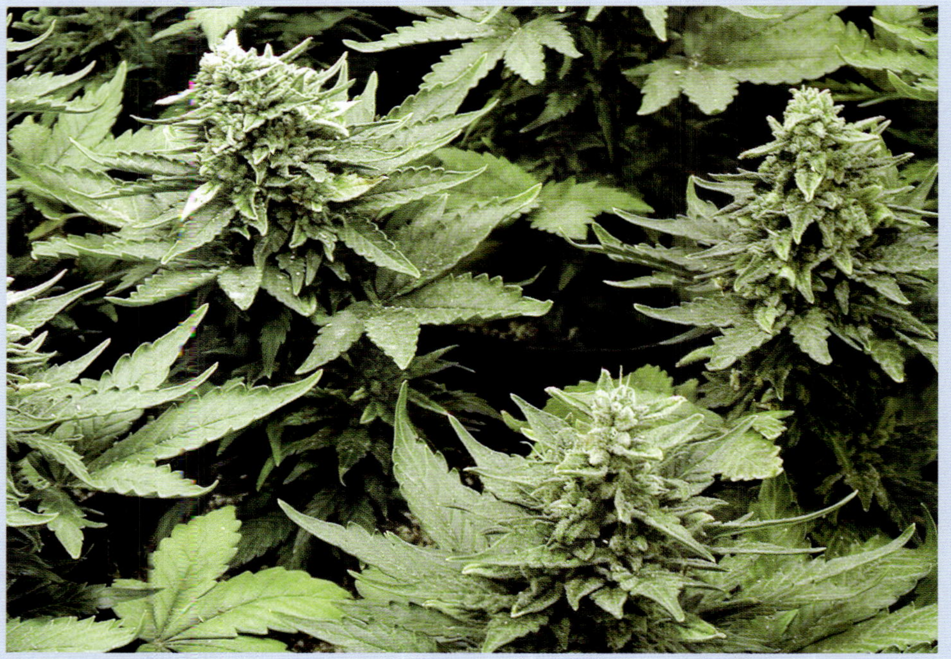

The Lowryder 2 offers stability and size.

In my excitement, I had already gabbled out "We need to pollinate these!" before I turned to see the best male already in his hands. On his face was a grin of youthful exuberance. His question, clearly, had been rhetorical.

The Joint Doctor took the seeds from those plants back to his place and got into the real work: Creating a variety, not just a cross. The autoflowering trait had appeared during the creation of the F1 generation, but it needed to be stabilized. This is where the true breeding occurs. A stable cross is closer to a P1 stock than an F2, as a good breeder will avoid the randomness that can occur in an F2. The Lowryder's unique autoflowering trait was the one we needed to isolate, but the process was no different than the process to maintain the smell or taste of your favorite variety.

When a regular variety is crossed with an autoflowering one, the F1 generation of seeds is going to be fast but will not exhibit the autoflowering trait. This won't show up until the F2 generation, when about 25% of plants show the trait. That's why it wasn't noticed in the original Northern Lights cross. When a female receives pollen from a male and both have the autoflowering characteristic, about 50% of the next generation will exhibit autoflowering. When a female and a male from this generation are bred together, approximately 75% of the seeds will have the autoflowering trait, then 87.5%, and so on. By inbreeding generations of the same variety like

PHOTOS: DAVID STRANGE

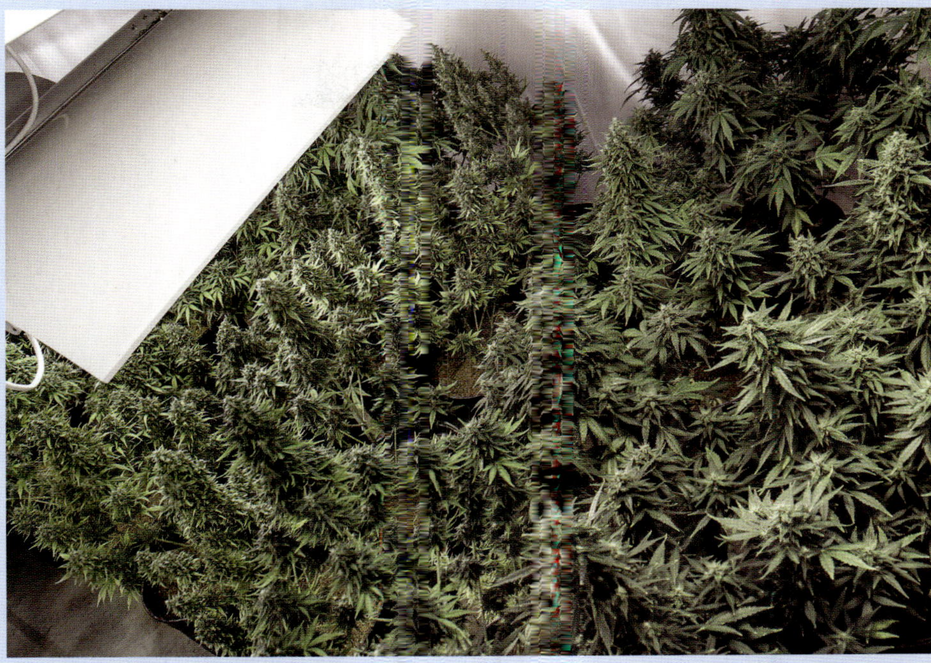

Bird's-eye view of an Ogre seed crop.

this, you create an inbred line, or IBL. This effectively breeds out certain characteristics and selects for others until the stability of that characteristic is achieved.

Once the Joint Doctor had gotten the Lowryder to the point of true breeding for the autoflowering trait, the next stage could begin. The IBL work over several generations had left him with a variety that was now uniformly age-determinate instead of light-determinate. All the plants went to bud according to how old they were (which was young!) rather than in response to a change in their lighting schedule. The plants matured in about 40-55 days from germination, had a deep musky smell, and smoked quite respectably. They were also only yielding about 7-14 grams on the larger end. With his IBL technique, the Joint Doctor had seemingly hit a plateau for size. It was eating into his confidence, making him unsure how far his new variety could go. Something was clearly going to have to be done about that.

That was the original Lowryder. But the project wasn't over. It was back to the drawing board and back to another F1 generation to add the things that seemed lacking in our original variety. A little more nose and a chunk more size. Some speed could be sacrificed. With the autoflowering trait stabilized, a batch of new crosses was created. The one that stood out as the earliest—and, handily, also the most stable—was the cross with Santa Maria. This was then put through the aforementioned IBL technique until I stabilized, and voila! Lowryder #2 was born. This plant would go to bud automatically under any light regime, just like the original, but it now had much more kick, had a smell that could sell a bag, and was getting into the ounce-per-plant range. The most popular growing method of the time was a SOG with fairly young clones, and this plant fitted that set up perfectly. It was also a perfect plant for those growing in limited space, producing just for themselves.

Any serious smoker knows that smoking the same strain over time makes you build up a tolerance, which makes you fall out of love with that strain a little. That's where Joint Doctor was at with Lowryder #2. I had recently returned from a trip to the Cannabis Cup in Amsterdam and he had been gathering some new gems, so we did the seed exchange thing again. Some of his most prized Lowryder seeds were traded for some of the first generation of NYC Diesel given me by Soma and some Mazar from Sensi Seeds.

With these genes in hand, it was back to the F1 table. The cycle began again. We grew, looked out for the best traits, and inbred the plants to stabilize those traits. When we bred the NYC Diesel with Lowyder, we selected mainly for the distinctive smell and flavor. This plant became the DieselRyder. An AK-47 from Serious Seeds was bred with Lowryder, while selecting for size and solidity, and this became the EazyRyder. This strain came in at 19% THC, making it the most potent autoflower to date. A few generations of inbreeding later, the Mazar would show its colors; this

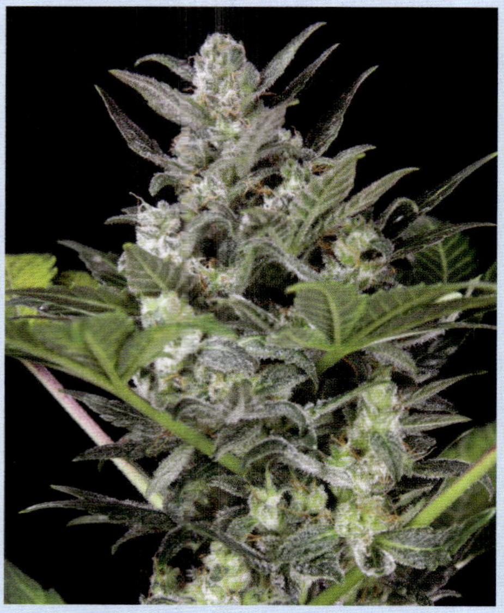

The DieselRyder is a soaring high and smells of all that gasoline.

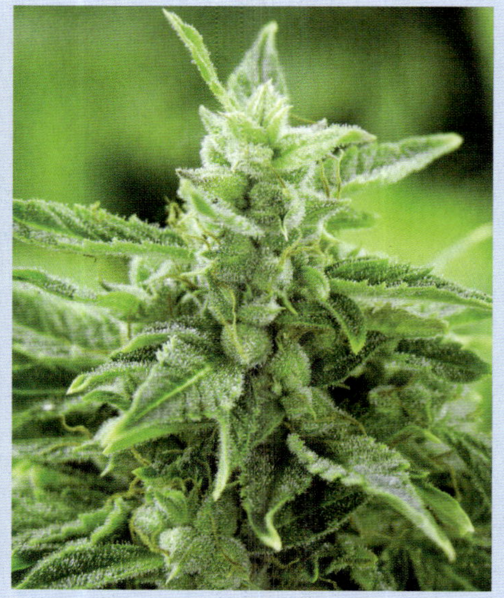

The EazyRyder utilizes some of Serious Seeds' AK-47.

PHOTOS: DAVID STRANGE

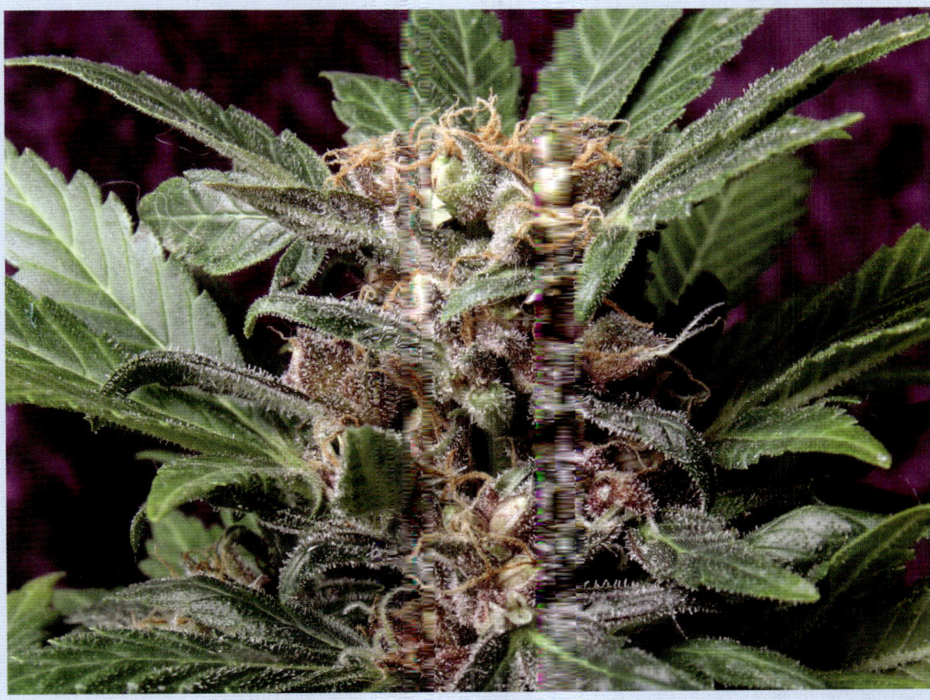

The range of colors and flavors available is seemingly endless.

variety became stabilized as the PurpleRyder. Another line of the Mazar would be bred for a distinctive musk, speed, and a relaxed high to become the Betty Boo. The Lowryder magic just kept on coming.

There's a difference between chucking pollen at your plants and actually breeding. The latter isn't difficult, but it is a skill. Hopefully this story explains to you why this breeding chapter is not to be feared, and should in fact inspire you on to great things.

Over the span of his breeding journey Joint Doctor has learned and likely utilized almost every technique in this chapter to achieve something great. At the beginning, however, he didn't know any of them. He also started in a room that you could set up affordably in a weekend in almost any house in North America. You can do great things, just as he did.

Autoflowering genetics now account for 60-70% of all European seed sales. This all began with Lowryder. I hope you can see how the special plant in your grow room has the potential to be something truly revolutionary. Hell, with enough devotion and a little luck you might have the next Diesel or OG or even Lowryder. It sounds like a cliché, but you actually can change the world—one seed at a time.

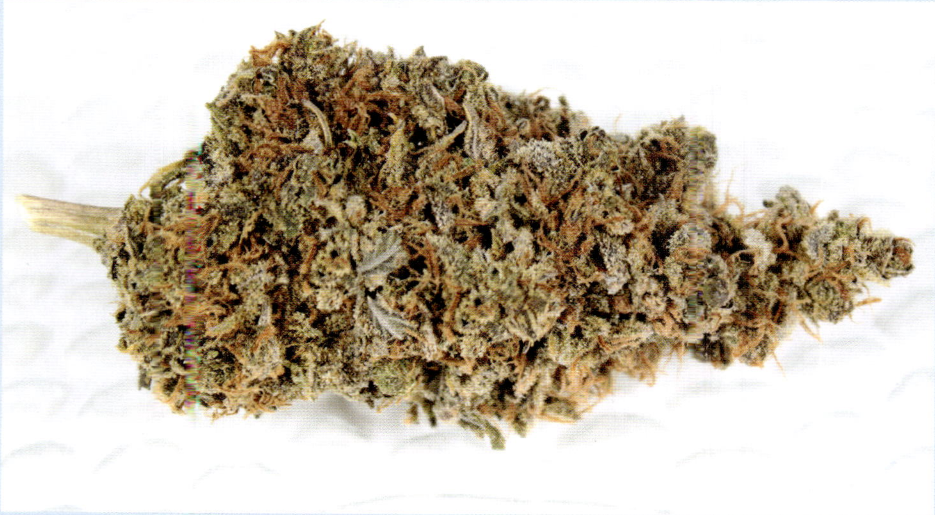

A True Living Organics (TLO) Breeding Run
by The Rev

Welcome! I'm The Rev and I have been growing cannabis for just about half a century. I have been breeding cannabis for about 40 years. For the last 20 years, I have been an all-natural style, True Living Organics (TLO) grower. In my past I have grown using almost every style; I used to be an expert hydroponics grower but I would never grow that way these days. Personally, I can't stand the low-quality product that synthetic nutrients produce.

When you're growing for seeds, the plant's flowers aren't as large as sinsemilla (seedless) flowers would be. This is because the flowers are laden with seeds, making them much denser and heavier, and the plant is using its energy to produce seeds

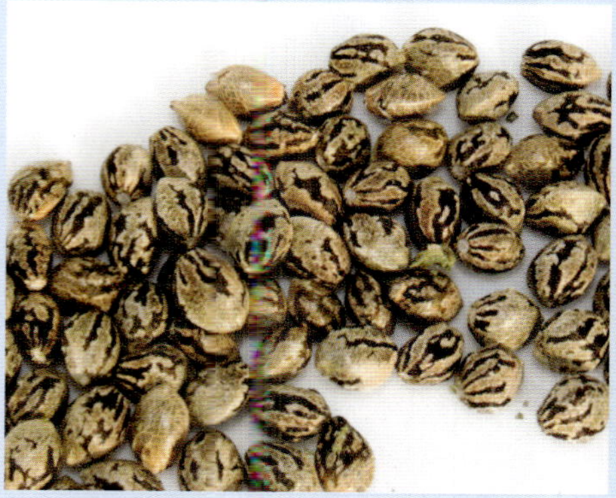

It all starts with my decades-old collected seeds.

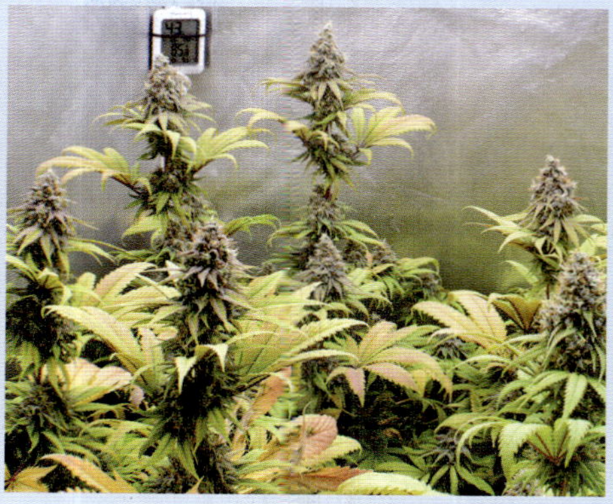

I make sure to grow plenty of sinsemilla plants from my seeds.

PHOTOS: THE REV

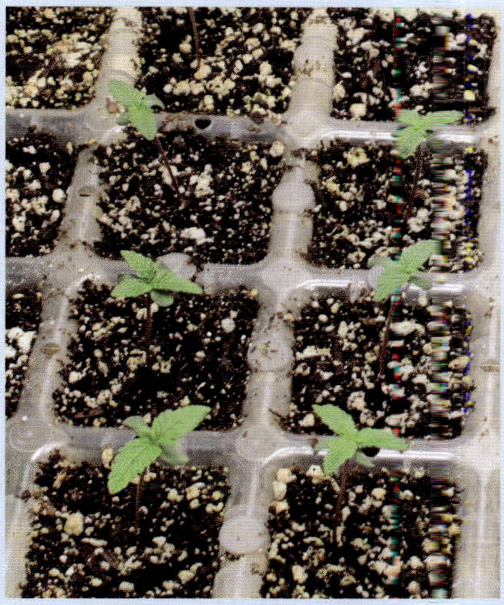

My standard seed germination method.

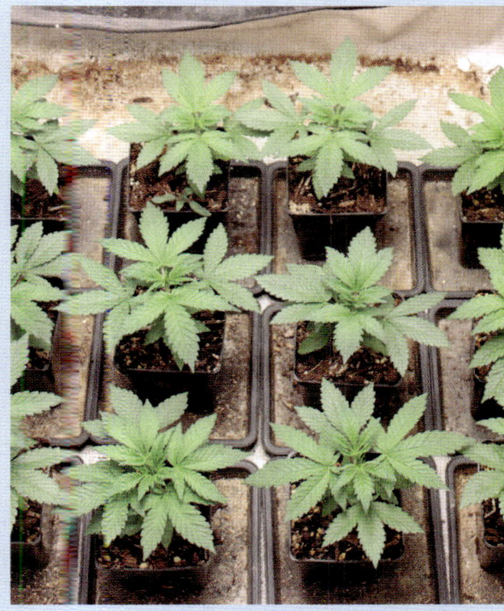

My selected 12 plants.

instead of growing buds. I am very familiar with most of the cannabis genotypes I work with, which gives me a big advantage because I am already familiar with their marker expressions, tendencies, and phenotypes. The key to successful breeding is choosing good genetics.

My main flowering room is a 10 x 10-foot bedroom. It houses two 3 x 3-foot grow tents and a couple of workstations for things like the Churn (a concentrated living tea), top dressings, water reservoirs, etc. I vent my tents directly. In the summer months when it's warmer, I run 400-watt LED lights, lately 420h LEDs, because my metal halide lamps get way too hot. But in the winter months, those HID metal halide lamps are both lights and heaters.

I normally use two germination trays for every run. I use a 16-unit tray for my main project seeds. I find this is a good number to start with to make sure I end up with high-quality breeder plants. I also use an eight-unit tray and plant eight seeds of a strain that has low viability; my 16-unit tray is for the more "sure thing" plants I want to work with. In the photo, you can see that out of the eight seeds I planted of a 30-year-old South American strain, only one sprouted. These trays are on a 16/8 photoperiod using a 250-watt Eye Hortilux Blue metal halide light.

I normally get 15 or 16 seeds to sprout from viable stock in the 16-unit flat. 20 days after they have sprouted, I will remove any unfavorable plants. Usually, I end up with around 12 plants at this point.

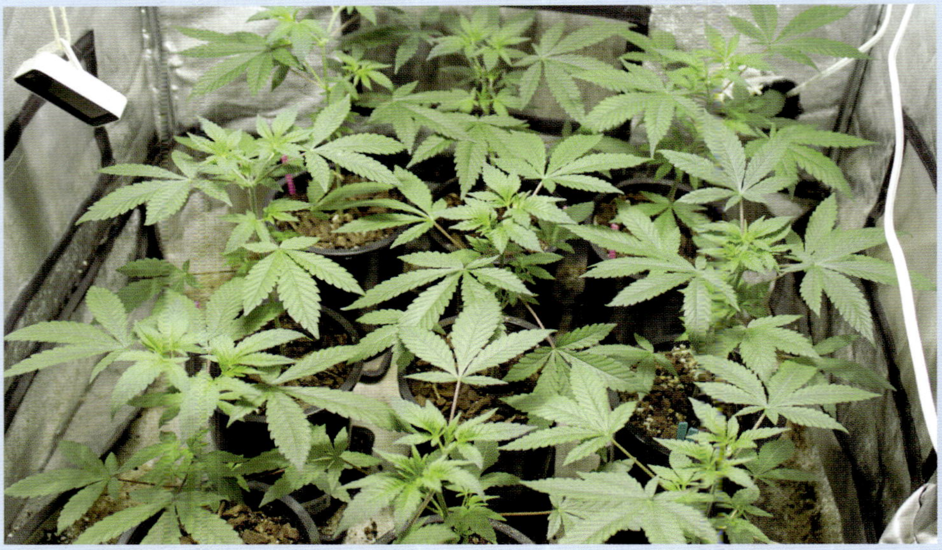

At 30 days old, only nine plants remain.

Once the plants have hit about 30 days above ground, I have culled additional plants from the herd and am usually down to 9 or 10 plants. Normally they are topped by this time. I flower in two Gorilla Grow Tents that are 3 x 3 foot. Indoor tents are extremely useful when you are flowering "special needs" genetics such as long inbred lines, longer flowering landrace strains, or cultivar sativas and sativa dominants. I can flower four females per tent if I keep my males small and I place them in the center. By the time I get to flowering, I am down to something like six total selected females.

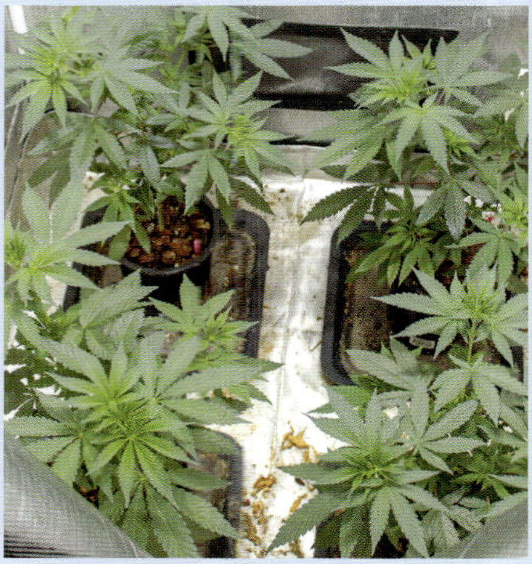

At about 40 days above ground, topped male and females are placed into flowering tents.

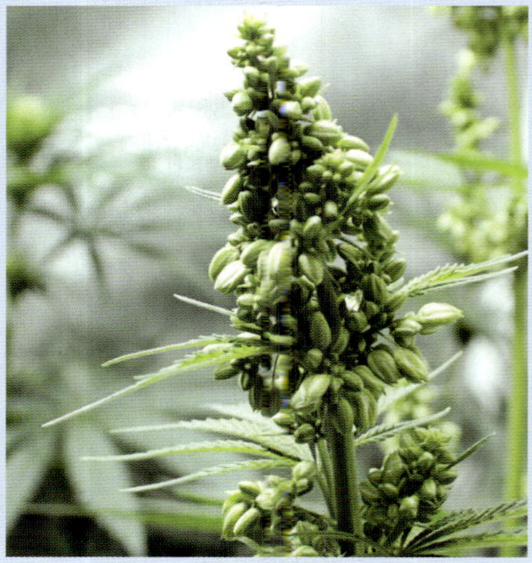

Male flower, within days of throwing viable pollen.

PHOTOS: THE REV

Once the plants are moved into the flowering tents at about 40 days old, the photoperiod is set to 15/9 under a 400-watt Eye Blue Hortilux metal halide lamp. This lets them know flowering time is approaching, but still gives them plenty of light to grow vigorously. I keep them under this photoperiod until they are big enough to start flowering, normally about 12 inches in height. This way they will finish just under 3 feet tall: Perfect for my environment. At about 18 inches tall and 50 days old, I switch the photoperiod to 12/12.

After about two weeks of the 12/12 photoperiod, flowers appear, both male and female. Once the male starts throwing pollen, I let him blow for about a week before removing him. His job is done.

When I am cultivating seeds, I allow more apical branches on the plants for more buds. Apical branching is when a branch splits off into two. During the seed removal process, I keep notes of the yield, resin production, and terpenes, keeping all the females labeled and likewise keeping all the seeds separated and labeled per plant. I also keep all the deseeded, trichome-rich flower debris separate and labeled.

I love smoking hash made from deseeded buds. I dry-sift the plant matter and hand-pack the trichomes to make temple balls. I also smoke the flower debris using my PAX Plus floral vaporizer. This way I can take note of the flavors, effects, and potency. This ultimately decides which female seeds I will be using for my next

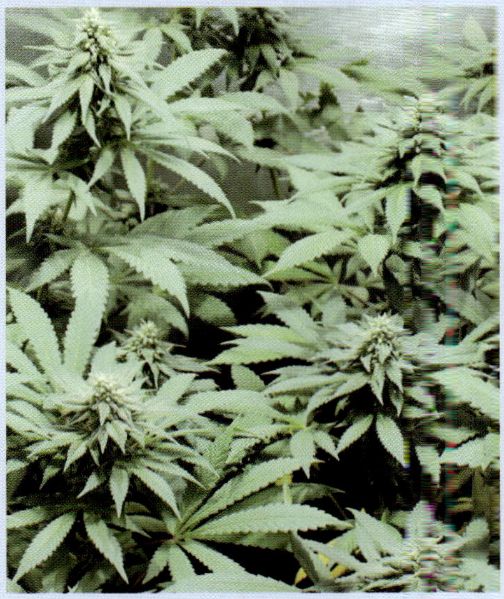

The tents fill up with seed-heavy buds after 30 to 40 days of flowering.

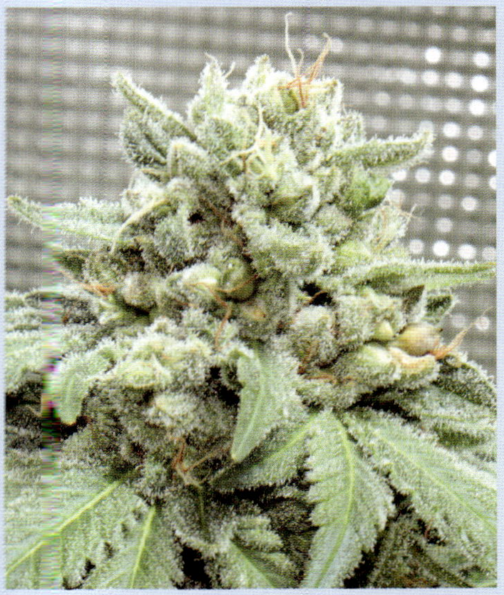

Killer KOS bud full of seeds.

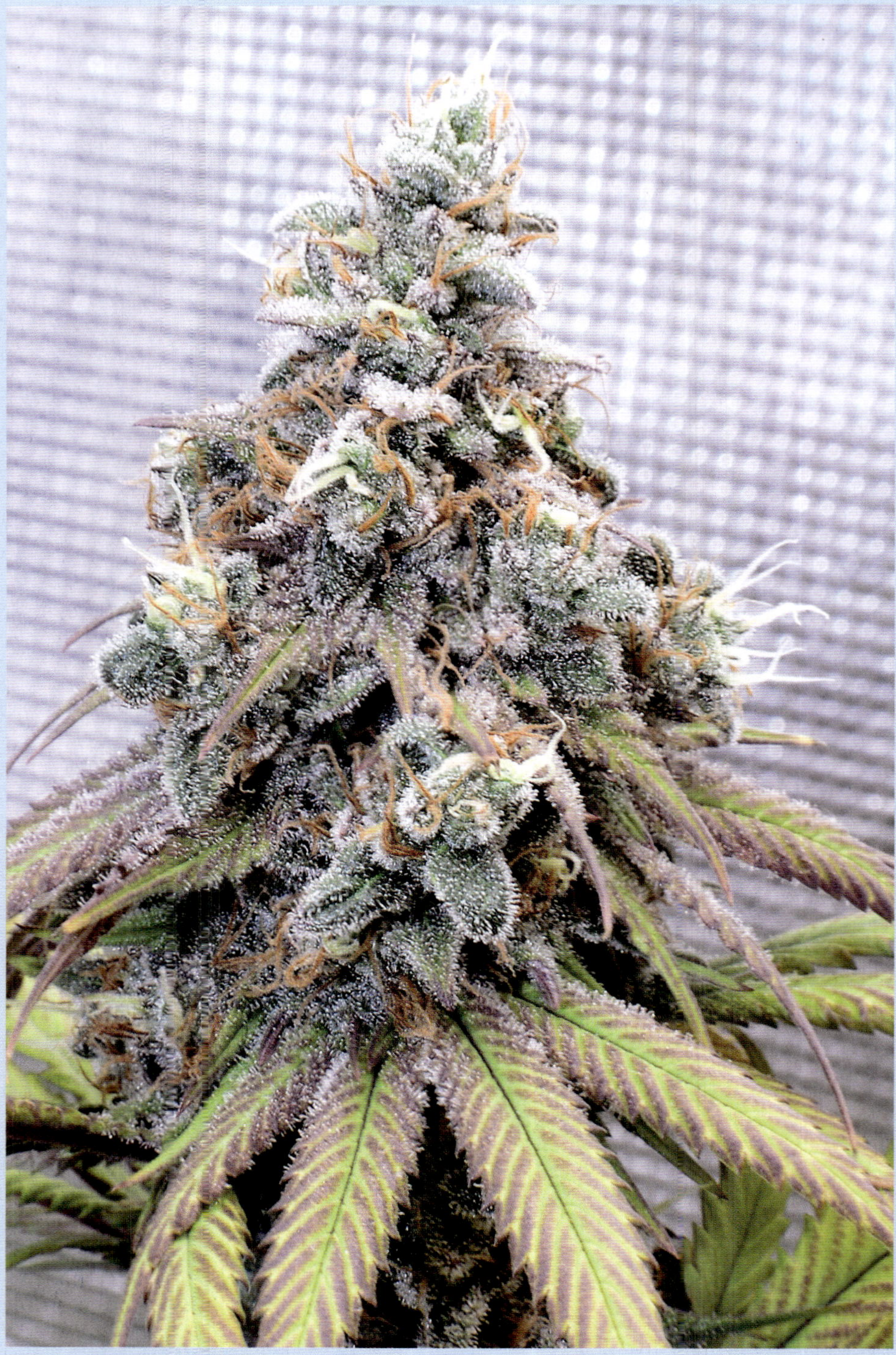

PHOTOS. THE REV

I love flowering sinsemilla plants from KOS Genetics.

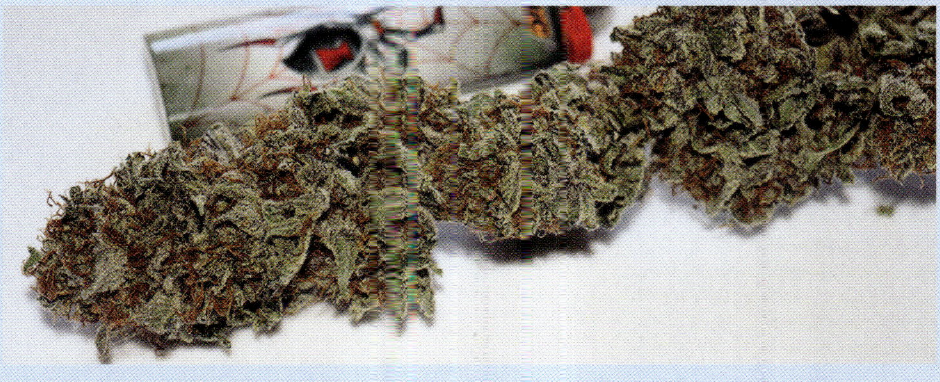

Seedless harvested Thai bud that flowers in 13 weeks

round of breeding. The process of smoking the different plants and taking note of their effects takes time but it allows me to see which strains give me a good high. I love sampling diverse strains from all around the world.

Flowering highly exotic cannabis strains using True Living Organics produces some of the most mouthwatering and deadly versions of unusual genetics. Grab a copy of my latest book, *True Living Organics: Druid Edition*, and learn the ways of the TLO Druid. My book teaches you how to grow without the need for bottled nutrients and shows you how to recycle your soil. Recycled soil is like fine wine: It just gets better with age.

That's all for this journey today, my green friends. I hope you enjoyed this breeding run. Drop by SKUNK Magazine online if you want to keep up to date with my latest all-natural growing articles, and for sure visit Kingdom Organic Seeds. I think you'll love what you find there.

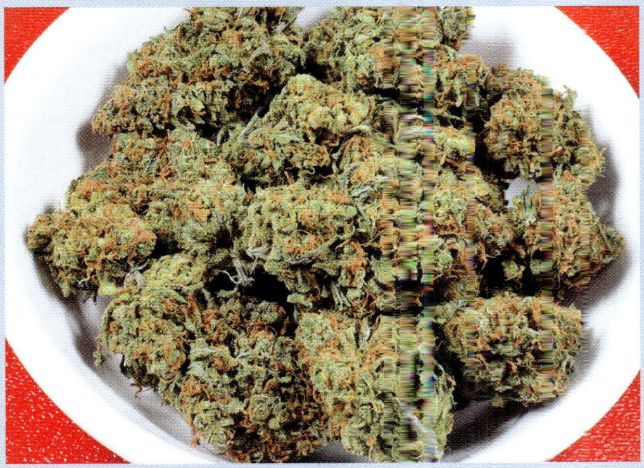

A bowl of acrid hashish smelling TLO-grown Bhutanese.

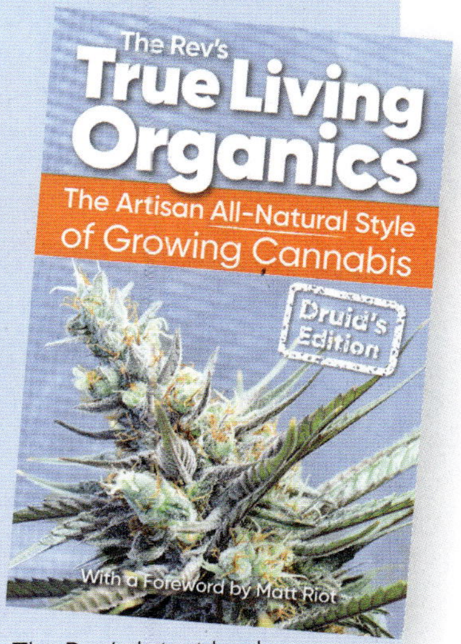

The Rev's latest book.

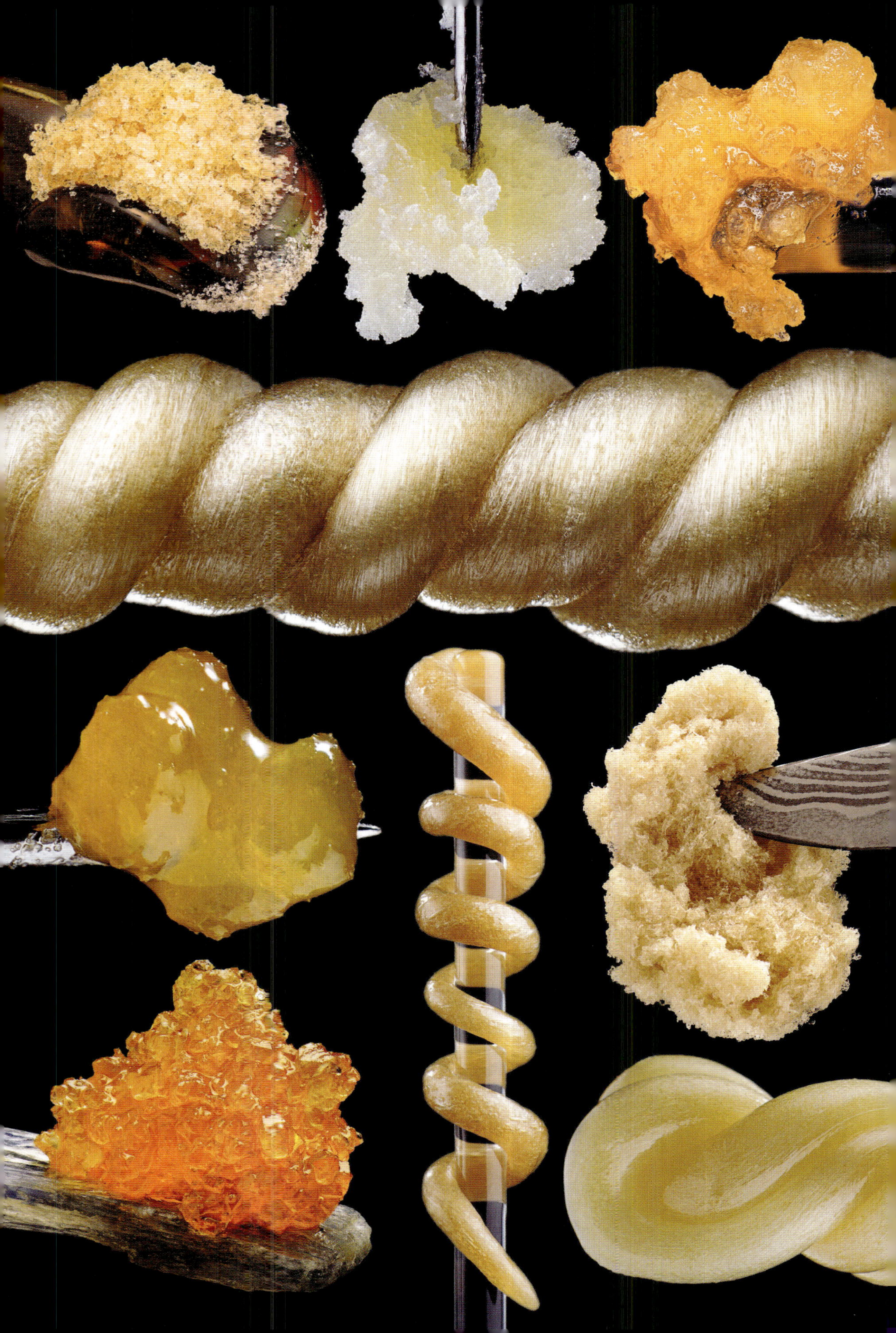

18

Extractions

The female cannabis plant primarily produces THC in its trichomes, found on pistils, calyxes, or leaves, especially near and within its flowers. Cannabinoids can be found elsewhere in the plant, though usually in smaller quantities, and are rarely extracted from anywhere other than the trichomes. The cannabis resin gland heads, the rounded tips of the trichomes, contain cells that secrete the major cannabinoids in an oil-like substance, often referred to as resin, to serve the evolutionary purpose of providing protection for the plant's flowering system. This resin is extremely sticky and can be easily removed by rubbing your fingers over the bud.

A cured bud contains plant tissue, chlorophyll, and other trace elements in addition to cannabinoids. Curing helps reduce the presence of unwanted elements, but further separation can be accomplished through resin extraction and/or filtration. What distinguishes the two is that extraction typically targets cannabinoid oils for purity, while filtration segregates resinous plant material into different grades for further processing.

Get Your Harvest Right First

When harvesting, try to disturb your flowers as little as possible. Trichomes on pistils can rupture, which will decrease the number of viable flowers available for hash making. It is more important to keep the secretory cell heads on top of the trichomes safe than the stalks, which do not produce as many cannabinoids. It is important to optimize your cultivation methods to achieve the best results possible for extraction and purification. Good growing conditions and harvesting techniques will yield many trichomes. Poorly harvested and improperly manicured buds, on the other hand, will lose their trichome heads and are not ideal. Regardless of your technique, you can't get good-quality hash from poor-quality harvests. In addition to your harvesting skills, the quality of your hash is also largely determined by the genetics you started with. Growing a strain suitable for hash production will ensure better results. Breeders typically recommend selecting an indica strain for its resinous characteristics, but you can still make hash from low-yielding sativa. You can produce a small amount of nice hash from a subpar harvest, but optimizing and honing your harvesting skills is essential for producing high-quality hash.

PHOTOS: DANKSHIRE PHOTOGRAPHY AND RUSSELL-HOWLAND PHOTOGRAPHY

Observing different strains of cannabis flowers reveals that not all trichomes are equal. Scientifically, they fall into three classifications: *Stalked* (with a shape similar to a mushroom, having a head and stalk); *bulbous* (lacking a head, only a stalk, and possibly warped); and *sessile* (having a head with a very short stalk). You can categorize them by appearance into *regular* (stalked), *head-only* (bulbous) or *stalk-only* (sessile). If the entire structure is missing and only resin remains, this is due to *burst trichomes*. These types can appear on the same plant at different stages of flowering. Use a magnifying aid to identify regular trichomes by their typical round heads on the stalks. Burst trichomes, which release resin in a viscous state, are usually just trichomes that have ruptured. You can identify these as ones where the outer structure has burst and the oils have been released. The oils will be sticky to the touch. Trichome rupture is the primary defense response against insects and predators; physically interacting with them can cause rupturing. High temperatures can also cause rupturing, so honing your growing setup is important. Sometimes, the strain itself is prone to trichome ruptures. In strains that are rich with resin, like Afghani #1, this explosive gland action appears automatic in the last stages of flowering. These strains also seem to produce curled pistils that may appear withered but are still sticky. Many ruptured trichomes do not mean that the plant cannot be used for extraction. As long as the trichome structures on another part of the plant are good and the cannabinoids are still on the pistils, the plant is suitable for resin extraction.

Another key indicator that growers use when growing for hash making is the color of the trichomes themselves. As the cannabis plant reaches later stages of flowering the trichomes will go from a clear color to an amber shade as the cannabinoids inside mature and concentrate. Depending on the type of hash you aim to produce, trichome color is a good indicator for when a plant is ready to be harvested. Traditionally hash would have been produced from cannabis that was harvested at full maturity with a high proportion of amber trichomes. Newer types of extracts on the market utilize the moniker "live", such as live resin or live rosin, to indicate that the cannabis plant was harvested and frozen immediately (without drying or curing) to capture the full chemo profile of the plant at the time of harvest. Growers for this type of hash will typically harvest their plant before the majority of trichomes have turned amber, opting for a higher proportion of milky-white trichomes. This causes live resins and live rosins to have a lighter color compared to extracts from cured buds.

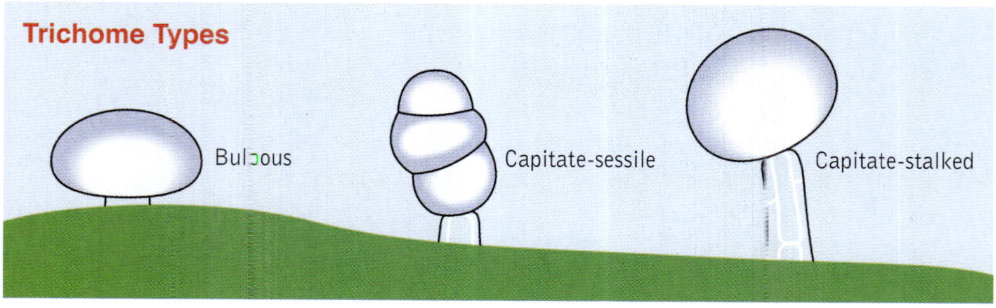

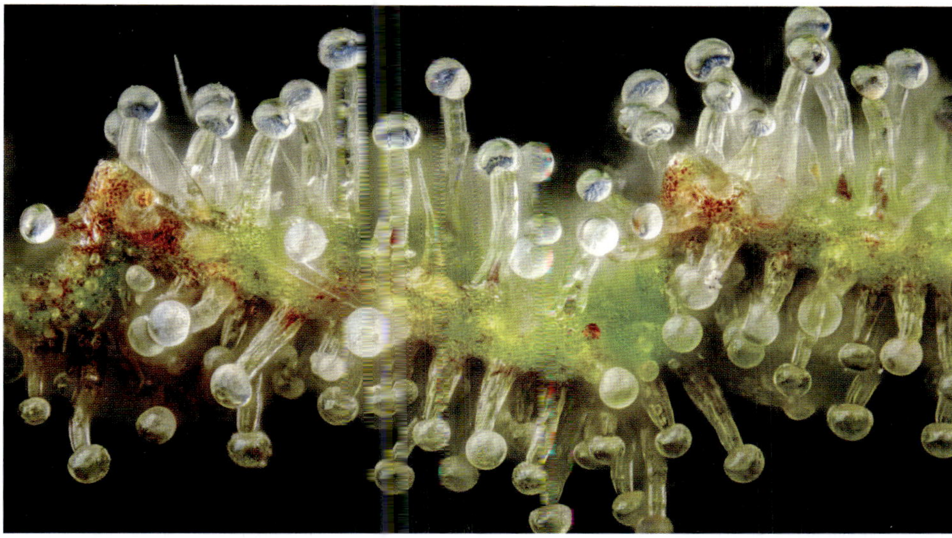

Mostly clear/milky trichome heads.

PHOTO: ROB BRAMHILL

Screening Trichomes: Dry Sifting

Hash is made primarily from collected resin, preferably from stalked capitate trichomes, heads, and stalks. Through filtering and pressure techniques, the collected resin is transformed into a blocky mass known as hashish. There are various methods and scales of doing this, ranging from bulk hash production to rolling small, finger-sized quantities, which each produce hashish of different quality or grade. Some methods gather only the trichome cannabinoids, while others collect trichomes and other subsidiary elements, such as leaf particles and branch shavings. These variations affect the purity of the final product. Higher-grade hashish contains fewer unwanted plant materials and a higher concentration of glandular trichome heads, rich with resin. It is possible to obtain multiple grades of hash from the same sample by using different purification methods or changes in filter sizes.

Screening is used to separate trichomes from other plant matter. The recommended screen pore size for collecting high-quality sift is 125 microns (120 lines per inch). Increasing the pore size can allow more unwanted plant material to pass through; however, smaller pores can allow only smaller immature trichomes or some burst resin to get through, leaving behind larger trichome heads which have reached maturity and are full of cannabinoids and terpenes. Coarse screening is often the first stage of purification, where dried cannabis flower or trim is broken up over a larger pore sized screen (180 μm) to yield a rough/farm-grade kief, which can be further screened to remove plant matter and isolate trichome heads. By using smaller pore screens, we purify better by filtering out the unwanted plant material. This significantly improves the quality of the final product, with many connoisseurs considering full-melt drysift to be one of the highest quality forms of solventless extracts.

Trichomes to Hash

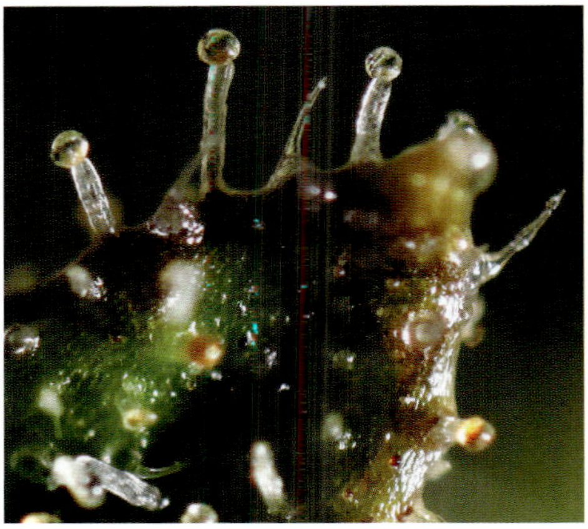

Mid-process resin with untouched trichomes.

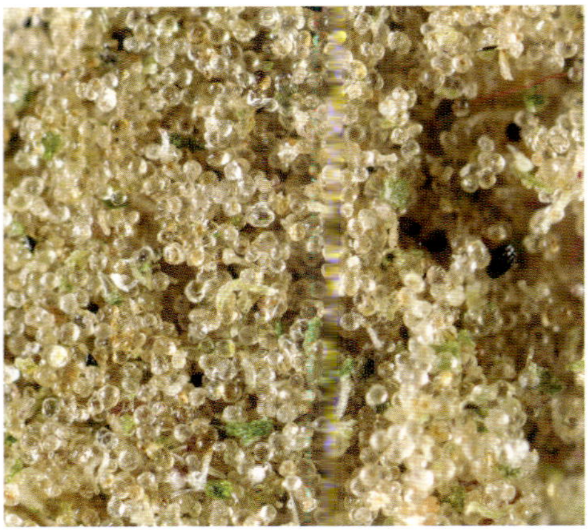

First pass of drysift which is still impure.

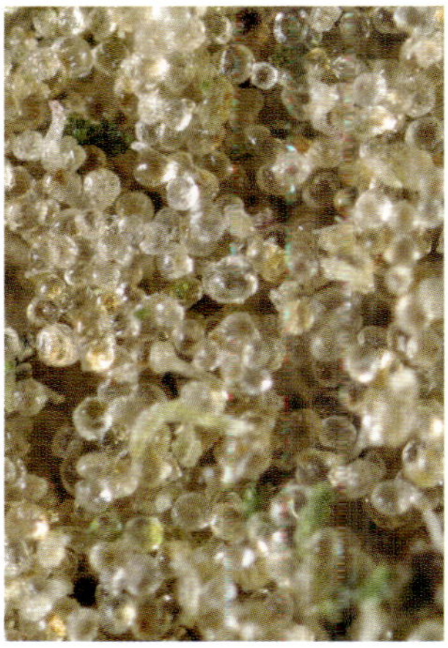

Dense trichome clustering.

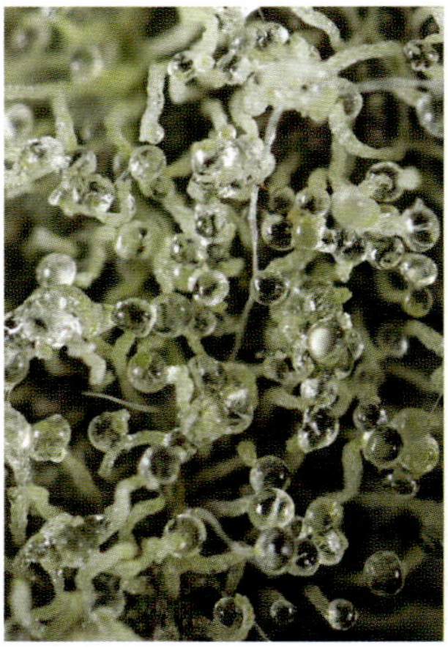

Trichomes are fusing together.

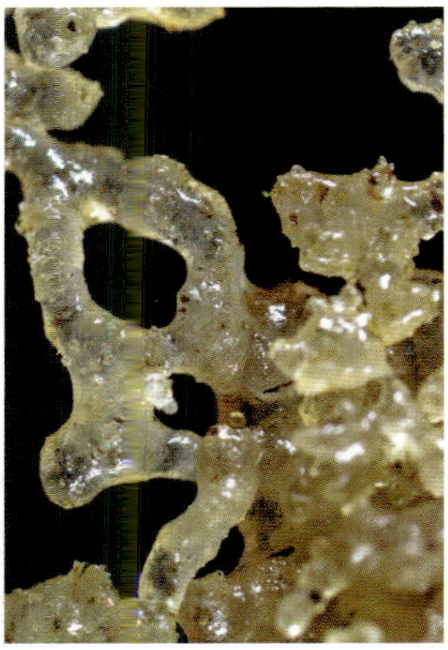

Fused trichomes.

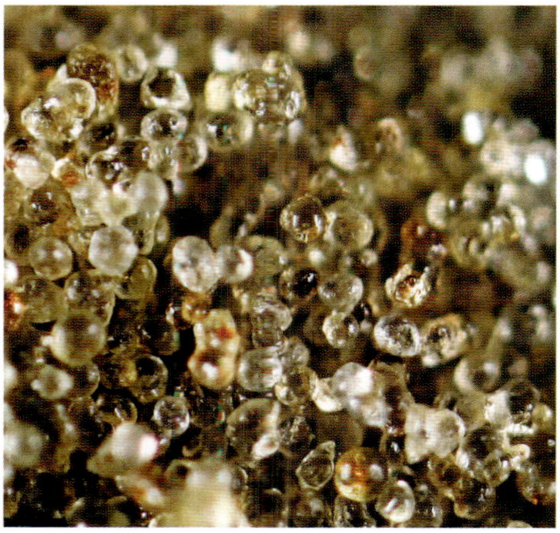

Trichome maturity can vary by color.

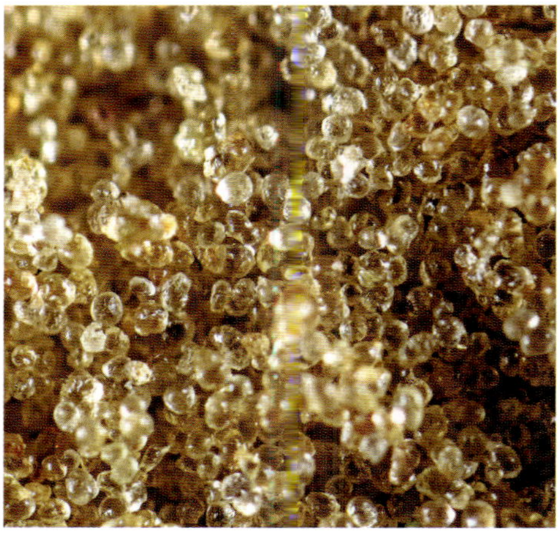

Trichomes with uniform color, shape, and size.

PHOTOS: BUBBLEMAN

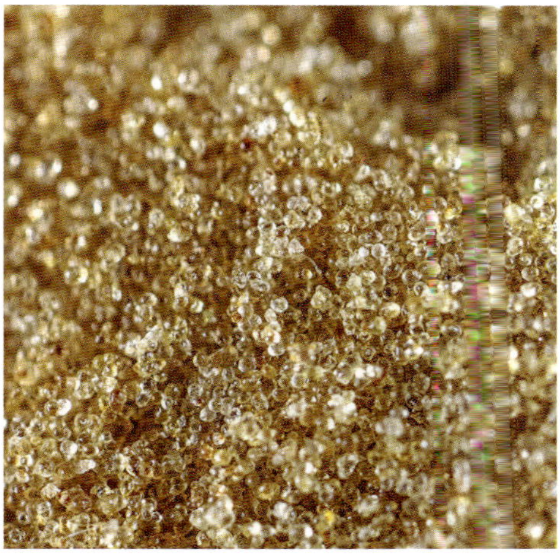

This extraction is so pure that plant matter is nearly nil.

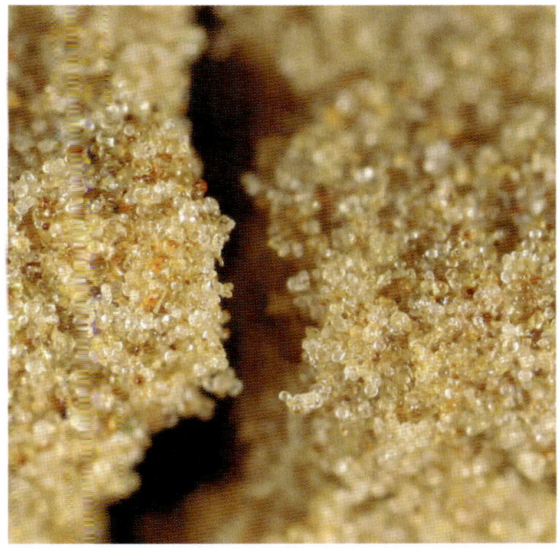

At broader resolutions this collection looks more like a solid.

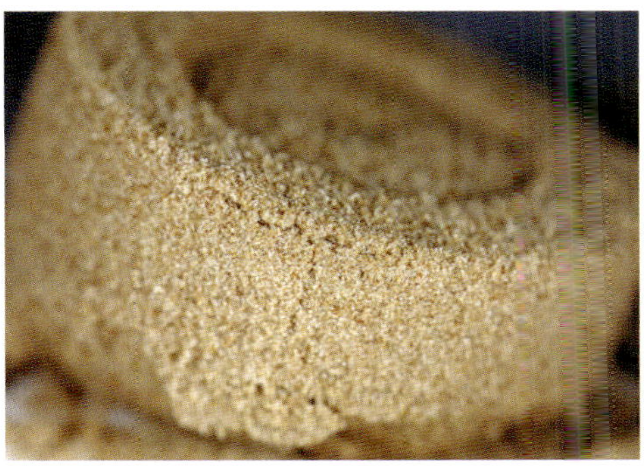

The more extract added, the more mass gained.

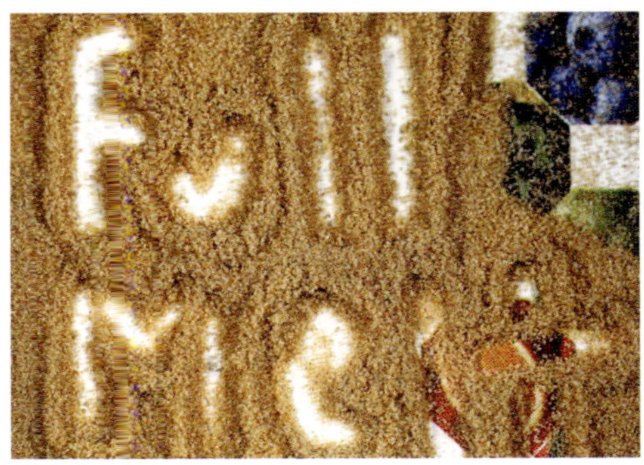

When dried, resin extract can become powdery.

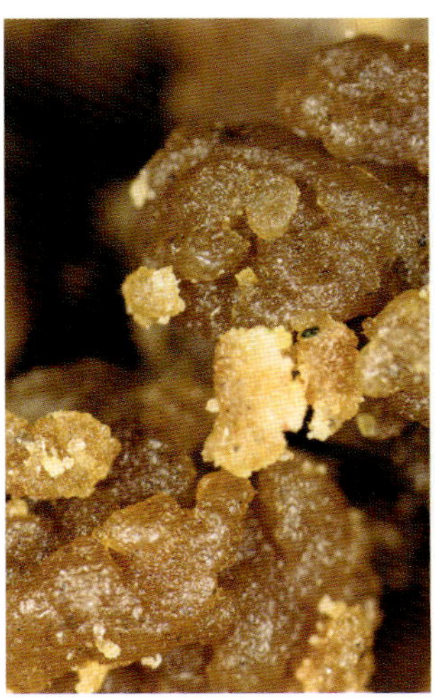

Hash becomes a semisolid with further processing.

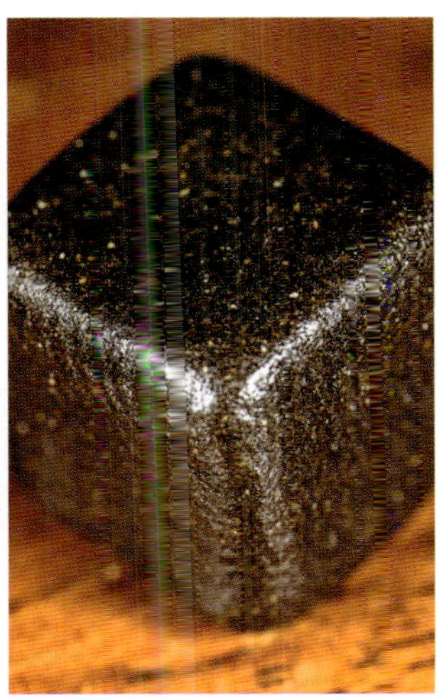

Pressing results in a denser hash.

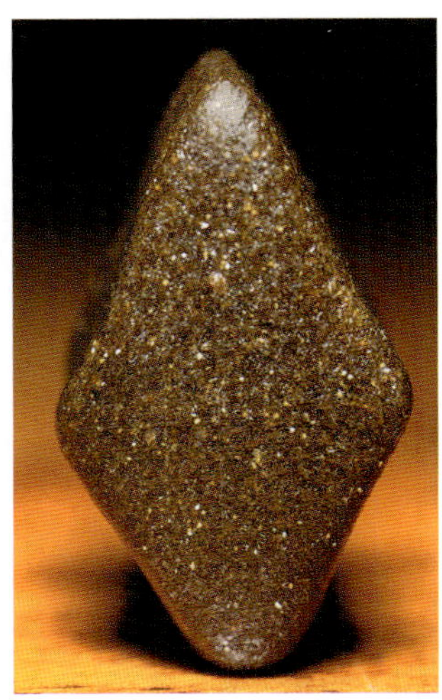

Hash comes in all shapes, sizes, and quality.

Traditional Hash

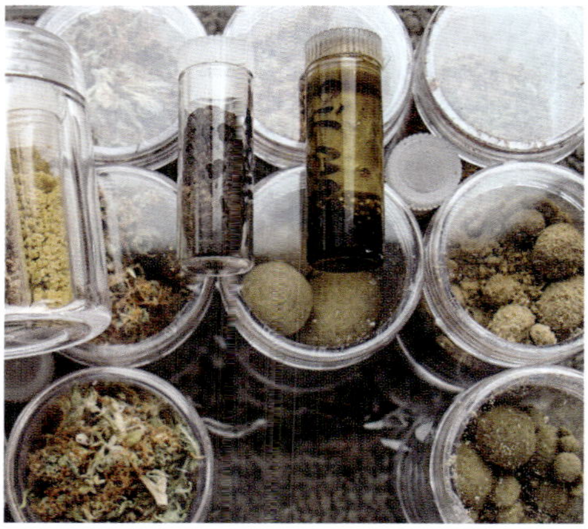

An assortment of bud, kief, and resin.

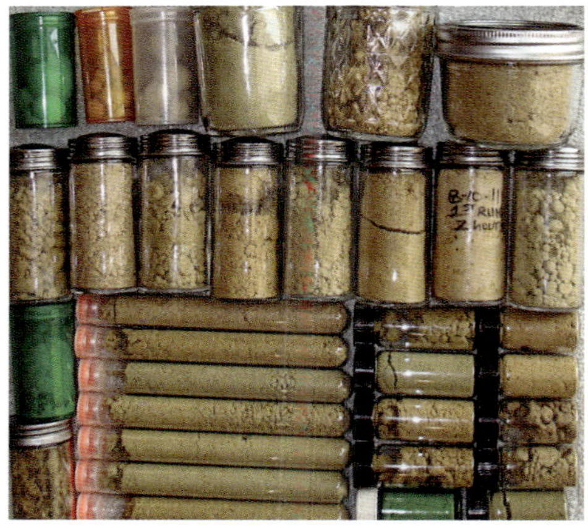

Various grades of kief from screening.

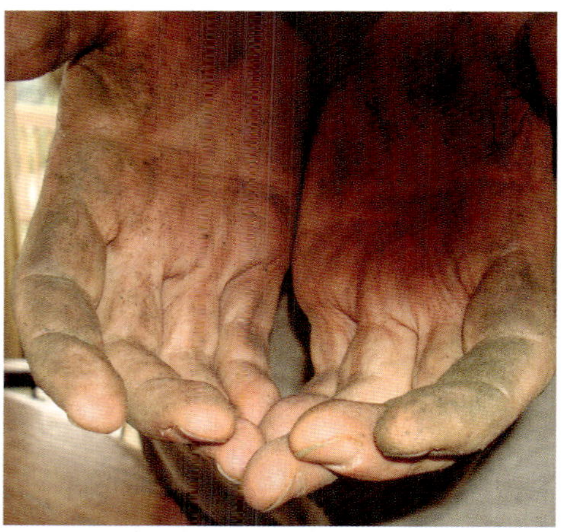

Resin will stain your hands and items.

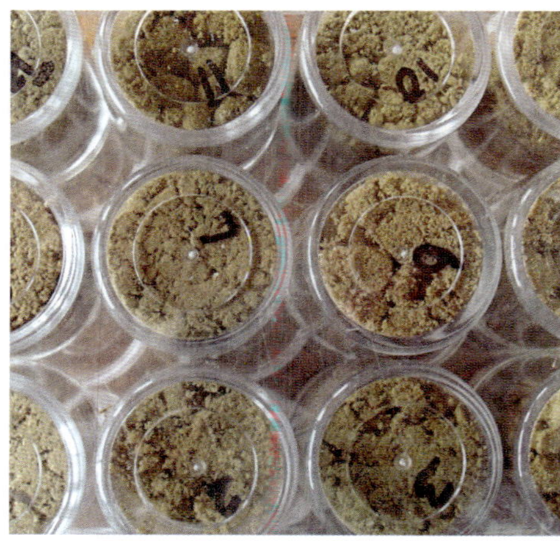

Label/reference your screenings.

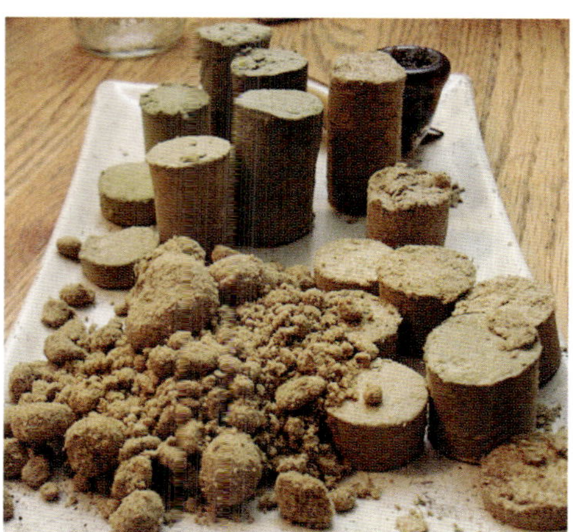

Press kief with presses or compact storage.

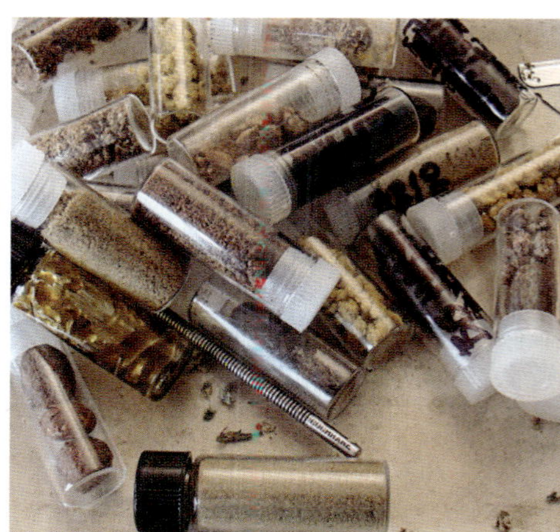

Pressing into tubes can also compact kief.

PHOTOS: MAX BORTNICK

Easy Hash Making

Water extraction is the best method for home growers to achieve an extract with a high purity of trichome heads. We'll describe this in more detail later. Many processing techniques have been improved with better technologies, often available online or at your local headshop. Investing in high-quality equipment yields better results but requires maintenance and cleaning, as resin processing can be messy work.

Freezing and Grinding

Growers have found that freezing buds makes it easier to separate trichomes and resin from unwanted plant matter. This causes the trichomes to become brittle and break off as a solid instead of rubbing off in a sticky, viscous state. Resin from any burst trichomes will also break off in a similar way but in clumps. By placing cured buds and other prepared resinous materials in the freezer for an hour or so before extraction, you can work much more effectively, as there is less resistance to trichome and resin removal, and a reduced amount of the unwanted plant matter that comes with it.

Before placing your bud in the freezer you can grind it into a container. The ground, frozen trim can then be spread on the screen, and you can tap the screen lightly instead of dragging, letting trichome particles dance around before passing through, while the unwanted plant matter remains. This method involves less work overall but does require initial grinding, and will have a lower yield than more vigorous screening techniques; however, the quality of hash will be high since less plant material will pass through the screen, due to the gentle extraction method.

Skuff/Trim/Shake

When harvesting your bud, you'll typically trim the leaves from the bud. These trimmed leaves are referred to as fresh skuff, trim, or shake.

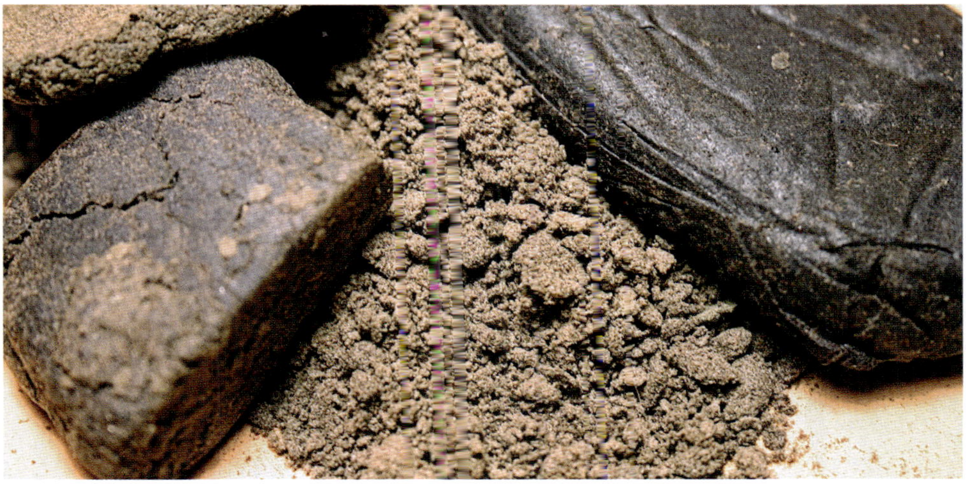

PHOTO: DAVID STRANGE

Hash can have various textures, from a solid to semi-solid to a crumble.

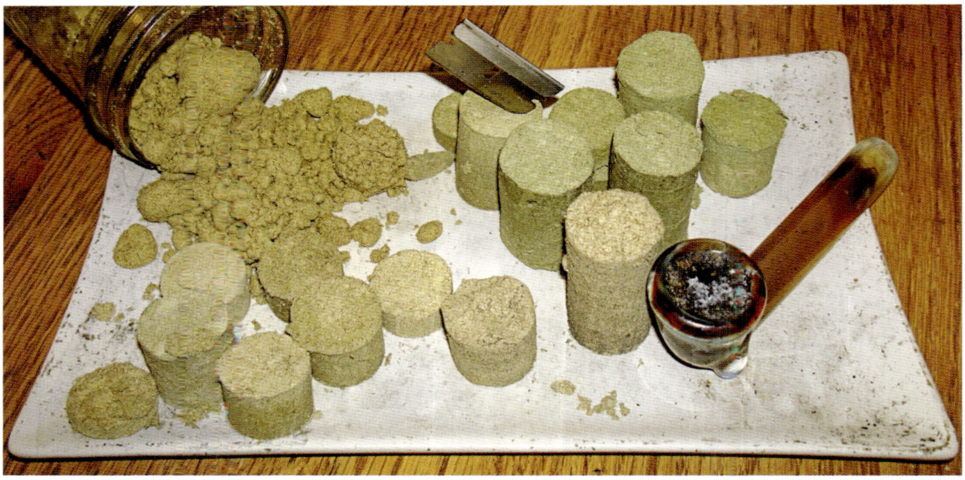

Packing kief in tubes can shape a block.

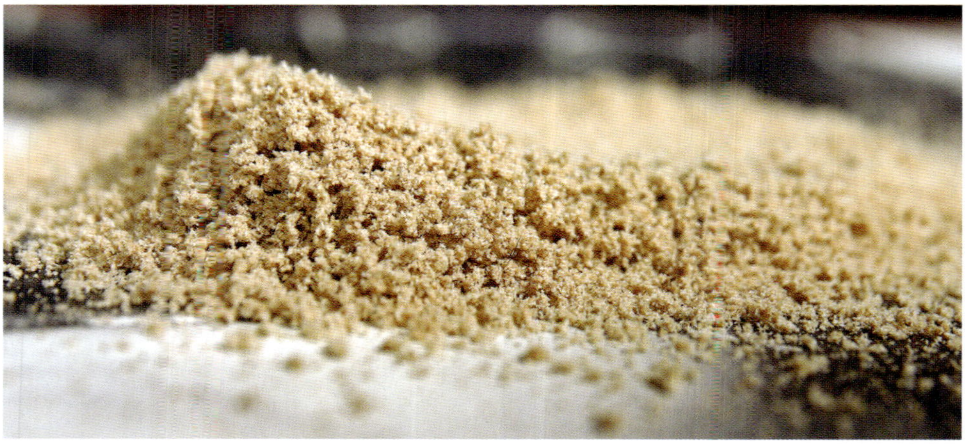

Skuff that has been recently screened.

PHOTOS: MAX BORTNICK (TOP), DAVID STRANGE (BOTTOM)

Skuff is more a subjective term and less a classification, a designation for unwanted material that still has the potential for resin extraction. This includes plant matter collected on the bottom of an herb box or jar, the trimmings after manicuring, or bits fallen into a canvas bag. When dealing with separated parts of the plant after it has been cut up, you should try to get something out of these leftovers. Different grades of skuff can be used in a vaporizer, for example, or to make hash later.

Wherever its source on the plant, skuff should be sticky. As long as it feels tacky, it has the potential to be used for resin extraction. Examine skuff with your magnifying aid for the presence of trichomes, which indicates better quality skuff. Make at least two piles of skuff, one with trichomes and one without, possibly further dividing them into different grade piles. Before labeling and storing the skuff, trim away the parts without any stickiness. Store your skuff for three to six weeks to cure, similar to curing canned bud, before using one of the extraction methods. Once the skuff is cured, examine its quality. Greener skuff contains more plant matter; browner skuff has a higher concentration of resin and is therefore higher quality.

Screening (Basic Methods)

Screening resembles grating cheese, but on a finer level.

Dry Sift Screening

Dry sift screens come in many formats. A popular one is a silkscreen with a pore size of 120 to 180 microns across a rectangular wooden or aluminum frame, secure but not overly tight. Smaller microns yield higher quality but lower quantities of hash, while larger microns produce more but may allow some leaf matter and branch trim through, which decreases hash quality. Smaller pore screening results in hash that is more refined than typical street hash. If you are unsure of the size of the pores you can look up 'mesh micron conversion charts' to help pick the right one.

Avoid stretching the screen excessively while attaching it to the frame. Stretching the screen, especially a poorer quality one, can increase pore size. Take photos with a camera phone and zoom in to compare stretching sizes to the base observations. Apply minimal pressure when pressing down the skuff on your screen, as greater pressure can also enlarge the pore size.

Place the bud on the screen and drag across it either manually or by tumbling. Manual screening works well for smaller quantities of bud, but larger quantities may require an automatic tumbling machine, which will be explained later. Place a sheet of glass, a mirror, or a piece of parchment paper under the screen to collect the material that falls through the screen and ensure the system works. After the screening is complete, tap the screen to shake off any remaining sift stuck to its pores.

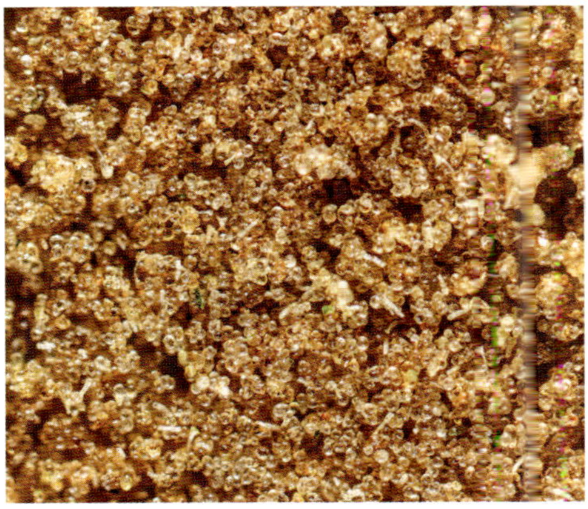

Resin needs to be dried during curing for easy screening.

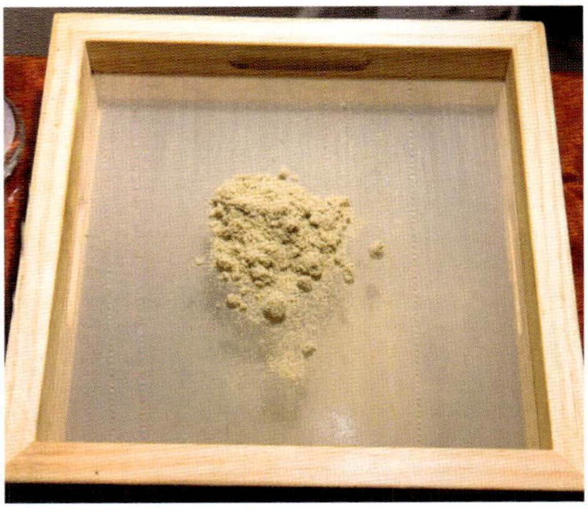

After screening dried buds through multiple filters you end up with fine powdery kief.

PHOTOS: BUBBLEMAN

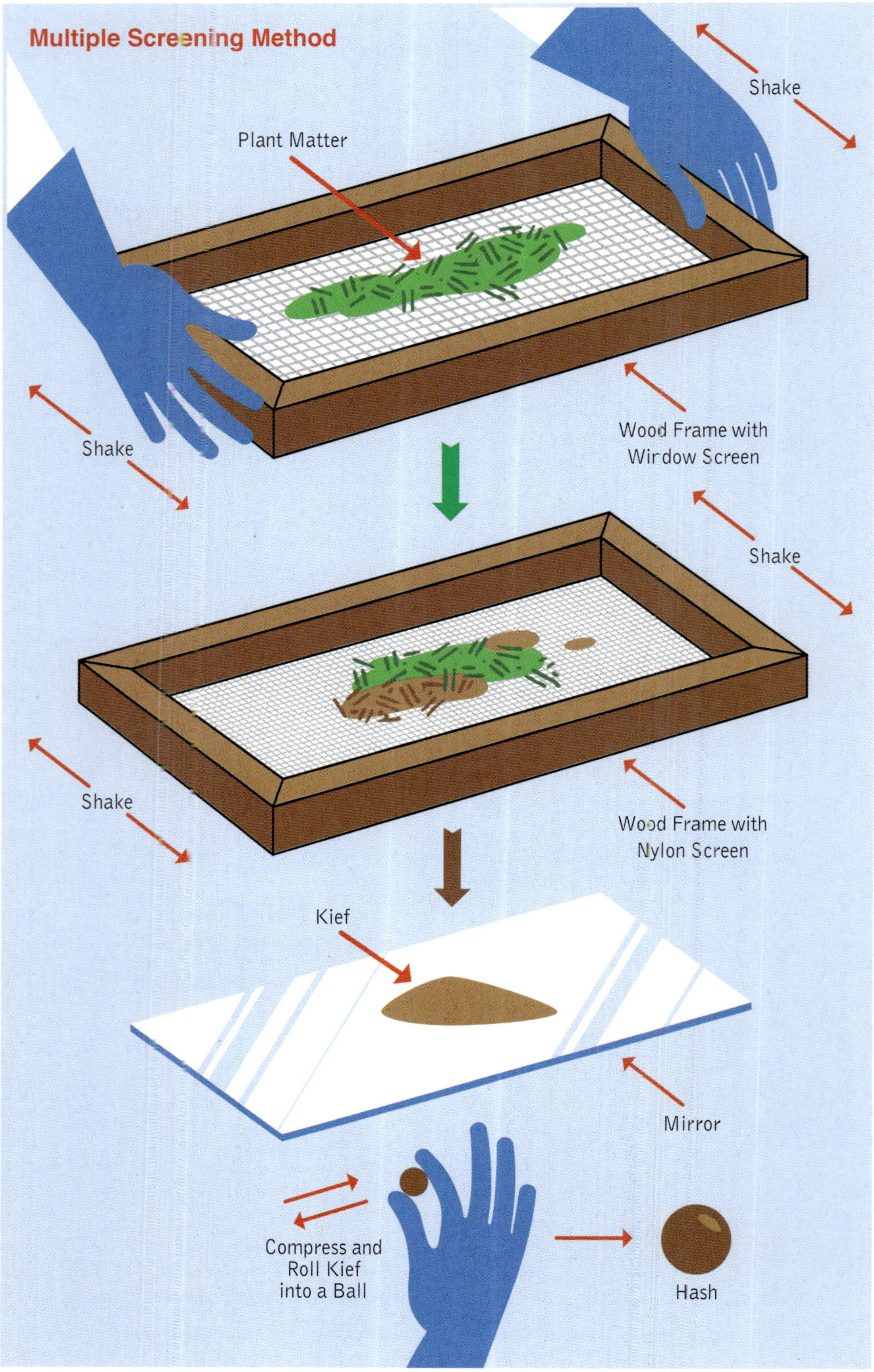
Multiple Screening Method
Shake
Plant Matter
Shake
Wood Frame with
Window Screen
Shake
Shake
Wood Frame with
Nylon Screen
Kief
Mirror
Compress and
Roll Kief
into a Ball
Hash

Flat Metal Screening

Before any screening, cured bud can undergo an optional grating process. A grate, made of sturdy nylon or stainless steel, has pores the same size as the silk screen. This step removes more matter from the skuff than a silk screen. Material that passes through the metal screen can be sieved through the silkscreen, resulting in two grades of sieved bud residue. Some metal screening methods resemble grating, particularly metal hand-turned ice makers/grain grinders. To use a hand-turned ice maker, first, insert the skuff into the top of the unit, then rotate the cylindrical metal grate inside by turning the handle, and the refined skuff will tumble out. Anything left inside the cylinder needs to be tapped out. These dry systems can be suspended by a hoist so that you can easily move in and out boxes. There are several devices that follow this theme, which may also be called sifters, pollen, or kief tumblers.

Multiple Screens

A typical setup uses three to four screens. Each screen should have a different micron measurement, beginning with the largest and ending with the smallest silk screen. The screens do not need to be attached and can just be shaken over each other while ensuring there is something, such as a mirror or glass, under the last screen to catch the resin. If you are doing larger batches, then metal or plastic screens are safer than silk screens to avoid stretching. The process should be repeated with each new screen until most of the matter has passed through. You should end up with multiple grades of refined skuff across several screens down to the finer trichomes and resin on the last one. It is an excellent way to achieve great results.

Trichome Shakers

Screens and water extraction bags are now widely available on the internet, but some growers prefer to experiment with a more minimal setup. The challenge lies in finding an appropriate pore size that prevents plant matter from passing through and allows only trichomes. Nylon, typically used in tights, socks, stockings, and other thin clothing articles, can be stretched to create "pores." Various nettings and linings are available at fabric craft stores. Determining the right pore size may require some trial and error. Begin by filling a jam jar with skuff, ideally chopped with scissors. Stretch the nylon over the top of the jar, making sure it's not so tight that it might rip. Shake the jar as you would a salt shaker over a glass surface. After some time, trichomes will start to fall through. If the collected material is very green, the pore size is too large, so loosen the nylon and shake the jar again. This process requires considerable shaking to see results. The idea is to shake as vigorously as possible for several minutes, stop, gather the material into piles, and repeat the process. The piles will vary in color, with lighter ones containing smaller trichomes, and greener ones containing a higher plant matter content. The disadvantage to this method is that some resin particles may not land directly on the surface because it is not a contained system.

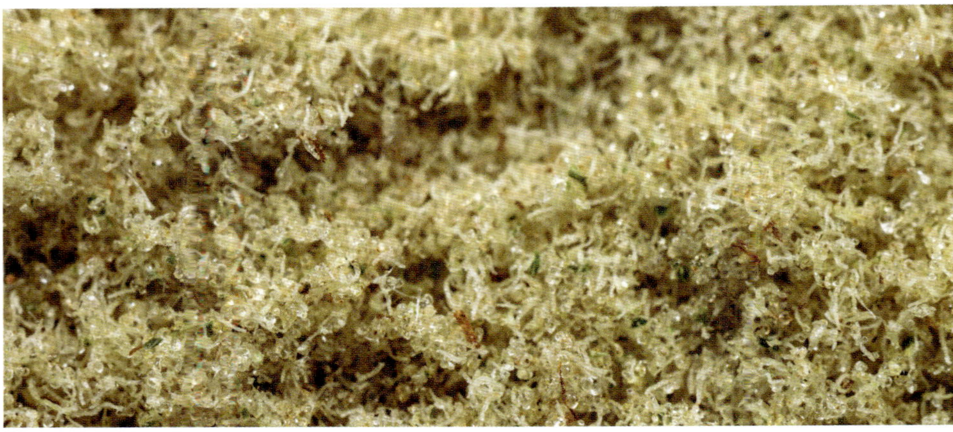

Collection of trichome stalks and cystolythic hairs, with few heads.

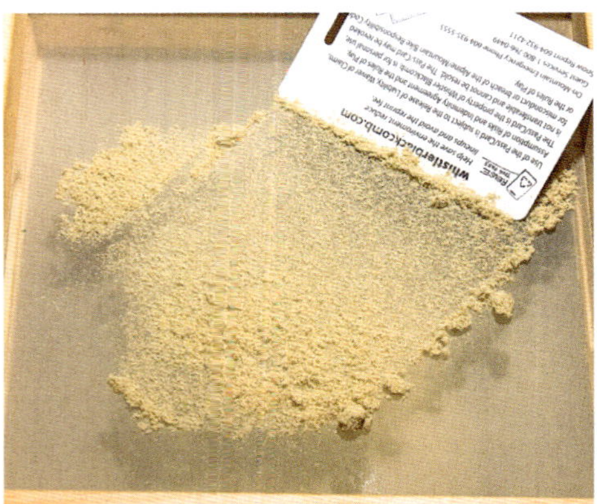

Kief is screened over and over by rubbing a card gently against it.

Remove the top screen and repeat the process with a smaller micron screen.

Advanced Screening

Now we delve into advanced screening techniques. This one can be applied to the described screening methods.

You use a metal or nylon screen first, followed by a silk screen. Steel fabrics are available with much smaller pores than even the finest silk screen. Typically, a metal or nylon screen of 105 to 140 microns is preferred; home hash makers commonly use a screen with 125 microns. A wooden frame can be constructed to hold the screen.

Advanced screening method:

1. First, make a square of four small wooden blocks on a sheet of glass or a mirror.
2. Position the screen over the blocks, with a block under each corner, leaving an inch gap between the glass and the screen, and place a small amount of skuff on the screen.

PHOTOS: BUBBLEMAN

3. Tap the screen to see if anything falls through. Continue tapping as long as resin or trichomes are falling through.
4. Collect the falling resin onto the glass and use a card to sweep it onto another surface.
5. When tapping is no longer effective, gently roll the skuff/trim/biomass back and forth across the screen using a card or similar tool. Do this with minimal pressure, repeating the process as many as 100 times until you see resin glands accumulating on the mirror below.
6. As you progress, apply more pressure after each repeat to create different piles.

Eventually, when the piles become green, you can stop to compare them. Each time, the extra force removes any resin glands that didn't fall through the last time, but will also push through some less valuable material, such as small branch shavings and leaf particles, hence the greener tint. As such, each round of screening results in lower-quality skuff.

You can consume the different grades of resin immediately, but you may notice difficulty with the smaller grade screenings from the initial piles. Since this powder is of an extremely fine particle size, it can easily fall through the pores of a vaporizer filter. Instead, you can compress this resin into hashish. We will discuss hash pressing later in the chapter.

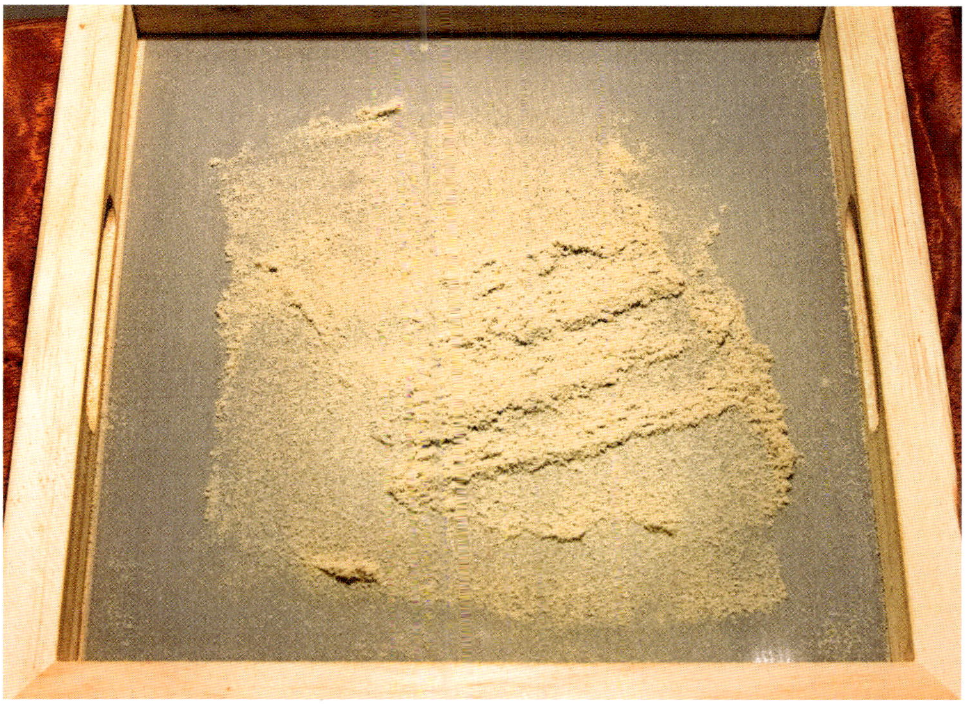

PHOTO: BUBBLEMAN

Eventually you end up with the finest screened kief.

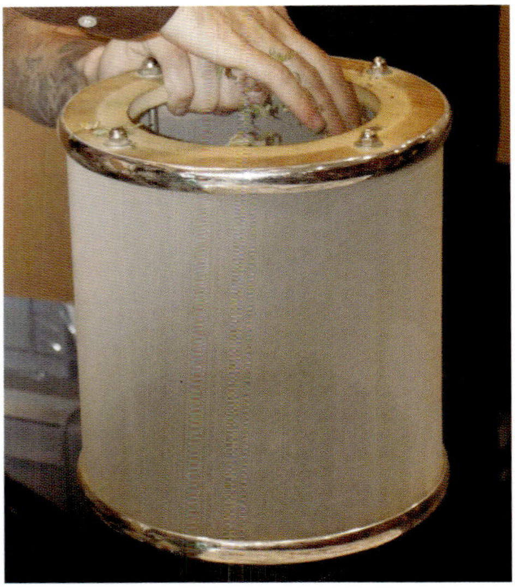

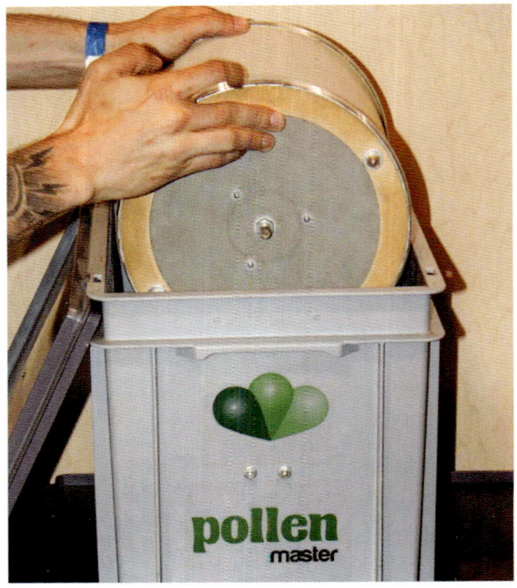

Dry sift tumblers are a quick and easy way to turn your homegrown trim or flower into a fine quality hash that can be pressed into bricks or refined further through screening techniques.

PHOTOS: GCP

Drum Machines/Tumblers

The most basic tumbler is a DIY hand-turned system; much more advanced is an automatic centrifugal force vortex extraction. Most drum machines have a 1.5- to 2-foot diameter, though the size you choose depends on how much cannabis you wish to sieve at a time.

For a basic DIY tumbler, a screen is placed between two wooden cylinders, and the cannabis trim is placed inside this screen. The drum can be hand cranked or rotated by a small motor attached to the side, at about two rotations per minute to cause the trichomes to drop through the sieve. A simple mirror or sheet of glass can be used to catch the skuff, placed between the legs of the drum. The tumbler can be left to rotate for up to one hour to get the most from your skuff without applying pressure. YouTube has many videos of DIY tumblers in action if you want to see the methods people have come up with to tumble.

You can also place a small wooden ball, or anything slightly heavy with a smooth rounded surface, inside the drum barrel to apply more pressure as the drum rotates. Different-sized screens can additionally be used to extract different qualities of skuff.

Kief (Screened Skuff)

Kief is the fine powdery dried resin you get after sifting, which can be compressed into bricks of hash or consumed as a powder by sprinkling onto bowls or used for cooking. Because the powder is so fine, it is often best to compress it into hashish, a process that involves applying heat and pressure to it to form a solid mass. We will cover this later.

Dry Sift Tumbler

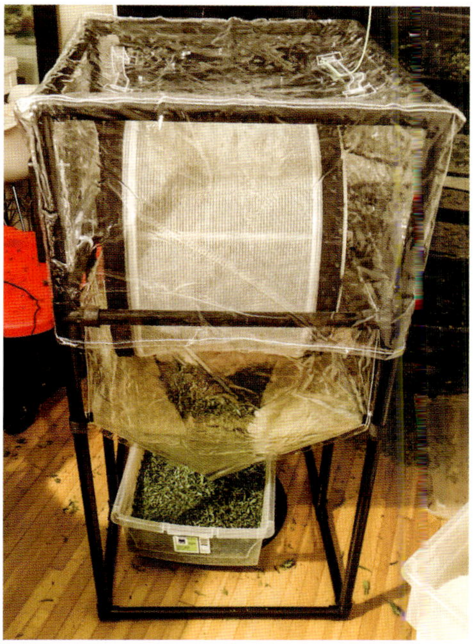

Flowers are loaded into the tumbler to collect trim. Run time is approximately 5 minutes.

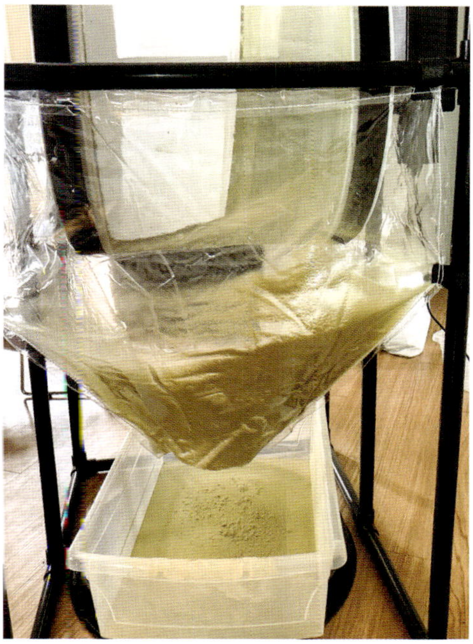

The trim is then loaded into the tumbler to collect resin. The screen used is 150 micron.

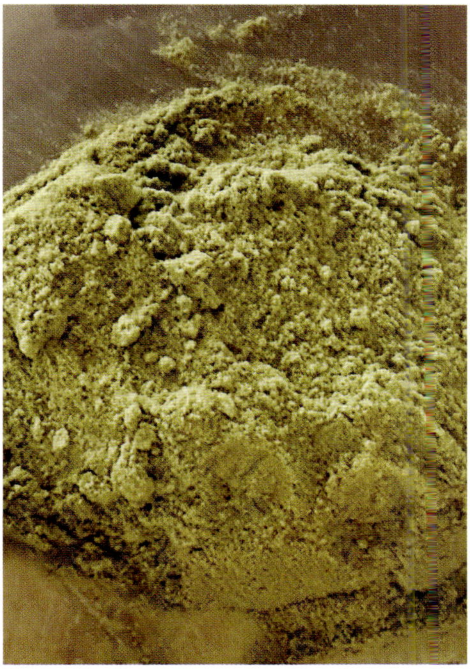

Resin is collected in a container at the base of the machine. This stage is very exciting!

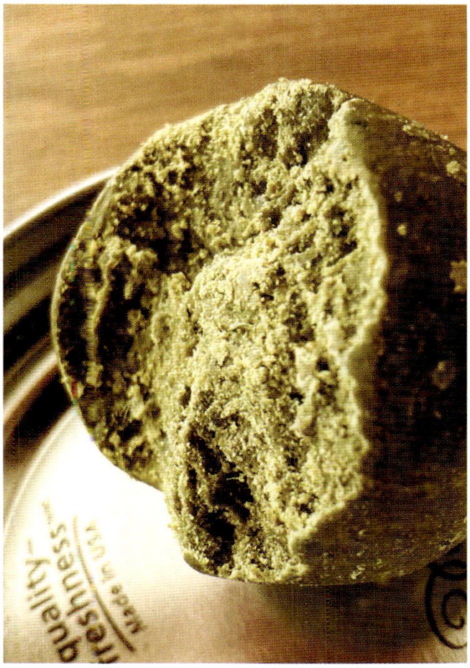

Resin is pressed into balls for sustainability. This hash was formed with pressure, not heat.

PHOTOS: FATHER NATURE, ROBERT BUTTS

Commercial Extraction Equipment From Hashtek

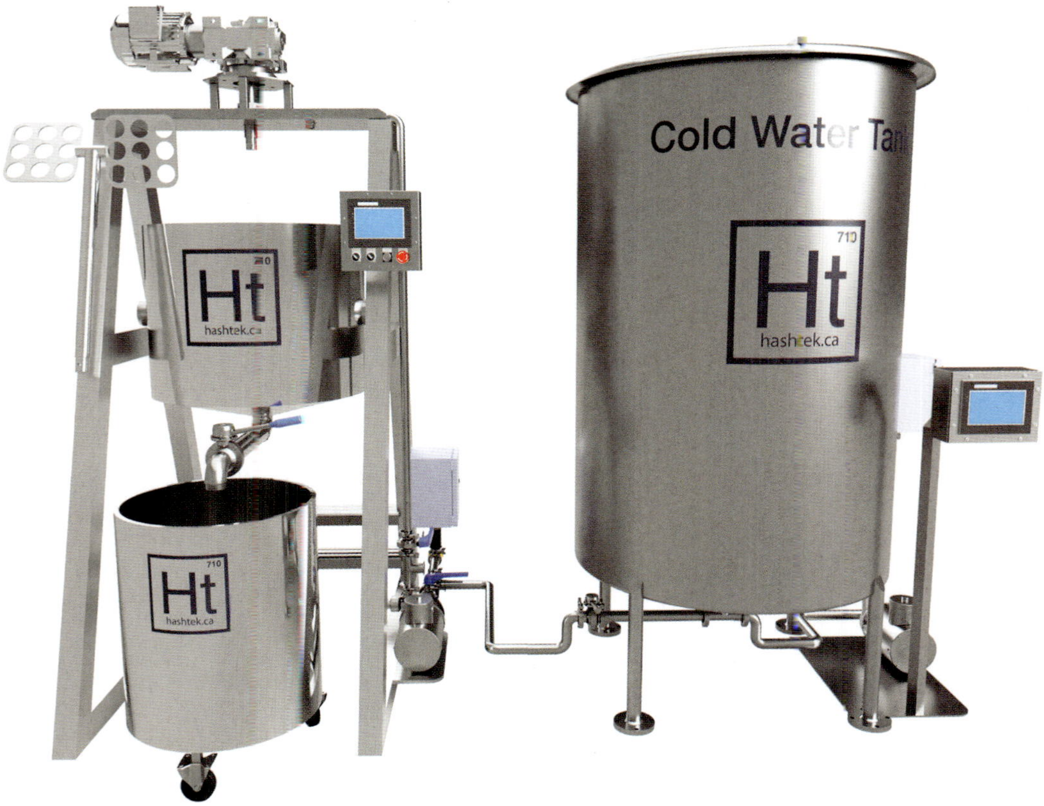

This setup includes an 85-ton, 250-gallon cold water tank and a 5 HP chiller, creating a truly ice-free, turnkey washing system. It can produce 20-100 kg of rosin per month

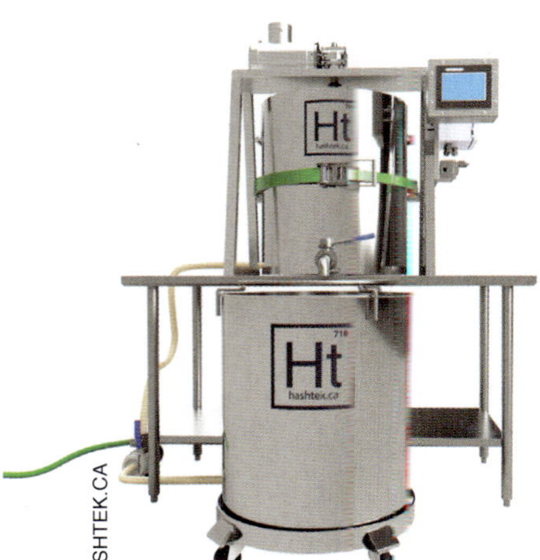

Agitator combined with a 50-gallon collection tank.

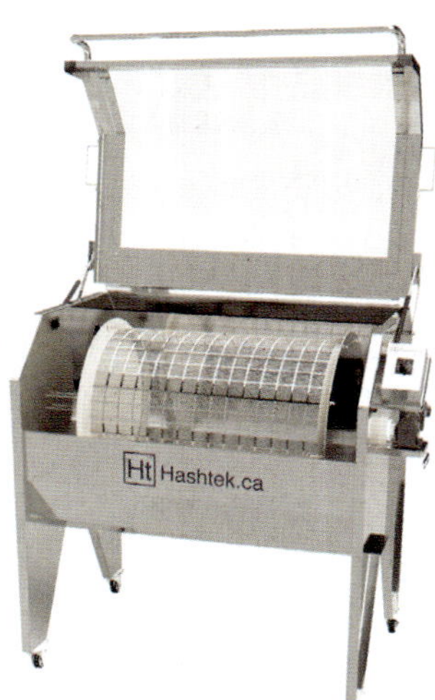

Cannabis Tumbler.

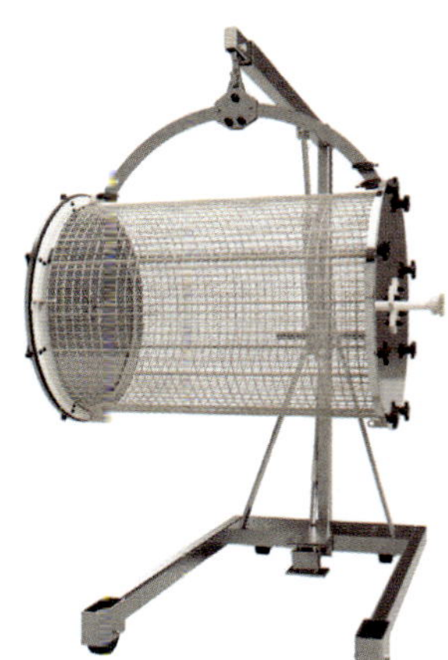

Tumbler Hoist.

PHOTOS: HASHTEK.CA

Extraction Freezing Process

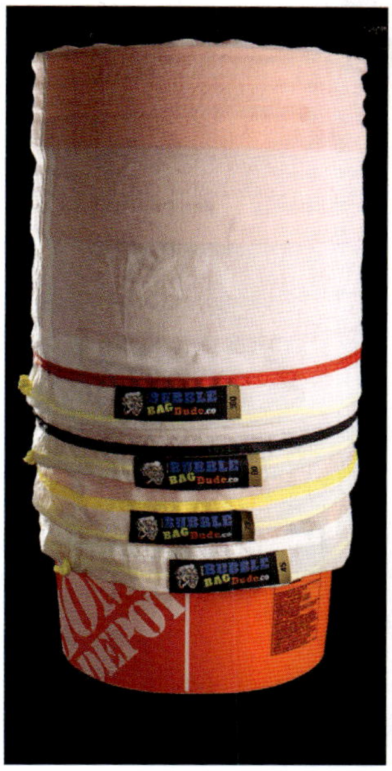

Buckets lined with bubble hash extraction bags. Lined from smallest micron to largest.

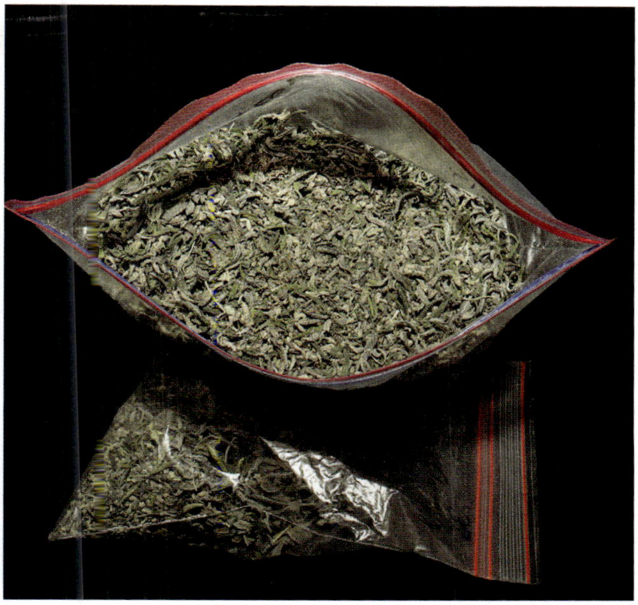

This unique indica-dominant hybrid strain is the result of crossing the powerful Oreoz with Mendo Breath F2.

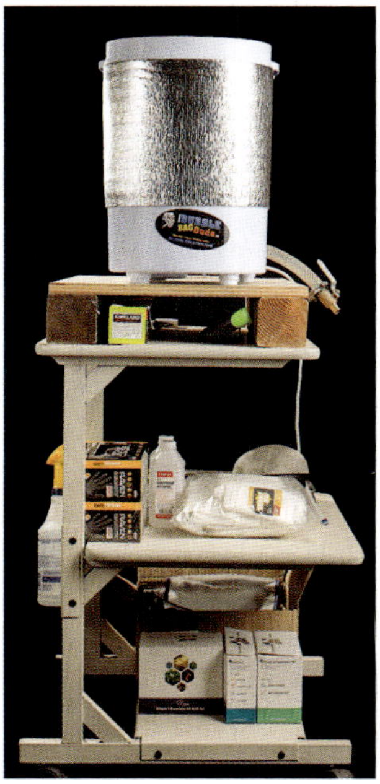

Hash cart with washer elevated for easy drainage during hash collection.

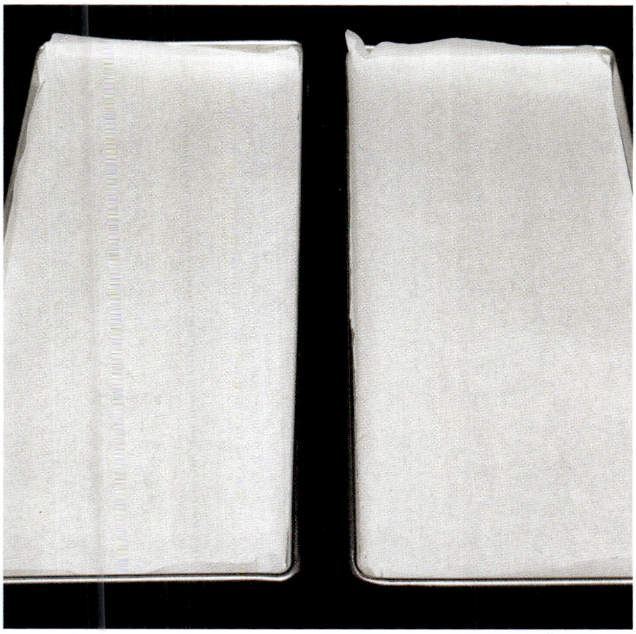

Freeze Dryer trays should be prepared ahead of time, by lining them with parchment paper for the collection of wet hash.

continues...

PHOTOS: RUSSELL-HOWLAND PHOTOGRAPHY

Extraction Freezing Process *continued*

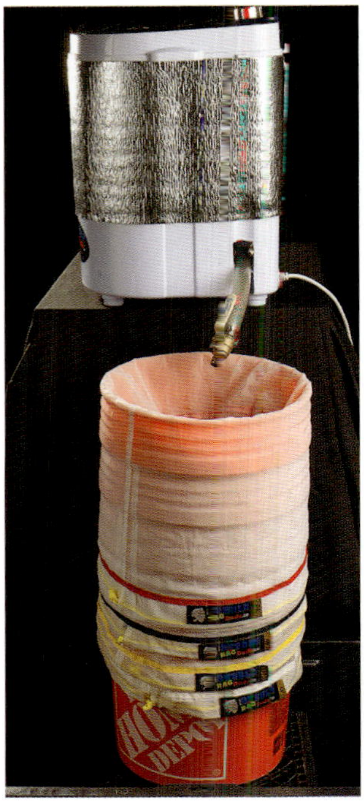

Full wash setup.

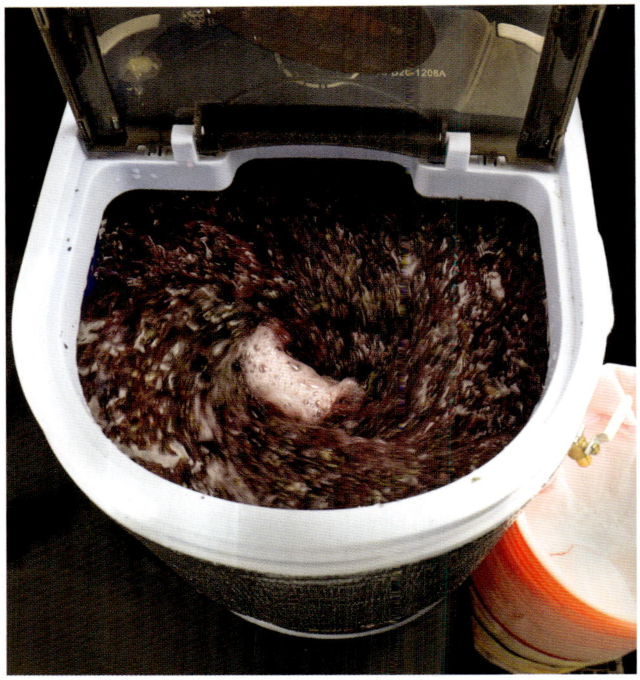

Extraction water can change color due to water soluble terpenes, flavonoids, and even chlorophyll.

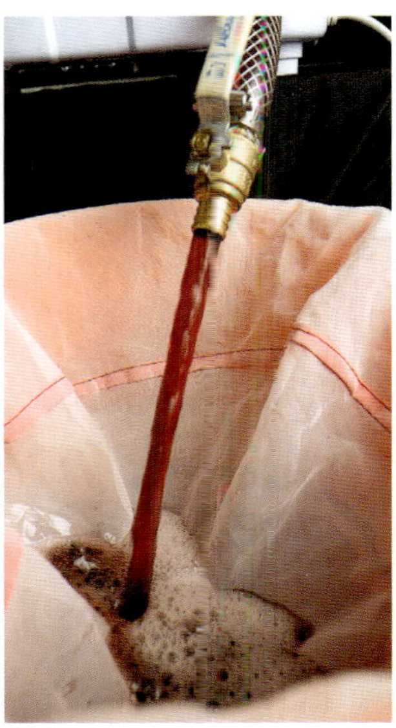

After wash cycle is complete, open drain valve and begin filtering out the hash.

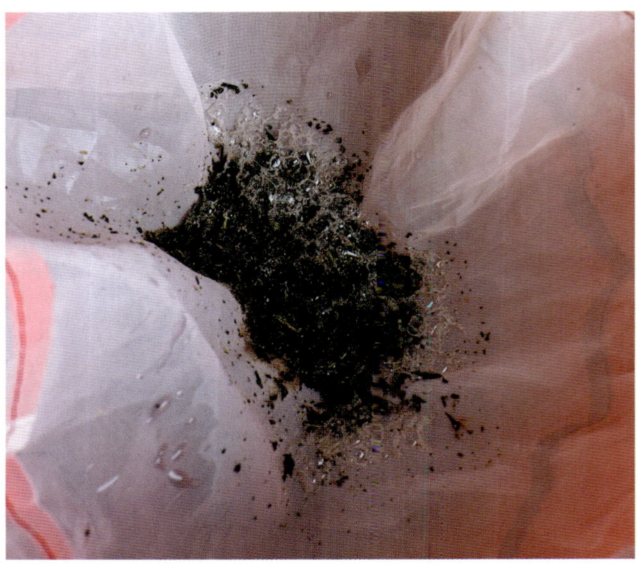

Some plant material will be caught in the first extraction bag. Using a 220 μm work bag helps prevents this plant material from mixing and contaminating the hash collected in the subsequent bags.

PHOTOS: RUSSELL-HOWLAND PHOTOGRAPHY

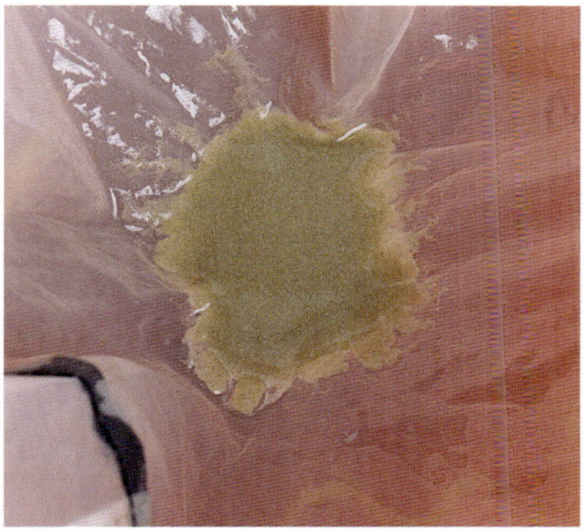

Spray the hash down the sides of the bags with water and allow it to pool in the center.

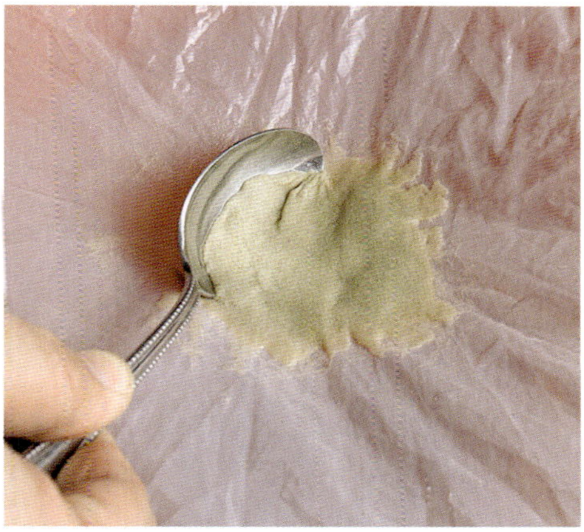

Once the water has drained from the pooled hash, it can be scooped up with a spoon.

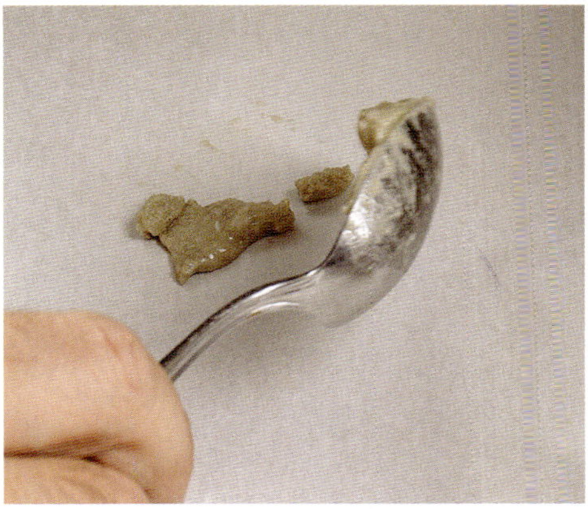

Place the wet hash on the Freeze Dryer trays. It is good to keep the different-micron-size bags separated. This is the 90 µm hash.

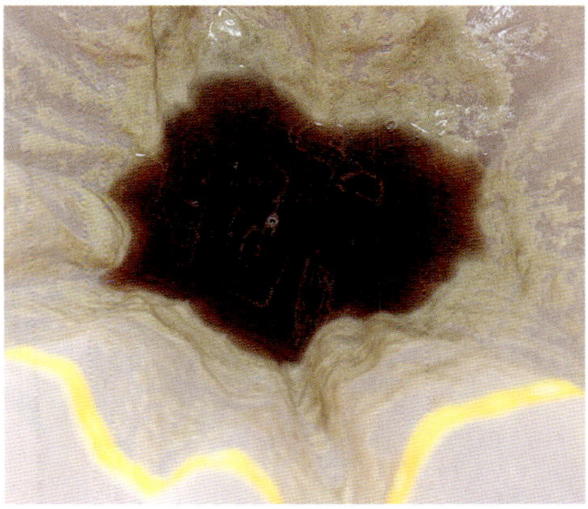

Repeat the steps of spraying and pooling the hash in the next bag before collecting. Here is the 73 µm hash being pooled before collection.

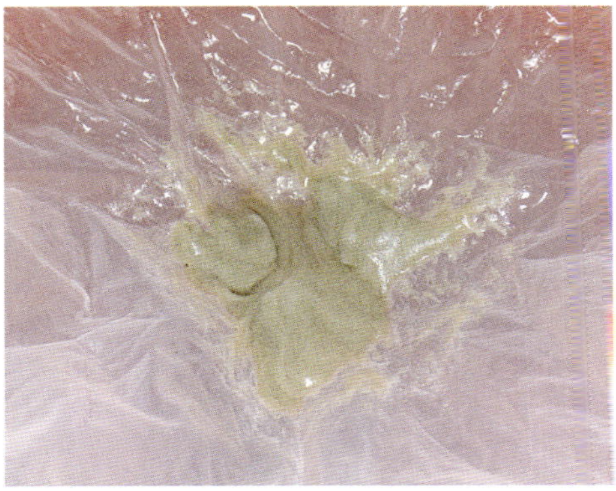

73 µm hash almost ready to be scooped. Notice the different textures of hash in each micron

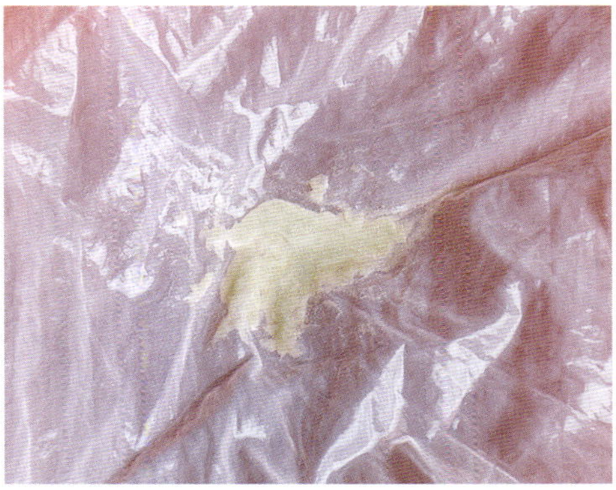

73 µm hash drained and ready to be collected.

continues...

Extraction Freezing Process *continued*

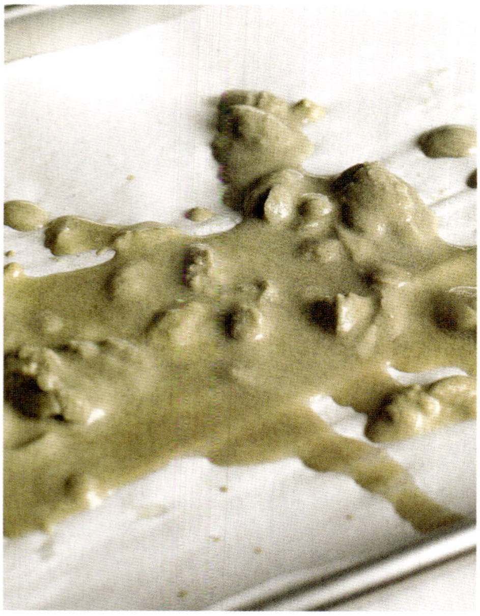

Spread the wet bubble hash out on the Freeze Dryer tray to increase surface area, which helps the drying process.

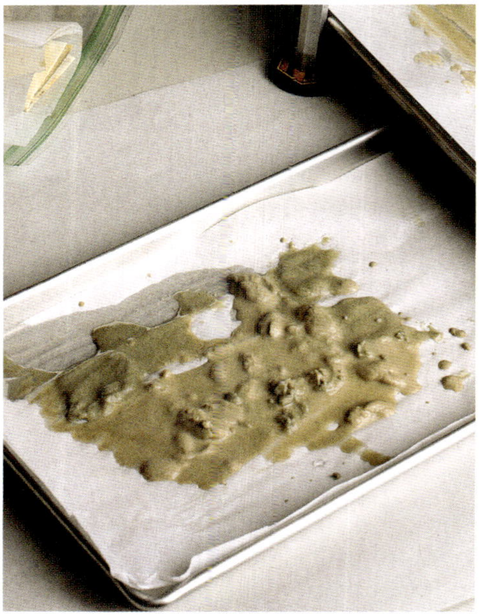

Wet bubble hash can sometimes have the consistency of wet beach sand.

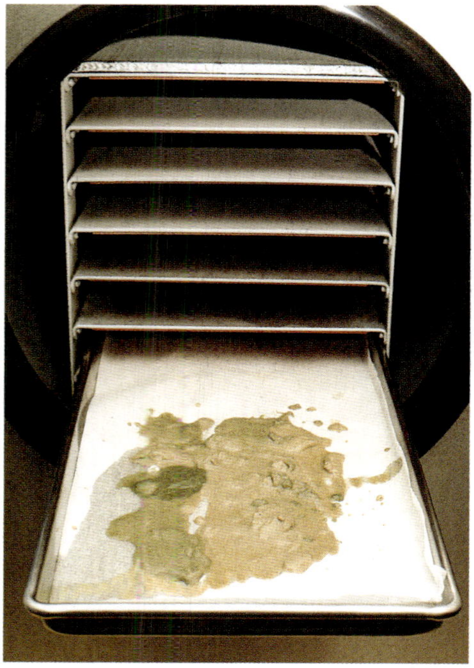

Load the trays of wet bubble hash into the Freeze Dryer.

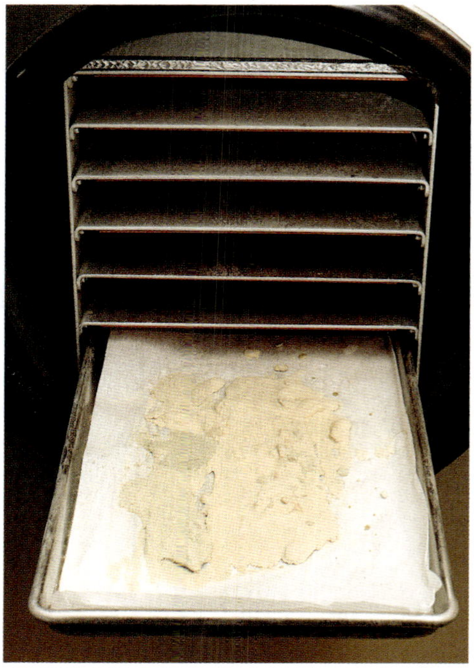

After Freeze Dryer cycle is complete, check to ensure hash is fully dry.

PHOTOS: RUSSELL-HOWLAND PHOTOGRAPHY

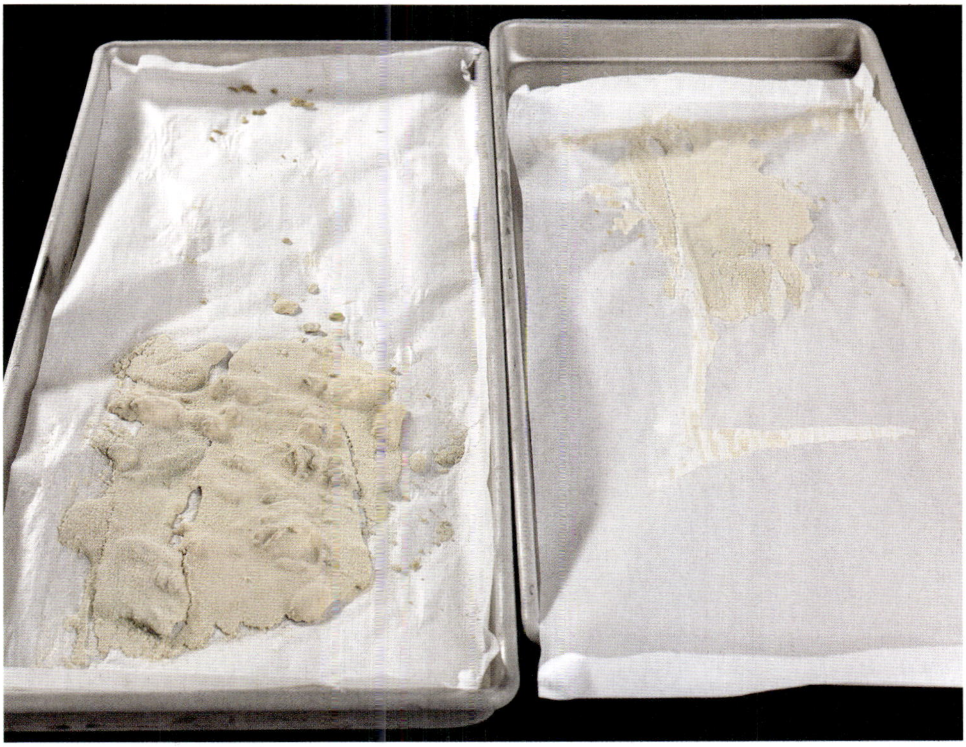

Dry bubble hash will have a loose sandy consistency while it is still cold/frozen.

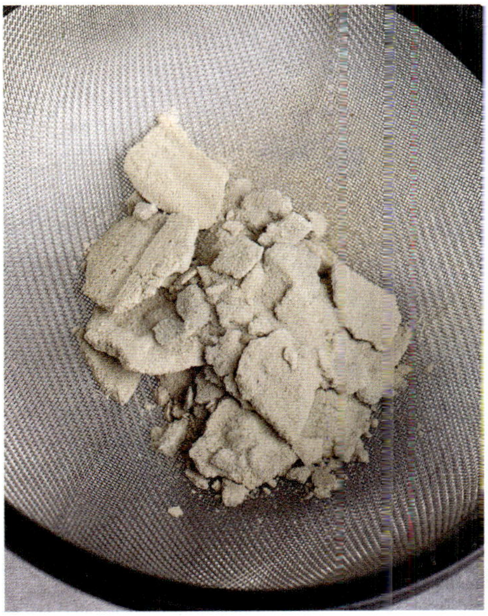

Once your hash is dry, it's time to lightly sieve it to break it up into finer particles and ensure there are no ice chunks.

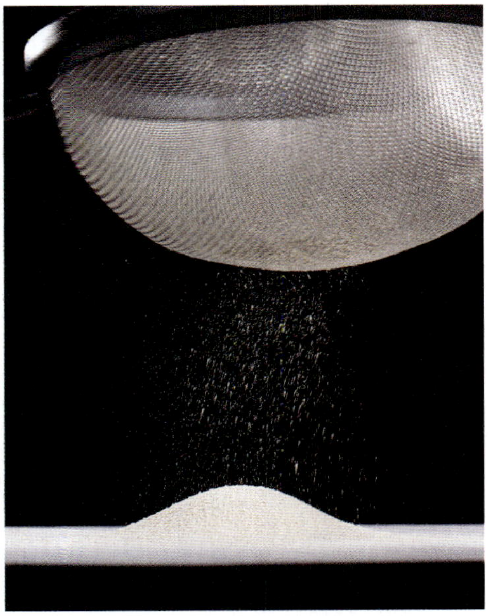

Shake and toss the bubble hash to allow it to break down naturally or use a spoon to press it through the mesh.

continues...

Extraction Freezing Process *continued*

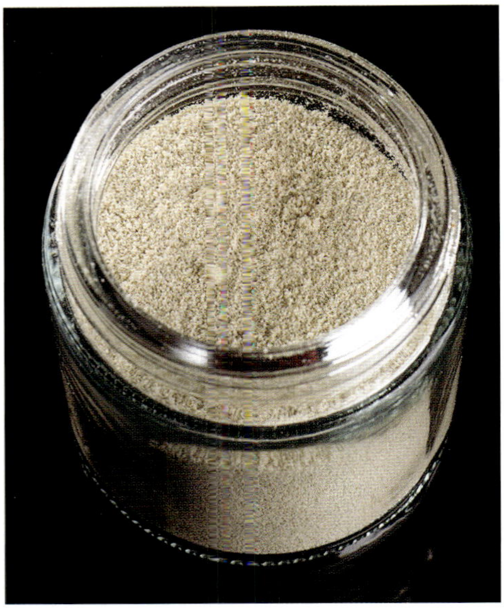

Loose bubble hash is best stored in the freezer, especially if it's of very high quality. It will melt and self-press if kept at room temperature.

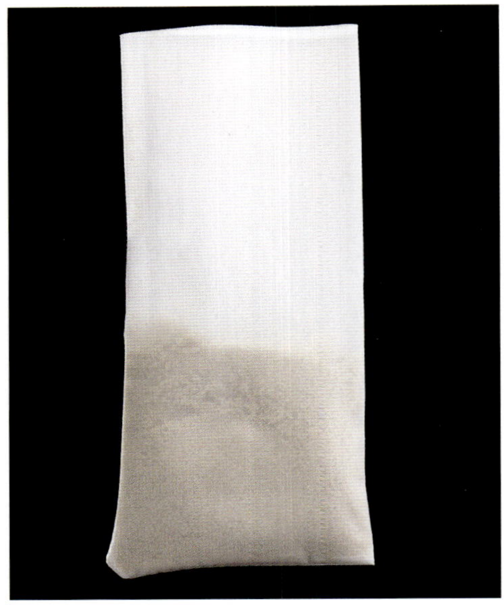

Bubble hash loaded into a rosin bag ready to be pressed into hash rosin.

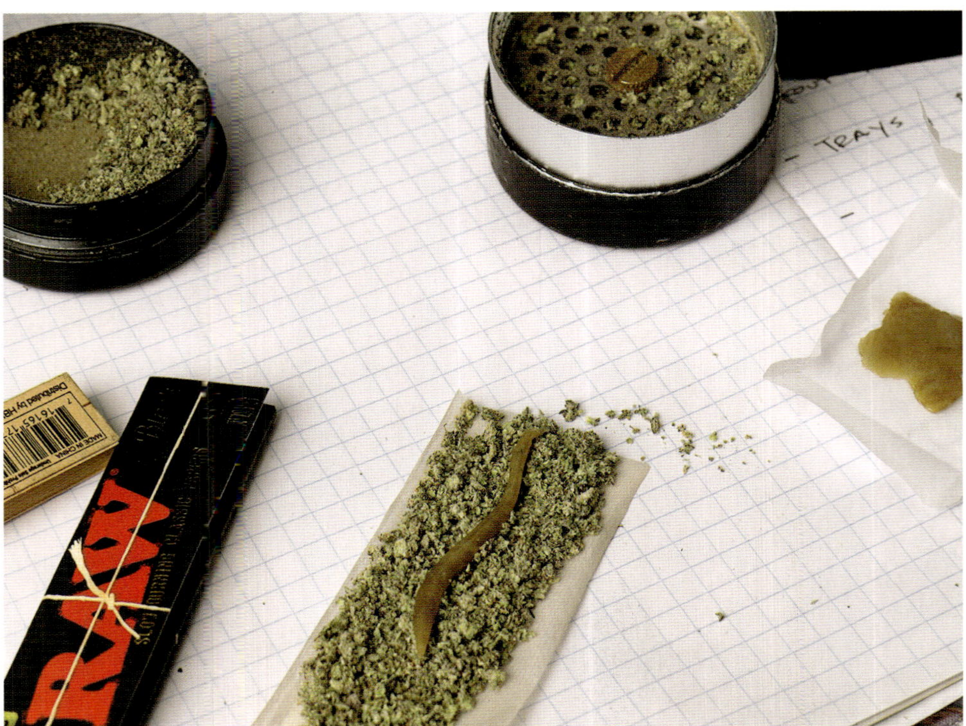

A hash hole pre-roll with a snake of hash rosin ready to be rolled up.

PHOTOS: RUSSELL-HOWLAND PHOTOGRAPHY

Basic Water Extraction

Resin glands can be removed from the cannabis plant by agitating the trim or flowers in ice water or water chilled in a fridge overnight.

Water extraction:

1. Place the trim in a bucket, fill it with cold water, and mix it all together with a tool like a large spoon or electric whisk.
2. Let the mixture sit for a few minutes before scooping out the skuff floating on the surface.
3. Strain the remaining liquid through a coffee sieve to collect most of the remaining trichomes.
4. Once this has dried, you can use the trichome extract to make hash.

This method uses cold water to break the trichomes away from the leaf matter, causing the glands, which are heavier than water, to eventually sink to the bottom of the bucket. The bulk leaf matter will stay afloat and can be scooped away. Water Extraction is a great way for home growers to make some very high-quality hash with their harvest, either using full flowers or just the small buds, trim or sugar leaves. Here is a simple one-bucket procedure for utilizing bubble bags such as the ones mentioned below.

Input Material

As mentioned previously, the right growing and harvesting techniques must be used to ensure the cannabis is suitable for extraction. If aiming to produce Live Rosin, you will need to harvest your cannabis and freeze the buds immediately. This is called fresh-frozen cannabis. If going for traditional bubble hash you can use dried and cured bud, but it is still a good idea to freeze this cannabis before extracting.

Preparation

The real Bubblebags, produced by BC Cannabis Pioneer Bubbleman, come as a full eight-bag set with pore sizes 25, 45, 73, 90, 120, 160, 190, and 220 μm. This allows you to extract a wide array of different trichome sizes and qualities. Using all eight bags gives you a great understanding of how that particular cultivar produces and yields trichomes and can also be an indicator of proper or improper growing/harvesting techniques. A healthy plant should produce the majority of trichomes in the 45-160 μm range, however capturing the hash from the other fractions (25, 160 and 190 μm) is a good idea, especially if you plan to produce edibles or topicals, or just want to capture as much of the resin as possible.

Preparing the Bubblebags:

1. Get a bucket and line it with your Bubblebags, starting with the smallest micron size first then placing the next larger sized Bubblebag on top, finish with a 220 μm bag to hold the cannabis and ice during filtration.

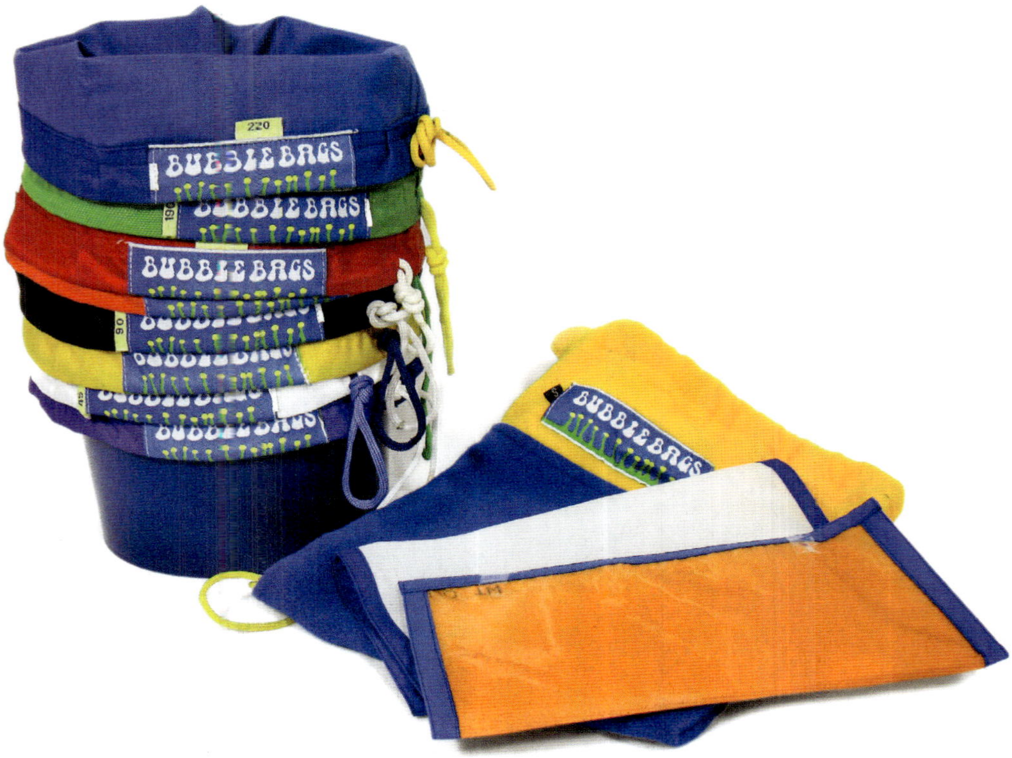

BC Bubbleman's 8-bag 1 gallon kit, containing some of the highest quality water extraction bags on the market.

2. Fill the bucket with cold water and ice.
3. Allow the water to chill to a temperature of 32°F (0°C) before putting your cannabis in.
4. While your bucket is chilling, get some clean, empty pizza boxes and line the bottom with parchment paper. This is how we will dry the wet bubble hash once it's been extracted.

Washing the cannabis:

1. Once your water temperature has reached 32°F (0°C) or as close as possible, pour your cannabis into the bucket and mix lightly to allow all the buds to get wet and saturated. Often it is a good idea to allow your cannabis to pre-soak in the water for a few minutes (5-30 mins depending on quantity of bud), especially if you are using dried/cured bud, as this allows the water to soak into the whole bud.
2. After pre-soak, you can begin agitating the cannabis by stirring it around in the bucket with a large spoon or paddle.
3. Agitate the cannabis vigorously and allow the ice to break down larger buds, exposing more trichomes and causing them to become brittle and fall off the plant. Agitate for 10-30 minutes depending on quantity and desired output quality.

PHOTO: BUBBLEMAN

4. Once you are finished washing/agitating, allow the material to rest for a couple minutes. This will allow the heavier trichome heads which have been knocked free of the buds to sink to the bottom of bucket.
5. Pull out the first bag (220 μm), which will hold your cannabis and ice. Allow this bag to drain all the hash water into the bucket and then place the bag aside for further washing.
6. Pull out the next bag and scoop any extracted hash off the screen with a spoon. Pre-freezing your spoon will help with collecting the hash off the bubblebag screen, especially if it is very high quality and sticky.
7. Use a spray bottle with chilled water to spray the hash down the sides of the bags into a small pile in the middle of the screen that can be scooped easily with a spoon.
8. Place the collected hash on the 25 μm dabmat to further wick away any water.
9. Place the hash into the parchment-lined pizza box once wicked.
10. It is a good idea to keep your hash piles clearly separate to ensure the higher quality microns of hash do not mix with the lower quality hashes from the coarse screens.
11. Pull out the next sequential bag and repeat the above steps to scoop the hash from the screen and place into pizza box to dry. Place the pizza box into a freezer in between collections.
12. Once all bags have been collected you can reline the bucket with the extraction bags and put the 220 μm bag with the cannabis back into the bucket for further washing. Continue washing until there is a noticeable reduction in yield or quality; often it will take more than three washes to collect the majority of the available resin.

Drying the Bubble Hash:

1. After all the hash has been collected, place the pizza box in the freezer for a few minutes to freeze the hash before proceeding.
2. Now the hash needs to be sieved or grated into a loose powder to allow it to dry properly. Take a metal cheese grater or sieve and place in the freezer for a few minutes. This will allow the hash to pass through the metal more freely and not melt and stick.
3. Take the frozen hash chunks and grate them over the sieve until all has passed through and there is a loose pile on the parchment-lined pizza box. Note: It is often a good idea to have several pizza boxes on-hand to allow you to keep different grades of hash separate during drying.
4. Continue sieving the frozen hash until completed. If the hash begins to smear on the sieve you can place it back into the freezer which will loosen the hash and allow more to pass through easier.
5. Now place your pizza boxes in a clean, dry area for several days and allow the hash to air dry.

Dry bubble hash will have a loose, sandy consistency, which can then be collected and consumed as is, or pressed into rosin or hash-bricks or hand-rolled into temple balls.

Bubble Hash

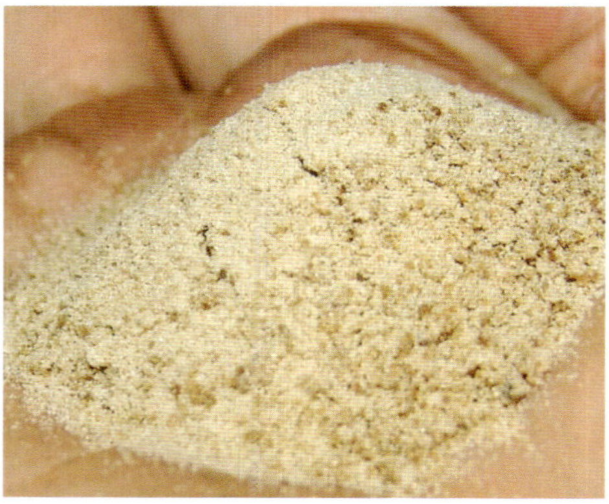

You can test the quality of your bubble hash by using a lighter to apply heat to a small pile and see how much it melts.

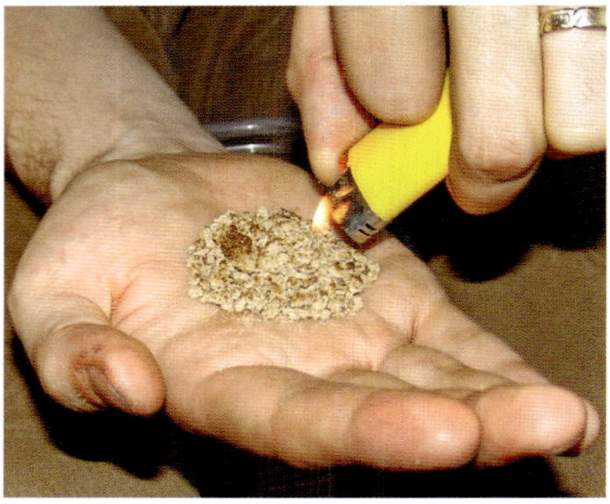

The idea is to apply heat exclusively to the top of the pile.

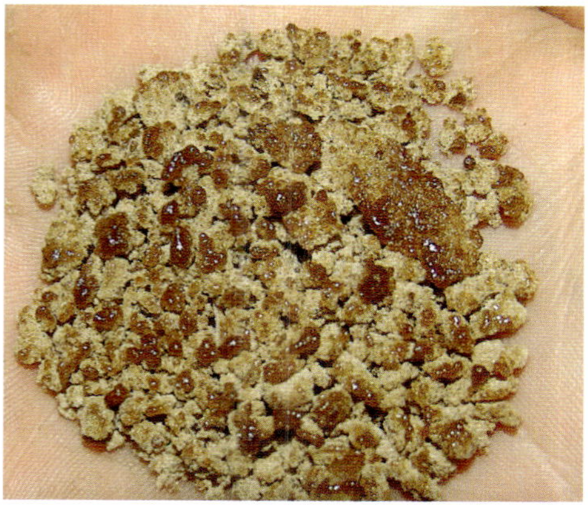

You don't want to heat a lot. Just some.

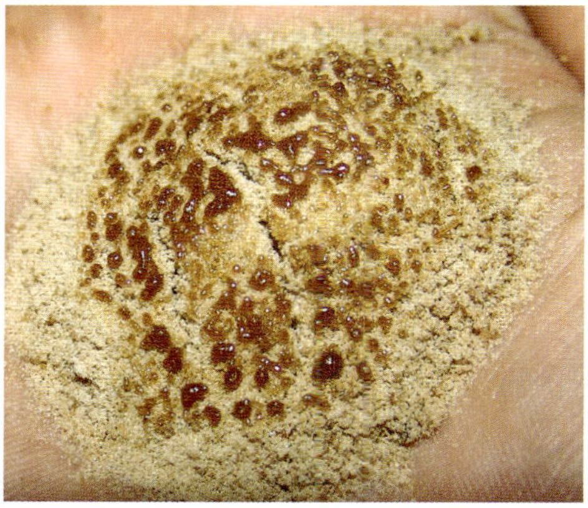

Bubble hash gets it name from the way it bubbles and melts when heat is applied to it.

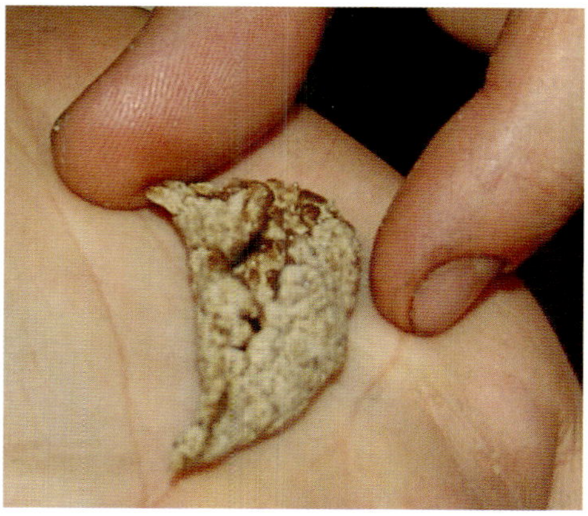

Now compact it like a small piece of dough.

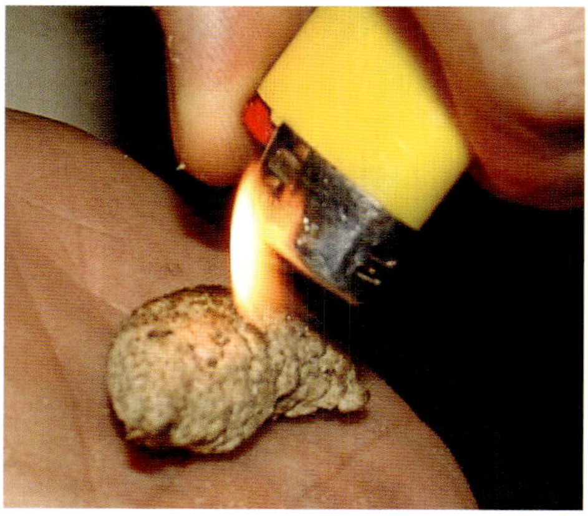

Heat more to bind it.

PHOTOS: BUBBLEMAN

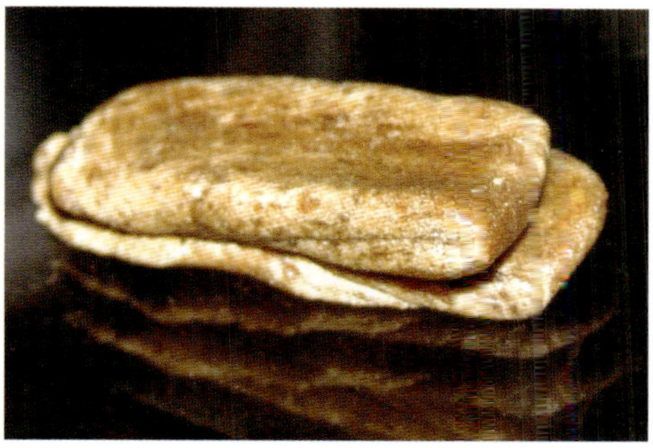

When it's semisolid you can shape it.

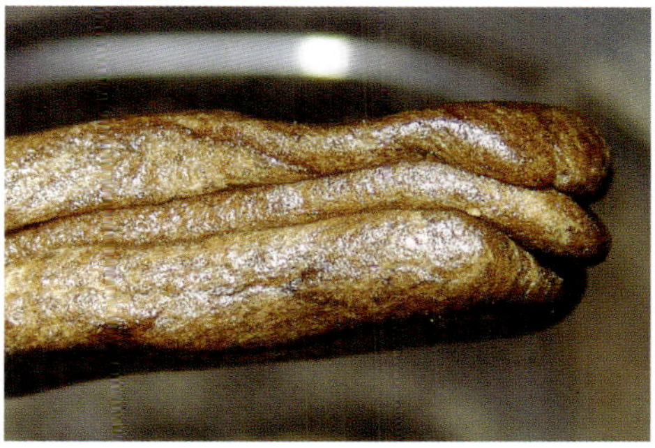

You can roll or flatten it.

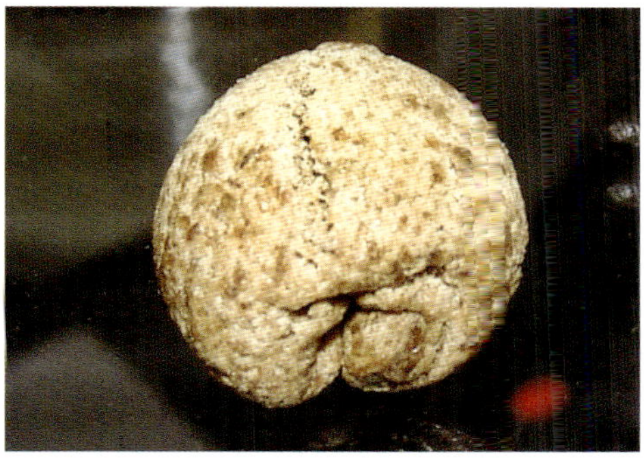

Prepare a cool sample to use.

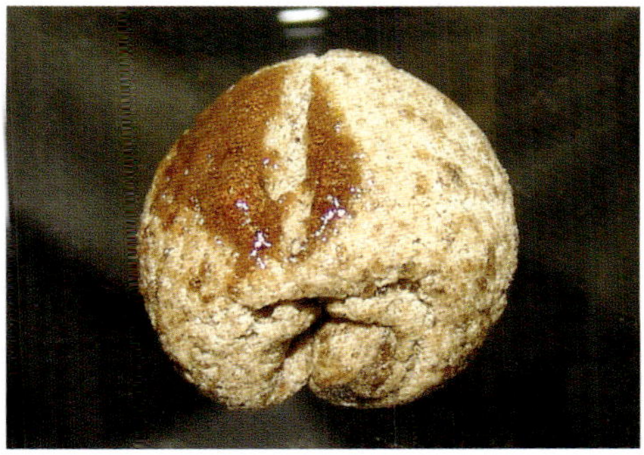

Heat a piece.

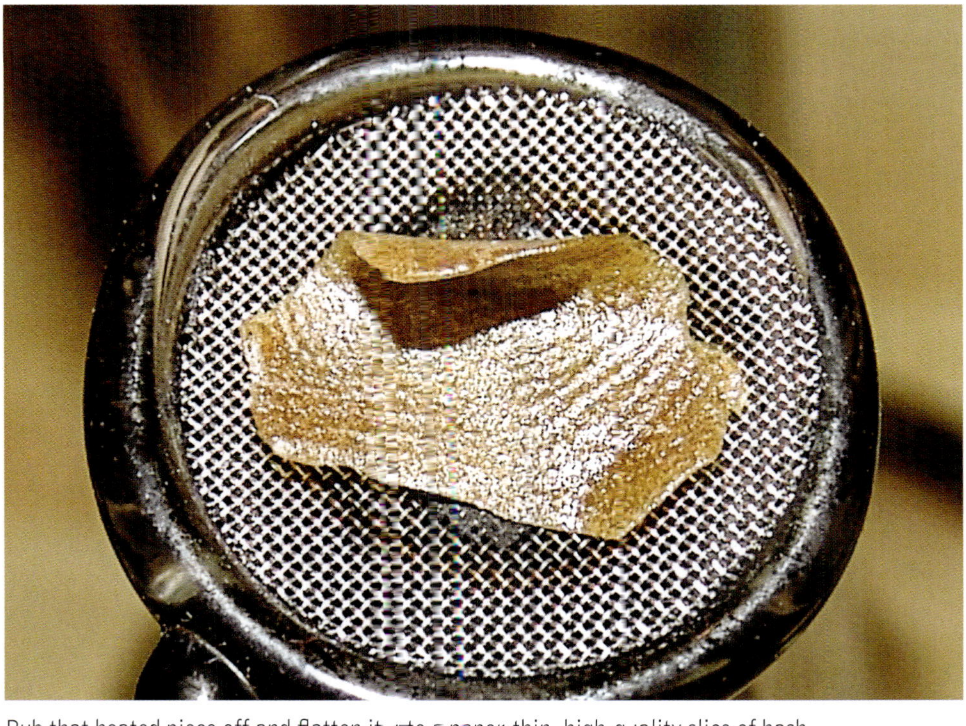

Rub that heated piece off and flatten it into a paper-thin, high-quality slice of hash.

Ice Extraction with AEG

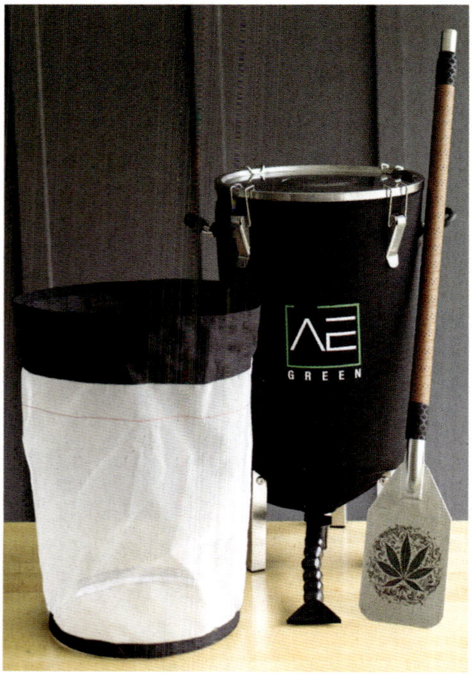

AE Green's insulated wash vessel, extraction bag, and paddle.

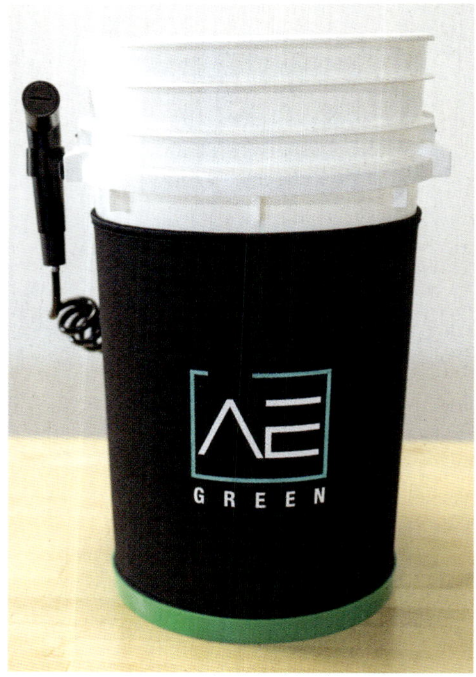

Insulated extraction buckets with hose for rinsing. Extraction buckets have been insulated to maintain cold temperature during the wash.

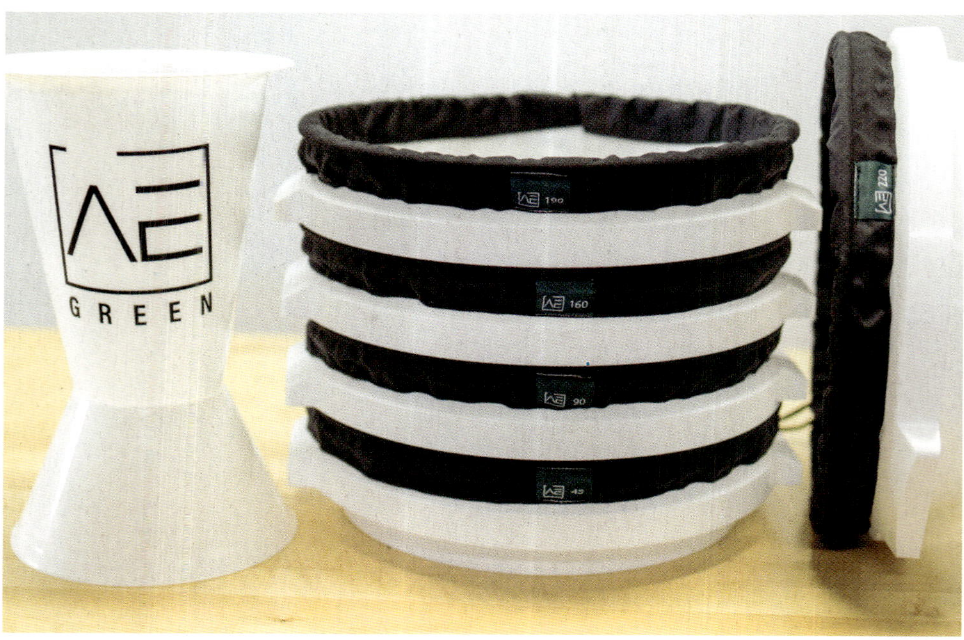

Extraction bags with bucket top fittings.

PHOTOS: AETHERGREEN.COM

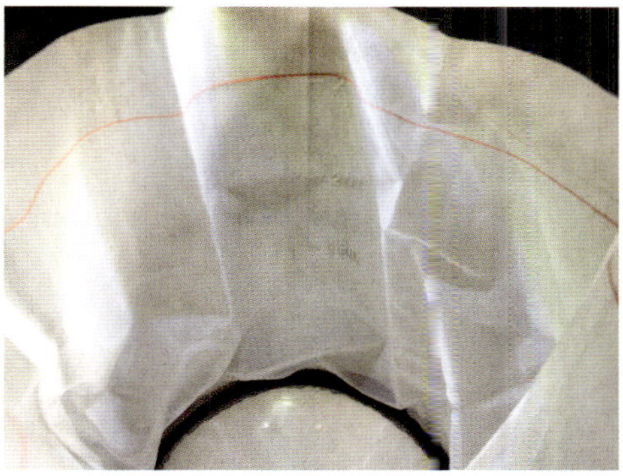

Begin filling wash vessel with cold water.

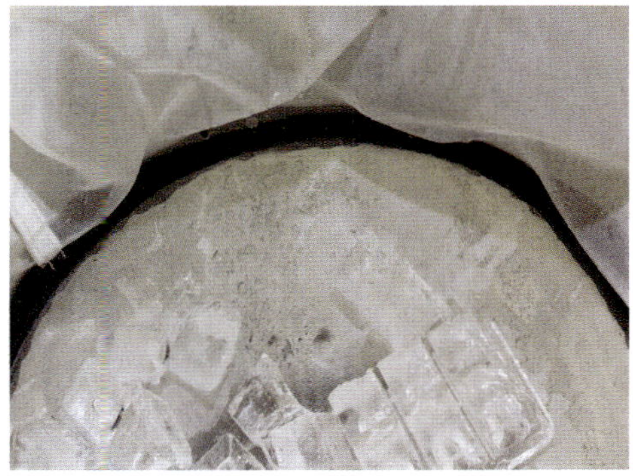

Add ice to bring water temperature down.

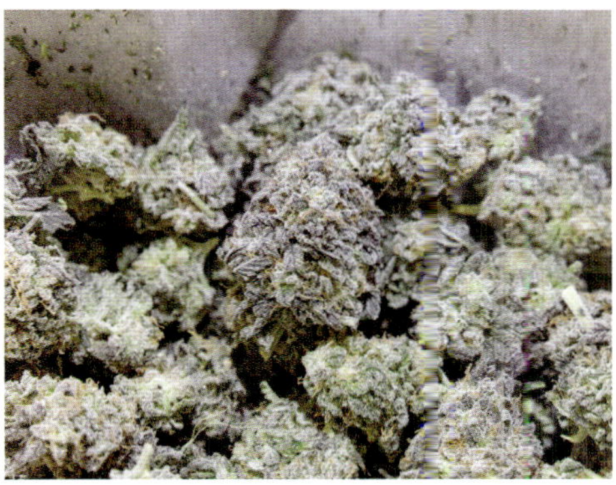

Add your cannabis into the wash vessel.

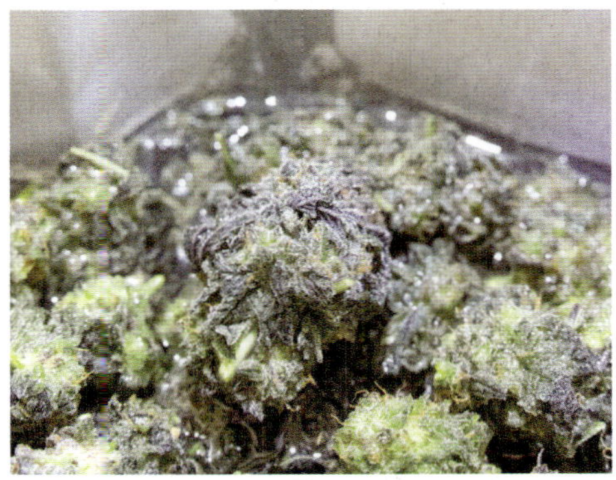

Continue to fill vessel with water and ice.

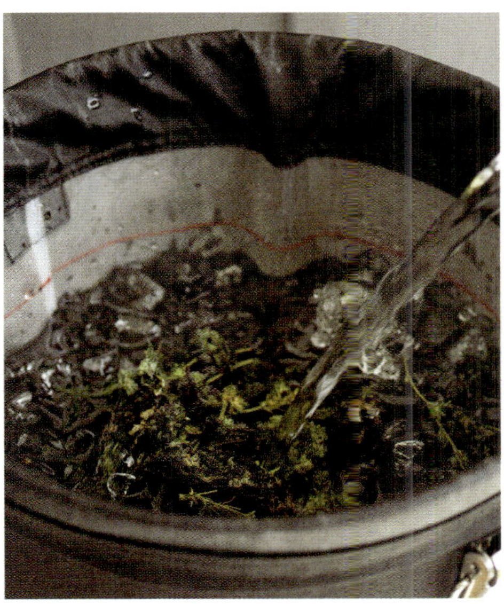

Fill wash vessel with water up to the marked red line.

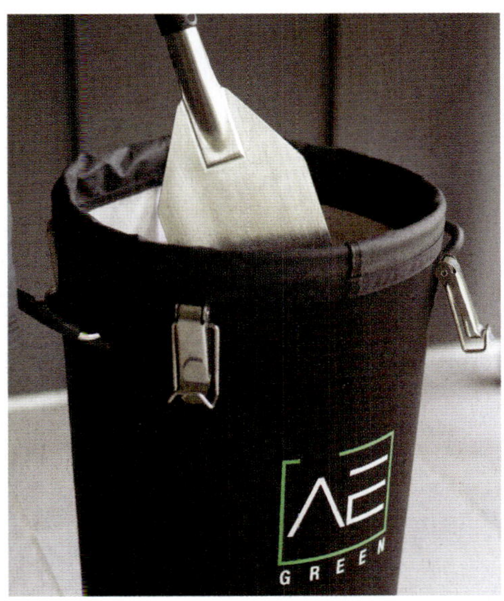

Use the paddle to ensure cannabis is fully submerged. Push ice on top of buds to sink them down if needed.

continues...

Ice Extraction with AEG *continued*

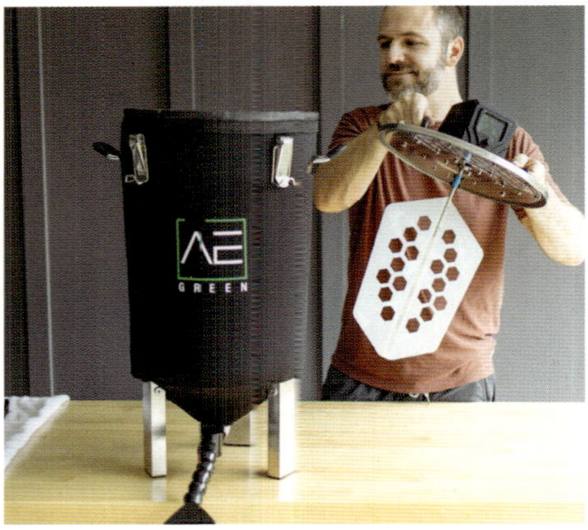

Once cannabis is submerged, grab the lid.

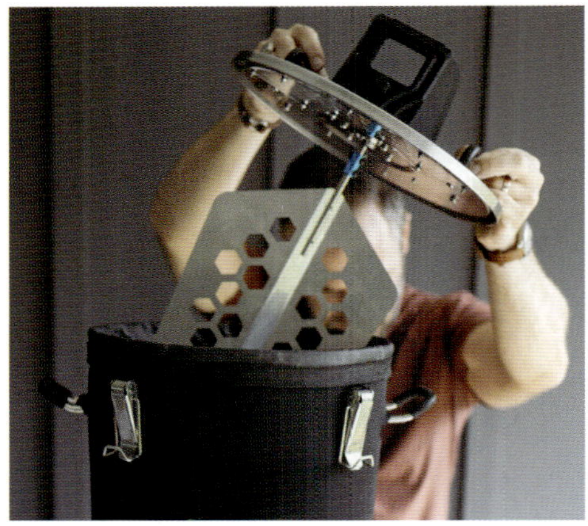

Place agitator/impeller lid onto wash vessel.

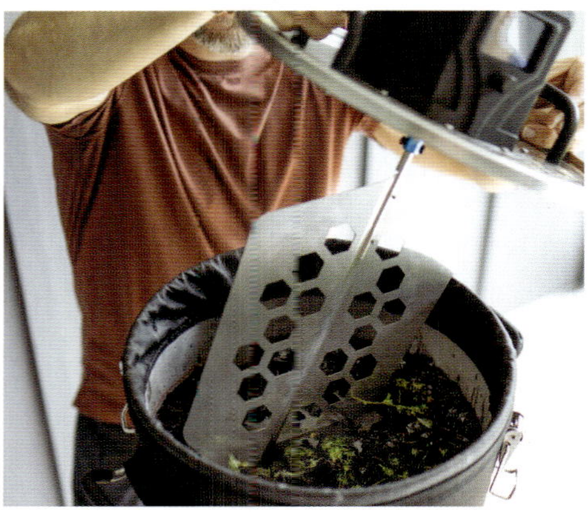

Make sure agitator/impeller is placed in the center and clear from extraction bag.

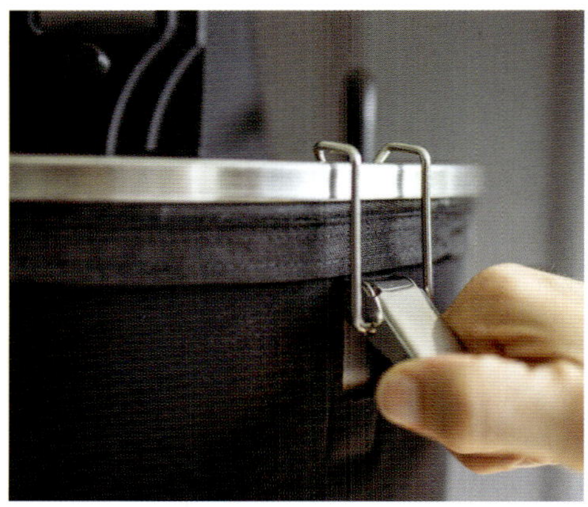

Lock lid down with side clamps.

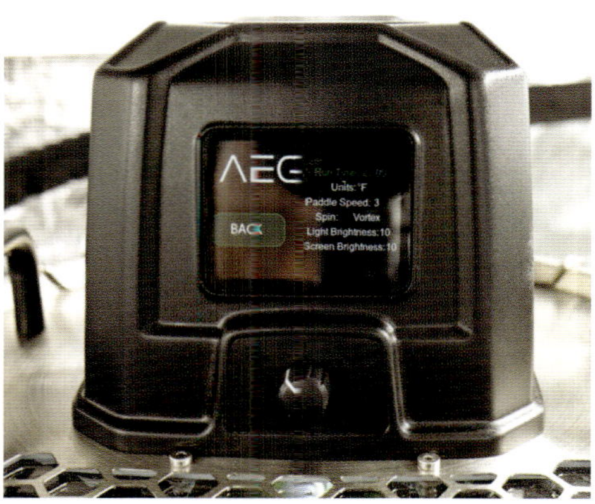
AEG
Units: °F
Paddle Speed: 3
Spin: Vortex
Light Brightness:10
Screen Brightness:10
BACK

Set desired wash program.

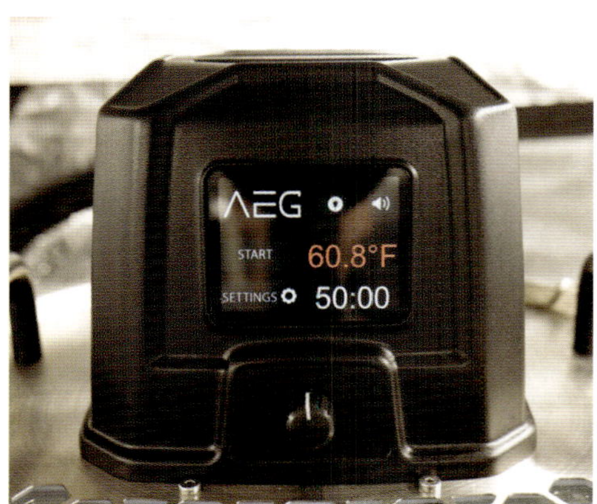
AEG
START
60.8°F
SETTINGS
50:00

Set desired wash temperature and other parameters.

PHOTOS: AETHERGREEN.COM

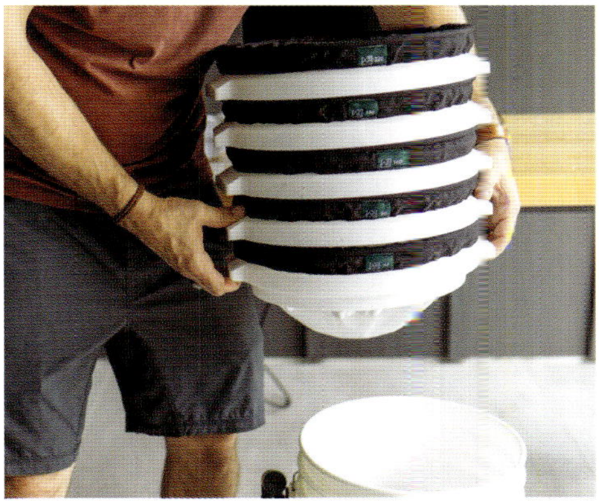

Place collection bags on bucket.

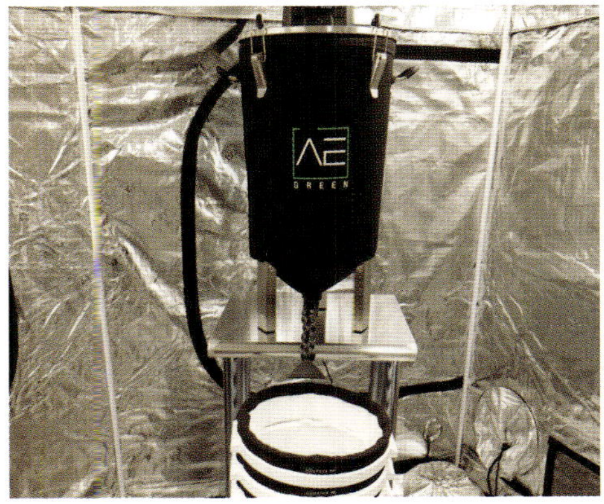

Place wash vessel above the collection buckets for easy drainage.

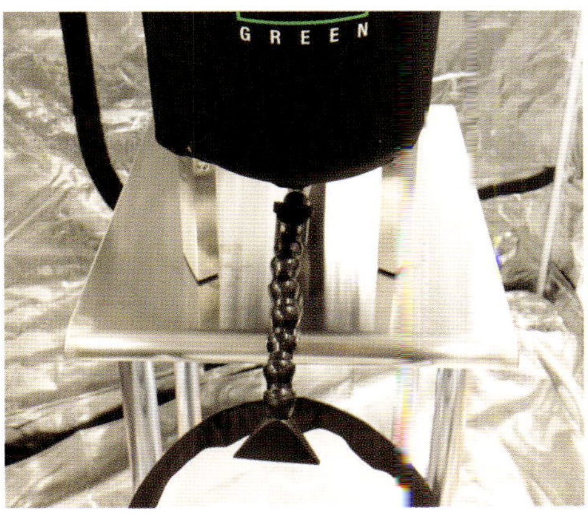

Ensure drainage hose is directed into collection buckets.

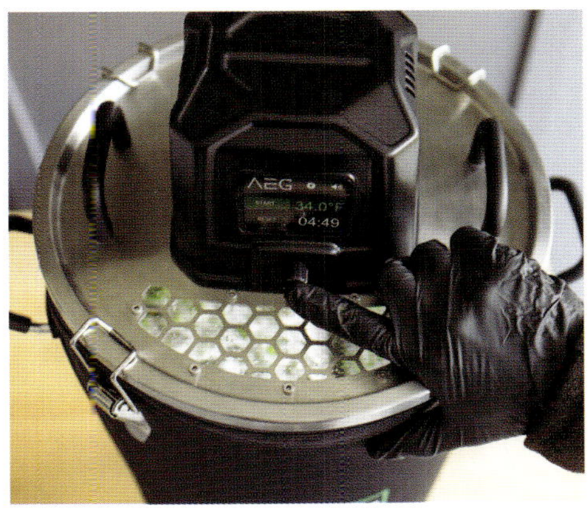

Begin wash cycle.

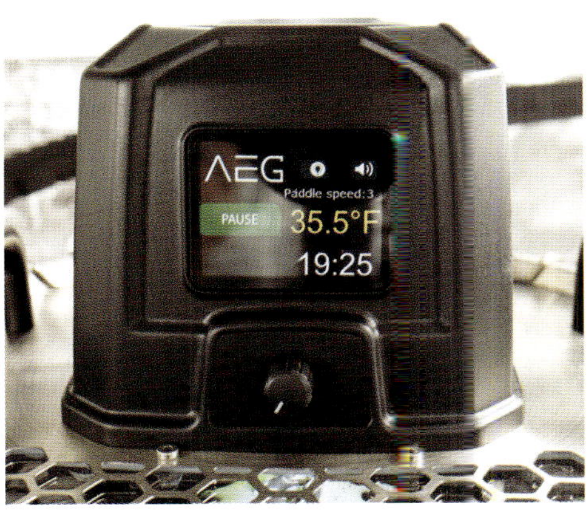

Wash temperatures and other parameters displayed.

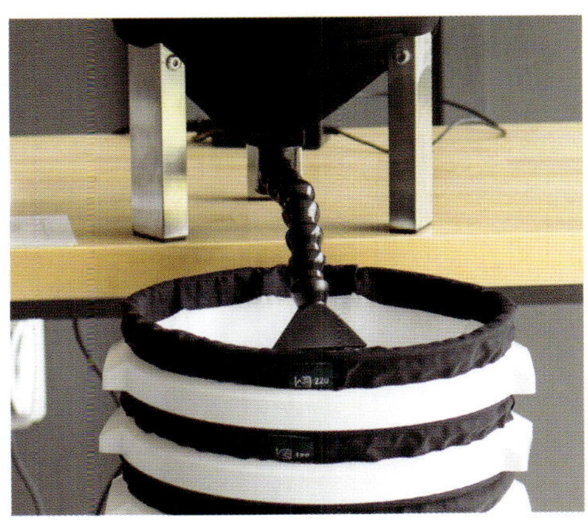

When wash cycle is complete, position the collection bucket under the drain hose before opening the valve.

continues...

Ice Extraction with AEG *continued*

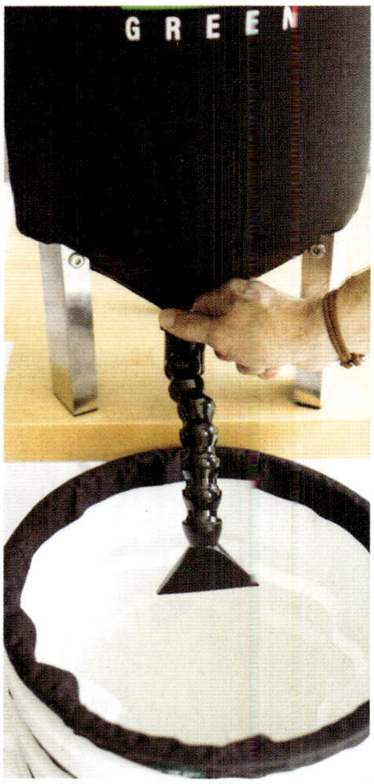

Position valve over the bucket.

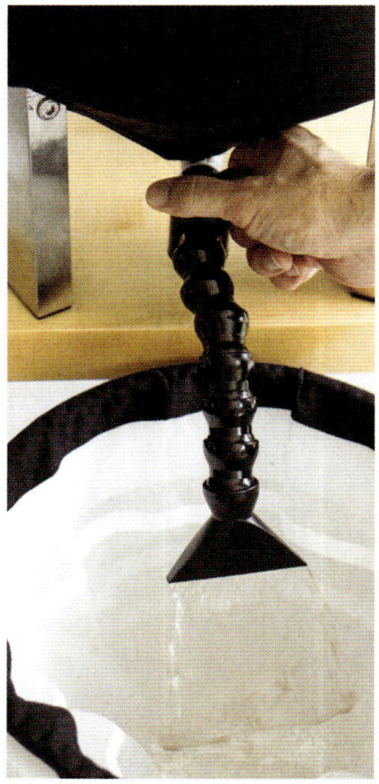

Open valve slowly.

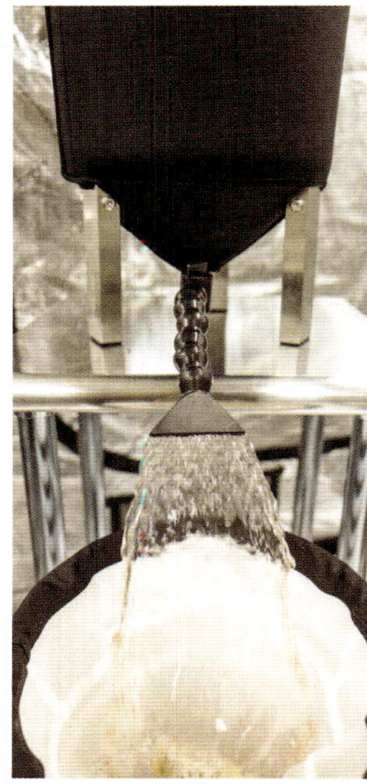

Allow water to flow into collection bucket.

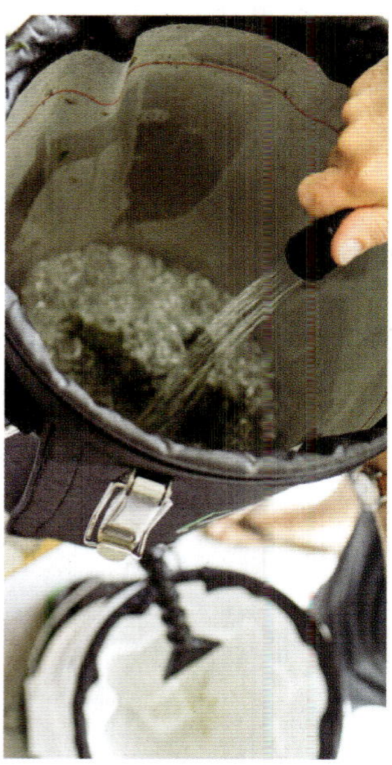

Turn on the hose and direct the water back into the wash vessel.

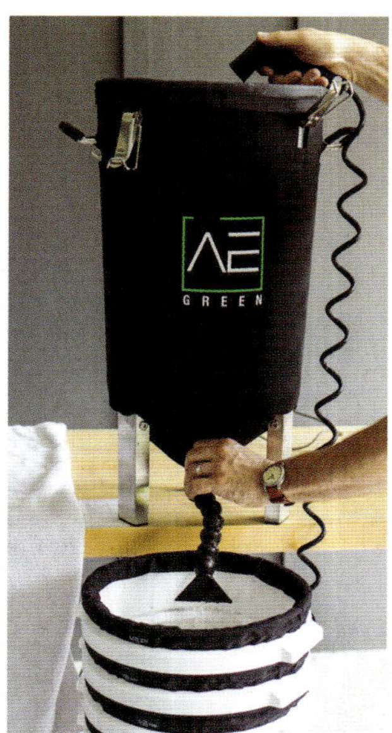

Continue spraying down through the top of the wash vessel to keep flowing water through the collection buckets.

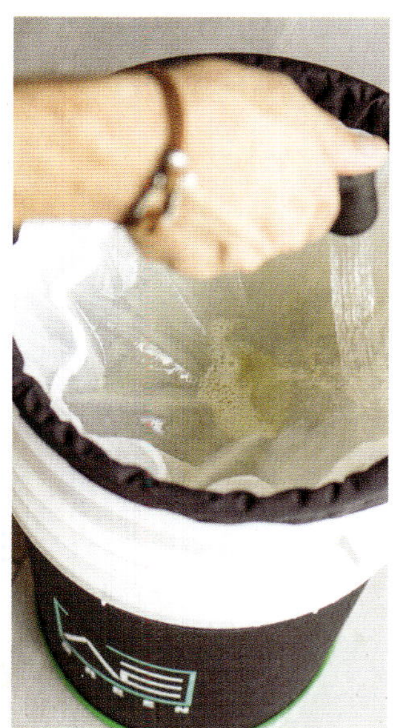

Use the hose to spray the hash down the sides of the bags and pool in the center.

PHOTOS: AETHERGREEN.COM

Pressing Resin into Hash

There are many variations on hash making technologies. They may use different methods, but their results inevitably condense into a solid hash material.

The plant and resin gland qualities determine the properties of the hash: Quality in equals quality out. Hashish grade is based on the ratio of cannabinoids to other plant material, from high concentration to low. Better extraction and pressing techniques result in hash with a high concentration of cannabinoids. Hash grading used to run from 00, or Zero Zero, to five, which is the lowest. Legal hash and extracts are analytically tested to determine potency of major cannabinoids. This is done through HPLC at certified labs. Typically most forms of dry sift/blonde hash range from 20-40% THC, where bubble hash can be as high as 70% THC due to the high purity and concentration of trichome heads. Bubble hash potency can go as high as 77%, which is in the same range as low grade THC distillate potencies

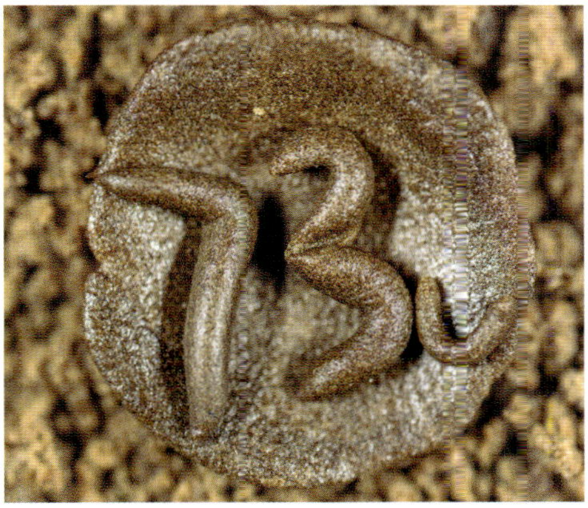

At 73 microns, this malleable hash looks shiny because of cannabinoids.

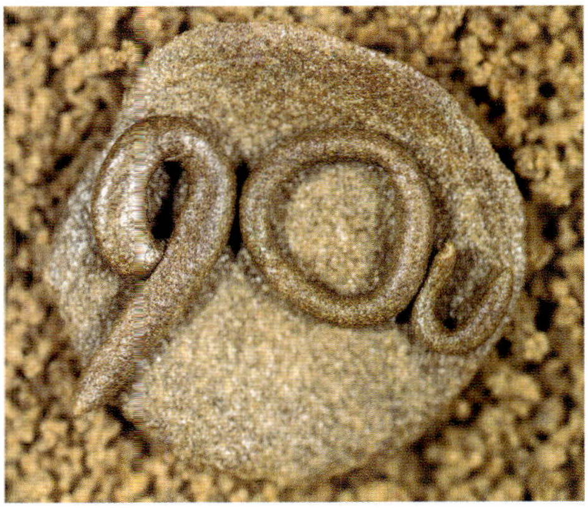

At 90 microns, less malleable and less shiny because of more plant matter.

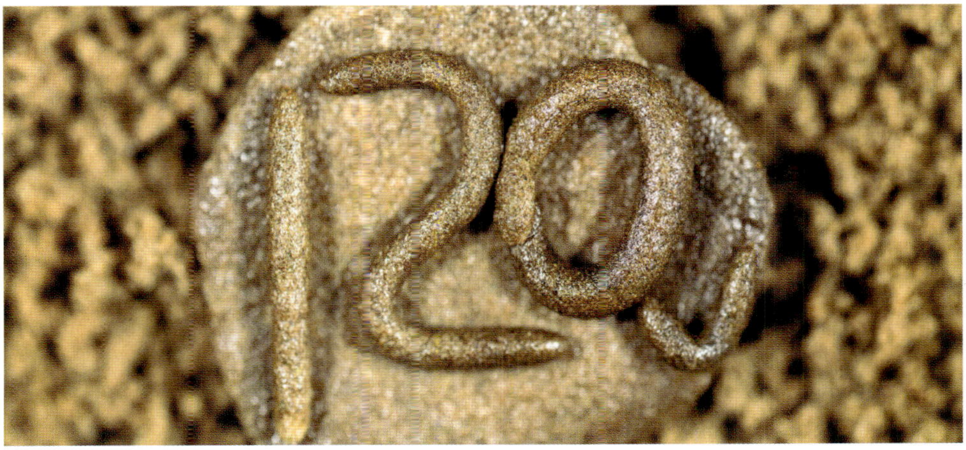

At 120 microns, even less malleable and even less shiny because of even more plant matter.

PHOTOS: BUBBLEMAN

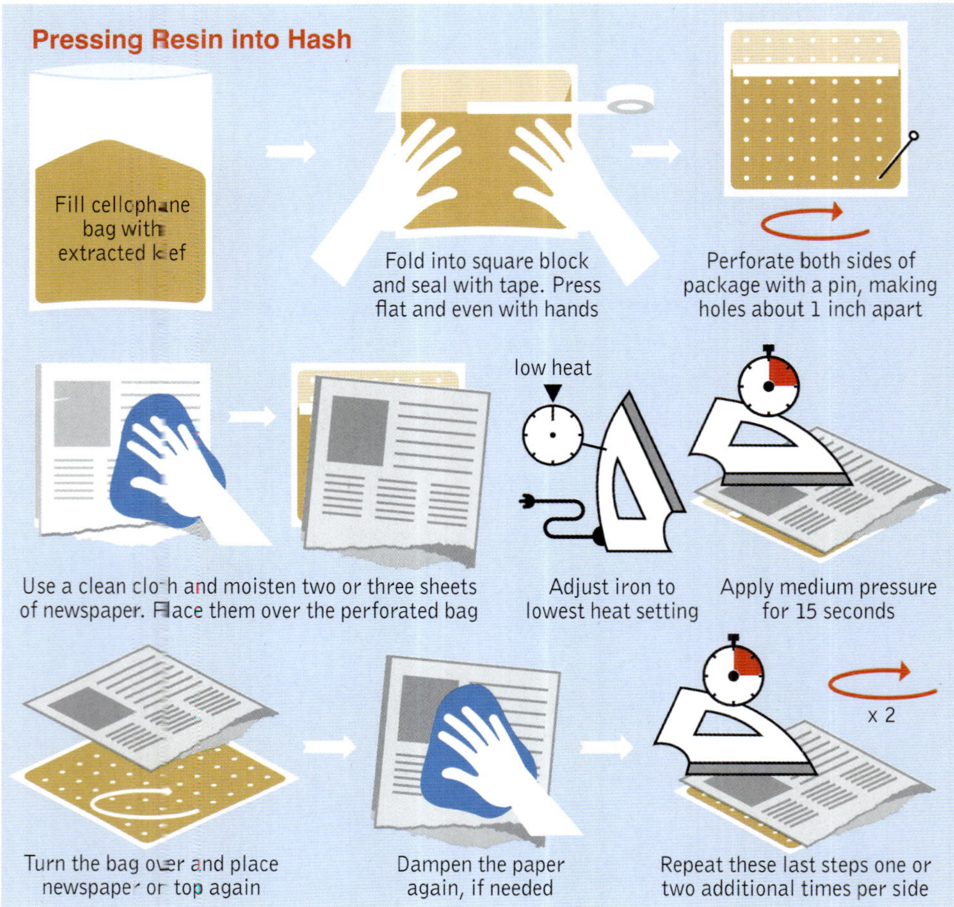
Pressing Resin into Hash
Fill cellophane bag with extracted kief
Fold into square block and seal with tape. Press flat and even with hands
Perforate both sides of package with a pin, making holes about 1 inch apart
low heat
Use a clean cloth and moisten two or three sheets of newspaper. Place them over the perforated bag
Adjust iron to lowest heat setting
Apply medium pressure for 15 seconds
x 2
Turn the bag over and place newspaper on top again
Dampen the paper again, if needed
Repeat these last steps one or two additional times per side

Pressing resin into hash:

1. Put your extracted kief or bubble hash into a food-grade cellophane bag or wrap.
2. Fold the material into a flat block shape, tape the ends of the cellophane to create a package, and press it flat with your hands, taking care to make it even.
3. Next, make some holes with a pin, about one hole per square inch, on both sides of the bag.
4. Then moisten two or three newspaper sheets with a clean damp cloth, making sure not to overly saturate or tear the paper, and place them over the cellophane bag.
5. Put an iron on the lowest heat, hold it over the paper, and press it down with medium pressure for about 15 seconds.
6. Turn the bag over and place the newspaper on top again. Dampen the paper again if needed. Repeat the pressure for the same amount of time. This should be repeated once or twice per side. Let the bag cool for five minutes, remove the cellophane and you should have a nice block of hash.
7. The combination of dampness and low heat will have prevented the cannabinoids from vaporizing.

Hot-Bottle Tech

A simple way to make pressed black hash is similar to above.

Hot-bottle tech:

1. Place your extracted kief or bubble hash into a food-grade cellophane pouch or bag.
2. Fold the cellophane edges to seal in the kief and not allow it to escape during pressing.
3. Fill a glass wine bottle with hot water (from a kettle). Be careful not to spill while filling. Use oven mitts or heat-resistant gloves to handle the filled bottle, and do not use boiling water, which can cause the bottle to smash.
4. Place the rounded edge of the bottle onto the cellophane pouch and apply some pressure to the kief for a minute or two before you roll it out. This heat will burst trichome heads and begin decarboxylation processes.
5. Press firmly and roll the kief out, as if using a rolling pin on some pizza dough.
6. Continue pressing and rolling the kief; you will notice a color change and some hash will begin to liquify as the trichomes burst and release the resin.

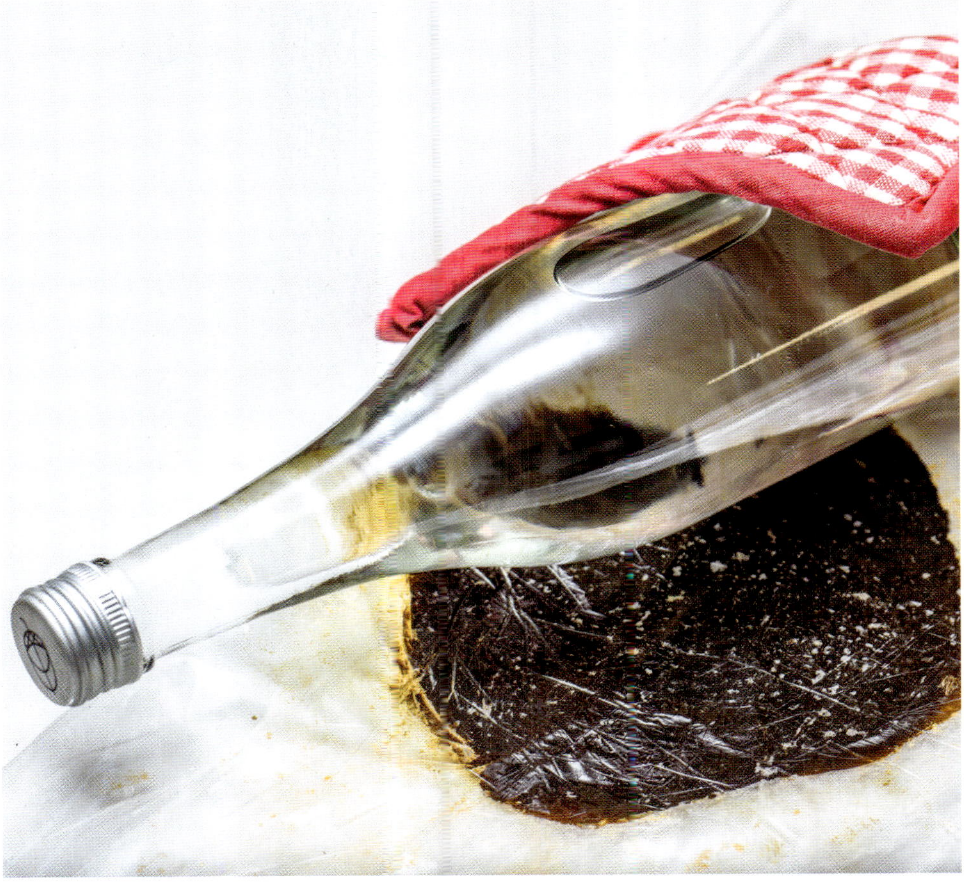

PHOTO: ERIC PALMER

Rolling a hot bottle onto kief in cellophane releases resin from trichome heads.

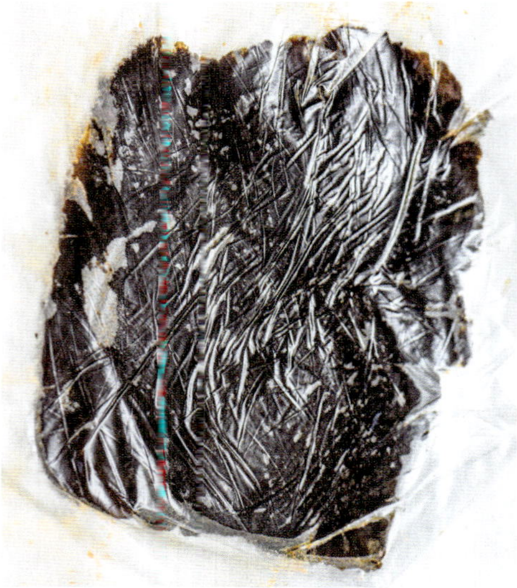

You will observe changes to the color and texture of the kief.

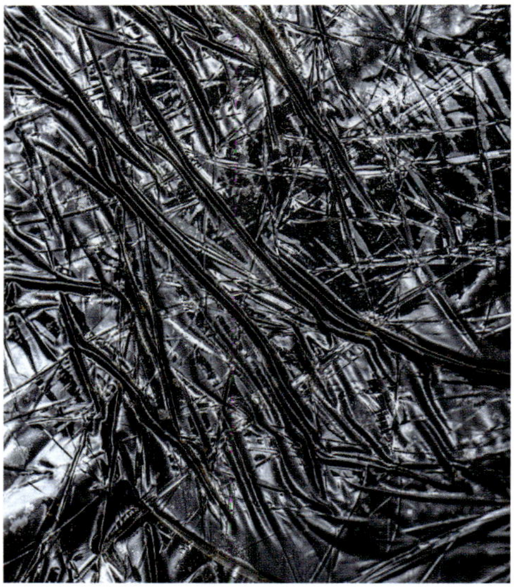

The heated kief now resembles hashish and is more solid.

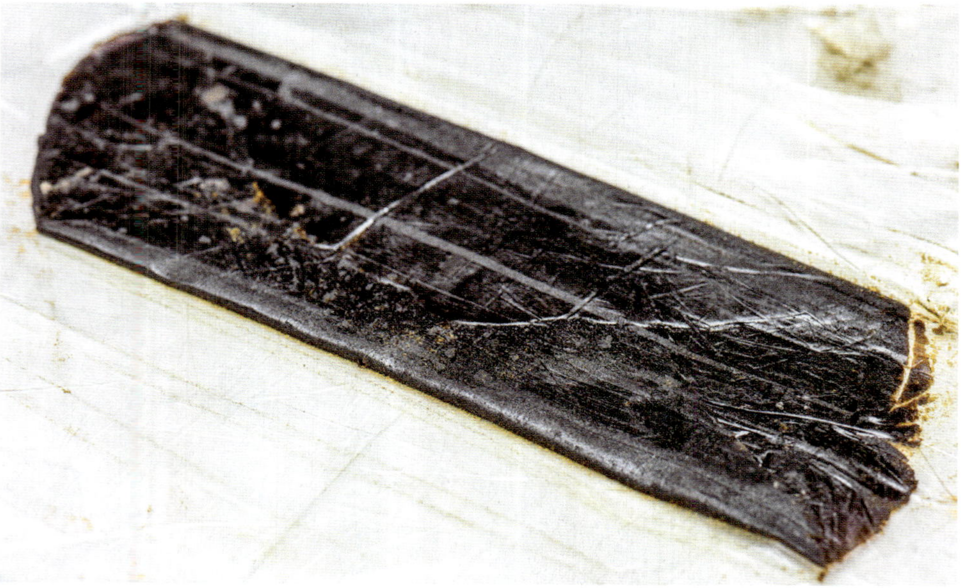

Rolling on the hash more ensures nothing powdery like kief is left and that what remains is shapable like plasticine.

PHOTOS: ERIC PALMER

7. After rolling for a few minutes, open the cellophane pouch and take the pressed hash out.
8. Now fold the hash back onto itself several times and form a small block or ball with the hash.
9. Put this back into the cellophane and repeat the rolling process.

After rolling a few times the hash will begin to take on a soft gummy consistency and can be hand rolled into a ball. If the hash is still powdery, then continue the above rolling techniques until the desired consistency is reached.

10. Now remove the hash from the cellophane and use your hands to form the hash into a ball.
11. Roll it around between your palms to smoothen out the surface and create a spherical temple ball.

This can now be smoked as is, or it can be wrapped back in cellophane and stored in a cool dry place for several months to age and mature.

Note: If the kief you're working with is low quality then it will not have enough resin to create a soft gummy hash, and would be better suited for pressing into bricks of blonde hash.

This will be of much better quality than street hash, which tends to be made from lower quality material to make more or bigger blocks. If you use homemade hash, you'll learn why 90% of street hash is sold at rip-off prices. Those big-ounce chunks tend to contain only a small percentage of cannabinoids, mostly plant matter, and often adulterants.

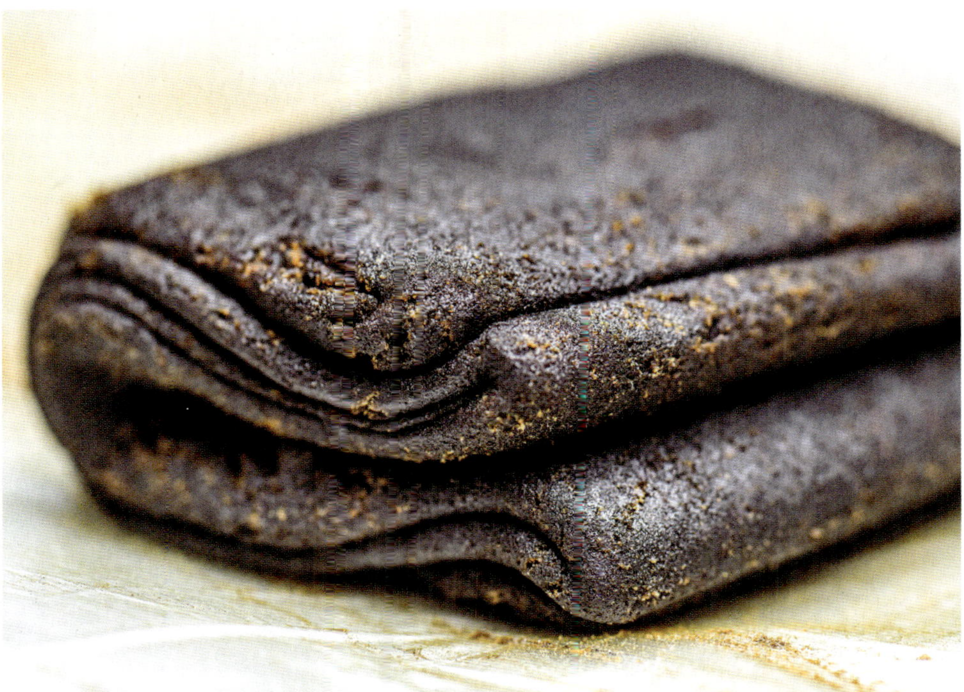

PHOTO: ERIC PALMER

The results are foldable and pressable. You can leave it as thin strips or fold and press it into a block or ball.

Temple Balls

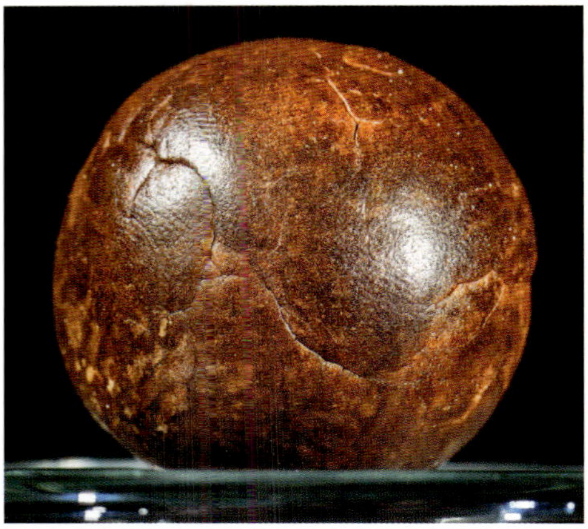

Fastbuds Mix Hash.

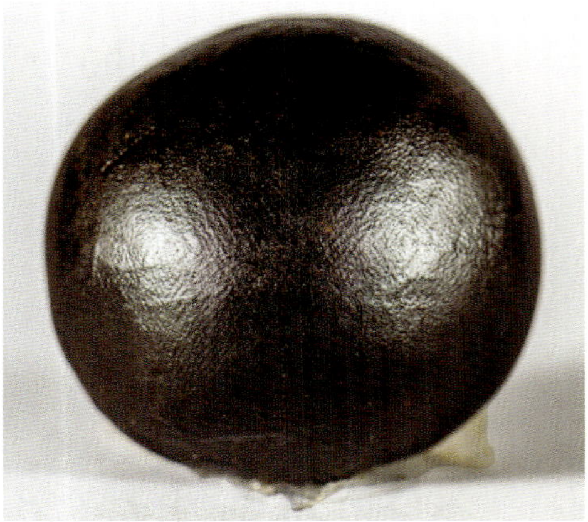

Auto Mix Hash.

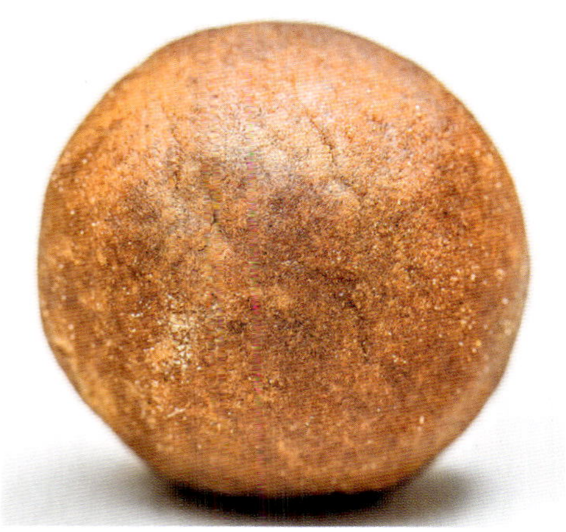

Champawat X Tangie by Loud.

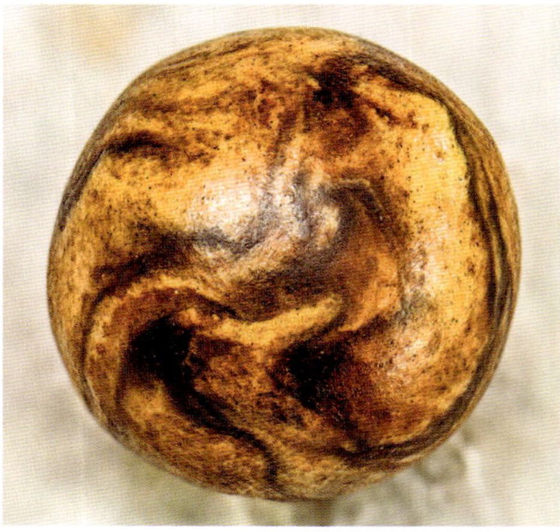

Terple and Divine Storm from In.

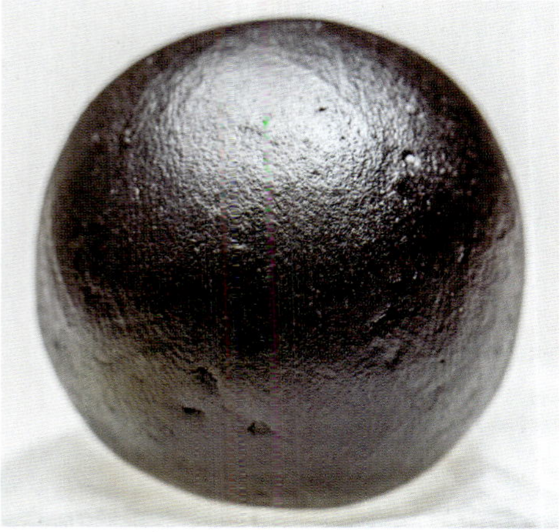

Dog Biscuits by Shinsimilla.

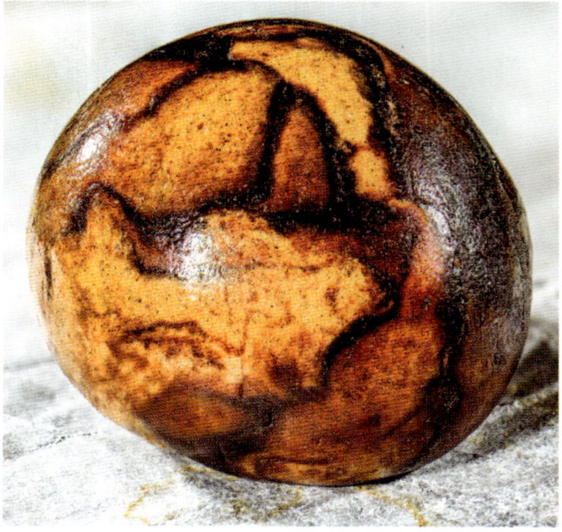

Terple and Divine Storm from In.

PHOTOS: ERIC PALMER

Rosin Press

A rosin press is any method that uses heat and pressure applied to cannabis flowers, bubble hash or kief to produce oil. A press can be anything from a weight to a hand-held or table-mounted pressing device, to a full-scale industrial-sized press, as long as the plates are hot.

Modern rosin presses are pneumatic or hydraulic presses about the size of a microscope, with two heated metal plates that compress together to extrude resin from cannabis flower, bubble hash or kief. The flower or bubble hash is packed into mesh bags and then placed into a folded parchment paper pouch, which gets pressed between the two heated metal plates. Smaller table-mounted devices produce the best results for home users, but a hair straightener can also be used as a press.

You start by placing the cannabis flower or bubble hash in a mesh rosin bag; kief is not recommended unless it's of very high quality and purity of heads, as it tends to have lower yields and produce a darker extract. Rosin bags come in a variety of different mesh sizes. If you are pressing bubble hash you should double bag it, with either two small micron bags (35 μm), or a small one to hold the hash and a larger sized bag outside (90 μm). This will help prevent the bag from ripping or breaking during pressing.

Using a rosin press:

1. Place the cannabis flower or bubble hash in a mesh rosin bag.
2. Turn on the rosin press and set your desired temperature for pressing. Flower pressing temperatures range from 180-220°F (80-105°C), bubble hash 140-200°F (60-90°C) and kief/dry sift 140-200°F (60-90°C).
3. Cut and fold a piece of parchment paper in half and place between the heated plates. You can secure the open ends to the top and bottom of the rosin press with magnets, which will allow you to place the filled rosin bag onto the plates, between the parchment paper.
4. Begin lowering the plates down to compress the rosin bag, allow the plates to preheat the rosin bag for 30-60 seconds, before compressing further.
5. As you apply more pressure you will see the rosin begin to flow out of the bag and run down the parchment paper. When you near the end of extraction, the rosin will stop flowing as quickly and you can use this as a good indicator of when to stop pressing.
6. Release the pressure, separating the plates and remove the parchment paper and bag together. It is a good idea to let this cool before opening and trying to scoop up the rosin.
7. Place the parchment paper on a cool surface or directly in the freezer for a few minutes. This will freeze the rosin making it much easier to lift off the parchment paper with a dab tool.

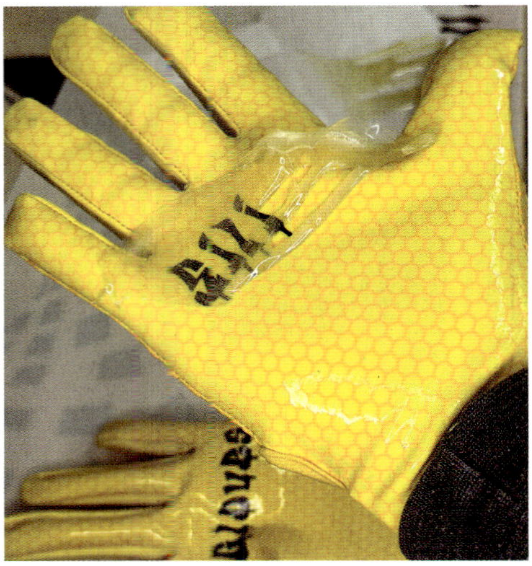

Non-stick, reusable gloves designed for the cannabis industry. Perfect for harvest or extraction work. Wipe with alcohol to clean.

Make sure enough paper is left free on the outside of the plate when the paper is folded over the kief, as the oil will be squeezed onto this area. Press the kief "sandwich" in a vise grip between the two hot plates for around five seconds. The timing and temperature may vary between units, and you can also experiment to determine what works best for you. Start by using small quantities of flower, bubble or kief, since it may require some trial and error at the start.

Don't open the parchment immediately after it has been pressed or it will come away like hot glue; instead, let it cool. You can chill a plate in the fridge and cover the parchment with it for a few minutes to reduce heat exposure. Remove the cold plate and peel the paper open. You will see the shape of your plate in the middle with oil surrounding it. Use a dab tool to remove the cannabis oil, which is very pure.

Fresh rosin is a sticky, viscous, honey-like liquid, making it hard to work with. However, you can change the consistency by using a process known as air curing. Rosin flavor, texture, and potency can be improved by curing freshly pressed rosin concentrate in a glass jar and storing it between 70-85°F (21-29°C) in a cool, dark place. Then, once a day, open each jar for a few minutes for air exchange, to prevent mold. This is called burping the jars. After a week or two, the rosin should have changed slightly in composition into a butter-like substance. It can be stirred with a stick if it requires more exposure to air in the jar. The longer you cure the rosin, the more buttery it will become, and it should eventually be easier to work with. Cannabinoid content will shift, and potency usually increases as a result. As terpenes mature, new flavors will also emerge. Some people wait for months to enjoy these changes. This is what air curing rosin does. It changes the rosin concentrate.

If you harvest more than 10 plants, it is worthwhile to use one or two to make a nice chunk of hash or oil. However, to produce bulk amounts of hash, you would need to use a lot of cannabis material. The purest hash is devoid of leaf matter and other foreign elements. Making your own hash, you can control for the presence of other content, guaranteeing better results. Cannabis connoisseurs regard homemade hash as an excellent way of getting the "best" from the plant. You may even end up producing a load of homemade hash instead of buds. Give it a whirl; you will be pleased with the results.

PHOTO: SILIGLOVES.ORG

Rosin Pressing

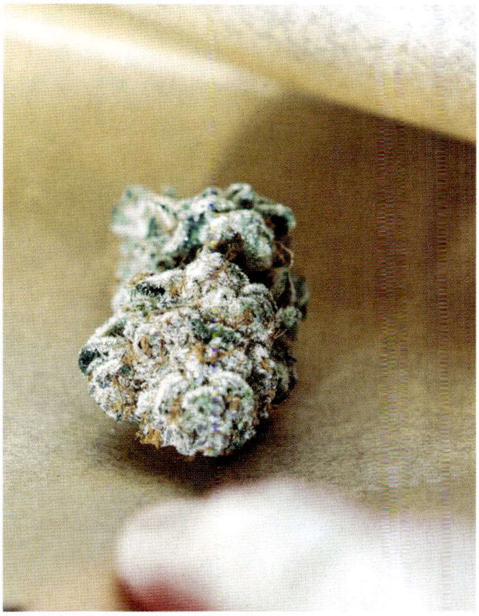

A bud is placed between parchment paper.

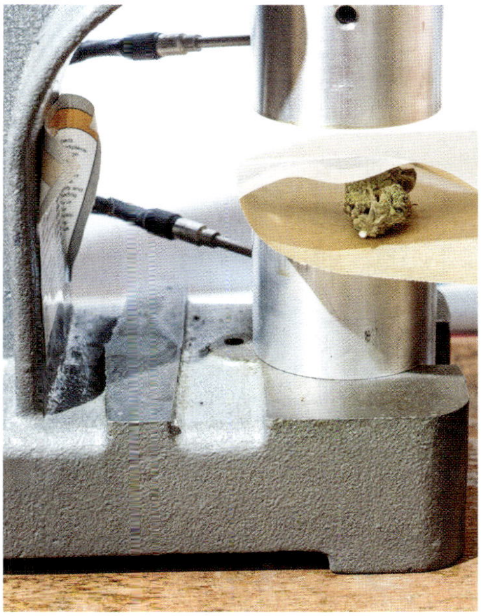

The parchment paper with bud is placed between the clamps of a Medisun Press.

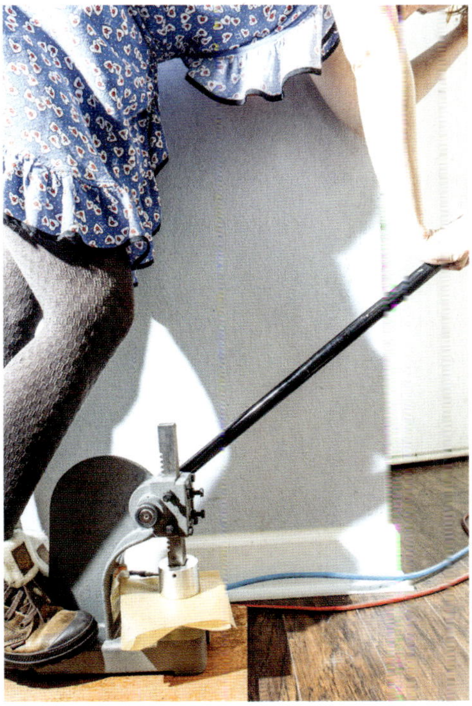

Allie Butler, of The Hepburns, stands on top of the press to create pressure.

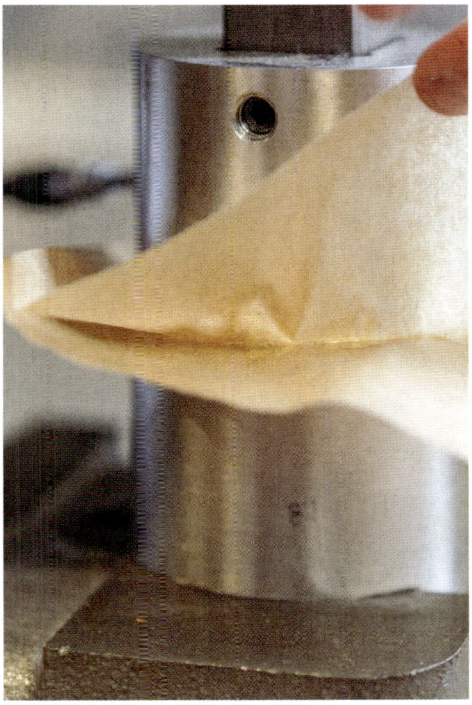

The bud is squashed by the press.

continues...

PHOTOS: GRACIE MALLEY, CANNABIS NOW

Rosin Pressing *continued*

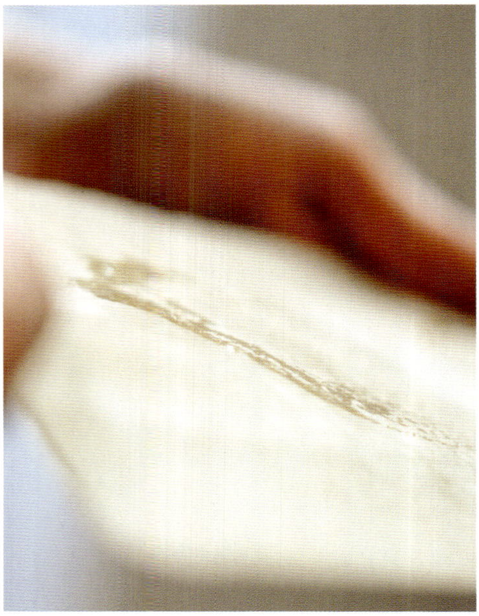

The freshly pressed rosin shines on the parchment paper after the bud has been pressed.

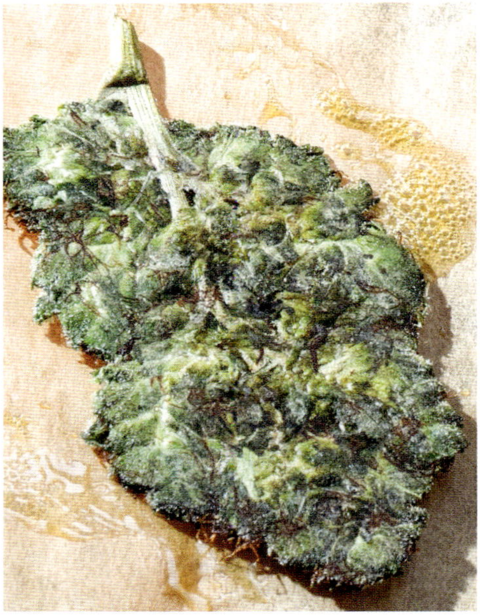

The flattened bud is surrounded by the rosin it has secreted.

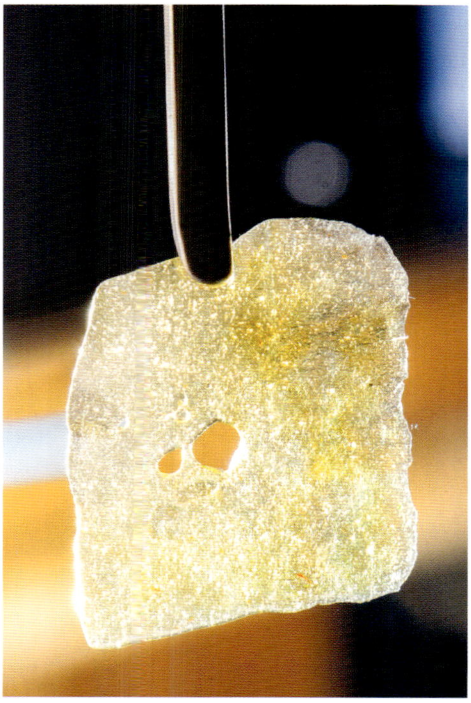

Rosin pressed from a bud glistening in the sunlight.

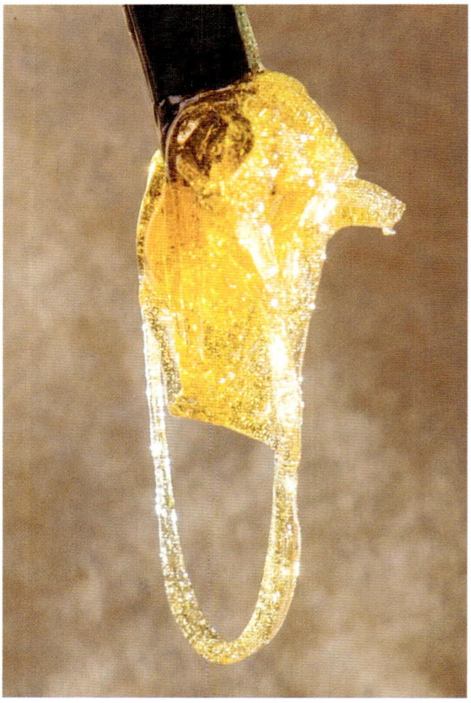

Rosin from the bud is collected and placed onto a dab tool.

PHOTOS: GRACIE MALLEY, CANNABIS NOW

Modern Rosin Pressing

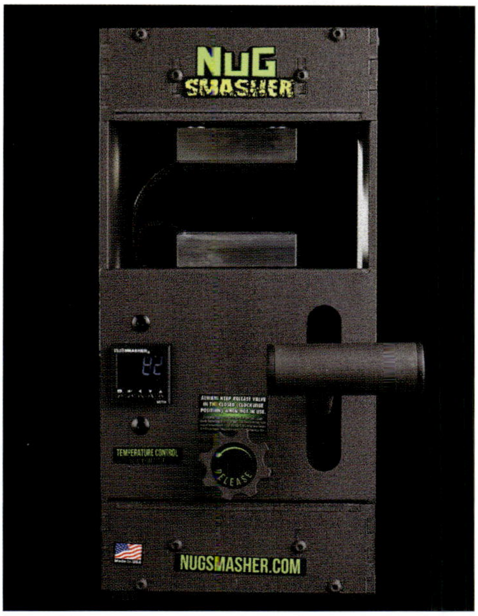

Place the press on a stable surface and set the plate temperature. The bags can hold up to 7 grams.

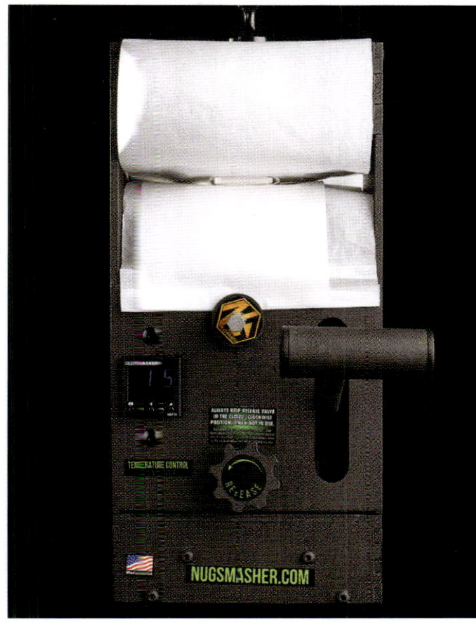

With a piece of parchment paper between the plates, add the bag and compress the plates until they hold it. Preheat for 30-90 seconds.

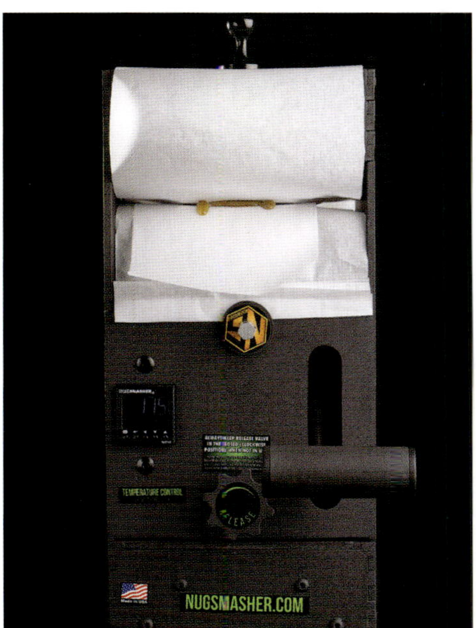

Push down on the lever to begin compression. Only minimal pressure is needed to begin extraction.

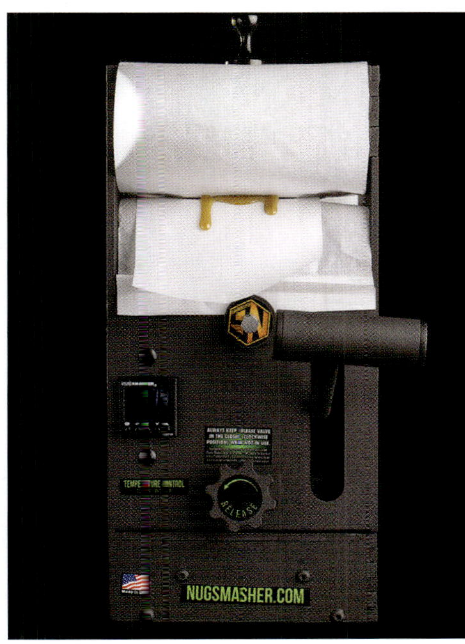

Increase the pressure slowly. If using a pressure gauge, go up in increments of 500–1000 psi at a time.

continues...

PHOTOS: RUSSELL-HOWLAND PHOTOGRAPHY

Modern Rosin Pressing *continued*

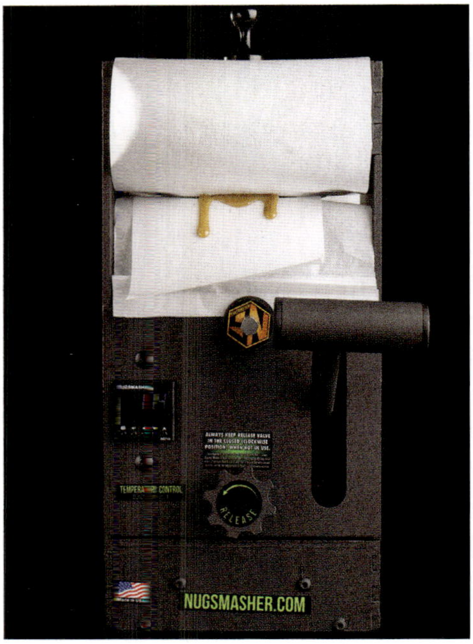

Increase the pressure to the maximum. As the flow of the rosin slows, try to add even more pressure.

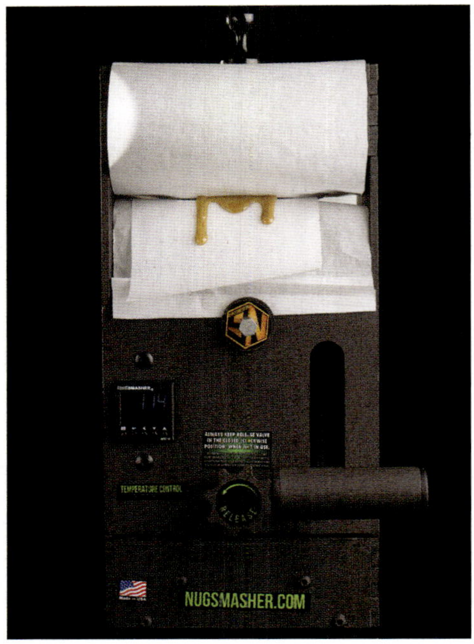

When the flow is almost finished, release the pressure, then remove the parchment paper and rosin bag.

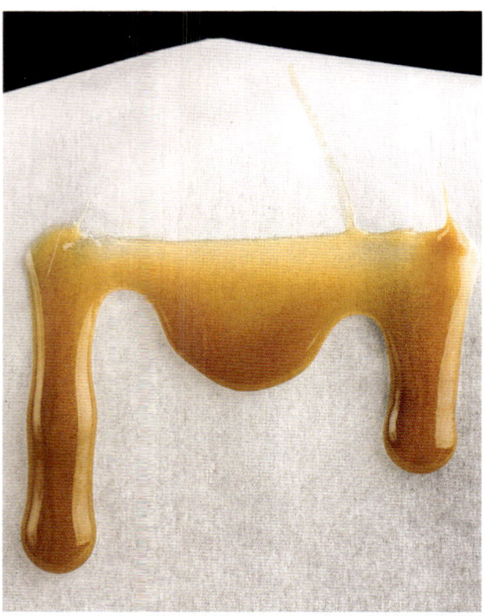

Open the parchment paper and remove the rosin bag. Scoop up the extracted rosin with a dab tool.

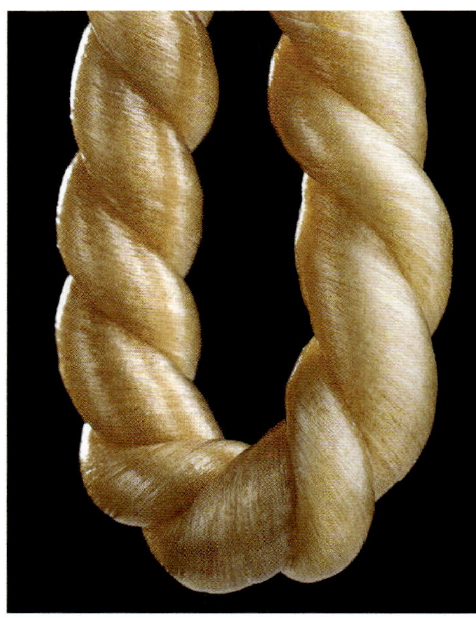

Rosin should be cured in a sealed jar for several days after pressing. It can be whipped or twisted into braids.

PHOTOS: RUSSELL-HOWLAND PHOTOGRAPHY

Rosin Air Curing with Hashtek

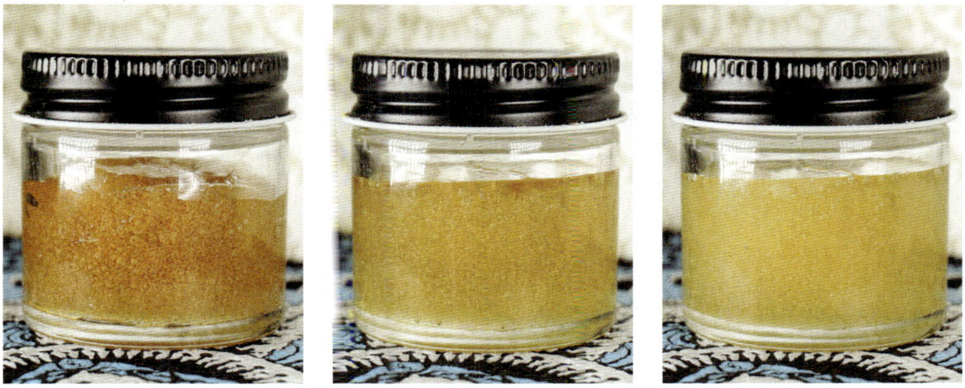

Day 1, 2, and 4 (left to right): Freshly pressed hash rosin is placed into a sealed jar and left to cure over several days.

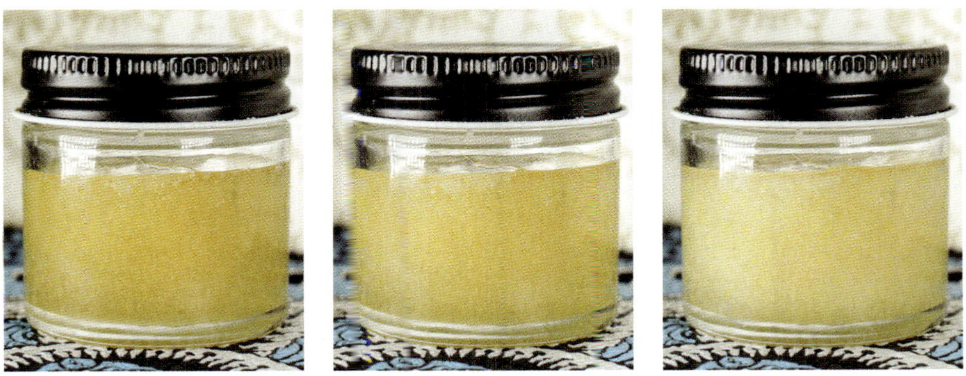

Day 5, 6, and 8 (left to right): After five days curing, the color and consistency of the rosin begins to change from a clear sappy form to a more semi-opaque creamy texture.

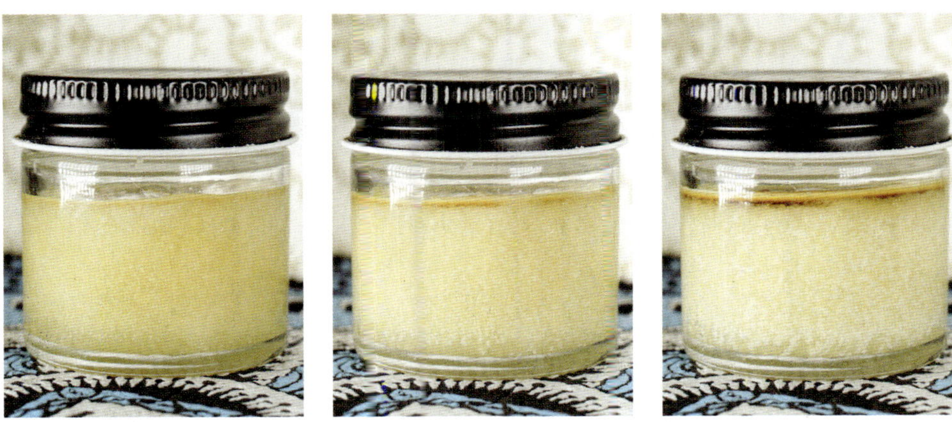

Day 10, 11, and 12 (left to right): By day 10, the rosin has begun to budder up and the terpenes are beginning to come out of phase and separate from the rest of the rosin. Note the layer of terpenes on top of the rosin by day 12

PHOTOS: HASHTEK.CA

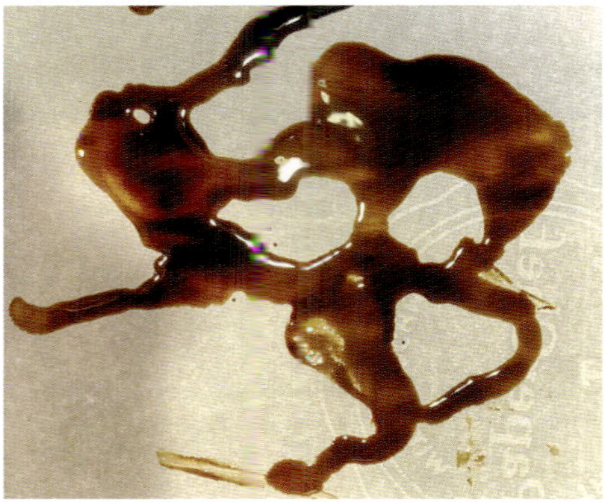

Hash oil is a sticky, viscous liquid, which often has a darker color due to the presence of decarboxylated cannabinoids.

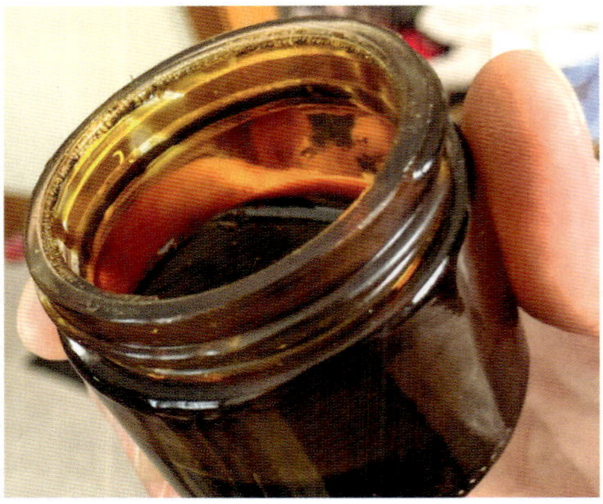

Hash oil can be consumed by spreading it on rolling papers or dropping it on a bong bowl. It can also be used as a feedstock for further refinement into distillates and isolates.

Hash Oils

Trichome resin is naturally in a viscous state, but is kept in a solid state by being contained within the waxy cuticle of the trichome membrane, which can be used in hash-making through techniques such as freezing and heat pressing. Freezing and screening can be used with burst trichomes to help break off fine particles of solid resin. Hash oils can also be screened, but their oleoresin stickiness makes the process more awkward. Resin can be poured through materials such as cheesecloth even in its viscous state. However, if possible, a purer extraction method should be used to produce a desirable final product. Hash oils have numerous uses, including as a tincture for medical applications. Items used during the process, such as the cheesecloth, can be placed in the freezer to extract any oils left behind.

Solvent Extraction

Isopropyl and ethanol are popular solvents for hash oil extraction, but the process for each is time-consuming, costly, and material-intensive. In addition, when done at home, it can often result in smaller amounts of lower-quality hash oil. Butane extraction is a much easier and more affordable way to produce cannabis oil as it produces better results in a shorter time frame. Butane was often the first choice of domestic cannabis oil makers due to its availability and ease of use; however, it is very flammable. CO_2 extraction is also popular (in commercial extraction settings) and safer, but it requires more expensive technology. Butane extraction can be performed indoors, with a closed-loop extraction system and a controlled ventilation system. When making butane hash oil (BHO) at home, it is far safer outdoors where gases can be naturally vented. Accidents with butane can and do happen, so have someone else nearby to oversee the procedure and step in if needed. Always wear gloves, safety goggles, and a mask to avoid inhaling any fumes, and have a fire blanket accessible. It can't be stressed enough how

PHOTOS: FATHER NATURE, ROBERT BUTTS

important it is to do this type of extraction outside in an open ventilated area, free from spark or static hazards. Don't smoke a joint nearby, and allow all of the butane to evaporate off the extraction surface before bringing it indoors to scrape up the oil.

In these procedures, a solvent is used as extraction fluid, and it separates raw cannabis oil from the harvested cannabis flowers. Raw cannabis oil contains psychoactive cannabinoids, terpenes, flavonoids, waxes and some plant tissue including chlorophyll in low percentages, and trace elements, such as non-psychoactive water-soluble matter in low percentages.

Cannabis oil is best extracted from highly resinous strains like Afghani. The best-quality plant materials, such as cured buds, tend to be used for oil extraction, although skuff/trim can also be used. The end material of a strain that isn't considered very resinous is still a very high-grade form of hash oil. However, strains not considered resinous or dry due to poor techniques are inadequate for cannabis oil extraction as not enough oil can be extracted to justify the procedure. The extraction process would need to be repeated several times with a plant like this before producing a substantial amount of psychoactive or medicinal oil.

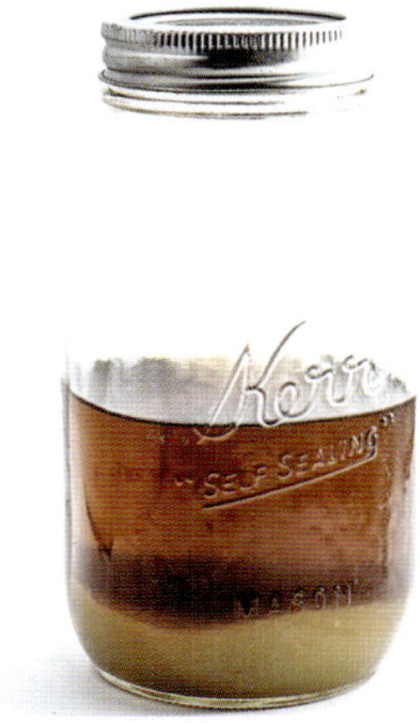

Ethanol extraction.

Every ounce of good-quality resinous plant material, such as cured bud, should produce 5 to 10 grams of hash oil. Every ounce of trim or skuff should produce about 0.5 to 2 grams, depending on its quality. However, all this is highly dependent upon the strain and quality of the grow. 20% THC should yield in that range depending on extraction method.

Butane Extraction

Butane extraction, based on industrial supercritical fluid extraction (SFE), is very easy to perform, but can be extremely dangerous if not done properly and with caution. Use only butane fuels that have been filtered several times, such as those recommended for flameless lighters or jet torch fuel. These types of butane are much cleaner and more efficient at extracting raw hash oil than butane fuel types commonly found at the drugstore or fuel depot. Flameless lighter butane is usually stocked by hardware stores and newsagents as well as headshops. Butane separates cannabis oils from most unwanted plant matter by dissolving the non-polar cannabis oil, producing a filtered oil like amber honey, for which it is sometimes nicknamed "honey oil." SFE can produce highly pure cannabis oil from resinous strains by separating cannabis oils from plant tissue, chlorophyll, and other trace elements. The final weight of the butane-extracted oil will be about the equivalent of the total weight of anything sticky or oily on the plant. You can purchase most home butane extraction equipment from a local headshop or online.

PHOTOS: DANKSHIRE PHOTOGRAPHY

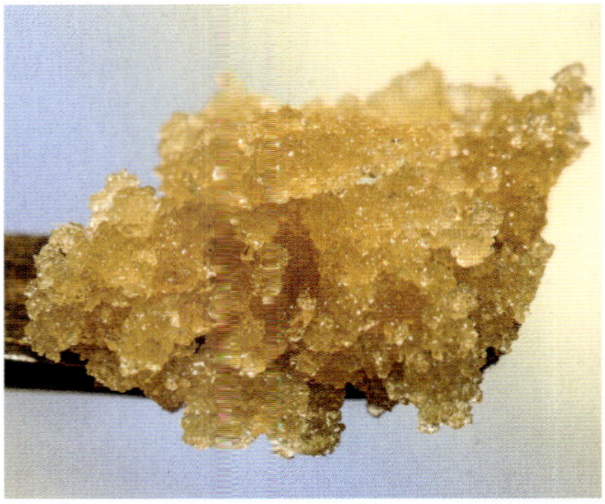

BHO sugar wax.

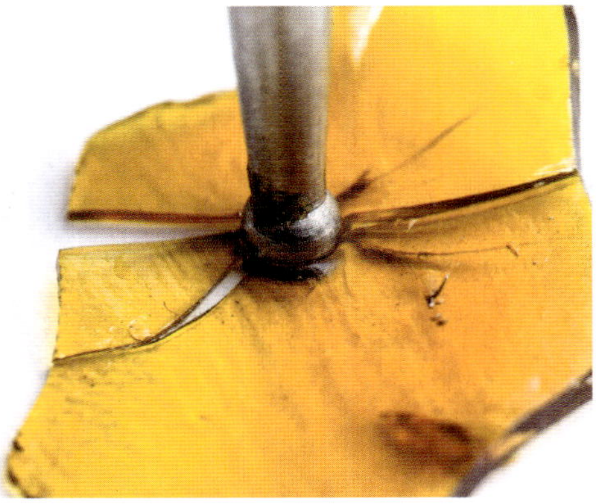

BHO shatter.

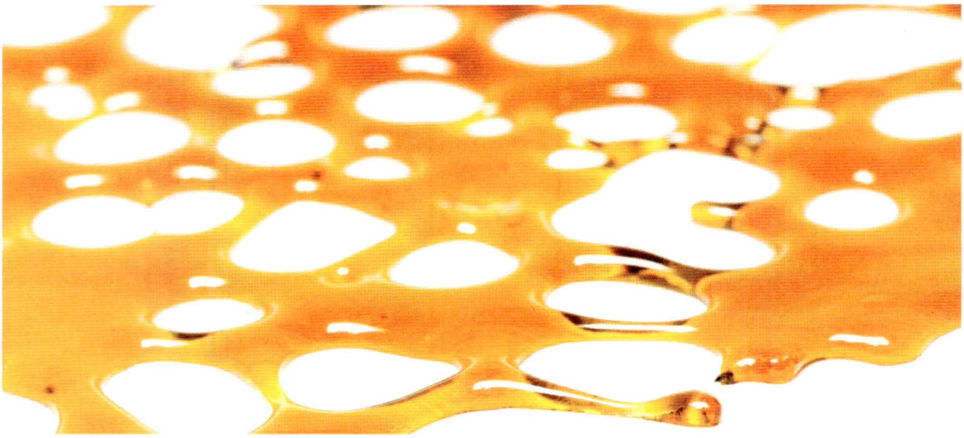

Shatter can be glass-like or pull-and-snap consistencies.

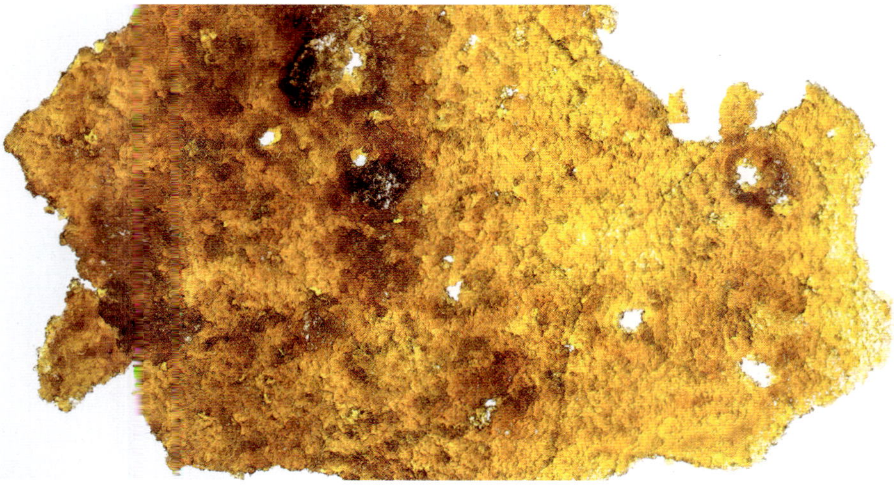

Resin can "sugar" up during shatter production due to improper purging temperature or resin agitation.

PHOTOS: DANKSHIRE PHOTOGRAPHY

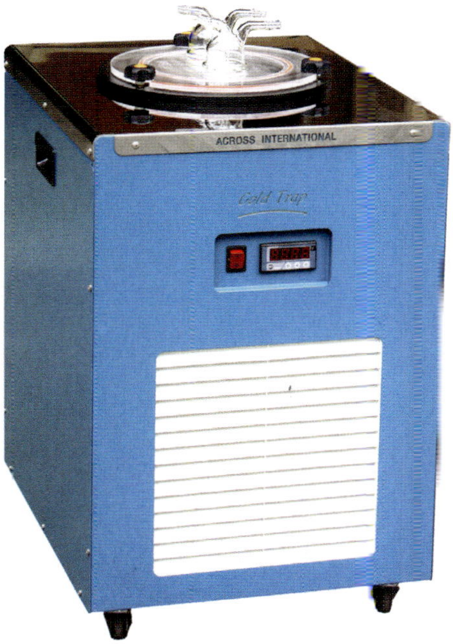

A cold trap for vacuum purging condenses vapors, capturing terpenes for reintroduction to cannabis extracts or for refinement into pure terpenes.

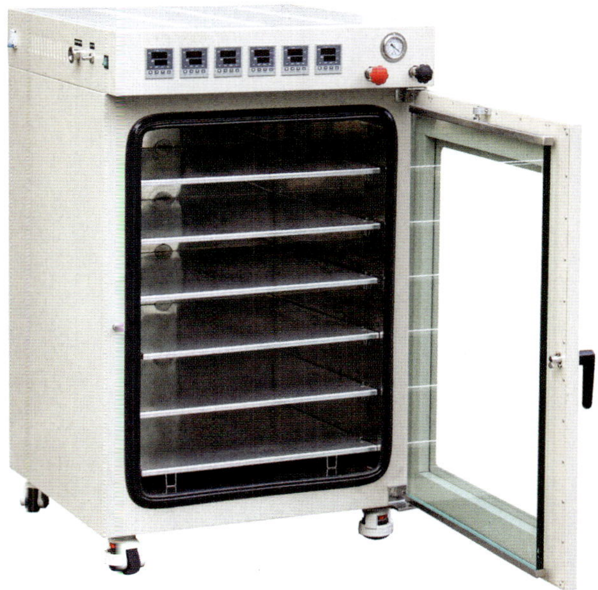

Digital vacuum oven to process large amounts of materials.

PHOTOS: ACROSS INTERNATIONAL

With butane, you'll need a pipe 1.5-2 inches in diameter, 16-24 inches long, made from either polypropylene (PP) or polyethylene (PE), as well as a cap for each end, which can be found in any home improvement store. If you cannot find suitable caps, you can use large bottle caps and Blu Tack to hold them in place.

Metal and glass blast tubes can be purchased from most head shops for $50-100 depending on size. They come tapered at the top with a small opening that fits the butane cap, and a larger opening at the bottom that can be filled with cannabis. Tubes typically range from the smaller 1 oz to larger ¼ lb sizes. Once the tube is filled with cannabis, you can take two coffee filters or some low-micron steel mesh and cover the bottom opening. Secure this with a hose clamp or other fastener.

The bigger the pipe, the more bud it can hold. PVC piping should never be used as it can be a health hazard.

You will also need a stand to hold the pipe off the ground, such as a lab or a microphone stand with a clamp arm. You will also need a filter—a cloth filter, like screening cloth, cheesecloth, bandage wrap with pores, or fine pipe gauze—to allow oil to drop through but leave the plant matter in the pipe; coffee filters will not work well unless they have a large pore size. Finally, you will need a clear plastic measuring cup, a clean wooden stick, such as a craft stick, and of course, nicely manicured skuff or bud.

The diagram below shows the parts in alignment without the stand. The whole unit should snap into place. The procedure will take about one hour, including two 20-minute breaks. Wear gloves and protective glasses. Never bring a flame or anything that can spark near the apparatus, ever.

Butane extraction procedure:

1. Drill a hole at the end of the first cap that allows the nozzle of the butane canister to fit neatly into it.
2. Drill six small holes near the center of the second cap.
3. Place the filter in the second cap.
4. Attach the second cap to the bottom of the pipe.

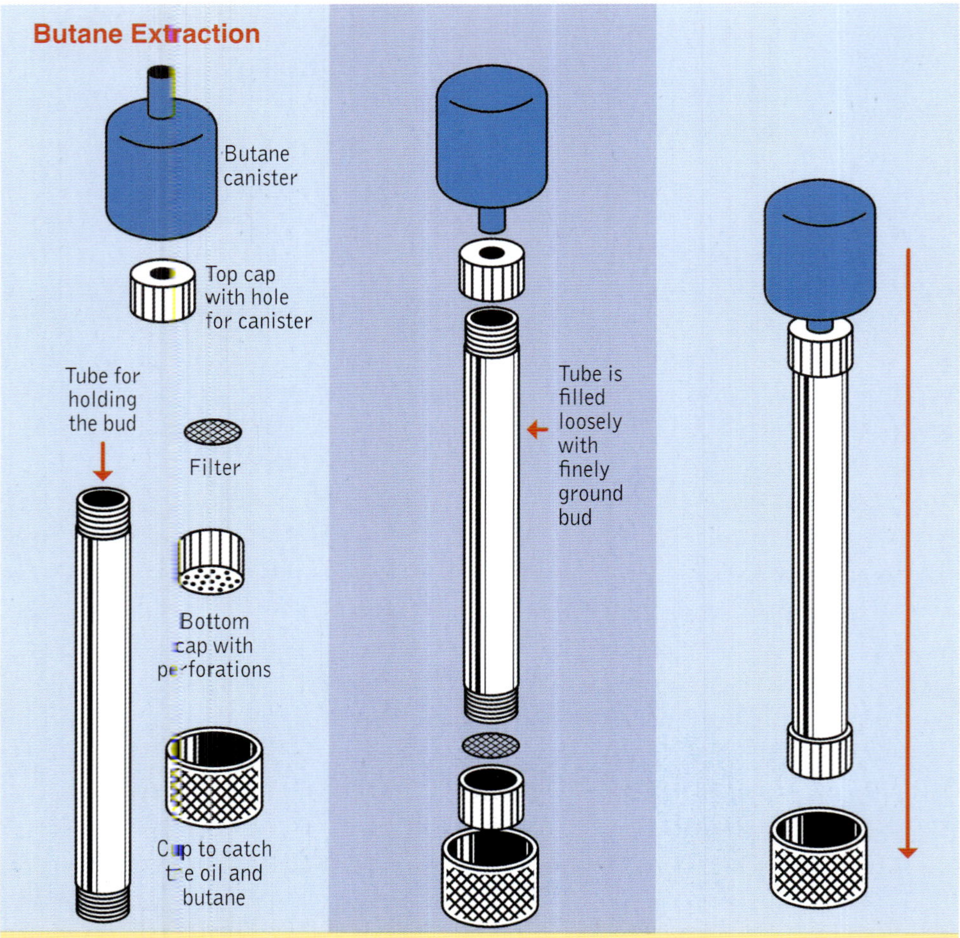

SAFETY NOTE: Butane is a volatile fuel and will combust when ignited by a spark. Unless you have a professional SFE unit with proper ventilation, perform butane extraction only outdoors, away from buildings and other people. Wear a face mask to avoid inhaling butane or the exhaust from butane extraction.

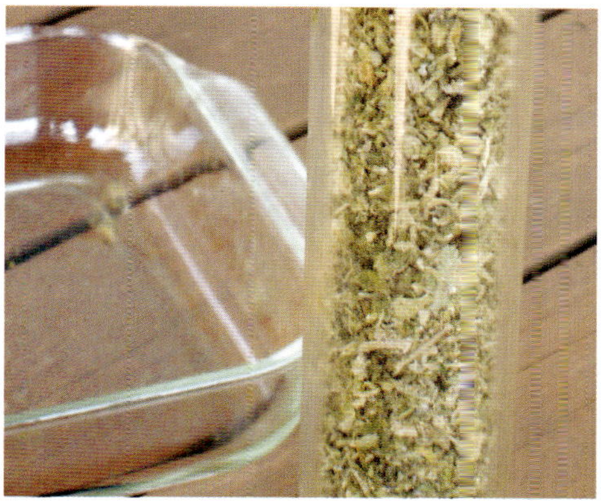

Glass extraction tube loaded with cannabis material to be extracted.

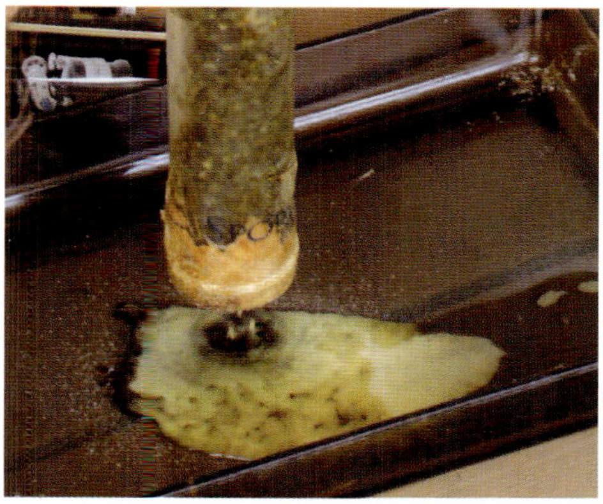

Butane flows through the top of the extraction tube, soaking the cannabis material, and exits the bottom

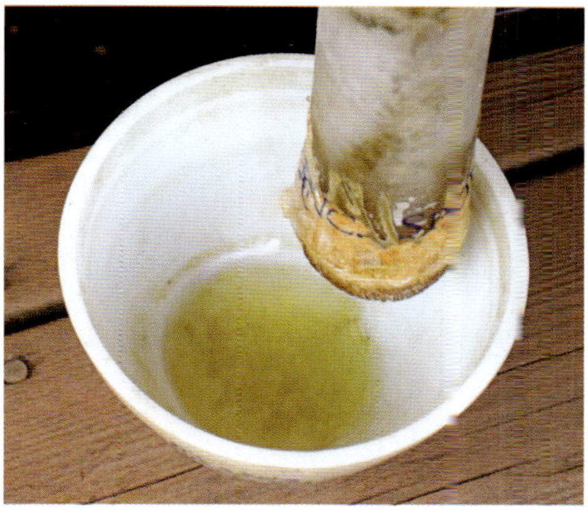

Allow all of the butane to exit the bottom of the extraction tube to ensure maximum yield.

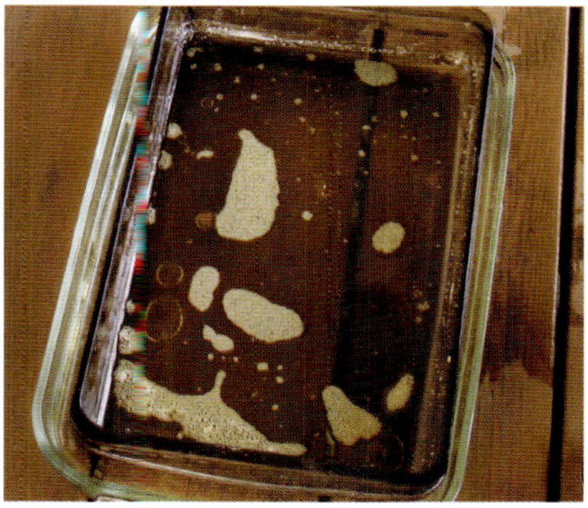

Collected butane, full of the extracted cannabinoids, needs time to finish evaporating, before further processing.

5. Fill the pipe loosely with your bud or skuff. Do not cram the skuff in.
6. Attach the first cap to the pipe.
7. Place the pipe on your stand over your clean measuring cup.
8. Open the butane can and turn it upside down, placing the nozzle in the top cap. Fill the pipe slowly, allowing the butane to draw the oils down through the tube.
9. Remove the butane canister when it is empty, and move a safe distance away.
10. Wait 20 minutes before approaching the apparatus, even if the top cap has not given any visible signs of fume release. The butane should have evaporated, leaving a mixture of oil and butane in the cup.
11. Open the top cap to allow all fumes to escape. Butane will still be active in the cup and bud in the pipe, so leave these two alone for another 20 minutes. The remaining oil in the cup is raw hash oil with some butane.

PHOTOS: MAX BORTNICK

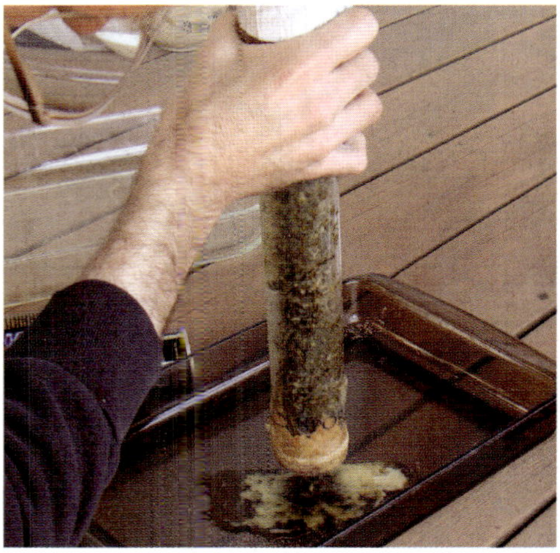

The less packed, the better the extraction.

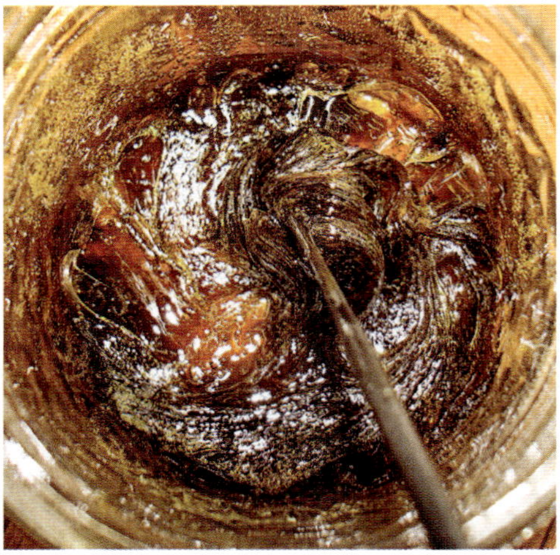

Cannabis oil from butane.

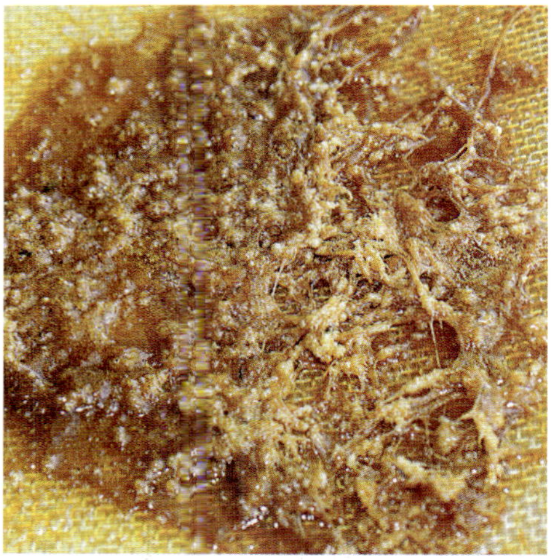

Butane honey oil yield of 16 grams from 175 grams of powdered bud.

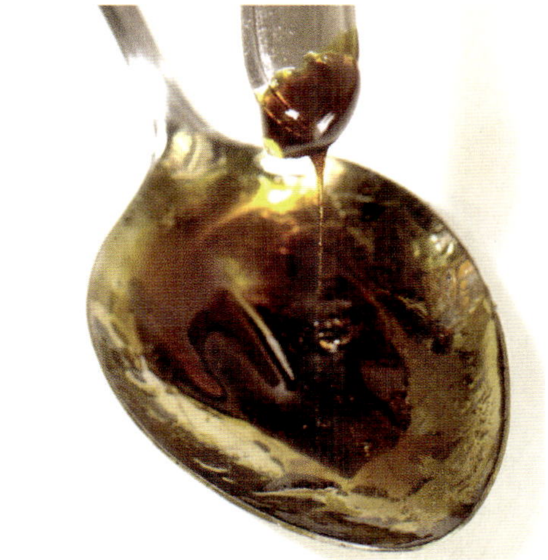

Hash oil is like a thick syrup.

12. Any remaining butane can be evaporated by placing the cup into a dish of hot water.
13. The raw hash oil you have just made should be ready to smoke in a few hours.
14. You can place this cup on a heat pad or hot plate to speed up final evaporation and ensure all solvent is gone.
15. The oil can also be whipped during heating to create nucleation points and cause the oil to change to a buttery consistency.
16. Further processing of the oil can be done by placing into a vacuum oven and purging the remaining solvent out. Vacuum ovens will also allow you to manipulate the phase state of the oil and you can create hard glass like resin (shatter), or waxy honeycomb states, by using different purging temperatures and techniques.

PHOTOS: MAX BORTNICK

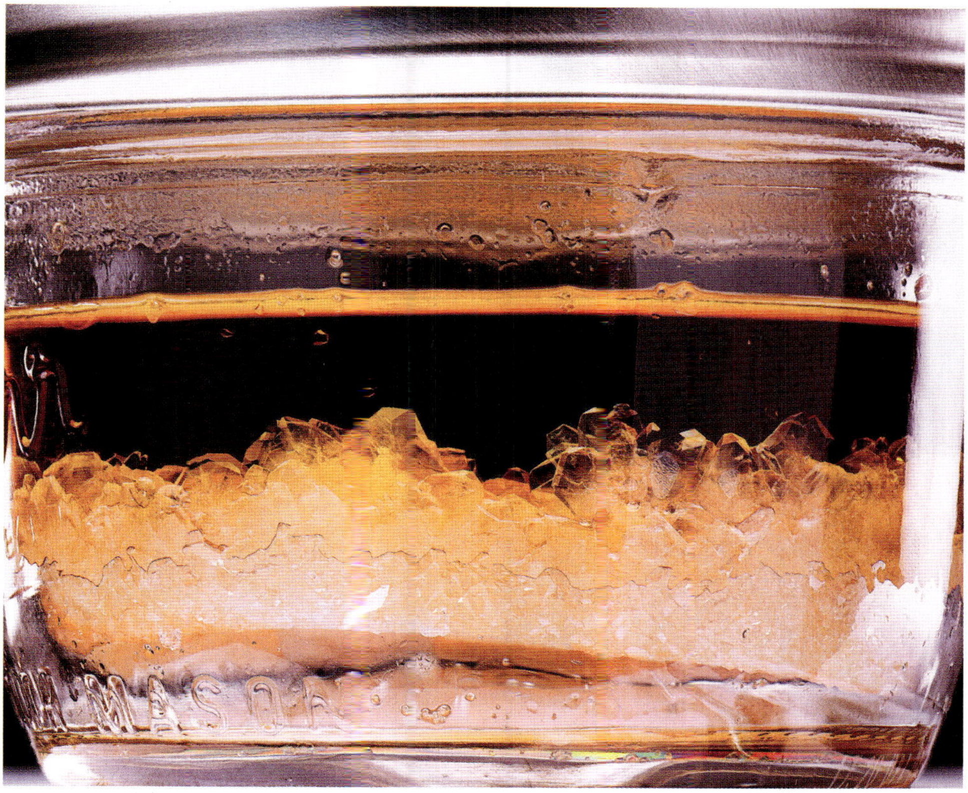

THCA Diamonds form under pressure in a sealed mason jar. Note the separate layer of terpenes on top of the crystal layer.

PHOTO: DANKSHIRE PHOTOGRAPHY

BHO Diamonds

BHO diamonds are a highly concentrated extract known for their crystalline structure and transparency. These crystals primarily contain non-psychoactive THCA, which converts to psychoactive THC when heated. The production process involves butane extraction, an additional crystallization step, and purging in a vacuum oven.

After butane extraction, the crude cannabis concentrate is allowed to evaporate. The concentrate is then placed in a jar and stored in a cool place for several weeks, allowing THCA crystals to form. During this period, the crystals separate from the liquid terpenes and other compounds. These THCA crystals are then removed from the liquid and placed in a vacuum oven to purge any residual butane and impurities.

Following purging, the remaining product consists of pure THCA diamonds. The separated liquid terpenes and other compounds can be reintroduced to the THCA diamonds to create a product known as "diamonds and sauce." Due to their high potency and concentration, BHO diamonds are typically consumed through dabbing and other vaporizing techniques in small quantities.

BHO Diamonds

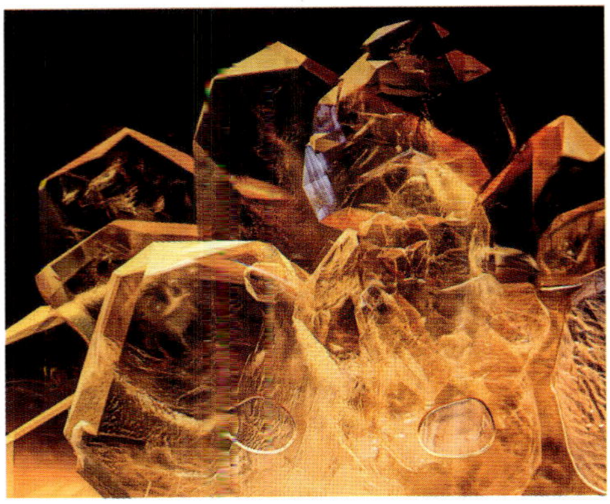
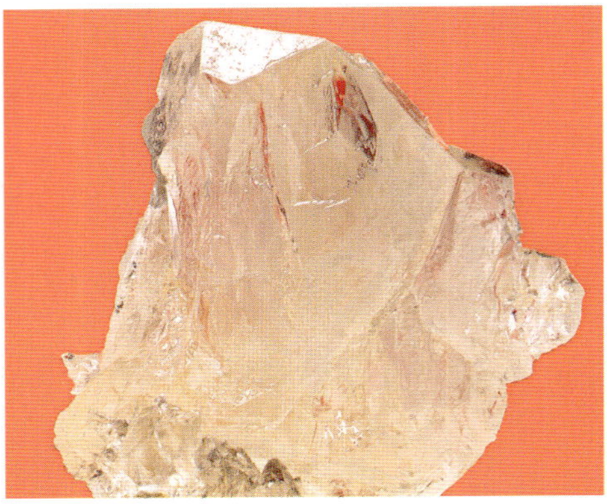

THCA diamonds can range in color from an amber to clear white, depending on extraction method and level of refinement.

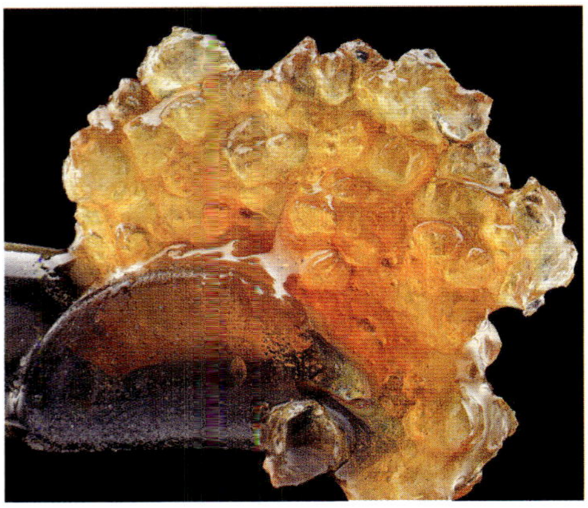
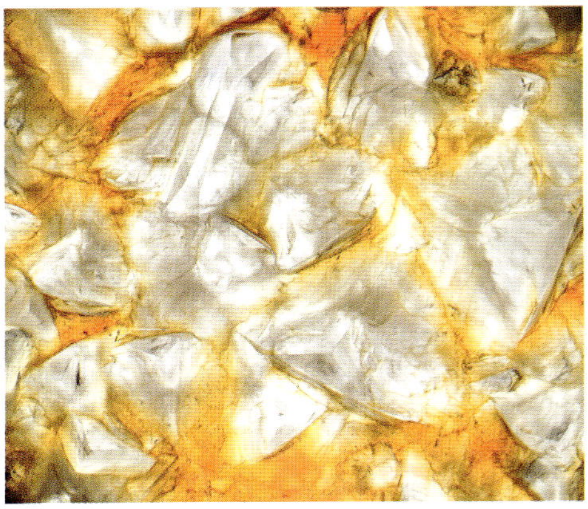

A dabber scoop full of diamonds and sauce. As you zoom in you can see that a single diamond is formed by many small crystallizations.

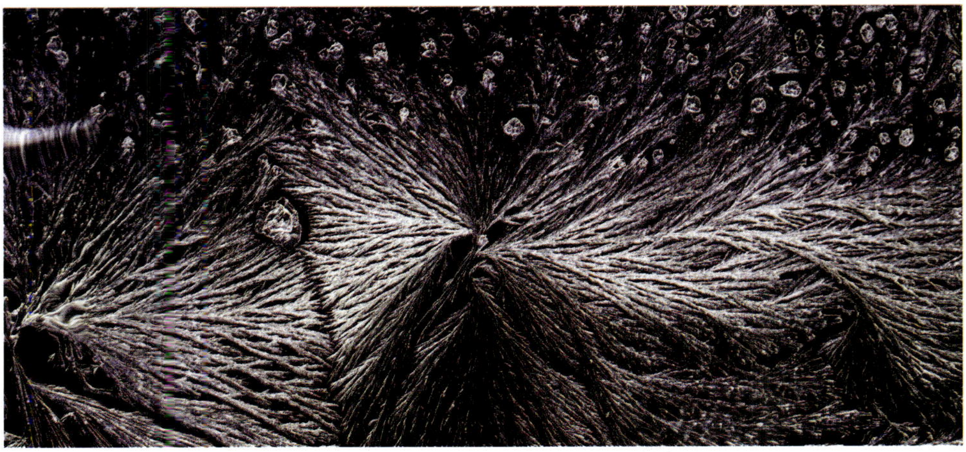

Electron scanning microscope image of the pattern of crystallization of a forming THCA diamond.

PHOTOS: DANKSHIRE PHOTOGRAPHY

Tips for Butane Extraction

SFE accidents caused by butane are not uncommon. Most occur when the pipe is full and butane is dripping into the cup below, or while the solvent is evaporating out of the extracted oil. During this stage the solvent is vaporizing and becoming a gas, which can be easily ignited by a flame or even small spark. It is crucial that you do not extract indoors and you do not bring your extracted oil indoors before it has fully purged the solvent. Any flame, spark, or ignition will cause that butane to combust. Almost all the accidents I have heard about occurred because a flame or spark ignited the butane. In most cases, it was caused by smoking near the pipe; however, even small static electric sparks from faulty electronics or old wiring can ignite the gas. Never smoke when you are performing butane extractions.

As the butane drains into the cup, it collects raw hash oil. It must be left untouched to drain completely. During this process, vapor and fumes will escape through the top of the cap and the cup.

After about 20 minutes, the butane will have passed through the pipe. Some remaining butane or oil extract may remain near the filter and end cap. You can give the pipe a brief shake to allow this to fall into the cup; forcing this through the tube by blowing, tapping, or pushing may add unwanted materials to your oil extract and is not recommended.

Use a silicone spatula or stainless steel scraper to wipe away any of the oil and butane mixture from the base of the filter. The butane will continue to evaporate as part of the SFE process, leaving behind only oil.

Butane has a low boiling point and evaporates at room temperature. If there is excess butane in the cup, place the cup into a bowl of hot, but not boiling, water and watch the butane entirely evaporate This is one reason why butane extraction should always be done outdoors, where butane will evaporate into the atmosphere instead of into your home, where it can become a fire hazard. You should eventually be left with amber-colored high-grade hash oil in the cup.

High-grade hash oil is sticky and best used in small quantities because it is very pure. As a result of this purity, cannabis oil is excellent for medicinal use. Cannabis oil can be best enjoyed by vaporizing, through which the user can enjoy a pure form of cannabis without carbon monoxide.

Some additional tips for butane extraction:
After the hash oil is removed from the cup, use 99% isopropyl alcohol to collect any residual oil. Add a small amount to the cup, enough to just swirl it around, and heat the cup at no more than 200°F (90°C) to evaporate the isopropyl but not the THC.

Hot Water Butane Evaporation

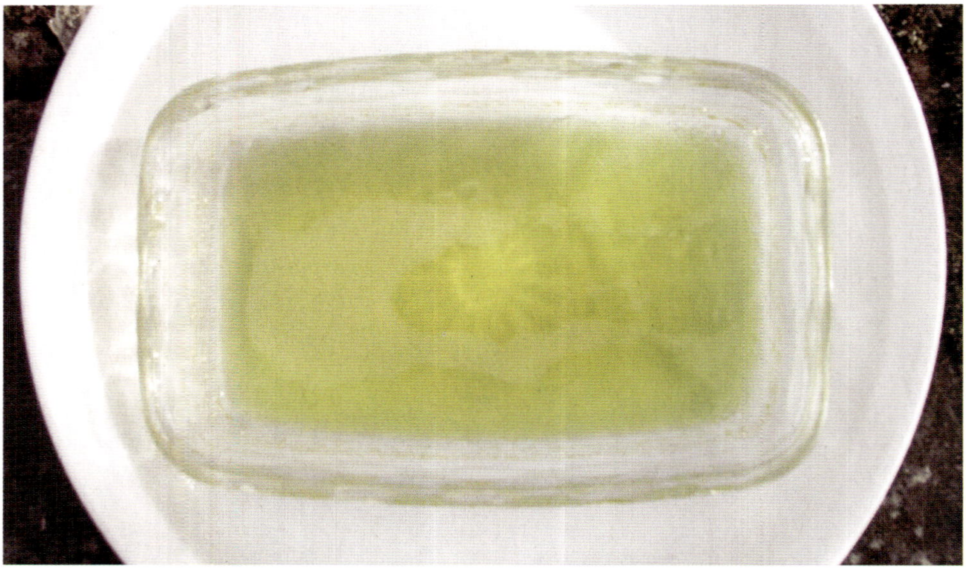

Allow butane in the collection tray to evaporate until only sticky, viscous hash oil remains.

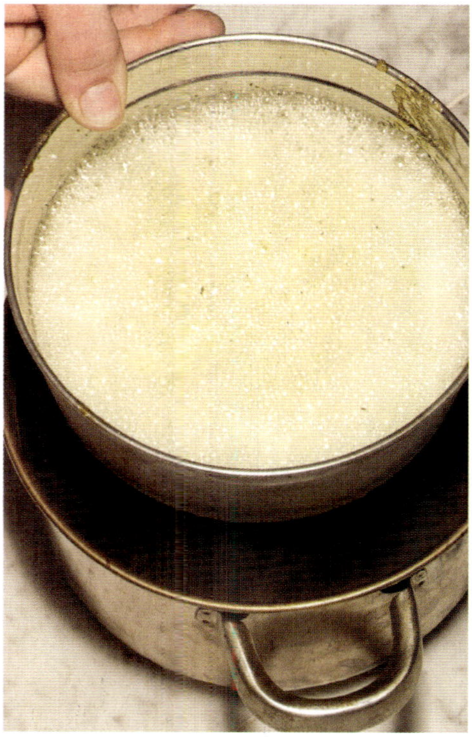

When first in a hot water bath, butane boils vigorously. Avoid overheating to prevent terpene loss.

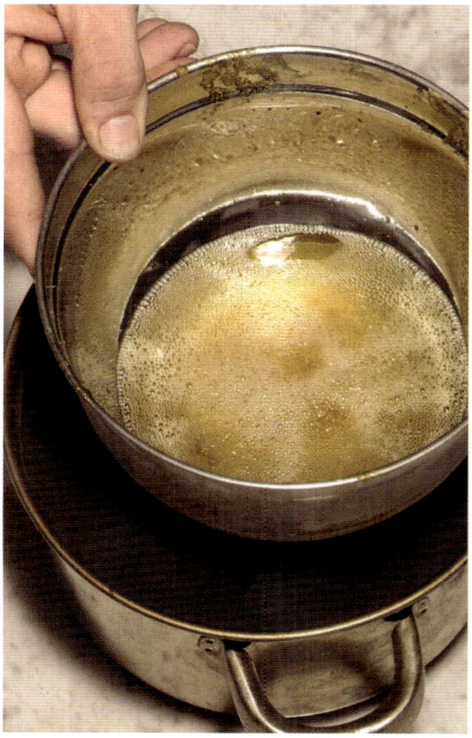

Continue evaporating until most butane has boiled off and the solution turns into thick, viscous, sticky oil.

PHOTOS: MAX BORTNICK

BHO Further Evaporation

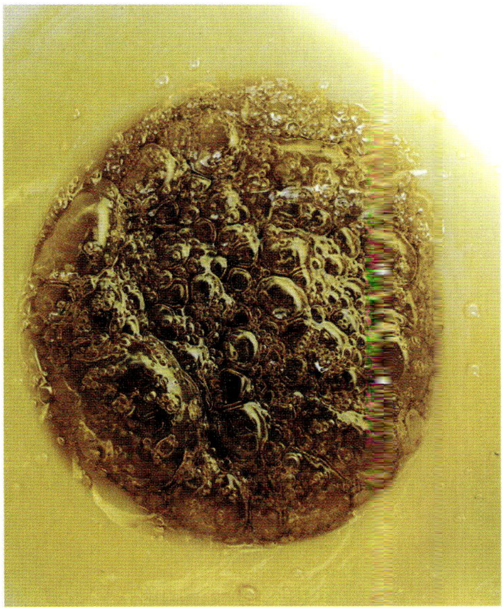

After removing butane, heat the BHO in a jar or under vacuum to further process and stabilize the oil.

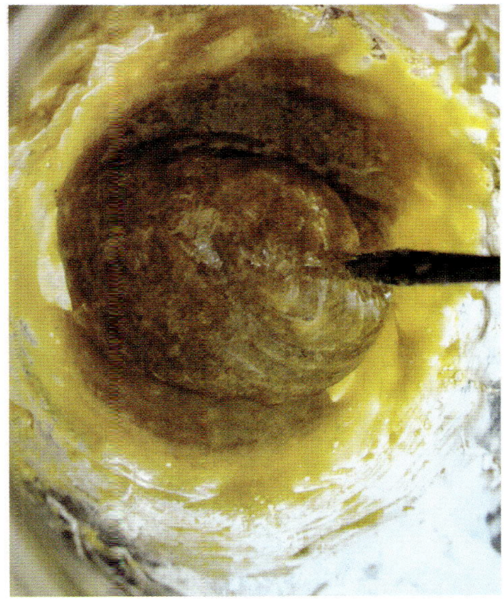

Heating and stirring the BHO purges more solvent and causes the oil to nucleate, changing its state.

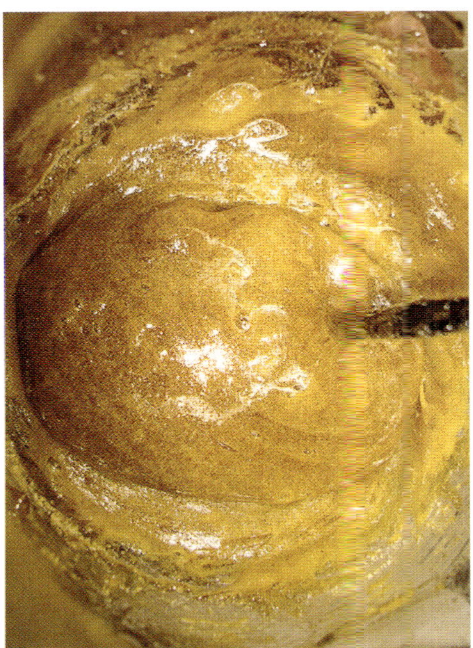

Stirring promotes remaining reactions. It's good to do this for a while.

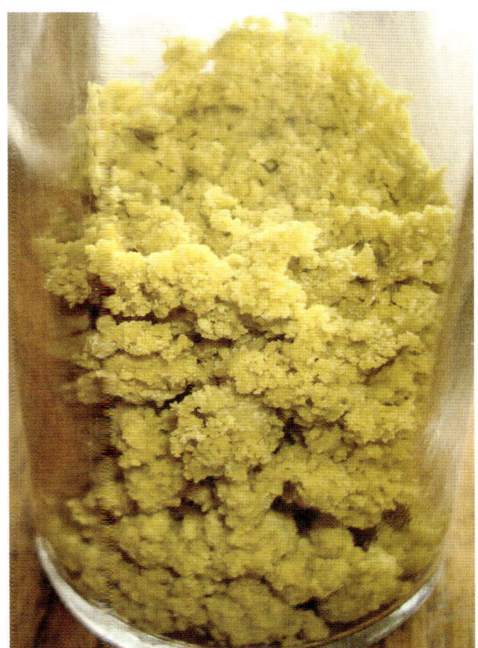

With the right temperature and stirring, you can turn sappy BHO into a crumble or wax-like consistency.

PHOTOS: MAX BORTNICK

You can also perform a second extraction using the same procedure to remove any excess oil still left in the buds. Whatever plant matter remains should then be mostly devoid of cannabinoid compounds. Do not force all the butane through quickly; slow release of butane into the pipe allows sufficient time for the SFE to occur, which improves the quality of the final extract.

Most bottled butane is not pure, as it is usually mixed with chemicals to indicate gas leaks. These chemicals can interfere with the SFE process, so ensure the butane purchased is as pure as possible. Before extraction, grind the buds or skuff to a fine powder.

Resin or oleoresin is essentially composed of starches and fat stores from fat-related molecules in the cell membranes of chloroplasts, amyloplasts, and mitochondria. These products may also contain minimal parts of the cell, such as organelles' components, which is completely natural. If these starches and fats are completely separated from the cannabinoids, what would be left is an absolute oil.

Butane is not the only solvent able to extract oils from cannabis, but butane and other non-polar solvents extract less chlorophyll from the plant matter and therefore yield a lighter colored and nicer crude extract than polar solvents. Professionals use closed-loop extraction for SFE, which is generally expensive. However, low-end models of closed-loop extraction setups are available at more affordable prices. The unit resembles laboratory-grade equipment made from metal. They are available unassembled, to be put together by the user. Building a closed-loop extraction unit requires both metalwork skills and an understanding of PSI-rated parts to tolerate pressure-related stress.

Closed-Looping

SFE is a dynamic system of chemical changes. The system of solvent extraction discussed above is an open system, in which elements, such as when the gas evaporates, are not under our control. Closing the system means all aspects of the system's dynamic need to be controlled, which entails error correction in design and operation for optimal systems.

Closed-loop cannabis oil extraction systems consist of metal containers, pipes, valves, measuring systems, solvent recovery and cooling systems. The device is vacuumed to remove oxygen, which not only takes up space that butane can occupy but also can cause vapor lock, blocking the looping of the system. Thus, closed-loop systems must contain a vacuum port that can be opened and closed to manage the presence of oxygen.

A metal container acts as the butane chamber. For gravity-based systems, this chamber is placed on top, while flat systems make use of pumps to fill the chamber with butane. To help with calculations, a pressure-measuring device is used to indicate the pressure inside the chamber. As the chamber fills, the pressure increases. Pressure gauges can be used to measure the PSI. Expert systems will lower the pressure of butane by chilling the chamber and remove any residual oxygen with additional vacuuming. The less oxygen, the better the extraction process. Cooling the chamber can be accomplished with ice or professional coolants.

To achieve a higher density of plant material, experts put different sizes of chopped material in the plant material chamber, which they place under the butane chamber in gravity-based systems; flat systems pump from the butane chamber to the material chamber. Finely chopped material can be packed in to fill the chamber, but it will take longer to process. In this way, closed systems, unlike open systems in which densely packing the chamber is suboptimal, can work through it if given the extra time. The butane will leave its chamber, pass through the material chamber, and then be recondensed into a liquid before returning to the butane chamber again hence the term closed-looping.

The butane begins its loop by condensing on the cold walls of the butane chamber. A valve opens, allowing the liquid to flow from the butane chamber into the plant material chamber, where it turns it into a gas, which increases the pressure. When the used butane returns to its initial chamber, the coolness causes it to condense. The process repeats, forming the loop. While butane evaporates into the air in an open system, the pressure in the closed system is regulated by the design of the apparatus and measured with readers.

Any leaks that occur contaminate the closed-loop system with air. The butane remains as a gas instead of liquid, which prevents the looping of butane back into the chamber. This vapor-locking the system causes the extraction to stop. Because of this, error correction in design is essential for optimal performance. Once it works, it works well. When you have a loop, you can continuously extract until everything is isolated.

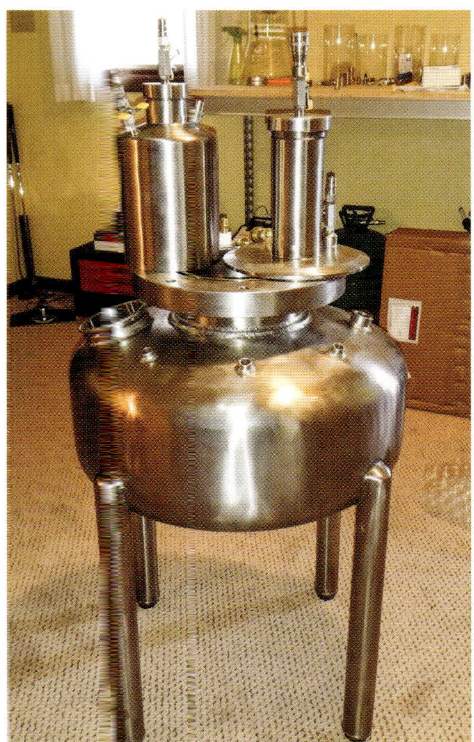

Closed-loop extraction system.

PHOTO: TAMISIUM EXTRACTORS

To stop the extraction process in a closed-loop system, the butane must be drained, along with the oil extract, from the material chamber to a third gathering chamber. Gravity helps to push the extract into this chamber. As this third chamber fills, the butane extraction slows down. A tube runs from the third chamber up to the butane chamber, allowing for a quicker evacuation of the gaseous butane so that the extracted

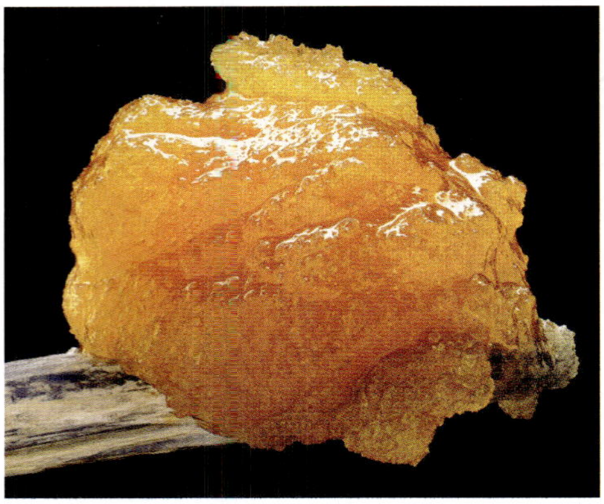

Live resin: High in cannabinoids and terpenes.

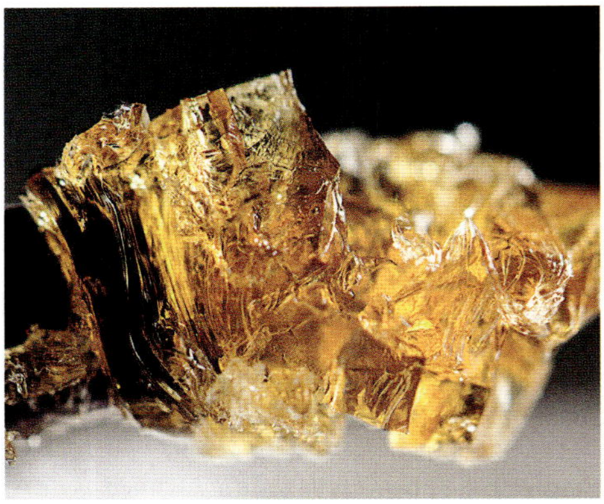

THCA diamonds can have potencies higher than 85% THC.

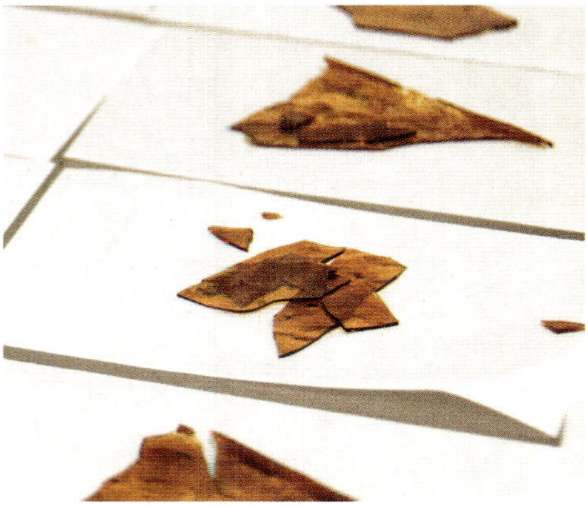

Pieces of shatter laid out for packaging.

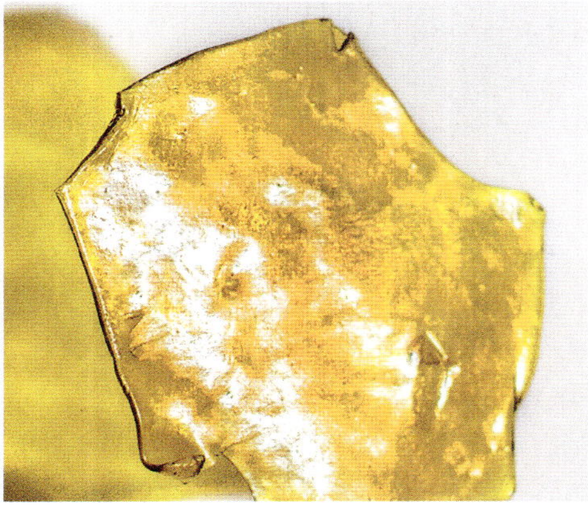

A small piece of shatter produces effects.

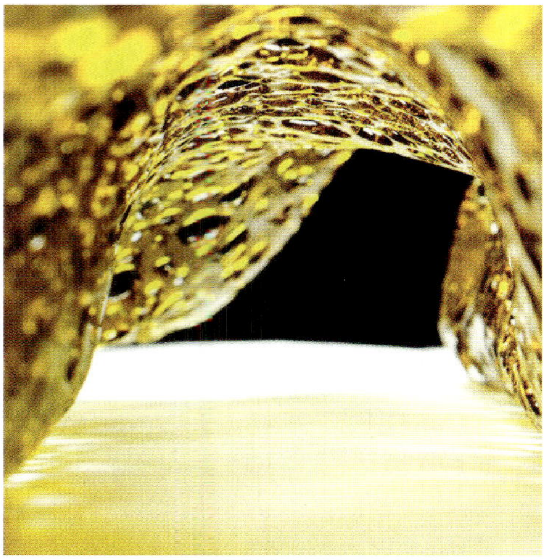

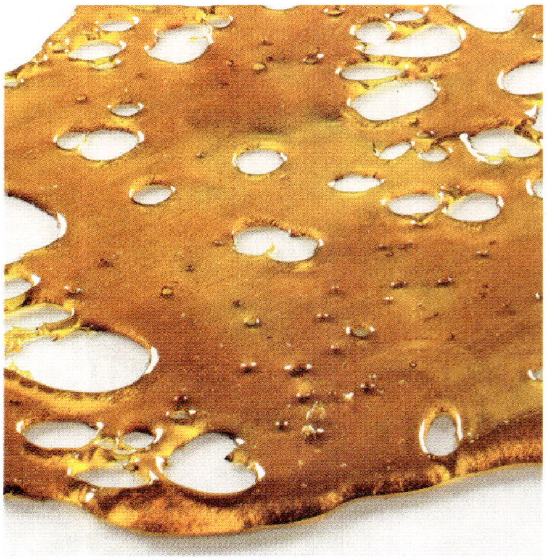

The color of the extract depends on the strain or age of the material. Older material tends to produce darker extracts

PHOTOS: DANKSHIRE PHOTOGRAPHY (TOP ROW), CRAFT CONCENTRATES (MIDDLE ROW), TRICHOME ART (BOTTOM ROW)

oils flow more quickly. The valve between the butane and plant chambers is closed, and the now-chilled butane chamber recovers butane from the other two chambers. Because of the lower pressure in the butane chamber, the butane transforms into a liquid. Warm water surrounding the gathering chamber creates a pressure difference between the chambers.

The amount of butane recovered can be measured. If you recover all that you started with, you are looking at a 100% recovery. This is why it is recommended, even necessary, to measure PSI for expert systems. Cooled butane will have a lower PSI, so it is essential to measure your butane while cooled as well.

Whichever port was opened for vacuuming must be reopened for oxygen to re-enter the system. Otherwise, the system will remain in a vacuum. At this point, the extract should be in the gathering chamber and can be tested through spectroscopy for quality analysis of cannabinoid content and ratio.

All professional systems base their designs on parameters determined through applied SFE processes. These are mainly concerned with the size of each chamber and the quality of pipes used between chambers. Quality pipes for SFE can be very expensive, but good results depend on the quality of the materials used. The SFE operator measures the size of the pipes and extraction timing of the chopped pieces to compare graphed plots of the amount extracted over time for each technique to determine what produces the best result.

Engineering a system like this requires an understanding of pressure and the dangers of using sub-quality metals that cannot withstand stress. Never allow the system's pressure to pass the PSI it was built to manage, or you risk the setup blowing up. That means using metals rated for SFE and parts that are flame resistant and won't spark. Gaskets should be used to allow the gas to evacuate. In professional setups, this evacuated gas is released through an emergency ventilation hood in an area away from the operator. If you are unsure or do not understand the PSI of any system, do not use it.

The system must be tested with butane before any plant material is added. The engineer and operator should measure the butane amount as it transforms from a liquid to a gas to a liquid again. If the system works, the reclaim of that gas should be 100%.

Closed-looping systems can be as simple as three chambers and some piping, and as complex as a sophisticated piece of apparatus with target pressures met through monitoring the device. The more control you have over each closed loop part, the more control you have over the results. You gain control by using heating elements instead of warm water, professional vapor lines, rupture discs, active pumps, timers, and LCD readers. Scaling up your closed-loop system can take you from a device the size of three pots to an operation the size of a pharmaceutical plant, with each step carried out on different floors that are connected with pipes and monitored by chemical engineers.

The Original Resinator Post-Harvest Processing

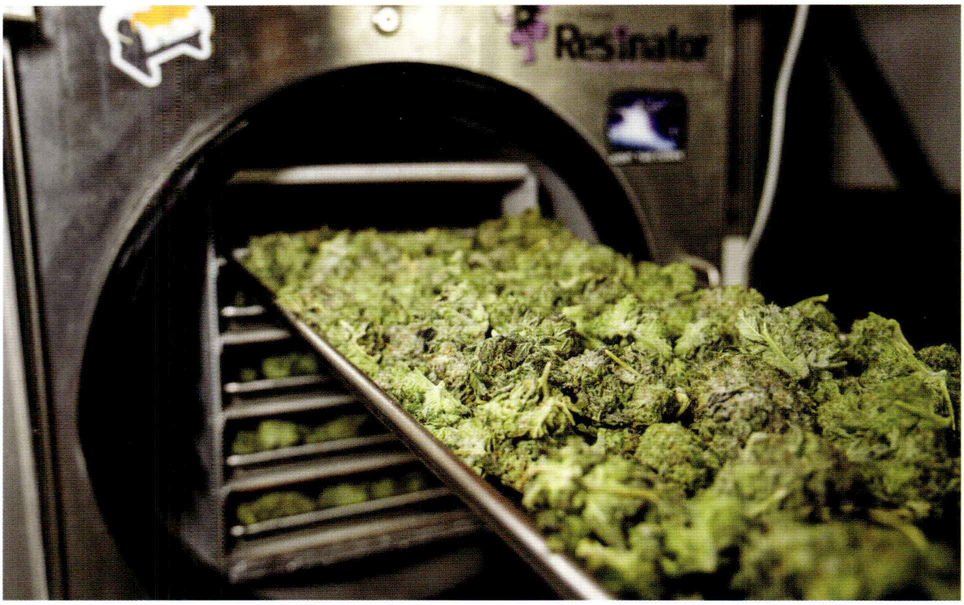

Fresh frozen buds that have undergone the Cryo-Trim® process in an Original Resinator and are heading to the freeze dryer to complete the Crop-to-Cure® process, which dries and fully cures flowers in 48 hours using a specialized lyophilization technique.

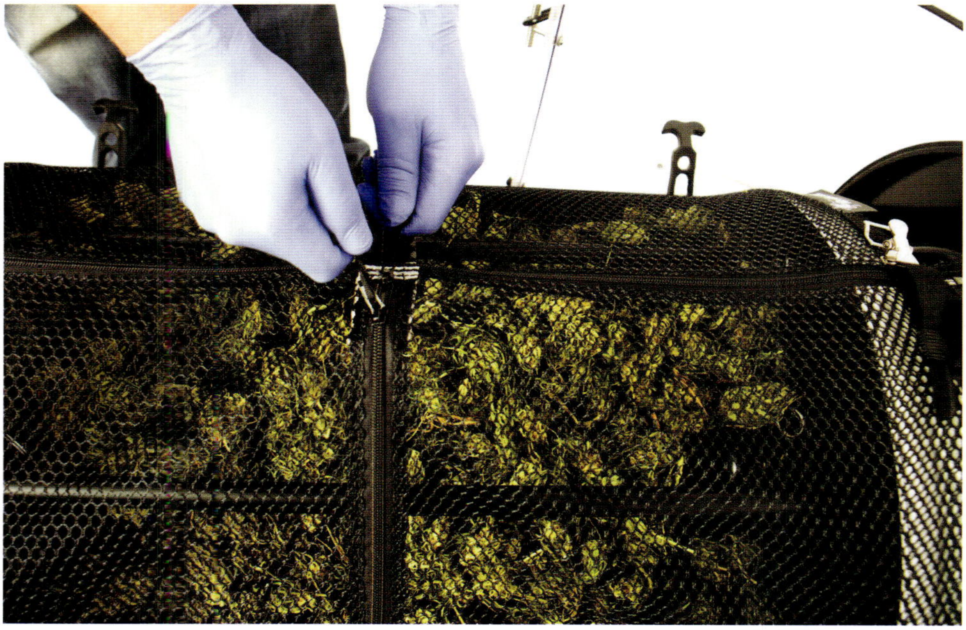

Previously hang-dried cannabis buds that have been loaded into an Original Resinator XL to be trimmed by one of their bladeless drum screens using patented liquid CO_2 technology known as Cryo-Trim®.

PHOTOS: THEORIGINALRESINATOR.COM

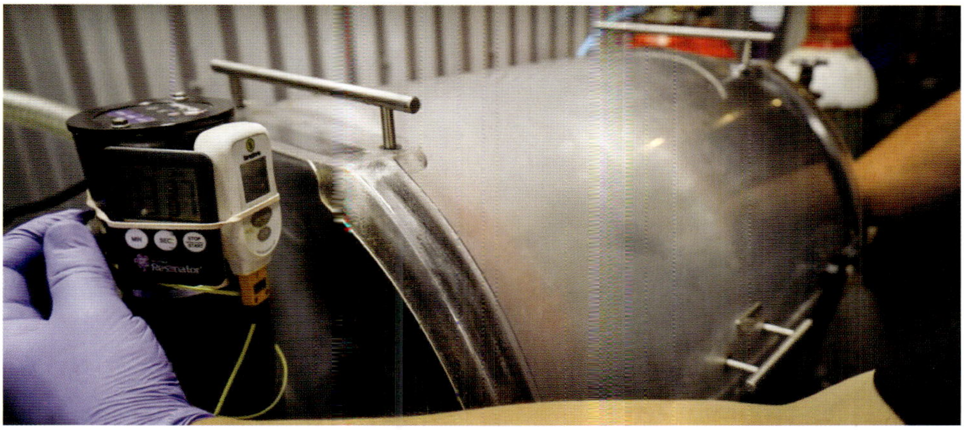

The Cryo-Trim® runs in the Original Resinator XL and extracts resin by sifting it with liquid CO_2. The goal here is to extract as many resin glands as possible while leaving leaf matter behind. The result will be a very pure level of resin extraction.

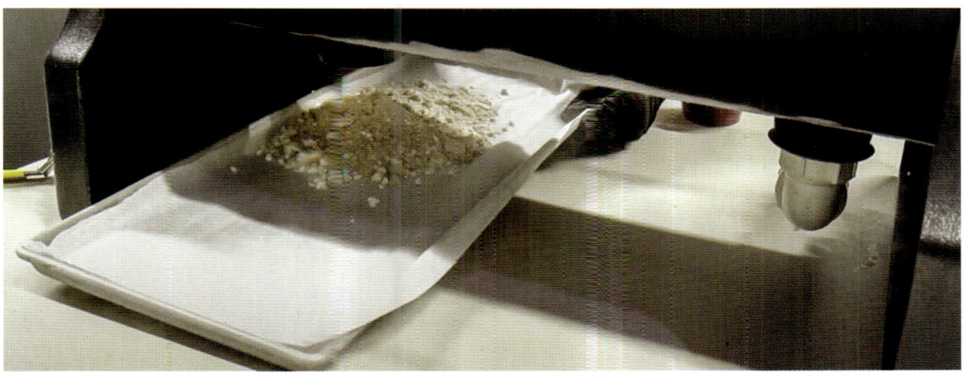

A fresh-frozen trim containing residual unevaporated CO_2, called the live sift, will appear in the collection tray under the Original Resinator XL. The live sift will appear as white chunks which are not as golden as regular screened resin.

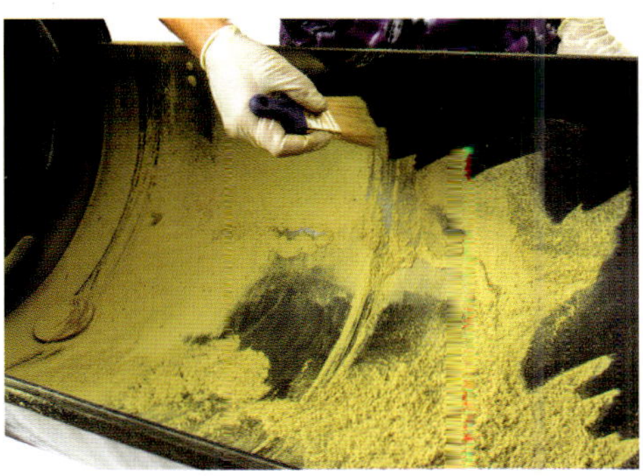

A brush is used inside the Original Resinator XL to collect the dry sift. This resin will be more golden than the live sift.

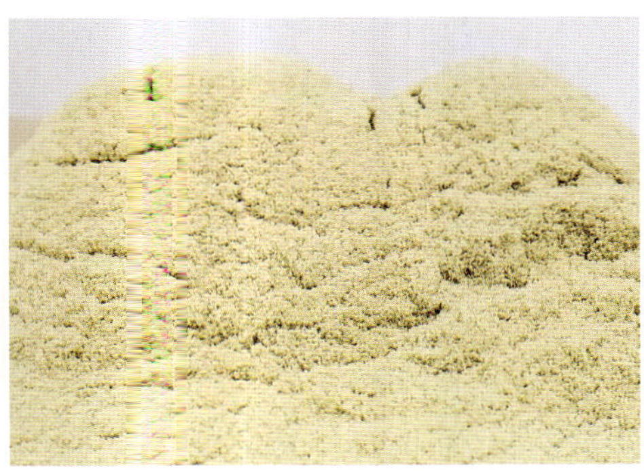

This is a sift made with fresh-frozen trim material that was then freeze-dried like ice water hash. A very pure resin results.

CO_2: Subcritical Fluid Extraction

CO_2 oil is typically used to produce a crude extract that is then further refined into distillates for vape pens. Butane extracts are of much higher quality than CO_2 extracts. Butane produces shatter, live resin, diamonds, crumble/honeycomb and honey oil. While butane is popular, CO_2 is safer. We are all familiar with gaseous and frozen CO_2; excess gaseous CO_2 in the atmosphere is responsible for climate change, and frozen CO_2 (dry ice) is used on stage for smoke effects. Other forms, subcritical and supercritical CO_2, occur when the pressure and temperature are outside standard conditions. These form a fluid with the physical properties of liquid that moves like a gas. Cannabis extraction with subcritical CO_2 is run for several hours at 50°F (10°C) and 950 PSI, while supercritical CO_2 is run for slightly less time at 104°F (40°C) and 230 PSI. Many growers use CO_2 for other purposes, so it makes sense to also use it for extraction, but they are still expensive devices.

Similar to butane, a CO_2 extraction system contains a CO_2 chamber, a plant material chamber, and an extract chamber. The system can be looped or not. Many closed-loop units available on the market are expensive because they can handle upwards of 10,000 PSI for industrial extraction. While CO_2 is an excellent solvent even when used alone, the CO_2 subcritical fluid extraction operator can combine CO_2 with other co-solvents for desired results. Using CO_2 opens up more possibilities, while butane is more restrictive with co-solvents.

This system is capped, but it does not need to be looped. Pressure regulation is essential with CO_2 extraction. The material chamber, for example, needs to handle 2,000 PSI. A regulator is usually placed at the material chamber for back pressure. Thus, when the top of the tube is capped, the pressure is regulated even in a non-looped system. Beneath the CO_2 chamber is the area of the tube that will contain plant matter, under which is the part of the tube for the dry ice. The base of the pipe is where the

CO_2 Extraction Process

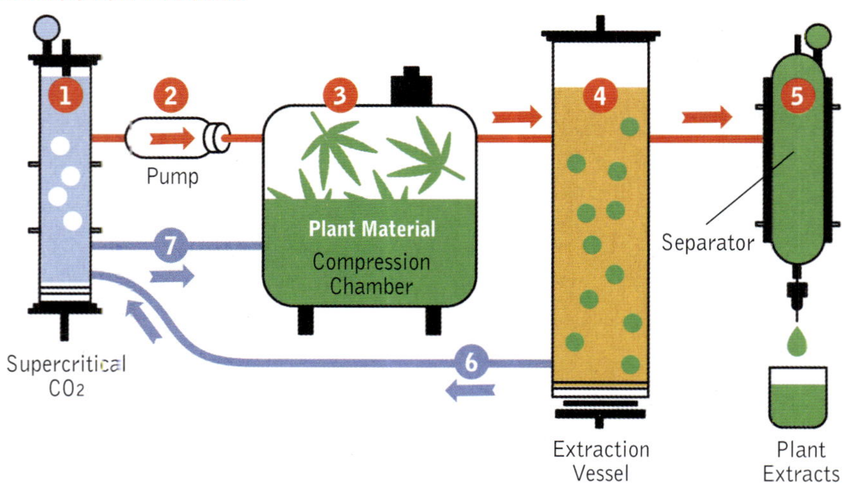

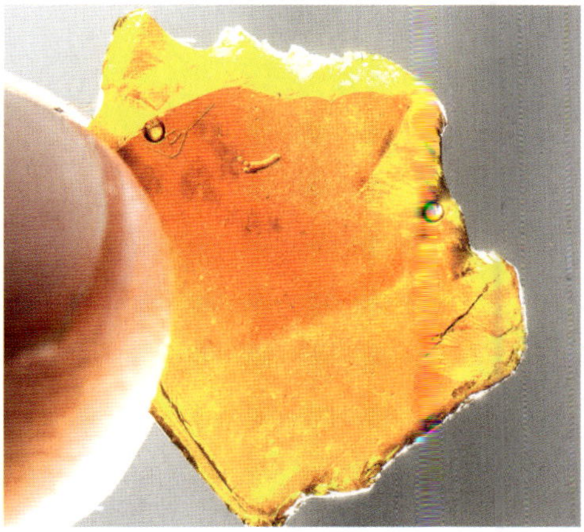

CO_2 extraction. Only a fraction of this piece is used for its effects.

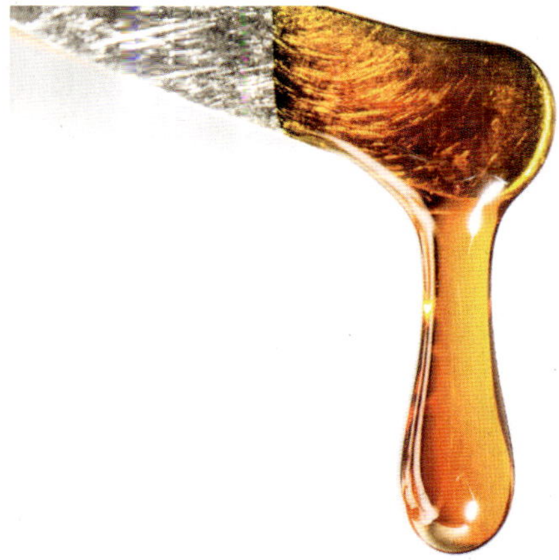

Dabbing from CO_2 extraction. Again only a drop is used for its effects.

extraction takes place. After the tube is filled with CO_2, it is tilted up so that the plant matter is released into the CO_2 by gravity. The desired temperatures and pressures are achieved by surrounding the unit with a heated coil and using the pressure regulator. Although the system described is a basic non-looped extraction system, it can be looped and the CO_2 recycled. The most crucial component of this unit is the blockage-resistant back pressure regulator on top of the separation chamber.

Tank-to-Tank CO_2 Extraction

A tank that can hold CO_2 is usually able to withstand higher PSIs and so can be heated. Some domestic users have managed to use CO_2 tanks in place of the CO_2 and plant chambers, as plant matter in one tank can be flooded with CO_2 from the other. This method can use either supercritical and subcritical CO_2, and is a way for domestic users to get into CO_2 extraction on a budget.

Smaller systems for domestic users tend to take about one hour to operate. More extensive systems run for four to six hours, and use a compressor. At the time of writing, CO_2 is considered an industry standard for extracting cannabis oil. With the steady rise of vaporization use and technology, oils are becoming as popular and plentiful as hashish, a significant development in the cannabis community.

Cleaning

Cannabis produces sticky resin. Parts of extraction systems that deal with sticky oils need regular cleaning and maintenance. The extraction chamber needs to be unclogged after every use. As you clean a unit, you can retrieve more resin, a nice bonus. Cleaning these systems is not only necessary work but is essential for getting purer results. If you plan to buy an extraction system, first ask about replacement parts and their costs, and compare your options.

PHOTOS: DANKSHIRE PHOTOGRAPHY

Types of Extractions

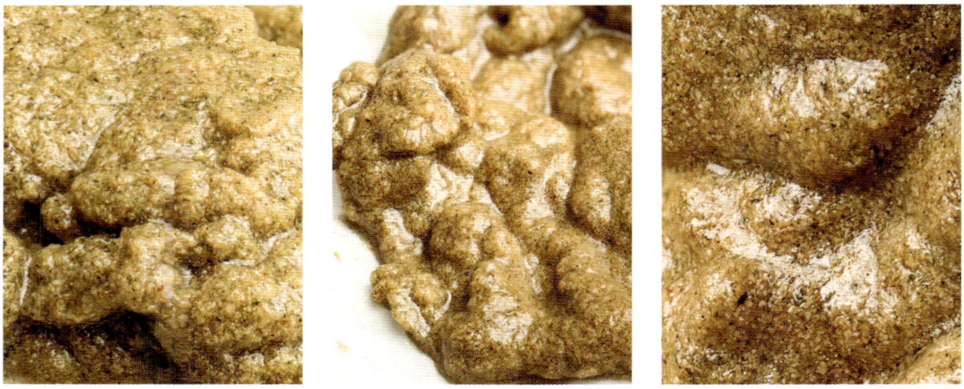

Wet Bubble Hash.

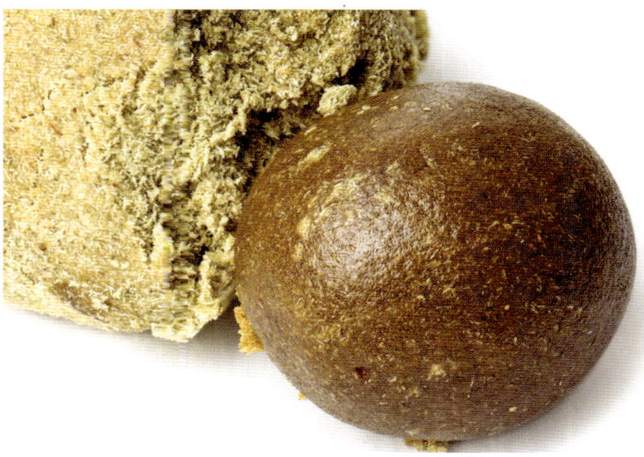

Frenchy Temple Ball.

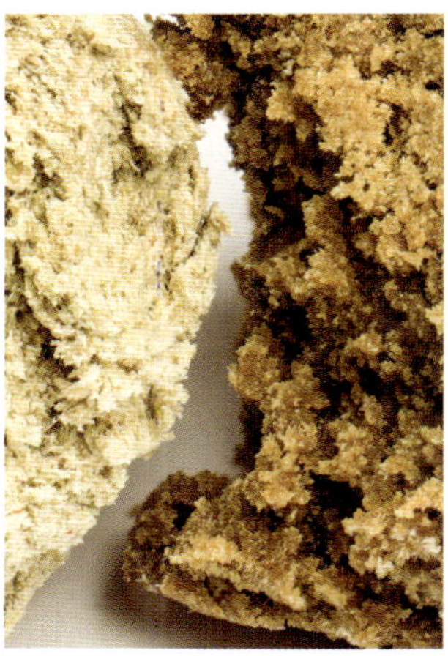

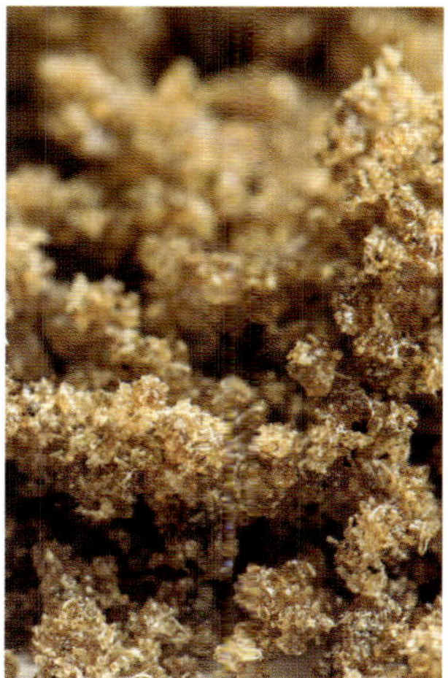

3-star water hash.

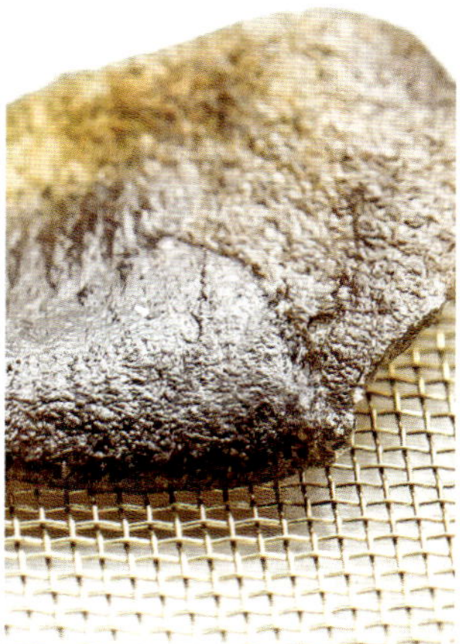

3-star water hash pressed.

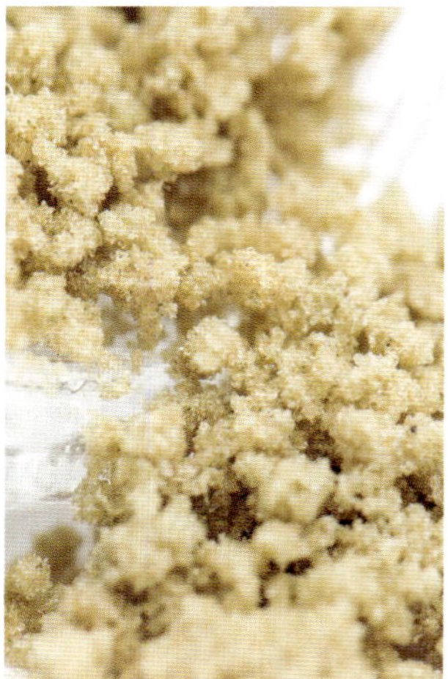

4-star ice wax.

PHOTOS: TRICHOME ART (TOP AND MIDDLE ROW), DANKSHIRE PHOTOGRAPHY (BOTTOM ROW)

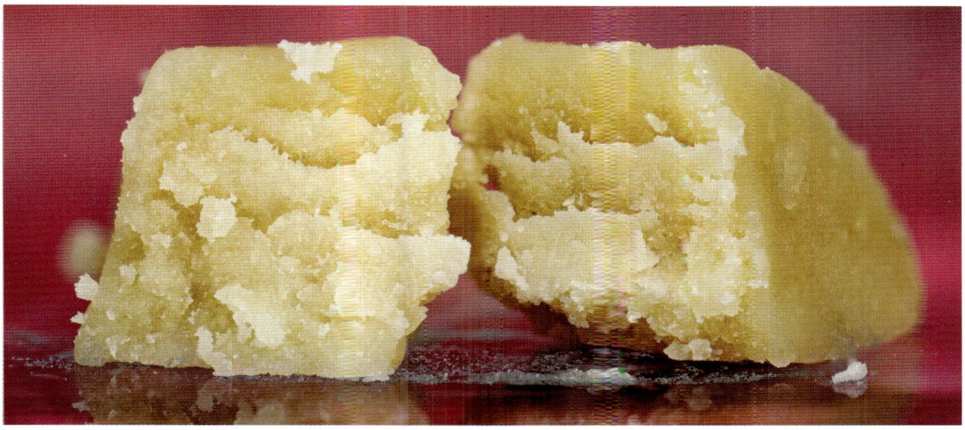

Live rosin.

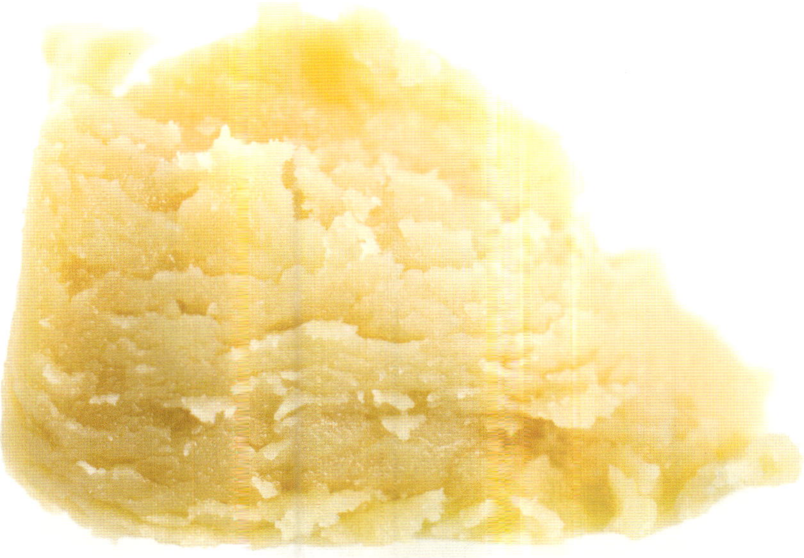

Live hash rosin.

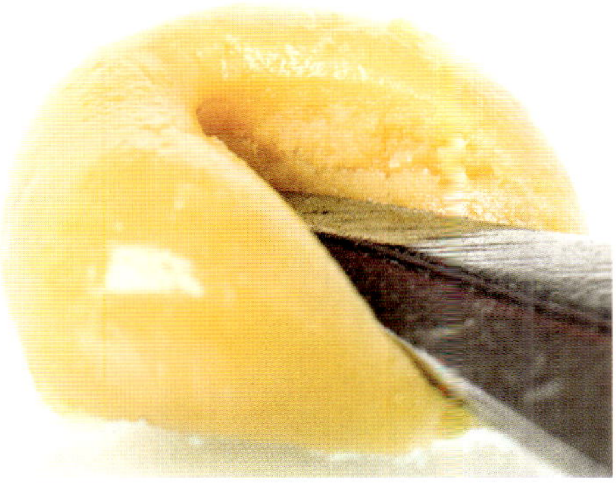

Live hash rosin

Live hash rosin

PHOTOS: TRICHOME ART

continues...

Types of Extractions *continued*

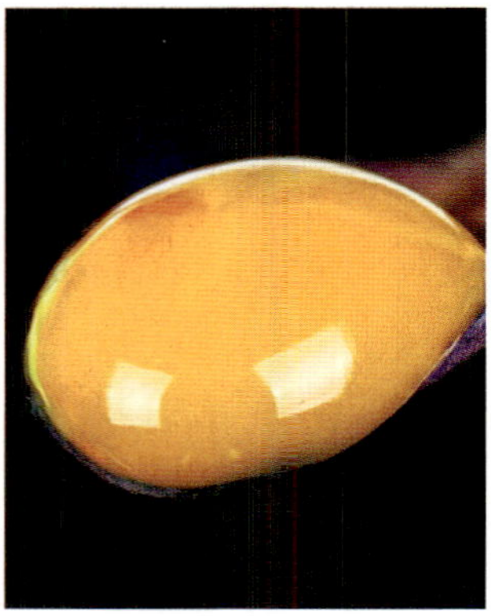
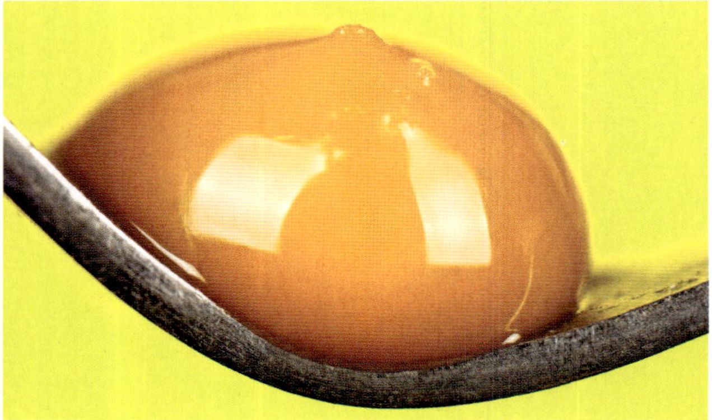

Flower rosin.

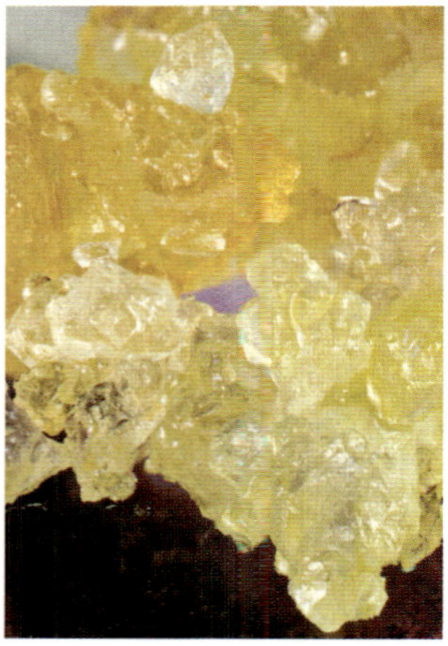

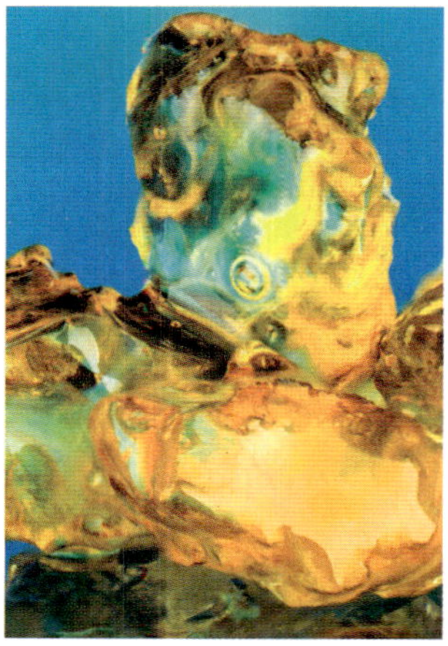

Live resin.

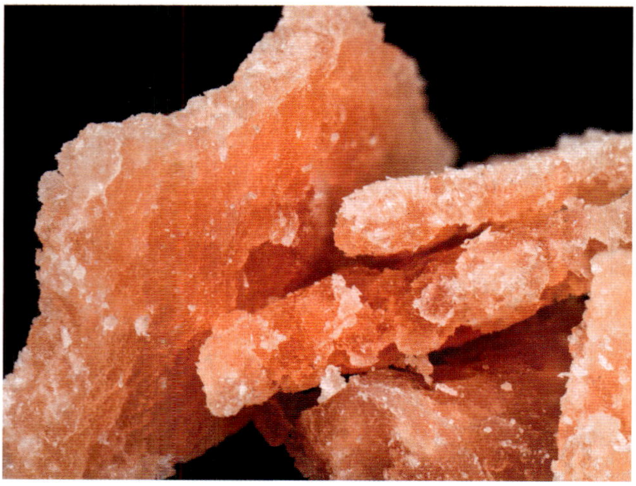
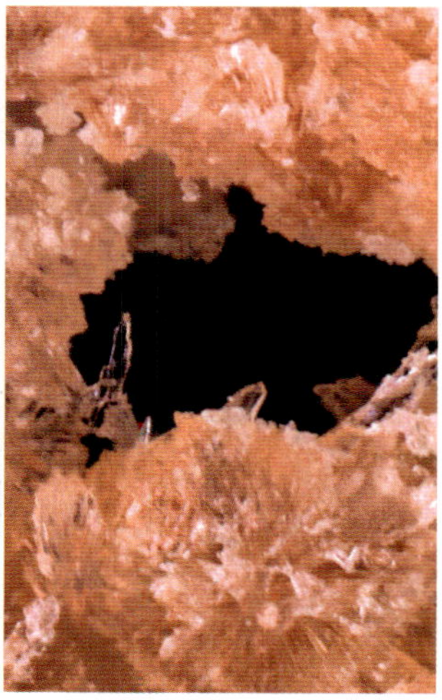

BHO crumble.

PHOTOS: TRICHOME ART

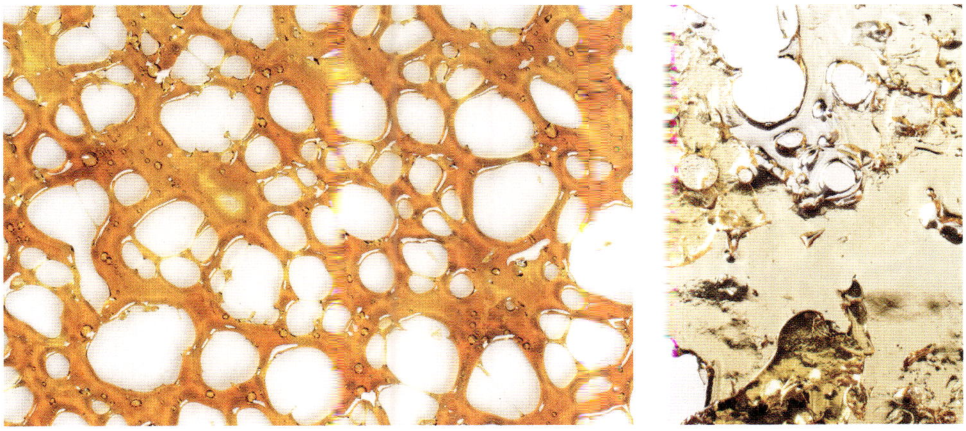

Shatter.

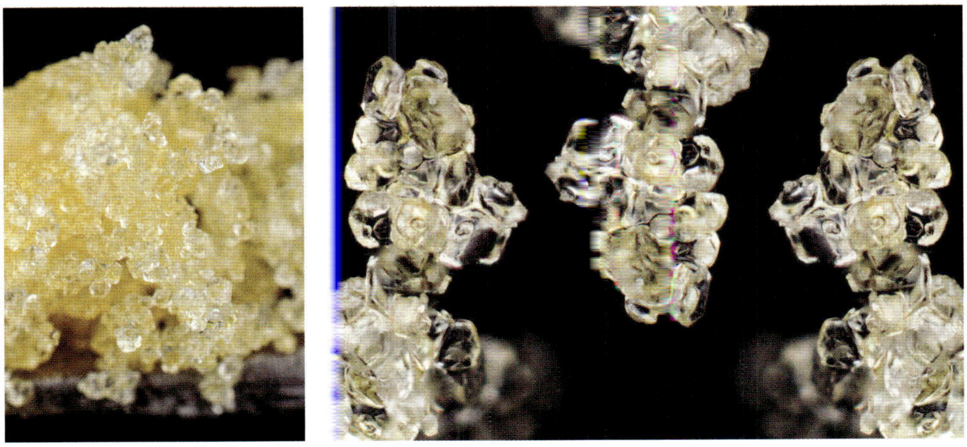

Live resin diamonds.

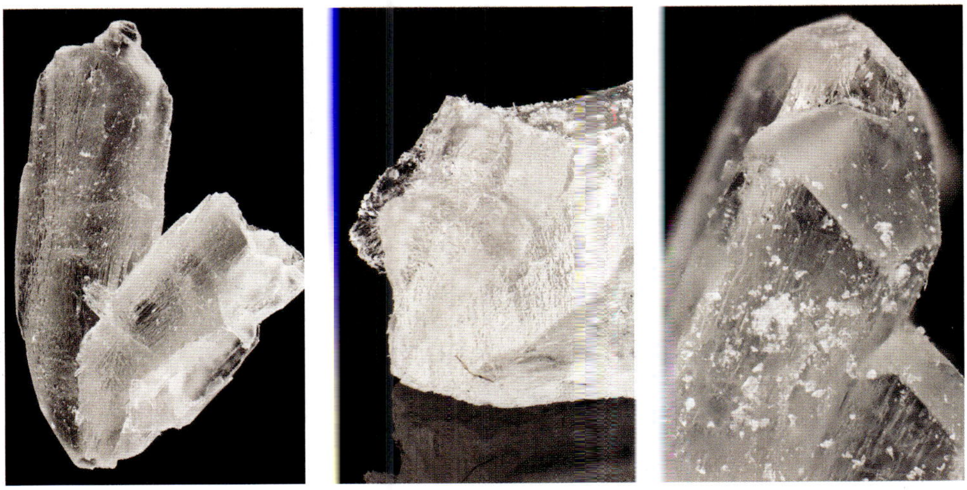

THCA diamonds.

Cooking with Cannabis

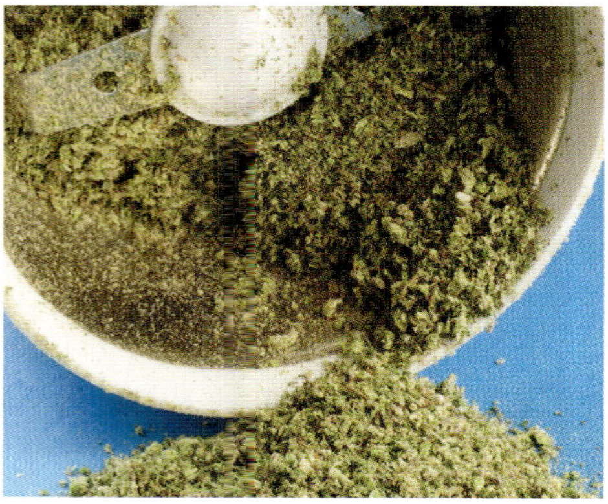

A simple coffee grinder is enough to prepare your weed for butter-making.

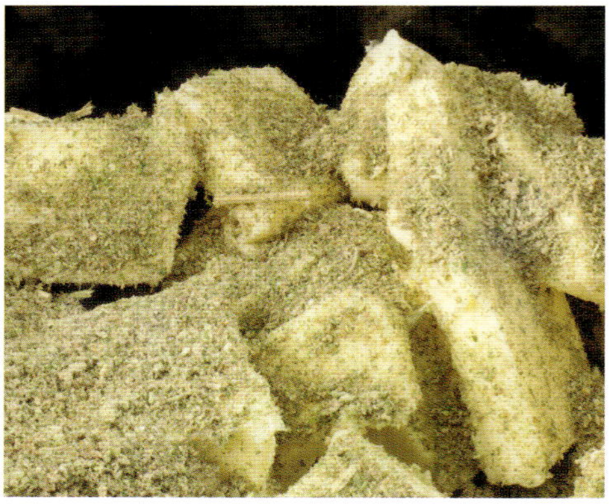

All you need is butter and weed—no additional ingredients!

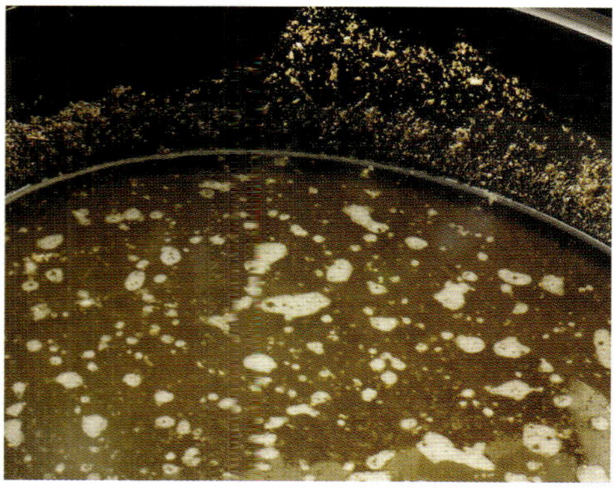

Don't overcook the butter; just three hours in a crock pot is fine.

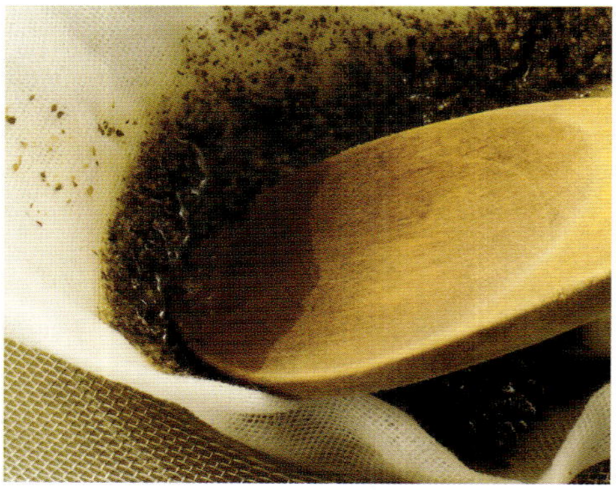

Strain well for a smooth and clear finished product that's ready for consumption!

Cannabis Butter

Cannabis butter can be used in any number of recipes, from desserts to entrees and appetizers. For best results, cannabis butter should be prepared one full day before using.

Directions

1. Grind the cannabis up well, using a coffee grinder if possible.
2. Combine the butter and cannabis in a large crock pot.
3. Add enough water to cover the bud and butter by a couple of inches.
4. Turn the crock pot on low and allow the butter to melt, then stir.
5. Simmer on the lowest heat for 3 hours or longer to attain maximum extraction.
6. Turn off the crock pot and allow mixture to cool slightly.
7. Pour the mixture through a fine mesh strainer lined with cheesecloth into a glass bowl.
8. Press the remaining liquid from the cannabis.

PHOTOS: VIRGINIA HAZE

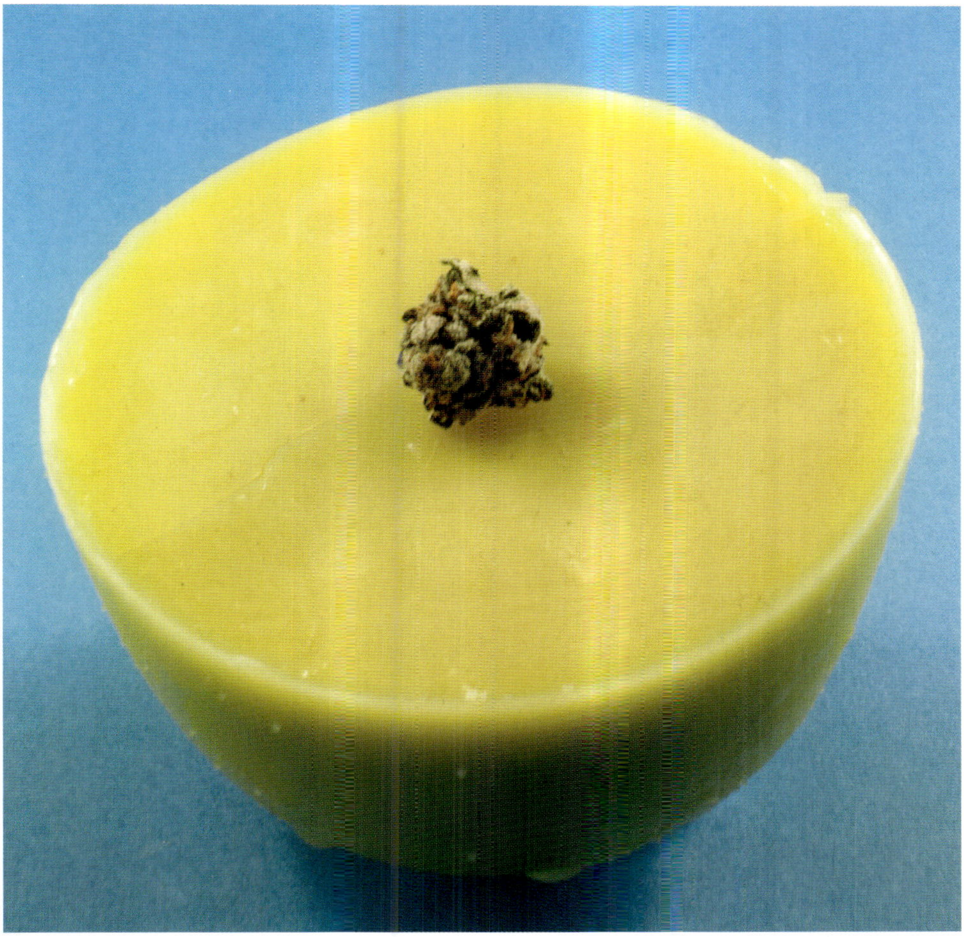

Making cannabis butter is quicker and easier than you might think.

9. Refrigerate for a few hours or overnight, until the butter has solidified on top of the water.
10. Lift the butter away from the water and drain the water away, then remelt the butter gently in a crock pot or pan.
11. Divide into several smaller containers ready for use.
12. Freeze until needed.

Recommended Dosage

Approximately 1/2 ounce of bud for every 1 pound of butter

Preparation Time

5 minutes

Cooking Time

3 hours

Sweet Sentations Sugar Cookies

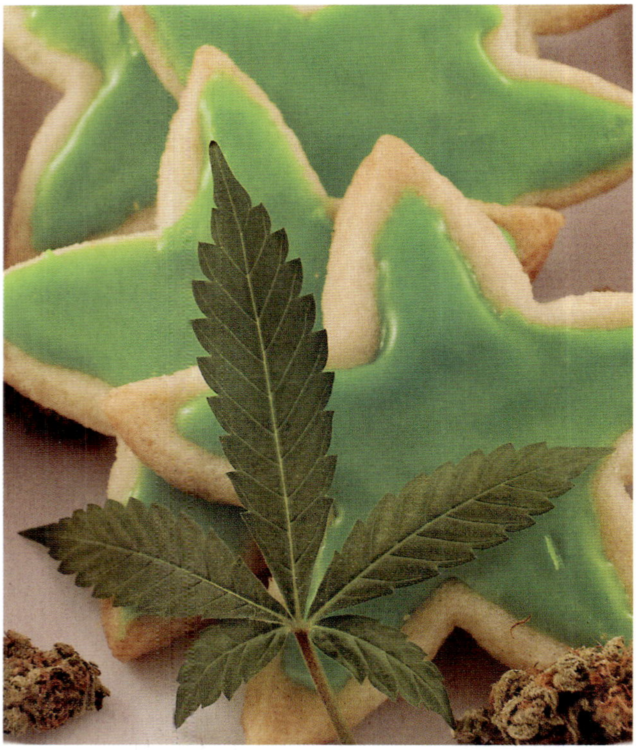

Ingredients

6 tablespoons of cannabis butter (page 826)
2 tablespoons of unsalted butter
2 cups of all-purpose flour
1/4 teaspoon of salt
1/2 teaspoon of baking powder
1 cup of sugar
1 large egg
2 tablespoons of milk
1/2 teaspoon of vanilla extract

Servings

24 cookies

Recommended Dosage

1 cookie

Preparation Time

15 minutes

Cooking Time

1 hours to chill, 10 minutes for cooking

Directions

1. Preheat oven to 350°F (175°C).
2. In a mixer or with a fork or whisk, cream together the cannabis butter, unsalted butter and sugar until light and fluffy.
3. Add in the egg, milk and vanilla extract and mix until combined.
4. In a separate bowl, sift together the flour, salt and baking powder.
5. Stir the flour mixture into the butter mixture until just combined.
6. Transfer the dough onto a floured surface and work into a ball.
7. Cover with plastic wrap and place in the refrigerator for 1 hour.
8. Remove the dough from the refrigerator and allow it to soften slightly.
9. Pinch off teaspoon-sized pieces of dough and roll into a ball, then place onto a cookie sheet lined with parchment paper and flatten slightly. Repeat for all the dough.
10. Alternatively, roll out to ¼-inch thickness and use cookie cutters to cut into shapes, then place on the cookie sheet.
11. Bake for 8 to 10 minutes, until lightly browned, then transfer to wire racks to cool.
12. Decorate with icing or just serve as they are.

PHOTOS: VIRGINIA HAZE

"Choc-ful-'o-Pot" Chocolate Chip Cookies

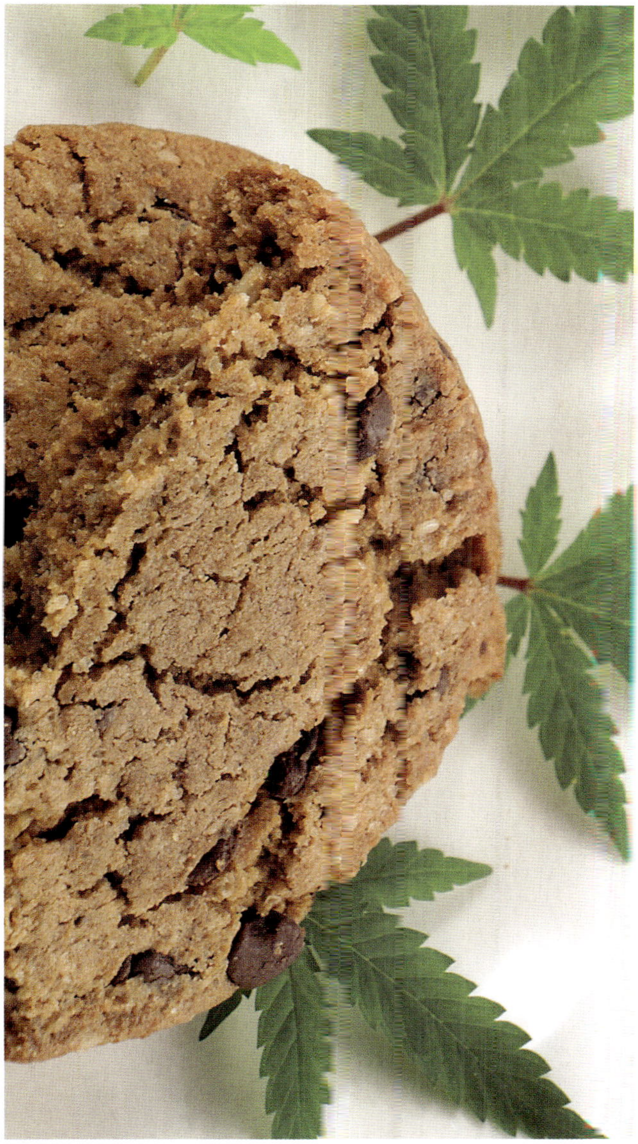

Ingredients

- 1/[illegible] cup of butter, softened
- 1/[illegible] cup of cannabis butter (page 826)
- 1 cup of packed brown sugar
- 1 cup of white sugar
- 2 eggs
- 2 teaspoons of vanilla extract
- 3 cups of all-purpose flour
- 1/2 teaspoon of salt
- 1 teaspoon of baking soda
- 2 teaspoons of hot water
- 2 cups of semisweet chocolate chips
- 1 cup of chopped walnuts (optional)

Servings

[illegible] cookies

Recommended Dosage

1 cookie

Preparation Time

20 minutes

Cooking Time

10 minutes

Directions

1. Preheat oven to 350°F (175°C).
2. Cream the butter, cannabis butter and sugars together until smooth.
3. Beat in the eggs one at a time, with a pinch of the flour.
4. Stir in the vanilla.
5. Dissolve the baking soda in the hot water and add it to the batter, with the salt.
6. Stir in the flour, chocolate chips and nuts (if using).
7. Drop large spoonfuls of batter onto an ungreased baking tray.
8. Bake for about 10 minutes, or until the edges are slightly browned.

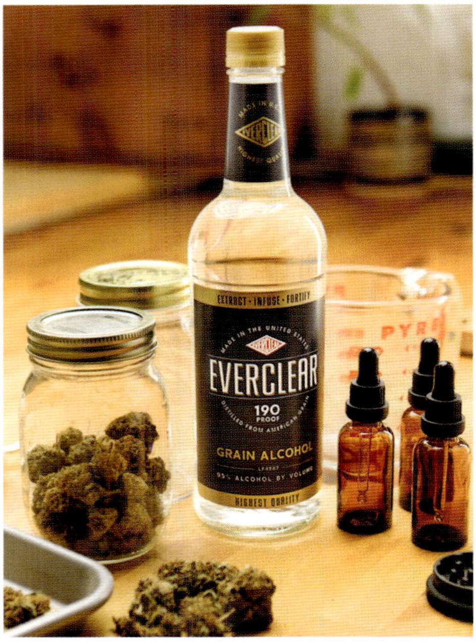

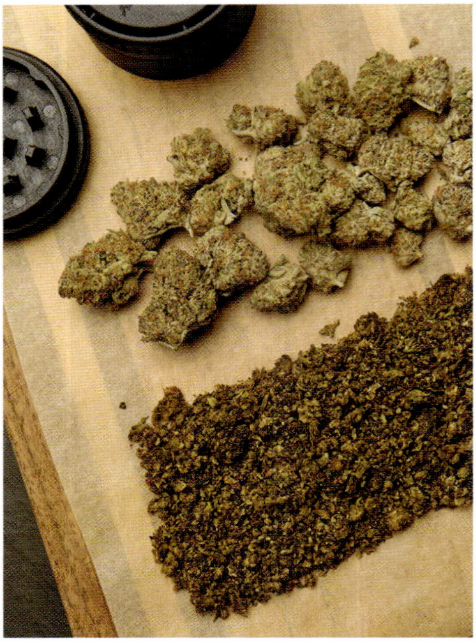

Cannabis Tincture

A cannabis tincture is created when we extract the cannabinoids from cannabis into alcohol. Here's a basic recipe to make one of your own:

Directions

Decarboxylation

1. Preheat oven to 240°F (115°C).
2. Grind the cannabis coarsely.
3. Spread the ground cannabis evenly on a baking sheet lined with parchment paper.
4. Bake for 30-40 minutes, stirring halfway. This process activates the THC and CBD in the cannabis.

Infusion

5. Place the decarboxylated cannabis into a Mason jar.
6. Pour enough high-proof alcohol to cover the cannabis completely. Seal the jar tightly with the lid.

Extraction

7. Store the jar in a cool, dark place (for e.g., a cupboard) for at least 2 weeks. Shake the jar gently every day. The alcohol will gradually extract cannabinoids from the cannabis.

Ingredients

Cannabis: About 7-10 grams of dried cannabis bud (adjust based on potency preference)

High-proof alcohol: Everclear or another high-proof alcohol with at least 60-80% alcohol content

Equipment

Grinder
Mason jar with lid
Fine mesh strainer or cheesecloth
Funnel
Amber glass dropper bottles for storage

PHOTOS: THOMAS WHITCOMB

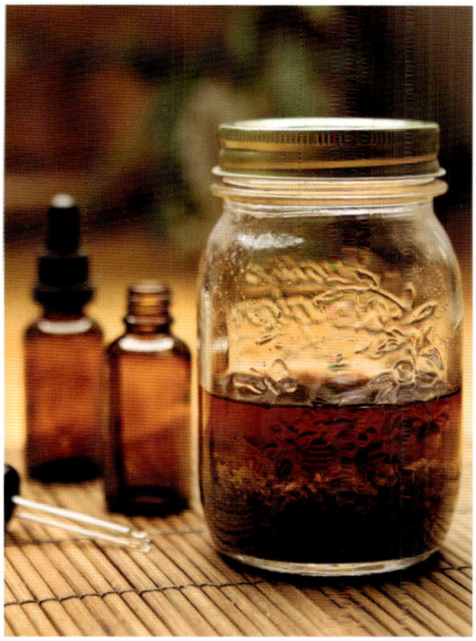

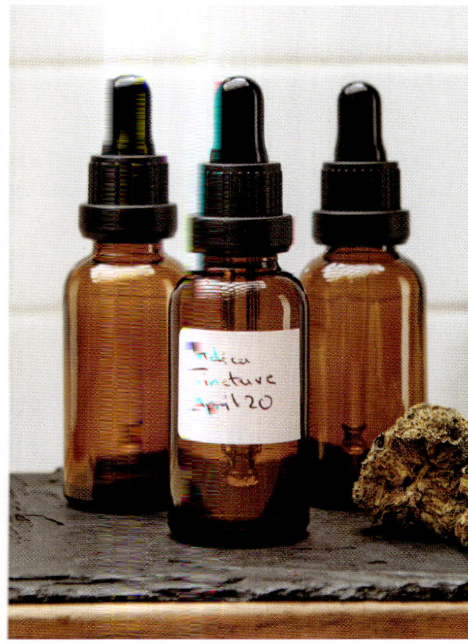

Straining

9. After 2 weeks (or longer for a stronger tincture), strain the mixture through a fine mesh strainer or cheesecloth into a clean bowl.
10. Squeeze the cheesecloth tightly to extract all the liquid. Discard the leftover bud.

Storage

11. Use a funnel to pour the tincture into amber glass dropper bottles for storage. Amber bottles help protect the tincture from light.
12. Label the bottles with the date and potency (if known).

By following these steps, you can make your own cannabis tincture at home. Adjust the dosage and potency according to your personal preferences and experience level with cannabis products.

TIPS

Dosage

Start with a small amount (like one dropperful) to assess potency before increasing.

Potency

The longer you let the cannabis infuse, the stronger the tincture will be.

Safety

Work in a well-ventilated area due to the alcohol fumes.

Storage

Store your cannabis tincture in a cool, dark place, away from children and pets.

Dosed Gummy Bears

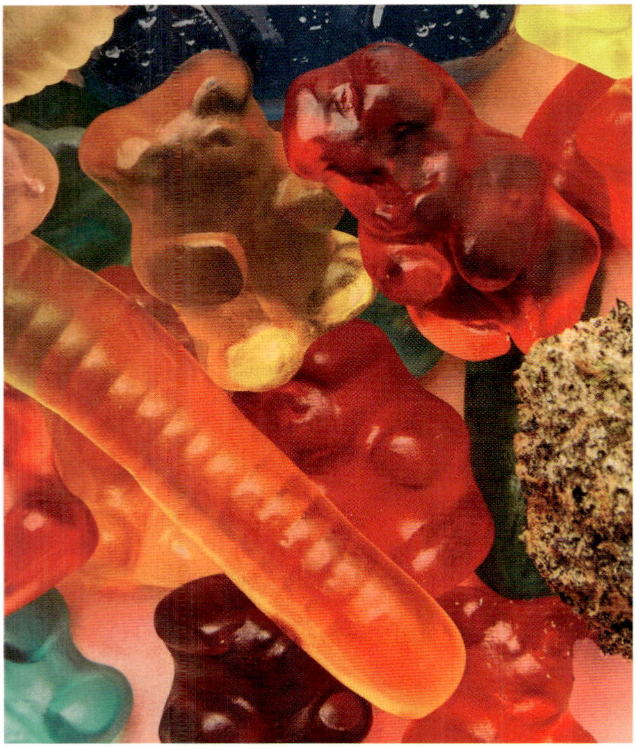

Ingredients

1½ cups pure fruit juice – orange, pomegranate, apple or whatever juice you prefer
½ teaspoon lemon juice
4 tablespoons gelatine (vegan if you are)
3 tablespoons honey, agave or another liquid sweetener
4 teaspoons of cannabis tincture (page 830)

for sour gummies:
½ cup caster sugar
2 teaspoons citric acid

Servings

Bears: 28 to 34
Worms: 20,
depending on your molds

Recommended Dosage

1 worm or 2 bears, depending on cannabis tincture strength

Preparation Time

5 minutes

Cooking Time

10 to 15 minutes

Directions

1. Place the fruit juice and lemon juice in a medium saucepan and gently heat until warm. Do not bring to a boil.
2. Add in the cannabis tincture and stir.
3. Add in the gelatine super slowly and whisk until combined.
4. Add in a tab espoon of the sweetener and taste. Add more until it has reached your desired sweetness.
5. Carefully pour or spoon the mixture into your gummy molds, or if you have a cooking syringe, use that. It's a lot easier.
6. Refrigerate for 4 hours.
7. If you're making sour gummies, mix the citric acid and sugar in a bowl. Pop the gummies out of the molds and roll them in the mixture.
8. Give one a try. Wait an hour. This will give you an idea of how strong they are, and whether you need to take more.
9. Store in an airtight container in the fridge, away from children. Consume within 2 weeks.

PHOTO: THOMAS WHITCOMB

Cinnamon Canna Rock Candy

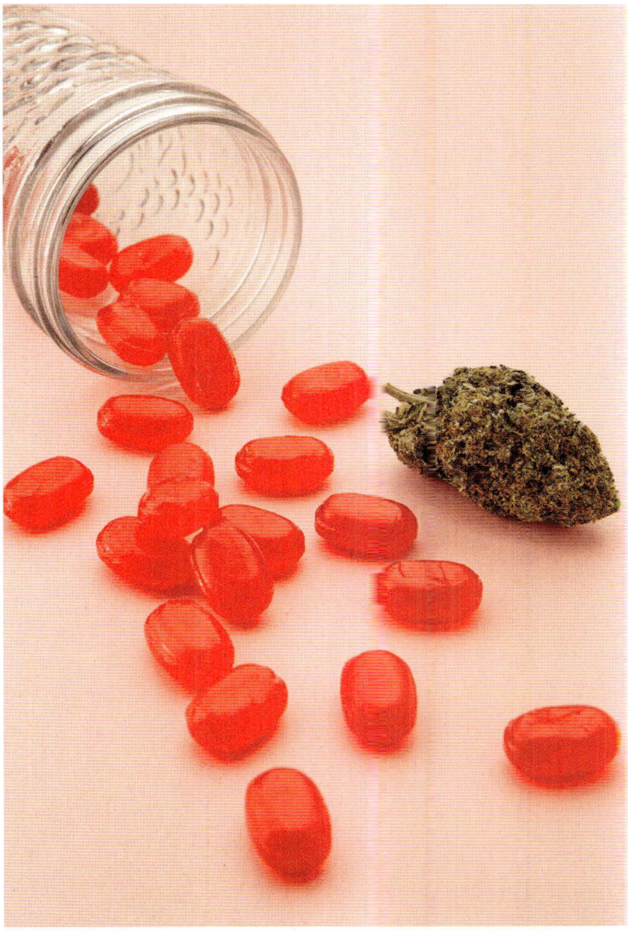

PHOTO: THOMAS WHITCOMB

Ingredients

2 cups sugar
1 cup water
½ cup light corn syrup
½ teaspoon cinnamon oil
½ teaspoon red food coloring
3 teaspoons of cannabis tincture (page 830)

Servings

23

Recommended Dosage

1 or 2 pieces

Preparation Time

5 minutes

Cooking Time

25 minutes

Directions

1. Combine the sugar, corn syrup and water in a medium saucepan over a medium-high heat.
2. Stir until the sugar is totally dissolved and bring to the boil. Stop stirring when it starts to boil.
3. Place your candy thermometer in the pan and when it reaches 300°F (149°C), pull the pan immediately from the heat.
4. Watch until the temperature cools until 250°F, then add in the cinnamon oil, the food coloring and the cannabis tincture. Stir to combine. Note: Alcohol is flammable, so make sure the pan is NOT near any heat at this point.
5. Pour onto a greased cookie sheet with a lip (not a totally flat one) or one covered in parchment paper.
6. Allow to cool at room temperature for up to an hour.
7. Break into pieces and store in an airtight container away from children, for up to a month.

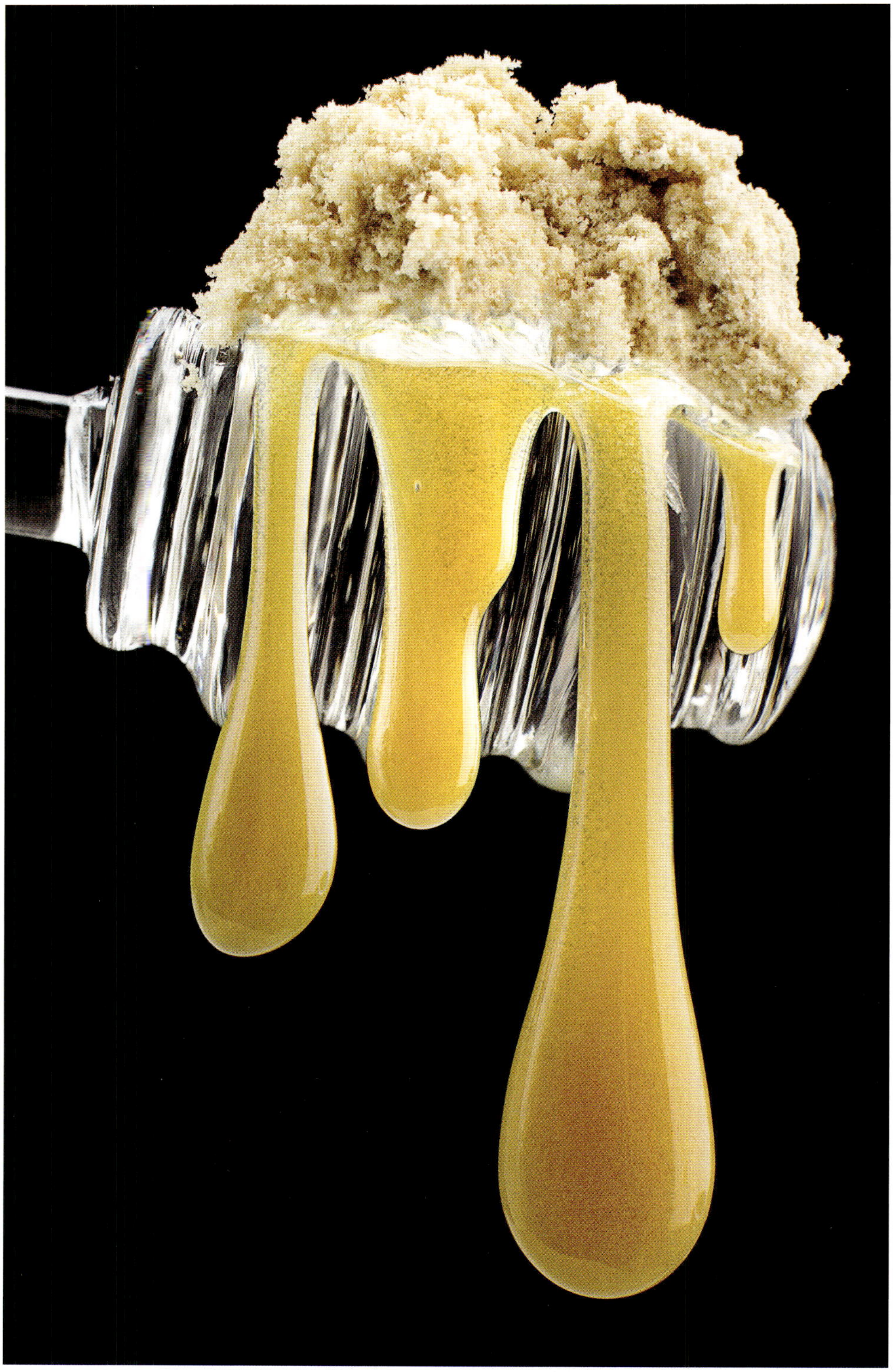

PHOTO: DANKSHIRE PHOTOGRAPHY

A honey dipper can be used to collect viscous extracts for movement from one location to another.

Thin Film Evaporators

Thin film evaporators are used to further separate cannabinoids. A thin film evaporator is composed of a pipe with an internal heated rotor. Cannabis oil is fed to the pipe's top, into the heated rotor, and forced to the inner sides of the pipe. The rotor blade creates a wave inside the fluid that flows downwards. Depending on application, evaporation can occur at the top or bottom of the pipe. What evaporates can be collected, and the extracted oils will flow from the bottom of the evaporator. The result is the segregation of THC from all other cannabinoids. Using different temperatures in purification can target different cannabinoids. Other professional systems use flash chromatography to accomplish the same thing. These professional units are not DIY and are usually bought by science departments and labs. However, as the field of cannabis research grows, so does access to these units for research.

What is thin film evaporation? Sample extractions can be performed in chromatography with the results stained on a test slip that contains samples of each substance. Thin film evaporators work similarly, except more sample sizes and usable amounts of the extracted material are produced. This same methodology is carried out in graduate and post-graduate-level biochemistry, so thin film evaporation is used only by those experienced in advanced extraction. The segregation of cannabinoids at such a level of purity is also usually reserved for experiments due to the high costs involved and small quantities yielded. As a result, most medical cannabis products may contain many cannabinoid compounds, but in desired ratios. For example, many CBD products contain less than one percent THC.

Terpenes

Terpenes are oils that produce the aromas and flavors of cannabis plants as well as flowers, fruit and trees like conifers. They can also significantly modify and enhance the effects of cannabinoids. Scientists theorize that their function is to attract birds for seed dispersal, as well as provide protection against predators. Some terpenes have anti-fungal and insecticidal properties, which indicates a potential use in pesticide application.

Cannabis terpenes vary throughout flowering. The most significant change is the aroma intensity as flowers bloom and produce trichomes containing VOCs (volatile aromatic compounds). These aromas can also be the result of selective breeding or pheno-hunting, where breeders will select strains with specific characteristics and crossbreed them to enhance or alter these flavors, thereby creating new strains. Aromas are hugely influential in variation between strains, as they are among things that breeders look to control, the other elements being potency and yield. There is a big difference between spicy, citrus, and forest aromas. Aromas can also leave the plant as airborne molecules, drifting around the environment. Thus, controlling the aroma traits can reduce unwanted smells.

Terpenes are part of the cannabinoids' biosynthesis pathway, which also includes isoprenoid diphosphates such as the building blocks of cannabinoids, geranyl diphosphate (GPP). Terpenes combine with phenols for the cannabinoid production of cannabichromene (CBC), cannabidiolic acid (CBDA), cannabigerol (CBG), cannabinol (CBN), cannabidivarin (CBDV), cannabidivarinic acid (CBDVA), cannabigerolic acid (CBGA), cannabicyclol (CBL), delta 8-THC, tetrahydrocannabinolic acid (THCA), and tetrahydrocannabivarin (THCV). We came across these at the beginning of the book and learned how cannabinoid compounds combine and change form. For example, compounds like Delta 9-THC and CBD are derived by vaporization.

Monoterpenes, diterpenes and sesquiterpenes are the three important terpenes found in the analysis of cannabinoid pathways. Monoterpenes contain limonene, β-myrcene, α-pinene, linalool, and small amounts of α-terpinolene and trans-ocimene. Sesquiterpenes contain (E)-caryophyllene, caryophyllene oxide, *E*-β-farnesene, and β-caryophyllene.

These terpene components are responsible for the aromas of cannabis plants. β-myrcene gives cannabis its baseline herbal smell, which is described scientifically as hops. Myrcene is the most abundant terpene in Skunk #1 strain and can often give cannabis the "skunky" smell we have all grown to love. Increased amounts of β-myrcene can cause indica-type body effects, while low amounts result in a sativa-type cerebral effect. Pine smells come from α-pinene and β-pinene. β-caryophyllene, when present with limonene, produces a citrus-lime aroma, while β-caryophyllene alone produces a spice smell. Limonene is responsible for citrus aromas in cannabis as well as lemon plants. Terpinolene also creates a citrus aroma, like orange. Combining these compounds can produce combined aromas. For example, one combination may produce a mostly citrus aroma with a woody, herbal hop undertone.

There are over 200 terpenes, not including all their possible combinations and changes through chemical processes, resulting in a staggering landscape of aroma opportunities. Terpene aromas are closely related, and these relationships can be expressed in a "terpene color wheel" which organizes the smells as color hues. The color wheel is used for organization because terpenes combine in a similar manner to colors, resulting in the emergence of another aroma that cannot be present without them. However, as the wheel depends on descriptions of the aroma experience, it is fairly subjective. In the center of the wheel are the "primary colors." These are surrounded by descriptions like "fruity," "woody," "spicy," "earthy," "floral," and "herbal," with each adjective in individual sections. Each of these segments is then subdivided into more categories, which then divide more into precise aroma descriptions. You can work backward from a smell to the primary aroma (or aromas), which corresponds to one or more terpenes. The wheel demonstrates how many combinations of terpenes can exist. However, you will likely pick a strain and its aroma based on the breeder's description of its traits.

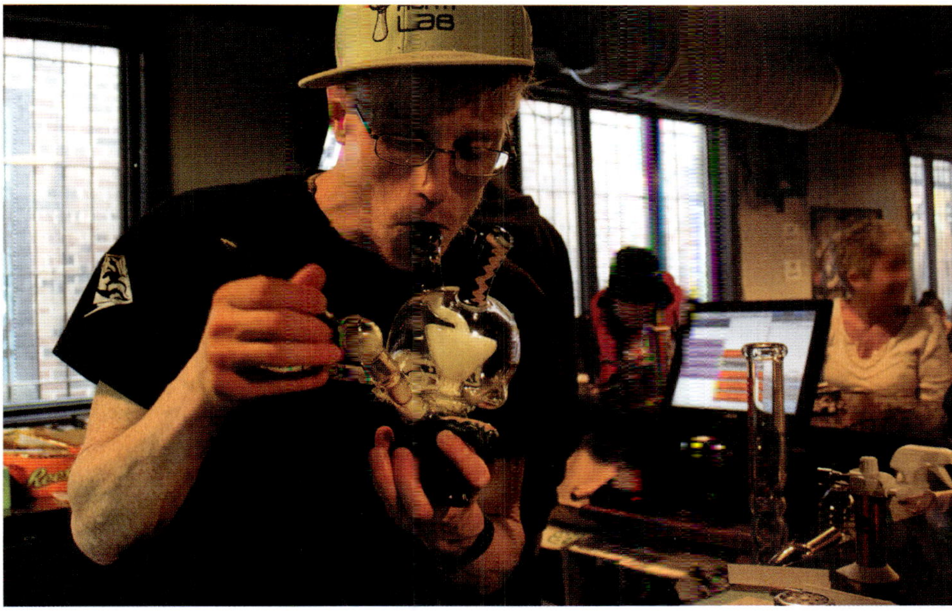

A dome is quickly placed over the preheated nail before dabbing to help contain the vapor and allow it to be inhaled through the rig, instead of escaping.

Dabbing

Dabbing is the process of ingesting zero-residue, vaporizable cannabis concentrates by "dabbing" some on a heated surface attached to a small bong-like unit. Dabbing allows you to inhale the vapor in one big powerful hit, similar to smoking a bowl from a bong.

There are many forms of concentrate or dabs, and just as many types of hardware, or dab rigs. You can also vaporize cannabis concentrate using hardware similar to e-cigs known as "dab," "concentrate," or "shatter pens." Traditional dabbing is analogous to hitting a bong; using pens is analogous to using a vape cartridge or smoking a joint. Pens can also be used with prefilled cartridges, allowing for standardization in the medicinal and legal recreational markets.

The high purity of concentrates or extracts makes for an extremely potent and fast-acting hit. High doses can be consumed rapidly, making dabbing popular with medical and recreational tokers who have developed a high tolerance to cannabis flowers. Dab Pens are also a much more discreet form of cannabis consumption, thanks to a lack of potent odor when smoking and storing the concentrate. A pen is easily used without attracting attention, and can be pocketed quickly, ready for use again whenever necessary, whereas trying to stash part of a joint for later is usually a bit of a mess.

Dabbing, once an underground phenomenon, has quickly gained traction in the last 20 years, aided by the establishment of online forums and information sharing between glass

PHOTO: SEAN BRADY

artists, as well as by the expansion of medical and recreational legalization of cannabis in Canada and multiple American states. As its popularity has increased, so has investment in the science of cannabis concentrate extraction and refinement, as well as in functional glass art and technology for its ingestion. Around 2011 these markets exploded, and dabbing is now beyond mainstream. In many areas, dabbing has practically taken over as the preferred ingestion method, with high-end dab rigs and vaporizers dominating headshops. Dispensaries also now offer a wide range of extracts and pre-loaded pens.

Any zero-residue concentrate can be dabbed, including butane honey oil (BHO), shatter, hash oil, bubble hash, CO_2 extracts, THC distillate, THCA diamonds, and rosin.

Equipment

Cannabis concentrates have existed for several decades, and people have smoked them in a bong, joint or cigarette or using a hot knife. While effective, many methods are often messy, cumbersome, and harsh. In response, glassblowers began to create oil-specific smoking tools and accessories. The dab straw is an oil pipe where the bowl has been replaced by a plate of glass and heated with a blowtorch. As the internet slowly became the indispensable communication tool, glass artists began sharing ideas on online forums such as Toke City, selling their products directly to a rapidly expanding customer base. The curve design, which became popular in the 1990s, incorporated

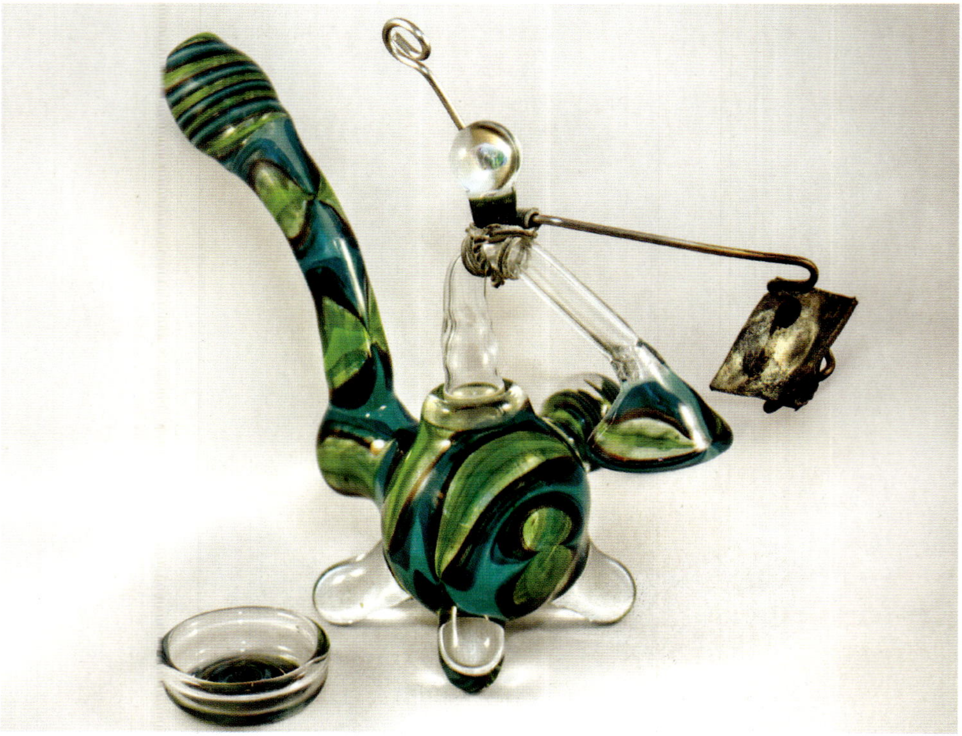
PHOTO: SEAN BRADY

A swing oil rig by Hashmasta Kut with matching dish.

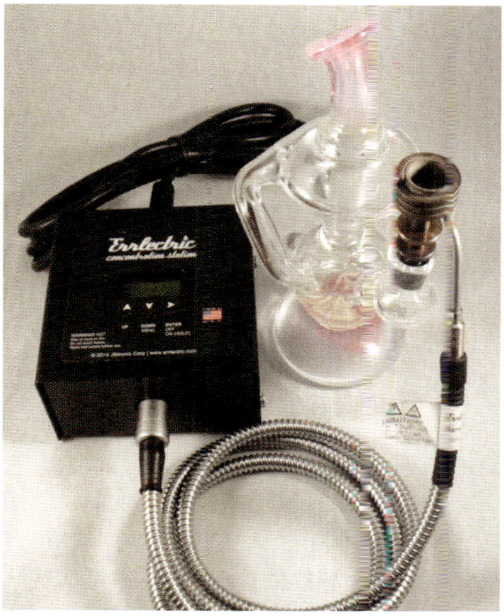

A titanium e-nail with a Klein-style oil rig. The electronic controller uses a metal coil to maintain a constant temperature on a domeless nail.

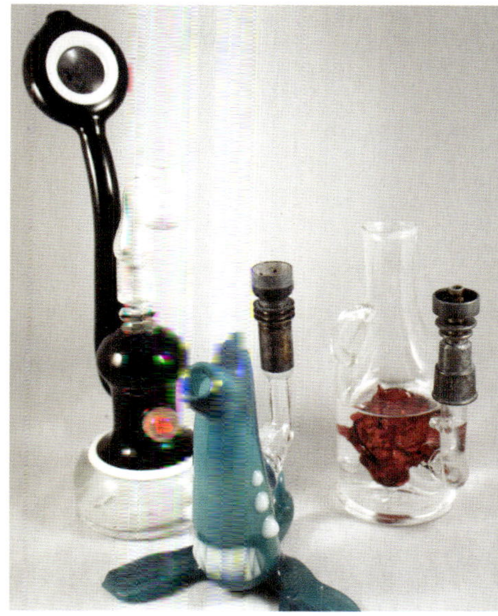

Three examples of domeless nail styles: A quartz bucket/banger, a titanium wok and hollow titanium.

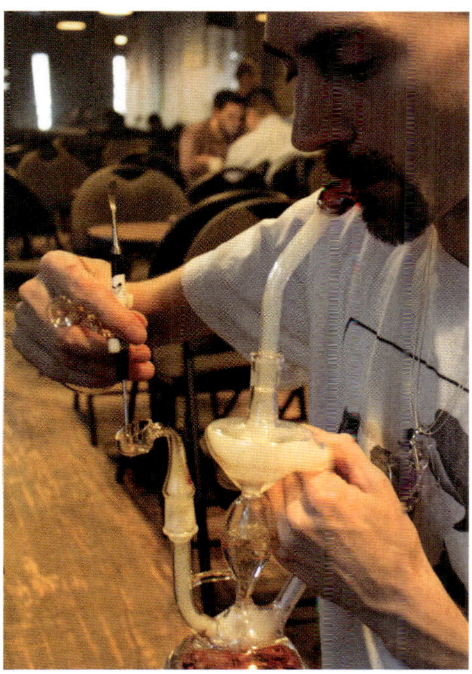

Start firmly inhaling just before touching a dab to the hot nail, or most of it will be lost to the environment before you've even started.

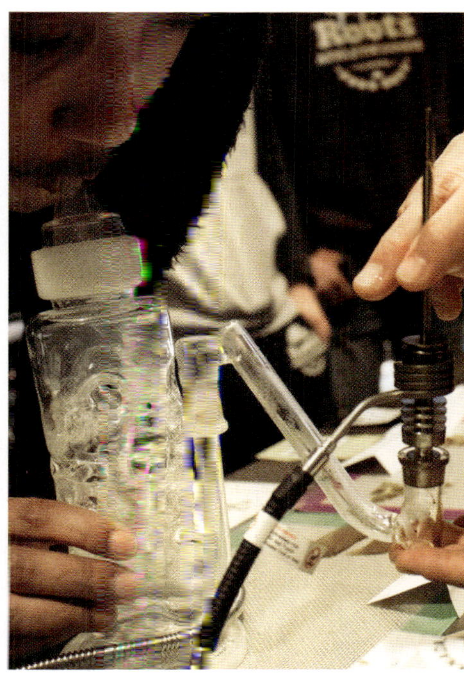

Using a carb cap will also help avoid vapor loss while dabbing on a domeless nail, especially if you inhale slowly or need to take a second pull.

PHOTOS: SEAN BRADY

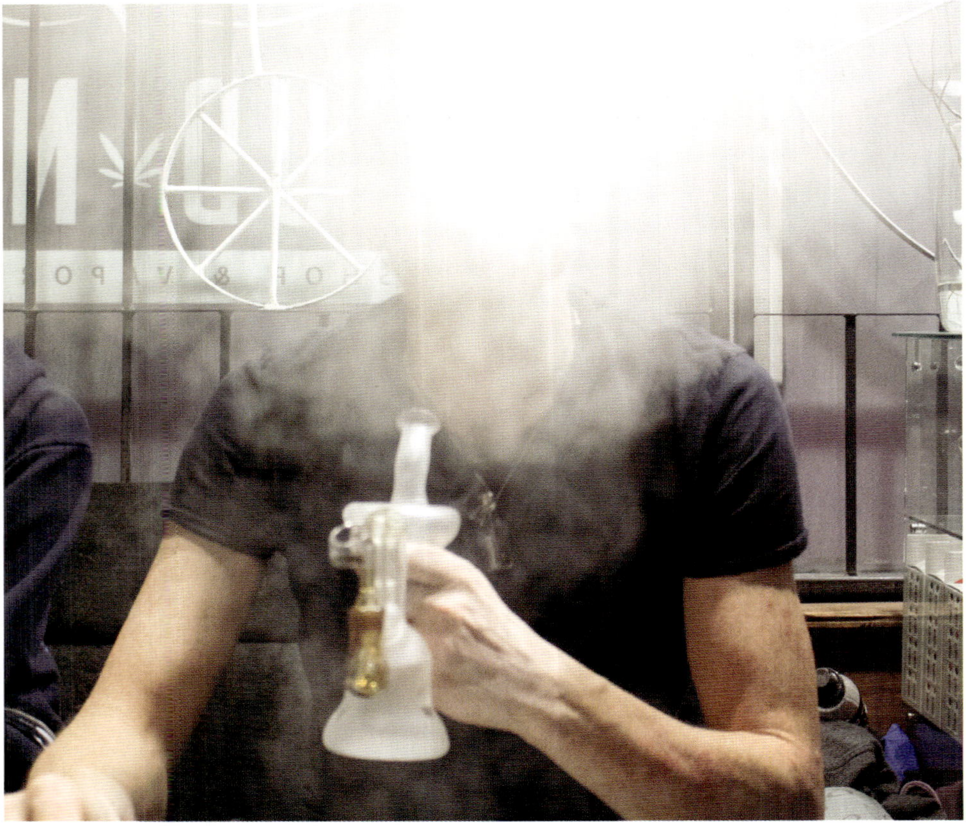

And finally, exha e!

the water filtration of a typical bong into a tiny glass unit with a downward-facing hood in place o- a bowl, which could be used in place of a straight tube to mellow hoots of cannabis oil off hookah hot rocks.

Hashmasta Kut (HMK) expanded upon this design to develop and popularize what are widely considered the first commercial dab rigs by adding a titanium plate that could "swing" to the side to be heated with a blowtorch and then swing back directly under the curve to be dabbed on. The vapor is then inhaled through the unit. The design was widely adopted and dominated the market for about a decade.

The "nail and dome" design, which incorporates glass-on-glass joints, was quickly considered a simpler and more effective method than the swing, as it required less precision to use and provided a more concentrated hit. This design is still in use, with titanium nails favored by some because of their durability and high heat retention, and quartz nails favored by others because of taste. The nail is heated with a blowtorch and then the dome is placed over and around the nail to help contain the vapor, which is drawn through the unit as the nail is dabbed on. There are several styles of

PHOTO: SEAN BRADY

domeless nails made in titanium, quartz, and ceramic for both male and female glass-on-glass joints. The surface is heated with a blowtorch then dabbed on, and the vapor is drawn through the center, edges, or top of the nail. A "carb cap" can also be used to help contain the vapor, much like a dome with a traditional nail. These may help concentrate the hit and reduce waste from vapor loss but aren't fully necessary.

Buckets/bangers are another newer progression in the dabbing world. As the name indicates, it is a fairly deep bucket shaped bowl, with an opening near the top which leads to the typical glass on glass bong bowl connection to your pipe. The bucket, made of quartz, is heated with a blowtorch and then extract is dropped in the top of the bucket, with a carb cap placed on top to brew the hit.

Terp Slurpers are an advancement on the bucket style, which consists of a elongated bucket with a saucer at the base with small holes to allow airflow. Inside the elongated bucket tube you can place marbles or spinners. Once you place your dab onto the saucer and begin pulling, the spinners will help move your dab up the surface of the slurper, providing an even greater flavor and dab experience.

E-nails apply consistent heat to a domeless nail with a metal coil, ensuring it is always ready and at the correct temperature, which can vary greatly depending on personal taste. While there are still risks of being burned if the unit is mishandled, it eliminates the fire risk that's associated with a blowtorch. Some manufacturers also make a heated coil that a quartz bucket/banger sits in. The metal coil surrounds the bottom and sides of the bucket providing heat without any blowtorches.

Another form of e-rigs are the portable dab units like the Puffco Peak and Focus V Carta 2. These small battery operated units are basically small water pipes with an electronically heated bowl, which you drop your dab into. Perfect for camping or on the go when you don't want to bring your whole rig.

Dabbing Safety

Three simple rules must be followed to dab safely:

1. Start slow. Dabs are far more potent and less harsh than cannabis smoke, so it is easy to overindulge without realizing it. Many seasoned tokers have accidentally greened out during their first dab session. Take your time and enjoy the process.
2. Don't burn yourself or your surroundings. Exercise extreme caution when handling a blowtorch and/or hot nail. Fires are far easier to start than to put out, and burns are best avoided.
3. Know your source. Poorly flushed flowers can leach dangerous chemicals into extracts and concentrates. Improperly purged solvents can damage the nervous system. Purchase your dabs from a reliable source or make your own in a safe fashion.

A Closer Look at Terpenes with Trichome Technologies
by Kenneth Morrow

Terpenes are natural compounds found in many animals and plants. As of 2017, more than 560 unique chemical constituents have been identified in cannabis, with more than 100 unique cannabinoids and more than 150 individual terpenes reported. Data presented in a 1996 paper titled "The Volatile Oil Composition of Fresh and Air-Dried Buds of Cannabis Sativa", by Samir A. Ross and Mahmoud A. Elsohly, "show that fresh bud oil is mainly composed of monoterpenes (92%), with 7% sesquiterpenes and approximately 1% made up of other chemical classes such as simple ketones and esters."

The authors also found that "not unexpectedly, drying the plant material resulted in overall reduction in the percentage of the oil recovered. Most of the loss appears to take place during the first week of drying.... [Drying] the plant material results in a significantly greater loss of monoterpenes than sesquiterpenes. However, qualitatively speaking, none of the major components of the oil (>0.1% of the total) completely disappeared in the drying process."

Regarding most of the terpenes available in the market today, multiple sources are available:

- Organic food-grade (derived from plants and fruits)
- CO_2-extracted, fractionalized (derived from cannabis)
- Steam-distilled, hydrodistilled, and steam/hydrodistilled (utilizing cannabis)
- Thin film distilled (utilizing cannabis)

Each of these terpene-extraction and isolation methods carries its own potential problems.

The Science of Distillation and Extraction

The cannabis-derived terpenes sold to extractors are not what consumers—and sometimes manufacturers—think they are. Hydrosols are not pure cannabis terpenes in composition, but rather a byproduct derived from distillation. Most true essential oils are produced by distillation.

The term distillation is derived from the Latin word *distillare*, which means "trickling down." In its simplest form, distillation is the evaporation and subsequent condensation of a liquid and typically produces artifacts of the original composition caused by oxidation, thermal degradation (i.e., heat), chemical degradation and chemical conversion.

The term "essential oil" is a contraction of the original *quintessential oil*. This definition stems from the Aristotelian idea that matter is composed of four elements, namely fire, air, earth and water. The fifth element, or quintessence, was then considered to be the spirit or life force. Distillation and evaporation were thought to be processes of removing the spirit or life force from the plant. This is also reflected in our language since the term "spirits" is used to describe distilled alcoholic beverages such as brandy, whiskey and eau de vie. The last of these (from French: "Water of life") again makes reference to the concept of removing the life force from the plant.

There are multiple distillation processes used, but in all of them, water is heated to produce steam, which carries the most volatile chemicals (terpenes are classified as volatile organic compounds) and essential oils of the plant material with it. Then, the steam is cooled in a condenser, with the resulting distillate collected in a separate container. Whether using steam distillation or hydrodistillation or a combination of the two, the resulting hydrosols are basically the same and are equally problematic.

Steam versus Hydro Distillation

Steam distillation is the most efficient form of distillation and the most versatile. (For an in-depth explanation, I suggest reading "Hydrosols or Distillation Waters: Their Production, Safety, Efficiency, and the Sales Hype" by Martin Watt.) Although many oils are produced by steam distillation, they all lack the vibrancy of the oils collected without being exposed to heat, as sensitive compounds could be thermally degraded and/or hydrolyzed.

One of the many disadvantages of water or steam distillation is oxygenated compounds such as phenols. Phenols have a tendency to dissolve in distilled water, so their complete removal by distillation is not possible. Essential oils with high solubility in water and those susceptible to damage by heat cannot be separated through steam distillation. The compounds also must be steam-volatile for steam or water distillation to be feasible. Therefore, essential oil obtained by distillation does not represent the natural oil as it originally occurs in plant material. Another disadvantage of steam or water distillation is that complete extraction is not possible, and that certain esters are only partly hydrolyzed, and sensitive substances like aldehydes, which are highly reactive, tend to polymerize or form undesirable byproducts. Proper extraction of essential oils occurs only by the process of expression or solvent extraction.

Before discussing the basic principles of essential oil production, it is important to understand that the essential oils people have in bottles or drums are not necessarily identical to what is present in the plant. With a few rare exceptions, it is wishful thinking to consider an essential oil to be "the soul" of the plant, and thus an exact replica of what is present in the plant. Only expressed oils that have not come in contact with heat or aerial oxidation may meet the conditions of a true plant essential oil. The chemical composition of distilled essential oils is not the same as that of the contents of the oil cells present in the plant or with the odor of plants growing in their natural environment.

A great example is rose oil. A non-professional individual examining pure natural rose oil, even in distillation, will not recognize the plant from which it was sourced. The alterations caused by hydrodistillation are remarkable: As the plant material comes into contact with steam, it undergoes many chemical changes. Hot steam will decompose terpenes, and aldehydes and esters may be formed from acids generated during the vaporization of certain essential oil components. Some water-soluble molecules may be lost by solution in distillation water, thus altering the oil's fragrance profile.

Distillation produces essential oils and a byproduct called floral water, or hydrosol, hydrolate, herbal water and essential water, which are aqueous byproducts of distillation. They are colloidal suspensions (hydrosols) of essential oils as well as water-soluble components obtained by steam or hydrodistillation from plants and herbs. Distillates are used for flavorings, pharmaceuticals and cosmetics. Herbal distillates are produced in the same or similar methods as essential oils, but the appropriate term for the resulting product, essential water, is more descriptive and appropriate.

In the past, these essential waters were considered a byproduct of distillation. Today, they are considered co-products. The science of distillation is based on how different compounds vaporize at different temperatures. Unlike other extraction techniques based on the solubility of a compound in either oil or water, distillation will separate a multitude of compounds from the plant matter (although some will be lost in the water). The distillate will contain compounds that vaporize at or below the temperature of distillation. The actual chemical components of any distillate have not yet been fully identified, but distillates will contain some essential oil compounds as well as organic acids and other water-soluble plant compounds.

Compounds with a higher boiling point will remain behind and will include many of the water-soluble plant pigments and flavonoids. Herbal waters contain diluted essential oils. In addition to aromatic chemicals, these distillates also contain many more plant acids than pure essential oils, making them skin-friendly.

Cosmetics and toiletries manufacturers have found many uses for herbal distillates, but floral water (hydrosols) are unfit for human consumption via inhalation. (Do not vaporize, smoke or "dab" hydrosols.)

Challenges with Food-Grade Terpenes

As of yet, it is impossible to recreate the odor and flavor of the 150+ terpenes that exist in various cannabis cultivars or cultigens using food sources such as fruits and plants. It's also unclear how many of these food-grade terpenes are safe to inhale—the data does not exist regarding vaping or dabbing.

The CO_2 extraction process typically utilizes dried plant material, where a percentage of terpenes are lost to evaporation. Then, processors extract the dry material using pressurized CO_2 gas. Any remaining moisture in the plant material contributes to the formation of carbolic acid and a phenol, an aromatic organic compound that tends to homogenize the odor and flavor of whatever terpenes remain. Some extractors super-dry their material, destroying and evaporating even more terpenes.

Steam and/or hydrodistillates are not whole terpene compositions. Some are simply hydrosols being sold for $10 per drop. These hydrosols contain minimal percentages of terpenes and only a small percentage of the available 150+ terpenes available in cannabis. Steam and/or hydrodistillates produce destroyed, converted artifacts of the original terpene composition from the original plant material, which includes any true distilled terpenes, as well.

Thin film distillation units can process and distill many forms of extract ranging from cold-fluid extraction to CO_2 extraction to ethanol extracts and so on. But terpenes are lost and converted by heat in this distillation process, creating artifacts and fractions. Therefore it is impossible to produce a distillate that has the odor and flavor of the original plant material.

The Advantages of Heat-Free Extraction

Headspace technology is a unique method allowing for the capture of the volatile constituents of oil cells, providing additional information about the plants. Clive Christian, a British perfume company, describes headspace technology as "a process used to capture the odor compounds present in the air surrounding an object. This provides perfumers with the data needed to recreate a synthetic scent from something in nature that isn't extractable via traditional methods." In other words, this method has made it possible to detect the volatile components of the plant's "aura."

I suspect the phytochemical percentages cited in Ross and ElSohly's 1996 paper would be very different if researchers looked at modern-day cultivars using a heat-free extraction and analytical method, such as cold headspace trapping. Existing data comes from U.S. cannabis labs that often lack more effective terpene testing capabilities, such as cold headspace trapping. (Cold headspace trapping is almost exclusively used in the fragrance industry.)

The chief benefit of hydrocarbon, ethanol and CO_2 extraction is that a consistent temperature can be maintained during the process. This allows extracted oils to have a more complete odor profile. For example, very delicate aromatics like jasmine and linden blossom cannot survive the process of distillation. To capture their magical aromas, processors use a solvent extraction process.

The most aromatic extractions occur at or below ambient temperatures, which prevents thermal degradation of the compounds. The solvent extraction process uses the selectivity of the solvent with no heat application, oxidation, degradation conversion or destruction of the original composition.

Terpenes and the Future of Pharmaceuticals

Effective drug development depends on multidisciplinary collaborations, such as those among botanical, phytochemical and biological disciplines. Worldwide sales of terpene patent-based pharmaceuticals in 2002 were approximately US$12 billion ("Terpenes and Derivatives as a New Perspective for Pain Relief: A Patent Review Expert Opinion"). With the real medicinal value of cannabis compounds, such as cannabinoids and terpenoids, just beginning to be explored, expect a multi-billion-dollar cannabis pharmaceutical industry to emerge someday.

So, Are Terpenes Safe?

The extracts of cannabis, both cannabinoids and terpenes, are very complex, and very little is known regarding consumption in concentrated form. I believe that cold-solvent extraction yields far superior products than steam or hydrodistillation with respect to terpene extraction, isolation and preservation. Also, I think terpenes derived from pure cannabis are higher in quality, and represent a fuller terpene profile and composition than simple hydrosol or floral water. Hydrosols, again, are not fit for heated inhalation.

That being said, I have not yet found correlating data that unequivocally states that elevated or concentrated levels of terpenes are healthy to inhale, and too many questions remain to make safe assumptions about concentration levels and toxicity thresholds of each terpene. Again, these questions are in regard to pure terpenes, not hydrosols, which contain only small percentages of terpenes.

It should be possible to relate the intake of high doses of the substances to observed toxicity, yet efforts to evaluate the safety of a natural product based on its chemical composition and the variability of that composition's phytochemistry for the intended use are in their infancy. The chemical constitution of a natural product is fundamental to understanding the product's intended use and factors affecting its safety.

Recent advances in analytical methodology have made intensive investigation of the chemical composition of a natural product economically feasible and even routine. High-throughput instrumentation necessary to perform extensive qualitative and quantitative analysis of complex chemical mixtures and to evaluate the variation in the composition of the mixture is now a reality. In fact, analytical tools needed to chemically characterize these complex mixtures are becoming more cost-effective, while the cost of traditional toxicology is becoming more cost intensive.

Based on the wealth of existing chemical and biological data on the constituents of essential oils and similar data on essential oils themselves, it is possible to validate the safety of a natural mixture based on its chemical composition. By looking at the interaction between one or more molecules in the natural product and macromolecules, such as proteins and enzymes, we can understand the biological response, regardless of whether it is a desired functional effect, such as a pleasing taste or a potential toxic effect, such as lung damage.

The most disturbing issue regarding the sale, formulation and heated inhalation of concentrated essential oils and hydrosols is that there is no correlating data supporting either a pro or con for use related to inhalation at elevated temperatures in part or as a whole composition of a matrix of terpenes. A healthy threshold must be established for the industry to confidently sell its products without worrying about getting patients and consumers sick. As it stands, people who are dabbing or inhaling hydrosols for which they pay $10 a drop are being used as test subjects.

From all substantiated data above, it's clear that cold-solvent extraction—such as the cold expression of fresh, undried plant material—produces the highest-quality terpene extracts and that hydrosols and formulations of a few food-grade terpenes can't completely recreate the flavor or odor of living plant characteristics. (A mixture of many cannabis terpenes also has an inevitable color tone. Purified compounds and mixtures of a few, such as hydrosols and floral waters, can be clear in color, but mixtures of many terpenes have color.)

Research and recent lessons are reminders that we as an industry should be mindful of how we present our products to ensure we're not misrepresenting the contents or the safety of our patients' and consumers' favorite products.

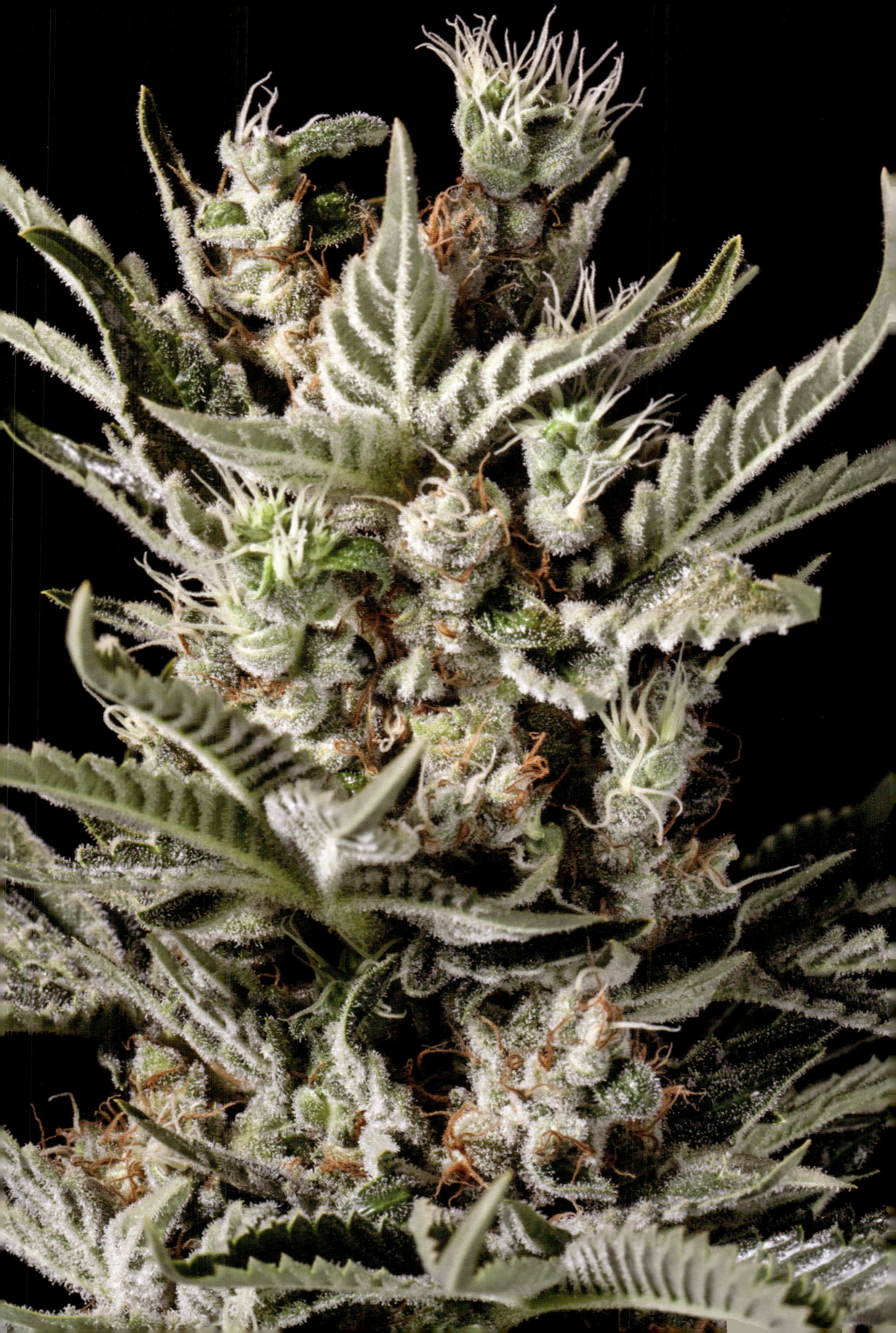

19

The Cannabis Grow Bible Checklist

We are pampered with choices when it comes to cannabis genetics and the many ways we can grow this wonderful and rewarding plant.

This book will help you switch from a dependency on middle-of-the-road product from large companies to the "blatant self-sufficiency" of growing your own top-notch weed. And if you haven't realized it yet, growing your own can be a lot of fun.

You will save so much money. It will take you out of whatever loop you have been in, and give you complete control over your cannabis. Learning "blatant self-sufficiency" is the challenge that, once overcome, opens doors that were previously shut. You can apply this same principle anywhere.

This final chapter serves as a checklist summarizing the most important points for superior cannabis growth results. These factors are:

- Good Genetics
- Proper Lighting
- The Right Growing Medium
- Optimal Pot Size
- Quality Safe Fertilizers
- Air Circulation and Ventilation
- Carbon Dioxide (CO_2)
- 12/12 Photoperiod
- Avoiding Plant Stress
- Labeling

PHOTOS: DINAFEM SEEDS (OPPOSITE PAGE), JOE'S CANNA GROWS (THIS PAGE)

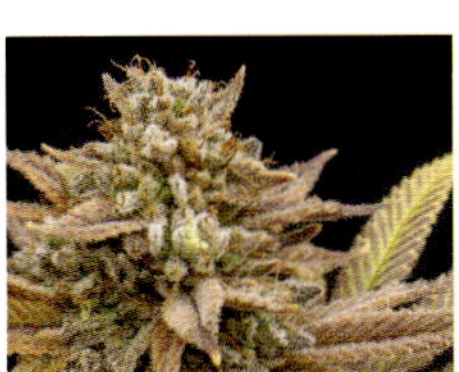

√ Good Genetics

Good genetics are the way. If you start with bad genetics, you'll have poor results, no matter what you do or how skilled a grower you may be. A plant genetically predisposed for low bud production and potency will not produce an outstanding crop. You should get your seeds from reputable breeders advertised on seed banks to ensure you obtain good genetics. Many breeders enter competitions, such as The High Times Cannabis Cup and the Emerald Cup, which showcase some of the best current strains available. Most of the cannabis pictures in this book are of well-known strains produced by breeders that can be bought through seed banks.

Selecting a good clone mother is also essential as obtaining good genetics is crucial for good growing results. By selecting a good mother plant, you can create a population of clone mothers that increases your overall yield.

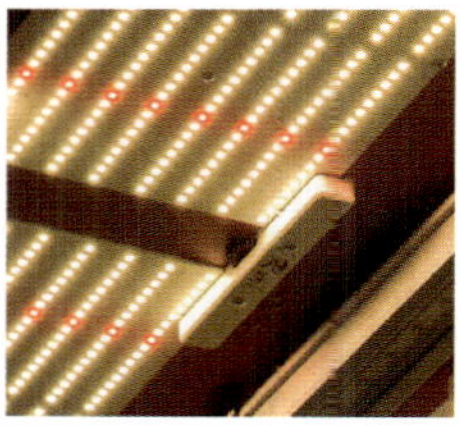

✓ Proper Lighting

Next to genetics, lighting is probably the most critical factor in plant growth and bud production. LEDs are more economical to use, and can compete with high-wattage HIDs, so it is best to upgrade from low-wattage HIDs to LEDs. The future is here, and LEDs are the way.

It is essential to conserve light. Reflectors, white walls, and Mylar should be used to keep the spread of light even and contained in your grow room or tent. Any light leaks mean that usable light is being lost. Deal with this lost light and your plants will love you for it.

Keep lights as close to the plants as possible without burning them. Proximity increases overall yield and reduces internode length development. Keep those internode lengths down, and you will get much better results.

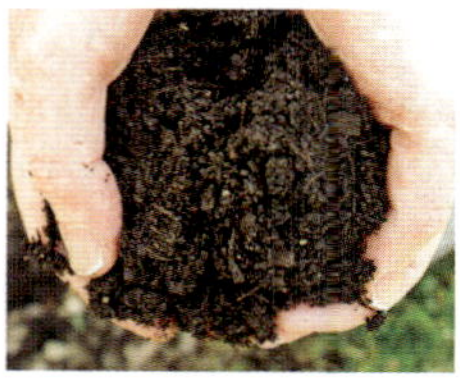

✓ The Right Growing Medium

Soil is the most popular choice of medium. Never underestimate the importance of using the right soil; if the soil isn't suitable for growing cannabis, no matter how skilled a grower you are, your plants will not reach their optimum potential. Ensure the pH is neutral and the nutrients your plant requires are present. Soils should hold some water but drain well—you don't want muddy or fast-draining soils. Aim for the middle ground and choose a soil that does both well. For this purpose, balanced loam makes the most sense.

Hydroponics require more maintenance than soil growing, but can have improved yields and considerably faster growing times. If you have the time and money, give hydroponics a shot as it can be a fantastic way to optimize results.

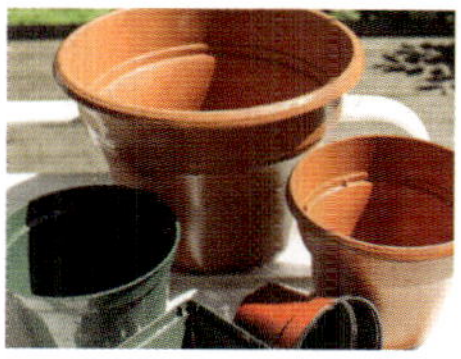

✓ Optimal Pot Size

Cannabis tends to do most of its rooting during the vegetative stage of growth. As soon as flowering begins, root development slows down considerably. A four-inch-square pot may be suitable for clones or SOG-type growing situations, but anything less

PHOTOS: HORTICULTURE LIGHTING GROUP, HLG.COM (TOP), STONED ROSIE (MIDDLE AND BOTTOM)

than that can stunt plant growth. "Pot-bound" or "root-bound" plants also experience nutrient deficiencies. For these reasons, most growers prefer to use a 3-gallon bag or a 3-gallon nursery pot. This size permits enough root growth to allow the plant to flourish. If you want indoor plants to achieve maximum sizes, try increasing to 5-gallon pots. These will help produce sturdy, robust plants with thick stems and plentiful node development. The problem with 5-gallon pots is that they take up quite a bit of space, so fewer plants will fit into the grow room. The plants also take longer to grow as cultivators hold back on flowering to push that extra vegetative growth. For this reason, 3-gallon is a good standard if not extending vegetative growth.

For hydroponic systems, net pots usually range between 2- and 8-inches square. The most common net pot is the 5- or 6-inch type. This net pot size suits simple hydroponic systems like The Bubbler. For large sativa plants, an 8-inch net pot is more suitable.

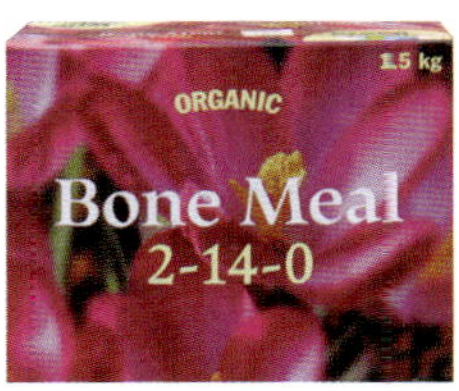

√ Quality Safe Fertilizers

If you provide the food your plants require, they will provide you with good results. Cannabis plants like food, but do not give them too much. Only use feeding solutions designed for food plants, never for ornamental plants; avoid the kind used for roses. Some non-food plant fertilizers contain ingredients beyond the standard primary, secondary, and micronutrients which can often be toxic; a warning label on the side of the fertilizer container should indicate this. The same goes for pest sprays. This is another good reason to grow your own bud: You can control what sprays and fertilizers your plant is exposed to.

When you get your feeding mixtures right, you'll boost the overall performance of your plants and keep them healthier, too.

Keep notes of feeding times and amounts to help you gauge your feeding routines. It is sometimes easy to forget when you last fed your plants and what mixtures you used. And make sure to keep these notes safely hidden from prying eyes.

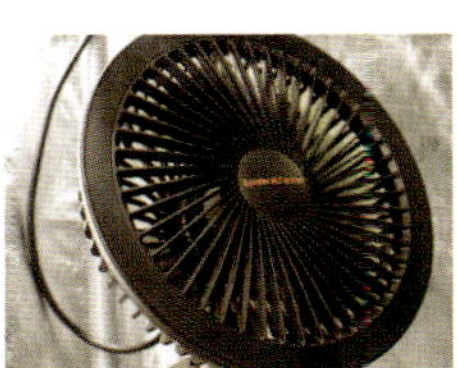

√ Air Circulation and Ventilation

Air circulation is crucial. Outdoor plants don't have this problem, but indoor plant growth can sometimes be stunted or slowed if the plants don't receive enough fresh air. Fresh air is essential to replenish gases. The percentage of different compounds that make up air can change or fluctuate if new air isn't introduced into the grow room, which can cause problems with your grow. Heat can also build up in spaces that don't have good air ventilation, and a temperature rise can cause stunted plant growth. Try to keep fresh air always moving around your grow room for the best results.

PHOTOS: GCP (TOP), @TREETRUNK422 (BOTTOM)

Air circulation also brings a mild wind to your grow, which is essential for stem and branch robustness. The wind will cause the plant to respond with a thicker stem and branch growth by stressing it slightly. This is important for bud production; the plant will be thicker, stronger, and healthier overall.

Dust is also a problem for indoor growers, as it can come with mold in high humidity. In a grow room, you must use ventilation to keep dust from settling on your sticky bud. Those tiny pistils are producing the resin that you want. A big blob of dust on a pistil will stunt its growth and reduce the bud's overall effect when sampled.

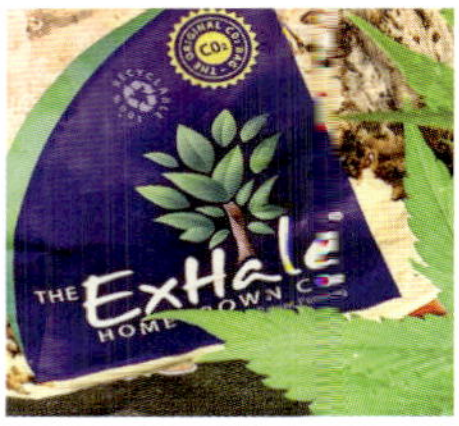

✓ Carbon Dioxide (CO_2)

CO_2 supplements boost yields and should be employed if you have the resources. CO_2 supplements are generally considered inconsequential to climate change compared to CO_2 produced by upstream energy providers, where the bulk of the problem resides. My experience has shown that CO_2 can naturally enhance yields to almost double that of a similar grow without a CO_2 supplement.

Although you can produce great results without using CO_2, it can make all the difference. Growers who use CO_2 rarely ever turn away from it. It is a wonderful way to achieve high yields with the right genetics.

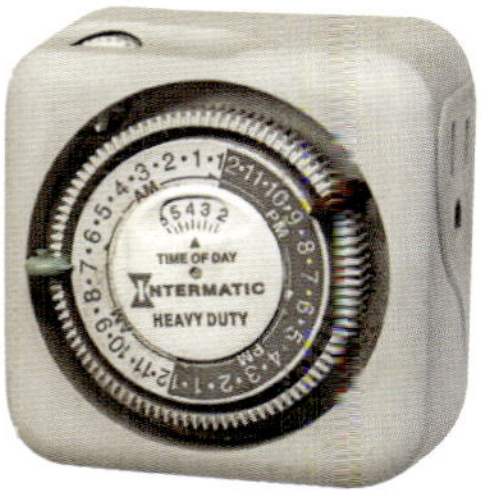

✓ 12/12 Photoperiod

Using a 12/12 photoperiod and keeping your flowering room completely lightproof will improve your overall yield. Total darkness is vital to your plants during the flowering stage of the life cycle; a 100% lightproof room will increase yields by as much as 30% more than a room that is only 99% lightproof.

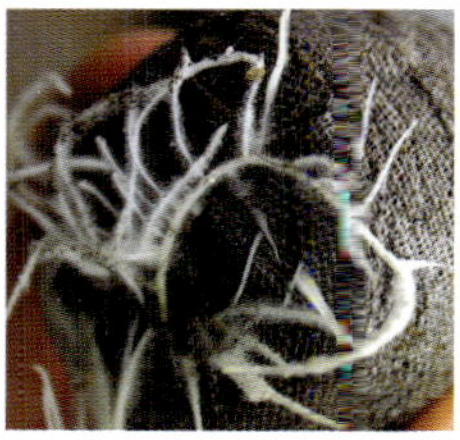

✓ Avoiding Plant Stress

You should avoid doing multiple transplants of the same plant to minimize plant stress. You will get much more effective results by solving problems quickly and caring for your plants. Stress-related disorders are often responsible for lower yields and hermaphrodites.

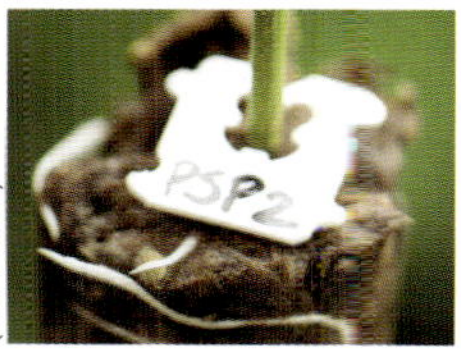

✓ Labeling

Never underestimate the importance of labeling. Label everything you can, including seeds, seedlings, vegetative plants, flowering plants, clones, harvest, manicured bud, plants you're testing nutrients with and all end products in storage.

PHOTOS: TANYA PETERSEN (TOP), JUSTINCANNABIS.COM (2ND FROM TOP), PEACE NATURALS (3RD FROM TOP), ERIC PALMER (BOTTOM)

Labeling prevents mix-ups from occurring. If you mix up your plants, you will have to guess the correct flowering times and strain type.

My experience as a grower has taught me that the cannabis plant is so diverse that no one country, seed bank, or breeder can claim to have all the best genetics. In fact, most high-quality genetics are available to any grower through the right seed bank, so there is nothing preventing good growers from obtaining what they need.

If you can understand and control the above points, then you will be able to grow superior bud. We hope that this book has helped in some way and that you will continue to refer to it in the future.

If you know people who have an interest in cannabis, tell them about this book. They need this kind of information to grow their own high-quality bud. The results are cheaper and better, as you will see!

Remember: Do not break the law. Check your country's laws before you get seeds or clones, or grow cannabis, to ensure that your actions are not illegal. As much as we would like you to grow cannabis, we do not want you to get into legal trouble.

Have fun, and thanks for reading this book.

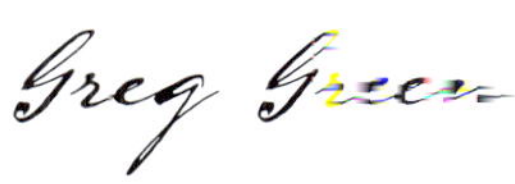

Endnotes

Introduction

1 To see the Tree of life, visit https://timetree.org/.

2 This classification changes depending on the species of rose.

Page xxi

3 Forest, Félix, and Mark W. Chase. "Eurosid I." *The Timetree of Life*, April 23, 2009, 188–96. https://doi.org/10.1093/oso/9780199535033.003.0020.

Page xxii

4 Not the idea of a designer, but that organisms had somehow appeared spontaneously complex. Darwin, in fact, didn't comment on a designer in his publications, but he did omit using one in his explanations.

5 Molluscs, like the common octopus *Octopus vulgaris*, have blood vessels passing behind their retina.

6 Technically moles are not completely blind, as their eyes retain some very subtle ability to detect daylight from night. This does not dispute our statement because it shows that eyes can vary in complexity from good vision, like in humans and molluscs, to poor vision, as per moles. If we can show examples of gradual improvements in sight among currently present organisms, this undermines the view that good vision must appear spontaneously complex.

7 Not "survival of the fittest," which is not a biological term and has nothing to do with evolutionary biology. That is a political/social term that misunderstood Darwinian evolution.

8 Two plants give rise to four which give rise to 16... and so on, until the world can't sustain them anymore.

Page xxiii

9 This is a simplistic view of the situation. In evolutionary biology, there are many more complex variables to consider.

10 Healthy individuals that can reproduce and fitness in biological terms has a much stricter definition, but this will do for now.

Page xxiv

11 Evolutionary biologists actually use phylogenetic trees.

12 Note the term "combination," not "mixture." Blending doesn't happen. What occurs is Mendelian inheritance.

13 In some organisms, it is RNA.

Page xxv

14 The situation of how genes recombine is a lot more complex, but this example is fine for now.

15 Both are mechanisms that can bring about speciation, where a gene pool becomes separated and both evolve separately to the point that hybridization is no longer possible. This does not appear to have happened with cannabis, which can hybridize, but reproductive isolation can be a powerful barrier between indica and sativa strains.

16 The gene pool is the total number of genes from any selection that we make. If we took cannabis species as a whole, that would be an example of a gene pool. If we just took a smaller sample from a grow room that would be a gene pool also.

CHAPTER 2

The Cannabis Plant

Page 25

1 Fleming, Michael P., and Robert C. Clarke. "Physical Evidence for the Antiquity of *Cannabis Sativa* L." *Journal of the International Hemp Association* 5, no. 2 (January 1998): 80–92.

2 Ren, Guangpeng, Xu Zhang, Ying Li, Kate Ridout, Martha L. Serrano-Serrano, Yongzhi Yang, Ai Liu, et al. "Large-Scale Whole-Genome Resequencing Unravels the Domestication History of *Cannabis Sativa*." *Science Advances* 7, no. 29 (July 2021). https://doi.org/10.1126/sciadv.abg2286.

Page 27

3 Harlan, Jack R. "The Possible Role of Weed Races in the Evolution of Cultivated Plants." *Euphytica* 14, no. 2 (June 1965): 173–76. https://doi.org/10.1007/bf00038984.

4 Saxena, Sanjeev, and Anuruddh K. Singh. "Revisit to Definitions and Need for Inventorization or Registration of Landrace, Folk, Farmers' and Traditional Varieties." *Current Science* 91, no. 11 (2006): 1451–54. http://www.jstor.org/stable/24093836.

5 Friis-Hansen, Esbern, and Bhuwon Sthapit. *Participatory approaches to the conservation and use of Plant Genetic Resources*. Rome, Italy: IPGRI, 2000.

Page 28

6 Wyse, Joseph, and Gilad Luria. "Trends in Intellectual Property Rights Protection for Medical Cannabis and Related Products." *Journal of Cannabis Research* 3, no. 1 (January 6, 2021). https://doi.org/10.1186/s42238-020-00057-7.

Page 30

7 Busta, Lucas, Ismail Dweikat, Shirley J. Sato, Haolin Qu, Yong Xue, Bangjun Zhou, Lu Gan, et al. "Chemical and Genetic Variation in Feral *Cannabis Sativa* Populations across the Nebraska Climate Gradient." *Phytochemistry* 200 (August 2022). https://doi.org/10.1016/j.phytochem.2022.113206.

Page 33

8 "Cannabinoid." Wikipedia, July 31, 2024. https://en.wikipedia.org/wiki/Cannabinoid.

9 Sideris, Alexandra, Justas Lauzadis, and Martin Kaczocha. "The Basic Science of Cannabinoids." *Anesthesia & Analgesia* 138, no. 1 (December 15, 2023): 42–53. https://pubmed.ncbi.nlm.nih.gov/38100799/.

Page 34

10 Zlebnik, Natalie E., and Joseph F. Cheer. "Beyond the CB1 Receptor: Is Cannabidiol the Answer for Disorders of Motivation?" *Annual Review of Neuroscience* 39, no. 1 (July 8, 2016): 1–17. https://doi.org/10.1146/annurev-neuro-070815-014038.

11 Vučković, Sonja, Dragana Srebro, Katarina Savić Vujović, Čedomir Vučetić, and Milica Prostran. "Cannabinoids and Pain: New Insights from Old Molecules." *Frontiers in Pharmacology* 9 (November 13, 2018). https://doi.org/10.3389/fphar.2018.01259.

12 Fathordoobady, Farahnaz, Anika Singh, David D. Kitts, and Anubhav Pratap Singh. "Hemp (*Cannabis Sativa* L.) Extract: Anti-Microbial Properties, Methods of Extraction, and Potential Oral Delivery." *Food Reviews International* 35, no. 7 (April 22, 2019): 664–84. https://doi.org/10.1080/87559129.2019.1600539.

Page 38

13 Nelson, Kathryn M., Jonathan Bisson, Gurpreet Singh, James G. Graham, Shao-Nong Chen, J. Brent Friesen, Jayme L. Dahlin, Matthias Niemitz, Michael A. Walters, and Guido F. Pauli. "The Essential Medicinal Chemistry of Cannabidiol (CBD)." *Journal of Medicinal Chemistry* 63, no. 21 (August 17, 2020): 12137–55. https://doi.org/10.1021/acs.jmedchem.0c00724.

Page 45

14 Gittleman, John L. "Species." Encyclopædia Britannica, June 21, 2024. https://www.britannica.com/science/species-taxon.

Page 46

15 The date that Lamarck described C. indica is commonly reported as 1783. Breistroffer (1948) and Stafieu (1967) have noted that in fact Lamarck's description was published in 1785. Small, E. "American Law and the Species Problem in Cannabis: Science and Semantics." *Bull Narc* 27, no. 3 (July 1975): 1-20. PMID: 1041693.

Page 47

16 Hillig, Karl William. "A Systematic Investigation of Cannabis," 2005. https://doi.org/10.13140/RG.2.1.2648.3680

Page 50

17 Hirata, K. "Cytological Basis of the Sex Determination in *Cannabis Sativa* L." *The Japanese Journal of Genetics* 4, no. 4 (1929): 198–201. https://doi.org/10.1266/jjg.4.198.

18 Schaffner, John H. "Heredity and Sex." *Ohio Journal of Science* 29, no. 1 (January 1929): 289–300. hdl:1811/2398.

19 Schaffner, John H. "The Fluctuation Curve of Sex Reversal in Staminate Hemp Plants Induced by Photoperiodicity." *American Journal of Botany* 18, no. 6 (June 1931): 424–30. https://doi.org/10.2307/2435878.

Page 51

20 Galoch, Elżbieta. "The Hormonal Control of Sex Differentiation in Dioecious Plants of Hemp (*Cannabis Sativa*). the Influence of Plant Growth Regulators on Sex Expression in Male and Female Plants." *Acta Societatis Botanicorum Poloniae* 47, no. 1–2 (1978): 153–62. https://doi.org/10.5586/asbp.1978.013.

21 Dellaporta, S L, and A Calderon-Urrea. "Sex Determination in Flowering Plants." *The Plant Cell* 5, no. 10 (October 1993): 1241–51. https://doi.org/10.1105/tpc.5.10.1241.

22 Hall, Jack, Surya P. Bhattarai, and David J. Midmore. "Review of Flowering Control in Industrial Hemp." *Journal of Natural Fibers* 9, no. 1 (January 2012): 23–36. https://doi.org/10.1080/15440478.2012.651848.

23 Punja, Zamir K., and Janesse E. Holmes. "Hermaphroditism in Marijuana (*Cannabis Sativa* L.) Inflorescences – Impact on Floral Morphology, Seed Formation, Progeny Sex Ratios, and Genetic Variation." *Frontiers in Plant Science* 11 (June 25, 2020). https://doi.org/10.3389/fpls.2020.00718.

24 Flajšman, Marko, Miha Slapnik, and Jana Murovec. "Production of Feminized Seeds of High CBD *Cannabis Sativa* L. by Manipulation of Sex Expression and Its Application to Breeding." *Frontiers in Plant Science* 12 (November 1, 2021). https://doi.org/10.3389/fpls.2021.718092.

Page 52

25 Adal, Ayelign M., Ketan Doshi, Larry Holbrook, and Soheil S. Mahmoud. "Comparative RNA-Seq Analysis Reveals Genes Associated with Masculinization in Female *Cannabis Sativa*." *Planta* 253, no. 17 (January 2021). https://doi.org/10.1007/s00425-020-03522-y.

CHAPTER 3

Seeds: Selection, Banks, and Storage

Page 64

1 While pollen from other strains can be used, the hybridizing will be quite unstable because it is a different male donor.

Page 76

2 If a breeder aims for their strain to go viral, they have to account for the high demand and produce enough seeds.

CHAPTER 4

Germination and Propagation

Page 85

1 "An Update of the Angiosperm Phylogeny Group Classification for the Orders and Families of Flowering Plants: APG II." *Botanical Journal of the Linnean Society* 141, no. 4 (April 2003): 399–436. https://doi.org/10.1046/j.1095-8339.2003.t01-1-00158.x.

Page 87

2 Harvey, R. "Growing Ferns from Spores." Australian Plant Information. Accessed August 12, 2024. https://www.anbg.gov.au/ferns/fern.spore.prop.html.

3 Single cotyledons are produced by monocotyledons and gymnosperms may have two or more.

Page 93

4 Some germination soils are unsuitable for cannabis because they contain higher amounts of P and K than N. Most growers find that ordinary loam soil is just as good for germination as long as the N values are equal to or higher than the P and K values.

5 See pages 103-115 on transplanting.

Page 98

6 Propagation kits can also be used with growing media besides rockwool.

Page 99

7 Seeds take up to three weeks to germinate. If no seeds have germinated after this time, check your seeds and germination method. Usually, seeds germinate together within a few days of one another. If all the seeds fail to germinate and your method is good, then report this to the seed bank to see if their batch is faulty. Reputable seed banks keep records of germination rates and failures.

8 See page 215 and pages 258-260 for details on temperature.

Page 102

9 Charles Darwin, using experiments in his back garden, examined birds' feet and left seeds in water for months to simulate animal trekking and ocean transport. Darwin concluded that these methods allowed fauna to spread from island to island and this successfully explained how the same fauna species could appear in areas separated by obstructions.

CHAPTER 7

Grow Lights

Page 163

1 Professional growers choose lighting kits with an external ballast because they are easier to move and keep temperatures cooler. Internal ballasts make the light system heavier and cause unwanted heat on your plants. External ballasts are highly recommended.

Page 177

2 Fluorescent lights tend to produce buds that are airy and less dense than buds produced under HID and LED lights.

Page 192

3 Most bulbs have a lifespan of approximately two to four grows. This depends heavily on the bulb type and how long the bulbs are left on. After the third grow, the bulb's quality tends to reduce.

4 Generally, HID grow bulbs come in the following wattages: 250, 400, 600, and 1000.

Page 194

5 The conversion of electricity to light has been one of the great modern environmental catastrophes because of its inefficiency. Previously, lights lost around 90% of the energy used to operate them. Energy-saving bulbs helped reduce that, and the LED revolution has further reduced the waste factor.

Page 202

6 Westmoreland, F. Mitchell, Paul Kusuma, and Bruce Bugbee. "Elevated UV Photon Fluxes Minimally Affected Cannabinoid Concentration in a High-CBD Cultivar." *Frontiers in Plant Science* 14 (August 11, 2023). https://doi.org/10.3389/fpls.2023.1220585.

7 Chmielinski, Maximilian J., Patricia O. Ehrlich, Martin Cohen, Tania M. Isaksen, and Christopher D. Simpson. "Ultraviolet Radiation Exposure in Cannabis-Growing Facilities." *Journal of Occupational and Environmental Hygiene* 20, no. 7 (July 3, 2023): 268–78. https://doi.org/10.1080/15459624.2023.2207616.

CHAPTER 9

Pre-Flowering and Flowering

Page 292

1 Although some growers can manipulate the photoperiod without sexual dysfunctions emerging, it is not worth the risk. Once a dysfunction appears, it cannot be reversed.

Page 301

2 Punja, Zamir K., and Janesse E. Holmes. "Hermaphroditism in Marijuana (*Cannabis Sativa L.)* Inflorescences – Impact on Floral Morphology, Seed Formation, Progeny Sex Ratios, and Genetic Variation." *Frontiers in Plant Science* 11 (June 25, 2020). https://doi.org/10.3389/fpls.2020.00718.

CHAPTER 10

Indoor Grow Methods

Page 313

1 It's a good idea to weigh the top cola of each plant and compare it to the yield of all the side-branched buds together. Figure out if the top colas weigh more than the total weight of these

side-branched buds. If the top colas weigh more, you have an excellent strain for canopy methods like SOG growing. If not you should consider pruning them for a ScrOG-type grow.

CHAPTER 11

Hydroponics

Page 380

1 Mylar is an excellent material for patching light leaks because of its high reflectivity.

CHAPTER 12

Outdoor Growing

Page 429

1 Sometimes, roots can grow through the bottom pot pores if a vacuum is created between the pots and the dish/tray. Pots with short and raised bases help prevent this.

CHAPTER 13

Caring for Mature Cannabis Plants

Page 483

1 F1 hybrids and non-uniform plants tend to exhibit more of this range than stable stains and IBLs (inbred lines).

Page 494

2 Cannabis plants rarely fail after losing around 50% of their leaves sometime after the seedling phase, but they will be stunted. Most strains will fail if no leaves are left on the plant.

Page 508

3 The exceptions to this rule are Ruderalis plants and their hybrids with autoflowering properties. These stains can only be continued with seed and cannot be reverted to vegetative growth.

Page 521

4 It does not matter if you rejuvenate a seeded or sinsemilla female. The results will be the same.

CHAPTER 14

Organic Growing

Page 538

1 Steiner, Rudolf. *Agriculture: Spiritual Foundations for the Renewal of Agriculture*. Kimberton, PA: Bio-Dynamic Farming and Gardening Association, 1993.

2 Ibid. Look up various Biodynamics Associations around the world.

3 Paull, John. "The Farm as Organism: The Foundational Idea of Organic Agriculture." *Journal of Bio-Dynamics Tasmania*, July 1, 2006: 14–18.

4 Northbourne, Lord. *Look to the Land*. London: J.M. Dent & Sons, 1940.

Page 541

5 Organic farms produce the same corn and soybean yields as conventional farms, but consume less energy and use no pesticides. Maeder, Paul, Andreas Fliessbach, Dariid Dubois, Lucie Gunst, Padruot Fried, and Urs Niggli. "Soil Fertility and Biodiversity in Organic Farming." *Science* 296, no. 5573 (May 31, 2002): 1694–97. https://doi.org/10.1126/science.1071148.

Page 543

6 "What Is Climate Change?" United Nations. Accessed August 8, 2024. https://www.un.org/en/climatechange/what-is-climate-change.

Page 582

7 Summers, Hailey M., Evan Sproul, and Jason C. Quinn. "The Greenhouse Gas Emissions of Indoor Cannabis Production in the United States." *Nature Sustainability* 4, no. 7 (March 8, 2021): 644–50. https://doi.org/10.1038/s41893-021-00691-w.

CHAPTER 17

How to Breed Cannabis

Page 699

1 An IBL (inbred line) doesn't mean the strain has been backcrossed to the parents. IBLs are stabilized strains with homologous genes that become so stable that the parent and offspring are identical enough to just cross them as if they were any individuals in a population. They will still produce identical offspring because most of their traits are identical. Backcrossing can occur to produce seeds quickly.

Page 719

2 BB or bb is not BB "and" bb.

CHAPTER 18

Extractions

A Closer Look at Terpenes: References

Breitmaier, Eberhard. *Terpenes: Flavors, Fragrances, Pharmaca, Pheromones.* Weinheim: Wiley-VCH, 2006.

Brenneisen, Rudolf. "Chemistry and Analysis of Phytocannabinoids and Other Cannabis Constituents." In *Marijuana and the Cannabinoids*, pp. 17-49. Totowa, NJ: Humana Press, 2007.

Handa, Suckdev Swami, Suman Preet Singh Khanuja, Gennaro Longo, and Dev Dutt Rakesh. *Extraction Technologies for Medicinal and Aromatic Plants.* Trieste (Italy): International Centre for Science and High Technology, 2008.

Heusler, Friedrich. *Chemistry of the Terpenes.* Philadelphia , PA: P. Blakiston's Sons and Co, 1902.

Higley, Connie, and Alan Higley. *Reference Guide for Essential Oils.* Spanish Fork, UT: Abundant Health, 2017.

Hüsnü Can Başer, K., and Gerhard Buchbauer. *Handbook of Essential Oils: Science, Technology, and Applications.* Boca Raton, FL: CRC Press, 2009.

Newman, A. A. *Chemistry of Terpenes and Terpenoids.* London: Academic Press, 1972.

Pinder, A. R. *The Chemistry of the Terpenes.* New York: Wiley, 1960.

Ross, Samir A., and Mahmoud A. ElSohly. "The Volatile Oil Composition of Fresh and Air-Dried Buds of *Cannabis Sativa*." *Journal of Natural Products* 59, no. 1 (January 1, 1996): 49–51. https://doi.org/10.1021/np960004a.

Sell, Charles S. *A Fragrant Introduction to Terpenoid Chemistry.* Royal Society of Chemistry, 2003.

Sell, Charles S. *Chemistry and the Sense of Smell.* Hoboken, NJ: Wiley, 2014.

Watt, Martin. "Hydrosols, Their Production, Safety, Efficacy, and Sales Hype." Natural Ingredient Resource Center, September 9, 2015. https://naturalingredient.org/?p=2072.

Index

Photography Credits

Photographs © Across International, Abramoff/ShutterStock.com, AdvancedSeeds.com AetherGreen.com, Alex, Alpine Seeds, Andre Grossman, AnnibaleSeedShop.com, Barriography/ShutterStock.com, BC Northern Lights, @BEAN401, Bodhi Seeds, BonsaiBudsRI.com, Brendan Brown, Bubbleman, Budtrainer.com, Bumboklot Seeds, Cannanetics (Medicinal Clones 694), Cap, Centennial Seeds, CH9 Female Seeds, Chikamasa, Craft Concentrates, Czechbayarea, Dankshire Photography, David Grau Forografia, David Strange, Deep Roots/ShutterStock.com, Delta9Labs.com, Dinafem Seeds, DNAGenetics.com, DoctorsChoice.farm, Dosatron.com Dr. Atomic Seedbank, Dr. Grow's Fem Seeds, DrGreenThumb.com, Dutch Passion, Ed Borg, Emerald Triangle Seeds, Eric Palmer, Father Nature Robert Burns, Franz Janyr, Freebie, Gavita, GCP, Gibridov, GorillaGrowTent.com, Gracie Malley, Cannabis Now, GrandmasterLeds.com, Green Haven Genetics Green Thom, Greenhouse by Issac Pabst and Henri Van Den Bos, Greenrush LLC, Grubbycup Stash, Hanna Bliss, HashTek.ca, Hemp Solutions, Henry Woodward (Marijuana Daily Gardening), Hip2TheCrop, Horticulture Lighting Group, HLG.com, HumboldtNutrients.com, HydroFarm.com, HydroGarden.com, Ian C., JB Haze / Cannabis Regeneration, Jeff Goldberg, Joe's Canna Grows, JulieK2/ShutterStock.com, Kaliman Seeds, Kanga Seeds, Kaya, Keystone Life, KindLedGrowLights.com, Kristen Angelo, JUSTINCANNABIS.COM, LotusNutrients.com, Luke Sparrow, Macrolife/ShutterStock.com, MammothLighting.com, Mandala Seeds, Mark Heinrich, Master Thai Seeds, Max Bortnick, Mel Thomas, MG Imaging MiamiMangoca.com, MM Jars, Monica Griffin, MNice.nl, Nathan Guillard, NMS, Northern Scrogger, Optimize Horticulture Consulting Original Seeds, Paradise-seeds.com, Paulo Ferreira, Peace Naturals, Peter Alva, Philosopher Seeds, Pong Pong/ShutterStock.com, Praphat Louilarppraserl/ShutterStock.com, Preston Bjornson, Protasov An/ShutterStock.com, Pure Bred Growers, RemoNutrients.com, ResinSeeds.net, Riot Seeds, Rob Bramhill, Roberto Michel/ShutterStock.com, RootPouch.com, RoyalQueenSeeds.com, Russell-Holland Photography, Sean Brady, SecretJardin.com, Seeds of Africa, SensiSeeds.com, ShopFreeGrow8.com, SiliGloves.org, Sjamaan.com, Travis Hoellerer @sofakinghigh, Solis Tek, Soilder-farmer.com, SpliffSeeds.nl, Stoned Rosie, SuiteLeaf.com, Sweet Seeds, Tanisium Extractors, Tanya Petersen, Tee Roberts, The Rev, TheHouseofHydro.com, TheHydroBucket.com, TheOriginalResinator.com Thomas Whitcomb, Tomasz Klejdysz/ShutterStock.com, Tommy L. Gomez, TreeTownSeeds.com, @TreeTrunk422, Trichome Art, Trichome Tech, TrimPro.com, Tropical Seeds, Tweed, TwisterTrimmer.com, Tyler J. Markwart and Danielle Halle, Vinicius R. Souza/ShutterStock.com, Virginia Haze, Weado, Weed.co.za, Zenzy Photo/ShutterStock.com